Care of the GERIATRIC PATIENT

in the tradition of E.V. Cowdry

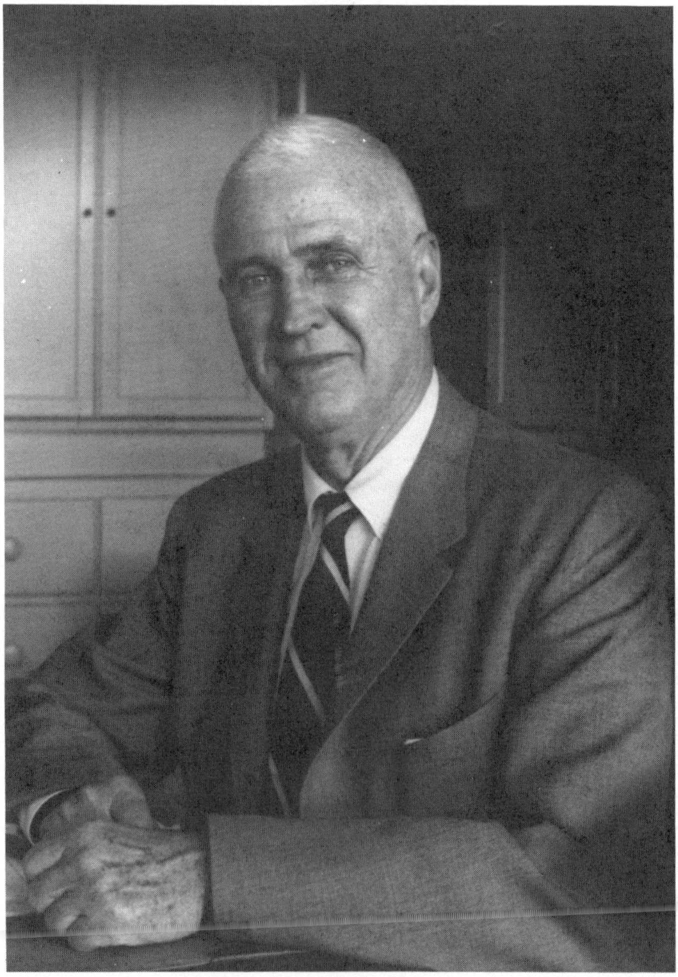

E.V. Cowdry, Ph.D.

1888–1975

Care of the GERIATRIC PATIENT

in the tradition of E.V. Cowdry

Edited by

FRANZ U. STEINBERG, M.D., F.A.C.P.

Professor of Clinical Medicine, Associate Professor of Preventive Medicine,
Washington University School of Medicine; Director,
Department of Rehabilitation Medicine, and
Physician, Department of Medicine,
The Jewish Hospital of St. Louis;
Assistant Physician, Barnes Hospital,
St. Louis, Missouri

SIXTH EDITION

with **86** *illustrations*

The C. V. Mosby Company

ST. LOUIS • TORONTO • LONDON 1983

MOSBY

A TRADITION OF PUBLISHING EXCELLENCE

Editor: Karen Berger
Assistant editor: Terry Van Schaik
Manuscript editor: Mary Dolan, Carol Claverie
Production: Margaret B. Bridenbaugh, Linda R. Stalnaker

SIXTH EDITION

Printed in the United States of America

The C.V. Mosby Company
11830 Westline Industrial Drive, St. Louis, Missouri 63141

Library of Congress Cataloging in Publication Data

Cowdry, E.V. (Edmund Vincent), 1888-1975.
Care of the geriatric patient.

Rev. ed. of: Cowdry's The care of the geriatric patient. 5th ed. 1976.
Bibliography: p.
Includes index.
1. Geriatrics. I. Steinberg, Franz U., 1913-
II. Title. [DNLM: 1. Geriatrics. WT 100 C271]
RC952.C6 1983 618.97 82-8088
ISBN 0-8016-4775-4 AACR2

GW/CB/B 9 8 7 6 5 4 3 2 01/A/031

CONTRIBUTORS

LOUIS V. AVIOLI, M.D.

Professor of Medicine, Department of Medicine, Washington University School of Medicine and The Jewish Hospital of St. Louis, St. Louis, Missouri

PHILLIP M. BERMAN, M.D.

Clinical Associate Professor of Medicine, Department of Internal Medicine, Abraham Lincoln School of Medicine, University of Illinois; Director, Rebecca and Harry Port Gastroenterology Laboratory, Louis A. Weiss Memorial Hospital, Chicago, Illinois

AARON BIRENBAUM, M.D.

Medical Director, Division of Home Care, Instructor of Clinical Medicine, Washington University School of Medicine; Attending Physician, The Jewish Hospital of St. Louis, St. Louis, Missouri

HERMAN T. BLUMENTHAL, Ph.D., M.D.

Research Professor of Gerontology, Aging and Development Program, Department of Psychology, Washington University; Adjunct Professor, Department of Community Medicine, St. Louis University School of Medicine; Medical Director and Pathologist, International Clinical Laboratories, St. Louis—Midwest, Missouri

†MONICA D. BLUMENTHAL, M.D., Ph.D.

Professor, Department of Psychiatry, University of Pittsburgh School of Medicine; Director of Geriatric Psychiatry Program, Western Psychiatric Institute and Clinic, Pittsburgh, Pennsylvania

ROSE E. BOYARSKY, Ph.D.

Research Associate, Department of Surgery (Urology), Washington University School of Medicine; Clinical Psychologist in Private Practice at Boyhill Center, St. Louis, Missouri

RUBIN BRESSLER, M.D.

Professor and Head, Department of Internal Medicine; Professor of Pharmacology and Clinical Pharmacology, The University of Arizona Health Sciences Center, Tucson, Arizona

MICHAEL H. BROOKE, M.D.

Professor, Department of Neurology, Washington University School of Medicine; Director, Jerry Lewis Neuromuscular Research Center; Medical Director, IWJ Rehabilitation Institute, St. Louis, Missouri

IRENE BURNSIDE, R.N., M.S., F.A.A.N.

Assistant Professor, Department of Nursing, San Jose State University, San Jose, California

MITCHEL P. BYRNE, M.D.

Clinical Assistant Professor of Surgery, Loyola University Stritch School of Medicine; Associate Attending Surgeon, St. Francis Hospital, Evanston, Illinois

RODNEY M. COE, Ph.D.

Professor, Department of Community Medicine, St. Louis University School of Medicine; Education Coordinator, Geriatric Research Education and Clinical Center, Veterans Administration Medical Center, St. Louis, Missouri

KENNETH A. CONRAD, M.D.

Assistant Professor, Departments of Internal Medicine and Pharmacology, The University of Arizona Health Sciences Center, Tucson, Arizona

PHILIP E. CRYER, M.D.

Professor of Medicine; Program Director, Clinical Research Center, Washington University School of Medicine, St. Louis, Missouri

OCTAVIO de MARCHENA, M.D.

Assistant Professor of Clinical Neurology, Washington University School of Medicine, St. Louis, Missouri

MICHAEL DEVAS, M. Chir., F.R.C.S.

Professor, Department of Orthopaedics, School of Medical Sciences, Universiti Sains Malaysia, Minden, Penang, Malaysia; Formerly Consultant Orthopaedic Surgeon, Royal East Sussex Hospital, Hastings, England

†Deceased.

ROBERT B. DODD, M.D.

Clinical Professor, Department of Anesthesiology, Southern Illinois University School of Medicine; Chairman, Department of Anesthesia, Memorial Medical Center, Springfield, Illinois

MARTI FIGLIOLI, B.S.N.

Administrative Director of the Division of Home Care, The Jewish Hospital of St. Louis, St. Louis, Missouri

FRED C. GAU, M.D.

Instructor in Surgery, Loyola University Stritch School of Medicine; Attending Surgeon, St. Francis Hospital, Evanston, Illinois

ROBERT GOLDSTEIN, Ph.D.

Professor of Communicative Disorders, Department of Communicative Disorders, The University of Wisconsin College of Letters and Science, and Department of Rehabilitative Medicine, The University of Wisconsin School of Medicine, Madison, Wisconsin

ARNOLD W. GUREVITCH, M.D.

Associate Professor and Chief, Division of Dermatology, Department of Medicine, Harbor-UCLA Medical Center, Torrance, California, UCLA School of Medicine, Los Angeles, California

BEVRA H. HAHN, M.D.

Associate Professor of Medicine; Director, Multipurpose Arthritis Center, Department of Medicine, Washington University School of Medicine, St. Louis, Missouri

WILLIAM B. HARDIN, Jr., B.A., M.D.

Assistant Professor of Clinical Neurology, Department of Neurology, Washington University School of Medicine, St. Louis, Missouri

JACQUELINE HARTMAN, M.A., CCC-SP/A

Research Associate, Instructor in Rehabilitation, Department of Preventive Medicine and Department of Neurology, Washington University School of Medicine, St. Louis, Missouri

ARTHUR E. HELFAND, D.P.M.

Professor and Chairman, Department of Community Health, Pennsylvania College of Podiatric Medicine; Adjunct Professor of Medicine, Thomas Jefferson University, Jefferson Medical College; Chief, Department of Podiatry and Director of Podiatric Education, James C. Giuffré Medical Center; Consultant, Philadelphia Veterans Administration Medical Center; Consultant, Philadelphia Department of Public Health, Philadelphia, Pennsylvania

WEBB S. HERSPERGER, M.D.

Clinical Assistant Professor of Surgery, Pennsylvania State University College of Medicine, Hershey, Pennsylvania, Staff Member, Carlisle Hospital, and Consultant, U.S. Dunham Army Hospital, Carlisle, Pennsylvania, Lecturer, Medical Aspects of Exceptional Children, Shippensburg State College, Shippensburg, Pennsylvania

ROBERT J. HICKOK, B.S., M.H.A.

Assistant Vice Chancellor for Medical Affairs; Assistant Professor, Program in Physical Therapy; Assistant Professor, Program in Health Administration and Planning, Washington University School of Medicine, St. Louis, Missouri

SAUL KAMEN, B.A., D.D.S., F.A.C.D.

Chief of Dental Service, Jewish Institute for Geriatric Care, New Hyde Park, New York; Professor of Dental Health, State University of New York at Stony Brook; Chief, Pediatric Dentistry, Long Island Jewish-Hillside Medical Center, New Hyde Park, New York

JOSEPH B. KIRSNER, M.D., Ph.D.

Louis Block Distinguished Service Professor of Medicine, Department of Medicine, Gastroenterology Section, University of Chicago, Chicago, Illinois

ROBERT E. KLEIGER, M.D., F.A.C.C.

Professor of Medicine; Director, Graphics Lab, The Jewish Hospital of St. Louis, Washington University School of Medicine, St. Louis, Missouri

ALVIN J. LEVENSON, M.D.

Associate Professor and Chief, Section on Geriatric Psychiatry, Department of Psychiatry, The University of Texas Medical School at Houston; Lecturer in Psychopharmacology and Aging, Baylor College of Medicine, Texas Medical Center, Houston, Texas

MARVIN E. LEVIN, M.D.

Associate Professor of Clinical Medicine and Associate Director, Diabetes Metabolism Clinic, Washington University; Attending Physician, The Jewish Hospital of St. Louis, St. Louis, Missouri

WILLIAM C. MANN, O.T.R., Ph.D.

Director of Graduate Studies/Associate Professor, Department of Occupational Therapy, State University of New York at Buffalo, Buffalo, New York

JAMES H. MASON, M.D.

Chairman, Department of Surgery, St. Francis Hospital, Evanston, Illinois; Clinical Professor of Surgery, Loyola University Stritch School of Medicine, Evanston, Illinois

DAVID W. MELTZER, Ph.D., M.D.

Assistant Professor of Ophthalmology, Department of Ophthalmology, Washington University School of Medicine, St. Louis, Missouri

RICHARD M. PEARSON, M.D.

Assistant Clinical Professor, Department of Urology, University of Tennessee Center for the Health Sciences; Staff Urologist, Baptist Memorial Hospital, Memphis, Tennessee

THOMAS L. PETTY, M.D.

Professor of Medicine; Head, Division of Pulmonary Sciences, Department of Medicine, University of Colorado Health Sciences Center, Denver, Colorado

†BEN H. SENTURIA, M.D.

Professor Emeritus of Clinical Otolaryngology, Washington University School of Medicine; Director Emeritus, Department of Otolaryngology, The Jewish Hospital of St. Louis; Co-Editor, *Annals of Otology, Rhinology and Laryngology* and *Annals of Head and Neck Medicine and Surgery*, St. Louis, Missouri

IAN M. SMITH, M.D., FRCP (G) FRCPath

Professor, Departments of Internal Medicine and Family Practice, University of Iowa Hospitals & Clinics, Iowa City, Iowa

SAMUEL D. SOULE, M.D.

Clinical Professor, Emeritus, Department of Obstetrics and Gynecology, Washington University School of Medicine; Director, Emeritus, Department of Obstetrics and Gynecology, The Jewish Hospital of St. Louis, St. Louis, Missouri

†Deceased.

FRANZ U. STEINBERG, M.D., F.A.C.P.

Professor of Clinical Medicine, Associate Professor of Preventive Medicine, Washington University School of Medicine; Director, Department of Rehabilitation Medicine, and Physician, Department of Medicine, The Jewish Hospital of St. Louis; Assistant Physician, Barnes Hospital, St. Louis, Missouri

MARTHA STORANDT, Ph.D.

Associate Professor, Department of Psychology, Washington University, St. Louis, Missouri

JOHN R. WALSH, M.D.

Professor of Medicine; Head, Division of Gerontology, Oregon Health Sciences University; Chief, Geriatric Medicine Section, Veterans Administration Medical Center, Portland, Oregon

EDWARD M. WOLIN, M.D.

Medical Oncologist, Colima Internal Medical Group, Whittier, California; Formerly Chief of Oncology, The Jewish Hospital of St. Louis; Assistant Professor of Medicine, Washington University School of Medicine, St. Louis, Missouri

JESS R. YOUNG, M.D.

Head, Department of Peripheral Vascular Disease, Cleveland Clinic, Cleveland, Ohio

VERNON R. YOUNG, Ph.D.

Professor of Nutritional Biochemistry, Department of Nutrition and Food Science, Massachusetts Institute of Technology, Cambridge, Massachusetts

PREFACE to sixth edition

The need to publish a new edition of this book after only 6 years indicates the rapidly growing interest in the medical problems of the aged and in their management. This interest is timely and appropriate. The aged constitute 11% of the total population, but their health care expenditures are 28% of that of all Americans. Approximately 5% of all persons over the age of 65 are disabled to an extent that they need to be confined to nursing homes. It should be the overriding goal of geriatric medicine to keep aged individuals in a satisfactory state of health for as long as possible and to prevent physical and mental disabilities so that they may continue living in the community.

The care of the geriatric patient requires a special body of knowledge. Some diseases are more prevalent in old age, and others present different clinical pictures. The aged who so often suffer from multiple chronic diseases require long-term health care of high quality in addition to the management of periodic acute problems. Also the aged, more than any other group, need care from associated health care professionals, such as nurses, therapists, and social workers. The authors of the new edition have attempted to present up-to-date information that should be available to all those who are responsible for the care of the geriatric population.

The sixth edition has maintained the structure of the previous editions. New chapters have been added on the biology of aging, age changes in organ systems, infections, clinical pharmacology, endocrinology, muscle diseases, home care, and education in geriatric medicine. The chapters on cancer, hematology, dermatology, nutrition, urology, dental surgery, psychiatry, occupational therapy, and nursing have been rewritten by new authors. All other chapters have been updated and revised.

It is in the nature of a book with many contributors that there will be some lack of uniformity in the approach to the problems of the aged and in the style of writing. This is a distinct disadvantage, but it is outweighed by the fact that each chapter has been written by an expert in that field. No attempt has been made to curtail the bibliographies. The reader should have the opportunity to pursue subject matters of his choice in depth.

In closing I would like to express my sincere appreciation to the many contributors who have given so generously of their time and who have allowed us to benefit from their expertise in their chosen specialty.

Franz U. Steinberg

PREFACE to fifth edition

Dr. E. V. Cowdry opened the preface to the first edition with the sentence: "There is a large gap between advances in our knowledge of the problems of aging and the practical utilization of that knowledge." In the intervening eighteen years this gap has certainly not become smaller. Rapid advances in all areas of medicine and social science have added greatly to our knowledge, but they have also made it more difficult to apply what we now know in the everyday care of our elderly patients. This book, as the previous editions, is intended for the physician and other health personnel who are responsible for the primary health care of the aged. We hope that it will contribute to closing the gap.

The decision concerning what material to present in a text on geriatric medicine is difficult. The emphasis should be on diseases that are most commonly encountered in the geriatric population and on those that present a distinctive pathologic and clinical picture in the aged. By necessity, this selection must be somewhat arbitrary.

The book has been organized into five major sections: medical care, surgical care, disorders of the nervous and sensory systems, geriatric rehabilitation, and special aspects of geriatric care. New chapters have been added on evaluation of the geriatric patient, diabetes mellitus, osteoporosis, care of the foot, physical therapy, occupational therapy, and speech pathology. Various chapters of the previous edition dealing with health care delivery have been consolidated into a single new chapter. Seven other chapters have been completely rewritten by new contributors; the other chapters have been revised and updated.

I would like to express my sincere appreciation to the contributors whose splendid cooperation has made it possible to prepare this edition in a relatively short peroid of time.

This edition is dedicated to the memory of Dr. E. V. Cowdry, Sr., who died on June 25, 1975 at the age of 86. Dr. Cowdry, Professor Emeritus of Anatomy at Washington University School of Medicine, was one of the early leaders of cancer research. His outstanding work, which took him to many distant parts of the world, brought him many distinguished honors and awards. His students will remember him as a most stimulating teacher whose interests ranged over a wide field of biologic and social sciences. In 1971 he asked me to assist him with the preparation of the fourth edition of this book and to take on the fifth edition as my sole responsibility. To work with Dr. Cowdry has been an inspiring experience and a great privilege. Even though he did not actively participate in the preparation of this edition, his thoughts and advice during the early planning phase have been invaluable.

Dr. Cowdry, coming from research and teaching in the biologic sciences, conceived this book out of a deeply felt concern for the welfare of the aged. This humanitarian spirit will remain an incentive to all who have had the privilege of working with Dr. Cowdry.

Franz U. Steinberg

CONTENTS

PART III

DISORDERS OF THE NERVOUS AND SENSORY SYSTEMS

PART IV

REHABILITATION

PART V

SPECIAL ASPECTS OF GERIATRIC CARE

PART I MEDICAL CARE

CHAPTER 1 · THE AGING OF ORGANS AND ORGAN SYSTEMS

Franz U. Steinberg

Morphologic and functional changes from youth through maturity to old age are continuous but affect organs and organ systems at different rates and at different times of life. The physician who cares for an aged patient may find it difficult to determine if a given abnormality is due to aging or to disease; this consideration may well affect the diagnostic and therapeutic approach. Aging alters the response to disease. The aging process and the stress of previous diseases cause the body to respond to the same noxious stimulus in ever changing ways. Bürger has dramatized this point with the statement that just as nobody can bathe twice in the same river, no individual can become ill twice in exactly the same manner.[1] As time goes on, degenerative changes and altered immune responses increasingly weaken the defense mechanisms and the ability of the aging body to cope with disease.

In this chapter a brief review is given of some of the physiologic changes that accompany aging. Several monographs are available that treat this subject in greater depth.[2-4]

Different body functions decline at different rates; the pertinent data on this have been summarized by Shock.[5] The internal environment of the body is protected by homeostatic processes. Core temperature, acidity, and electrolyte composition of body fluids and their osmotic pressure are rigidly maintained and vary little from youth to old age. However, according to Shock, it is the recovery of this homeostatic balance, once it has been disturbed by disease or environmental factors, that is significantly delayed in the aging organism. Thus hypothermia, from which a young individual may recover without complications, may be fatal to an aged person. Changes in plasma pH and electrolyte composition are much more difficult to correct in an older individual than in a young patient.

Body functions that involve only one organ system may change little from youth to old age. There is almost no change of the fasting blood sugar level from age 30 to age 80,[5] and the nerve conduction velocity declines by less than 20%. However, functions that require the integrated activity of several organ systems decline at a much more rapid rate. As a result, vital capacity and renal blood flow decrease by 50% from age 30 to age 80, the maximum breathing capacity by 60%, and maximal work rate and maximal oxygen uptake by 70%. Shock states that aging in the total animal "may be more a function of the breakdown in integrative mechanisms than of changes in individual cells, tissues, or organs."[5]

Calloway,[6,7] who has written extensively on the biologic characteristics of aging, found that most functions decline in a hyperbolic curve rather than in a linear fashion if changes during the early phases of life are taken into account. Basal metabolic rate and percentage of body water, for instance, decrease steeply during the first 10 years of life. Thereafter the decline can be represented by a gradually descending straight line, the asymptote of a hyperbola. As a result the half-life of biologic functions occurs early in life. In other words, as times goes on the rate of aging decreases.

BODY COMPOSITION AND STRUCTURE

Mitotic cells are capable of reproduction during an individual's life span. However, as

Hayflick[8] has shown and as is now recognized, the proliferative capacity of mitotic cells is finite for human diploid fibroblasts. These cells are capable of only about 50 divisions, after which the strain perishes. Postmitotic cells cannot reproduce, and once lost they cannot be replaced. Thus neurons and muscle cells, which are postmitotic, may last through the lifetime of the individual, but they undergo gradual degenerative changes.

The corollary to the Hayflick phenomenon is a decrease of body cells over the life span of an animal. It is estimated that by the age of 65 an individual will have lost 30% of the body cells.[9] Since cells become somewhat larger with age, the total cell mass does not decline as much as the number of cells. The total cell volume can be estimated by determining total body water or, more specifically, intracellular water. Since extracellular water varies little with age, the total body water can be taken as a fairly precise measure of cell mass.

From young adulthood to old age total body water of males decreases from 61% of body weight to 54%.[10] The intracellular water declines from 42% to 35%.[9] The extracellular water approximates 20% of body weight. It remains constant with advancing years or shows a slight increase in males over the age of 60.[11] Body fat increases from 15% to 30% from ages 30 to 80. However, since water is only 15% of adipose tissue, fluctuations of body fat contribute little to changes in extracellular water mass.

There is no evidence that the metabolic activity of body cells declines with age. It is true that the basal oxygen consumption falls by about 15% from age 30 to age 80. However, if the oxygen consumption is calculated per liter of body water, which serves as a measure of cellular mass, it turns out to be constant throughout the life span. It may be concluded that the metabolism of individual cell remains constant and that the decline in basal oxygen consumption is due to a reduction in the number of body cells.

Total body potassium is another useful measure of the cellular mass of the body. Potassium is a cellular electrolyte. Cell water contains 150 mEq of potassium per liter, 30 times more than the extracellular compartment. Earlier studies determined exchangeable potassium by injecting the isotope ^{42}K. More recently total body potassium has been estimated by measuring the naturally occurring isotope ^{40}K, which amounts to about 1/100 of total body potassium. In the young adult male the potassium of fat-free body mass is 72 mEq/kg; in the female it is 50 mEq/kg.[12] The decrease due to the aging process amounts to 30% in the male and 25% in the female. This steady decline can be temporarily arrested by vigorous exercise programs, which lead to muscle cell hypertrophy.[13]

The steady decline of total body potassium with aging indicates a loss of cells, particularly of skeletal muscle, which contains about one half of the body potassium. A decrease in the size of cellular organs such as liver, kidneys, brain, spleen, and pancreas adds further to the loss of potassium. Sex differences in the total body potassium and its decrease with advancing age are explained by the heavier muscle mass in males and the greater percentage of fat-containing tissue in the adult female.

Fat and body weight

Body weight increases slowly until 45 to 55 years, and thereafter it declines gradually. In women the peak is reached later in life and the decrease in old age is less pronounced than in men. Although actuary tables give normal weights related to height, Shephard[14] has pointed out a number of pitfalls inherent in the collection and interpretation of such data. Since many of these samples have been collected for insurance purposes, they are biased toward a special selected population group. Skeletal and muscle mass may substantially affect body weight. An athletic person with a heavy skeletal frame and hypertrophic muscles may have a higher than normal weight without being obese. In an aged person with osteoporosis and atrophic muscles, body weight may underestimate the amount of adipose tissue. Also obese individuals have a higher mortality. They may die younger and as a result lightweight individuals may predominate in the older age groups.

A number of mathematical formulae have been developed to express the relation of normal body weight to height.

Broca's index[15] (100 years ago):

$$\text{Normal weight (in kilograms)} = \text{Height (in centimeters)} - 100$$

Body mass (or obesity) index:

$$\text{Weight} \div \text{Height}^2$$

Ponderal index:

$$\text{Height} \div \sqrt[3]{\text{Weight}}$$

This latter index defines body shape. It is based on the assumption that "weight is a measure of volume and that volume increases according to the cube of linear dimensions."[16] According to Seltzer the Ponderal index relates to mortality in an exponential curve.

Body fat can be measured by methods that are more specific than the height/weight ratio. Skinfold measurement is simple but has to be done with care to avoid error. Shephard[17] collected skinfold measurements in aged individuals from the literature and compared them to measurements taken in young adults. Taking samples from 10 different sites of the body he found that between the ages of 25 and 65 average skinfold thickness increased by 25% in males and by 51% in females. Women showed a particularly large accumulation of fat over chest, waist, hips, thighs, and shins. In men adipose tissue was deposited mostly over the waist, lower abdomen, and chest. Women maintain fat deposits to an older age than men. In the seventh and eighth decades subcutaneous fat decreases, first in distal portions of the extremities and last over the trunk. At the same time some of the parenchyma of inner organs is gradually replaced by fat.

Total body fat can be estimated indirectly by measuring ^{40}K and total body water, since fat contains almost no potassium and less water than other soft tissues. The reliability of these procedures is uncertain.[17] Body fat can also be estimated by measuring the specific gravity of the body. This procedure, which involves total body immersion in water, is not easily carried out especially in older individuals. From a review of the pertinent literature, Shephard[17] concludes that the percentage of body fat is 26% in elderly men and 38% in elderly women. This compares to 19.8% for sedentary young men and 28.4% for sedentary young women.

Stature and body contours

It is well-known that older individuals become shorter, but this observation is difficult to quantify. Cross-sectional determinations are in part invalidated by the fact that succeeding generations are taller than those that preceded them. Longitudinal studies of individuals are difficult and have pitfalls of their own. Height and its decline will be affected by the racial composition of a given population, the extent of the physical activity of individuals, nutrition, and the effects of illness. This may explain the considerable divergence of reported data. A detailed summary has been given by Rossman.[18] Most studies agree that loss of height begins past the age of 50. In the female the loss of height over her lifetime amounts to approximately 5 cm, in males to 3 cm. Most of this loss is due to shortening of the spinal column, caused in turn by shrinkage of the intervertebral discs and in some individuals by the collapse of osteoporotic vertebrae. The length of the long bones remains fairly constant over a lifetime, and differences in cross-sectional studies probably reflect secular trends.[19]

Other bony contours change with age. Shoulder width, the biacromial diameter, diminishes with age. In contrast the bony pelvis becomes wider both in males and females. Span, the distance from fingertips to fingertips of horizontally raised arms, changes little through the adult lifetime. It is closely related to height, and a decrease of the height/span ratio with advancing years indicates shrinkage of the spinal column.

The spine, in addition to becoming shorter, assumes abnormal contours. Kyphosis of the thoracic spine increases. As a compensation the neck is held in extension. The extensor muscles of the neck become thicker while the anteriorly located flexors become shortened and atrophic. Associated with kyphosis of the thoracic spine is an abduction, that is, a forward displacement of the scapulae. In the sacrolumbar area the normal lordotic curve usually diminishes with age and the low back looks flat. Moll and Wright,[20] who measured true low back mobility by a method that eliminates hip motion from the overall calculation, found that forward flexion decreases by 27% in aged males and by 23% in aged females. Extension is reduced by 52% in males and by 44% in females. The pelvis becomes wider in the transverse diameter so that the distance from trochanter to trochanter is increased. The angle between the femoral neck and the femoral shaft becomes larger, resulting in a valgus deformity of the hips. Particularly in old women the knees may develop varus deformities leading to a narrow-based insecure gait. Postural changes in very old age evoke the picture of an old man or woman walking or standing with a stoop, the head forward, the knees in varus position, the ankles turned outward, and the arches of the feet flattened.

Kyphosis of the thoracic spine leads to an increase in the anterior-posterior diameter of the chest, giving it a barrel chest appearance. The chest also becomes wider in the transverse diameter. This configuration of the thorax does not indicate the presence of chronic obstructive pulmonary disease, and the term "senile emphysema" has been abandoned.

Freeman[21] has constructed a scenario in which he describes how postural changes with advancing age affect the overall function of the body. Barrel chest deformity flattens the diaphragm and diminishes the efficiency of inspiration. The low position of the diaphragm predisposes to development of a hiatal hernia with all its discomforts and complications. The abnormal position of the cervical spine contributes to the narrowing of neural foramina and to the development of uncomfortable radicular symptoms. The abnormal posture of the neck may interfere with the ability to swallow and to cough effectively. The shortening of the thoracic spine may displace the innominate artery into the neck and cause it to buckle. These changes in posture can lead to significant functional abnormalities.

Changes of bone structure are discussed in Chapter 9. The aging of the skin is discussed in Chapter 12.

CARDIOVASCULAR SYSTEM

Diseases of the cardiovascular system are major causes of illness and death in the aged population. To separate the effects of aging of heart and blood vessels from the consequences of disease is a difficult task. Blumenthal in Chapter 2 of this book has examined the very complex interrelationship of disease and aging. The most common abnormality encountered in the aging circulatory system is atherosclerosis-arteriosclerosis and its sequelae. To what extent atherosclerosis can be viewed as an aging process remains problematic. Many risk factors contribute to its pathogenesis, even though aging remains the most important. Associated diseases such as diabetes mellitus, hypertension, and hyperlipidemia are additional major risk factors, and as a result atherosclerosis may occur much earlier in life than at senescence. This section will deemphasize the effects of atherosclerosis and concentrate on other aspects of the aging cardiovascular system.

The most common pathologic abnormality of the aging heart, other than those caused by atherosclerosis, is a brown pigmentation of the myocardium. Its appearance is not related to sex, race, or cardiovascular disease, and it is not found in young or middle-aged individuals. The pigmentation is due to an accumulation of lipofuscin granules at the poles of the myofiber nuclei.[22] There is no evidence that these granules interfere with myocardial function. On the other hand, the myocardial atrophy frequently encountered in association with brown pigmentation, the "brown atrophy," appears to be the result of disease.

Other age-related changes of heart and blood vessels are due to an alteration of collagen. With aging this structural protein becomes less soluble and stiffer. (See Balazs[23] for a discussion of the chemical processes underlying these changes.) In addition, with advancing years the amount of collagen increases at the expense of muscle. This process is more pronounced in the subepicardial and subendocardial layers than in the central myocardium.[24] Ito et al. have reported a positive correlation between age and the content of hydroxyproline, a constituent of collagen, in autopsy specimens of hearts of individuals without overt evidence of heart disease. The hydroxyproline accumulation was most marked in the subendocardial layers of the left ventricle and in the papillary muscles.[25] The endocardium of the atria and of the atrioventricular valves thickens with age. A nodular thickening also appears at the valvular closure lines, and lipids are deposited in the collagen of the valvular cusps.[26]

The conduction system of the aging heart has been studied by Davies.[27,28] The number of pacemaking cells, the P-cells, diminishes with age, particularly after the age of 60; and after age 75 their number may be reduced to 10% of nodal cells. This decrease may be a significant factor in the development of the "sick sinus syndrome" in old age. No age changes of the atrioventricular node have been identified. Left fascicles of the bundle of His are commonly lost after the age of 60, and eventually more than 50% of the fascicles may disappear. One theory has it that the fascicles are compressed and distorted as they pass through the upper interventricular septum, an area which is under a constant mechanical strain and becomes fibrotic as a result.[29] This process is accentuated by hypertension. The distal bundle branches show an increase of fine fibrous and elastic tissues with advancing age.

It is apparent that the structural changes which the heart undergoes with aging are not spectacular. However, as Kohn has pointed out,[30] myocardial cells do not have the capacity to divide and endothelial and smooth muscle cells divide only under exceptional circumstances. They are stable and last through a lifetime, but they undergo progressive morphologic and chemical changes. The collagen and elastin components are metabolically inert but are under a constant mechanical strain and also must be expected to progressively degenerate with age.

Changes in the structure and function of arteries associated with aging are difficult to separate from those engendered by atherosclerosis, and often the distinction may be arbitrary. The most striking changes in senescent arteries are thinning and fragmentation of the elastic lamellae, deposits of lipid and calcium in the media, and an increase of collagen. All these changes contribute to an increasing rigidity of arterial walls. The functional corollary to the anatomic changes is a diminished compliance of the large arteries, which appears to be independent of vessel wall thickness or peripheral vascular disease. Bader[31] subjected autopsy specimens of human aortas to passive stretch. In the aortas of 20-year-old subjects a pressure of 100 mm Hg increased the volume by 190%; in octogenarians it increased the volume by only 40%. Mozersky et al.[32] determined the elastic properties of femoral and brachial arteries of living subjects by a transcutaneous ultrasonic method, which demonstrated increasing stiffness with age.

Due to its elastic properties the normal human aorta stores one half of the stroke volume during systole and ejects it gradually during diastole. Because of the loss of elasticity this buffering effect gradually declines with aging. Up to the age of 60 the volume of the aorta increases as a compensatory mechanism. In later years, as the ability of the aorta to store blood during systole is further decreased, systolic blood pressure rises. Furthermore, since pressure receptors in the aortic wall depend on elastic stretch, their function also diminishes as the aortic wall becomes more rigid. As a result the diastolic pressure may increase also.[31]

Changes in the small arteries have been less extensively investigated. The walls become thicker while the lumen is reduced. Kilo et al.[33] studied the muscle capillaries in diabetics and in normal controls by electron microscopy. In both groups the basement membrane thickens progressively with age. In the normals this process was more marked in males than in females. The sex difference was not demonstrable in diabetics.

Changes in cardiovascular function with age are of particular interest to the clinician. During rest the function of the aging heart differs little from the heart of the young or middle aged, but significant differences are brought to the fore by stress. Dock has appropriately drawn an analogy from the aging eye to the aging heart, comparing presbycardia to presbyopia:

> Just as distant vision is well maintained while ability to adjust for close vision is lost, so the aging heart maintains its ability to deal with its usual burden, while progressively losing ability to adapt to sudden increase in rate, venous return or in arterial resistance. Presbycardia like presbyopia, is only manifest when an unusual strain is imposed.[34]

Although resting heart rate does not change with age, the effect of age on stroke volume and cardiac output at rest is not clear. Brandfonbrener[35] found that resting cardiac output decreased by 1% per year from age 19 to age 86. During the same period the stroke volume fell from 85.6 ml to 60.1 ml, and the cardiac index, which relates cardiac output to body surface diminished by 0.8% for each year of life. Granath,[36] who measured cardiac output by catheterization, reported a decrease of 25% at age 71 compared to young men in their twenties. However, this reduction was present only when the examination was done in the supine position, and there was no difference when the subjects were examined while sitting. In a critical review of this subject, Gerstenblith et al.[37] questioned whether an examination done by cardiac catheterization truly depicts a resting state, since it is a stressful invasive procedure. They cite a study by Proper and Wall[38] who determined stroke volume and cardiac output by a noninvasive method, using a precordial counter after the injection of radionuclide material. These investigators found no age-related differences in a group of 500 men age 20 to age 70.

Age-associated electrocardiographic changes are minor and of questionable significance.[39] Some authors have reported a prolongation of the ventricular ejection time,[40] but other investigations have failed to confirm this observation. Montoye et al.[41] have reported a slowing of the systolic preejection phase in over 600 healthy aged men and women, even after the data had been corrected for heart rate. They found no age-related slowing of the ejection phase. Montoye's findings suggest that with age the systolic tension of the myocardial fibers develops more slowly. However, it is quite possible that an increasing rigidity of the wall of heart and arteries also contributes to the slowing of the systolic preejection phase. Ventricular relaxation during diastole also becomes slower with aging.[41] Gerstenblith et al.[37] have pointed out that both the slowing of contraction and relaxation need not indicate changes of myocardial function but may be partly or totally due to changes in the compliance of cardiovascular structures and of the work load imposed upon the heart.

Age-associated changes occurring during exercise are more significant. During submaximal exercise the heart rate of aging individuals rises to the same extent as it does in younger individuals. However, the oxygen pulse, the ratio of oxygen consumption ($\dot{V}O_2$) to heart rate, at submaximal work loads does not change with advancing years.[42] The maximal attainable heart rate, however, declines with age in a linear fashion. Roughly it equals 220 minus the age. This formula is not universally applicable, and higher maximal heart rates in aged subjects have been reported.[43] Shephard[43] postulates that a decreased sympathetic drive to the pacemakers may be the possible cause. However, as mentioned before, degenerative changes appear in the sinus node with aging, and it is quite possible that as a result this pacemaker becomes less responsive to sympathetic stimulation.

Maximal oxygen consumption ($\dot{V}O_2$ max) is the definitive measure of the ability of the cardiovascular and respiratory systems to respond to maximal physical stress. Numerous studies have shown that the maximal oxygen consumption decreases with age parallel to the decrease in the maximal heart rate. This decline can be retarded by improving physical fitness but it cannot be abolished. The literature contains a large number of studies on the effects of aging on maximal oxygen consumption. The data have been summarized by Shephard.[43] For example, Astrand[44] found that the maximal oxygen uptake of 65-year-old men was 70% that of 25-year-old men. Dehn and Bruce[45] reported a decrease of $\dot{V}O_2$ max of 0.56 ml/kg per minute per year of life for active men and of 1.62 ml/kg per minute per year of life for inactive men. Decrease in maximal oxygen uptake parallels decline of maximal work capacity.

Cardiac output and stroke volume during exercise decline with aging. This subject has been reviewed by Strandell.[46] The cardiac output rises with increasing work loads in a linear fashion, and the slope of this line is not affected by age. However, at the same work load cardiac output is lower in elderly men than in young men. As expected, maximal stroke volume is lower in aged individuals and is reached at a lower work load expressed as percentage of $\dot{V}O_2$ max.[46]

Several factors contribute to an age-related decrease in the stroke volume. Systolic pressure load on the left ventricle increases with age, since peripheral vascular resistance rises and since rigidity of the large arteries reduces their function as compression chambers. This increased pressure load on the ventricles tends to lower its output with each systole. Furthermore, ventricular walls, including the pericardium, become more rigid with age and their compliance is diminished. All these factors have an impact, and it is impossible to determine to what extent a loss of contractile myocardial power contributes to reduced exercise stroke volume.

One of the main functions of circulation is distribution of oxygen to the tissues. To compensate for the reduced cardiac output, extraction of oxygen by the tissues is increased. As a result the arteriovenous oxygen difference increases with age,[46-48] except for the maximal arteriovenous oxygen difference which declines. Shephard[43] lists a number of reasons to explain this decline, such as reduced arterial oxygen saturation, lower hemoglobin level, changes in peripheral blood distribution with a relatively greater blood flow through the skin with exercise, and reduced tissue enzyme activity.

Peripheral blood flow

Total peripheral resistance, as expressed by the ratio of mean arterial pressure to cardiac output, rises with age. It is not clear whether the increased resistance is due to a decrease in the size of the arteriolar bed or due to a decreased capacity of the small arteries and arterioles to dilate. In any case increased resistance leads to increased diastolic blood pressure. In aged individuals peripheral resistance does not fall during exercise to the same extent as it does in younger persons. The aorta and large arteries become more rigid and lose their elastic recoil. As a result systolic pressure rises in aged individuals, both at rest and during exercise, more precipitously than in young individuals. The effect of this loss of buffering capacity on the heart has been discussed. The rigidity of arterial walls adversely affects the baroceptor reflexes and contributes to increased relative constriction of the small arteries. All this enhances the prevalence of hypertension in the aged.

The distribution of peripheral blood flow changes with age. Earlier studies have been summarized by Bender.[49] Later studies have confirmed most of the early data. Cerebral and coronary blood flow changes are minimal. The blood flow through the kidneys, the splanchnic vascular bed, and the skin (at rest) is decreased, but Shephard[43] has reported that blood flow through the skin of aged individuals rises above normal during exercise. The reduction in blood flow through the inner organs is greater than can be explained by decreased cardiac output; therefore peripheral vascular changes must play a significant role.

Summary

In summary, as individuals age heart and blood vessels become more rigid due to changes of the physicochemical properties of the collagen. In the myocardium collagen is increased at the expense of muscle tissue. The elastin of the arteries undergoes degenerative changes. Functional abnormalities are most obvious when the cardiovascular system is stressed by exercise. Both stroke volume and cardiac output rise with increasing work loads, but for the same work load they remain lower than in younger individuals. Maximal oxygen consumption, exercise stroke volume, heart rate, and cardiac output all decline with age. Peripheral vascular resistance increases, and with exercise it does not fall to the same extent as it does in young individuals.

All these observations indicate that the capacity of the aging cardiovascular system to respond to stress declines significantly.

RESPIRATORY SYSTEM

Aging is accompanied by morphologic changes of the thorax and lungs. The alveolar walls become thinner and the number of capillaries is reduced. The total number of alveoli remains unchanged, but the internal alveolar surface area decreases from adolescence to old age, indicating a decline of the surface area of individual alveoli.[50] At the same time the alveolar ducts and small bronchioles enlarge in volume at the expense of the alveolar volume. The number and thickness of the elastic fibers that form the supportive tissue of the lung are reduced. Pulmonary arterial walls thicken with age, both in the intimal and the medial layers. Hernandez et al.[51] have reported an increase of bronchial mucous glands in an aged population of nonsmokers who lived in the same geographic area and were therefore exposed to the same atmospheric environment.

The costal cartilages become more rigid with advancing years, and eventually they may calcify. This loss of elasticity may lead to a barrel chest deformity and an increasing kyphosis. Pierce and Ebert[52] have shown that these structural changes, while resembling those encountered in emphysema, are not accompanied by the functional changes of chronic obstructive pulmonary disease, and they recommended that the term "senile emphysema" be abandoned. The intercostal muscles tend to become atrophic and weaker.

The elastic recoil of the lungs declines with aging. This decline has been estimated to amount to 0.25 mm H_2O per year of life (at 50% of total lung capacity) in nonsmoking normal adults. As a result the pressure needed to distend the lung to a given volume decreases.[53,54] In physiologic terms, static lung compliance increases with age. These findings have been confirmed more recently.[54,55] Knudson et al.[54] found the age-related decrease of elastic recoil to be more pronounced at higher lung volumes. There were no sex differences if lung sizes were taken into account. In contrast compliance of the chest wall diminishes with age, and this reduction is greater than the increase in compliance of the lung. As a result total compliance of the respiratory system is reduced with age, and the work needed to overcome the elastic forces of chest wall and lungs combined, according to Turner et al.,[53] is 20% greater in a 60-year-old than in a 20-year-old.

The elastic fibers maintain the patency of the small airways against increasing expiratory pressures. This function declines with aging, and as a result "the closing volume," the lung volume at which airways collapse during expiration, becomes larger with advancing years.[56-58] Airway closure occurs earlier during the expiratory phase in supine than in seated subjects. In individuals over the age of 65 airway closure occurs at an expiratory volume that exceeds the expiratory reserve and lies within the tidal range. The tendency of small airways to close during expiration is enhanced by exercise. Closure affects mostly the dependent portions of the lung. The pulmonary circulation remains unchanged so that blood continues to flow through relatively unaerated portions of the lung. As a result the alveolar-arterial oxygen difference increases.

The effect of aging on lung volumes has been extensively studied. Available data have been summarized by Shephard[43] and Muiesan et al.[59] In addition to age and sex, body height correlates most closely with the vital capacity. The interpretation of available data is complicated by the fact that both in population cross-sections and in longitudinal studies body height decreases with age. Nevertheless, it is apparent that the vital capacity decreases with age. The average decrease amounts to 26.4 ml/per year for males and 21.6 ml per year for females.[59] Bühlmann has constructed a nomogram based on the examination of over 1100 men and women between the ages of 19 and 70 years and of over 700 men and women between the ages of 71 and 90 years.[60] These nomograms indicate normal values for age and body height. However, the decline of vital capacity with age is not linear. For all age groups a value more than 20% below normal is considered pathologic.

Total lung capacity changes with age are insignificant. Since vital capacity decreases, residual volume must be increased. The ratio of residual capacity to total lung volume rises from 20% at age 20 to 35% at age 60.[59] Most investigators have found that functional residual capacity increases with age. This increase, however, is proportionally less than the rise of residual volume.

Studies also show a deterioration in airflow with age. Maximal voluntary ventilation, peak expiratory flow rate, and maximal midexpiratory flow rate all decrease with age. The 1-second forced expiratory volume (FEV_1) declines with age.[61] Bühlmann[60] reported a reduction of the FEV_1/vital capacity ratio to less than 70% in men and women over the age of 71. Schmidt et al.[62] reported similar results. In men over 55 years and in women over 60 years, the ratio of FEV_1/forced vital capacity varied from 70% to 75% in contrast to younger persons in whom it was greater than 80%. On the other hand, Milne and Williamson[63] reported that their data on FEV_1 and FVC did not fit the regression equations developed for a younger population. These and other discrepancies in the literature may be due to the different characteristics of the test populations selected by the various authors. The mechanism by which expiratory airflow is decreased with aging has not been fully explained. Black and Hyatt[64] reported a decrease in the maximal inspiratory and expiratory pressure with aging. This decrease is most likely caused by a weakness of the respiratory muscles. Another factor may be the loss of elastic recoil, which becomes increasingly prevalent as individuals age. There is no evidence that pulmonary resistance increases in the absence of obstructive pulmonary disease.

At rest the minute volume of respiration changes little, but with effort it rises more rapidly in aged individuals than in young adults. To a large extent this may be due to diminished physical fitness, loss of joint mobility, or simply to poor coordination. Sidney and Shephard[65] found that the ventilatory equivalent, that is, the minute volume of respiration per liter of consumed oxygen, is increased above normal when aged individuals exercise on a bicycle but not when they walk on a treadmill.

The increase in alveolar-arterial oxygen difference with age is entirely due to a decrease of the arterial oxygen pressure, since the alveolar oxygen tension remains unchanged. The decline in PaO_2 may be at least partly caused by a decrease of diffusion of oxygen from the alveoli to the blood. Another factor may be a mismatch of ventilation and perfusion. As pointed out before, closing volume increases with age and as a result the dependent portions of the lung may remain underventilated especially during quiet effortless breathing. Since the rate of perfusion remains normal, inadequately oxygenated blood may flow from poorly ventilated segments of the lung.

The respiratory system undergoes structural and functional changes with aging. However, in the absence of disease these changes do not appear to interfere significantly with gas exchanges in aging individuals.

GASTROINTESTINAL TRACT
Teeth and oral mucous membranes

Dental enamel shows evidence of wear with advancing years. It also becomes somewhat darker because staining substances to which the teeth are exposed over a lifetime are absorbed into its substance and because the darker dentin shows through the thinning enamel covering. Attrition is variable and depends on dietary habits and on the mechanics of chewing, which in turn is affected by the structure of the jaws and the loss of other teeth. Dentin is structurally related to bone. Odontoblasts, the cells that produce dentin, diminish in number with advancing years and may be replaced by undifferentiated pulpal cells. Secondary (or reparative) dentin is formed throughout the lifetime of a tooth mostly in response to noxious stimuli. It encroaches on the pulpal cavity, which becomes smaller. Blood vessels of the pulp undergo atherosclerotic changes often at a very early age; nerves also show signs of degeneration.[66,67] Cementum decreases with age even though new cementum continues to be formed. As the gums recede cementum becomes exposed and vulnerable to chemical and mechanical injuries. The recession of the gums deprives the cementum of its supply of nutrients.

The salivary glands undergo degenerative changes such as fibrosis and fat deposits. Secretion is reduced, and many old individuals complain that their mouth is dry much of the time. The dry mucous membrane in turn becomes subject to injuries and infections.

Decreased taste sensation, a common complaint of the very old, is usually associated with structural changes of the tongue. From childhood to old age 65% of the taste buds of the circumvallate papillae are lost.[68] A large proportion of the remaining taste buds are atrophic. Taste sensitivity to sweet, sour, and bitter is lost earlier than taste sensitivity to salt. Hughes studied taste sensation by applying a direct electric current to the oral mucous membrane; he found that the threshold increased fivefold from age 20 to age 80.[69]

Decreased taste sensibility may also be caused by loss of smell sensation, which also diminishes with old age. Neurologic lesions, either central in the parietal lobe or peripheral in the facial, glossopharyngeal, or vagus nerves and their nuclei may also be responsible for this loss.

Esophagus

The esophagus is a muscular organ. The upper quarter is striated muscle; the lower one-third is smooth muscle. The intermediate segments are composed of a variable mixture of the two muscle types. The upper sphincter lies opposite the larynx. It is closed in its resting stage and opens only to permit a bolus of food to pass. In this fashion the upper sphincter prevents the aspiration of food into the respiratory tract. The food bolus is transported by peristaltic waves. In addition the lower one half of the esophagus may exhibit ringlike nonperistaltic so-called tertiary contractions. The lower sphincter separates the esophagus from the stomach. It opens during swallowing, and it remains open until after the peristaltic wave has passed through it. Its tone is decreased by gastric and other acids, alcohol, iced beverages, and anticholinergic drugs. It is increased by alkali, cholinergics, and the hormone gastrin, which acts on the postganglionic cholinergic nerves.

With aging the nonperistaltic contractions increase, and this may interfere with the propulsion of food through the esophagus. Peristaltic waves are reduced, and the lower sphincter fails to relax in about one half of the swallows.[70] This delays the emptying of the esophagus, a condition which has been given the name of *presbyesophagus*.

Gastroesophageal reflux is due to inadequate lower sphincter closure, and the suggested cause is gastrin deficiency.[71] It may occur in the presence or absence of a hiatal hernia. In other words, sphincter function is not materially affected by its location above or below the diaphragm. A study of the motility of the esophagus in aged individuals free of other disease showed only decreased amplitude of the peristaltic contractions.[72] The authors concluded that all other disorders of motility may be due to associated diseases.

Difficulties in swallowing, commonly seen in the elderly, may also be due to dysfunction of the pharyngeal musculature, particularly of the cricopharyngeal muscle.[73,74]

Stomach

The secretion of acid decreases with advancing years. The anatomic corollary is an atrophy of the gastric mucosa and its glands. Both mucosa and muscular wall become thinner. The atrophy of the mucosa may be patchy or may be confined to either the antrum or the fundus. Atrophic lesions of the antrum tend to cause gastrointestinal symptoms more frequently and are precancerous. The secretion of pepsin and of intrinsic factor is also diminished. Whether or not gastric motility and emptying of the stomach are affected by aging is not known.

Small intestine

The secretion of enzymes is diminished with aging. Nevertheless, normal amounts of pancreatic amylase are available after stimulation to digest carbohydrates, which so often are the major dietary staple of the aged. Trypsin secretion is also reduced. In general enzyme production, although diminished, is adequate for the digestion of normally ingested foods.

Absorption does not appear to be affected by age alone. The surface area of the small intestine is enormous and provides a generous reserve of absorptive potential. The absorption of certain materials is adversely affected by the gastric achlorhydria of the aged. Thus the absorption of calcium and of iron may be reduced.

The capacity of the intestinal mucosa to absorb carbohydrates has been tested with the D-xylose absorption test. Xylose is a pentose, the absorption of which requires no amylase or other pancreatic enzymes. Failure to absorb xylose therefore, indicates an abnormality of the small intestinal mucosa. Under normal circumstances 25% of the ingested xylose is excreted by the kidney in 5 hours. Guth studied the effect of age on the D-xylose absorption test.[75] He found a decrease of renal xylose excretion after a loading dose in individuals 70 years old or older. It is not clear, however, if this reduction was caused by decreased absorption or renal abnormalities. It may be concluded that age does not critically affect either enzyme production or absorption. The malnutrition so frequently encountered in the aged is mostly due to disease or to poor dietary habits.

Colon

Constipation, so commonly experienced by aged individuals, is almost always caused by external factors such as low dietary bulk, inadequate fluid intake, or laxative abuse. Only rarely do organic factors contribute to the development of constipation; possible causes are neurologic disease or endocrine disorders such as hypothyroidism or Hirschsprung's disease.

Diverticulosis is a frequent disorder of old age. Diverticula appear in only 8% of adults under the age of 60. Over the age of 70 the incidence is 40%.[76] Diverticula arise by herniation between the bands of the taeniae coli, associated with an increase of intraluminar pressure. It has been suggested that a low residue diet narrows the lumen of the colon, increases intracolonic pressure, and thereby predisposes to the development of diverticula. It has not been clearly determined to what extent the motility of the colon is altered in diverticulosis. Parks' studies suggest that the colon muscle function is abnormal in diverticulosis and that this abnormality precedes the development of diverticula.[77]

Liver

Liver size declines with age. Calloway,[78] who examined 400 livers at autopsy, found that livers of 70-year-old persons weighed 27.5% less than those of 30-year-old individuals. Liver weight remained constant at 2.5% of body weight until age 80 when it fell to 1.9%. Cellular changes which have been described in animals consist of variations of cell size with a general increase of the size of the centrolobular hepatocytes. Hyperchromatic giant nuclei and clear perinuclear zones may appear.[70,79-81] Connective tissue is not increased. Enzyme changes have been found in animal models, particularly in those enzymes concerned with oxidation and reduction. That they also occur in aged humans can be surmised but has not been demonstrated. Liver function tests remain normal. The Bromsulphalein test has been studied by several investigators. In spite of conflicting reports there seems to be no clear-cut evidence that this test is affected by age alone.[79] Serum albumin production declines with age, but total serum protein level does not change significantly.

Whatever enzyme changes may occur in the aging liver affect the metabolism of drugs more than any other function (Chapter 15). The oxidation of anticonvulsant drugs, psychotropic drugs, and oral anticoagulants is impaired in old age, but the oxidation of ethanol remains unchanged.[80] Drug acetylation appears to remain normal.

Gallbladder

Diseases of the gallbladder are discussed in Chapter 8. The evidence that the prevalence of gallstones increases with age is overwhelming. In individuals over the age of 70 the prevalence has been estimated to be above 40%. In a recent autopsy series gallstones were found in 36% of men and 63% of women above the age of 70.[82] The formation of gallstones appears to be related to an increase of hepatic cholesterol and increased excretion of cholesterol in bile. Much of the evidence is based on animal experimentation, but one recent human study demonstrated that over 41% of aged woman excrete bile supersaturated with cholesterol compared to 8.3% of young women.[83] Bile acid metabolism does not appear to change with age.

In summary, age-conditioned changes of the alimentary tract have not been as extensively studied as those of other organ systems. In the absence of disease, changes due to aging appear to have little effect on overall alimentary tract function.

EXCRETORY SYSTEM

Numerous studies spanning several decades of research have demonstrated the decline of renal function with age. Details of these investigations have been summarized in a number of publications.[84,85]

Weight of the kidneys decreases by about 20% from young adulthood to old age.[84] At birth each kidney contains approximately one million nephrons. By the age of 80 this number will have decreased by about 30%. The filtering surface of the glomeruli in individuals over the age of 16 is 1.6 m^2. Between the ages of 66 to 73 years it declines to 0.9 m^2.[86] The number of glomerular and tubular cells is reduced. The length of the proximal tubules decreases by 35% from youth to very old age; the volume of the tubules declines by 31%.[87] The basement membranes both of the glomeruli and tubules thicken with age.

Degeneration of the renal vascular system is an obvious manifestation of aging. As the glomeruli become atrophic their blood vessels degenerate. In the cortical area the arterioles end blindly but remain patent. It is assumed that blood from these arterioles is carried to the peritubular vascular bed.[88] In the juxtamedullary zone a shunt develops between the afferent and efferent arterioles of degenerating glomeruli. The interlobular and arcuate arteries become tortuous. The muscle of the medial layer of arteries becomes fragmented and is interspersed with collagen, which gradually replaces the smooth muscle. The elastic laminae split and may partly calcify. The interstitial tissue becomes less cellular.

Renal function decline parallels anatomic changes. Davies and Shock[89] determined glomerular filtration rates by inulin clearance in 70 men who were free of renal disease. They found a steady age-related regression that was almost linear. Wesson[90] compiled data from 37 reports in the literature and calculated glomerular filtration rates and effective renal plasma flow per 1.73 m^2 of body surface in normal men and woman. For both sexes the filtration rate declined slowly from age 15 to 45 and more rapidly thereafter. In males the filtration rate was 140 ml per minute at age 15 and 125 ml per minute at age 45. At the age of 60 it had decreased to 105 ml per minute, at age 70 to 88 ml per minute, and at age 80 to 75 ml per minute. Shock[91] reported on a longitudinal study of creatinine clearances in 600 males who were examined at intervals of 18 to 20 months. He found only a slight decline up to the age of 50 but a significant steady reduction thereafter. More recently Rowe et al.[92] reported on the relation of age to 24-hour creatinine clearances in 884 subjects with an age range from 17 to 96 years. Of these, 293 individuals underwent repeated serial examinations. All subjects were active community-dwelling men, free of renal disease, and not taking any medication that might affect renal function. The results of the cross-sectional and longitudinal studies were the same. In 30-year-old subjects the creatinine clearance averaged 140 ml per minute. It began to decline after age 34; the rate of decline increased after age 65. At age 80 the creatinine clearance averaged 97 ml per minute. The authors constructed a nomogram that relates creatinine clearance to age. Various authors have reported decreased urea clearance with age, associated with a rise of the blood urea concentration. However, since blood urea concentration is partly dependent on protein intake, this association is not close.

The effective renal blood flow is measured by determining the clearance of either Diodrast or para-aminohippuric acid. At low arterial concentrations 92% of these substances are cleared with one passage through the kidneys. Most studies have reported a decrease in renal blood flow with age. Wesson's previously noted compilation of data from the literature demonstrated a value of 670 ml per minute for healthy young males. By the age of 45 this had declined slightly to 610 ml per minute, by age 60 to 520 ml per minute, and by age 75 to 350 ml per minute.[90]

The portion of the blood plasma perfusing the kidney that is filtered by the glomeruli is defined as the *filtration fraction*. It is calculated as the ratio of the glomerular filtration rate to effective renal blood flow. Since the glomerular filtration rate declines less rapidly with age than the effective renal blood flow, the filtration fraction rises with advancing years.

The aging kidneys receive less of a share than the normal 20% to 25% of the cardiac output. The question of whether the reduced blood flow through the kidneys in old age is due to structural vascular changes or due to a state of relative functional vasoconstriction has remained unresolved. McDonald et al.[93] found that after the administration of a pyrogen as vasodilator the effective renal blood flow increased almost evenly in all age groups. This suggested a state of relative vasoconstriction in the aging kidney but no fixed vascular changes. Hollenberg et al[94] determined renal blood flow by a washout technique after injection of radioactive xenon into the renal artery. Their 207 subjects, ranging in age from 17 to 76 years, were healthy potential kidney donors. Hollenberg and his coworkers injected acetylcholine as a vasodilator into the renal artery and found, in contrast to McDonald's earlier findings, that there was less vasodilatation in aged individuals than in the young. However, the response to the injection of a vasoconstrictor angiotensin was not affected by age. These studies suggest that the kidneys of older individuals are less capable of vasodilatation than those of younger subjects. Further studies are needed to resolve these contradictions.

Hollenberg's experiments yielded other interesting data. The ^{133}Xe washout technique measures blood flow per unit tissue. Results indicate a reduction of renal blood flow with aging above and beyond the decrease of kidney mass. The ^{133}Xe technique is capable of measuring flow to the rapid-flow compartment separately, that is of the outer cortical area. Results show that, in addition to the overall reduction of renal blood flow, the percentage of blood perfusing the outer cortex is further diminished with age.

Renal tubular function is measured by the maximal tubular excretion of para-aminohippuric acid or Diodrast or by the maximal tubular reabsorption of glucose. All these functions decline with age. The rate of decline of these functions per year of life is almost identical and parallels the decrease of the glomerular filtration rate.[95] This suggests that the decline is due to a loss of nephrons as functional units. However, other experimental data also suggest alterations in the metabolism of tubular cells, and it is possible that the reduction of renal function with age may have multiple causes.[85]

The ability of kidneys in old age to maximally dilute urine is diminished. However, Lindeman[85] has shown that the free water clearance remains normal if corrected for glomerular filtration rate and solute excretion. He postulated that as nephrons are lost with age the remaining nephrons have to excrete a larger solute load and that this explains the impaired ability to form a dilute urine. However, additional data have shown that loss of diluting capacity outstrips the decrease in the glomerular filtration rate.[84] The capacity to form a concentrated urine with increased solute loads or dehydration is also diminished in old age. The response to vasopressin is unchanged.

The aging kidney continues to do its share of maintaining the acid-base balance of tissue fluids. However, the response time is prolonged. The pH and bicarbonate adjustments to a load of either 20 gm of sodium bicarbonate or 10 mg of ammonium chloride require 24 to 48 hours in the aged compared to 8 to 10 hours in the young.[96]

The removal of one kidney causes a hypertrophy of the other kidney. This compensatory hypertrophy occurs in the old as well as in the young, but the increase of kidney size and function becomes slower in the aged as time passes. Boner et al.[97] studied the function of the remaining kidney of kidney donors between the ages of 21 and 63 years. In the first 3 weeks after nephrectomy, the function of the remaining kidney increased at the same rate in both young and old donors. However, during a 4-year follow-up the glomerular filtration rate of aged donors had increased considerably less than that of young donors. The compensatory enlargement is not due to an increase of the number of nephrons but to hypertrophy and to some extent to a hyperplasia of the remaining glomeruli and tubules.

Various diseases commonly seen in the aged tend to decrease renal function. Hypertensive disease, as expected, lowers renal blood flow beyond the decline usually expected in old age. Chronic bacteriuria lowers maximal urine osmolality, renal plasma flow, and glomerular filtration rate.[98] Alwell[99] reported that pyuria with or without bacteriuria reduced maximal concentrating ability. Chronic urinary obstruction due to prostatic hypertrophy also reduces renal function.

In summary, the size of kidneys and the number of functioning nephrons decrease with age. There is a parallel decrease in glomerular filtration rate, tubular excretion, and tubular reabsorption. Since these functions decline at the same rate, the reduction is best explained by a loss of nephrons. The blood flow to the kidneys decreases with age. This occurs to a greater extent than can be accounted for by the loss of kidney mass. The aging kidney receives a smaller share of the cardiac output. It is not clear to what extent the reduction of renal circulation is due to structural blood vessel changes versus a functional vasoconstriction.

The aging kidney's capacity to form diluted urine in response to an increased water load or to produce concentrated urine in response to dehydration or an increased load of solutes is diminished. The kidneys of older individuals are still capable of maintaining the acid-base balance of tissue fluids. However, the response time is markedly prolonged, a delay that may become critical. Changes in renal function have important implications for the administration and dosage of those drugs that are removed from the body primarily by renal excretion. This subject is discussed in Chapter 15.

The effect of old age on bladder structure and function is discussed in Chapter 20.

REFERENCES

1. Bürger, M.: Altern und Krankheit, ed. 3, Leipzig, 1957, Georg Thieme Verlag.
2. Finch, C.E., and Hayflick, L.: Handbook of the biology of aging, New York, 1977, Van Nostrand Reinhold Co.
3. Goldman, R., and Rockstein, M., editors: The physiology and pathology of human aging, New York, 1975, Academic Press, Inc.
4. Holle, G., editor: Handbuch der allgemeinen Pathologie. IV. Altern, vol. 6, Berlin, 1972, Springer Verlag.
5. Shock, N.W.: System integration. In Finch, C.E. and Hayflick, L.: Handbook of the biology of aging, New York, 1977, Van Nostrand Reinhold Co.
6. Calloway, N.O.: The basic laws of biologic senescence, J. Am. Geriatr. Soc. **17**:638, 1969.
7. Calloway, N.O.: The concept of biologic half-life in relation to senescence, J. Am. Geriatr. Soc. **17**:974, 1969.
8. Hayflick, L.: The limited in vitro life-time of human diploid cell strains, Exp. Cell. Res. **37**:614, 1965.
9. Goldman, R. Speculations on vascular changes with age, J. Am. Geriatr. Soc. **18**:765, 1970.
10. Edelman, I.S., et al.: Further observations on total body water. I. Normal values throughout the life span, Surg. Gynecol. Obstet. **95**:1, 1952.
11. Schwab, M., Dissmann, T., and Schubert, W.: Der Einfluss des Alters auf die Flüssigkeitsräume des Körpers, Klin. Wochenschr. **41**:1173, 1973.
12. Pierson, R.N., Jr., Lin, D.H.Y., and Phillips, R.A.: Total body potassium in health: effects of age, sex, height and fat, Am. J. Physiol. **226**:206, 1974.
13. Misner, J.E., Boileau, R.A., Massey, B.H., and Mayhew, J.L.: Alterations in the body composition of adult men during selected physical training programs, J. Am. Geriatr. Soc. **22**:33, 1974.
14. Shephard, R.J.: Physical activity and aging, Chicago, 1978, Year Book Medical Publishers, Inc., pp. 53-54.
15. Broca, D. In Holle, G., editor: Handbuch der allgemeinen Pathologie. IV. Altern, vol. 6, Berlin, 1972, Springer Verlag, p. 234.
16. Seltzer, C.C.: Some re-evaluation of the build and blood pressure study, 1959, as related to the ponderal index, somatotype and mortality, N. Engl. J. Med. **274**:254, 1966.
17. Shephard, R.J.: Physical activity and aging, Chicago, 1978, Year Book Medical Publishers, Inc., p. 56.
18. Rossman, I.: Anatomic and body composition changes with aging, In Finch, C.E., and Hayflick, L.: Handbook of the biology of aging, New York, 1977, Van Nostrand Reinhold Co.
19. Hertzog, K.P., Garn, S.M., and Hempy, H.O., III.: Partitioning the effects of secular trend and aging on adult stature, Am. J. Phys. Anthropol. **31**:111, 1969.
20. Moll, J.M.H., and Wright, V.: Normal range of spinal mobility, Ann. Rheum. Dis. **30**:381, 1971.
21. Freeman, J.T.: Posture in the aging and aged body, J.A.M.A. **165**:843, 1957.
22. Strehler, B.L., Mark, D., Mildvan, A.S., and Gee, M.V.: Rate and magnitude of age pigment accumulation in the human myocardium, J. Gerontol. **14**:430, 1959.
23. Balazs, E.A.: Intercellular matrix of connective tissue. In Finch, C.E., and Hayflick, L.: Handbook of the biology of aging, New York, 1977, Van Nostrand Reinhold Co.

24. Lenkiewicz, J.E., Davies, M.J., and Rosen, D.: Collagen in human myocardium as a function of age, Cardiovasc. Res. **6:**549, 1972.
25. Ito, A., Yamagiwa, H., and Yasaki, R.: Effects of aging on hydroxyproline in human heart muscle, J. Am. Geriatr. Soc. **28:**398, 1980.
26. Pomerance, A.: Aging changes in human heart valves, Br. Heart J. **29:**222, 1967.
27. Davies, M.J.: Pathology of the conduction system. In Caird, F.I., Dall, J.L.C., and Kennedy, R.D.: Cardiology in old age, New York, 1976, Plenum Press.
28. Davies, M.J., and Pomerance, A.: Quantitative study of aging changes in human sinoatrial node and internodal tracts, Br. Heart J. **34:**150, 1972.
29. Lev, M., Unger, P.A., Rosen, K.M., and Bharati, S.: The anatomic substrate of complete left bundle branch block, Circulation **50:**479, 1974.
30. Kohn, R.R.: Heart and cardiovascular system. In Finch, C.E., and Hayflick, L.: Handbook of the biology of aging, New York, 1977, Van Nostrand Reinhold Co., p. 302.
31. Bader, H.: Dependence of wall stress in the human thoracic aorta on age and pressure, Circ. Res. **20:**354, 1967.
32. Mozersky, D.J., Sumner, D.S., Hokanson, D.E., and Strandness, D.E.: Transcutaneous measurement of arterial wall properties as a potential method of estimating aging, J. Am. Geriatr. Soc. **21:**18, 1973.
33. Kilo, C., Vogler, N., and Williamson, J.R.: Muscle capillary basement membrane changes related to aging and diabetes mellitus, Diabetes **21:**881, 1972.
34. Dock, W.: How some hearts age, J.A.M.A. **195:**148, 1966.
35. Brandfonbrener, M., Landowne, M., and Shock, N.W.: Changes in cardiac output with age, Circulation **12:**557, 1955.
36. Granath, A., Johnson, B., and Strandell, T.: Circulation in healthy old men studied by right heart catheterization at rest and during exercise in supine and sitting position, Acta Med. Scand. **176:**425, 1964.
37. Gerstenblith, G., Lakatta, E.G., and Weisfeldt, M.L.: Age changes in myocardial function and exercise response, Prog. Cardiovasc. Dis. **19:**1, 1976.
38. Proper, R., and Wall, F.: Left ventricular stroke volume measurements not affected by chronologic aging, Am. Heart J. **83:**843, 1972.
39. Simonson, E.: The effect of age on the electrocardiogram, Am. J. Cardiol. **29:**64, 1972.
40. Willems, J.L., et al.: The left ventricular ejection time in elderly subjects, Circulation **42:**37, 1970.
41. Montoye, H., Willis, P.W., III, Howard, G.E., and Keller, J.B.: Cardiac preejection period: age and sex comparisons, J. Gerontol. **26:**208, 1971
42. Hanson, J.S., Tabakin, B.S., and Levy, A.M.: Comparative exercise performance of normal men in the third, fourth and fifth decades of life, Circulation **37:**345, 1968.
43. Shephard, R.J.: Physical activity and aging, Chicago, 1978, Year Book Medical Publishers, Inc.
44. Astrand, P., and Rodahl, K.: Textbook of work physiology, ed. 2, New York, 1977, McGraw-Hill Book Co., pp. 318-325.
45. Dehn, M.M., and Bruce, R.A.: Longitudinal variations in maximal oxygen uptake with age and activity, J. Appl. Physiol. **33:**805, 1972.
46. Strandell, T.: Cardiac output in old age. In Caird, F.I., Dall, J.L.C., and Kennedy, R.D.: Cardiology in old age, New York, 1976, Plenum Press.
47. Strandell, T.: Circulatory studies in healthy old men, Acta Med. Scand. (Suppl.) **141:**1, 1964.
48. Wahren, J., Saltin, B., Jorfeldt, L., and Pernow, B.: Influence of age on the local circulatory adaptation to leg exercise, J. Clin. Lab. Invest. **33:**79, 1974.
49. Bender, A.D.: The effect of increasing age on the distribution of peripheral blood flow in man, J. Am. Geriatr. Soc. **13:**192, 1965.
50. Thurlbeck, W.M.: Internal surface area and other measurements in emphysema, Thorax **22:**483, 1967.
51. Hernandez, J.A., et al: The bronchial glands in aging, J. Am. Geriatr. Soc. **13:**799, 1965.
52. Pierce, J.A., and Ebert, R.V.: The barrel deformity of the chest, the senile lung and obstructive pulmonary emphysema, Am. J. Med. **25:**13, 1958.
53. Turner, J.M., Mead, J., and Wohl, M.E.: Elasticity of human lungs in relation to age, J. Appl. Physiol. **25:**664, 1968.
54. Knudson, R.J., Clark, D.F., Kennedy, T.C., and Knudson, D.E.: Effect of aging alone on mechanical properties of the normal human lung, J. Appl. Physiol. **43:**1054, 1977.
55. Colebatch, H.J.H., Greaves, I.A., and Ng, C.K.Y.: Exponential analysis of elastic recoil and aging in healthy males and femles, J. Appl. Physiol. **47:**683, 1979.
56. LeBlanc, P., Ruff, F., and Milic-Emili, J.: Effects of age and body position on "airway closure" in man, J. Appl. Physiol. **28:**448, 1970.
57. Anthonisen, N.R., Danson, J., Robertson, P.C., and Ross, W.R.D.: Airway closure as function of age, Respir. Physiol. **8:**58, 1969/70.
58. Begin, R., Renzetti, A.D., Bilger, A.H., and Watanabe, S.: Flow and age dependence on airway closures and dynamic compliance, J. Appl. Physiol. **38:**199, 1973.
59. Muiesan, G., Sorbini, G.A., and Grassi, V.: Respiratory function in the aged, Bull. Physio-Pathol. Respir. **7:**973, 1971.
60. Bühlmann, A.A.: Normalwerte für die Vitalkapazität und die expiratorische Sekundenkapazität der Lungen im höheren Alter, Schweiz. Med. Wochenschr. **109:**677, 1979.
61. Morris, J.F., Koski, A., and Johnson, L.C.: Spirometric standards for healthy non-smoking adults, Am. Rev. Respir. Dis. **103:**57, 1971.
62. Schmidt, C.D.W., Dickman, M.L., Gardner, R.M., and Brough, F.K.: Spirometric standards for healthy elderly men and women, Am. Rev. Respir. Dis. **108:**933, 1973.
63. Milne, J.S., and Williamson, J.: Respiratory function tests in older people, Clin. Sci. **42:**371, 1972.
64. Black, L.F., and Hyatt, R.E.: Maximal respiratory pressures: normal values and relationship to age and sex, Am. Rev. Respir. Dis. **99:**696, 1969.
65. Sidney, K.H., and Shephard, R.J.: Maximum and submaximum exercise tests in men and women in the seventh, eighth and ninth decade of life, J. Appl. Physiol. **43:**280, 1977.

66. Tonna, E.A.: Aging of the skeletal-dental systems and supporting tissues. In Finch, C.E., and Hayflick, L.: Handbook of the biology of aging, New York, 1977 Van Nostrand Reinhold Co.
67. Bernick, S.: Age changes in the blood supply to human teeth, J. Dent. Res. **46**:544, 1967.
68. Arey, L.B., Tremain, M.J., and Monzingo, F.L.: The numerical and topographical relation of taste buds to human circumvallate papillae throughout the life-span, Anat. Rec. **64**:9, 1935.
69. Hughes, G.: Changes in taste sensitivity with advancing age, Gerontol. Clin. **11**:224, 1969.
70. Bhanthumnavin, K., and Schuster, M.M.: Aging and gastrointestinal function. In Finch, C.E., and Hayflick, L.: Handbook of the biology of aging, New York, 1977, Van Nostrand Reinhold Co.
71. Lipshutz, W.H., Gaskins, R.D., Lakush, W.M., and Sode, J.: Hypogastrenemia in patients with lower esophageal sphincter incompetence, Gastroenterology **67**:423, 1974.
72. Hollis, J.B., and Castell, D.O.: Esophageal function in old men, Ann. Intern. Med. **80**:371, 1974.
73. Kilman, W.J.: Disorders of pharyngeal and upper esophageal sphincter motor dysfunction, Arch. Intern. Med. **136**:592, 1976.
74. Palmer, E.D.: Disorders of the cricopharyngeus muscle: a review, Gastroenterology **71**:510, 1976.
75. Guth, P.H.: Physiologic alteration in small bowel function with age. The absorption of D-xylose, Am. J. Dig. Dis. **13**:565, 1968.
76. Manousos, O.N., Truelove, S.C., and Lumsden, K.: Prevalence of colonic diverticulosis in general population of Oxford area, Br. Med. J. **3**:762, 1967.
77. Parks, T.G.: Natural history of diverticular disease of the colon, Br. Med. J. **4**:639, 1969.
78. Calloway, N.O.: Uncertainties in geriatric data. II. Organ size. J. Am. Geriatr. Soc. **13**:20, 1965.
79. Carr, R.D., Smith, J.J., and Keil, P.G. The liver in the aging process, Arch. Pathol. **70**:15, 1960.
80. Earnest, D.L., and MacGregor, I.L.: Therapy for gastrointestinal disease. In Conrad, K.A., and Bressler, R. editors: Drug therapy for the elderly, St. Louis, 1982, The C.V. Mosby Co.
81. Schmucker, D.L., Mooney, J.S., and Jones, A.L.: Age related changes in hepatic fine structures: a quantitative analysis, J. Gerontol. **31**:135, 1976.
82. Coyne, M., Marks, J., and Schoenfield, L.: Mechanisms of cholesterol gallstone formation, Clin. Gastroenterol. **61**:129, 1977.
83. Lindstrom, G.C.: Frequency of gallstone disease in a well-defined Swedish population: a prospective necropsy study in Malmo, Scand. J. Gastroenterol. **12**:341, 1977.
84. Goldman, R.: Aging of the excretory system: kidney and bladder. In Finch, C.E., and Hayflick, L.: Handbook of the biology of aging, New York, 1977, Van Nostrand Reinhold Co.
85. Lindeman, R.D.: Age changes in renal function. In Goldman, R., and Rockstein, M., editors: The physiology and pathology of human aging, New York, 1975, Academic Press, Inc.
86. Dunnill, M.S., and Halley, W. Some observations on the quantitative anatomy of the kidney, J. Pathol. **110**:113, 1973.
87. Darmady, E.M., Offer, J., and Woodhouse, M.A.: The parameters of the aging kidney, J. Pathol. **109**:195, 1973.
88. Davidson, A.J., Talner, L.B., and Downs, W.M.: A study of the angiographic appearance of the kidney in an aging normotensive population, Radiology **92**:975, 1969.
89. Davies, D.F., and Shock, N.W.: Age changes in glomerular filtration rate, effective renal plasma flow, and tubular excretory capacity in adult males, J. Clin. Invest. **29**:496, 1950.
90. Wesson, L.G.: Physiology of the human kidney, New York, 1969, Grune & Stratton, Inc., pp. 96-102.
91. Shock, N.W.: Current trends in research on the physiological aspects of aging, J. Am. Geriatr. Soc. **15**:995, 1967.
92. Rowe, J.W., et al.: The effect of age on creatinine clearance in man: a cross-sectional and longitudinal study, J. Gerontol. **31**:155, 1976.
93. McDonald, R.K., Solomon, D.H., and Shock, N.W.: Aging as a factor in renal hemodynamic changes induced by a standardized pyrogen, J. Clin. Invest. **30**:457, 1951.
94. Hollenberg, N.K., et al: Senescence and the renal vasculature in normal man, Circ. Res. **34**:309, 1974.
95. Watkin, D.M., and Shock, N.W.: Agewise standard value for C_{In}, C_{PAH} and Tm_{PAH} in adult males, J. Clin. Invest. **34**:969, 1955.
96. Papper, S.: The effects of age in reducing renal function, Geriatrics **28**:(5)83, 1973.
97. Boner, G., Shelp, W.D., Newton, M., and Rieselbach, R.E.: Factors influencing the increase in glomerular filtration rate in the remaining kidney of transplant donors, Am. J. Med. **55**:169, 1973.
98. Dontas, A.S., Papanayiotou, P., Marketos, S., and Papanicolaou, N.: The effect of bacteriuria on renal function patterns in old age, Clin. Sci. **34**:73, 1968.
99. Alwell, N.: Aging kidney, Lancet **2**:635, 1978.

CHAPTER 2 · BIOLOGY OF AGING

Herman T. Blumenthal

It is important, if not critical, to an understanding of those disorders prevalent among geriatric patients to determine which derive directly from intrinsic biologic aging and which are induced primarily by environmental factors. The currently dominant view is that many nonlethal infirmities prevalent in the elderly are a direct consequence of biologic aging, whereas the diseases that account for the vast majority of mortalities in the aged are largely the consequences of environmental factors. Specifically, biologic aging is generally regarded as being genetically programmed, whereas pathologic aging is considered to be nonprogrammed.[1,2]

The diseases that currently account for almost all disease-related mortalities in the aged, and designated here as the diseases of aging, include atherosclerosis-arteriosclerosis and its sequelae (heart attack, stroke, renal vascular disease with uremia, and gangrene of the lower extremity or intestinal tract), cancer, and chronic obstructive pulmonary disease (COPD). Although diabetes, hypertension, and senile dementia are usually included in this list, most elderly diabetic and hypertensive patients die of the consequences of an intensified or accelerated atherosclerosis-arteriosclerosis, and patients with Alzheimer's dementia have a reduced life expectancy but die of the same spectrum of diseases as other elderly subjects.[3] In many elderly the immediate cause of death is pneumonia, either secondary to some other disease process or as a single postmortem finding, and in a small number of cases senile amyloidosis may be the cause of death; these are attributable to failure of the immune system.

Current thinking also holds that these diseases, with the possible exceptions of senile dementia and amyloidosis, are the consequences of exposure to a spectrum of risk factors, the most common of which are a high intake of certain dietary constituents, cigarette smoking, environmental or psychogenic stresses, hypertension, viral infections, and aging. This risk factor concept is based on statistical associations rather than on a cause-and-effect relationship. In this regard it is important to note that the best statistical correlations among these various risk factors are those between age and these diseases. On a plot of log mortality versus age (Fig. 2-1) there is a straight line correlation between each of these diseases and age.[4] However, this association is generally ignored because it is assumed that nothing can be done to retard biologic aging.

The list below shows several ways in which the aging-disease relationship may be considered.

1. Diseases prevalent in the elderly are caused by environmental factors, which must act continuously over many years, or by periodic repeated insults.
2. Diseases may be accelerators of aging in the sense that they add injury to the insult of senescence.
3. Biologic aging involves changes that confer a state of increased susceptibility to disease.
4. There may be a fundamental intrinsic relationship between biologic and pathologic aging.

In the first aging is regarded as incidental to the requirement of a long latent period during which the risk factors must act. It should be pointed out, however, that in those disorders which are considered to be caricatures of aging such as progeria, Cockayne's syndrome, Down's syndrome, Werner's syndrome, and others, the causes of death are the same diseases as for the elderly, even though the shortened life span does not permit prolonged application of risk

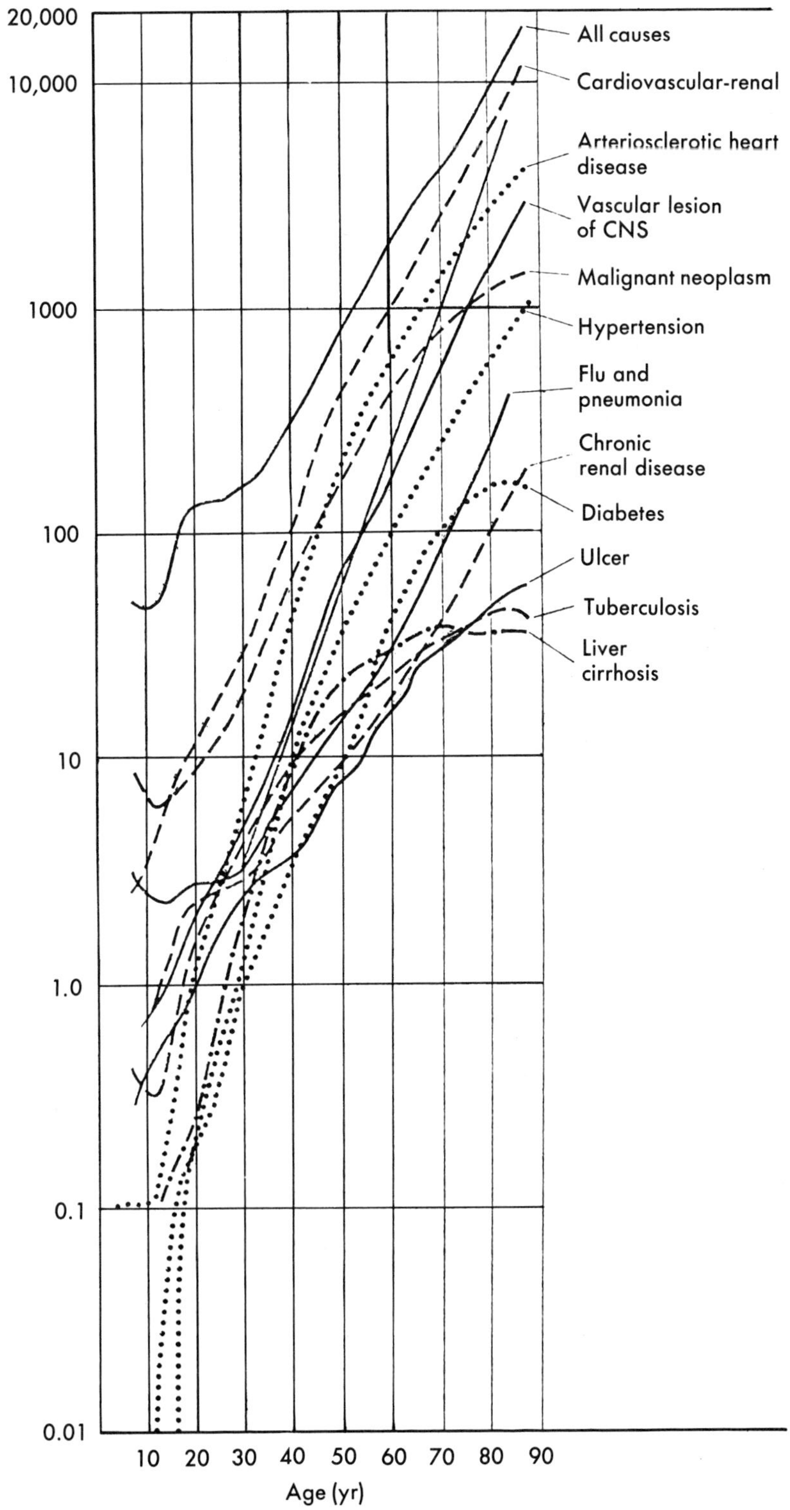

Fig. 2-1. Plot of age-specific death rates for a number of diseases. The unlabeled line corresponds roughly to the original Gompertz[11] plot in which the vertical axis represents log mortality rate. (Modified from Kohn, R.R.: J. Chronic Dis. **16**:5, 1963.)

factors. Moreover, as in the elderly, patients with such disorders of precocious aging are concomitantly afflicted with more than one of these diseases. Such clinical observations suggest that there may be a more fundamental relationship between biologic aging and the diseases of aging than the currently dominant view reflects, and indeed in respect to the genesis of cancer this concept of the role of aging has been regarded as "simplistic."[5] The second concept reflects the impact of diseases on aging; they add injury to the insult of senescence. That disease can have such an effect is generally not in dispute. The third concept, although still separating biologic and pathologic aging, does away with the requirement of a long latent period for risk factor action. And the fourth holds that biologic aging and the diseases of aging are inextricably linked. The basis for considering the latter two possibilities are explored in this chapter.

Medicine's current model is, in principle, ecological. It derives from the discovery that identifiable microorganisms or dietary deficiencies cause specific diseases.

> Contemporary medicine (therefore), attempts to cure or prevent damage wrought by the environment. It achieves this by neutralizing pathogens or by compensating for the lack of something the environment normally supplies.[6]

This has recently been extended to developing strategies for the eradication of certain infectious diseases (smallpox, poliomyelitis, measles, and yaws).[7] In respect to the risk factor concept (and even genetic disease), the ecological model attempts to intercept some environmental trigger. The new model would regard the diseases of aging as either the consequences of particular vulnerabilities of aging cells and associated aging homeostatic mechanisms, or as having a primary intrinsic genesis with external factors having only an accelerating effect. In the context of the "new pathology," the diseases of aging may have a common substrate.[8] The new model proposes that both biologic aging and the diseases of aging may be directly due to the loss of "fidelity of (genetic) information flow" associated with aging.[9]

DEFINITION AND DEMOGRAPHY

An encompassing definition of aging, although of profound concern, has yet to be forthcoming despite some four decades of particularly intensive research in gerontology. Perhaps such a definition is not possible because of the diversity of phenomena associated with the passage of time. Nevertheless, these criteria are generally accepted as characterizing biologic aging: universal, intrinsic, progressive, and deleterious.[10] The criterion of universality expresses the principle that aging phenomena occur in all members of a species who live long enough, while that of intrinsicality excludes environmental factors except possibly as having a secondary influence. These two separate aging from disease, the first by virtue of the fact that old people die of a variety of diseases and the second because disease is regarded as due primarily to environmental causes. To the extent that diseases may lack prolonged prodromal symptoms, they may also lack progressiveness in the context intended by this criterion. Cured disease may be only minimally deleterious.

Aging has also been defined in terms of "force of mortality" as originally proposed by Gompertz (1825) and plotted as a composite of the diseases associated with mortalities shown in Fig. 2-1.[11] Another plot expressing the aging-disease relationship is that shown in Fig. 2-2. In the latter the vertical axis represents survivorship rather than mortality. The progressive improvement in survivorship between "ancient times" and the present can be attributed, in large part, to public health measures such as improved nutrition, better prenatal and maternal care, the purification of water supply, and improved sewage disposal. The introduction of immunizations and antibiotics in the control of infectious diseases has also contributed to this improvement. It is noteworthy, however, that recent so-called biomedical breakthroughs have only minimally improved survival since 1950. Almost all the improvement in life expectancy has taken place at the front end of the life span since, as illustrated in Fig. 2-3, life expectancy at birth has improved from 47 years in 1900 to 73 years today, but remaining life expectancy after age 75 has changed only minimally during these eight decades.

Keyfitz,[12] among many others, has pointed out that if general cures for the diseases of aging could be discovered, life expectancy would be increased only by an additional 7 years—to about age 80. Approaching the same problem

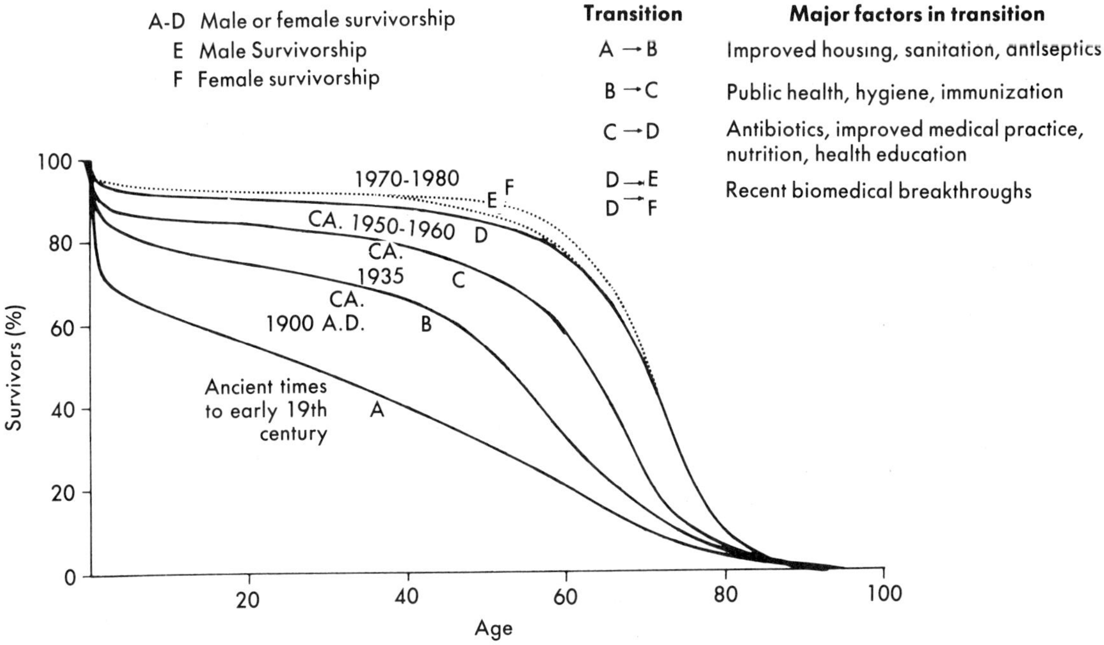

Fig. 2-2. Human survivorship curves showing progressive improvement in life expectancy from ancient to modern times and illustrating the approach that has been taken since about 1950 to the limiting rectangular (ideal) survivorship curve. (From Strehler, B.L.: Implications of aging research for society. In Thorbecke, G.J., editor: Biology of aging and development, New York, 1975, Plenum Press.)

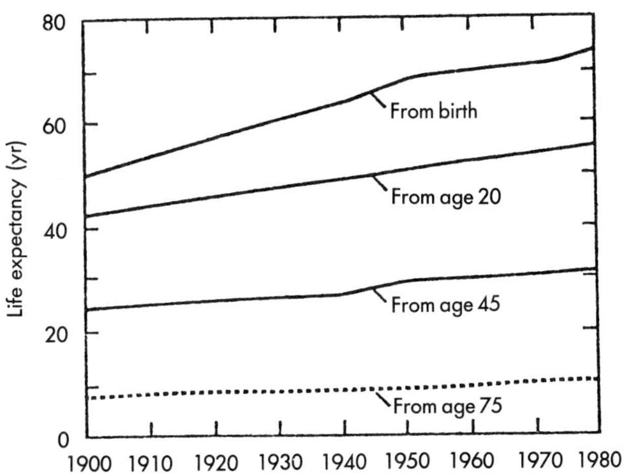

Fig. 2-3. Life expectancy changes in the United States between 1900 and 1980 showing that life expectancy at birth has increased by 28 years, whereas at age 75 it has increased by only 3 years. (From Fries, J.F.: N. Engl. J. Med. **303:**130, 1980. Reprinted, by permission of The New England Journal of Medicine.)

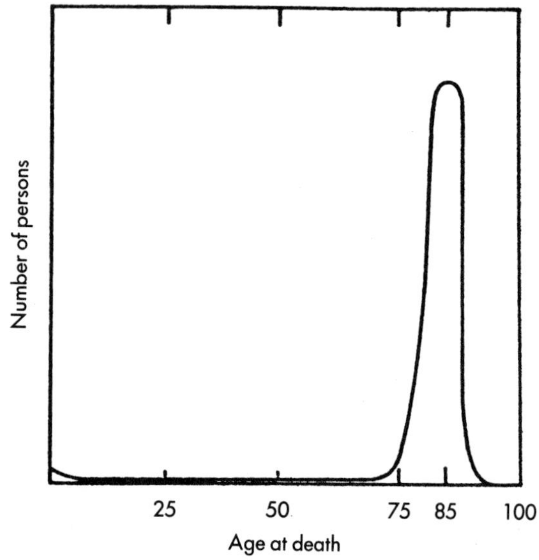

Fig. 2-4. Morbidity curve to about age 75 has been made rectangular, and shape of curve after age 75 has been detailed. (From Fries, J.F.: N. Engl. J. Med. **303:**130, 1980. Reprinted, by permission of The New England Journal of Medicine.)

from a somewhat different perspective in which it is assumed that an effective health maintenance strategy can be developed, Fries[13] has constructed the plot shown in Fig. 2-4. Conceptually, the latter does not differ fundamentally from the ideal or rectangular survival curve traditionally proposed by biogerontologists. Fig. 2-4 expresses the hypothesis that the elimination of the diseases of aging would permit a given population cohort to live to advanced old age, when in a few years the life span of that cohort would be terminated as a consequence of biologic failure. Fries simply proposes that this terminal event would take the form of a bell-shaped curve rather than a precipitous decline.

Inherent in the concept of an ideal survivorship curve is the separability of biologic and pathologic aging, currently accepted as valid by the vast majority of biomedical scientists. On the other hand, an historical review of opinions on this separatist issue,[14] which begins with those offered by Bernard in 1865 and Charcot in 1881, reveals that there has always been something less than unanimity. Recently Ludwig[6] stated, "Man will never die of old age alone but always from disease. However, terminal disease of the future will be different from that we are faced with now and presumably more diversified."

An initial consideration is whether or not the diseases of aging, like biologic aging itself, are genetically programmed. Fig. 2-5 identifies the various diseases responsible for the present survivorship curve.[15] Strehler points out that in a heterogeneous population such as the human species, different maximum longevities are to be expected in a universal environment, or even in an ideal one, "because different genetic endowments lead to death from inherent defects at different times." This survivorship curve, as Strehler points out further, can be construed as consisting of a composite of genetically limited rectangular curves. However, even this model leaves open the possibility that there is a very small percent of any population cohort, which represents a genetically elite group that dies in extreme old age of "general failure without specific disease." Presumably a plot of the latter would yield the ideal survivorship curve.

Strehler's hypothesis has recently been considered from a somewhat different perspective.[14] On the assumption that there are diseases of genetic or congenital origin expressed either in childhood or somewhat later in life and that there are diseases of aging involving the same or associated genes, but altered as a consequence of aging, the following list of diseases has

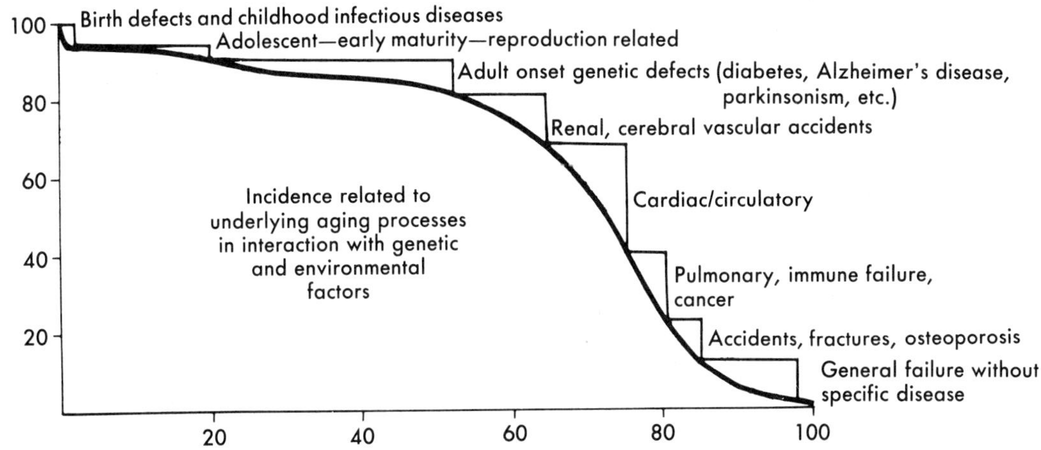

Fig. 2-5. Origins of survivorship curve in the United States, showing genetic predispositions to specific causes of death, which express themselves during different epochs of the human life span. (From Strehler, B.L.: Implications of aging research for society. In Thorbecke, G.J., editor: Biology of aging and development, New York, 1975, Plenum Press.)

been compiled which have juvenile and senescent counterparts.

Cancer
Atherosclerosis-arteriosclerosis
Diabetes
Hypertension
Rheumatoid arthritis
Osteoporosis
Alzheimer's dementia
Hirschsprung's megacolon
Paget's disease

This, in all likelihood, is not a complete list, but it does contain the diseases that are prevalent in the aged. Although some of the common forms of childhood cancer are different from those of the adult years (e.g., Wilm's tumor, neuroblastoma, rhabdomyosarcoma), a number are similar, including lymphoid tumors, the leukemias, and testicular tumors. Cancer of the colon, which is common in late life, has an earlier counterpart associated with familial polyposis. Similarly atherosclerosis-arteriosclerosis, which is predominantly a disease of late life, has its juvenile counterpart associated with familial hypercholesterolemia and with a defect in low density lipoprotein receptors.[16] Although diabetes is now subdivided into insulin-dependent and non–insulin-dependent forms, both are found in juveniles and adults. Hypertension and rheumatoid arthritis are also predominantly diseases of adults but have counterparts in children.[17,18] On the other hand, Hirschsprung's disease (aganglionic megacolon), a disease predominantly of newborns and infants, also has an adult-onset form.[19] The senile plaques associated with senile dementia are found in mongoloids in their twenties and thirties.[20] Finally, some cases of Paget's disease of bone which occur in middle life can be traced to an inborn error, while others not so clearly inherited emerge in late life.[21]

As already noted, one common characteristic of the diseases of aging is that two or more occur concomitantly. Or as Ingelfinger[22] pointed out: if one disease is cured, another shortly arises to take its place. This characteristic is commonly referred to as the *polypathy of aging*. At the same time that mortality from cardiovascular disease is declining, mortality from cancer continues a slow, steady ascent. Measures, such as replacing saturated with polyunsaturated fats, that appear to be successful in reducing mortality from coronary occlusion do not result in a significant increase in longevity; rather there seems to be a trade-off between death from a heart attack and death from cancer. Whether polyunsaturated fats are conducive to cancer development or whether the data simply reflect the polypathy principle is not clear.[23]

An observation that probably influences a separation of aging and the diseases of aging is that lower animals do not die of disease (at least as the latter is defined for higher species), although they also show a Gompertz type of mortality curve. On the other hand some pathologists, at least, would agree with the statement of Wisniewski and Terry[24] that "biological age is the integrated expression of disease". As Sonneborn pointed out, the biologic and physiologic bases of aging need not be identical or even similar in different species in spite of the widespread existence of aging and death. Each species has undergone selection for a particular life span. "The thing selected is the end result, not the means of achieving it." Sonneborn[25] concludes that the search for a single fundamental aging process and mechanism "may well be doomed to eternal failure".

MOLECULAR-CELLULAR BIOLOGY OF AGING

The past four decades have witnessed an unprecedented revolution in the biologic sciences. Molecular biologists can now provide molecular maps of genes and their products and can excise genes from one organism and splice them into the genetic program of another. Comparable developments have taken place in immunology and neuroendocrinology. But perhaps most important has been the application of cybernetic principles to biologic phenomena. As a consequence, life is now operationally defined in cybernetic terms "as an information processing system—a structural hierarchy of functioning units—that has acquired through evolution the ability to store and process the information necessary for its own accurate reproduction."[26] As Davis[27] explains, "DNA stores a program like a computer on a one dimensional tape; and cells use this information to specify the structures of their working machinery."

The input to this information processing system is the gene—the base sequence of double-stranded DNA—and the printout is the assembly of amino acids in proper sequence and steric configuration specifying each protein. In between is a complex transfer system involving transcription and translation and governed by delicately balanced control mechanisms. The genes are replicated enzymatically, maintain extraordinary fidelity, but occasionally mutate. They are transformed into messenger RNA (mRNA) and expressed as protein sequences under the control of transfer RNA (tRNA). The synthetases involved in transcription are generally controlled by the concentration of end product, which at appropriately high levels, inhibits further catalytic activity.

In the context of the computer analogy the operation of the genetic program may be viewed as follows: the DNA consists of four different bases or letters, the order or the sequence of which provides the meaning. When DNA replicates, the helix opens up and the strands separate. The single strands then act as templates for the construction of mRNA, which is complementary to the original strands. The DNA in one human cell has been estimated to contain 5 million base pairs or letters, or the equivalent of about 1000 two-thousand page volumes.[28] The mRNA also consists of four bases, one different from those of the DNA. Their letters consist of triplets, with each triplet specifying an amino acid; in addition, one triplet signals "start" along the ribosome designated to print out the protein, and another triplet signals "stop" and "release the protein." The right amino acid finds the right mRNA triplet by means of an adapter tRNA. There are 20 different amino acids and a corresponding 20 families of tRNA. This process is depicted in Fig. 2-6.

The major machinery of the cell consists of hundreds of different proteins with an infinite variety of specific combining sites involving such entities as enzymes, hormones, antigens, antibodies, regulatory proteins, membrane transport proteins, and the structural proteins that bind cells together and that also constitute the cytoskeleton of individual cells. Included in the latter is the microtubular-microfilamentous system utilized for the intracellular transport of nutrients and hormones, as well as for the movement of chromosomes during mitotic division. To account for these specific sites it is necessary to know not only how one-dimensional information is translated from a nucleic acid sequence into a polypeptide sequence, but also how such information creates specific three-dimensional shapes. The one-dimensional polypeptide folds spontaneously into its final three-dimensional form because the chain contains in itself the information in the form of attractions and repulsions between the side chains of the 20 different amino acids. The protein chains can form an alpha helix, which is flexible, and side chains can interact at any angle, providing extraordinary plasticity.[27]

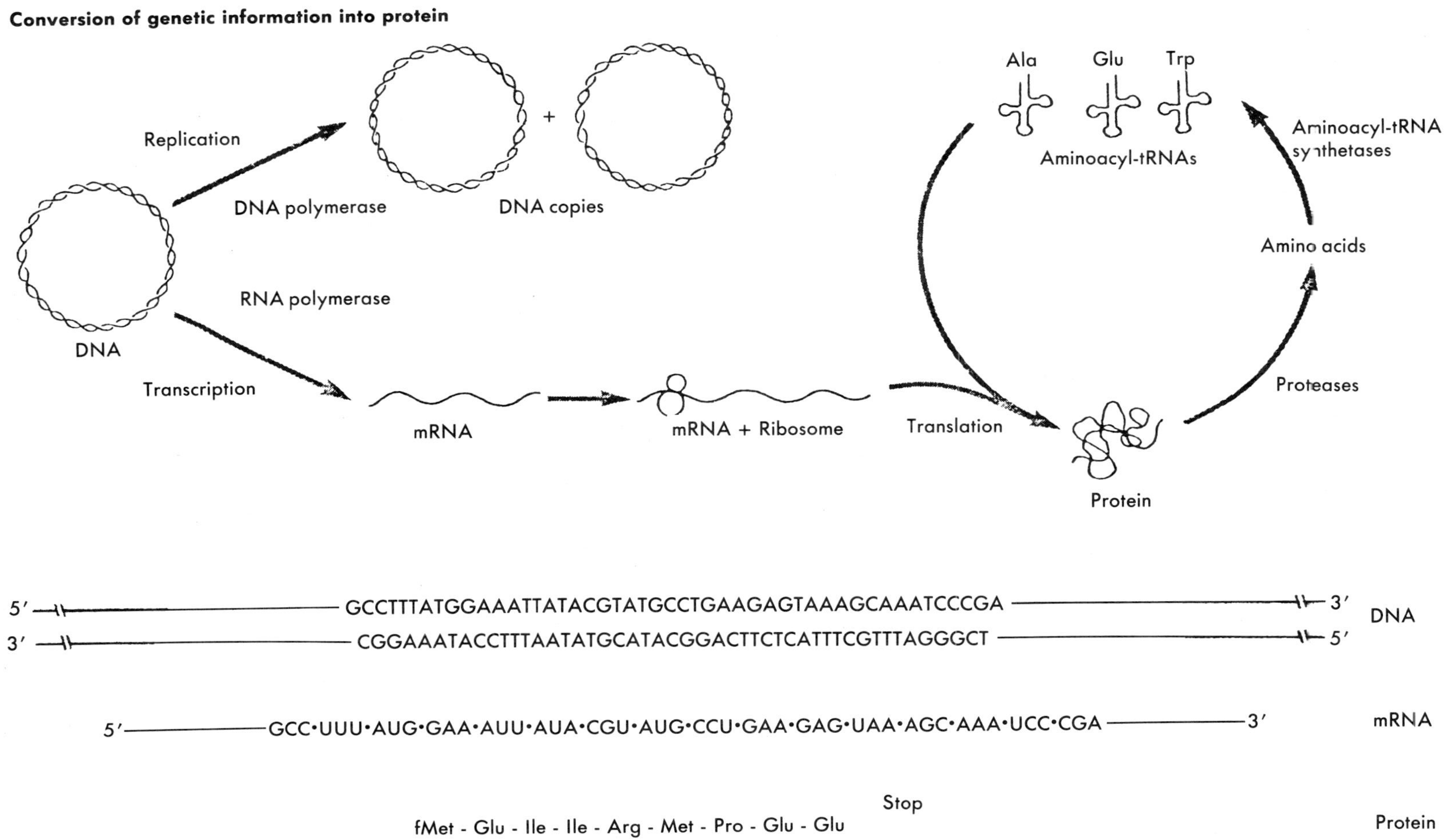

Fig. 2-6. Schematic representation of conversion of genetic formation into protein. (From Rich, A.: The Sciences **20:**10, 198C.)

Carbohydrates also carry biologic information by virtue of the fact that a large number of structures can be formed from a small number of monomers. In other words, monosaccharides can also serve as letters in a vocabulary of biologic specificity, where the words are formed by variations in the nature of the sugar present, the type of linkage to proteins, and the presence or absence of branch points. The specificity of many polymers is written in terms of sugars rather than amino acids or nucleotides. This is particularly applicable to sugars on cell surfaces, which appear to determine the organ specificity of cells as well as the life span of circulating cells and their distribution through the body. For example, the sugar on a lymphocyte serves as a "zip code," directing it where to go. These specificities can be removed simply by enzymatic digestion. Important to matters discussed in this chapter is the fact that cell surface sugars may determine the specificity of receptors for various other physiologic substances such as hormones and that pronounced changes in cell-surface sugars take place in the transformation of normal to malignant cells.[29]

The purpose in recounting the elements in this now well-established cybernetic system is to point out that information does not always flow perfectly and to use it as a frame of reference for pointing out where errors may occur that are relevant to molecular-cellular aging. One estimate gives an error frequency for DNA replication as one in 30,000 letters and for mRNA as one in 10,000.[30] Another estimates only one mistake in over 100 million letters in DNA replication.[31] It is doubtful, however, that either of these has considered the possibility of an increase in error frequency as a consequence of aging. The mispairing of bases resulting in an amino acid substitution (misspelling) is one possible source of error. Perhaps a more common source is that of "frame shift" resulting from a misalignment of DNA strands during replication. This gives rise to a protein printout, designated as "gibberish," or to premature termination in the distal part of the printout. Moreover, it has long been recognized that there is more DNA than the organism uses in its lifetime. This redundant DNA has been regarded as a reservoir for the replacement of damaged DNA, with the size of this reservoir in a particular species determining the latter's characteristic life span.[32] The intervening sequences of redundant DNA are first transcribed to mRNA and then excised, leading some investigators to suggest that it provides spaces between words or sentences.[30] This redundant DNA has also recently been designated as "selfish" DNA[33,34] because its replication is perpetuated even though it may serve no useful function. Nevertheless, the transcription-excision process constitutes a potential source of error.

Another recent discovery is that there are two molecular forms of DNA, a right-handed BDNA and a left-handed ZDNA. Most of the DNA in a cell is of the right-handed variety. The DNA with the reverse twist has exposed segments that are normally hidden in the right-handed form. There is some evidence that these exposed segments may be where carcinogens bind, as well as evidence suggesting that high rates of mutation may occur in sequences with the left-handed configuration.[28] There is, as yet, no information regarding possible changes with aging in the ratio of BDNA to ZDNA.

For most of the approximately 40 years that gerontology has operated as an organized discipline much of the research has been largely descriptive in the sense of systematically identifying morphologic and physiologic decrements accumulating over time and in measuring the rates at which they occur. Although earlier studies on the effects of radiation on the rate of aging suggested a role for some mutagenic phenomenon, it was Szilard[35] who first proposed that mutations accumulated in the genomes of somatic cells, gradually inactivating chromosomes until ultimately the functional capacity of the chromosome was destroyed and the cell died. However, Szilard's proposal, based on aging as a consequence of cell attrition, is applicable only to postmitotic cells such as neurons and skeletal and myocardial muscle, since organs with a capacity for mitotic division have cells capable of replacing dead ones, and most if not all organs possess considerable redundancy.

Nevertheless, Szilard's proposal appears to have led to a consideration of mechanisms that may bring about the synthesis of altered proteins which would be inactive or would exhibit a degeneration in specificity. The estimates of inherent error in the fidelity of information flow, as with somatic mutations, did not appear to occur with sufficient frequency to account for the multitude of molecular-cellular changes associated with aging. Accordingly, Orgel[36,37] proposed the error catastrophe concept on the basis that if mutations or errors occurred in the enzymes involved in translation and transcription (since these synthetases are proteins that are also vulnerable to misspecification), there would be an exponential amplification of production of altered proteins.

Although studies, too numerous to review here, have been carried out to test the error catastrophe hypothesis, they have yielded equivocal results; evidence has nevertheless accumulated supporting a progressively increasing heterogeneity of enzyme proteins,[38] hormonal polypeptides,[39] and antibody proteins[40] with advancing age and with a resulting spectrum of activity ranging from completely inactive to partially active to normally active components in these entities in old subjects. Klug et al.[39] have classified the origins of this heterogeneity as shown below.

1. Failure to complete posttranslational modification such as conversion of precursors to appropriate products
2. Conversion of polypeptide into a partially degraded or conformationally altered form
3. Release of incomplete polypeptide or substitution of individual amino acids
4. Selective gene expression by selective gene transcription and translation

It is evident that the heterogeneity may be due not only to errors which occur in the cybernetic system of the cell as discussed before, but also to posttranslational modification in which carbohydrate and lipid moieties may be involved as well as to deficiencies in the processes of degradation associated with the metabolism of these proteins.

In sum, as Goldstein has observed, "Cells undergoing aging accumulate a multiplicity of abnormal gene products that almost certainly represent molecular mischief one or more steps removed from the primary events."[41]

Fidelity assurance mechanisms

The organism is not without defenses against the potential interference of such errors with biologic functions. Following are the mechanisms that assure fidelity of information flow:

Kinetic proofreading
Selective enzymatic degradation
DNA repair mechanisms
Immune inactivation

There are kinetic proofreading systems that monitor the flow of genetic information and assure its fidelity.[31] Cells also possess enzymes that can selectively degrade misspelled proteins.[42] However, changes with age in the reliability of these mechanisms have not yet been studied.

Perhaps most important to fidelity assurance is the DNA repair mechanism. In this process the damaged or erroneous DNA segment is enzymatically excised and a new one synthesized by its complementary segment; the new segment is then spliced into the excised area. Species showing the greater DNA repair capacity live longer; among vertebrates the maximum life span of different species and the DNA repair capacities show a log-linear relationship.[43] However, the reliability of this mechanism progressively deteriorates with age, perhaps because of the mis-specification of enzymes involved in the process, and this then permits an accumulation of mis-specified proteins.

Finally in respect to fidelity assurance is the protection afforded by the immune system. The latter possesses an array of cell-mediated and humoral surveillance mechanisms for either destroying misspecified cells or inactivating them so that they cease to interfere with normal physiologic functions. It is not within the scope of this chapter to detail these mechanisms and their changes with age; however, several sources provide this information.[44-47] Suffice it to point out here that the operation of the immune system involves a number of regulatory interactions that include processes leading to degradation and elimination of the offending antigen. Such regulation includes maintenance of an appropriate balance of action between helper and suppressor T cells, the latter providing feedback suppression of production of antibody molecules. It is an imbalance of this regulatory mechanism that largely accounts for the aging-related failure of the immune system rather than an attrition of essential cells which make up the system. It is noteworthy that a reciprocal relationship exists between the progressive failure of the immune system with advancing age and the progressively increasing incidence of the diseases of aging as illustrated in Fig. 2-7. Smith and Walford[48] point out that the master genetic control for immune system function is expressed

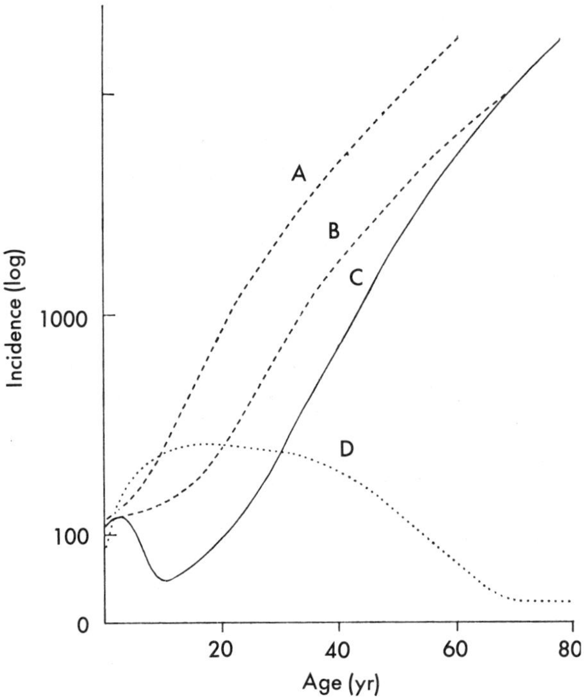

Fig. 2-7. Reciprocal relation between cancer incidence and capacity for immune surveillance. *A*, Hypothetical curve in the absence of immune surveillance; *B*, with immune surveillance deteriorating over time; *C*, actual curve; and *D*, change in immune capacity with advancing age. A similar plot for other diseases of aging would give comparable curves. (From Burnet, F.M.: Intrinsic mutagenesis. A genetic approach to ageing, New York, 1974, John Wiley & Sons, Inc.)

in the cell surface histocompatibility complex (HLA or MHC) and that longevity in different inbred strains of mice, with HLA differences being the only genetic differences between the various strains, can be attributed to differences in this complex. Walford et al.[46] point out that the HLA complex determinants, which in the human reside on chromosome 6, are associated with such phenomena as immune regulation, cancer susceptibility, development, and aging. They point out that there are now several hundred papers reporting a linkage between the HLA complex and a variety of diseases, particularly diseases associated with autoimmune phenomena.

There is an increasing frequency of autoimmune phenomena associated with aging-linked failure of the immune system, and on an individual basis this has a negative prognostic value for further survival, even though in many instances the presence of autoantibodies has no associated disease. Listed below are the conditions necessary for autoantibodies to be associated with pathologic manifestations[49]:

1. The individual must be genetically predisposed.
2. The individual must be in an immunologically hypoactive state.
3. The magnitude of the autoimmune response must be relatively high and sustained.
4. The target antigen must be accessible to autoantibody, macrophage, and/or cytologic effector cell.
5. Autoantibody must be of the type that activates macrophages and antibody-dependent cytolytic cells.

In addition to the directly destructive effects of pathologic autoimmunity, two other phenomena are associated with failure of the immune system: immune complex diseases characterized by a complement-dependent deposition of antigen-antibody complexes and amyloidosis in which there are tissue deposits of either misspecified immunoglobulin, partially formed immunoglobulin, or incompletely degraded immunoglobulin.[50] Two sites of amyloid deposits are particularly relevant to the diseases of aging; they form the core of the senile plaque in senile dementia, and they obliterate the islets of Langerhans in diabetes. Nevertheless, it should also be pointed out that the presence of nonpathologic autoantibodies may be indicative of an adaptive or protective immune response.

BIOLOGY OF SYSTEMS AGING

A fundamental well-established principle of aging on a systems level is that over time there is a progressive loss of capacity of homeostatic systems to return to a steady state following displacement by an environmental challenge. A classic example of this phenomenon is the change with age in the glucose tolerance test; there is a progressive slowing of the return to the basal serum glucose level following the challenge of a glucose load. The studies of Sacher,[51] which show that, from an evolutionary perspective, the life span of mammals is fundamentally related to a specific measure of relative brain size (index of cephalization) and a measure of

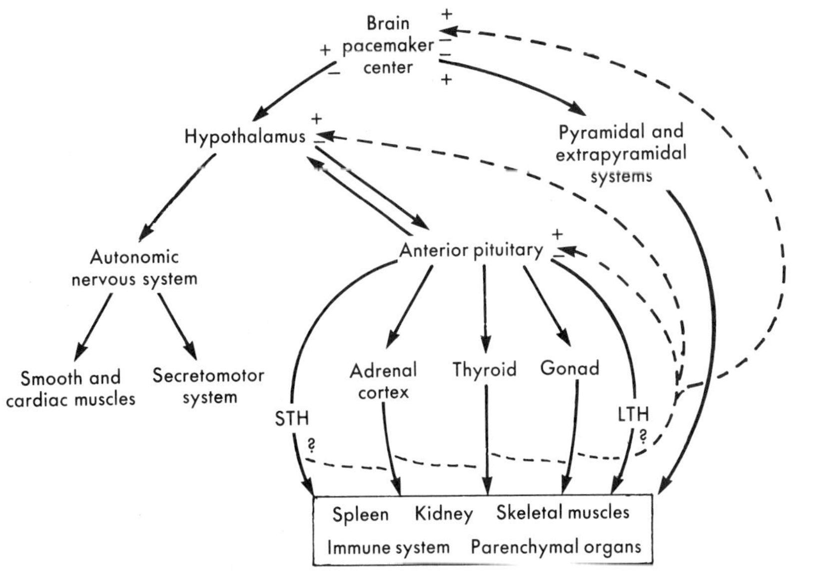

Fig. 2-8. This diagram hypothesizes an aging pacemaker in the higher brain centers, the neurons of which either stimulate (+) or inhibit (−) the neurosecretory cells of the hypothalamus. It shows feedback loops between the hypothalamus and the anterior hypophysis, between the endocrine target organs and the anterior hypophysis, between the endocrine target organs and the hypothalamus, and between the endocrine target organs and the higher brain centers. It also shows the hypothalamic regulation of secretomotor functions and the activities of smooth muscle via the autonomic nervous system and the control of skeletal movement by pacemaker neurons in the pyramidal and extrapyramidal systems. (From Timiras, P.S.: Am. Sci. **66:**605, 1978.)

lifetime metabolic activity, carry the implication that the brain may have an important influence on the capacity of many of the homeostatic systems of the organism. The neuroendocrine system is particularly important to a consideration of systems aging because it not only regulates cell function, but also integrates and coordinates the functions of other organ systems.

As Timiras[52] has pointed out, the sequence of events in the operation of the neuroendocrine system includes the detection of stimulus by higher brain centers, the response of the hypothalamic-hypophyseal system, the action of a target tissue, and finally a return to the resting level generally by means of a negative feedback loop. As depicted in Fig. 2-8, several feedback loops are involved. There is a long loop between the target organs and the higher brain centers, which Timiras proposes as an aging pacemaker. There are somewhat shorter loops between the target organs and the hypothalamus, as well as between the target organs and the anterior pituitary gland. And there is a short loop between the hypothalamus and the pituitary gland.

Timiras points out that the long-standing notion that aging is associated with a general reduction in hormone output is no longer tenable and that for most endocrine glands the output continues at a normal or even elevated level. Instead, as detailed by Timiras[52] and by Klug et al.,[39] the literature now contains many examples of the fact that polypeptide hormones are first synthesized as large precursor molecules and then by enzymatic cleavage they are converted to the active form. They may be misspecified or incompletely or incorrectly cleaved, the latter giving rise to a circulating hormone that is "incompletely sculptured" and less active than the normal hormone.

At the target end of the system are the receptors for hormones and neurotransmitters. Hormone receptors are specialized protein molecules that bind the hormone and subsequently mediate its intracellular response. Baxter and Funder[53] designate two roles for receptors: (1) they distinguish a particular signal from the jumble of hormones that impinge on the cell, and (2) they relay the signal internally in such a way that the appropriate cell response follows. In most cases where cell surface receptors are involved, internalization of the signal activates cyclic AMP, and the latter then effects the discharge of the target cell hormone. The latter is applicable to the binding of peptide hormones, catecholamines, and hypothalamic-releasing factors. Steroid hormones are bound in the soluble intracellular compartment of the cell and attach to the chromatin of the target cell nucleus. For thyroid hormones the primary intracellular binding sites are also found on the chromatin of target cells.

Roth[54] points out that for some systems receptor and hormone may contribute approximately equal information, whereas for other systems the information is in the hormone and the receptor serves only to concentrate and process it and to expedite its translocation to the site of action. In still other cases, the full program of information is within the receptor, and the hormone acts only to cause the receptor to express its program. Receptors may vary in number, affinity, and capacity.

Although receptor research has only recently attracted attention in respect to aging, there is already some relevant information. Abnormal receptors (presumably structural) are present in androgen insensitivity states involving a genetic male who is phenotypically female, and a comparable receptor abnormality to insulin may account for the insulin resistance in acanthosis nigricans. Other receptor abnormalities are present in several neoplastic diseases, in myasthenia gravis, in Graves' disease, and in receptors to a number of other hormones. There is also some evidence suggesting an aging-related loss of receptor function. Important here also is the fact that receptors may be subject to competitive binding between prohormone with reduced or absent physiologic activity or of its metabolites on the one hand and normal hormone on the other. Carnegie and Mackay[55] have proposed that autoimmune responses to receptor sites require a failure of immunologic tolerance such as occurs in various autoimmune diseases and in aging, and they believe that this phenomenon is also applicable to many endocrinopathies.

Thus aging-related loss of information flow at the cellular level translates into phenomena that impair information flow at the systems level; conceptually this may be regarded as the introduction of "noise" into the system. Yockey[56] has proposed a cybernetic theory of aging in which the failure of homeostatic systems occurs when the ratio of noise to proper signal exceeds a certain critical value.

DIABETES MODEL

Galton et al.[57] have proposed that errors in protein synthesis, consisting of amino acid substitutions or conformational changes, may give rise to faulty enzymes, carrier proteins, receptors, and protein and polypeptide hormones and that these phenomena may give rise to a variety of metabolic diseases. *Diabetes is considered here as a possible model, exemplifying the principles inherent in this proposal but placed in an aging context.*

Andres and Tobin[58] point out that there has been an "uninterrupted flow of publications" for about 50 years providing an overwhelming consensus that there is a progressive deterioration in glucose tolerance (GT) throughout the adult life span. They note further that this phenomenon is so prevalent that about half the older subjects "lie above an arbitrary mean +2 SD cut-off point of data derived from young adults." By this standard some reports show only a slight change with age, but other reports indicate that virtually 100% of older subjects are abnormal. To avoid recognizing diabetes as possibly a universal disease of human aging, separate normal distribution curves have been constructed for each decade of life, and only the most deviant subjects are considered to have diabetes. Nevertheless, such considerations have led to the proposal by Blumenthal[59] that the differences between the diabetes of most older subjects and age-linked deterioration in GT may be quantitative rather than qualitative.

There are dangers in adopting a strategy that adjusts norms by age. While it is generally recognized that diabetes is associated with about a fivefold increase in myocardial infarction, a twofold increase in stroke, and an 18-fold increase in the risk of gangrene of the lower extremity,[60] it is also true that a lesser age-linked deterioration in GT also incurs a significantly increased risk for these sequelae of athero-arteriosclerosis, although perhaps not to the same degree. There is also some evidence supporting an increased risk for certain neoplastic diseases such as lymphomas and endometrial cancer. Frequently associated with the deterioration in GT is hyperinsulinemia and aberrations in lipid metabolism and platelet function, so that it is not certain whether the elevated glucose or hormone levels or other abnormalities are the primary offenders. Nor is it clear whether or not these associations are simply examples of the polypathia of aging noted above.

The older classification of diabetes into juvenile and adult onset types has recently been replaced by a division into insulin dependent (type 1) and noninsulin dependent (type 2) forms. This change has been brought about by the recognition that both types can occur in young and old. To complicate the matter further, there are evidently cases which early on are of the noninsulin dependent type that later become hormone dependent. Type 1 constitutes about 10% of diabetics and type 2 about 90%.

Type 1 diabetics, as the designation indicates, have low or absent serum insulin levels; in type 2 diabetes hormone levels are either normal or elevated. However, various abnormalities of the insulin response to a glucose load have been reported in type 2 diabetes. Some researchers stress a delay in the acute-phase response with age and in diabetes, which may be attributed to a defect in the glucose receptor on the beta cell or to the internalization of the glucose signal.[62,63] On the other hand, studies by Malaisse et al.[64] suggest that this delay may be caused by a defect in the microtubular-microfilamentous system of the beta cell along which the insulin containing granules are delivered to the cell surface for secretion. Other investigators emphasize an insulin glucagon imbalance or a change in the insulin-proinsulin glucagon imbalance or a change in the insulin-proinsulin ratio indicative of a relative increase in less active proinsulin at the expense of normal insulin.[65,66] The latter is indicative of an incomplete or faulty enzymatic cleavage in the molding of the most active form of insulin.

There is also evidence for the synthesis of a "mutant" hormone. On a morphologic level there are several lines of supporting evidence. There are studies that report polyploidy of the nuclei of islets restricted to the beta cells,[67,68] a phenomenon that occurs with progressively increasing frequency with age and has a higher frequency in diabetics age-matched with control subjects.[69] In addition ultramicroscopic studies reveal that unlike in several other species, the beta cell granules of the human sometimes exhibit several different forms; some are round, some irregular in shape, and some resemble crystalline bars.[70] Some of these forms may represent an altered macromolecular configuration of insulin or are of an amino acid composition different from normal insulin. Significantly, some of these granules do not bind an antibody to normal insulin.

Several investigators have reported on amino acid analyses of insulins derived from diabetic subjects that show a variety of amino acid substitutions; an example of this phenomenon is shown in Fig. 2-9.[71-76] Some of these amino acid interchanges result in insulins similar to those found in some animal species and are therefore presumed to provide normal physiologic competency. Others are variants not found in any species and are presumed to have reduced or absent activity. In some cases there is a familial distribution of the abnormality, and the studies of Kanazawa et al.[76] suggest inheritance of an autosomal dominant gene. In general, these cases are hyperinsulinemic. As Gabbay[77] points out, these patients do not become diabetic until adulthood, and he speculates that the output of a mix of normal and abnormal insulins may maintain normal glucose homeostasis until the aging process creates an imbalance. An aging-related failure of DNA repair might also account for the late appearance of diabetes. This amino-acid sequencing technique has evidently not been carried out on a sufficiently large scale to determine the prevalence of "mutant" insulins in diabetes more generally.

Andres and Tobin[58] pose two basic questions in respect to diabetes: (1) Is the beta cell response to hyperglycemia decreased with advancing age and in diabetes? (2) Is the sensitivity to insulin reduced with age and in diabetes?

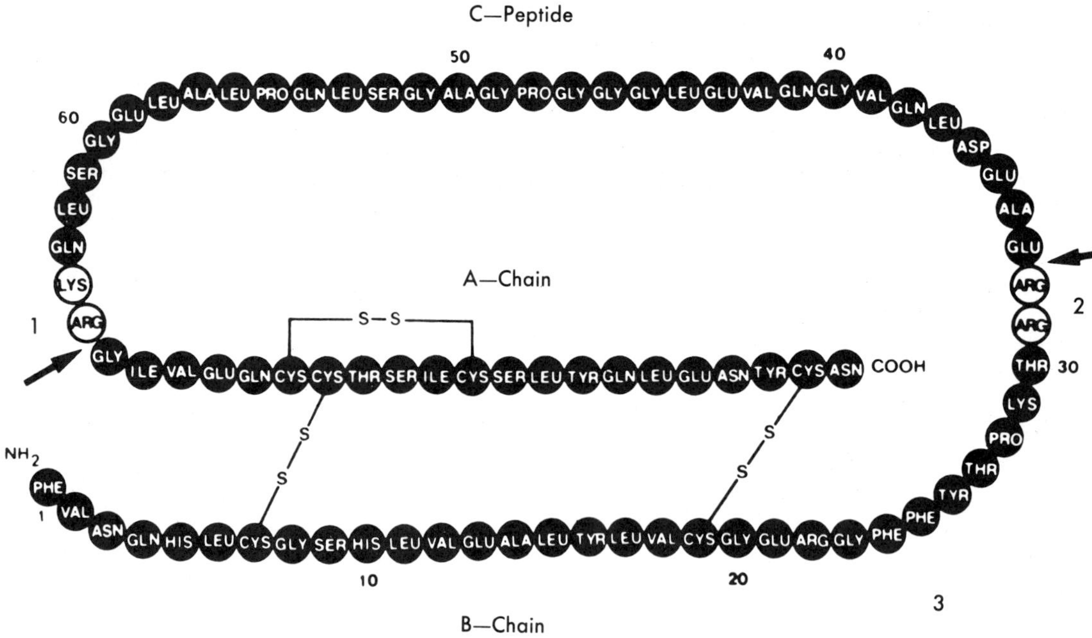

Fig. 2-9. Human proinsulin. Arrows indicate two sites of normal cleavage. The ARG-31 and 32 residues are subsequently removed to yield insulin and C peptide. The cleavage sites (*1* and *2*) and the receptor site (*3*) are known or suspected mutation sites. (From Gabbay, K.H.: N. Engl. J. Med. **302:**165, 1980. Reprinted, by permission of The New England Journal of Medicine.)

Both questions relate to receptor function—the first to the glucoreceptors (GRs) on beta cells and the second to the insulin receptors on peripheral tissue cells. In regard to GRs, Niki and Niki[78] have presented studies that suggest a direct receptor for glucose on the plasma membrane of islet cells that is stereospecific to the alpha configuration of D-glucose. Other studies indicate a similar defect in the taste buds of the tongue and of the neurons of the satiety center of the hypothalamus.[79] The studies of Cerasi et al.[80] suggest a decrease in sensitivity of GRs in diabetes. Much more study is obviously needed to determine changes in GRs in aging and in diabetes.

There are peripheral receptors to all of the glucoregulatory hormones. Those for insulin, glucagon, and the catecholamines are on the plasma membrane. The receptors for steroid hormones are in the cytosol fraction, and nonsuppressible insulin-like factor, growth hormone, and somatomedin are bound by intracellular membrane receptors. Moreover, different glucoregulatory hormones may elicit the same physiologic response but in different ways. Most glucoregulatory hormones exert their intracellular effect through the cyclic AMP system, although insulin appears to be an exception to this rule. Insulin receptors may be of two types, a low affinity, high capacity receptor with a rapid dissociation rate which does not degrade insulin and a high affinity, low capacity receptor with a slow dissociation rate which mediates insulin degradation.[81-83]

Elevated insulin levels result in a decrease in insulin receptors, so-called down regulation, which may be a mechanism by which the cell is protected from excess insulin activity. While most investigators believe that this down regulation by adipocyte receptors accounts for the insulin resistance in obesity and in obese diabetics, other investigators believe that insulin resistance may also be caused by a metabolic abnormality beyond the receptor level.[84-86]

In a review of changes in insulin receptors with age, Roth[54] cites studies reporting a decrease, others that report an increase, and still others that report no change. He concludes that in some species and in some cells receptor function may decline with age. Kinetic studies indicate that in aging there is an increase in insulin in the interstitial spaces or bound to receptors in proportion to plasma hormone levels, while in type 2 diabetes there is a decrease in binding by this compartment relative to plasma hormone level.[87] This observation suggests a change or progression beyond that attributable to aging.

In another review Roth presents evidence that suggests that in type 2 diabetes there is either an abnormality of insulin receptor function or some process "downstream" from it, that is, of some intracellular receptor-triggered events. Receptor malfunction is prevalent in obesity and in obese diabetics who make up about 70% of the diabetic population. In another small group of diabetics with hyperinsulinemia, receptor function appears to be normal and the defect is probably intracellular. There is also a group of thin hyperinsulinemic diabetics in whom an autoantibody to receptors has been discovered. However, the binding site of antibody on the receptor is not the same as for insulin, but an adjacent one. This binding, nevertheless, changes the receptor structure in such a way that it can no longer bind insulin rightly, and these patients have extremely high serum insulin levels.

To complete the analogy between the aging-related loss of fidelity of genetic information flow and diabetes it is necessary to examine immune phenomena associated with this disease. While most of what has been discussed above relates to type 2 diabetes, most of the immunologic manifestations are relevant to the 10% of cases that make up the type 1 category.

Axioms established in early research on autoimmune disorders hold that (1) there is a progressive increase in a spectrum of serum autoantibodies with age, and (2) when one autoantibody is detected there is a high probability of others being present concomitantly.[88,89] The second axiom has been extended to hold that when there is a disease associated with the presence of a spectrum of autoantibodies unrelated to the disease, the latter is likely to have an important autoimmune component. This extension would appear to apply to both types of diabetes, since in both the associated autoantibodies include those against thyroid, adrenal, parathyroid, gastric parietal cell, gastric intrinsic factor, liver mitochondria, double-stranded DNA and antinuclear antibody (ANA). This association in respect to juvenile diabetes has prompted Whittingham et al.[90] to propose that type 1 diabetes is associated with premature aging.

It is now well established that type 1 diabetes is associated with an islet lesion characterized by an infiltrate of lymphocytes (insulitis).[91,92] This is generally interpreted as a manifestation of cell-mediated immunity, and there are now many studies purporting to show that this lesion can be caused by a variety of viruses. However, LeCompte and Legg[93] found this lesion in a few cases of type 2 diabetes, and the lesion can be produced in animals by immunization with insulin in Freund's adjuvant, and by subdiabetogenic doses of streptozotocin (SZ).[94,95]Moreover, the transfer of lymphocytes from mice with SZ insulitis to athymic nude mice results in diabetes,[96] and the same effect can be produced in guinea pigs by the transfer of lymphocytes from animals immunized with insulin. A spectrum of tests for cell mediated immunity to insulin or for islet cell antibodies in human diabetes has also been carried out (for review, see Blumenthal[13]). Such tests are positive in a high percent of type 1 cases, but also in some type 2 diabetics; in both types tests were positive in a significant number of individuals who had not received exogenous insulin.

Three types of circulating (humoral) antibody are under study in respect to diabetes, including insulin antibody, islet cell antibody, and insulin receptor antibody. In earlier studies it was shown that the angiopathies of diabetes bind insulin and complement, and therefore, presumptively at least, contain insulin antibodies; in some cases there was no history of injections of exogenous insulin.[97,98] These angiopathies were induced in animals by the injection of insulin in Freund's adjuvant. Such studies as well as some by others demonstrating serum insulin antibodies by the complement consumption test did not receive general acceptance because the techniques used were regarded as lacking specificity. However, over the past decade about 20 cases have been reported in which serum insulin antibodies have been identified in patients with no history of exogenous insulin using techniques of generally accepted specificity.[99-104] These patients characteristically display a normal fasting glucose level, postprandial hypoglycemia, a diabetic GT curve followed by reactive hypoglycemia, hyperinsulinemia, hypertrophy of the islets, and a high antibody titer of IgG class with kappa light chains. Moreover, there appears to be some association with Graves' disease suggesting a more general immune endocrinopathy. To date this syndrome appears to be rare, although the awareness it has created may prompt the discovery of additional cases.

Serum islet cell antibodies appear to be of several types. One type binds all islet cells—alpha, beta and delta—but does not bind insulin, glucagon, somatostatin, or pancreatic polypeptide. There are two species of this antibody, one that fixes complement and one that does not. The complement fixing antibody has been shown to be cytotoxic. Patients with these antibodies are, for the most part, of particular HLA types and this may be indicative of some defect of the immune response genes. The antibody is transient, occurring in about 80% of cases at the time of onset of diabetes, declining to about 50% by 6 months, to about 20% to 25% of cases at the end of the first year of disease, to about 5% after 10 to 20 years. These ICAs are present in about 8% to 10% of patients with type 2 diabetes, in 5.6% of patients with other autoimmune disorders but not diabetes, in 2.5% of first degree relatives of diabetics, and in 0.5%-1.7% of the general population. There is still another serum antibody that binds to the cell membrane of islet cells, the import of which is yet to be determined. The foregoing information derives largely from a review by Doniach and Bottazzo,[105] and a monograph by Galbraith.[106]

There are some aspects of immune phenomena associated with diabetes that require clarification. Do the ICAs represent a cause or an effect of diabetes? The fact that they bind to all types of islet cells and not to islet cell hormones suggest an antibody to some structural component common to all islet cells. What is the relation, if any, of the long recognized islet amyloid to these immune phenomena? Many years ago it was shown that the incidence of islet amyloid increases progressively with age, and on an age matched basis its incidence is higher in diabetes than in nondiabetic controls.[107] This association suggests a link with maturity-onset (type 2) diabetes rather than with the type 1 form. In this regard it has been suggested that the amyloid may be derived from an aging-related defect in the microtubular-microfilamentous system, since the plaques of senile dementia containing abnormal microtubular-microfilamentous structures have an amyloid core, and as noted above, there is some evidence for a similar defect in the beta cells of the islets of Langerhans.[108] Our earlier suggestion in respect to the angiopathies of diabetes would comply with current concepts of immune complex disorders, and this might also be applicable to islet amyloid.

Table 2-1 provides a summary of phenomena which are linked with both aging and diabetes, but occur earlier or in a more intense form in diabetes. They include some of the phenomena discussed in this chapter, as well as others not specifically considered here. As Bierman[109] has pointed out, they suggest that diabetes is somehow associated with accelerated aging.

Table 2-1. Comparison of aging and diabetes

Phenomenon	*Present in aging*	*Accelerated or intensified in diabetes*
Glucose intolerance	+	+
Hyperinsulinemia	+	+
Hyperglycagonemia	+	+
Hormonal (polypeptide) heterogeneity	+	+
Islet hyperplasia	+	+
Islet amyloidosis	+	+
Finite replicative life span of cultured fibroblasts	+	Reduced
Basement membrane thickening	+	+
Atherosclerosis-arteriosclerosis	+	+
Osteoporosis	+	+
Increased autoantibodies	+	+
Renal immune complex disease	Nephrosclerosis ?	Nodular glomerulosclerosis?

CONCLUSION

Several writers have commented on the plethora of theories of aging,[110-112] and no attempt has been made here to present an analysis of them. Most gerontologists now agree that there is probably no single cause of aging, and Finch[113] believes that a universally applicable theory is not likely to emerge because some species appear to lack an exponentially increasing mortality or maximum life span and because the physiologic and pathologic changes associated with aging vary significantly between species.

Nevertheless, it is noteworthy that aging theories generally fall into the following two categories: (1) Developmental concepts attribute aging to a series of orderly programmed genetic events that terminate or slow down essential physiologic phenomena when postreproductive age is reached. Such theories are, therefore, based on the concept that age changes, like developmental changes, are programmed into the original pool of genetic information and are "played out" in an orderly sequence just as are developmental changes. (2) Stochastic, or random, concepts hold that functional failures over time are the consequence of the random accumulation of "noise" in vulnerable parts of the system. To accommodate the regularity and predictability of aging phenomena are such concepts as "mean time to failure"[112] or programmed mutagenic genes,[114] which may regulate the activities of polymerases responsible for the fidelity of information flow.

Because of accumulating evidence supporting a progressive loss of fidelity of information flow with advancing age, concepts of aging now seem to be focused on explaining the origin of the genetic instability that gives rise to a progressive accumulation of faulty copying in dividing cells or on the accumulation of errors in information-containing molecules and the possible sources and effects of such phenomena.

At the molecular-cellular level possible changes in nucleic acids and in enzymes as well as in other specific proteins, including posttranslational modification, have been considered. Changes at the latter level translate into effects at the systems level involving homeostatic mechanisms, particularly those involving functions of the neuroendocrine system such as the molding and secretion of hormones, as well as changes in receptor function and in postreceptor (intracellular) activities.

Since the validity of the traditional separation of biologic aging and disease continues to be challenged, this chapter also considers how one disease, diabetes mellitus, may represent a direct extension of biologic aging. It attempts to accomplish this by discussing the origin of this disease in the context of an aging-linked loss of fidelity of information flow insofar as the latter involve glucose homeostasis. Although there is considerably more information in respect to the application of this principle to diabetes than to such other diseases of aging as cancer and atherosclerosis-arteriosclerosis, there remains a need to develop more information of this type in respect to other diseases of aging.

The primary emphasis in this chapter has been that basic intrinsic biologic aging phenomena can directly give rise to disease, although superimposed environmental agents including viruses may have similar effects. If this is a valid concept, then the current "ecological model" and its implications regarding therapy and prevention may be inappropriate. A new model based on an intrinsic genesis of the diseases of aging suggests that there may be a need to expand research on the development of techniques for retarding aging. Such a strategy, if successful, would result in a postponement of the time of onset of these diseases, and some of them might even be postponed out of the life span of some individuals.[115]

REFERENCES

1. Sobel, H.: Ageing and age-associated disease, Lancet **2:**1191, 1970.
2. Hayflick, L.: The cellular basis for biological aging. In Finch, C.E., and Hayflick, L., editors: Handbook of the biology of aging, New York, 1977, Van Nostrand Reinhold Co., p. 159.
3. Kay, D.W.K.: Outcome and cause of death in mental disorders of old age: a long-term follow-up of functional and organic psychoses, Acta Psychiatr. Scand. **28:**249, 1962.
4. Kohn, R.R.: Human aging and disease, J. Chronic Dis. **16:**5, 1963.
5. Good, R.A.: Editorial. Cancer and aging. Hosp. Pract. **15:**10, 1980.
6. Ludwig, F.C.: What to expect from gerontological research, Science **209:**1071, 1980.
7. Stetten, De W., Jr.: Eradication, Science **210:**1203, 1980.
8. Stoddard, L.D.: Toward a new human pathology. I.

Biopathological populations or sets: a substitute for the old pathology's diseases, Hum. Pathol. **11:**228, 1980.
9. Cutler, R.G., editor: Cellular Ageing: concepts and mechanisms. Interdisciplinary topics in gerontology, vol. 9-10. Basel, Switzerland, 1976, S. Karger.
10. Strehler, B.L.: Time, cells and aging, ed. 2, New York, 1977, Academic Press, Inc.
11. Gompertz, B.: On the nature of the function expressive of the law of human mortality and on a new mode of determining life contingencies, Philos. Trans. R. Soc. Lond. Ser. A. **115:**513, 1825.
12. Keyfitz, N.: Improving life expectancy: an uphill road ahead, Am. J. Public Health **68:**954, 1978.
13. Fries, J.F.: Aging, natural death, and the compression of mortality, N. Engl. J. Med. **303:**130, 1980.
14. Blumenthal, H.T.: The aging-disease connection in retrospect and prospect. In Blumenthal, H.T., editor: Handbook of the diseases of aging, New York, Van Nostrand Reinhold, Co. (In press.)
15. Strehler, B.L.: Implications of aging research for society. In Thorbecke, G.J., editor: Biology of aging and development, New York, 1975, Plenum Press, p. 3.
16. Goldstein, J.L., and Brown, M.S.: Familial hypercholesterolemia: pathogenesis of a receptor disease, Johns Hopkins Med. J. **143:**8, 1978.
17. Voors, A.W., et al.: Racial differences in blood pressure control, Science **204:**1091, 1979.
18. Suciu-Foca, N., et al: HLA-DR5 in juvenile rheumatoid arthritis confined to a few joints, Lancet **1:**40, 1980.
19. Lesser, P.B., et al.: Adult-onset Hirschprung's disease, J.A.M.A. **242:**747, 1979.
20. Schochet, S.S., Jr., Lampert, D.W., and McCormick, W.F.: Neurofibrillary tangles in patients with Down's syndrome: a light and electron microscopic study, Acta Neuropathol. **23:**342, 1973.
21. Cheung, H.W., Singer, F.R., Mills, B., and Nimni, M.E.: In vitro synthesis of normal bone (type 1) collagen by bones of Paget's disease patients, Proc. Soc. Exp. Biol. Med. **163:**547, 1980.
22. Ingelfinger, F.J.: Medicine: meritorious or meretricious, Science **200:**942, 1978.
23. Pearce, M.L., and Dayton, S.: Incidence of cancer in men on a diet high in polyunsaturated fat, Lancet **1:**464, 1971.
24. Wisniewski, H.M., and Terry, R.D.: Neuropathology of the aging brain. In Terry, R.D., and Gershon, S., editors: Neurobiology of aging, vol. 3, New York, 1976, Raven Press, p. 265.
25. Sonneborn, T.M.: The origin, evolution and nature and causes of aging. In Behnke, J.A., Finch, C.E., and Moment, G.B.: The biology of aging, New York, 1978, Plenum Press, p. 361.
26. Gatlin, L.L.: Information theory and living systems, New York, 1972, Columbia University Press.
27. Davis, B.D.: Frontiers of the biological sciences, Science **289:**78, 1980.
28. Rich, A.: Bits of life. How information is handled in living systems, The Sciences **20:**10, 1980.
29. Sharon, N.: Carbohydrates, Sci. Am. **243:**90, 1980.
30. Correspondent: Accuracy of the transmission of biological information, Nature **276:**442, 1978.
31. Gueron, M.: Enhanced selectivity of enzymes by kinetic proofreading. Am. Sci. **66:**202, 1978.
32. Medvedev, Z.A.: Repetition of molecular-genetic information as a possible factor in evolutionary changes in the lifespan, Exp. Gerontol. **7:**227, 1972.
33. Doolittle, W.F., and Sapienza, C.: Selfish genes, the phenotype paradigm and genome evolution, Nature **284:**601, 1980.
34. Orgel, L.E., and Crick, F.H.C.: Selfish DNA: the ultimate parasite, Nature **204:**604, 1980.
35. Szilard, L.: On the nature of the aging process, Proc. Natl. Acad. Sci. USA **45:**30, 1959.
36. Orgel, L.E.: The maintenance of accuracy of protein synthesis and its relevance to aging, Proc. Natl. Acad. Sci. USA **49:**517, 1963.
37. Orgel, L.E.: The maintenance of accuracy of protein synthesis and its relevance to aging. A correction, Proc. Natl. Acad. Sci. USA **67:**1426, 1970.
38. Gershon, D., et al.: The accumulation of faulty enzyme molecules in aging cells. In Shaltiel, S., editor: Metabolic interconversion of enzymes, New York, 1975, Springer-Verlag New York, Inc. p. 227.
39. Klug, T.L., Obenrader, M.F., and Adelman, R.C.: Heterogeneity of polypeptide hormones during aging, Adv. Exp. Med. Biol. **113:**59, 1978.
40. Walford, R.L.: Antibody diversity, histocompatibility systems and aging, Lancet **2:**1226, 1970.
41. Goldstein, S.: Biological aging. An essentially normal process, J.A.M.A. **230:**1651, 1974.
42. Goldberg, A.L., and Dice, J.F.: Intracellular protein degradation in mammalian and bacterial cells, Annu. Rev. Biochem. **43:**835, 1974.
43. Hart, R.W., and Setlow, R.B.: Correlation between deoxyribonucleic acid excision repair and lifespan in a number of mammalian species, Proc. Natl. Acad. Sci. USA **71:**2165, 1974.
44. Makinodan, T., and Yunis, E., editors: Immunology and Aging, New York, 1977, Plenum Medical Book Co.
45. Walford, R.L.: The immunologic theory of aging, Copenhagen, 1969, Munkssgaard.
46. Walford, R.L.: Immunology and aging, Am. J. Clin. Pathol. **74:**247, 1980.
47. Segret, D., and Smith, I., editors: Immunological aspects of aging, New York, Marcel Dekker, Inc. (In press.)
48. Smith, G.S., and Walford, R.L.: Influence of the main histocompatibility complex on ageing in mice, Nature **270:**727, 1977.
49. Kay, M.M.B.: Immunological aspects of aging. In Kay, M.M.B., Galpin, J., and Makinodan, T., editors: Aging, immunity and arthritic disease, vol. 11, New York, 1980, Raven Press, p. 33.
50. Glenner, G.G.: Amyloid deposits and amyloidosis, N. Engl. J. Med. **302:**1283, 1980.
51. Sacher, G.A.: Longevity, aging and death. An evolutionary perspective, Gerontologist **18:**112, 1978.
52. Timiras, P.S.: Biological perspectives on aging, Am. Sci. **66:**605, 1978.
53. Baxter, J.D., and Funder, J.W.: Hormone receptors, N. Engl. J. Med. **301:**1149, 1979.

54. Roth, G.S.: Hormone action during aging: alterations and mechanisms, Mech. Ageing Dev. **9**:497, 1979.
55. Carnegie, P.R., and Mackay, I.R.: Vulnerability of cell-surface receptors to autoimmune reactions, Lancet **2**:684, 1975.
56. Yockey, H.P.: The use of information theory in aging and radiation damage. In Strehler, B.L., editor: The biology of aging: a symposium, Washington, D.C., 1960, American Institute of Biological Sciences, p. 338.
57. Galton, D.J., Higgins, J.M.F., and Reckless, J.P.D.: Errors in metabolic regulation. A common group of metabolic disorders, Lancet **1**:1224, 1975.
58. Andres, R., and Tobin, J.D.: Endocrine systems. In Finch, C.E., and Hayflick, L., editors: Handbook of the biology of aging, New York, 1977, Van Nostrand Reinhold Co., p. 357.
59. Blumenthal, H.T.: Aging: biologic or pathologic, Hosp. Pract. **13**:127, 1978.
60. Blumenthal, H.T.: The relation of microangiopathies to arteriosclerosis, with special reference to diabetes, Ann. N.Y. Acad. Sci. **149**:834, 1968.
61. Ganda, O.M.P.: Review. Pathogenesis of macrovascular disease in the human diabetic, Diabetes **29**:931, 1980.
62. Reaven, G.M., Shen, S.W., Silvers, A., and Farquhar, J.W.: Is there a delay in the plasma insulin response of patients with chemical diabetes mellitus? Diabetes **20**:416, 1971.
63. Fujita, Y., Herron, A.L., and Seltzer, H.S.: Confirmation of impaired early insulin response to glycemic stimulus in nonobese mild diabetics, Diabetes **24**:17, 1975.
64. Malaisse, W.J., Malaisse-Lague, F., Walker, M.O., and Lacy, P.E.: The stimulus-secretion coupling of glucose-induced insulin release. V. The participation of a microtubular-microfilamentous system, Diabetes **20**:257, 1971.
65. Unger, R.H.: Alpha and beta cell interrelationships in health and disease, Metabolism **23**:581, 1974.
66. DeHaën, C., Little, S.A., May, J.M., and Williams, R.W.: Characterization of pro-insulin intermediates in human plasma, J. Clin. Invest. **62**:727, 1978.
67. LeCompte, P.M., and Merriam, J.C.: Mitotic figures and enlarged nuclei in the islands of Langerhans in man, Diabetes **11**:35, 1962.
68. Ehrie, M.G., and Swartz, F.J.: Diploid, tetraploid and octaploid beta cells in the islets of Langerhans of the normal human pancreas, Diabetes **23**:583, 1974.
69. Blumenthal, H.T.: The aging-disease connection in retrospect and prospect. In Blumenthal, H.T., editor: Handbook of the diseases of aging, New York, Van Nostrand Reinhold Co. (In press.)
70. Lacy, P.E.: Pathology of the islets of Langerhans, Pathology annual **1**:352, 1966.
71. Kimmel, J.R., and Pollock, H.G.: Studies of human insulin from nondiabetic pancreas, Diabetes **16**:687, 1967.
72. Tager, H., et al.: A structurally abnormal insulin causing human diabetes, Nature **281**:122, 1979.
73. Given, B.D., et al.: Diabetes due to secretion of an abnormal insulin, N. Engl. J. Med. **302**:129, 1980.
74. Gabbay, K.H., et al.: Familial hyperinsulinemia: an autosomal dominant defect, N. Engl. J. Med. **294**:911, 1976.
75. Gabbay, K.H., et al.: Familial hyperproinsulinemia: partial characterization of circulating proinsulin-like material, Proc. Natl. Acad. Sci. USA **76**:2881, 1979.
76. Kanazawa, Y., et al.: Familial proinsulinemia: a possible cause of abnormal glucose tolerance (Abstract.), Eur. J. Clin. Invest. **8**:327, 1978.
77. Gabbay, K.H.: Editorial. The insulinopathies, N. Engl. J. Med. **302**:165, 1980.
78. Niki, A., and Niki, H.: Is diabetes mellitus a disorder of the glucoreceptor, Lancet **2**:658, 1975.
79. Asplund, J.: Glucoreceptor deficiency in diabetes, Lancet **1**:418, 1976.
80. Cerasi, E., Luft, R., and Efendic, S.: Decreased sensitivity of the pancreatic beta cells to glucose in prediabetic and diabetic subjects, Diabetes **21**:224, 1972.
81. Herzberg, V., Boughter, J.M., Carlisle, S., and Hill, D.E.: Evidence for two insulin receptor populations on human erythrocytes, Nature **286**:279, 1980.
82. Sonksen, P.H.: Probing the insulin receptor, Nature **282**:11, 1979.
83. Olefsky, J.M., Kobayashi, M., and Chang, H.: Interactions between insulin and its receptors after the initial binding event, Diabetes **28**:460, 1979.
84. Wigand, J.F., and Blackard, W.D.: Downregulation of insulin receptors in obese man, Diabetes **28**:287, 1979.
85. Misbin, R.I., O'Leary, J.P., and Pulkkinen, A.: Insulin receptor binding in obesity: a reassessment, Science **205**:1003, 1979.
86. Beck-Nielsen, H.: The pathogenic role of an insulin-receptor defect in diabetes mellitus of the obese, Diabetes **27**:1178, 1978.
87. McGuire, E.A., Tobin, J.D., Berman, M., and Andres, R.: Kinetics of native insulin in diabetic, obese and aged men, Diabetes **28**:110, 1979.
88. Mackay, I.R., and Burnet, F.M.: Autoimmune disease, Springfield, Ill., 1963, Charles C Thomas, Publisher.
89. Mackay, I.R., Whittingham, S.F., and Mathews, J.D.: The immunoepidemiology of aging, In Makinodan, T., and Yunis, E., editors: Immunology and aging, New York, 1977, Plenum Medical Book Co., p. 35.
90. Whittingham, S.F., et al.: Diabetes mellitus, autoimmunity and aging, Lancet **1**:763, 1971.
91. LeCompte, P.: "Insulitis" in early juvenile diabetes, Arch. Pathol. **66**:450, 1958.
92. Gepta, W.: Pathologic anatomy of the pancreas in juvenile diabetes, **14**:619, 1965.
93. LeCompte, P.M., and Legg, M.A.: Insulitis (lymphocytic infiltration of pancreatic islets) in late-onset diabetes, Diabetes **21**:762, 1972.
94. Renold, A.E., Soeldner, J.S., and Steinke, J.: Immunological studies with homologous and heterologous pancreatic insulin in the cow, Ciba Found. Colloquia. Endocrinol. **15**:122, 1964.
95. Lee, J.C., Grodsky, G.M., Caplan, J., and Craw, L.: Experimental immune diabetes in the rabbit, Am. J. Pathol. **57**:597, 1969.
96. Buschard, K., and Rygaard, J.: Passive transfer of streptozotocin induced diabetes mellitus with spleen cells, Acta Pathol. Microbiol. Scand. **85**:469, 1977.
97. Blumenthal, H.T., and Berns, A.W.: Autoimmunity

and aging. In Strehler, B.L., editor: Advances in gerontological research, New York, 1964, Academic Press, Inc., p. 289.

98. Blumenthal, H.T., Goldenberg, S., and Berns, A.W.: Pathology and pathogenesis of the disseminated angiopathy of diabetes mellitus. In Leibel, A.S., and Wrenshall, G.A., editors: On the nature and treatment of diabetes, Excerpta Med. Internat. Congr. Ser. No. 84, Amsterdam, 1965, Elsevier Publishing Co., p. 397.
99. Hirata, Y., et al.: Insulin autoimmunity in a case with spontaneous hypoglycemia, Jpn. J. Diabetes **13**:312, 1970.
100. Hirata, Y., Tominago, M., Ito, J., and Noguchi, A.: Spontaneous hypoglycemia with insulin autoimmunity in Graves' disease, Ann. Intern. Med. **81**:214, 1974.
101. Ichihara, K., et al.: Mechanisms of hypoglycemia observed in a patient with insulin autoimmune syndrome, Diabetes **26**:500, 1977.
102. Folling, I., and Norman, N.: Hyperglycemia, hypoglycemic attacks and production of anti-insulin antibodies without previous immunization. Immunological and functional studies in a patient, Diabetes **21**:814, 1972.
103. Ohneda, A., et al.: Hypoglycemia due to apparent autoantibodies to insulin. Characterization of insulin-binding protein, Diabetes **23**:41, 1974.
104. Hirata, Y.: Spontaneous insulin antibodies and hypoglycemia, Proc. IX Congr. Internat. Diabetes Fed., p. 278, 1978.
105. Doniach, D., and Bottazzo, G.F.: Autoimmunity and the endocrine pancreas. In Ioachim, H.L., editor: Pathobiology annual, New York, 1977, Appleton-Century-Crofts, p. 327.
106. Galbraith, R.M.: Immunological aspects of diabetes mellitus, Boca Raton, Fla., 1979, CRC Press.
107. Bell, E.T.: Hyalinization of the islets of Langerhans in nondiabetic individuals, Am. J. Pathol. **35**:801, 1959.
108. Nordensen, I., et al.: Chromosomal abnormality in dementia of Alzheimer type, Lancet **1**:481, 1980.
109. Bierman, E.L.: Diseases of carbohydrate and lipid metabolism, Annu. Rev. Gerontol. Geriatrics, p. 154, 1980.
110. Marx, J.L.: Aging research. I. Cellular theories of senescence. II. Pacemakers of aging. Science **186**:1105, 1974.
111. Moment, G.B.: The Ponce de Leon trail today. In Behnke, J.A., Finch, C.E., and Moment, G.B., editors: The biology of aging, New York, 1978, Plenum Press, p. 1.
112. Hayflick, L.: Future directions in aging research, Proc. Soc. Exp. Biol. Med. **165**:206, 1980.
113. Finch, C.E.: The regulation of physiological changes during mammalian aging, Q. Rev. Biol. **51**:49, 1976.
114. Burnet, F.M.: Intrinsic mutagenesis. A genetic approach to ageing, New York, 1974, John Wiley & Sons, Inc.
115. Comfort, A.: Measuring the human ageing rate, Mech. Ageing Dev. **1**:101, 1972.

CHAPTER 3 · EVALUATION AND TREATMENT OF THE GERIATRIC PATIENT

Franz U. Steinberg

The clinical evaluation of the aged patient is complicated by three factors. First, a geriatric patient is likely to suffer from more than one disease at a time. Williamson et al.[1] undertook a random sampling of 200 persons over the age of 65 years and found a mean of 3.26 disabilities in men and 3.42 disabilities in women. In over 2200 autopsies of patients in the age range of 65 to 84 years, Howell[2] found an average of 7.02 significant lesions. The physician therefore cannot be satisfied with having diagnosed one disease but must search for additional diseases, which may have unrelated causes that will obviously interact and affect the diagnosis and treatment program.

Second, age changes the individual's response to disease. Many of the guideposts that help in diagnosing disease in young and middle-aged persons may not be apparent. Pain may be diminished or absent. A myocardial infarction may be silent or become manifest only by circulatory collapse. Abdominal diseases such as acute appendicitis, acute cholecystitis, or perforation of a viscus may produce little or no pain. Infections may not be accompanied by fever or by leukocytosis. Furthermore, social and emotional factors may have a greater impact on the health of the elderly than on any other age group.

Third, it is difficult to separate the effects of aging from the consequences of disease. This is a hazard both to patient and physician. The patient may fail to report important symptoms because he may consider them natural signs of aging and as such not worth mentioning. For similar reasons the physician may omit important diagnostic procedures, and remediable conditions may thus remain undiagnosed.

The evaluation of the aged patient requires a great deal of diagnostic acumen. The patient's problems must be approached systematically and thoroughly. A second or third look may yield additional facts that were not apparent initially.

MEDICAL HISTORY TAKING

Taking the medical history of an aged patient presents particular pitfalls. Deafness, memory deficits, and confusion are common obstacles. The leading complaint that brought the patient to the physician may be relatively trivial. Other, more significant symptoms may go unmentioned; the physician must search for them by tactful probing. For instance, the patient may complain of painful feet but may fail to mention that he must sleep on four pillows to get his breath. Important symptoms may not be reported, either because patients are afraid to face the implications or because they believe them to be the result of age and therefore not relevant. The physician, after eliciting specific complaints, must embark on a careful historic review of all the patient's organ systems, making sure that the questions are fully understood. Some terms need to be elucidated. Indigestion may mean anything from chest pain to heart burn or gas pain. Constipation may simply mean that the patient has no daily bowel movement. Terms such as *diarrhea*, *dizziness*, and *fainting* have to be qualified by a careful detailed description.

Taking such a systemic history may be difficult and time-consuming because many elderly patients are vague and tend to drift from one subject to another. The physician should hear them out as best as possible. At the same time, however, he must keep them to the subject at hand, clarify contradictory statements, and try to put the information in order. The duration of given symptoms is important, but this information may be difficult to obtain since aged individuals are often vague about time relationships.

Questions about the patient's everyday activities will help to clarify some symptoms. It may be important to know, for instance, when a patient gave up independent shopping trips or stopped going out unescorted. If this information can be correlated with the onset of specific symptoms, important diagnostic clues can be obtained. The use of leisure time, past and present, may give vital information about the patient's mental acuity or sight and hearing defects.

As discussed in Chapter 15, the elderly person's response to many drugs is altered, and a history of their drug usage is important. This must include not only those drugs that the patient takes on medical prescription but also those taken on the patient's own initiative. The physician must not take for granted that medications are used as directed. Errors are common but often can be avoided by better communication between physician and patient. For example, if a physician prescribes a drug to be taken after each meal, it is assumed that the patient eats three meals a day and that the medication will therefore be taken three times a day. However, many old people eliminate one meal, and so the medication is taken only twice a day. Such errors will come to light only on specific inquiry.

Various studies have demonstrated the frequency of medication errors in the aged. Schwartz et al.[3] investigated the medication habits of 178 elderly, chronically ill patients and found that 59% of them made medication errors; in 26% of the patients the errors were potentially serious. As a precaution, all medications should be labeled by name. The physician should ask the patient to bring all medications to the office, regardless who prescribed them or if purchased over the counter, so their use can be reviewed at each visit. It is important to remember that the incidence of drug reactions increases with age. Hurwitz,[4] in a prospective study of over 1000 hospitalized patients, found a 15.4% incidence of drug reactions in patients over the age of 60, compared with 6.3% in patients under 60. The entire subject of drug therapy of the aged has been discussed in two monographs[5,6] and several recent papers.[7,8]

Nutrition also requires close scrutiny. Nutritional deficiencies are common and are not limited to those living under economic stress. Inquiries about diet must be detailed. Elderly patients with little appetite may honestly believe that their diets are adequate. Only specific questioning will reveal if their intake of protein, fresh fruit, vegetables, and bulk is sufficient. Many aged persons develop a particular dislike for meat, and as a result they subsist on a protein-deficient diet. This information is difficult to come by since geriatric patients rarely admit to dietary inadequacies. A quick inspection of pantry and refrigerator, if the occasion arises, will often provide a valuable insight into patients' dietary habits.

Alcoholism in aged men and women is more common than is generally realized. The patient will rarely admit to the physician or to themselves that they have a drinking problem. Yet over a day's time their alcohol consumption may be significant. It may enhance confusion and forgetfulness and contribute to the tendency to falls. It also contributes to nutritional deficiencies. Tactful questioning and inquiries with family members may bring this problem to light.

The physician must also inquire about the patient's social circumstances. A recent social decline may have a profound impact on an aged person's well-being. Retirement, with its accompanying changes in daily routine; a decline in social status and income; a recent change in dwelling place; illness or death of family or friends; tension between patients and their children may all cause depression and greatly affect the patient's physical well-being. The aged patient may not volunteer any of this information; the physician must bring it out by gentle and tactful questioning.

PHYSICAL EXAMINATION AND LABORATORY TESTS

The physical examination of the geriatric patient must be complete and thorough. The physician must probe particularly into areas that are likely to show abnormalities.

Skin, oral mucosa, and the tongue may give important clues to the patient's state of hydration and nutrition. The condition of teeth or dentures must be assessed, since poor mastication will obviously contribute to nutritional deficiencies.

The neck, as usual, is examined for palpable lymph nodes or an abnormal thyroid gland. The carotid arteries must be palpated and examined for bruits. The range of motion of the cervical spine should be evaluated. Cervical spondylosis is common in the aged. It may be responsible not only for neck pain but also for occipital headaches and pain in the upper extremities and chest area. More rarely, cervical spondylosis may cause neurologic abnormalities, including long tract signs.

The breasts should be palpated. The configuration of the chest should be noted even though a barrel chest deformity as such does not denote chronic pulmonary disease. The mobility of the diaphragm should be noted. During the auscultation of the lung bases the patient should be asked to cough lightly; this maneuver may bring out rales that had not been apparent before. The heart auscultation should be done both in a sitting and supine position. The abdominal examination should include a search for asymptomatic hernias.

A rectal examination is mandatory, especially for men in whom cancer of the prostate may thus be discovered in an early phase. Guinan et al.[9] have reported that of 10 tests evaluated, the rectal examination was the most efficient in detecting cancer of the prostate. In women, pelvic examinations should be done, especially if there is a history of bleeding, discharge, or ulceration (see Chapter 22).

The back must be inspected for structural abnormalities and loss of motion. In old age an increase of the kyphotic curve of the thoracic spine is common and is associated with a reduction of the lordosis of the lumbosacral spine. Range of motion should be determined by having the patient bend forward with the knees extended. The examiner should observe the motions of the lumbosacral spine as the patient flexes and then returns to the erect position. All major joints are inspected, palpated, and tested for range of motion and for pain. The pain of arthritic hip joints is often referred to the thigh or knee but can be produced by movements of the hip joint.

The feet are inspected for evidence of circulatory impairment, such as atrophy of nails and loss of hair over the toes. The arterial pulses of the lower extremities should be palpated in all geriatric patients. If the pedal pulses cannot be felt, an oscillometer or Doppler ultrasound equipment should be used to assess the arterial circulation of the legs.

The neurologic examination can be kept brief if the patient has no symptoms of a neurologic disorder. Much can be learned by watching a patient walk, arise from a chair, and get on and off the examination table. The patient should be made to stand still with eyes closed to test the equilibrium. The patient should be asked to stand on toes, then heels, and on one leg at a time. The cranial nerves must be examined, followed by a brief evaluation of upper and lower extremity muscle function, sensation, and reflexes. Tests for ataxia are indicated, particularly if the patient complains of clumsiness and poor coordination.

All patients in the geriatric age group should have an ophthalmologic examination for glaucoma at least once every 2 years.

Annual laboratory examinations should include urinalysis, blood count, and biochemical profile. These examinations are not costly and provide a great deal of information. Many laboratories have recently replaced the blood urea nitrogen determination with a determination of serum creatinine, from which a rough estimate of the creatinine clearance can be calculated.[10] Patients taking diuretic medications should have periodic serum electrolyte determinations.

A chest radiograph should probably be done at least once every 2 years. For any patient above the age of 50, at least one electrocardiogram should be in the physician's file to serve as a base of comparison in case the patient develops chest pain or other symptoms at a later date.

Steel et al.[11] have reported that laboratory examinations in the aged have a high yield of abnormal findings. Even though many tests may at first show normal results in the asymptomatic, well aged, they will serve as a valuable baseline for comparison with later examinations and after symptoms have developed.

COMMON COMPLAINTS

A variety of complaints are common in old age. Since they are not specific to any one disorder, they require careful evaluation.

Fatigue and weakness

If the patient complains of excessive fatigue and weakness, the physician must determine if these symptoms have developed recently or if they have been present for some time. If they have appeared suddenly in an aged person who had been active and vigorous, they may point to an acute illness. In the very aged, a myocardial infarction may be painless, and extreme weakness, sometimes with syncope, may be its only manifestation. Anemia caused by blood loss or a hemolytic process, infections with little or no fever, a cerebral vascular thrombosis without localizing signs, or adverse drug reactions may all be present with no more than the nonspecific complaint of weakness. If an elderly person suddenly takes to his bed, refuses to eat, or becomes incontinent, the physician must search for a definite and possibly remediable cause.

A gradual and undefined onset of chronic lassitude requires a different assessment. Chronic fatigue may be the result of several hidden causes such as anemia of various origins, arteriosclerotic heart disease with reduced cardiac output, chronic pulmonary disease with hypoxia, or chronic infection with insignificant temperature elevations. Patients who are receiving diuretics may develop hypokalemia, which can cause profound weakness. The physician must obtain an accurate medication history. Many aged patients take sedatives that they do not need and that may keep them drowsy through much of the day. Others who believe that they cannot sleep at night may take excessive doses of hypnotics that have a cumulative effect. The patient may not see the relationship of his drug habits to his fatigue. Rather, he will express the belief that his insomnia, which is often more imaginary than real, keeps him tired through the day. Depression and boredom are common causes of fatigue.

Disorders of the thyroid gland must always be considered as a possible cause of extreme weakness and fatigue. Signs and symptoms may be atypical in the aged. Hypothyroidism is more common in the aged than is thyrotoxicosis. Lloyd and Goldberg[12] found hypothyroidism in 1.7% and thyrotoxicosis in 0.5% of 3417 new patients referred to a geriatric service. Jefferys[13] found an incidence of hypothyroidism in 3.8% and of thyrotoxicosis in 2.3% of 300 patients consecutively admitted to a geriatric hospital.

Hypothyroidism may have an insidious onset. Mental and physical slowing, cold intolerance, and apathy may be the leading symptoms. The skin is coarse and dry; face, neck, wrists, and ankles may be puffy. Weight gain without increase in appetite is common. The patient may complain of joint pain and muscle aches. A normocytic anemia may be present. The diagnosis must be made early, since mental changes are not always reversible.

Rosenbaum and Barzel[14] have coined the term "failing thyroid syndrome." These patients are not yet clinically hypothyroid, but an elevated blood level of thyroid stimulating hormone (THS) indicates an impending failure of thyroid function. The authors observed this condition in a number of aged subjects who had been treated previously for Graves' disease or Hashimoto's thyroiditis. Early administration of thyroxine prevented the development of frank hypothyroidism.

Thyrotoxicosis in the aged often has atypical symptoms. The hyperactivity characteristic of young thyrotoxic patients may be absent. To the contrary, the patient may be apathetic, and often the condition is misdiagnosed as old-age depression.[15] The incidence for men and women is about equal; while in younger individuals thyrotoxicosis is much more common in women. The thyroid gland is not enlarged to the same extent as it is in younger patients, but it may be multinodular. Tachycardia is also not as marked in older individuals, but arrhythmias such as atrial fibrillation and ventricular ectopic beats are common. Muscular weakness and weight loss are prominent signs in aged thyrotoxic patients. The increases of serum levels of T4 and T3 may be only marginal.[16] The aged thyrotoxic patient does not tolerate stress, and any intercurrent illness may lead to rapid decline and death.[17] For this reason an early diagnosis is important.

In evaluating the weak and tired patient the physician must distinguish between general lassitude and true muscular weakness. Muscle strength declines with age but usually not to the point of seriously interfering with common day-to-day activities. Muscle atrophy seen in the very old is often not associated with profound weakness. True muscle weakness can be demonstrated by physical examination. The hand grip may be unduly weak. Pelvic girdle muscle weakness may make it impossible for an elderly patient to arise from a chair without help. A patient with shoulder girdle weakness cannot hold the arms up for any length of time and cannot work on high shelves. A patient with calf muscle weakness cannot stand on his toes. Proximal muscle weakness may indicate polymyositis, not infrequently associated with malignancies. Disorders of joints may cause weakness of the adjacent muscle groups. The weakness in turn adversely affects the condition of the joints.

Various metabolic disorders may cause muscle weakness. Thyrotoxicosis has been mentioned previously. Hypokalemia, often the result of the use of diuretics, may cause true weakness, which is rapidly relieved by potassium administration. Judge and Cowan[18] reported that muscle weakness in the aged may be related to an inadequate intake of potassium. However, their findings have been disputed by Burr et al.[19] Aged individuals whose dietary intake did not exceed 45 mEq of potassium were placed in a controlled study. At the end of 2 weeks those subjects who had received 48 mEq of supplementary potassium had not improved their grip strength any more than the placebo group.

Other metabolic disorders causing muscle weakness may include hypercalcemia of various causes, diabetic amyotrophy, and the prolonged administration of adrenocortical steroids. Polymyalgia rheumatica, a disease of the older age group, causes muscle pain rather than weakness. In any case, if a patient complains of weakness, the physician must try to demonstrate loss of strength through objective testing. Often this is not easy, since muscle tests require the patient's cooperation. Functional testing such as having patients hold their arms extended in front of them, arising from a chair, stepping on a stool or chair, and standing on one leg at a time may be quite informative.

Electromyography is a valuable tool that distinguishes neurogenic weakness from primary muscle disorders and localizes the lesion within the peripheral nervous system.

Syncope

The physician is rarely present to witness a syncopal attack. The patient himself will usually be unable to contribute much information, and witnesses may be too excited to provide worthwhile observations. For these reasons a clear description of the fainting attack is often impossible to obtain.

This section is limited to attacks of fainting from which the patient recovers fairly promptly without neurologic sequelae. The transient ischemic attack does not fall into this category, since by definition it leaves the patient with a temporary neurologic deficit.

Cerebral vascular disease is a common cause of fainting in the aged. Constricted atherosclerotic carotid arteries may become partially blocked by certain movements of the head, such as hyperextension of the neck. Elderly men complain at times that they become dizzy and faint while shaving. A tight collar can have the same effect.

Fainting may be the symptom of a myocardial infarction or of acute anemia caused by blood loss. Adams-Stokes attacks or other dysrhythmias must be considered as a possible cause of loss of consciousness. If this is suspected, a Holter monitor test should be done.

Postural hypotension is frequently encountered in the aged. The baroceptor reflexes become less efficient with age, and a sudden change to the upright position may cause hypotension and fainting. On the other hand, Gross[20] has concluded from tilt-table experiments that postural hypotension of the aged is caused by vascular rigidity rather than insufficiency of the baroceptors. Certain drugs such as phenothiazines, alpha-adrenergic blocking agents, tricyclic antidepressants, and levodopa enhance the tendency to postural hypotension. The diagnosis is easily made by taking the patient's blood pressure in the recumbent, sitting, and standing position. A drop of the systolic pressure by more than 20 mm Hg is significant.

Idiopathic orthostatic hypotension is an entity of its own. It is associated with other autonomic deficits, such as lack of sweating, impotence, and disorders of bladder and bowel function. In later stages, signs of basal ganglia disorders, such as rigidity, tremors, and paucity of movements, are common.[21] The pathologic cerebral findings have been described by Shy and Drager,[22] who first identified this syndrome. Hickler et al.[23] and Fine[24] have shown that idiopathic orthostatic hypotension is often associated with excessive renal excretion of sodium and may be treated with sodium chloride and fluorohydrocortisone.

In any case of orthostatic hypotension, patients should be advised to arise slowly from a recumbent position and to remain sitting on the edge of the bed for a few moments before they stand up or walk.

True epileptic seizures may be caused by idiopathic epilepsy that may produce only a few attacks in a lifetime. Epileptic seizures that appear for the first time in old age may be caused by vascular disease or by a space-occupying lesion such as a tumor or a subdural hematoma. Hypertensive vascular disease rarely causes seizures in the aged and should not be accepted as an explanation without a thorough search for other causes.

Hysterical attacks of fainting may occur in the elderly as well as in the young.

Vertigo

True vertigo must be differentiated from giddiness and faintness. The physician must seek a careful description of the attack of dizziness. Vertigo may be caused by a lesion of the cerebellum or brain stem or of the arteries that supply these structures, such as the basilar artery or the posterior inferior cerebellar artery. Afflictions of the labyrinth or eighth nerve, often associated with inner ear deafness, can cause recurrent and disabling attacks of vertigo. Wax in the ear canal or diseases of the middle ear can be responsible for intense dizziness. Postural hypotension from various causes may result in dizziness and at times true vertigo (see Chapter 29).

Falls

Aged persons at times experience falls that are not accompanied by a loss of consciousness or changes in heart rate or blood pressure. The patients report that while standing, or more often while walking, their legs suddenly give way and they find themselves on the ground. In many patients these attacks remain unexplained after the more obvious causes such as neuropathy, cerebral vascular disease, parkinsonism, drug effects, or alcohol have been excluded. At times the falls may be caused by inattentiveness, the patients simply may not watch where they are going, the house may be cluttered with throw rugs or other obstacles, or unsuitable footwear may not give adequate support. In other cases the patients may have lost the ability to rapidly coordinate back and lower extremity movements. Normal walking, after all, consists of an alternating loss and recapture of body balance. While walking the aged subjects may have moved their center of gravity too far ahead of their supporting leg and are then unable to retrieve their balance quickly enough to remain upright. Sheldon has postulated that a tendency to drop attacks may be associated with a loss of cerebellar Purkinje cells and a resulting dysfunction of the cerebellar cortex.[25] More recently, Stevens and Mathews reported that most subjects with "cryptogenic drop attacks" were women and that the falls often first appeared before the subjects were 50 years old. The authors were unable to attribute the drop attacks to any one particular cause but concluded that the characteristics of their gait predisposed women to unexplained falls.[26] Azar and Lawton found that the most common gait abnormality of older women was associated with varus deformities of the knees. As a result the gait was narrow, predisposing the women to a loss of balance and to falls.[27]

Headache

Migraine headaches often disappear as the sufferers reach old age. Only occasionally does one encounter an aged patient who still has typical attacks of migraine. Tension headaches also are less common in the aged. Headaches that appear suddenly in an elderly patient must be taken seriously and should be investigated. They may indicate a space-occupying lesion, or they may foreshadow a cerebral vascular catastrophe. Giant cell arteritis of the temporal arteries is accompanied by severe throbbing headaches. It is a disease of middle and old age, and it must be considered in the differential diagnosis of headache with sudden onset. Tender and hardened arteries can often be palpated, and an examination of the eyegrounds may reveal retinal hemorrhages and beginning optic atrophy. The erythrocyte sedimentation rate is elevated. A prompt diagnosis, which may require a biopsy of the artery, is mandatory so that treatment with cortical steroids can be initiated before eyesight is irretrievably lost.

Occipital headaches may be caused by osteoarthritic changes in the cervical spine with nerve root encroachment. The headache may be dependent on body position. It is usually associated with hyperesthesia of the occipital skin.

Glaucoma may have headache as the initial symptom. Herpes zoster of the fifth nerve may cause severe headache before the appearance of a skin eruption establishes the diagnosis.

Insomnia

Complaints of sleeplessness need to be evaluated by careful questioning. Often patients who complain that they do not sleep a wink can be observed sleeping quite peacefully for several hours in succession. However, the sleep may indeed be interrupted by dreams or by brief periods of awakening. They will leave the patient with the impression of not having slept at all while actually the total sleeping time may be sufficient. Some patients may be awakened by physical discomforts such as back or neck pain, being too cold or too warm or by the need to make frequent trips to the toilet. These patients should be given mild analgesics for pain. They may need advice about the regulation of room temperature and the restriction of fluids in the evening may reduce the need to urinate at night. Some patients nap a great deal during the day or go to bed early out of boredom. As a result they are unable to sleep well at night. Cutting down on the number of naps or going to bed later may solve the problem. Coffee or tea should be avoided in the evening or late afternoon.

Inability to go to sleep may be caused by anxiety, while early awakening, as in all age groups, may be a sign of depression. In the long run sympathetic counseling may be much more effective than hypnotics, which should be avoided if at all possible. Sleeping medications, particularly barbiturates, will make the patient listless and drowsy during the day and may add to confusion and depression. If the patient is depressed, a tricyclic antidepressant given at bedtime may help the patient to sleep more soundly. Phenothiazines taken at bedtime will help the patient whom anger or anxiety tend to keep awake.

Dysphagia

Difficulties in swallowing rarely are of functional origin and must be investigated. They may be caused by a lesion of the brain stem; in that case other neurologic abnormalities will establish the diagnosis. Organic diseases of the esophagus occur frequently with advancing years. A barium swallow will aid in the diagnosis of diverticula, carcinoma of the esophagus, or tumors of adjacent structures. Another common cause of dysphagia is a hiatal hernia with reflux esophagitis. The peristalsis of the esophagus changes with advancing age, and this too will make swallowing increasingly difficult. (Diseases of the esophagus are discussed in Chapter 8.)

Loss of appetite

A sudden loss of appetite may indicate an acute illness such as an infection or congestive heart failure. Liver disease or renal failure with uremia are usually accompanied by profound anorexia. Intoxication by a variety of drugs such as digitalis or sedatives is a common cause of loss of appetite and nausea.

Long-term anorexia may be the result of depression or apathy. (Anorexia nervosa does not occur in the aged.) The sensations of taste and smell are diminished in old age and this takes away the pleasure of eating. Elderly people often do better with highly seasoned foods. Those who live alone and have little interest in food do not like to cook for themselves. Often they subsist on a deficient diet, which in turn aggravates the anorexia.

Stomach disease, such as carcinoma or atrophy of the gastric mucosa, may occur with anorexia and a particular dislike for meat. Often the aged are unaware of their poor appetite and deficient diet and will not mention it without specific inquiry.

Constipation and diarrhea

Constipation is a frequent complaint. Loss of abdominal muscle tone, relaxation of the pelvic floor, and insufficient intake of bulk-producing foods and fluids combine to interfere with defecation. Aged patients may exhibit undue anxiety over constipation. They may become habitual users of laxatives, and, as time goes on, more and stronger medications are needed to bring results. Better dietary habits, stool softeners, and reassurance may remedy the situation, unless the laxative habit has become ingrained over many years. In that case it is best to permit the patient to continue with the accustomed use of laxatives.

Hypothyroidism may cause constipation. More frequently a variety of drugs may be responsible. Codeine, an ingredient of many cough mixtures, may cause constipation, as do other opiates, anticholinergic drugs, and salicylates. Weakness of the abdominal muscles may be an important contributory factor. Depression, which tends to slow many autonomic functions, may cause constipation.

If the problem is of recent origin, the physician should search for organic lesions of the colon, such as a carcinoma of the left colon or diverticulosis. Diarrhea, alternating with constipation, is particularly suspicious. A fecal impaction is usually discovered by rectal examination. Occasionally a flat film of the abdomen must be obtained to discover a high impaction, out of the reach of the examining finger.

Diarrhea may be caused by infection, diverticulitis, or malignancies. In older individuals, laxative abuse must be considered as a possible cause. Fecal impaction may cause oozing of liquid stool around the obstruction: this can easily be mistaken for true diarrhea.

Drugs such as broad-spectrum antibiotics, iron preparations, or, occasionally, digitalis may cause diarrhea. Food poisoning must be suspected in elderly people who live alone and who are not alert enough to recognize that food has spoiled.

CONCLUSION

In the geriatric population different diseases may have similar or identical symptoms that are often vague and do not point to definitive diagnoses. Fatigue, weakness, dizziness, poor appetite, and so on are not characteristic of any one disease; single or in combination these symptoms may lead the physician, intent on making the correct diagnosis, into a variety of different directions. Symptoms that are characteristic for certain diseases in the young and middle aged may be absent in the old. The diagnostic process in aged patients therefore is a difficult task that requires thoroughness, patience, and mature clinical skills.

REFERENCES

1. Williamson, J., et al.: Old people at home, their unreported needs, Lancet **1**:1117, 1964.
2. Howell, T.H.: A student's guide to geriatrics, ed. 2, Springfield, Ill., 1970, Charles C Thomas, Publisher.
3. Schwartz, D., Wang, M., Zeitz, L., and Goss, M.E.W.: Medication errors made by elderly, chronically ill patients, Am. J. Public Health **52**:2018, 1962.
4. Hurwitz, N.: Predisposing factors in adverse reactions to drugs, Br. Med. J. **1**:536, 1969.
5. Hall, M.R.P., editor: Evaluation of drug therapy in the elderly, Gerontol. Clin. **16**:1, 1974.
6. Drugs and the elderly, Los Angeles, 1973, Ethel Percy Andrus Gerontology Center, University of Southern California.
7. Vener, A.M., Krupka, L.R., and Climo, J.J.: Drug usage and health characteristics in noninstitutional retired persons, J. Am. Geriatr. Soc. **27**:83, 1979.
8. Hale, W.E., Marks, R.G., and Stewart, R.B.: Drug use in a geriatric population, J. Am. Geriatr. Soc. **27**:374, 1979.
9. Guinan, P., et al.: The accuracy of the rectal examination in the diagnosis of prostate carcinoma, N. Engl. J. Med. **303**:499, 1980.
10. Gral, T., and Young, M.: Measured versus estimated creatinine clearance in the elderly as an index of renal function, J. Am. Geriatr. Soc. **28**:492, 1980.
11. Steel, K., Williams, T.F., Fairbank, M., and Know, K.: Laboratory screening in the evaluation and placement of geriatric patients, J. Am. Geriatr. Soc. **22**:538, 1974.
12. Lloyd, W.H., and Goldberg, I.J.L.: Incidence of hypothyroidism in the elderly, Br. Med. J. **2**:1256, 1961.
13. Jefferys, P.M.: The prevalence of thyroid disease in patients admitted to a geriatric department, Age Ageing **1**:33, 1972.
14. Rosenbaum, R.L., and Barzel, U.S.: Clinical hypothyroidism in the elderly—a preventable disorder? J. Am. Geriatr. Soc. **29**:221, 1981.
15. Thomas, F.B., Mazzaferri, E.L., and Skillman, T.G.: Apathetic thyrotoxicosis: a distinctive clinical entity, Ann. Intern. Med. **72**:679, 1970.
16. Kawabe, T., et al.: Hyperthyroidism in the elderly, J. Am. Geriatr. Soc. **27**:152, 1979.
17. Lazarus, J.H., and Harden, R.M.: Thyrotoxicosis in the elderly, Gerontol. Clin. **11**:371, 1969.
18. Judge, T.G., and Cowan, N.R.: Dietary potassium and grip strength in the older people, Gerontol. Clin. **13**:221, 1971.
19. Burr, M.L., St. Leger, A.S., Westlake, C.A., and Davies, H.E.F.: Dietary potassium deficiency in the elderly: a controlled trial, Age Ageing **4**:148, 1975.
20. Gross, M.: The effect of posture on subjects with cerebrovascular disease, Q.J. Med. **39**:485, 1970.
21. Thomas, J.E., and Schirger, A.: Neurologic manifestations in idiopathic orthostatic hypotension, Arch. Neurol. **8**:204, 1963.
22. Shy, G.M., and Drager, G.A.: A neurological syndrome associated with orthostatic hypotension, Arch. Neurol. **2**:551, 1960.
23. Hickler, R.B., Thompson, G.R., Fox, L.M., and Hamlin, J.T.: Successful treatment of orthostatic hypotension with 9-alpha–fluorohydrocortisone, N. Engl. J. Med. **261**:788, 1959.
24. Fine, W.: Some common factors in the causation of postural hypotension, Gerontol. Clin. **11**:206, 1969.
25. Sheldon, J.H.: On the natural history of falls in the aged, Br. Med. J. **2**:1685, 1960.
26. Stevens, D.L., and Mathews, W.B.: Cryptogenic drop attacks: an affliction of women, Br. Med. J. **1**:439, 1973.
27. Azar, G.J., and Lawton, A.H.: Gait and stepping as factors in the frequent falls of elderly women, Gerontologist **4**:83, 1964.

CHAPTER 4 · ARTHRITIS, CONNECTIVE TISSUE DISORDERS, AND EXTRAARTICULAR RHEUMATISM

Bevra H. Hahn

Pain in articular and periarticular structures is a common problem among geriatric patients. Exact diagnosis of the disorders underlying these symptoms is desirable if optimal therapeutic results are to be achieved. Patients with various forms of arthritis can usually obtain relief of pain and protection from severe crippling and disability if managed with appropriate medical, physical, and surgical therapies. In this chapter, the diagnosis and therapy of the most common forms of rheumatic diseases affecting the elderly are reviewed.

ARTHRITIS

Degenerative joint disease (osteoarthritis, osteoarthroses)

Of the many different types of arthritis, degenerative joint disease (DJD) is by far the most common, affecting 50% of people in their sixth decade of life and 78% in their eighth decade. This disease is characterized by deterioration of articular cartilage and formation of new bone at the joint surfaces. Predisposing factors include advanced age, trauma, mechanical stresses, and genetic predisposition. Patients complain of gradually increasing pain in the affected joints, usually exacerbated by using the joint and relieved by resting it. The involved joints usually stiffen with disuse but can be limbered up by a few minutes of mild exercise. There are no systemic complaints.

In early disease, examination of the involved joints may reveal tenderness under local pressure, pain on motion, and mild heat. Although inflammatory changes are usually unimpressive, there are exceptions, and some patients have periarticular heat, erythema, and effusion or soft tissue swelling on examination. (Erosive osteoarthritis is a hereditary form of DJD that affects middle-aged women. It is accompanied by considerable pain and erythema in the distal and proximal interphalangeal joints of the hands and is characterized by bony hypertrophy, erosions of affected joint margins, and deformities of the involved hand joints.) Crepitation during joint motion is often present, but this may be detected in some normal joints. In later stages, bony hypertrophy is visible and/or palpable in distal interphalangeal (DIP) and proximal interphalangeal (PIP) joints of the hands, in the knees and in the first metatarsophalangeal (MTP) joints of the feet. In advanced disease, deformities may occur, such as subluxation of DIP and PIP joints, genu varus or valgus, and coxa varus. Frequently involved in the disease are the DIP and PIP joints of the hands; the first carpal-metacarpal joints (base of the thumbs); the cervical, thoracic, and lumbar spine; hip and knee joints; and the first MTP joints of the feet.

X-ray films show narrowing of the joint spaces caused by a loss of cartilage, sclerosis of subchondral bone, bony hypertrophy at joint margins, subchondral bone cysts, and, in advanced cases, deformities. Other laboratory tests, including the erythrocyte sedimentation rate, are normal, unless there is additional disease.

Treatment of DJD includes measures to reduce mechanical stress on joints, physical therapy to preserve joint motion, analgesics, antiinflammatory drugs, and surgery in selected cases. Decreasing mechanical stress on involved joints is extremely important in promoting control of pain and decreasing progression of the disease. The patient should be advised to alter his activities to favor involved joints. For example, patients with involvement of the hands should avoid scrubbing and the use of vibrating tools. Patients with lumbar spine disease should avoid lifting heavy objects. Patients with back, hip, or knee involvement should relieve those joints of weight bearing as much as possible by taking rest periods, sitting instead of standing, avoiding impact loading of cartilage, such as that associated with running or contact sports, and using appliances such as canes, crutches, or a walker. Supporting collars are useful in cervical arthritis for decreasing motion and for relieving pressure on nerve roots. A hard plastic Thomas collar is often helpful; four-poster steel braces provide firmer support but are often more uncomfortable than the Thomas collar. Lumbar corsets with steel stays are sometimes helpful in the management of lumbar spine degenerative disc or joint disease. Muscle-relaxing drugs such as diazepam (Valium), chlorzoxazone-acetaminophen (Parafon Forte), methocarbamol (Robaxin), and carisoprodol (Soma) are sometimes useful in relieving pain and stiffness associated with paravertebral muscle spasm. However, use of these agents may be limited by their propensity to cause drowsiness and confusion, especially in older patients.

Physical therapy is important for relieving stiffness and preserving joint function. Heat offers temporary relief of pain and is especially useful when followed by exercises designed to improve or maintain a full range of motion and to strengthen supporting muscles. For example, a patient with arthritis involving the knee should be instructed in a home exercise program that puts the knee through a full range of motion and that strengthens the quadriceps muscle group without increasing the load on the cartilage. Straight leg raising in a supine position is usually a good exercise for such a patient.

Analgesics are often required. Salicylates are useful in most patients and have antiinflammatory as well as analgesic properties. Initial doses of 600 mg of aspirin three or four times a day are recommended. The dose should then be altered to obtain the maximum beneficial effects with minimal toxicity. Doses should be taken with meals or with antacids to minimize gastric irritation. Preparations of salicylates with enteric coatings are associated with fewer gastrointestinal side effects.[1] Magnesium salicylate, sodium salicylate, and choline salicylate have less gastrointestinal toxicity than acetylsalicylic acid; they also have weaker antiinflammatory effects. One preparation, Trilisate, has the advantage of a long half-life and can be given at 12-hour intervals (1000 mg or two tablets every 12 hours). The salicylates have two major therapeutic advantages—they are inexpensive, and a readily available laboratory test can be used to adjust the dosage to a therapeutic range (15 to 25 mg/100 ml is the desired serum salicylate level).

However, salicylates have two major disadvantages—a relatively high incidence of gastrointestinal intolerance, including bleeding, and a high incidence of tinnitus, especially in the elderly. Other side effects include hearing impairment, headaches, vertigo, irritability, and confusion. Patients with asthma, especially those with nasal polyps, may have severe allergic reactions to salicylates; the drug should not be administered to those patients. All salicylates potentiate the anticoagulant effects of coumarin drugs; therefore salicylates should not be administered to patients receiving sodium warfarin (Coumadin) or dicumarol.

Since salicylates have a relatively high incidence of undesirable side effects, this author agrees with Huskisson's[2] view that nonsteroidal antiinflammatory drugs (NSAID) of the nonsalicylate group are better first-line drugs than salicylates, even though they are three to four times more expensive. NSAID available at the time of this writing include propionic acid derivatives—ibuprofen (Motrin), fenoprofen calcium (Nalfon) and naproxen (Naprosyn); indoleacetic acid derivatives—tolmetin sodium (Tolectin), sulindac (Clinoril), and indomethacin (Indocin); phenylbutazone (Butazolidin); oxyphenbutazone (Tandearil); and the carboxylic acid derivative meclofenamate sodium (Meclomen). All are antipyretic, analgesic, and antiinflammatory, probably in part because of their inhibition of prostaglandins. All are equivalent to full therapeutic doses of salicylates in controlling pain, inflammation, and stiffness associated with DJD and rheumatoid arthritis. All are less likely than aspirin to produce gastrointestinal discomfort, bleeding, and tinnitus. All except phenylbutazone can be used with warfarin sodium anticoagulants, although some have a mild effect by displacing the drug from plasma proteins; prothrombin times should be checked frequently if the drugs are used with warfarin. However, important adverse effects can occur with any of the NSAID, including dyspepsia, peptic ulcers, gastrointestinal bleeding, headaches, confusion, depersonalization, salt retention (occasionally severe enough to precipitate hypertension or even congestive heart failure in individuals with organic heart disease), allergic reactions in patients with asthma and nasal polyps (the same group with allergic reactions to salicylates), hepatitis, and, rarely, nephrotic syndrome or interstitial nephritis. The NSAID may also cause elevations in serum creatinine levels. All reduce platelet adhesiveness, but unlike aspirin the effect is reversible. Although the efficacy and toxicities of all these preparations are similar, a few important differences should be noted (Table 4-1). Naproxen and sulindac have longer half-lives than the other NSAID and can be given in two daily doses 12 hours apart. Such a dosage regimen may improve compliance. Ibuprofen has been associated with a few cases of aseptic meningitis. Meclofenamate may cause diarrhea and bone marrow suppression. Phen-

Table 4-1. Nonsteroidal antiinflammatory drugs (NSAID)—preparation, dosage, and precautions

Preparation					
Generic name	*Trade name*	*Dosage (mg)*	*Dosage schedule*	*Maximal daily dose (mg)*	*Side effects*
Propionic acid derivatives:					
Ibuprofen	Motrin	300 400 600	t.i.d. to q.i.d.	3000	GI toxicity (low incidence); salt retention; renal, hepatic, and CNS effects; aseptic meningitis Better tolerated than aspirin both long- and short-term
Fenoprofen calcium	Nalfon	300	t.i.d. to q.i.d.	2400	GI toxicity; salt retention; renal, hepatic, CNS effects
Naproxen	Naprosyn	250 375	q.12hr.	750	Same effects as fenoprofen calcium
Indoleacetic acid derivatives:					
Indomethacin	Indocin	25 50	t.i.d. to q.i.d.	150	More GI toxicity than propionic acid derivatives
Tolmetin sodium	Tolectin	200 400	t.i.d. to q.i.d.	1800	Same effects as indomethacin: less GI and CNS toxicity
Sulindac	Clinoril	150 200	q.12h.	400	Same effects as tolmetin
Others:					
Meclofenamic acid	Meclomen	500	t.i.d. to q.i.d.	2000	Same effects as fenoprofen plus diarrhea; slight interference with warfarin sodium and oral hypoglycemics
Phenylbutazone	Butazolidin	100	t.i.d. to q.i.d.	600	Same effects as fenoprofen plus agranulocytosis, thrombocytopenia, aplastic anemia, especially in elderly; interferes with warfarin sodium
Oxyphenbutazone	Tandearil	100	t.i.d. to q.i.d.	600	Same effects as phenylbutazone

ylbutazone and oxyphenbutazone are occasionally associated with fatal bone marrow suppression, especially agranulocytosis, which limits the usefulness of these drugs. Since this reaction may be more frequent in older individuals, it may be wise to avoid administering butazones to elderly individuals. Several additional NSAID are soon to be released but with two exceptions (benoxaprofen and flufenamic acid, which can be administered once daily) will probably offer no advantages over the preparations currently available. Several good reviews of the pharmacology, efficacy, and toxicity of the NSAID are available.[2,3]

Table 4-1 lists the dosages and some characteristics of each NSAID.

Other analgesic agents that do not have antiinflammatory properties but may be useful in relieving the pain of DJD include acetaminophen (Tylenol), propoxyphene hydrochloride (Darvon), ethoheptazine citrate (Zactirin), and pentazocine (Talwin). Narcotic analgesics should be avoided since therapy for DJD must be extended for long periods of time.

Local intraarticular administration of corticosteroids is effective in many patients with DJD, although the effects are temporary and repeated injections are usually required. This therapy is particularly useful in the management of DJD of the knees. An injection of 20 to 40 mg of triamcinolone acetonide will relieve pain from several days to several months in the majority of patients,[4] and injections can be repeated every few months. If care is taken to administer injections in a sterile fashion, the hazards of such treatment are minimal. Systemic complications of this form of steroid therapy do not occur. Local infection is the major complication (1 in 16,000).[4] Subcutaneous atrophy can also occur along the needle tract. Rabbits receiving frequent steroid injections in their joints have accelerated deterioration of cartilage; whether these observations are applicable to humans is unknown.

Systemic use of glucocorticoids is rarely necessary in DJD. An occasional patient, usually with significant inflammatory and erosive components of DJD, will receive substantial relief from low doses of prednisone (5 to 10 mg daily). When inflammation subsides, prednisone administration should be tapered and discontinued. Although such low doses are relatively safe, the undesirable side effects of corticosteroids administered over a period of years are considerable. The use of systemic steroids may be particularly hazardous in older individuals who may already have osteopenia, diabetes, hypertension, congestive heart failure, cataracts, or glaucoma. A more extensive discussion of systemic steroid therapy appears later in this chapter under Rheumatoid arthritis.

Since there are no drugs available that alter the progression of DJD, the usual course of the disease is one of gradual worsening. Fortunately, several excellent surgical procedures are available for patients who are significantly disabled by DJD in spite of medical and physical therapy. These include fusion of the first carpometacarpal joint of the wrist, total hip replacement, total knee replacement, and arthroplasty of the first MTP joint of the foot. Advanced age is not a contraindication to these procedures unless significant disease of major organs is present. We have seen many gratifying surgical results in patients with DJD who are in their seventies and eighties. The surgical procedures available to patients with various arthropathies are discussed in Chapter 15.

In summary, therapy for DJD consists of reducing mechanical stress on involved joints; exercise to preserve joint function; administration of salicylates or NSAID and analgesics; and intermittent intraarticular injections of corticosteroids. Surgical intervention is eventually necessary in some patients.

Rheumatoid arthritis

Rheumatoid arthritis (RA) is a common arthropathy that can appear at any age but is frequently seen in the geriatric age group. In general, it is far more disabling than DJD and usually requires more aggressive therapy. RA is characterized by inflammation in the synovial membranes that form the lining of joints and tendons. The inflamed synovium hypertrophies and invades surrounding tissues—cartilage, bone, tendons—causing the most damage to those tissues. The etiology of the inflammatory reaction is unclear; an immunologic reaction is probably involved.[5] Immune complexes consisting of IgG and anti-IgG (rheumatoid factors) are deposited in synovial membranes and phagocytized by leukocytes in synovial fluid. These complexes are capable of activating complement and of releasing lysosomal enzymes from leukocytes; both reactions result in inflammation.

Patients with RA usually experience either an insidious or an explosive onset of symmetrical, progressive polyarthritis, characterized by painful, swollen, warm joints. Morning stiffness lasting for 1 hour or more is characteristic. RA should be regarded as a systemic illness that is often associated with increased fatigability, malaise, and low grade fever.

Physical examination reveals heat, synovial thickening, tenderness, and effusions in several joints. The involvement is usually symmetric; swelling of PIP and second and third MCP joints of the hands is quite common. Other joints frequently involved include the temporomandibular, shoulder, elbow, wrist, hip, knee, and ankle joints; the MTP joints of the feet; and the cervical spine. Approximately 20% of patients develop subcutaneous nodules near the elbows and around tendon sheaths. Characteristic deformities appear as the disease progresses, including swan-neck (DIP-flexion contractures, PIP-extension contractures) or boutonniere (DIP-extension contractures, PIP-flexion contractures) deformities of the fingers; ulnar deviation at the MCP joints; subluxation of wrists; flexion contractures of elbows, hips, and knees; genu valgus or varus; hallux valgus; and hammer toes. Cervical spine involvement in patients with long-standing RA often results in subluxation of C1 on C2; clinical manifestations include occipital headaches, pain radiating to the back of the eye, and neurologic deficits if spinal cord or nerve roots are compromised.

X-ray films of involved joints show periarticular demineralization and soft tissue swelling in early stages, then erosions of marginal bone and loss of cartilage, and finally the deformities that occur as the disease advances.

Approximately 80% of patients have IgM rheumatoid factors circulating in their serum. Testing for rheumatoid factor has prognostic as well as diagnostic value. In general, patients who are seronegative have milder disease that progresses less rapidly than those who are seropositive. High titers of rheumatoid factor tend to correlate with resistant, severe disease as well as with complications of rheumatoid arthritis, such as vasculitis, interstitial lung disease, pleural effusions, pericarditis, skin ulcers, and Felty's and Sjögren's syndromes. Elevated erythrocyte sedimentation rates and mild normochromic normocytic anemia are usually present. Ten percent to 20% of patients have positive serum tests for antinuclear antibodies (ANA) and/or L.E. cells. Some patients are antinuclear antibody (ANA)-positive and rheumatoid factor-negative; their disease follows the pattern of the rheumatoid factor-positive patient.

Therapy for RA includes antirheumatic, antiinflammatory drugs; physical and occupational therapy; and surgery. Patients with mild disease may do well with administration of salicylates or NSAID and with physical therapy and maneuvers to relieve mechanical stress on inflamed joints. (These therapies are discussed in detail in the preceding section on DJD.) To obtain optimal antiinflammatory effects of aspirin, a blood level of salicylate ranging from 15 to 25 mg/100 ml should be achieved. These levels should be checked periodically (specimens should be drawn 2 hours after routine aspirin administration). Doses required to maintain this level vary greatly in individual patients and range from 8 to 16 300-mg tablets daily. Salicylates should be given with meals to minimize gastric irritation. Some salicylate preparations are less likely to cause dyspepsia and bleeding than others. (These are also discussed in the preceding DJD section of this chapter.) NSAID are also antiinflammatory and may be substituted for or used in preference to aspirin in patients with RA as discussed in the DJD section.

Since RA usually continues to progress, sometimes at a rapid rate, many patients require antirheumatic agents that are stronger than aspirin. These include gold salts, antimalarial drugs, D-penicillamine, glucocorticoids, and cytotoxic agents.

Administration of gold salts results in significant improvement of the inflammatory component of RA in the majority of patients. The mechanism by which these compounds reduce inflammation is unknown. Their efficacy has been well established in controlled clinical trials.[7,8] Soluble preparations are recommended such as gold sodium thiomalate (Myochrysine) or aurothioglucose (Solganol). They are administered in weekly intramuscular injections, usually 50 mg weekly. Improvement usually begins and continues at a gradual rate after administration of 350 to 600 mg. Most patients stabilize at an improved level (complete remissions are occasionally achieved) after 800 to 1000 mg have been administered.

Drugs used in the treatment of rheumatoid arthritis

1. *Nonsteroidal antiinflammatory drugs* (rapid response, relatively low toxicity).
   a. *Nonsalicylates:* Increase to maximal doses recommended if tolerated.
   b. *Salicylates* and *enteric-coated salicylates:* Achieve serum level of 15 to 25 mg/100 ml if tolerated.

   If response to two or three different group 1 drugs is unsatisfactory after several weeks begin administration of the following drugs.

2. *Noncytotoxic remission-inducing drugs* (slow acting with relatively high toxicity).
   a. Hydroxychloroquine (Plaquenil): Administer 200 to 400 mg daily. Probably less effective than gold or penicillamine; also less toxic. Major toxic reaction in eye; ophthalmologic examination required every 6 months.
   b. Gold (Solganal or Myochrysine): Administer 50 mg intramuscularly once weekly up to 1000 mg; discontinue if ineffective. If effective, reduce dosage to one injection every 2 weeks; then every 3; then every 4 weeks if effect persists. Twenty percent of patients will not tolerate gold. Major toxic reactions are dermatitis, mouth ulcers, immune glomerulonephritis with proteinuria, and bone marrow suppression.
   c. D-penicillamine (Depen, Cuprimine): Begin administering 250 mg daily between meals; increase by 125 mg every 6 to 8 weeks until response. If no improvement after 1500 mg administered, discontinue use. Toxic reactions are related to dosage; doses greater than 500 mg daily produce unacceptable side effects in 40% of patients. Major toxic reactions are dermatitis (including pemphigus), loss of taste, mouth ulcers, immune glomerulonephritis with proteinuria, bone marrow suppression, myasthenia gravis, vasculitis, and lupus-like syndromes.

   If response to group 1 drugs is unsatisfactory, and rapid relief is essential, or if response to group 1 plus group 2 drugs is unsatisfactory, begin administration of the following drugs.

3. *Systemic glucocorticoids* (rapid acting, severe and increasing toxicities with time).
   Prednisone and methylprednisolone (Medrol): Administration of one dose in the morning every other day has lower incidence of side effects but often does not control RA satisfactorily. Daily administration of 15 mg of prednisone or less in the morning may not suppress adrenal gland and may not control morning stiffness. Two daily doses will usually suppress adrenal gland, even low doses, and is most likely to control disease.

   If responses to groups 1 and 2 drugs and to groups 1 and 3 drugs are unsatisfactory, or if there are major contraindications to glucocorticoids, begin administration of the following drugs.

4. *Cytotoxic drugs* (slow acting, high toxicity).
   a. Methotrexate: 7.5 mg orally once weekly or intramuscularly (see text).
   b. Azathioprine (Imuran): 0.5 to 2 mg/kg daily.
   c. Cyclophosphamide (Cytoxan): 0.5 to 2 mg/kg daily.

   Begin with low doses, increase if no response after 12 to 16 weeks if tolerated. Toxicities differ for each drug, but include GI intolerance, severe bone marrow suppression, liver damage (methotrexate and azathioprine), hair loss, mouth ulcers, sterility (cyclophosphamide), hemorrhagic cystitis and bladder cancer (cyclophosphamide), and increased risk of malignancy (azathioprine and cyclophosphamide).

5. *Experimental drugs and procedures* (not yet recommended or widely available but under study).
   a. Oral gold
   b. Levamisole hydrochloride
   c. Plasmapheresis[6]
   d. Lymphopheresis
   e. Extensive lymph node irradiation

When improvement has been achieved and the disease has been stable for 3 to 4 weeks, the gold dosage may be reduced to 50 mg every 2 weeks. If good results are maintained, reduction of the dosage to 50 mg every 3 weeks and eventually to once a month should be tried. If improvement is maintained and toxicity does not occur, gold therapy should be continued indefinitely. Most patients with RA respond to gold and are improved for a few years; then the disease process begins to escape control, and retreatment with weekly gold or other agents is needed. (In contrast, other patients experience total remissions after several years of disease, regardless of the form of treatment used.) Patients who do not improve after a total dose of 1000 mg of gold salts may be considered nonresponders, and administration of the drug should be discontinued.

Gold compounds are associated with significant toxic side effects. The most common is dermatitis, which occurs in 10% to 20% of patients. Various types of rashes may appear; they are invariably pruritic. Transient, mild rashes may occur after the first few injections; the weekly dose of gold may be reduced and therapy continued. More commonly the rash appears after 300 to 800 mg of gold salts have been administered. This is the most dangerous period for all types of gold toxicity, and administration of the drug should be stopped. In some patients gold can be restarted at a lower dose without the rash recurring, but in most patients the drug must be permanently discontinued. The most dangerous side effect of gold is suppression of any or all elements of the bone marrow—platelets, neutrophils, or erythrocytes; this reaction can be fatal. Fortunately, this complication is rare. Other adverse side effects include ulcerations of the mouth; immune complex nephritis (reversible), manifested usually as proteinuria and sometimes leading to nephrotic syndrome; vasomotor reactions; and, rarely, allergic pneumonitis. Administration of gold salts should be monitored by complete blood counts, platelet counts, and urinalyses at 1- or 2-week intervals. The interval between tests may be lengthened to once a month when a maintenance dosage is reached and eventually to once every 3 months. Any decrease in blood counts or the appearance of small amounts of proteinuria should arouse suspicion. The drug should be withheld until the abnormality disappears, then reinstituted cautiously at a lower dose, and discontinued if the adverse reaction recurs. Since most adverse reactions from gold occur within the first 6 months of therapy, patients who tolerate the drug during that period can usually be managed for many years with little hazard. In contrast, administration of glucocorticoids over a period of years may be associated with continually increasing side effects. Therefore, I usually choose gold rather than steroids to manage RA patients who fail to respond to aspirin or NSAID. An oral preparation of gold, auranofin, is currently being tested and may be available soon.

Antimalarial drugs are occasionally useful in the treatment of RA. Controlled therapeutic trials have shown that chloroquine (Aralen) and hydroxychloroquine sulfate (Plaquenil) both produce improvement in the majority of patients.[9] They are easy to administer since they are given in a single daily oral dose. They can be used in patients with RA who are not doing well on aspirin or NSAID and who cannot tolerate gold or cannot arrange weekly appointments for gold injections. The initial dosage is 200 mg daily (one tablet) of hydroxychloroquine sulfate. Responses appear slowly over a period of several weeks; if no benefit is achieved after 3 months of treatment, the dose can be increased by one half tablet. The dosage should not exceed two tablets daily (400 mg) because of the increased risk of retinal damage from higher doses. If the patient does not improve after 6 months of treatment, antimalarial drugs should be discontinued.

Undesirable side effects are uncommon but include nausea, weight loss, dermatitis (sometimes associated with striking photosensitivity), alopecia, loss of pigment in hair and skin, and peripheral neuropathy and myopathy. The most serious side effects are ocular. Chloroquine and hydroxychloroquine sulfate may be deposited in the cornea, where they interfere with vision. These lesions are reversible and resolve themselves after the drugs are discontinued. Both antimalarial agents have affinities for melanin and are deposited in pigmented tissues. Therefore, the retina, especially the macular region, is particularly susceptible to accumulation of these drugs and resultant injury. All patients receiving chloroquine or hydroxychloroquine sulfate should be examined at 6-month intervals by an ophthalmologist, who can often detect signs of retinal damage (usually loss of red vision) before the patient develops visual loss. Although retinal damage is usually halted by discontinuing therapy, cases have been reported in which the lesions have progressed, causing severe visual loss or blindness. Although retinal damage is reported to be rare, occurring in 1 out of 1000 patients,[9] in my experience the appearance of such lesions with either hydroxychloroquine sulfate or chloroquine is not unusual. Nevertheless, this class of drugs may be used with relative safety and considerable efficacy in some patients with RA.

D-penicillamine (Cuprimine, Depen) is another remission-inducing agent useful in the management of patients with RA who have persistent inflammatory synovitis during salicylate or NSAID therapy. Some patients who fail to respond to gold will respond to penicillamine, and vice versa. Its mechanism of action is uncertain, but the administered doses reduce cellular immune reactions[10] as well as serum levels of immunoglobulins, rheumatoid factors, and immune complexes.[11,12] Adverse side effects are frequent if high doses (750 to 1500 mg) are administered daily; most toxicities are dose related. Therefore, a low dose regimen with slow increases is recommended. Therapy is initiated with one 250-mg tablet or capsule; the dose is increased by 125-mg increments every 8 weeks until response is achieved. (Do not exceed 1500 mg daily.) Approximately one half of patients with early disease respond to a 500-mg dose, some require less and others more. Improvement begins a few weeks after the "critical" dose for an individual patient is reached and continues slowly. Most patients require 4 to 6 months to improve; others require as much as a year. Experience with D-penicillamine in RA is too limited to determine what proportion of individuals sustain prolonged improvement. Approximately two thirds of patients will improve.

Adverse side effects include allergic skin eruptions, pemphigus-like dermatitis, skin fragility, oral ulcerations, bone marrow suppression (thrombocytopenia is the most common hematologic side effect), immune complex nephritis (sometimes with nephrotic syndrome), and dyspepsia. Approximately 10% of patients lose their sense of taste or have it diminished. Usually sense of taste returns in 6 to 12 weeks even if the drug is continued. Uncommon side effects include vasculitis, a myasthenia gravis-like syndrome, a systemic lupus-like disease, and Goodpasture's syndrome. Indications for discontinuing D-penicillamine therapy include severe or persistent rash, pemphigus, a platelet count of less than 100,000/mm^3, a leukocyte count of less than 4000/mm^3, proteinuria of 1000 mg or more in 24 hours, rising serum creatinine level, vasculitis, myasthenia, or systemic lupus erythematosus (SLE).

The use of D-penicillamine is a major advance in the management of RA, since gold and cytotoxics were the only good remission-inducing agents available before. However, it has been used in RA for only a decade as opposed to 50 years of experience with gold. Physicians may need to revise their use of D-penicillamine as experience accumulates. (For reviews of this subject, see Jaffe.)[12]

Glucocorticoids are often dramatically effective in reducing the inflammation and consequently the pain, swelling, and stiffness of RA. They are potent antiinflammatory agents and probably would be used in most patients with RA if they were not associated with significant side effects, especially when used for a period of years. Improvement appears quickly, with most patients enjoying relief of their symptoms within 24 to 48 hours. There is conflicting evidence as to whether long-term therapy with steroids alters the course of the rheumatoid disease process. Once steroids are begun, it is difficult to discontinue them because synovitis usually flares. In general, it is desirable to reserve steroid therapy for patients who fail to do well on a more conservative regimen of salicylates, gold, antimalarial drugs, and/or D-penicillamine or for those patients who absolutely require immediate improvement. Many synthetic steroid preparations are available; prednisone is the least expensive, is quite effective, and will be used in this chapter as the reference glucocorticoid. Therapy may be begun with small daily doses, such as 5 mg of prednisone, and increased every few days until control of inflammation is achieved. As an alternative, relatively high doses, such as 40 mg, may be administered daily, and the dosage reduced by approximately 10% every 1 or 2 weeks until satisfactory maintenance levels are achieved. Most patients with RA can be maintained on a dosage varying from 5 to 15 mg daily.

Undesirable side effects of steroids are not as great at these low doses as they are in patients who require higher doses. Nevertheless, side effects are considerable in patients with RA and include fragility and easy bruising of the skin, osteopenia, myopathy, aseptic necrosis of bone (especially of the femoral heads), gastrointestinal bleeding, peptic ulceration, Cushingoid habitus, hirsutism, moon face, acne, hyperglycemia, hypertension, salt retention, cataracts, glaucoma, mental disturbances, and increased susceptibility to infection. There is recent evidence that the bone loss associated with long-term systemic glucocorticoid therapy can be diminished by administration of vitamin D (50,000 units 2 to 3 times weekly), 25-hydroxy vitamin D (Calderol), 50 μg daily, plus 500 mg of calcium daily.[13] This therapy partially reverses the malabsorption of calcium that accompanies administration of steroids. Hypercalciuria and hypercalcemia are possible complications. Twenty-four-hour urine specimens and serum calcium levels should be measured before and at 4 to 6 month intervals after instituting vitamin D or calcifediol (Calderol); urine calcium should not exceed 300 mg per 24 hours. The supplemental therapy should be discontinued if glucocorticoids are stopped.

Adrenal suppression is minimized when the daily dose of prednisone, given once in the morning, is 15 mg or less. However, some patients prefer dividing steroids into two daily doses to achieve better control of morning stiffness. Small doses of steroids given in the evening suppress the release of corticotropin releasing factor and therefore of adrenocorticotropic hormone (ACTH). Steroid preparations with a short half-life (methylprednisolone, prednisolone, prednisone) are less likely to suppress the pituitary-adrenal axis than steroid preparations with a long half-life (dexamethasone and betamethasone). Patients who receive daily doses of steroids for more than 2 weeks may have adrenal suppression and should be managed with increased steroid doses when under stress, such as surgery or a major infection. The pituitary-adrenal axis may also be protected by administering steroids once every other day. Recent reviews of the pharmacology, physiology, and cellular effects of glucocorticoids are available.[14,15] In my experience, most patients with RA cannot tolerate steroid administration every other day because of flares of arthritis on the day that steroids are omitted. In spite of their hazards, steroids are quite effective in the majority of patients with RA and should be administered to patients who are in danger of being disabled by their disease and are not responsive to more conservative regimens. They can also be used during the symptomatic period when gold or D-penicillamine therapies are being initiated and then tapered and withdrawn when those drugs take effect.

Cytotoxic agents are available for the small number of patients who do not respond well to the usual therapies for RA. These include azathioprine (Imuran), methotrexate, and cyclophosphamide (Cytoxan). Azathioprine is a cytotoxic agent that has also proven to be effective in severe RA that is unresponsive to conventional therapy, including glucocorticoids.[16] Therapy may be begun with as little as 1 mg of azathioprine per kilogram of body weight, given orally at bedtime (to reduce the incidence of nausea). The dose may be increased to a maximum of 2.5 to 3 mg/kg, if there is no response after several weeks. Objective and subjective improvement usually occur by 16 weeks of therapy. Toxic reactions include suppression of any or all bone marrow elements, nausea, diarrhea, and hepatocellular damage, usually manifested by elevation of serum transaminases.

Cyclophosphamide is a very potent cytotoxic and immunosuppressive drug that may be beneficial in patients with severe RA,[17] even in low doses. It is administered orally in doses of 0.8 to 2.5 mg/kg daily. It may be dramatically effective after several weeks of therapy (16 weeks is the median time for response to occur). I recommend beginning with low-dose therapy (1 mg/kg daily) and increasing gradually to 2.5 mg/kg daily after 16 weeks if improvement has not occurred. Cyclophosphamide is quite toxic; undesirable side effects include suppression of bone marrow elements (especially granulocytes), alopecia, sterility (which may not be reversible) in both men and women, nausea, diarrhea, hemorrhagic cystitis, fibrosing cystitis, and increased risk of infection. It should be administered in the morning with large amounts of fluid to minimize the risk of cystitis. There is evidence that patients with connective tissue diseases treated with either azathioprine or cyclophosphamide have an increased incidence of malignant tumors, especially lymphomas.[18]

Recently, some authorities[19] have reported that low weekly doses of methotrexate (7.5 to 15 mg) are efficacious in treating RA. This cytotoxic agent has not been associated with an increased risk of malignancy. However, oral ulcerations and bone marrow suppression are not infrequent, and methotrexate should be considered experimental at this time. Currently, azathioprine, cyclophosphamide, and methotrexate should be considered effective, but highly toxic agents and should be reserved for the small number of patients with RA who have active destructive synovitis despite therapy with adequate doses of salicylates, gold, antimalarial drugs, D-penicillamine, and steroids.

Extraarticular manifestations of rheumatoid arthritis. Before leaving the topic of RA, two fairly common complications of this disorder deserve special mention—cervical subluxation and vasculitis. Approximately 10% of patients with long-standing RA develop symptomatic subluxation of the first cervical vertebra on the second. If this complication is suspected, x-ray films of the cervical spine in full flexion and full extension should be taken to confirm the presence of the disorder. If neurologic symptoms or signs are present, the problem deserves special attention. If symptoms are confined to headache and mild cervical nerve root irritation, treatment should consist of mechanical devices that hold the cervical spine in extension. The hard plastic Thomas collar or a steel cervical brace should be prescribed. Pain is usually relieved. In some patients, these appliances can be removed after 6 weeks, and pain will not recur. In others, the cervical appliance will be required permanently. Evidence of spinal cord or brain stem disease constitutes an emergency situation; sudden death can occur. These patients should be managed by neurosurgeons and will require cervical traction and possibly surgical fusion of the affected vertebrae.

The second rather common complication of RA in the geriatric age group is vasculitis. Patients with this disorder usually have had RA for several years. They develop weight loss, increased fatigability, and peripheral neuropathy. They may also have fever, skin ulcers (usually around the ankles), gastrointestinal bleeding, angina pectoris, gangrene of the digits, and even central nervous system (CNS) disorders. The combination of gangrene of the digits and peripheral neuropathy is associated with a very poor prognosis and should be treated aggressively. Patients with life-threatening vasculitis may be managed with high doses of glucocorticoids. If no improvement results, cytotoxic agents (especially cyclophosphamide) or D-penicillamine may be added to the regimen. Patients with the life-threatening syndrome of digital gangrene and peripheral neuropathy should be treated quite aggressively with high doses of steroids (60 to 100 mg daily); penicillamine should be considered, beginning with 500 to 750 mg daily and increasing the dose every 5 to 6 days to a total daily dose of 1500 gm.[20] Intravenous cyclophosphamide (0.5 gm/m^2) and plasmapheresis are experimental therapies that may be considered instead of or in addition to D-penicillamine since their effect can be seen within days.[21] Patients who develop peripheral neuropathy as the major manifestation of vasculitis may be treated more conservatively. There is spontaneous improvement in approximately one third of these patients over a period of a few weeks. Another one third will remain relatively stable, and the remaining one third will develop progressive neuropathy and/or other life-threatening features of rheumatoid vasculitis. Only the latter group of patients should be treated aggressively.

Other extraarticular manifestations of RA include episcleritis, which can occasionally be severe and threaten vision; pericarditis; valvular heart disease; rheumatoid nodules in the lung; pulmonary interstitial inflammation and fibrosis; Felty's syndrome; sicca (Sjögren's) syndrome (keratoconjunctivitis sicca and xerostomia); myopathy; and compression of peripheral nerves (median, ulnar, and posterior tibial).

Gout and pseudogout

Gout and pseudogout are inflammatory arthropathies that are common in older age groups and result from formation of microcrystals of monosodium urate (gout) or calcium pyrophosphate dihydrate (CPPD) (pseudogout) in the joints and surrounding soft tissues. Pseudogout[22] may closely mimic gout, with acute, severe inflammation in one or a few joints that persists for several days then subsides spontaneously. However, it can also mimic chronic polyarticular RA or DJD. It may be associated with Charcot joints (severely destroyed joints with less pain than one would expect, such as those seen in patients with peripheral neuropathies, syringomyelia, or tabes dorsalis). In some patients, (CPPD) crystals are present in cartilage, producing chondrocalcinosis, but there are no associated symptoms.

In early gout and goutlike CPPD disease, the patient typically goes to bed feeling well and awakens with severe pain in one or two joints. The joints rapidly become swollen, erythematous, and hot and are so painful that it is impossible to bear weight or to bend them. In gout, the joints most commonly involved include the great toe, instep, ankle, knee, elbow, and wrist. In pseudogout, the same joints may be involved, with the exception that inflammation in the great toe is much less common. Although the patient is significantly disabled by the severe attack, the inflammation subsides over a period of several days, and the patient enjoys a symptom-free interval, which may last from a few weeks to several years. As time passes, the attacks occur more frequently and involve increasing numbers of joints. Eventually, if untreated, there is continual inflammation in multiple joints. At this stage, the patient has polyarthritis that may be symmetrical and associated with deformities. Chronic tophaceous gout may be confused with RA, with subcutaneous tophi being mistaken for rheumatoid nodules. Examination of patients in the acute stages of gout or pseudogout reveals hot, swollen joints that are quite tender and contain effusions. Striking involvement of periarticular tissues, including tendons, is usually present. Erythematous streaks may extend from joints into soft tissues, creating a clinical picture that mimics cellulitis. Fever is common in such an attack and leukocytosis is the rule. Patients in the chronic phase of these disorders usually have heat and swelling in multiple joints, often associated with deformities. In gout, tophaceous deposits are almost always present during this chronic phase and may be detected in ears, elbows, and in tendons, especially of the fingers and ankles. In pseudogout, deposits are confined to the joints and do not involve soft tissues. CPPD disease mimicking RA is associated with moderate joint inflammation; CPPD disease mimicking DJD produces only mild inflammation.

Disorders associated with gout include hypertension, cerebral and coronary arteriosclerosis, hypercholesterolemia, and diabetes mellitus. Disorders associated with pseudogout include hyperparathyroidism, diabetes mellitus, hypertension, arteriosclerosis, and hyperuricemia.

In gout x-ray changes consist of soft tissue swelling around the involved joints and punched out lesions in the surrounding bone. Chondrocalcinosis in the cartilages of involved joints is characteristic of pseudogout. However, chondrocalcinosis can occur in the absence of pseudogout as an isolated finding or in association with DJD.

Most patients with acute attacks of gout have hyperuricemia (greater than 8 mg/100 ml in males and 7 mg/100 ml in females); approximately one third of patients with pseudogout also have hyperuricemia. The only method of establishing these diagnoses with certainty is to identify crystals in synovial fluid or soft tissue deposits. Urate crystals are needle-shaped, strongly birefringent under polarized light, and negatively birefringent when studied with a red compensated polarized lens. CPPD crystals are pleomorphic, weakly birefringent under polarized light, and positively birefringent under red compensated polarized light.[23] The difference is important since therapies are different.

Therapy for gout consists of antiinflammatory drugs to treat acute attacks and the pain of chronic inflammation and drugs that lower the serum uric acid level to prevent further attacks of gout and formation of renal stones. Acute attacks of gout may be managed in one of three ways.[24] First, the physician may prescribe 0.5 mg of colchicine to be taken orally at the onset of the attack and repeated every hour until pain begins to subside. Although this method is time-honored, the dose of colchicine that produces pain relief may also produce diarrhea and abdominal cramps. A second course of oral colchicine should not be given until 3 days have passed, or severe gastrointestinal toxicity may ensue. Second, the physician may administer intravenous colchicine, administering 2 mg diluted in 20 ml of saline in the first dose and another 1 mg in 3 hours if necessary. Colchicine stimulates a more rapid response when administered intravenously. Furthermore, there are fewer gastrointestinal side effects with intravenous administration. There is a small danger of anaphylaxis and a larger danger of local tissue damage if infiltration occurs. Total dosage should not exceed 3 mg daily, and the intravenous dose should not be repeated for at least one week. Excessive doses of colchicine have been associated with sometimes fatal agranulocytosis.[25] Third, the physician may choose to treat gout with an antiinflammatory drug. Phenylbutazone (Butazolidin), 200 mg every 6 hours for the first 48 hours, and indomethacin (Indocin), 50 mg every 6 hours for the first 48 hours, are both effective in reducing the severe inflammation of acute gout. Newer NSAID have also been used, but there is less experience with those drugs. The incidence of gastrointestinal discomfort is lower with phenylbutazone, indomethacin, and other NSAID than with oral colchicine; dyspepsia and salt retention can occur with any of these drugs. When inflammation is clearly subsiding, usually after 48 hours of therapy, the dosage of phenylbutazone or indomethacin is gradually reduced and the drug discontinued after 7 to 10 days of administration. I prefer this last regimen because it provides rapid relief, usually beginning within 2 hours of the first dose, with minimal gastointestinal side effects. Since the drugs are discontinued after several days of therapy, the incidence of undesirable side effects is low. In patients with peptic ulcer disease, other upper gastrointestinal symptoms, or who may take nothing by mouth postoperative, I prefer intravenous administration of colchicine. It is useful to begin prophylactic doses of colchicine, 0.5 or 0.6 mg twice daily, shortly after phenylbutazone or indomethacin administration is begun or 3 or 4 days after administration of intravenous colchicine. Patients who do not respond to any of these regimens for an acute attack may be treated with intraarticular or systemic steroids; this is rarely necessary.

It is important to avoid manipulating serum levels of uric acid during acute gout attacks, since fluctuations of serum uric acid are associated with prolongation of current attacks and development of new ones. *After inflammation has subsided and small doses of colchicine have been administered for 2 or 3 days*, serum uric acid levels should be lowered. Drugs used for this purpose include allopurinol (Zyloprim), probenecid (Benemid), and sulfinpyrazone (Anturane).[24,26] Allopurinol decreases the synthesis of uric acid and lowers both serum and urine levels. Therefore, it is the drug of choice in patients with renal stones, hyperuricosuria (more than 700 mg per 24 hours), a glomerular filtration rate (GFR) less than 30 ml/minute, or with large tophi, since mobilization of urate will present a large load of urate to the renal tubules. This drug reduces gout attacks and prevents renal damage from elevated urinary uric acid. The initial dose of allopurinol is one 300-mg tablet daily. Serum uric acid levels should be lowered within 48 hours, the nadir occurring in 4 to 14 days (less than 7 mg/100 ml is the goal). The dose of allopurinol is then adjusted upward by 100-mg increments to as high as 600 mg or downward to 100 to 200 mg daily to determine the minimal dose necessary to maintain the uric acid level well within the normal range. Undesirable side effects of allopurinol include precipitation of acute gout attacks, allergic dermatitis (which occurs in approximately 10% of patients), bone marrow suppression, and hepatitis, the latter two being unusual. Severe vasculitis has been reported. Toxicity is more frequent in patients with renal insufficiency or when thiazides or ampicillin are given concurrently with allopurinol. Probenecid and sulfinpyrazone decrease urate resorption in the proximal tubules of the kidney and lower serum uric acid while increasing urinary uric acid. Use of these drugs is contraindicated in patients with significant renal disease (GFR less than 30 ml per minute) and in patients with a history of peptic ulcers. The initial dosage of probenecid is 0.25 gm twice daily (with high fluid intake to reduce the chance of renal stone formation), which may be increased by weekly 0.5-gm increments to as much as 3 gm daily if required to maintain a normal uric acid level. The initial dosage of sulfinpyrazone is 50 mg twice daily; this dose is increased gradually to control serum uric acid levels. The final maintenance dose averages 400 mg daily, but doses as high as 800 mg may be required. Sulfinpyrazone also reduces platelet adhesiveness, which may be desirable in some patients. Salicylates block the effects of uricosuric drugs and should not be used with them. Side effects of uricosuric agents include precipitation of acute gout attacks, formation of urate stones in the urinary tract, allergic dermatitis, gastrointestinal irritation, and peptic ulceration. In patients with tophaceous deposits that are disabling, either because of their location or their large size, combinations of allopurinol and uricosuric agents may be used to accelerate dissolution of tophi. As mentioned before, initial therapy with either allopurinol or a uricosuric drug may produce an acute attack of gout; this may often be prevented by maintaining the patient on 0.5 to 0.6 mg of colchicine administered twice daily. Colchicine may be discontinued after 6 to 12 months if serum uric acid levels are consistently normal and no acute attacks have occurred.

Patients with chronic gout have persistent inflammation in joints and need continual therapy with antiinflammatory agents in addition to colchicine, allopurinol, or uricosuric agents. Salicylates should not be used because in low to moderate doses they cause urate retention. All of the NSAID, including indomethacin, are useful in this group of patients.

The management of patients with pseudogout usually does not involve the use of drugs to lower the serum uric acid level. In general, pseudogout is more difficult to treat than gout. Some patients respond to NSAID, such as indomethacin administered in the usual doses of 25 mg three or four times daily. High-dose salicylate or low-dose corticosteroid therapy may be tried but is often not effective. Most patients with chronic pseudogout are not benefited by colchicine, but an occasional patient does obtain significant improvement; therefore a trial maintenance dose of colchicine (0.5 to 0.6 mg twice daily) may be worthwhile. During the acute attack of pseudogout, administration of intravenous colchicine, as for gout, is often effective.[27]

Psoriatic arthritis

Psoriasis is a common skin disorder that affects people in older age groups. Since DJD and RA are also common diseases afflicting geriatric patients, the coexistence of psoriasis with either of these arthropathies is not unusual. However, approximately 5% to 10% of patients with psoriasis develop an inflammatory arthritis that is distinctive and is designated *psoriatic arthritis*.

Patients with this disorder have either an insidious or explosive onset of pain, heat, and swelling that may be monarticular or polyarticular. Arthritis usually begins after psoriasis has been present for several years, but the dermatitis and arthritis may appear simultaneously, or arthritis may antedate the skin lesions by several months. Features that distinguish psoriatic arthritis from RA are as follows. First, involvement of the DIP joints of the hands and feet is common in psoriatic arthritis but unusual in RA. Second, involvement of the lumbar spine and sacroiliac joints is much more common in psoriatic arthritis than in RA. Third, exacerbations and remissions of the skin disease sometimes correlate with the flare-up of arthritis, whereas RA follows a slow progressive course unrelated to the presence of psoriatic skin lesions. Fourth, asymmetrical joint involvement is common in psoriasis and unusual in RA. Fifth, tests for rheumatoid factor are usually negative in patients with psoriatic arthritis. Sixth, the prognosis associated with psoriatic arthritis is usually better than the prognosis associated with RA. Patients with psoriasis tend to have more frequent and more complete remissions and are less likely to be crippled by their disease. However, there are exceptions, and a rapidly progressive, destructive form of arthritis mutilans can occur in patients with psoriasis. The severity of skin lesions and of arthritis are often not correlated. Most patients (80%) with psoriatic arthritis have abnormal finger and/or toe nails, with onycholysis being the most common and pitting second. The characteristics of psoriatic arthritis have been reviewed recently.[28]

Some changes that appear on x-ray films are suggestive of psoriatic arthritis. In early cases, soft tissue swelling can be seen in patients with psoriatic arthritis as in patients with RA. Periarticular demineralization of bone is less common in psoriatic arthritis than in RA. Erosions occurring in the DIP joints of hands or feet, especially if accompanied by x-ray evidence of sacroiliitis, are highly suggestive of psoriatic arthritis. Resorption of terminal phalanges can occur. In severe disease, bony ankylosis occurs.

Laboratory tests reveal a slightly elevated sedimentation rate, and many patients have mild hyperuricemia. This is sometimes confusing and leads the physician to make an incorrect diagnosis of gouty arthritis. Tests for rheumatoid factor are negative in 75% of patients; among the 25% with positive tests, many have coexisting psoriasis and RA.

Treatment of psoriatic arthritis requires the use of antiinflammatory drugs, gold, physical therapy, and surgery in selected cases. In some patients successful therapy for the skin lesions is associated with remissions in the arthritis, especially if the skin lesions are severe. In most patients, initial therapy should be directed toward care of the skin lesions. If synovitis persists, or if the dermatitis is refractory to therapy, treatment for inflammatory synovitis is necessary. High doses of salicylates are useful in mild disease. The methods of employing these agents, the various types of salicylates available, and their side effects are discussed in the section on DJD. Any of the NSAID are acceptable as initial therapy and may be substituted for aspirin in patients who cannot tolerate salicylates, since NSAID are in general less toxic than salicylates. Recommended doses of these agents and a discussion of their toxicities also appear in the section on DJD and are listed in Table 4-1. Local glucocorticoid injections are often useful in oligoarticular disease.

Gold salts for the treatment of psoriatic arthritis are effective and should be considered for patients with progressive arthritis in the face of control of the skin lesions and poor responses to NSAID or aspirin.[8] Approximately 70% of such patients respond to gold; some achieve complete remission. Toxicity rates are similar in patients with psoriatic arthritis and with RA. The use of gold is discussed in the preceding section on RA.

In patients with severe psoriatic arthritis who are in danger of being disabled, whose skin is resistant to therapy, or whose arthritis does not respond to conversative therapy nor to gold, glucocorticoids or cytotoxic drugs may be indicated. Since psoriatic arthritis often enters remission, the physician can plan to use relatively short courses of steroid therapy as opposed to the long-term therapy required for a patient with RA. Nevertheless, the decision to employ glucocorticoids in patients with psoriatic arthritis should be made cautiously, since dermatitis usually flares when the steroid dose is tapered. Most patients with psoriatic arthritis improve significantly on steroid therapy; they usually require 5 to 15 mg of prednisone daily or its equivalent. Methotrexate, a folic acid antagonist, is a cytotoxic drug that is often effective in the treatment of severe psoriatic dermatitis and/or severe psoriatic arthritis.[29] The use of this agent is hazardous because of bone marrow suppression and should be restricted to patients with disabling disease who have failed to respond to more conservative regimens. In the past, high doses have been used. Currently, the recommended dosage is 7.5 to 15 mg once weekly. The drug can be administered orally as three 2.5- or 5-mg doses given 12 hours apart[19] (since methotrexate is a cell-cycle dependent drug, the every-12-hour regimen may destroy larger number of cells, since more cells in proliferative phases will be affected), or as single 7.5 to 15 mg doses given orally or intramuscularly. Methotrexate may be administered intravenously, but veins are easily sclerosed by this agent; the oral and intramuscular routes are preferred for long-term treatment. Undesirable side effects include suppression of all the bone marrow elements (especially leukocytes), nausea, diarrhea, hair loss, oral ulcerations, and hepatic damage, which may ultimately lead to cirrhosis. Persistent markedly abnormal liver function tests, the appearance of hepatomegaly or symptoms of hepatic dysfunction are indications to discontinue therapy. Complete blood counts and platelet counts should be checked before administration of each dose. Most patients improve significantly after methotrexate therapy is instituted. However, there are usually exacerbations of both skin lesions and arthritis after the drug is discontinued, usually requiring reinstitution. Other cytotoxic drugs have been used in severe cases, including azathioprine and cyclophosphamide.

The mangement of psoriatic arthritis, as with other arthropathies, should include physical therapy to preserve joint function and to strengthen supporting muscles. Patients who develop joint destruction or have persistent synovitis in a few joints may benefit from surgical arthroplasty or joint replacement.

Septic arthritis

Infection is an important cause of arthritis in all age groups, including the elderly.[30] Patients with septicemia from any source can develop localization of microorganisms in one or more joints. Patients who already have arthritis are especially susceptible to infection in their damaged joints. There is an increased incidence of septic arthritis in patients with rheumatoid disease; patients with DJD, gout, any other arthropathy, or trauma to joints are also at risk. Prompt diagnosis and therapy are extremely important in this disorder. The most common offending organism in older age groups is staphylococcus, which causes approximately two thirds of nongonococcal infections. Pneumococcus, streptococcus, and gram-negative organisms are next in frequency. Gram-negative infections are especially frequent in debilitated patients with cancer or other diseases associated with suppressed immune responses. Mixed infections occur. Anaerobic bacteria, fungi, and various mycobacterial species are all capable of producing locally destructive and life-threatening septic arthritis.

Patients with pyogenic arthritis usually complain of considerable pain, heat, and swelling in one or more joints, which worsen rapidly over a period of a few days. Fever and chills usually accompany the onset of the arthritis. Polyarthritis occurs, but monarticular or oligoarticular involvement are more common. Physical examination reveals very tender, erythematous, hot, swollen joints, often with cellulitis in surrounding soft tissues. The picture is similar to that seen in patients with acute attacks of gout or pseudogout. Patients are usually febrile and have leukocytosis. A careful search for the source of infection should be made. Organisms most commonly disseminate from areas of pneumonia, from skin lesions such as carbuncles or traumatized areas, or from meningitis. Urinary and gastrointestinal tracts are increasingly common sources.

The most important laboratory information is obtained from study of the synovial fluid.[23,30,31] If septic arthritis is suspected, the physician should perform an arthrocentesis. Synovial fluid from septic joints is turbid or frankly purulent in appearance. The leukocyte count is quite high, usually greater than 50,000 cells per cubic millimeter. Polymorphonuclear leukocytes predominate, constituting more than 90% of the leukocytes in the effusion. The glucose content of the fluid is usually less than 50% of the glucose content of simultaneously drawn serum. Glucose levels are most helpful when synovial fluid is withdrawn while the patient fasts or at least 6 hours after the patient's last meal; this allows time for serum and synovial fluid glucose to equilibrate. Gram stains of the fluid are often positive and will provide the physician with enough information to help him select the correct antibiotic. Of course, the diagnosis of septic arthritis is proven by culturing the offending microorganisms from the synovial fluid. The majority of cultures are positive when the organism is a gram-positive coccus, gram-negative bacillus, or fungus. Mycobacteria, gonococci, and meningococci are more difficult to culture.

Antibiotic therapy should be begun immediately if septic arthritis is suspected, and altered later after cultures and drug sensitivities of the offending microorganism are available. Until the organism is identified, therapy should be directed against staphylococci and gram-negative organisms, for example, intravenous nafcillin or oxacillin and gentamicin. If nonstaphylococcal gram-positive cocci are likely causes of the infection, therapy may be begun with penicillin. If staphylococci are suspect or proven by the cultures, oxacillin, methicillin, cephalosporin, lincomycin, vancomycin, or nafcillin should be started intravenously. If gram-negative organisms are found on a smear of the synovial fluid, intravenous antibiotics such as gentamicin, cephaloridine or cephalothin should be begun. Most patients with septic arthritis show definite improvement within 4 to 7 days after institution of appropriate antibiotic therapy. Synovial fluid or serum antibiotic levels (minimal inhibitory concentrations) can be measured to determine if dose levels are adequate. Antibiotic therapy should be changed if the patient is not responding to initial therapy in the face of adequate antibiotic levels and if cultures continue to be positive. The presence of effusion in septic joints is harmful since it produces pressure on cartilage and soft tissues and interferes with antibiotic effectiveness. Therefore, septic joints should be aspirated frequently to keep them as dry as possible. If joint effusion accumulates repeatedly after several days of adequate antibiotic therapy or if the joint is relatively inaccessible, surgical drainage should be considered. Since high levels of antibiotics in synovial fluid are readily achieved in most patients with effective bactericidal blood levels, surgical intervention is not usually required.

In general, patients with staphylococcal and gram-negative arthritis have slower improvement than those with arthritis caused by other bacteria. They usually require intravenous therapy for 4 to 6 weeks.[31] In any form of septic arthritis, when significant improvement has occurred, antibiotics may be changed from parenteral to oral routes. If improvement continues or is maintained, the patient may be discharged from the hospital and maintained at home on oral antibiotics for a few weeks. X-ray films of the affected joints should be taken every few weeks to be sure that joint damage is not progressing and that osteomyelitis is not present, which would require a longer duration of antibiotic therapy and in some cases surgical debridement. Two or three weeks of infection are usually required before even the most virulent organisms produce obvious changes on the x-ray films, which consist of destruction of bone and cartilage with surrounding bony sclerosis.

The high mortality associated with some forms of septic arthritis is probably related to the failure to make a prompt diagnosis, especially in patients with other underlying arthropathies. It is extremely important for the physician to suspect this disorder whenever one or two joints in a patient with RA, gout, or DJD become especially troublesome, whenever there is an obvious source of septicemia in an elderly patient, or when severe inflammatory arthritis is present in one or two joints.

CONNECTIVE TISSUE DISORDERS

Connective tissue disorders, including systemic lupus erythematosus (SLE), dermatomyositis/polymyositis, scleroderma, polymyalgia rheumatica, and arteritic syndromes, such as polyarteritis nodosa and Wegener's granulomatosis, may occur in older age groups.

Dermatomyositis/polymyositis

Dermatomyositis/polymyositis (DM/PM) is the most common of these syndromes in the elderly. With each increasing decade of age, the incidence of malignancy associated with polymyositis increases. Some studies have reported that the majority of men over 50 with polymyositis have an associated malignancy that involves the lung, the gastrointestinal (GI) tract, the genitourinary (GU) tract, the larynx or lymphomas. The association also exists in women but is less impressive; reproductive tract and breast carcinomas are frequent, as well as those malignancies that appear in men.[32] In most series, malignancy is found in about 10% of patients with DM/PM.

Patients with polymyositis complain of weakness, especially in the proximal muscles. Those with dermatomyositis have a skin rash that is often situated over the knuckles and around the nail beds of the fingers. On physical examination, weakness is evident in the proximal muscle areas and sometimes also distally. In addition, muscle atrophy may be present, and some muscle groups may be tender. Additional features of collagen disease may be present, including Raynaud's phenomenon, polyarthritis, and interstitial lung disease.

Laboratory tests show elevation of muscle enzymes, including creatine phophokinase (CPK), lactic dehydrogenase (LDH), serum glutamic oxaloacetic transaminase (SGOT), and aldolase. One or all the enzyme levels may be abnormal. Antinuclear antibodies and rheumatoid factors may be present. Electromyography is usually abnormal. Muscle biopsy shows necrosis and muscle inflammation and confirms the diagnosis.

Patients with polymyositis without other disorders usually respond well to high dose glucocorticoid therapy; some patients respond well to alternate day steroid therapy such as 100 mg of prednisone every other day; this approach should be considered for individuals whose disease is not life-threatening. For those in greater danger, daily glucocorticoids, usually in divided doses (e.g., 30 to 50 mg of prednisone every 12 hours), should be started,[33,34] and the dosage tapered when the disease is controlled, as indicated by falling muscle enzymes and improved strength. Since glucocorticoids can induce myopathy, recurrence of weakness in the presence of normal serum levels of muscle enzymes should be managed by reducing glucocorticoids. If inflammatory myositis recurs or if steroids are ineffective (rising enzymes, tender muscles), cytotoxic drugs should be added. Methotrexate and cyclophosphamide are probably effective in DM/PM[33,34]; azathioprine is used by some authorities. Recommended doses of these agents in polymyositis are as follows:

- Methotrexate: 15 to 50 mg orally or intramuscularly every 7 to 14 days
- Cyclophosphamide: 1.5 to 2.5 mg/kg per day orally as tolerated
- Azathioprine: 2.0 to 3.0 mg/kg per day orally as tolerated

Several weeks of daily oral cytotoxic therapy are required in most cases before response is definite. More rapid improvement may be obtained by administering intravenous cyclophosphamide, 0.5 gm/m^2, with repeated doses once every 6 to 12 weeks if necessary to maintain remission. This aggressive, experimental therapy is associated with a high risk of bone marrow suppression and should be reserved for the critically ill. Undesirable side effects of methotrexate, cyclophosphamide, and azathioprine are discussed in preceding sections on RA.

In general, patients with associated connective tissue diseases or malignancies do not respond as well to glucocorticoids and are more likely to require cytotoxic agents. The prognosis for patients with polymyositis and malignancies is not good, with 50% 5-year survivals. Among patients without tumors, 5-year survivals approximate 80%. The disease is almost always chronic; therapy is required indefinitely.

Systemic lupus erythematosus (SLE)

SLE is uncommon in older age groups. However, cases do occur, especially in women. SLE is a multisystem disorder[35,36] associated with multiple autoantibodies and circulating immune complexes and manifested as any combination of photosensitive dermatitis, nondeforming polyarthritis, nephritis, pneumonitis, pleurisy, myocarditis, pericarditis, peritonitis, anemia, thrombocytopenia, leukopenia, CNS disorders, fever, and myositis. Involvement of the heart and lungs is more common in older patients than in patients in the younger age groups, but nephritis is less common.[35] Thus, the "typical" elderly patient with SLE has fatigue, arthritis/arthralgias, low grade fever, pleurisy/pericarditis, and often pulmonary infiltrates. Distinguishing the disease from an infectious process depends predominantly on laboratory tests (unless the typical skin rash is present over the face).

Laboratory abnormalities characteristic of SLE are listed in Table 4-2. ANA are positive in at least 95% of cases. However, 10% to 15% of healthy individuals over the age of 60 are ANA-positive, so the test must be interpreted with some caution in these individuals. Antibodies to native DNA, L.E. cells, and antibody to Sm-antigen are all more specific for the disease than ANA, but less sensitive.[36] SLE usually follows a course of intermittent exacerbations and remissions; sustained remissions are unusual. In most cases, SLE in the elderly is mild, but death can result from infections, renal failure, CNS involvement, or cardiopulmonary disease.

When mild and not life-threatening, SLE may be controlled by NSAID or salicylates. When dermatitis and arthritis are the major problems, some patients respond to 200 to 400 mg of hydroxychloroquine administered daily (see discussion under RA). Most patients eventually require daily glucocorticoid therapy. Indications for high dose glucocorticoid therapy of SLE are as follows*:

Table 4-2. Laboratory abnormalities in SLE

Test	*Percent positive during course of disease*
ANA by indirect immunofluorescence (includes anti-NP, anti-DNA, anti-histone, anti-RNP, anti-Sm)	95
Antibodies to native DNA	65
Hypocomplemememia (includes CH_{50}, Clq, C4, C2, C3, properdin, factor B)	80
Cryoglobulins	35
Antibodies to Sm and or RNP	67
L.E. cells	60
Antilymphocyte antibodies	70
Anticytoplasmic antibodies	25
Positive direct Coombs' tests	65
Rheumatoid factors	50
Polyclonal ↑ in gamma globulins (especially IgG)	50
Circulating anticoagulants	10
False positive VDRL	10
False positive FTA	10
Anemia	80
of chronic disease	70
hemolytic	10
Leukopenia	65
Thrombocytopenia	15
Elevated ESR	80
Renal abnormalities (↑ serum creatinine, abnormal urinalysis, ↑ 24-hour urine protein)	60

From Parker, C.W.: Clin. Immunol. **1**:615, 1980.

Life-threatening involvement

Glomerulonephritis

Organic brain syndrome, stroke, cord lesions, seizures unresponsive to anticonvulsants, focal brain damage, severe peripheral neuropathy, etc.

Hemolytic anemia (Hgb < 8.0 g/dl)

Thrombocytopenia (platelets < 50,000/cu mm)

Circulating anticoagulant with bleeding

Vasculitis—skin, retina, optic nerve, gastrointestinal tract

Pericarditis unresponsive to indomethacin or with large effusion

Myocarditis

*From Parker, C.W.: Clin. Immunol. **1**:624, 1980.

Pleurisy unresponsive to indomethacin or with symptomatic effusions
Lupus pneumonitis
Interstitial lung disease
Polymyositis
Lupus crisis

Involvement seriously compromising the quality of life

Diffuse dermatitis unresponsive to conservative therapy
Disabling polyarthritis, with or without deformity, unresponsive to conservative therapy
Extreme fatigue, malaise, anorexia, nausea

Management

a. Daily steroids: 60 to 100 mg prednisone (or equivalent) initially, until improved and stable, then taper over several weeks to maintenance dose, usually 15 to 25 mg daily.

   Higher initial doses (300 mg daily) may be needed for severe CNS involvement.

b. High dose "pulse" therapy: 1 to 2 grams of Solu-Medrol (or equivalent) intravenously each day for 3 to 6 days, then 100 mg prednisone daily; taper over several weeks to maintenance dose. For patients with rapidly deteriorating renal or CNS function.

c. Alternate day steroids: Offers advantage of decreased steroid toxicity. Usually not effective in severe, active disease. Occasionally effective after disease is controlled by daily steroids. Taper slowly down on one day, raising on alternate day (to move, for example, from 20 mg daily to 40 mg every other day), then taper the alternate-day dose to maintenance levels.

A major cause of SLE-like disease in the elderly is administration of lupus inducing drugs. Procainamide is the most common offender; hydralazine follows second. Some authorities list isoniazid, chlorpromazine, and hydantoins as lupus inducers. If the syndrome is mild (low grade fever, arthralgias, nondisabling serositis), withdrawing the drug is adequate therapy. If more severe, a short course of glucocorticoids is usually effective.[36]

Three therapeutic approaches are available for the minority of patients with life-threatening disease who do not respond to conventional high dose glucocorticoid therapy (60 to 100 mg of prednisone daily in divided doses). All these approaches should be considered experimental, since adequate controlled trials in large numbers of patients are not yet available. The three therapies are as follows: (1) a massive dose of intravenous glucocorticoids; (2) administration of cytotoxic drugs, and (3) plasmapheresis. Methylprednisolone sodium succinate (Solu-Medrol), 1000 mg administered intravenously daily for 3 to 5 days, followed by 100 mg prednisone administered orally daily, have been used in the treatment of severe lupus nephritis and life-threatening CNS disease.[37] It is postulated that response may be more frequent and faster than with conventional steroid doses, and low maintenance doses of prednisone (or its equivalent) may be attained more rapidly. We await results of controlled studies to confirm these opinions. Conflicting results have been reported regarding efficacy of cytotoxic drugs in SLE.[18,38] Some investigators have reported better survival and steroid-sparing effects in patients with SLE receiving azathioprine or cyclophosphamide; others have reported no benefit. This author feels that alkylating agents (chlorambucil or cyclophosphamide) are useful in patients with life-threatening diseases that are not responsive to steroids or in those patients with unacceptable steroid side effects. Recommended doses of cytotoxics are azathioprine 2 to 3 mg/kg per day, chlorambucil 0.1 mg/kg per day, and cyclophosphamide 1.5 to 2.5 mg/kg per day. (See discussions in RA section for side effects of these drugs.) There has been recent interest in using low doses of both azathioprine and cyclophosphamide together on a daily basis for control of lupus nephritis, or pulse therapy with a single dose of intravenous cyclophosphamide, 0.5 to 1 gm/m^2 administered once every 3 months, but these approaches are highly experimental.[38] Plasmapheresis[21] involves removing 2 to 3 liters of a patient's blood through a surgically placed arteriovenous shunt, returning the patient's cells but replacing his plasma with normal human plasma or plasma substitutes. This procedure is repeated three times a week for 3 weeks. Its purpose is to remove circulating immune complexes and undesirable autoantibodies; its complications are bleeding, clotting, and infections associated with arteriovenous shunts, hepatitis from foreign plasma, and an increased "rebound" synthesis or increased release of undesirable antibodies. Some investigators feel it is necessary to initiate cyclophosphamide therapy, with all of its hazards, during the last week of pheresis to prevent the rebound phenomenon. Plasmapheresis has been used in SLE with reported success,[21] but controlled trials of this expensive and cumbersome technique are needed before it can be recommended. At present, this therapy should be reserved for patients who are succumbing to SLE (or severe immune complex or antibody-mediated disorders of other types such as vasculitis, myasthenia gravis, etc.) in spite of more conventional aggressive therapies.

Scleroderma

Scleroderma is a systemic disease consisting of Raynaud's phenomenon and tightness and thickening of skin. Atrophy of gastrointestinal smooth muscle may occur with aperistalsis of the esophagus and resultant esophagitis, alternating constipation and diarrhea, and malabsorption. Interstitial pulmonary fibrosis as well as pulmonary hypertension may pose serious threats to life. Polymyositis and polyarthritis are frequent manifestations. A small number of patients develop severe hypertension and fatal renal failure. Patchy fibrosis of the myocardium is a frequent problem in scleroderma and may be associated with arrhythmias or heart failure.

Currently there is no therapy that is of proven benefit in this disorder. Therapy consists primarily of attempts to relieve symptoms and to improve function of the affected organs. Raynaud's phenomenon may be improved by vasodilating agents such as phenoxybenzamine, methyldopa, or prazosin hydrochloride (Minipress), but all such drugs produce postural hypotension and therefore must be used with extreme caution in the elderly. Polymyositis usually responds well to glucocorticoid therapy; polyarthritis responds to NSAID or low doses of prednisone; malabsorption with diarrhea may respond to broad spectrum antibiotics. Rigorous control of hypertension is absolutely essential and may be associated with improved survival.[39] Cytotoxic drugs and colchicine have each been used to treat scleroderma; there is little evidence that they influence systemic manifestations. A recent investigation in which D-penicillamine (750 mg daily) was administered to patients with early scleroderma suggested that progression to major organ involvement was reduced after a few years.[47] There is also recent evidence that treatment with captopril, an oral angiotensin-converting-enzyme blocker, preserves or improves renal function in some patients with renal scleroderma and/or severe hypertension.[48] A recent review of the clinical manifestations, pathogenesis, and treatment of scleroderma is available.[40]

Vasculitis

Syndromes in which necrotizing vasculitis occur, such as allergic vasculitis, polyarteritis nodosa (PAN), and Wegener's granulomatosis, appear in geriatric age groups. Two excellent reviews of vasculitis have been published recently.[41,42] The prognosis of these disorders varies; allergic leukocytoclastic vasculitis usually remits spontaneously; PAN is often fatal in spite of aggressive therapy.

Allergic or leukocytoclastic angiitis occurs in response to infections, drugs, or unknown antigens and is manifested by purpuric skin lesions, fever, and myalgias/arthralgias. Other major organ involvement can occur but is unusual. Features of PAN include vasculitic skin lesions (which often ulcerate), ischemia and gangrene of the digits, peripheral neuropathy, arthralgias, myalgias, gastrointestinal bleeding and infarction, hypertension, glomerulonephritis, cerebral vascular accidents, and myocardial infarction. Wegener's granulomatosis is a syndrome of necrotizing granulomas and vasculitis involving upper airways (sinuses, ears), lungs, and kidneys. Giant cell arteritis produces necrosis of large (including the aorta) and medium-size arteries, with a predilection for cranial and cerebral arteries. PAN and giant cell arteritis are usually serious and require treatment with high doses of glucocorticoids. Survival in Wegener's granulomatosis is greatly improved if cytotoxic agents with or without glucocorticoids are initiated at the time of diagnosis.[43] This author agrees with others[41,42] that patients with life-threatening PAN should receive both glucocorticoids and cyclophosphamide. As discussed below, patients with giant cell arteritis usually respond well to steroids alone.

Classification of Vasculitis in Elderly

- Leukocytoclastic (hypersensitivity) vasculitis
- Leukocytoclastic vasculitis associated with other systemic disease
  - Infection (such as hepatitis, subacute bacterial endocarditis [SBE]
  - Henoch-Schonlein purpura

- Connective tissue disease
  - SLE
  - RA
  - Sjögren's syndrome
  - Other
- Mixed cryoglobulinemia
- Intestinal bypass
- Serum sickness

Polyarteritis nodosa (includes allergic granulomatosis of lungs)
Wegener's granulomatosis
Giant cell arteritis
- Polymyalgia rheumatica
- Temporal arteritis
- Takayasu's arteritis

Other

Polymyalgia rheumatica and temporal arteritis

Polymyalgia rheumatica (PMR) is a disorder that characteristically affects patients who are over 55 years of age. It is more common in women than in men. Patients complain of severe pain in the neck, shoulder girdle, hip girdle, upper arms, and thighs. This is usually associated with considerable stiffness. The onset may be insidious or quite abrupt. This syndrome is associated with considerable fatigability and may be accompanied by weight loss and low grade fever, as well as mild anemia. Physical examination is usually normal with the exception that patients are reluctant to undergo muscle strength testing in the girdle areas. Muscle tenderness is not impressive, and muscle atrophy is usually not present. Most laboratory tests are normal, except for the erythrocyte sedimentation rate, which is quite high (in the range of 50 to 120 mm per hour [Westergren method]).

Some authorities believe that PMR is always a manifestation of systemic arteritis. In some studies, as many as 40% of patients with PMR have associated giant cell arteritis, usually involving the temporal arteries. This subgroup of patients may complain of temporal headaches, transient visual loss in one or both eyes, claudication of the jaw, or pain in the tongue when chewing. However, some patients with biopsy-proven temporal arteritis have no complaints that suggest the presence of PMR. Temporal arteritis is a serious disease since sudden loss of vision can occur. It responds dramatically to high dose glucocorticoids. PMR and giant cell arteritis have been reviewed by Ettlinger et al.[44]

There is controversy regarding both the treatment of PMR and the need to perform temporal artery biopsies in patients without symptoms of cranial arteritis. Some authorities recommend that all patients with diagnosed PMR have a temporal artery biopsy; others do not. Since the temporal arteries may be used in bypass procedures for cerebral arterial insufficiency, some thought is necessary before removing a portion of this vessel in asymptomatic patients, especially on the side of the dominant cerebral hemisphere. I recommend that all patients with PMR with any symptom suggestive of cranial arteritis have a temporal artery biopsy. In patients without such symptoms, the advisability of biopsy is an individual decision.

There is little consensus regarding therapy for PMR. If there are any symptoms of giant cell cranial arteritis, therapy with 60 to 100 mg of prednisone or an equivalent administered daily should be instituted immediately, even if temporal artery biopsy is negative, since areas of arteritis are patchy and can be missed. If there are no such symptoms (especially if the biopsy is negative), the patient may be placed on 10 to 20 mg of prednisone daily or even on NSAID. This author has had little success with NSAID in PMR, but some authorities regard them as the initial treatment of choice. Steroid therapy should be tapered when symptoms resolve and the sedimentation rate returns to normal, both of which usually occur within a week or two. For some patients, glucocorticoids can be tapered and discontinued over a period of 1 to 3 years without recurrence. In others, the PMR and/or arteritis symptoms return, and the sedimentation rate rises whenever steroids are reduced below a critical maintenance level. For those patients long-term therapy is required.

EXTRAARTICULAR RHEUMATISM

Fibrositis syndrome

Fibrositis or "the stiff-man syndrome" is common in the elderly. Patients complain of deep aching and marked stiffness, which they locate vaguely in areas around joints. There is usually aching in muscles and tendons and areas of marked local tenderness, referred to as "trigger points." This syndrome is usually mildly to moderately disabling and is often associated with increased fatigability. Laboratory data are completely normal, including the sedimentation rate. Psychogenic factors may be prominent, or the physician may be convinced that organic disease is present.

There is a recent study[45] suggesting that patients with fibrositis are deprived of deep (non REM) sleep. Normal individuals experimentally deprived of non-REM sleep developed the syndrome; patients improved when non-REM sleep was restored by phenothiazines. These observations require confirmation; this author has had some success with the use of mild sedatives that induce REM sleep, such as flurazepam hydrochloride (Dalmane).

Treatment of fibrositis syndrome can be tried with lidocaine (Xylocaine) and/or corticosteroid injections of the trigger points, salicylates, or other NSAID, all of which are discussed in earlier sections of this chapter. Sometimes patients who do not respond to these fairly conservative measures show dramatic improvement after administration of low doses of corticosteroids, such as 10 mg of prednisone daily. Significant crippling does not occur with fibrositis syndrome, and remissions after 1 to 2 years of discomfort are the rule. Therefore, patients may be treated with low doses of corticosteroids with relative safety, since the physician can plan to discontinue the drug after several months. Less potent antiinflammatory and sleeping agents are preferable if effective.

Carpal tunnel syndrome

Compression of the median nerve in the carpal tunnel of the wrist causes pain in the wrist and hand that may be misinterpreted as arthritis. This syndrome is usually idiopathic and may occur unilaterally or bilaterally. However, several diseases may be associated with carpal tunnel syndrome. These include any type of synovitis occurring in the wrist (especially RA), diabetes mellitus, amyloidosis, hypothyroidism, Raynaud's disease, and acromegaly. In addition, some patients have had trauma to the region of the carpal tunnel or have been engaged in occupations that require forced flexion of the wrist and fingers. Patients usually complain of pain in the thumb, forefinger, and middle finger associated with paresthesias. Pain may also occur at the wrist and radiate upward into the elbow or shoulder. Typically, pain is worse at night and wakens the patient. Atrophy of the abductor muscle of the thumb and of the thenar eminence may occur with weakness of thumb abduction and thumb-to-finger opposition. Physical examination reveals decreased sensation in the thumb, forefinger, middle finger, and medial side of the ring finger associated with atrophy of thumb abductors and of the thenar eminence. A sharp tap over the carpal tunnel reproduces the paresthesias (Tinel's sign); pain is reproduced by pressing the hands together with the wrists flexed (Phalen's sign). The diagnosis may be confirmed by nerve conduction studies. Treatment of the idiopathic disease consists of surgical release of the median nerve, which is achieved by dividing the rigid transverse carpal ligament overlying the carpal tunnel. In patients with synovitis, injections of small amounts of glucocorticoids (e.g., 5 mg of triamcinalone hexacetonide) into the carpal tunnel may provide temporary relief. Some patients respond to resting the carpus in a wrist splint.

If control of synovitis can be achieved with various antirheumatic drugs, the carpal tunnel syndrome may not recur. If the syndrome persists after steroid injections and antirheumatic drug therapy, surgery should be performed. However, when the syndrome is idiopathic or results from trauma or amyloidosis, surgery is indicated.

Bursitis and tendonitis

Pain in one or both shoulders is a common problem. The great majority of patients with this complaint have bursitis or tendonitis involving the shoulder. Actual synovitis of the joint is much less common than bursitis and tendonitis. Diseases of the cervical spine, especially DJD, with nerve root impingement are also common causes of pain referred to the shoulder. The shoulder-hand syndrome (reflex sympathetic dystrophy) is another important cause of shoulder pain in the elderly but is far less common than bursitis, tendonitis, synovitis, or cervical spine disease. Since DJD and synovitis have been discussed earlier in this chapter, the discussion of painful shoulder syndromes will be confined to bursitis and tendonitis and the shoulder-hand syndrome.

Bursitis and tendonitis of the shoulder. The shoulder joint contains several structures that can become inflamed or torn and result in

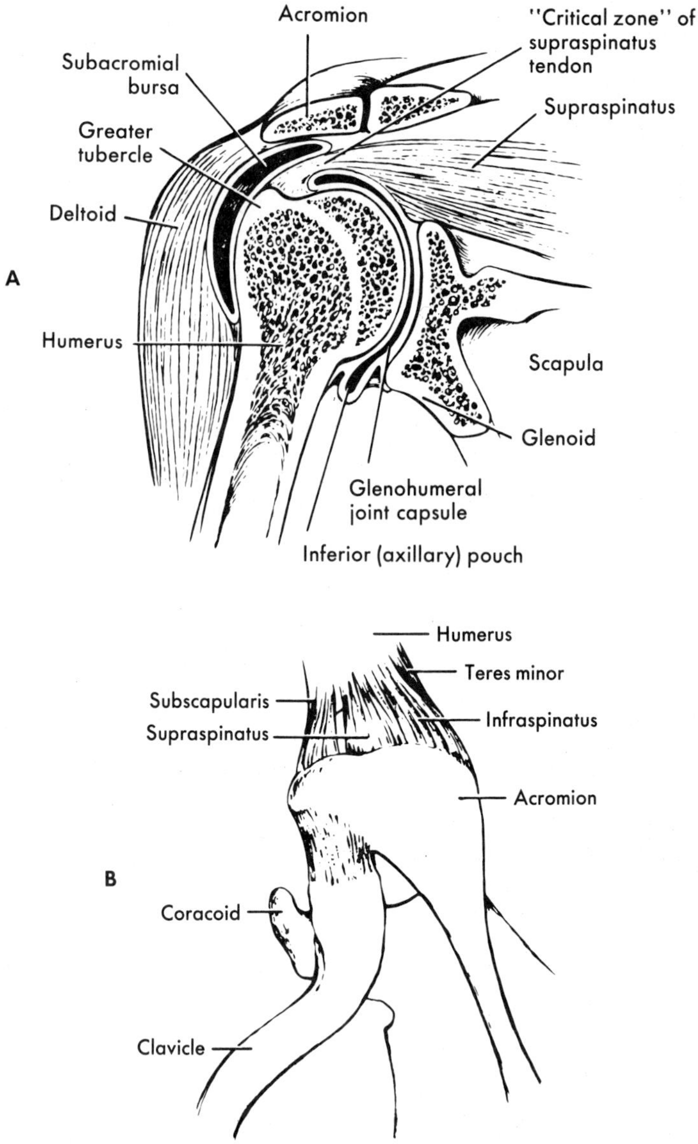

Fig. 4-1. A, Coronal section of the shoulder, illustrating relationships of glenohumeral joint, capsule, subacromial bursa, and rotator cuff (supraspinatus tendon). **B,** rotator (musculotendinous) cuff viewed from above.

pain and loss of motion (Fig. 4-1). The innermost structure subject to such changes is the joint capsule that lines the humero-glenoid joint. This structure is involved in many forms of synovitis. Inflammation beginning in the synovium can involve contiguous tissues, resulting in effusion and heat causing a swollen, tender, painful, anterior bulge below the acromion process. RA is the most common form of synovitis associated with this abnormality.

Immediately above the synovial lining of the shoulder is the musculotendinous cuff, which consists of the tendons of the rotator muscles joined in a connective tissue layer. Tears in the musculotendinous cuff are not uncommon; inflammation of this area with or without tears can also occur. Any abnormality of the musculotendinous cuff results in a frozen shoulder (i.e., restricted range of motion in the shoulder with extreme discomfort when motion exceeds a few degrees in any direction). Trauma is the most common cause of rotator cuff disease.

Above the musculotendinous cuff lies the supraspinatus muscle tendon, which is readily injured. Above the supraspinatus tendon lies the subacromial bursa. Inflammation of the supraspinatus tendon, usually associated with subacromial bursitis, is the most common cause of shoulder pain in adults.

Another important cause of shoulder pain is bicipital tendonitis, a disorder that is also usually related to trauma.

Clinically, all of these disorders have certain similarities, but there are features that permit the physician to distinguish between them. Pain in the shoulder occurs in all these disorders and is exacerbated by motion and relieved by rest. Shoulder motion is restricted, largely because of pain. In just a few days, inability to move the shoulder through a full range of motion results and may be permanent unless corrective exercises are begun promptly. In supraspinatus tendonitis and subacromial bursitis, pain is usually worse during abduction of the arm, when the inflamed structures are trapped under the acromion. There is usually point tenderness along the supraspinatus tendon and below the acromion. X-ray films may show calcification along the course of the tendon; however, a normal x-ray film is not unusual. In bicipital tendonitis, there is direct tenderness along the course of the biceps tendon and any motion that stretches that tendon is painful. Yergason's maneuver should be performed; the physician holds the patient's elbow close to the trunk, then has him supinate his hand against resistance. This puts considerable stretch on the bicipital tendon and causes pain along its course. Any disease of the rotator cuff is associated with significant reduction of range of motion of the shoulder and generalized tenderness around the shoulder joint. Synovitis of the shoulder joint itself is also associated with significant reduction of movement in all directions, and effusion may be palpable in the subacromial area.

Numerous therapies have been suggested for the management of these shoulder disorders. It is generally agreed that the patient should avoid mechanical stress on the shoulder but should exercise the involved shoulder regularly, beginning as soon as exercise can be tolerated. Exercises are designed to maintain or to increase the range of motion of the shoulder. The two exercises I most frequently recommend are wall-walking and arm-swinging. The first exercise is performed with the patient standing with his affected side at arm's length from the wall. He places his hand on the wall and walks his fingers upward, moving the trunk in toward the wall as he does so until he reaches the full extent of arm elevation that he can achieve. The second exercise is performed with the trunk flexed forward and the arm hanging down. The patient begins to swing the arm in an ever-increasing arc until the full range of motion is achieved. These exercises should be performed three times a day for approximately 10 minutes. They are better tolerated if either heat or cold is applied first, depending on the patient's preference. In general, injections of a combination of hydrocortisone and lidocaine into the affected areas are useful. Many patients obtain prompt significant improvement. In some, the improvement is short-lived; in others no further treatment is required. Sometimes a series of two to three injections given over a period of a few weeks are required to relieve pain and improve motion. In some patients no improvement results from this procedure, and in a few patients the pain is actually exacerbated. Corticosteroids administered in this fashion have few systemic side effects. Infection occurs in approximately 1 out of 16,000 joint injections.[4] Occasionally, atrophy of subcutaneous tissues along the injection site occurs. Hydrocortisone sodium succinate (Solu-Cortef) and 0.5 to 1 cc of 1% lidocaine can be injected into soft tissues along the course of the supraspinatus tendon, as well as into the area below the acromion process. The same dose of steroid and lidocaine can be injected into tender areas along the course of the bicipital tendon. For inflammation involving the joint space and synovium, 10 to 20 mg of triamcinolone hexacetonide (Arthrospan) and lidocaine should be injected directly into the shoulder joint. Care should be taken to keep injections sterile, especially if the joint cavity is entered. The reader is referred to Hollander[4] for details of methods and steroid preparations for joint and soft tissue injections. For patients who fail to respond to these injections, systemic antiinflammatory therapy may be prescribed with any of the NSAID, including salicylates. Use of these agents is discussed earlier in the chapter. Analgesics may be required in addition to antiinflammatory drugs, especially if the pain is acute and severe. If the rotator cuff is involved and does not respond to these measures, it is likely that there is a tear in the cuff; this is also true of the bicipital tendon. Such tears can be identified by arthrography. On occasion these tears can be repaired by surgery. Manipulation of the shoulder under anesthesia may be useful for improving range of motion in frozen shoulders that have not responded to more conservative therapies.

Bursitis and tendonitis of the shoulder has a variable course. Symptoms may resolve spontaneously, respond to therapy, or persist. Recurrences are common; patients with a history of bursitis should avoid twisting and lifting motions of the shoulder as much as possible. Likewise, bicipital tendonitis may occur once or recur at variable intervals. Shoulder synovitis is usually associated with synovitis in other joints and responds to therapy for generalized arthropathy. Rotator cuff lesions tend to be more disabling and chronic than other shoulder lesions. If a tear is present in the cuff, the patient tends to have chronic shoulder pain and loss of motion.

Bursitis and tendonitis of the elbow. Three conditions cause most painful elbow syndromes. First, the elbow may be involved in any type of synovitis. For example, gout attacks are not uncommon in the elbow joint or in the olecranon bursa. RA frequently involves this area. Traumatic arthritis can occur in the elbow. Pseudogout, psoriatic arthritis, and septic arthritis can also involve this joint.

More commonly, however, pain in the elbow is caused by epicondylitis or olecranon bursitis. Epicondylitis, or "tennis elbow," is usually seen in middle-aged or older individuals and is more common in men than in women. Inflammation occurs at the lateral epicondyle of the elbow joint, at the origin of the tendons of the extensor muscles of the wrist and fingers. Any activity that involves forceful pronation and supination of the hand or forceful extension of the wrist can produce tennis elbow. Pain may radiate upward from the elbow toward the shoulder and down into the dorsum of the hand or may be localized to the elbow. It is aggravated by any motion that stretches the extensor tendons. On physical examination there is point tenderness near the lateral epicondyle. There are no signs of inflammation, but forcing the patient to extend the wrist against pressure produces pain. This condition is treated by resting the area, avoiding activities that cause pain, and wearing an elbow guard pulled tight across the area (these are available at sporting goods stores). If resting the area for 2 weeks does not result in improvement, local injections of 25 to 50 mg of hydrocortisone may be tried, usually combined with a small amount of lidocaine. Two or three injections may be required for control of pain. Some patients do not respond to this form of therapy but improve during administration of NSAID such as naproxen, 250 to 375 mg twice daily, or indomethacin, 25 to 50 mg three to four times daily. It is important for the patient to avoid activities that put mechanical stress on the wrist and finger extensors until pain has been absent for several weeks. The patient may then cautiously resume such activities but runs a definite risk of reactivating the epicondylitis.

Olecranon bursitis appears as a boggy swelling along the tip of the ulna. Low grade inflammation is present. If an attack of gout, pseudogout, or infection involves the bursa, there is pain at rest as well as impressive signs of inflammation. Fluid should be removed from a swollen olecranon bursa and analyzed for crystals and infectious agents. Usually olecranon bursitis follows trauma and does not reflect a systemic arthropathy. In traumatic olecranon bursitis, draining the bursa and protecting it from further trauma are useful therapeutic maneuvers. Local steroid injections are occasionally helpful, and surgical excision is curative.

Other forms of bursitis. In the preceding paragraphs bursitis and tendonitis involving shoulders and elbows have been discussed. These conditions also constitute important causes of pain in the lower extremities.

Ischial bursitis occurs where the gluteus maximus crosses the ischial tuberosity. Patients complain of pain on sitting and have direct tenderness over the ischial tuberosity. There may be a history of trauma, such as a fall onto the buttocks or prolonged sitting on a hard surface. It is essential to rule out disorders involving the bones of the pelvis in patients with this complaint. Pelvic x-ray films should be taken. The disorders easily confused with ischial bursitis are Paget's disease and tumor replacement of bone.

If these conditions are ruled out and tenderness over the ischial tuberosities is persistent, injection of hydrocortisone and lidocaine into the affected area may provide significant relief of pain. Systemic NSAID may be tried if steroid injections do not provide relief.

Trochanteric bursitis is a fairly common cause of hip pain. There are several bursae in the region of the gluteal insertion on the greater trochanter of the femur. Any or all of these may become inflamed; a history of trauma is obtained in only a minority of cases. It is important to distinguish this disorder from intrinsic hip disease, since it is much less serious and is usually lessened by local therapy. Patients with trochanteric bursitis will complain of aching pain in the lateral portion of the hip, which is aggravated by motions that stretch the gluteal tendon, (such as climbing stairs), and rolling over on the affected side. The most important physical finding is the presence of point tenderness along the greater trochanter. Internal rotation of the hips as well as flexion and extension are all painless, suggesting that intrinsic hip disease is not present. External rotation of the hip stretches the gluteal muscles, as does abduction against resistance; therefore these motions produce pain in the area of the greater trochanter. Trochanteric bursitis is occasionally associated with calcification, visible on x-ray films. It usually responds to local steroid injections, but systemic antiinflammatory therapy with NSAID may be required. Some cases are refractory to therapy. It is important to reassure the patient that the disorder will not be associated with severe disability.

Prepatellar bursitis can cause knee pain and is readily distinguished from synovitis of the knee. In this disorder, swelling and effusion occur in front of or below the patella or around the patellar tendon. This bursitis may be produced by frequent kneeling. Effusions resulting from synovitis of the knee occur behind the patella and are readily distinguished from prepatellar bursitis. If the disorder is not troublesome, no treatment is required other than avoiding trauma to the prepatellar area. If there is tenderness in the area, fluid should be removed and cultured. If infection is not present, local steroid injection may be beneficial. Prepatellar bursitis is usually not a significantly disabling disorder.

There are several areas in the feet in which bursitis can develop and which cause discomfort on walking. Bursitis can occur in the region of the Achilles tendon, which becomes tender and slightly swollen. The patient must be fitted with appropriate shoes that do not rub this area. Calcaneal bursitis occurs where the plantar fascia attaches to the os calcis. The patient experiences pain on the bottom of the heel whenever he takes a step. Calcification or ossification may occur along the tendon insertions and can be seen on x-ray films as a calcaneal spur. Such spurs may be asymptomatic. This disorder is difficult to treat because walking produces continued trauma. Tender areas should be padded to protect them from the pressure of walking; heel inserts that will protect the calcaneus are available at orthotic shops. Steroid injections are occasionally helpful but usually of only transient benefit. If a bony spur has formed and pain continues, surgical excision of the spur should be considered.

Bunions are common abnormalities that occur in middle-aged and older individuals. The great toe is abducted, resulting in prominence of the first MTP joint. This joint is then irritated by shoes and weight bearing, with resultant bony enlargement of the medial aspects of the first MTP head. A bursa forms over this enlargement and becomes red, inflamed, and tender. If the condition is not severe, a patient may obtain relief of pain by padding the bunion and wearing shoes with soft, wide, anterior portions, arch supports, or metatarsal bars. If proper shoes do not provide significant relief, surgical procedures should be considered to correct the deformities. In my experience, results of such procedures have been good.

Shoulder-hand syndrome

This syndrome, also known as *Sudeck's atrophy* or *reflex sympathetic dystrophy*, consists of a rather abrupt onset of pain in one or both shoulders and/or hands. In addition, the hands become diffusely swollen and sweaty. Frequently, there are precipitating events such as physical or emotional trauma, stroke, or myocardial infarction, but many cases are idiopathic. X-ray films may be normal or show diffuse osteopenia of involved areas. Mobility of shoulders and fingers is rapidly lost, and the syndrome should be treated promptly. I usually begin patients on analgesics and NSAID as well as aggressive physical therapy; some authorities recommend 2 to 3 weeks of high dose prednisone followed by a slow tapering of the drug and aggressive physical therapy.[46] Most cases improve over a period of 2 months to 2 years. The goal of therapy is to prevent loss of motion during the period of active disease.

REFERENCES

1. Silvoso, G.R., et al.: Incidence of gastric lesions in patients with rheumatic disease on chronic aspirin therapy, Ann. Intern. Med. **91**:517, 1979.
2. Huskisson, E.C.: Anti-inflammatory drugs, Semin. Arthritis Rheum. **7**:1, 1977.
3. Dick, W.C., and DeCeulaer, K.: Nonsteroidal antirheumatic drugs. In Kelly, W.N., Harris, E.D., Ruddy, S., and Sledge, C.B., editors: Textbook of rheumatology, Philadelphia, 1981, W.B. Saunders Co., pp. 768-784.
4. Hollander, J.L.: Arthrocentesis and intrasynovial therapy. In McCarty, D., editor: Arthritis and allied conditions, Philadelphia, 1979, Lea & Febiger, pp. 402-414.
5. Johnson, J.S., Vaughan, J.H., and Hench, P.K.: Rheumatoid arthritis, Ann. Intern. Med. **78**:937, 1973.
6. Goldman, J.A., et al.: Limited plasmapheresis in rheumatoid arthritis with vasculitis, Arthritis Rheum. **22**: 1146, 1979.
7. Research Subcommittee of the Empire Rheumatism Council: A controlled trial of gold in rheumatoid arthritis, Ann. Rheum. Dis. **19**:95, 1960; **20**:315, 1961.
8. Dorwart, B.B., Gall, E.P., Schumacher, H.R., and Krauser, R.E.: Chrysotherapy in psoriatic arthritis. Efficacy and toxicity compared to rheumatoid arthritis, Arthritis Rheum. **21**:513-515, 1978.
9. Mackenzie, A.H.: An appraisal of chloroquine, Arthritis Rheum. **13**:280, 1970.
10. Lipsky, P., and Ziff, M.: The effect of D-penicillamine on mitogen-induced human lymphocyte proliferation, J. Immunol. **120**:1006, 1978.
11. Jaffe, J.A.: Penicillamine treatment of rheumatoid arthritis: effect on immune complexes, Ann. N.Y. Acad. Sci. **256**:330, 1975.
12, Jaffe, J.A.: D-penicillamine, Bull. Rheum. Dis. **28**:948, 1978.
13. Hahn, T.J., Halstead, L.R., Teitelbaum, S.L., and Hahn, B.H.: Altered mineral metabolism in glucocorticoid-induced osteopenia: effect of 25-hydroxyvitamin D administration, J. Clin. Invest. **64**:655-665, 1979.
14. Fauci, A.S., Dale, D.C., and Balow, J.E.: Glucocorticoid therapy: mechanisms of action and clinical considerations, Ann. Intern. Med. **84**:304, 1976.
15. Axelrod, L.: Glucocorticoid therapy, Medicine **55**:39, 1976.
16. Urowitz, M.B., et al: Azathioprine in rheumatoid arthritis. A double-blind, crossover study, Arthritis Rheum. **16**:411, 1973.
17. Cooperating Clinics of the American Rheumatism Association: Cyclophosphamide therapy of rheumatoid arthritis, N. Engl. J. Med. **283**:883, 1970.
18. Steinberg, A.D., Plotz, P.H., and Wolf, S.M.: Cytotoxic drugs in the treatment of non-malignant diseases, Ann. Intern. Med. **76**:619, 1972.
19. Willkens, R.F., Watson, M.A., and Paxson, C.S.: Low dose pulse methotrexate therapy in RA, J. Rheumatol. **7**:501, 1980.
20. Jaffe, J.A., and Smith, R.W.: Rheumatoid vasculitis—report of a second case treated with penicillamine, Arthritis Rheum. **11**:585, 1968.
21. Verrier Jones, J., et al.: Plasmapheresis in the management of systemic lupus erythematosus, Lancet **1**:709, 1976.
22. McCarty, D.J.: Calcium pyrophosphate dihydrate deposition disease, Arthritis Rheum. **19**:275, 1976.
23. McCarty, D.J.: Synovial fluid. In McCarty, D.J., editor: Arthritis and allied conditions, Philadelphia, 1979, Lea & Febiger, Chapter 5, pp. 51-69.
24. Kelly, W.N.: Gout and related disorders and purine metabolism. In Kelly, W., Harris, E., Ruddy, S., and Slege, C., editors: Textbook of rheumatology, Philadelphia, 1981, W.B. Saunders Co.
25. Carr, A.A.: Colchicine toxicity, Arch. Intern. Med. **115**:29, 1965.
26. Kelley, W.N.: Antihyperuricemic drugs. In Kelley, W., Harris, E., Ruddy, S., and Sledge, C., editors: Textbook of rheumatology, Philadelphia, 1981, W.B. Saunders Co.
27. Spilberg, I., McLain, D., Simchowitz, L., and Berney, S.: Colchicine and pseudogout, Arthritis Rheum. **23**:1062-1063, 1980.
28. Wright, V., and Moll, J.M.H.: Seronegative Polyarthritis, Amsterdam, 1976, Elsevier/North Holland, Biomedical Press.
29. Black, R.L., et al.: Methotrexate therapy in psoriatic arthritis, J.A.M.A. **189**:743, 1964.
30. Goldberg, D.L., and Cohen, A.S.: Acute infectious arthritis. A review of patients with non-gonococcal joint infections (with emphasis on therapy and prognosis), Am. J. Med. **60**:369, 1976.
31. Myers, A.R.: Septic arthritis caused by bacteria. In Kelley, W., Harris, E., Ruddy, S., and Sledge, C., editors: Textbook of rheumatology, Philadelphia, 1981, W.B. Saunders Co., Chapter 96, pp. 1551-1572.
32. Barnes, B.E.: Dermatomyositis and malignancy, Ann. Intern. Med. **84**:68, 1976.
33. De Vere, R., and Bradley, W.G.: Polymyositis: its presentation, morbidity and mortality, Brain **98**:637, 1975.
34. Bohan, A., Peter, J.B., Bowman, B.S., and Pearson, C.M.: A computer-assisted analysis of 153 patients with polymyositis and dermatomyositis, Medicine **56**:255, 1977.
35. Foad, B.S.I., Sheon, R.P., and Kirsner, A.B.: Systemic lupus erythematosus in the elderly, Arch. Intern. Med. **130**:743, 1972.
36. Hahn, B.H.: Systemic lupus erythematosus. In Parker, C.W., editor: Clinical immunology, Philadelphia, 1980, W.B. Saunders Co., Chapter 19, pp. 583-631.
37. Cathcart, E.S., Scheinberg, M.A., Idelson, B.A., and Couser, W.G.: Beneficial effects of methylprednisolone "pulse" therapy in diffuse proliferative lupus nephritis, Lancet **1**:163, 1976.
38. Decker, J.L., et al.: Systemic lupus erythematosus: evolving concepts, Ann. Inter. Med. **91**:587, 1979.

39. Wasner, C., Cooke, R.C., and Fries, J.F.: Successful medical treatment of scleroderma renal crisis, N. Engl. J. Med. **229:**873, 1978.
40. Rodnan, G.: Progressive systemic sclerosis (scleroderma). In Parker, C.P., editor: Clinical immunology, Philadelphia, 1980, W.B. Saunders Co., Chapter 26, pp. 784-814.
41. Fauci, A.S., Haynes, B.F., and Katz, P.: The spectrum of vasculitis: clinical, pathologic, immunologic and therapeutic considerations, Ann. Intern. Med. **89:**660, 1978.
42. Fan, P.T., et al.: A clinical approach to systemic vasculitis, Seminars in Arthritis Rheum. **9:**248, 1980.
43. Raitt, J.W.: Wegener's granulomatosis, treatment with cytotoxic agents and adrenocorticosteroids, Ann. Intern. Med. **74:**344, 1971.
44. Ettlinger, R.E., Hunder, G.G., and Ward, L.M.: Polymyalgia rheumatica and giant cell arteritis, Annu. Rev. Med. **29:**15, 1978.
45. Smythe, H., and Moldofsky, H.: Two contributions to understanding of the "fibrositis" syndrome, Bull. Rheum. Dis. **28:**928, 1977.
46. Kozin, F., McCarty, D.J., Sims, J., and Genant, H.: The reflex sympathetic dystrophy syndrome, Am. J. Med. **60:**321, 1976.
47. Steen, V.D., Medsger, T.A., and Rodnan, G.P.: D-penicillamine therapy in progressive systemic sclerosis, Ann. Intern. Med. (In press.)
48. Whitman, H.H., III, et al.: Variable response to oral angiotensin-converting-enzyme blockade in hypertensive scleroderma patients, Arthritis Rheum. **25:**241, 1982.

CHAPTER 5 · CANCER IN THE GERIATRIC PATIENT

Edward M. Wolin

Cancer represents over 100 clinically and biologically distinct diseases. A detailed knowledge of the natural history and available treatment of the common forms is essential to the practice of geriatrics. Although most patients with cancer will be referred to a medical, surgical, or radiation oncologist, the primary physician plays a continuing and critical role in the care of the elderly patient, providing supportive care during treatment programs and terminal care if treatment fails. Cancer is second only to cardiovascular disease as a cause of death in the elderly. One fourth of all Americans develop cancer, and the majority of these cases will be in the geriatric age group due to the extraordinary exponential increase in cancer incidence with age (Fig. 5-1).[1] For example, the death rate from colon cancer increases one thousand-fold between the ages of 30 and 80.

As Table 5-1 shows,[2] the three most common cancers and causes of cancer-related death are lung, colorectal, and breast and these remain common even in the elderly. But, as shown in Table 5-2, the incidence of other cancers increases dramatically in the elderly.[3] For example, prostate cancer increases until it is the leading cause of cancer death in men in the over-75 age group.

DIAGNOSIS AND STAGING OF CANCER

Diagnosis

An accurate histopathologic diagnosis is the first stage of treatment planning,[4] since frequently each of the many histologic subtypes of cancer in a particular site responds differently to chemotherapy and radiotherapy. Thus a biopsy procedure is always indicated prior to initiating therapy, unless the procedure itself would be more dangerous than the anticipated therapy, as in the case of gliomas located in critical areas of the brain or in life-threatening airway obstruction.

If a recurrence of cancer is suspected after primary treatment, it again becomes crucial to obtain a biopsy to determine whether the apparent recurrence is a metastasis of the original tumor, a second neoplasm, or a nonmalignant condition. The likelihood of recurrent cancer decreases markedly if a long cancer-free period (usually over 5 years) has elapsed.

Staging

For each site of origin of cancer, there are "low stage" cancers, which are localized and generally curable by surgery, and "high stage"

Table 5-1. Estimated new cases and deaths for major sites of cancer, 1974

Site	*Number of cases*	*Deaths*
Lung	83,000	75,000
Colon-rectum	99,000	48,000
Breast	90,000	33,000
Uterus*	46,000	11,000
Oral	24,000	8,000
Skin†	300,000	5,000
Leukemia	21,000	15,000

From American Cancer Society, Inc.: 1974 Cancer facts and figures, New York, 1974, The Society.
*If carcinoma-in-situ is included, cases total over 86,000.
†Estimates vary widely from 300,000 or more for superficial skin cancer.

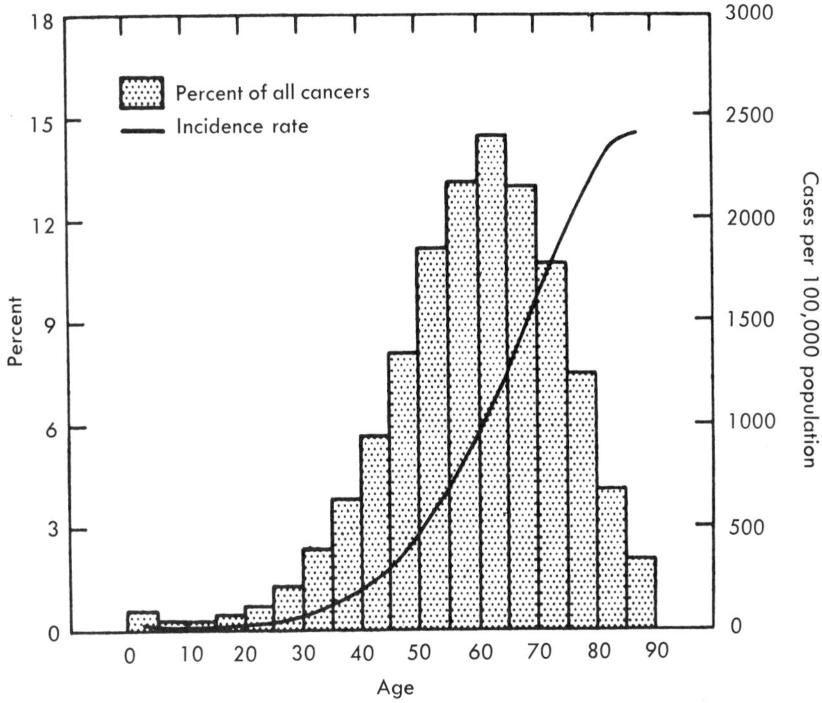

Fig. 5-1. Incidence of cancer as a function of age. (From Morbidity from cancer in the United States, Public Health Service Pub. No. 590, Public Health Monograph No. 56, Washington, D.C., 1959, U.S. Government Printing Office.)

Table 5-2. Mortality for the five leading cancer sites by age, sex, and site, United States, 1969

55 to 74 years		*75+ years*	
Male	*Female*	*Male*	*Female*
Lung 32,838	Breast 13,966	Prostate 9,184	Colon-rectum 9,307
Colon-rectum 11,915	Colon-rectum 11,057	Lung 8,342	Breast 5,805
Prostate 7,336	Lung 6,175	Colon-rectum 7,520	Stomach 2,808
Pancreas 5,777	Uterus 6,092	Stomach 3,379	Pancreas 2,802
Stomach 5,352	Ovary 5,146	Pancreas 2,678	Uterus 2,689

From Vital Statistics of the United States, 1969.

cancers, which are more extensive, less often curable, and usually treated with radiotherapy or chemotherapy. The staging of cancer thus expresses the extent of tumor in a manner useful for predicting the prognosis and approach to treatment and allows for accurate communication.[4] A unique staging classification has been developed for every primary site of tumor, which takes into consideration the tumor's natural history, pattern of spread, and reasons for treatment failure. The particular laboratory and x-ray tests used will therefore depend on the natural history of the primary tumor.[5-7]

There are two classification systems in general use. The TNM system, which is widely used for most nonhematologic malignancies, defines the extent of the primary tumor (T), the extent of lymph node spread (N), and the extent of distant metastases (M). The second major classification system catagorizes the extent of tumor in three or four large categories (called Stage A, B, C, D; or Stage I, II, III, IV) with the higher letters or higher numbers representing more advanced stages of cancer.

EARLY DETECTION OF CANCER

The importance of a careful medical history and physical examination cannot be overemphasized, since the presenting symptoms of cancer are often nonspecific, and it is frequently the careful history and physical examination that alerts the physician to the likelihood of cancer.

Procedures*

THE SKIN

Warning signs:
A sore that does not heal
Change in a wart or mole
A lump or thickening

The skin is the most frequent site of carcinoma. Fortunately skin lesions can be detected while they are small, for they arise as tumors that are visible and tangible. A definite plan of examination should be followed.

First, a history should be taken to determine if the patient has been exposed to known etiological factors. Excessive exposure to sunlight, radiation dermatitis, exposure to coal-tar derivatives, and ingestion of arsenic may be associated with skin cancer. The disease also may develop at the sites of old burn scars whether caused by heat, x-ray or radium. Chronic ulcers of the skin and sinus openings of long duration are likewise favorable sites for skin cancer to develop.

There are few humans who do not have at least one pigmented mole. The examiner should always inquire about moles or birthmarks and whether or not the patient has noticed any change in color, ulceration or enlargement of the lesions.

Second, the skin of the entire body should be inspected including the scrotum and penis or vulva, palms of the hands and soles of the feet. The scalp must be thoroughly palpated as inspection alone is insufficient for the region.

Third, every crusted or ulcerated lesion of the skin of three weeks' duration or more should be biopsied. Provided the lesion is not large, it should be removed *in toto* as an excision biopsy. If x-ray therapy is to be used, a biopsy should be made in order to ascertain if the tumor has the ability to spread to lymph nodes (basal cell carcinomas do not, while epidermoid carcinomas do). If the lesion is pigmented and shows signs of ulceration or enlargement, the problem should be attacked in the hospital and not in the office. Electric cauterization should not be used except in lesions that are unequivocally benign, such as senile keratoses or small pedunculated nevi. Benign lesions that are subject to irritation, such as those located about the waist, hands or feet, should be excised. It is always wise to obtain a histologic examination on any skin lesion that is removed for whatever cause.

Sarcomas of the soft tissue may occur as firm or soft lumps which may or may not be fixed to adjacent structures. With the exception of synoviomas, sarcomas are seldom sensitive or painful. Rhabdomyosarcomas may occur in the thighs and upper arms while malignant synoviomas occur about the knee joints and on the hands and feet. The regional distribution of fibrosarcomas is not specific but may develop on the extremities. If the soft tissue lesion is small, excisional biopsy is preferable to incisional biopsy. If the lesion is large or appears vascular, or is on an extremity, the biopsy should be done in a hospital under tourniquet control with rapid section diagnosis available.

THE HEAD AND NECK

Warning signs:
A sore that does not heal
Hoarseness or cough
Difficulty in swallowing

1. The examiner inspects the skin on the head and neck looking for lesions of the skin and lips. Visible swellings, especially in the region of the salivary glands and neck, should be noted.

2. Palpation of the neck is performed first with the examiner in front of the patient. The region of the

*Modified from American Cancer Society, Inc.: Cancer detection in the physician's office, New York, 1967, The Society.

parotid salivary glands is palpated, then the neck is searched for enlargement of the lymph nodes. The examiner then stands behind the patient and repeats the examination. The thyroid gland is best felt by displacing the larynx to the side of the lobe to be examined, so that it can be palpated between the fingers and thumb.

3. Examination of the oral cavity is then made. The mouth is inspected and the fit of any dentures present is noted and the patient is then asked to remove them. The buccal mucosa is inspected as well as the tongue, roof and floor of the mouth. The examiner looks for areas of leukoplakia, ulceration and tumor. Gentle retraction of the patient's cheek with a throat stick makes the procedure easy for the examiner and comfortable for the patient.

4. Palpation of the lips, floor of the mouth and entire tongue is next performed in search of areas of induration or thickening. Have the patient bend forward when the base of the tongue is palpated and he will not gag.

5. The anterior nares are inspected with a nasal speculum. The nasopharynx and larynx are then inspected with the laryngeal mirror. The laryngeal mirror is also an aid to the general inspection of the oral cavity.

6. Biopsy of any area of leukoplakia, ulceration or tumor is made. If the lesion is less than 1 cm. in size it should be excised *in toto*, otherwise a small sample of the lesion is removed.

7. If an enlarged cervical lymph node is present the primary lesion should be looked for prior to any surgical procedure on the lymph node.

THE LARYNX, LUNGS AND ESOPHAGUS

Warning signs:

Hoarseness or cough

Difficulty in swallowing

Larynx. The larynx, base of the tongue, hypopharynx and nasopharynx can be visualized by mirror examination. Biopsy of a suspicious lesion should be made, and the area of lymphatic drainage should be carefully examined. Carcinoma of the larynx tends to spread to the deep cervical lymph nodes in the mid or upper portion of the neck.

Lung. It is a rare occurrence to arrive at a diagnosis of primary carcinoma of the lung when the chest x-ray examination is negative. The fact that the death rate per 100,000 from lung cancer in the United States has risen from 2 in 1930 to 22 in 1963, makes it imperative that all adult patients have an annual x-ray examination of their lungs. The Report of the U.S. Surgeon General's Advisory Committee on *Smoking and Health* in 1964 states that, "Cigarette smoking is causally related to lung cancer. . . . The risk of developing lung cancer increases with duration of smoking and the number of cigarettes smoked per day, and is diminished by discontinuing smoking."

Cytologic smears of the sputum are easily made in the office using the same technique as for vaginal smears. A negative cytologic smear of the sputum does not exclude the possibility of cancer.

Bronchoscopy is a hospital procedure that requires special skill. Bronchoscopy not only enables the operator to remove a fragment of tissue for microscopic examination, but permits expert appraisal of the characteristics of the lesion which aids in the decision regarding treatment. The differentiation of primary from metastatic pulmonary neoplasms may be difficult. If the lesions are multiple, or if the patient has a known primary cancer elsewhere, the pulmonary lesion is probably metastatic. However, if the lesion is solitary even if the patient has had removal of a cancer in the past, consideration of a primary lung tumor should not be dismissed.

Esophagus. The symptomatology of esophageal cancer shows little variation from case to case, but the dysphagia may be intermittent and depend on the type of food ingested. The tentative clinical diagnosis should be reported to the roentgenologist so he will be alerted to the fact that an esophageal lesion is suspected, and his attention will then not be prematurely diverted to the stomach and duodenum when he performs his examination. Esophagoscopy requires hospitalization and services of an experienced observer. The procedure permits biopsy of the lesion and evaluation of its extent.

THE BREAST

Warning sign:

A lump or thickening in the breast

1. The breasts are first inspected and palpated with the patient in the sitting position. The examiner looks for puckering of the skin or change in level of the nipples as the patient raises or lowers her arms.

2. While the patient is in the sitting position, the examiner palpates both the axillary and supraclavicular regions in search for enlarged lymph nodes.

3. With the patient supine, each breast is carefully palpated first with the arm over her head and then at her side. Palpation of the axilla is repeated at this time. The quadrants of the breast are systemically examined. The condition of the nipple and areola are noted, and the presence or absence of abnormal discharge from the nipples is determined.

4. The breasts should be compared. A discrete spherical tumor is suggestive of fibroadenoma, while a discrete irregular mass is suggestive of carcinoma. Cystic disease of the breast frequently is bilateral, but may be unilateral and difficult to differentiate from carcinoma.

5. Biopsy is indicated in every instance of solitary

tumor of the breast or when any segment of the breast shows changes from the normal. Breast biopsy should be performed under general anesthesia in a hospital and, ideally, facilities should be available for rapid section examination of the tissue.

6. Mammography is of diagnostic value. Mammography is soft tissue radiography of the breast. No contrast media, either opaque or air or gas, are used. While mammography is presently not part of the routine physical examination it can be of help, especially in the following circumstances:

a. Indeterminate mass or nodule
b. Follow-up of remaining breast after mastectomy
c. In the large fatty breast and in pregnancy or lactation
d. Numerous previous breast biopsies; fibrocystic disease
e. Vague complaints related to the breasts
f. The unknown primary lesion

THE STOMACH

Warning sign:
Indigestion

1. A careful history of digestive habits and symptoms should be taken. Any digestive disturbance (even if of very short duration) should be investigated by x-ray examination.

2. It is important to emphasize that a long history of duodenal ulcer *does not exclude* coexisting cancer of the stomach, and that cancer of the stomach may masquerade as benign ulcer of the stomach.

3. Keep in mind that stomach cancer still accounts for an estimated 21,000 new cancer cases annually, in spite of the fact that the incidence rate has been declining in recent years.

4. Secondary anemia may be the only sign of a gastric or colonic cancer.

5. Do routine tests for occult blood in the stool on all patients. Occult blood in the stool may be the first clue of a gastrointestinal cancer.

THE LARGE BOWEL AND RECTUM

Warning signs:
Change in bowel or bladder habits
Unusual bleeding or discharge

1. The examiner should carefully palpate the abdomen with particular regard for the size and regularity of the liver edge and the presence of abdominal masses and distention.

2. The digital rectal examination is the next step (in the female it follows the vaginal examination). First, a polyp or carcinoma of the rectum may be palpated; the prostate gland is examined both for hypertrophy and tumor nodules. Second, the bimanual rectal examination in either sex may reveal unsuspected pelvic masses. If the patient is asked to strain down during the examination, an intraluminal lesion otherwise just beyond the examiner's finger tip may become palpable. Third, a specimen of feces is usually available when the examining finger is withdrawn and a test for occult blood should routinely be made on this gloved finger specimen.

3. The next step is proctosigmoidoscopy, the most important procedure in the examination of the rectum and colon. This procedure is not difficult to master. If the examiner is gentle in manipulating the instrument, no harm can befall the patient. Proper examination requires a clear lower bowel.

4. The final stage of investigation of the patient suspected of having a colonic lesion is a barium enema. A patient with a suspected lesion of the colon should not be given barium by mouth prior to the barium enema. If there is a question of an obstructing lesion of the colon, a scout film of the abdomen should be made prior to any barium studies. While barium studies aid in the diagnosis, they may compound an incipient intestinal obstruction or make the preparation for surgery difficult. Contrast air enema will be indicated when polyps are discovered or suspected to be present.

THE UTERUS AND URINARY TRACT

Warning sign:
Unusual bleeding or discharge

1. A careful history of the menstrual cycle and events since the menopause, if postmenopausal, must be obtained.

2. Any spotting or bleeding that cannot be considered characteristic of normal menstruation demands careful investigation.

3. Any postmenopausal spotting or bleeding should be considered to be caused by cancer until proved otherwise.

4. Abnormal vaginal discharge particularly of a watery nature may be a sign of uterine cancer.

5. A cytologic smear of the vaginal secretions should be made. The positive smear is very significant, but a negative smear does not rule out the possibility of cancer, especially if there are symptoms. The smear however, must be interpreted by an expert.

6. Routine pelvic examination should always be done. This includes inspection of the vulva for leukoplakia and ulceration, digital examination of the vagina and cervix, and bimanual palpation of the uterus and adnexa.

7. Speculum examination of the vagina and cervix uteri is the next step. Any suspicious lesion of the cervix should be biopsied. Schiller's iodine solution painted on the cervix will demonstrate abnormal or glycogen-free epithelium from which a biopsy should be taken.

8. Dilatation and curettage is the only method by

which adequate samples of the endometrium can be obtained for histologic examination. It is a procedure that demands hospitalization and general anesthesia.

9. The advanced uterine lesion, either cervical or endometrial, is easy to diagnose, but the examiner must persistently seek the asymptomatic and early lesion.

The patient of either sex should be questioned about gross hematuria and a routine urinalysis, including examination of the urinary sediment, should be done. The findings of gross or microscopic hematuria require further investigation that calls for the services of a urologist. Cancer may occur in any part of the urinary tract and hematuria is the critical signal of that disease. Bleeding may also be an early symptom of many other cancers such as breast, lung, mouth, skin or bowel.

Diagnostic mistakes

There are several common errors which can lead to unnecessary delay in cancer diagnosis. The American Cancer Society, Inc.,[8] has referred to them as "The Seven Tragic Diagnostic Mistakes";

1. Failure to make a diagnosis of intraoral cancer on the assumption that it is a "canker sore" is an error that is avoided simply by making a biopsy of the lesion.
2. Failure to diagnose carcinoma of the breast because the physician believes the lump is a benign lesion, such as fat necrosis or inflammation, should never occur. A lump in the breast must be assumed to be malignant until biopsy proves it otherwise.
3. To treat a patient with the conviction that his symptoms are due to a duodenal or benign gastric ulcer without radiologic or laboratory evidence of the disease is to miss a possible diagnosis of cancer of the stomach. Barium x-ray examination of the stomach, gastric analysis for acid content, and study of the feces for blood should be performed prior to beginning treatment of a suspected peptic ulcer.
4. Failure to recognize that an inguinal hernia, especially of long duration, which suddenly becomes symptomatic, may be associated with carcinomatous lesions of the prostate or colon, is a pitfall to be avoided. The dynamics of straining to void or defecate may be the cause of the sudden increase of the symptoms from the hernia. In such instances the physician should investigate the possibility of lesions of the prostate or colon and not devote all of his thought to the hernia.
5. To treat abnormal uterine bleeding caused by cancer, with hormones, without a histologic diagnosis of the cause of the bleeding, is an error that is easily avoided. These patients should not be given hormonal or other medication until cancer of the uterus has been excluded by adequate histologic examination.
6. Failure to recognize that bleeding piles may mask a coexisting rectal carcinoma is a tragic oversight. Thus, even in the presence of bleeding hemorrhoids, it is necessary to exclude the possibility of coexisting polyps or cancer of the rectum or colon, by digital rectal examination, proctosigmoidoscopy and barium enema.
7. To treat anemia without recognizing that cancer may be the primary cause of the blood loss is a serious error. Cancer anywhere in the body may be associated with anemia, and gastric and large bowel cancers are notorious for the anemia they cause.*

Conclusion

In the history special attention should be given to those predisposing factors and premalignant conditions that will increase the likelihood of particular types of cancer (Table 5-3).[9] These historical items will alert the physician to be especially vigilant in screening for those cancers for which a particular patient is at high risk.

A useful approach for the geriatric physician would be to follow the current recommendations of the American Cancer Society, which are summarized in Table 5-4 and which represent a useful screening program for all patients. Those with special predisposing factors and premalignant conditions could then have other studies as indicated.[10]

CARE OF PATIENTS WITH CANCER

Once a cancer has been accurately diagnosed and staged, an optimal treatment program can be designed using surgery, radiation therapy, and chemotherapy as needed. Whether or not a particular cancer is curable with current modalities, skillful supportive care is always necessary and patients must never feel deserted by their physicians because nothing more can be done.

Cancer surgery in the elderly

The decision as to whether or not a patient should undergo a major operative procedure should never be based entirely on chronological age. The physiologic age of the patient is often quite different from the chronological age and is a much better predictor of how a patient will withstand major surgery. However, the geriatric patient has less reserve than the younger patient in withstanding major stresses to the cardiovas-

*Modified from American Cancer Society, Inc.: Cancer detection in the physician's office, New York, 1967, The Society.

Table 5-3. Guide to higher cancer risks

Predisposing factor	*Premalignant condition*
Skin	
Excessive exposure to x rays, sun, elements, arsenic, tar, petroleum products	Arsenical, senile keratosis; junctional or compound nevi; burn scars; xeroderma pigmentosum; Bowen's disease; radiation dermatitis
Head and neck	
Oral cavity, pharynx, and larynx	Leukoplakia; Plummer-Vinson syndrome
Tobacco; alcohol; syphilis (tongue); nutritional deficiency; previous respiratory tract cancer	
Thyroid	
Excessive exposure to radiation; iodine deficiency; goitrogenic substances	Adenoma (may be associated with cancer rather than a precursor)
Lung	
Cigarettes; exposure to chromate, asbestos, radioactive ore, metal dust, etc.; air pollution	Cytologic atypias; bronchial adenomas
Breast	
Never married; nulliparous; absence of lactation; high familial incidence; previous breast disease	"Chronic cystic mastitis"
Upper gastrointestinal tract	
Esophagus	Plummer-Vinson syndrome
Nutritional deficiency; tobacco; alcohol	
Stomach	Atrophic gastritis; gastric polyps; gastric ulcer
Achlorhydria; pernicious anemia; high blood type A	
Other gastrointestinal	
Liver	
Parasites; nutritional deficiency	Cirrhosis; hemochromatosis
Gallbladder	
Gallstones	Adenomatous polyps
Rectum-colon	
Prior polyp or cancer; ulcerative colitis; familial polyposis; high familial incidence	Mucosal hyperplasia; adenomatous polyps; villous adenomas
Uterus	
Cervix	
Uncircumcised partner; early age of frequent coitus; multiple pregnancies; radiation therapy	Cytologic atypias; chronic cervicitis; leukoplakia
Endometrium	
Endocrine imbalance; obesity, infertility and/or diabetes; functioning ovarian tumors; Stein-Leventhal syndrome; radiation therapy	Endometrial polyps of hyperplasia
Urinary tract	
Bladder	
Cigarettes; excessive exposure to aniline dyes and related chemicals; schistosomiasis; exstrophy	Leukoplakia; papillomas
Male genitalia	
Penis	
Uncircumcised; poor penile hygiene; phimosis	Erythroplasia; Bowen's disease; leukoplakia
Testis	
Cryptorchidism	Not known
Blood-forming organs	
Leukemia	
Excessive exposure to x-radiation and toxic chemicals; ? familial factor	Polycythemia vera

From Day, E.: CA **13**:2, 1963.

Table 5-4. Protocol for the early detection of cancer in asymptomatic geriatric patients

	Sex	*Age, risk*	*Frequency*	*Previous recommendations*
Chest x-ray	—	Not recommended	—	High risk person*
Sputum cytology	—	Not recommended	—	Not recommended
Sigmoidoscopy	M and F	Over 50	Every 3-5 years†	Persons over 40 annually
Stool Guaiac slide test	M and F	Over 50	Every year	Persons over 40, annually
Digital rectal examination	M and F	Over 40	Every year	Every year
PAP test	F	20-65	Every 3 years‡	Annual
Pelvic examination	F	Over 40	Every year	Every year
Endometrial tissue sample	F	At high risk§ Menopause	At menopause	At menopause
Breast self-examination	F	Over 20	Every month	Every month
Breast physical examination	F	Over 40	Every year	Every year
Mammography	F	Over 50	Every year	
Health counseling and cancer checkup¶	M and F	Over 40	Every year	"Periodic"

From Williams, P.A.: Cancer **47:**1146, 1981.
*Persons over 40 who smoke or are exposed to other lung carcinogens.
†After two initial negative examinations a year apart.
‡After two initial PAP tests done a year apart are negative
§History of infertility, obesity, failure of ovulation, abnormal uterine bleeding, or estrogen therapy.
¶To include examination for cancers of the thyroid, testicles, prostate, ovaries, lymph nodes, oral region, and skin.

cular system and kidneys. Postoperative thromboembolic and pulmonary complications are common, although if early ambulation and change are encouraged, these complications may be minimized. Blood loss is tolerated poorly, and even short periods of hypotension may lead to fatal strokes or myocardial infarctions. Chronic urinary and respiratory infections should be treated vigorously preoperatively to minimize the risk of postoperative septic complications. Oral hygiene should be optimized preoperatively to minimize the chances of respiratory infection after intubation. Finally, the nutritional status should be optimized before, during, and after surgery, using enteral or parenteral hyperalimentation if necessary.

The risks of an operation in a given patient must be balanced against the anticipated beneficial results of the operation. If a patient cannot withstand a radical operation, a lesser operation may be superior to no surgery at all. There are also many cases in which an alternative local treatment modality such as radiation therapy may achieve local tumor control in the elderly patient with less morbidity than surgery. If surgery is used, local or regional anesthesia should be used whenever possible to avoid respiratory depression and intubation.

The basic principles of cancer surgery remain the same in the elderly as in younger patients and are designed to minimize the chances of local recurrence and dissemination to distant sites. Manipulation of the tumor should be minimal so that tumor cells are not forced into the circulation. Whenever possible, the vessels that supply blood to a tumor should be ligated prior to resection to prevent tumor embolization. When bowel resection is contemplated, the bowel is usually ligated proximally and distally to minimize dissemination.

Radiation therapy

Radiotherapy can cure localized cancers and effectively palliate other tumors.[11] Ionizing radiation is usually used therapeutically in the form of gamma rays (high energy photons emitted from radioactive isotopes such as radium or cobalt-60) or x-rays (high energy photons from a target bombarded with electrons in a linear accelerator or similar apparatus). However, electrons, neutrons, and other particles can also be used as sources of therapeutic radiation in specific circumstances. Megavoltage energy radiation has almost totally replaced kilovoltage energy radiation as a modality for cancer treatment. This has been a most important development in making radiotherapy safe and well-tolerated, while at the same time improving results of treatment. With modern supervoltage radiation, skin absorption is less than absorption by deeper tissues, so skin toxicity no longer limits the radiation dose that can be given. In addition, the higher beam energy, the more sharply demarcated margins of the irradiated field, and the greater depth of penetration, allow treatment of larger volumes of tumor to higher doses. Linear accelerators, because of their high beam energies (4 to 35 MeV) accomplish all of these objectives more effectively than the lower energy cobalt-60 machines.[12]

Electrons are commonly used to irradiate superficial tumors while sparing deeper normal tissues from radiation. They typically penetrate into tissues 0.25-0.5 cm/MeV of energy so that the depth of irradiation can be accurately limited. Neutrons, protons, helium ions, and negative pi-mesons deposit more energy in tissues (higher linear energy transfer) than photons and can destroy anoxic cells that are resistant to photon therapy.

Radiation doses are customarily expressed in the rad, which is a unit of absorbed energy per volume of tissue. It is important to note that the biologic effect of radiation depends on more than the number of rads administered—the other important variables are the total time period during which the radiation dose was delivered and the dose given with each daily fraction. Typically 1000 rads per week is administered in fractions of 150 rads to 250 rads.

Certain toxicities of radiation such as nausea, vomiting, mucous membrane inflammation, pneumonitis, and dermatitis occur during a treatment course and are usually worst near the end of the treatment period. Other toxicities, which have a more chronic course and are maximal months to years after radiation treatment, result from progressive microvascular inflammation and fibrosis and cause necrosis and ulceration, which heal as atrophy and fibrosis.

Table 5-5. Radiation doses tolerated by normal tissues*

Tissue	Dose
Lungs (both)	1500 rads
Kidneys (both)	2400 rads
Heart	3500 rads
Spinal cord	4000 rads
Intestine	5500 rads
Brain	6000 rads
Bone	4500 rads

*Radiation delivered by megavoltage equipment in usual fractionated schedules.

These microvascular injuries are often more serious in the geriatric patient because of underlying vascular damage from atherosclerosis. Radiation can cause what appears to be an acceleration of the aging process in the irradiated volume.

Normal tissues vary widely in their sensitivity to radiation. When the radiation doses shown in Table 5-5 are exceeded (when given by standard megavoltage sources with usual fractionation), significant toxicities tend to occur in the irradiated tissue. Toxicities may occur at much lower dosages if advanced atherosclerosis is present or if the patient has also received chemotherapy with anthracyclines (e.g., doxorubicin) or certain other chemotherapeutic drugs.

Whether or not a tumor can be cured by radiation depends on its size (small tumors require less radiation) and on the radiosensitivity of the normal tissues in the area. If the normal tissues can withstand twice the radiation of the tumor, then the tumor would probably be called *radiosensitive*. But if larger doses of radiation are needed to destroy the tumor than normal tissues can tolerate, then radiation would not be curative, and the tumor would be called *radioresistant*.

Chemotherapy

Chemotherapy, the treatment of cancer with chemical substances, is the most important modality of therapy for a cancer that has spread further than the anatomic region where it originated. At this point there are over 40 clinically useful and widely available chemotherapy drugs and more than twice that number being used investigationally. Each of these drugs has many side effects and is used near its maximal tolerated dose to achieve maximum antitumor effect.[13] These drugs are often given in combination to achieve a synergistic antitumor effect.[14] Physicians who use chemotherapy drugs should be specially trained in medical oncology. However, the physician caring for the elderly should be aware of the toxicities of commonly used drugs, since he is likely to be the primary doctor during the period of cancer treatment.

For those types of cancer for which chemotherapy is potentially curative, aggressive therapy is frequently definitive even in the elderly. In situations in which chemotherapy can only be viewed as palliative, the drugs are generally given only for the treatment of symptomatic disease and doses are not pushed to levels at which major toxicities are expected.

Psychosocial aspects of cancer care

Total care of the cancer patient is of highest priority, whether or not the treatment is successful in curing the patient and whether life expectancy can be measured in years or days. In this country, cancer is the most terrifying of diseases, even though approximately 40% of cancer patients can be cured, and most of the remainder can be palliated for varying periods of time. It is also important to remember that even those cancers most incurable in advanced stages can be cured regularly when diagnosed early.

Most patients with cancer become aware of their diagnosis, and if the physician is dishonest, a most serious breakdown in the trust between patient and physician is likely to occur. Furthermore, patients are not likely to agree to highly uncomfortable treatment programs aimed at cancer control if they do not realize the seriousness of their illness. Patients and their families must always be told of their diagnosis in a gentle and compassionate manner, and the physician must be careful not to take away all hope from the patient. In particular, one must remember that actuarial statistics apply to populations of patients and not to any particular patient. To tell a patient, "You have 3 months to live" is not only inaccurate but will rather cruelly destroy a patient's feeling of hope.

In the terminal phase of a patient's illness, a special effort should be made to consider the patient and family as a unit, to focus therapeutic efforts on supportive care, and to make a special effort to manage the patient at home or in home-like surroundings in the presence of friends, loved ones, children, and other things important to the patient.[15] Coordinating these efforts with social workers and home health care personnel is especially rewarding.

Nutritional support

Anorexia and weight loss are common in cancer patients. The maintenance of a good nutritional status appears not only to improve the quality of a patient's life, but to enhance significantly the response to chemotherapy and to lessen the toxicity of therapy.[16] In colon cancer, maintenance of excellent nutrition can increase the response rate threefold.

Whenever needed, supplemental alimentation should be given orally, if possible, either as a supplementation of an ordinary diet with high calorie, high protein mixtures or as a tube feeding. However, intravenous hyperalimentation does have a role when oral alimentation is not possible due to pain with deglutition, malabsorbtion, or intestinal obstruction. It is particularly useful to improve the nutritional status of cachectic patients when tumor control is possible with chemotherapy, surgery, or radiotherapy.[16] There is no evidence to suggest that hyperalimentation enhances the growth of tumors preferentially. Scrupulous care of the catheter is necessary to keep risk of sepsis at a very low level (2%). Hyperosmotic nonketotic coma occurs easily in the elderly, and insulin must be used as needed with hyperalimentation. Electrolyte balance must be carefully controlled as well.[17]

Many attempts have been made to treat cancer with dietary modification, but none of these have a proven benefit at this time, including high dose vitamin C therapy. In a carefully controlled randomized trial of Vitamin C versus placebo in the treatment of cancer, there was no advantage to high dose Vitamin C.[18] Similarly, a well-designed trial of Laetrile plus "vitamin therapy" showed no benefit to this type of treatment.[19]

Pain management in cancer

Skillful pain management is an important aspect of care of the patient with cancer.[20-22] Although 50% of cancer patients never experience cancer-related pain, the other half are not so fortunate, and pain and its management often become central issues. One fifth of cancer patients experience severe pain not relieved with ordinary doses of oral narcotics. Undermedication is a frequent error either due to a fear of addiction or to lack of knowledge about optimal prescribing of narcotics. To make life more comfortable narcotics given frequently (e.g., every 4 hours) should be used in terminal patients having severe pain. Oral morphine elixir and methadone are ideal drugs for patients in severe pain and usually are as effective as parenteral narcotics and even heroin (diacetylmorphine). For slightly less severe pain, oxycodone, hydromorphone, or levorphanol are ideal. Alcohol improves the absorption of narcotics and can contribute to subjective pain relief by relieving anxiety. Phenothiazines with or without tricyclic antidepressants may also contribute to the analgesic effect and prevent narcotic-induced nausea. Brompton's solution, a fixed combination of alcohol, morphine, prochlorperazine (Compazine), and cocaine, is not recommended in the geriatric patient. As the dose of Brompton's solution is escalated to achieve a high enough dose of narcotic to relieve pain, the dose of prochlorperazine becomes high enough to cause extrapyramidal symptoms and the dose of cocaine becomes toxic as well, resulting in an extremely wakeful state in which patients are more aware of their pain. This can progress to acute paranoid reactions or convulsions.

MANAGEMENT OF SELECTED TYPES OF CANCER

Lymphomas

The lymphomas are a heterogeneous group of malignancies, all highly treatable, but with treatment and prognosis dependent on histopathology and stage. For this reason the pathologic diagnosis must be carefully reviewed and careful staging should be done, including chest x-ray, CT scan of abdomen, liver function tests, bone marrow biopsies, and so on to establish the extent of disease. Staging laparotomies is not generally recommended in geriatric patients.[23,24]

Hodgkin's disease. Hodgkin's disease has an increased incidence in the elderly as well as the well-known peak incidence in young adults.[25] Hodgkin's disease that is not more extensive than Stage IIIA is best treated with radiotherapy in the geriatric patient. The principles of successful radiation therapy of Hodgkin's disease have been clearly established.[26] They include (1) using a tumoricidal dose of radiation (3500 to 4500 rads), (2) using large fields to encompass commonly involved lymphoid tissues ("mantle" or supradiaphragmatic field and "inverted Y" or infradiaphragmatic field), (3) using high energy (megavoltage) radiation, (4) prophylactic irradiation of lymphoid tissue that is not clinically involved but which is adjacent or contiguous by way of lymphatic channels, and (5) treatment given by a highly experienced radiation oncologist. Radiation alone can be used to provide primary therapy for elderly patients with Hodgkin's disease in Stage I, Stage II, and most Stage IIIA.[27] Chemotherapy is not recommended except in patients with more advanced presentations and with recurrent disease. Stage IIIB and Stage IV Hodgkin's disease must be treated with chemotherapy. The best established regimen is MOPP (nitrogen mustard + vincristine + procarbazine + prednisone), which has about a 70% complete response rate, with two thirds of the patients in complete remission, their disease permanently eradicated. This regimen is quite toxic with severe vomiting, peripheral neuropathy, pancytopenia, and constipation most common. In addition, procarbazine often causes transient changes in the mental status of the elderly patient. The toxicities of high dose prednisone in the elderly are often significant as well. If MOPP is not well tolerated, it is usually possible to treat effectively with a less toxic regimen. In patients who progress after MOPP, effective treatment is often possible using "salvage chemotherapy," consisting of different drugs than those used in MOPP.

Non-Hodgkin's lymphomas. Non-Hodgkin's lymphomas should be thought of as being of two general types[28]: (1) the indolent lymphomas of low malignant potential (e.g., the nodular lymphomas and well-differentiated small-cell lymphoma) and (2) the aggressive lymphomas of high malignant potential (e.g., diffuse large cell lymphoma).

The indolent lymphomas in the elderly can be viewed as chronic diseases, often running a 5- to 10-year course.[29] They are generally incurable, and therapy must be viewed as palliative. Most of these lymphomas present as Stage IV disease with the bone marrow positive. The rare patients presenting with Stage I and II disease can be treated with local radiotherapy. Otherwise, no therapy needs to be used until such time as the disease becomes symptomatic. If symptoms are referable to a single large lymph node mass, this can be treated with radiotherapy.

The radiation therapy approach to non-Hodgkin's lymphomas is similar to that described for Hodgkin's disease except consideration must also be given to more frequent involvement of such areas as Waldeyer's ring and the mesenteric lymph nodes. In general, radiation therapy is used in Stage I and II presentations of indolent lymphomas. It can also be used to palliate local symptoms of disease (see palliation).

However, if fever, weight loss, massive generalized adenopathy, or pancytopenia develops, or if organ function becomes compromised, then treatment with chemotherapy is reasonable. An alkylating agent such as oral chlorambucil is usually effective and well tolerated and can be used as needed. When this ceases to be effective, a combination such as CVP (cyclophosphamide + vincristine + prednisone) can be used. If several years after an indolent lymphoma has been diagnosed, a lymph node starts to grow rapidly, this node should be biopsied, since there may have been a change in histology to a more aggressive variety.[30]

The aggressive non-Hodgkin's lymphomas of high malignant potential will usually result in death within 1 to 2 years unless treated very aggressively with combination chemotherapy[31] (except for Stage I patients who can be treated with radiotherapy alone). These lymphomas usually present as rather localized, but extremely fast-growing, masses either in lymph nodes or in extranodal sites, particularly bone, gastrointestinal sites, testis, thyroid gland, and Waldeyer's ring. Bone marrow is usually not involved. Early symptoms are caused by local extension of masses to cause compression of the airway, veins, or nerves. Lung parenchyma, pleura, liver, skin, and central nervous system are also common sites of involvement. Intensive chemotherapy should be started immediately with such combinations as CHOP (cyclophosphamide + vincristine + doxorubicin + prednisone) or C-MOPP (cyclophosphamide + vincristine + procarbazine + prednisone) if cardiac disease contraindicates the use of doxorubicin. With this type of intensive therapy, 40% to 50% of patients will have a lasting complete remission and will appear to be cured. In general all relapses occur within 2 years of diagnosis. It is worth noting that a rare elderly patient will have a less aggressive form of this disease that will allow for the less intensive management program recommended for indolent lymphomas.

Carcinoma of the breast

This is the most common cancer in elderly women, occuring in about 5% of the female population. Staging procedures recommended at the time of diagnosis include bilateral mammography, chest x-ray, bone scan, alkaline phosphatase, and serum calcium. Estrogen receptors (ER) should be measured in all primary tumors and in newly detected metastases.

The primary treatment of localized carcinoma of the breast (Stage I, II) is with a modified radical mastectomy or with lumpectomy followed by local radiotherapy.[32] When the latter procedure is performed an axillary lymph node dissection is advisable to stage the degree of involvement in axillary lymph nodes.[33,34] The current recommendation is to first perform a lumpectomy and establish the diagnosis of breast cancer on permanent sections before discussing the therapeutic alternatives with the patient. When a modified radical mastectomy is performed, there is no evidence that cure or survival can be improved by postoperative radiotherapy, and this should not be routinely done. However, there is a role for radiotherapy in those Stage II patients who have a high risk of local recurrence (e.g., a large number of positive axillary nodes or extension of tumor through the lymph node capsule), with the goal of treatment being reduction of the high local recurrence rate.[35]

The presence of positive axillary lymph nodes is an important predictor of the development of distant metastases.[36] With one to three positive nodes, nearly one half of women will develop distant metastases by 2 years after diagnosis, and with four or more nodes, the risk of distant metastases is 80% at 2 years. Although in premenopausal patients, adjuvant chemotherapy can be clearly shown to reduce the chances of developing distant metastases, the situation is less clear in postmenopausal patients.[37] However, evidence is now accumulating that even in elderly patients, adjuvant chemotherapy (e.g., with cyclophosphamide + methotrexate + 5-

fluorouracil) can be useful, particularly in those women who can receive more than 80% of calculated drug dosage.[37] Adjuvant chemotherapy does not appear to be useful in elderly patients who are debilitated or who have inadequate bone marrow function and could not tolerate chemotherapy drugs in high dose.

The initial treatment of inoperable breast cancer (Stage III and IV) is generally with local radiotherapy; then chemotherapy and/or hormones are used, as in treating metastatic disease.

At present, metastatic carcinoma of the breast is incurable, and palliation is the goal of all treatment. As a general rule, if estrogen-binding receptor protein is absent or if advanced visceral metastases are present, chemotherapy is the treatment of choice (hormones have less than a 5% chance of benefit in this setting).

However, if bone or soft tissue metastases are present and if estrogen-binding receptor protein is present, the chances of responding to a hormonal treatment are about 50% to 75% and the toxicity of hormonal treatment is considerably less than with chemotherapy.[38,39] So in these patients, hormonal treatments are used initially, and chemotherapy is used as a last resort. The antiestrogen, tamoxifen, is probably the least toxic hormonal treatment in elderly patients.[40] For this reason it is usually used as the first hormonal manipulation in the ER positive patient. The duration of a hormonal response averages 12 to 16 months. After responding to hormonal treatment, the chances are good for responding to a second hormonal treatment. In women who are more than 5 years postmenopausal, oral estrogen is often used as the second hormonal treatment. It has a response rate comparable to tamoxifen but is more toxic in the elderly patient—strokes, myocardial infarctions, other thromboembolic events, and fluid retention leading to congestive heart failure being the most common toxicities encountered. Androgens can be used as a third line hormonal treatment.[41] They have a 30% response rate and carry with them the toxicities of virilization and toxic hepatitis. In ER positive patients who have progressive disease after a response to the oral hormones and antihormones listed above, an endocrine ablation is likely to result in additional tumor regression.[42] This ablation can be either an adrenalectomy or hypophysectomy. Ablation of adrenal function without surgery can also be accomplished with aminoglutethimide. When any hormonal treatment is started, there may be a transient tumor flare with bone pain and hypercalcemia, which may resolve as the patient goes on to have a good antitumor response. However, this hypercalcemia may be life-threatening and must be diligently searched for and treated. If it does not promptly resolve, the treatment must be stopped.

There are several cytotoxic chemotherapy drugs useful in treating metastatic breast cancer.[43,44] These include doxorubicin, alkylating agents, vinca alkaloids (vincristine and vinblastine), and several antimetabolites. However, single drugs result in responses in only 20% to 35% of patients. Combination chemotherapy is much more effective with 50% to 80% of patients responding and 25% having a complete response. The best responses are seen in visceral and soft tissue metastases. Although doxorubicin-containing combinations have the highest response rates, doxorubicin is a difficult drug to use in the elderly because of its cardiotoxicity, and CMF (cyclophosphamide + methotrexate + 5-flurouracil) is recommended as the first choice combination in the geriatric patient. Responses to cytotoxic chemotherapy generally last 6 to 12 months, a shorter duration of response than that seen with hormonal treatments.

Adenocarcinomas of the gastrointestinal tract

The adenocarcinomas of the gastrointestinal tract include those arising in the esophagus, rectum, colon, stomach, pancreas, liver, and biliary systems. For all these cancers, surgery, radiation, or both are the only potentially curative treatments, with chemotherapy being strictly palliative. Radiation therapy combined with surgery appears to be optional for local control of rectal cancer.[45] The pattern of metastasis is first to spread to the regional lymph nodes, then to liver and lungs. The first detectable metastasis is often a low left supraclavicular lymph node (Virchow's node) because of the pattern of thoracic duct drainage. Staging procedures recommended at the time of diagnosis include chest x-ray, contrast studies of the gastrointestinal tract, liver scan (or abdominal CT scan), and liver function tests. A serum carcinoembryonic antigen (CEA) level should also be drawn.[46]

The most widely used single drug in treating metastatic gastrointestinal malignancies is 5-fluorouracil.[47,48] A partial response can be achieved in about 20% of patients who have a good nutritional status. These responses last an average of 4 to 5 months, and responders appear to live longer than nonresponders. Complete responses are rare. Other single agents with activity against gastrointestinal cancers are the nitrosoureas[49] (lomustine [CeeNu], carmustine [BiCNU], methyl-CCNU) and mitomycin-C, although these agents are seldom active in 5-fluorouracil failures.[50] Debilitated patients should not be treated with chemotherapy, since drug toxicity tends to be severe and the response rate is much lower than in nondebilitated patients. A well-tolerated administration schedule of 5-fluorouracil is 15 mg/kg per week given as an intravenous push.[51] In those patients with pancreatic or gastric cancer who have the performance status and bone marrow reserve to tolerate a more aggressive chemotherapy regimen, the combination of 5-fluorouracil + adriamycin + mitomycin-C has approximately a 40% response rate, significantly better than 5-fluorouracil alone.

Cancer of the genitourinary system

Prostate cancer. Carcinoma of the prostate gland is the second most common cause of cancer deaths in men and a major health problem in the geriatric patient.[52,53] With local invasion, surgical care is seldom possible. Radiotherapy appears to be at least as effective as surgery in permanently controlling local disease and has a lower incidence of incontinence and impotence, making this the preferred local treatment in the elderly.[54] Systemic hormonal therapy is recommended only when symptomatic metastatic disease develops, since there is no survival advantage to early hormonal therapy. A 60% response rate is achieved with either orchiectomy or diethylstilbestrol (DES); however in elderly patients, orchiectomy is clearly preferable because of less toxicity.[55] (DES causes gynecomastia, hypertension, thromboembolic events, and worsening of congestive heart failure.) When DES is used, the dose should be 1 mg per day, since excessive toxicity is seen with higher doses. No therapeutic advantage is seen when orchiectomy and DES are used together, and there is less than 10% response rate of patients when DES failures are treated with orchiectomy or vice versa.[56] Acid phosphatase is a useful parameter of disease activity and usually falls when a satisfactory antitumor effect is being achieved. There is no established regimen of cytotoxic chemotherapy for hormone-resistant prostate cancer,[57] although occasional short-lived responses are seen with such drugs as cyclophosphamide, doxorubicin, and cis-platinum.

Carcinoma of the bladder. Low grade superficial papillomata can be treated with transuretheral resection or fulguration.[58] Topical chemotherapy may be instilled in the bladder when there are large numbers of polyps or when they recur frequently. This achieves control in about 30% of patients.[59] With bladder wall invasion (Stage B_2 or C), preoperative radiotherapy followed by radical cystectomy is optimal therapy, with about 50% of patients cured.[60] In those elderly patients who are poor operative risks, radiation alone may provide successful palliation. Metastatic disease can be treated with cis-platinum or a cis-platinum combination, with clear benefit in about one half of patients.[61] There is a lower response rate to several other drugs including doxorubicin, cyclophosphamide, and 5-fluorouracil.

Carcinoma of the kidney. Removal of the primary cancer is the treatment of choice only if the tumor is localized or if the local complications of severe pain, bleeding, or infection make nephrectomy necessary. Radical nephrectomy is a hazardous procedure in geriatric patients. Although nephrectomy has been done for metastatic disease with subsequent regression of metastases, this procedure is discouraged because the mortality of the operation is greater than the likelihood of improvement. When these tumors invade blood vessels and then metastasize to lung and bone, systemic therapy is of little benefit. Progestins cause regression of pulmonary metastases in less than 10% of patients but are usually used first because of their low toxicity. Cytotoxic agents (vinblastine, nitrosoureas) can cause tumor regression in 20% of patients, but this regression usually lasts only several months.[62] An important part of treating patients with these tumors is managing a variety of paraneoplastic syndromes, including fever, amyloidosis, erythrocytosis, and hypercalcemia.

Gynecologic cancer

Ovarian cancer. Epithelial carcinomas of the

ovary are common in the elderly due to an exponential increase of incidence with age. Even in the elderly, laparotomy should always be considered the first step of therapy unless the tumor has metastasized outside of the abdomen. Not only is this necessary for staging and grading the tumor, but a successful "debulking" greatly enhances the response to chemotherapy.[63] Surgery consists of hysterectomy, bilateral salpingo-oophorectomy, omentectomy, resection of as much tumor as possible (so that no mass remains with a greater diameter than about 1.5 cm), and finally inspection of the undersurface of the diaphragm (a frequent site of metastatic involvement). Most patients present with Stage III disease (tumor confined to the abdomen). In patients with Stage III or IV disease, chemotherapy should be started after adequate wound healing from the laparotomy. Although aggressive therapy with such combinations as cis-platinum + doxorubicin + cyclophosphamide can produce remissions in the majority of patients and significantly prolong survival,[64] such a regimen requires good cardiac and renal function. In women who cannot tolerate such an intensive regimen, oral melphalan is a satisfactory treatment with low toxicity. In general, chemotherapy should be continued until the disease progresses or until a "second-look" laparotomy or laparoscopy demonstrates a complete remission. If the disease progresses during treatment with melphalan, responses can be obtained with such drugs as cis-platinum and hexamethylmelamine.

Endometrial cancer. Endometrial cancer is most likely in postmenopausal women and is commonly seen in the geriatric patient.[65] It typically develops in a setting of atypical adenomatous hyperplasia (adenocarcinoma of the endometrium in situ). High risk patients are women who are obese, nulliparous, or have hypertension, diabetes, or a positive family history of endometrial cancer. If the cancer is nonmetastatic, surgery or radiotherapy are used, depending on the stage of disease. Metastatic endometrial cancer in elderly patients is best treated first with a progestational agent.[66-68] Although the response rate is only around 20%, therapy is rather nontoxic and may produce good responses, particularly in women with well-differentiated tumors and a long disease-free interval between diagnosis of the primary tumor and appearance of metastases. Pulmonary metastases appear particularly responsive. Typical regimens include hydroxyprogesterone caproate, 1 mg intramuscularly twice weekly for at least 2 months, or megestrol acetate, 100 to 200 mg per day orally. If this is not effective, metastatic disease can often be controlled with the combination chemotherapy cyclophosphamide + 5-fluorouracil + methotrexate (CMF). Combinations using doxorubicin and cis-platinum are more effective but also are more toxic.

Carcinoma of the cervix. Carcinoma of the cervix is the third most common cancer in women and accounts for 50% of gynecologic cancer. A major effort should be made to detect it early with the PAP test. Limited surgery is reasonable for in situ tumors, but more extensive tumors are best treated with radiation therapy,[69] as long as they remain confined to the pelvis. Metastatic disease will occasionally respond to chemotherapy, but there is no established or effective regimen at this time.

Carcinoma of the lung

Bronchogenic cancer is the leading cause of cancer deaths in men, and it is increasingly common in women. Non-oat cell lung cancers (squamous cell carcinoma, adenocarcinoma, and undifferentiated large cell carcinoma) are remarkably refractory to current chemotherapy for palliation if the lesion is too extensive to be curable.[70]

Small cell undifferentiated lung cancer (oat cell cancer) accounts for 20% to 25% of lung cancer. It is a fast-growing cancer, spreading quickly to regional nodes and is hematogenously disseminating. Bone marrow involvement is present in 50% of patients and brain involvement in 10%. It is generally fatal within a few months unless treated aggressively with chemotherapy, and this should be done even in geriatric patients unless the patient is too debilitated to tolerate treatment.[71,72] Prior to treatment, these patients should be carefully staged with chest tomograms or CT scan, bone scan, liver scan, CT scan of brain, bone marrow biopsy, liver function tests, serum calcium tests, and electrolyte tests. Aggressive drug combinations such as CAV (doxorubicin + cyclophosphamide + vincristine) produce a response rate of 60% to 100%, with nearly half the patients having complete responses. At present the average length of survival in intensively treated patients is about 15 months when the tumor is confined to one hemithorax and about 10 months when tumor is metastatic.[73] However, an increasing proportion of patients are surviving over 2 years without recurrent tumor and may represent cures. Since about 40% of patients develop brain metastases during the course of their disease, prophylactic brain radiation has now become a standard part of the treatment program, and the incidence of brain metastases has been reduced to 7%.

Head and neck cancer

Squamous cell carcinoma of the upper respiratory and digestive system makes up about 90% of head and neck cancers. These cancers make up 7% of cancer in men and 2% of cancer in women. The most important risk factors for developing head and neck cancer are smoking and drinking alcohol. Stage, grade, and site are the most important prognostic features of these tumors. Patients tend to do better with cancers of the anterior tongue, lips, and larynx; cancers of the floor of the mouth, posterior tongue, and nasopharynx have a less favorable prognosis. All these cancers are treated with surgery, radiotherapy, or a combination of both, depending on the stage, grade, and site.[74] When recognized early and treated aggressively, the cure rate is impressive. Biopsy of the preinvasive lesions of leukoplakia and erythroplasia is always recommended.

Distant metastases are usually seen at a time when the cancer has recurred locally as well, or when patients have advanced local disease. It is possible to effectively palliate these tumors with chemotherapy, although responses are usually not very long-lasting. Methotrexate, cis-platinum, and bleomycin are the most effective chemotherapeutic agents currently available for palliation of these tumors.

Miscellaneous tumors

Nearly every variety of cancer can be treated with chemotherapy, including the many rare tumors which have not been discussed. Consultation with a medical oncologist is always advisable before concluding that no specific therapy is available for a mestastatic cancer or before embarking on any new treatment program.

REFERENCES

1. Morbidity from cancer in the United States, Public Health Service Pub. No. 590, Public Health Monograph No. 56, Washington, D.C., 1959, U.S. Government Printing Office.
2. American Cancer Society, Inc.: 1974 Cancer facts and figures, New York, 1974, The Society.
3. Leis, H.P., Jr., Mersheimer, W.L., and Hirose, T.: Breast cancer in the ninth and tenth decades, J. Am. Geriatr. Soc. **12**:527, 1964.
4. Ultmann, J.E., and Golomb, H.M.: Approach to diagnosis and management in oncology. In Thorn, G.W., et al., editors: Harrison's principles of internal medicine, ed. 8, New York, 1977, McGraw-Hill Book Co., pp. 1737-1745.
5. Bassett, L.W., and Steckel, R.J.: Imaging techniques in the detection of metastatic disease, Semin. Oncol. **4**:39, 1977.
6. Davis, D.O.: CT in the diagnosis of supratentorial tumors, Semin. Roentgenol. **12**:97, 1977.
7. Gerber, F.H., Goodreau, J.J., Kirchner, P.T., and Fouty, W.J.: Efficacy of preoperative and postoperative bone scanning in the management of breast carcinoma, N. Engl. J. Med. **297**:300, 1977.
8. American Cancer Society, Inc.: Cancer detection in the physician's office, New York, 1967, The Society.
9. Day, E.: Early detection of cancer as a control measure, CA **13**:2, 1963.
10. Williams, P.A.: A productive history and physical examination in the prevention and detection of early cancer, Cancer **47**:1146, 1981.
11. Radiation oncology, CA **26**:258, 1976.
12. Kaplan, H.S.: Radiotherapeutic advances in the treatment of neoplastic disease, Isr. J. Med. Sci. **13**:808, 1977.
13. Calabresi, P., and Parks, R.E., Jr.: Chemotherapy of neoplastic disease. In Goodman, L.S., and Gilman, A., editors: The pharmacological basis of therapeutics, ed. 6, New York, 1980, Macmillan Inc., pp. 1249-1314.
14. Chabner, B.A., Myers, C.E., Coleman, C.N., and Johns, D.G.: The clinical pharmacology of antineoplastic agents, N. Engl. J. Med. **292**:1107, 1159, 1975.
15. Plant, J.: Finding a home for hospice care in the United States, Hospitals **51**(13):53, 1977.
16. Dudrick, S.J., et al.: Parenteral nutrition techniques in cancer patients, Cancer Res. **37**:2440, 1977.
17. Copeland, E.M., III, Daly, J.M., and Dudrick, S.J.: Nutrition as an adjunct to cancer treatment in the adult, Cancer Res. **37**:2451, 1977.
18. Creagen, E.T., et al.: Vitamin C (ascorbic acid) therapy of preterminal cancer patients, Proceedings of the American Association for Cancer Research and American Society of Clinical Oncology **20**:355, 1979.
19. Moertel, C.G., et al.: A phase II trial of amygdalin (Laefrile) in the treatment of human cancer, Proceedings of the American Association for Cancer Research and American Society of Clinical Oncology **22**:383, 1981.
20. Catalano, R.B.: The medical approach to management of pain caused by cancer, Semin. Oncol. **2**:379, 1975.
21. Marks, R.M., and Sachar, E.J.: Undertreatment of medical inpatients with narcotic analgesics, Ann. Intern. Med. **78**:173, 1973.

22. Twycross, R.B.G.: Choice of strong analgesics in terminal cancer: diamorphine or morphine, Pain **3:**93, 1977.
23. Brogadir, S., et al.: Morbidity of staging laparotomy in Hodgkin's disease, Am. J. Med. **64:**429, 1978.
24. Young, R.C., Anderson, T., and DeVita, V.T.: The treatment of Hodgkin's disease: emphasizing programs at the Clinic Center, National Institutes of Health, Curr. Probl. Cancer **1**(7):1, 1977.
25. Kaplan, H.S.: Hodgkin's disease, ed. 2, Cambridge, Mass., 1980, Harvard University Press.
26. Glatstein, E.: Radiotherapy in Hodgkin's disease. Past achievements and future progress, Cancer **39**(Suppl.): 837, 1977.
27. Kaplan, H.S., and Rosenberg, S.A.: The management of Hodgkin's disease, Cancer **36**(Suppl.):796, 1975.
28. Braylan, R.C., Jaffe, E.S., and Berard, C.W.: Malignant lymphomas: current classification and new observations, Pathol. Annu. **10:**213, 1975.
29. Portlock, C.S.: Management of the indolent non-Hodgkin's lymphomas, Semin. Oncol. **1:**292, 1980.
30. Jones, S.E., et al.: Non-Hodgkin's lymphomas. IV. Clinicopathologic correlation in 405 cases, Cancer **31:**806, 1973.
31. Fisher, F.I., et al.: Prognostic factors for advanced diffuse histiocytic lymphoma following treatment with combination chemotherapy, Am. J. Med. **63:**177, 1977.
32. Special report: treatment of primary breast cancer, N. Engl. J. Med. **301:**340, 1979.
33. Fisher, B., and Gebhardt, M.C.: The evolution of breast cancer surgery: past, present, and future, Semin. Oncol. **5:**385, 1978.
34. Fisher, B.: Breast cancer management: alternatives to radical mastectomy, N. Engl. J. Med. **301:**326, 1979.
35. Harris, J.R., Levene, M.B., and Hellman, S.: The rule of radiation therapy in the primary treatment of carcinoma of the breast, Semin. Oncol. **5:**403, 1978.
36. Bonadonna, G., et al.: Are surgical adjuvant trials altering the course of breast cancer? Semin. Oncol. **5:**450, 1978.
37. Bonadonna, G., et al.: CMF adjuvant chemotherapy in operable breast cancer. In Salmon, S.E., and Jones, S.E., editors: Adjuvant therapy of cancer II, New York, 1979, Grune & Stratton, Inc., p. 227.
38. Legha, S.S., Davis, H.L., and Muggia, F.M.: Hormonal therapy of breast cancer: new approaches and concepts, Ann. Intern. Med. **88:**69, 1978.
39. McGuire, W.L., et al.: Hormones in breast cancer: update 1978, Metabolism **27:**487, 1978.
40. Tagnon, H.J.: Antiestrogens in treatment of breast cancer, Cancer **39**(Suppl.):2959, 1977.
41. Goldenberg, I.S., et al.: Androgenic therapy for advanced breast cancer in women: a report of the Cooperative Breast Cancer Group, J.A.M.A. **223:**1267, 1973.
42. Ratzowski, E., Adler, B., and Hochman, A.: Survival time and treatment results of patients with disseminated breast cancer especially after adrenalectomy and hypophysectomy, Oncology **28:**385, 1973.
43. Carbone, P.P., et al.: Chemotherapy of disseminated breast cancer: current status and prospects, Cancer **39**(Suppl.):2916, 1977.
44. Haskell, C.M., Sparks, F.C., Graze, P.R., and Korenman, S.G.: Systemic therapy for metastatic breast cancer, Ann. Intern. Med. **86:**68, 1977.
45. Gunderson, L.L.: Radiation therapy; results and future possibilities, Clin. Gastroenterol. **5:**743, 1976.
46. Zamcheck, N.: The present status of CEA in diagnosis, prognosis and evaluation of therapy, Cancer **36**(Suppl.): 2460, 1975.
47. Woolley, P.V., MacDonald, J.S., and Schein, P.S.: Chemotherapy of malignancies of the gastrointestinal tract, Prog. Gastroenterol. **3:**671, 1977.
48. Moertel, C.G.: Clinical management of advanced gastrointestinal cancer, Cancer **36**(Suppl.):675, 1975.
49. Moertel, C.G.: Therapy of advanced gastrointestinal cancer with the nitrosoureas, Cancer Chemother. Rep. **4:**27, 1973.
50. Schein, P.S., Kisner, D., and MacDonald, J.S.: Chemotherapy of large intestinal carcinoma: current results and future prospects, Cancer **36:**2418, 1975.
51. Jacobs, E.M., Luce, J.K., and Wood, D.A.: Treatment of cancer with weekly intravenous 5-fluorouracil, Cancer **22:**1233, 1968.
52. Murphy, G.P., editor: Carcinoma of the prostate, Semin. Oncol. **3:**101, 1976.
53. Franks, L.M.: Etiology, epidemiology, and pathology of prostatic cancer, Cancer **32:**1092, 1973.
54. Ray, G.R., Cassady, J.R., and Bagshaw, M.A.: Definitive radiation therapy of carcinoma of the prostate: a report on 15 years of experience, Radiology **106:**407, 1973.
55. Scott, W.W.: Rationale and results of primary endocrine therapy in patients with prostatic cancer, Cancer **32:**1119, 1973.
56. Byar, D.P.: The Veterans Administration Cooperative Urological Research Group's studies of cancer of the prostate, Cancer **32:**1126, 1973.
57. Carter, S.K., and Wasserman, T.H.: The chemotherapy of urologic cancer, Cancer **36**(Supple.):729, 1975.
58. Whitmore, W.F.: Surgical management of low stage bladder cancer, Semin. Oncol. **6:**207, 1979.
59. Koontz, W.W.: Intravesical chemotherapy and chemoprevention of superficial, low grade, low stage bladder carcinoma, Semin. Oncol. **6:**217, 1979.
60. Cummings, K.B., Shipley, W.U., Einstein, A.B., and Cutler, S.J.: Current concepts in the management of patients with deeply invasive bladder carcinoma, Semin. Oncol. **6:**220, 1979.
61. Yagoda, A., Watson, R.C., and Whitmore, W.: Cis-platinum (DDP) regimens in bladder cancer, Proceedings of the American Association for Cancer Research and the American Society of Clinical Oncology, 1979, p. 347.
62. Sufrin, G., and Murphy, G.P.: Renal adenocarcinoma, Urol. Surv. **30:**129, 1980.
63. Griffiths, C.T., Parker, S.M., and Fuller, A.F.: The role of cytoreductive surgical treatment in the management of advanced ovarian cancer, Cancer Treat. Rep. **63:**235, 1979.
64. Ehrlich, C.E., Einhorn, L., Williams, S.D., and Morgan, J.: Chemotherapy for Stage III-IV epithelial ovarian cancer with cis-dichlorodiammine platinum (11), Adriamycin, and cyclophosphamide: a preliminary report. Cancer Treat. Rep. **63:**281, 1979.
65. Di Saia, P.J., Morrow, C.P., and Townsend, D.E.: Synopsis of gynecologic oncology, New York, 1975, John Wiley & Sons, Inc.
66. Morrow, C.P., Di Saia, P.J., and Townsend, D.E.: Cur-

rent management of endometrial cancer, Obstet. Gynecol. **42**:399, 1973.
67. Wait, R.B.: Megestrol acetate in the management of advanced endometrial carcinoma, Obstet. Gynecol. **41**:129, 1973.
68. Reifenstein, E.C.: The treatment of advanced endometrial cancer with hydroxy-progesterone caproate, Gynecol. Oncol. **2**:377, 1974.
69. Brady, L.W.: Advances in the management of gynecologic cancer—radiation therapy, Cancer **36**:661, 1975.
70. Livingston, R.B.: Combination chemotherapy of bronchogenic carcinoma. I. Non-oat cell, Cancer Treat. Rev. **4**:153, 1977.
71. Williams, C.J., et al.: Treatment of oat-cell carcinoma of the lung—Stanford experience, 1972-1976, Salmon, S.E., and Jones, S.E., editors: The adjuvant therapy of cancer, New York, 1977, Elsevier North-Holland, Inc., p. 237.
72. Bunn, P.A., Jr., et al.: Advances in small cell bronchogenic carcinoma, Cancer Treat. Rep. **61**:333, 1977.
73. Livingston, R.B.: Combined modality approaches in lung cancer. In Salmon, S.E., and Jones, S.E., editors: Adjuvant therapy of cancer, New York, 1977, Elsevier North-Holland, Inc., p. 191.
74. Del Regato, J.A., and Spjut, J.J.: Cancer of the respiratory system and upper digestive tract. In del Regato, J.A., and Spjut, H.J.: Ackerman and del Regato's Cancer diagnosis, treatment, and prognosis, ed. 5, St. Louis, 1977, The C.V. Mosby Co., pp. 224-363.

CHAPTER 6 · CARDIOVASCULAR DISORDERS

Robert E. Kleiger

Since the last edition many advances in diagnostic and therapeutic procedures have become available for the care of cardiac disorders in the aged. Particularly noteworthy are improved diagnostic procedures using nuclear scanning, such as radionuclide ventriculograms[1] and thallium stress testing; the continued development of ultrasound, particularly cross-sectional or two-dimensional echocardiography[2]; the increased use of unloading agents, such as hydralazine hydrochloride, prazosin hydrochloride, and oral and sublingual nitrates, in the treatment of heart failure; and the improvement and increased use of cardiac surgery in elderly patients for both valvular and coronary disease.[1,3]

Since the geriatric patient may suffer from all the various heart diseases, including congenital heart disease, that occur in younger individuals and also may be subject to unique disorders associated with great age, it becomes a Herculean task to describe all the ailments of the heart to which elderly patients are susceptible, plus the significant diagnostic and therapeutic advances that have made therapy more rational in its quality.[4] Hence in this chapter I have attempted to discuss those conditions that occur most frequently in the geriatric patient, those which are unique to the aged, and those that, although important at all ages, are difficult to diagnose or treat in the elderly. Naturally such a selection must be arbitrary.

PATHOLOGY OF THE HEART

Pathologic studies of aged hearts have shown that virtually all cardiac lesions occurring in younger age groups occur in the elderly. Pomerance's autopsy findings on examination of 370 patients over the age of 75 years, 162 with congestive heart failure and 208 without,[5] was an excellent study of the aged heart.

Thirteen conditions were found in significant numbers. These included ischemic heart disease, hypertension, rheumatic heart disease, cor pulmonale, syphilitic heart disease, bacterial endocarditis, calcific aortic stenosis, nonbacterial "marantic" endocarditis, calcification of the mitral annulus, aortic cusp calcification, mucoid degeneration of the atrioventricular valves, postinflammatory valvular thickening, and senile amyloidosis.

Ischemic heart disease was the most common condition in the patients, with congestive heart failure occurring in 48%, but it also occurred in 18% of the non-failure group. Over the age of 90 the incidence of ischemic disease fell. In the failure group, acute infarction was common.

Calcific valvular degenerative changes were almost as common as ischemic heart disease (45%) in the congestive heart failure group and was the most common pathologic lesion in the nonfailure group.

Hypertensive heart disease, with blood pressures greater than 210/110 mm Hg, occurred in 35% of patients with congestive heart failure and 11% of those without. The incidence of hypertension increased with age until 90 years and then decreased sharply.

Calcific aortic stenosis was found in 9% of patients with congestive heart failure, senile amyloidosis in 18%, cor pulmonale in 9%, and rheumatic heart disease in 8%. Six percent of patients with failure had nonspecific inflammatory changes of the mitral valve, and the same percentage had mucoid or myxomatous valvular degeneration. The incidence of these abnormalities increased with age.

Comparison of the group with congestive heart failure to the nonfailure group not only showed a much higher incidence of the preceding abnormalities but also the failure group usually had more than one cardiac abnormality, multiple abnormalities occurring in 65% of the patients with heart failure. Heart failure without apparent cause, so-called "senile myocardial degeneration" or presbycardia, occurred in only 2.5% of cases.

Another excellent study on the pathology of the aging heart was performed by Sugiura et al.[6] They studied 1000 consecutive cases aged 56 to 99 years, with an average age of 76 years in men and 80 years in women. Eighty-three percent of the patients were between ages 70 and 89. Of the 657 patients that showed cardiac abnormalities, the average number of disorders per patient was 1.6. There were 428 cases of coronary arterial narrowing with 137 patients exhibiting infarction. Over 10% of the cases showed valvular disease. Even at the ages studied by these authors there were eight cases of rheumatic mitral valve disease. Other valvular lesions included 37 cases of mitral insufficiency, 12 cases of calcified aortic stenosis, 26 cases of syphilitic aortic regurgitation, and 35 cases of degenerative aortic regurgitation. Congestive heart failure was frequently found in the rheumatic and syphilitic patients.

Forty-one patients had chronic cor pulmonale with right ventricular hypertrophy (RVH). Fifty-nine patients had conduction disturbances secondary to degenerative changes.

There were 237 cases of left ventricular hypertrophy (LVH), most often related to hypertension. Unlike Pomerance's study, senile cardiac amyloidosis was not found. The authors concluded that heart disease in old age could be divided into two broad categories, those found in younger individuals as well as older individuals, such as congenital, hypertensive, ischemic, rheumatic, and syphilitic heart disease, and those diseases peculiar to old age, such as mitral ring calcification and dilatation, ruptured chordae tendineae, calcific aortic stenosis, degenerative aortic regurgitation, and high grade conduction disturbances secondary to fibrosis or degeneration of the conduction system.

ELECTROCARDIOGRAPHIC (ECG) CHANGES IN THE ELDERLY

Several studies have confirmed that the incidence of ECG abnormalities increases with age. Campbell et al.[7] studied the ECGs of 2254 people aged 65 or over. Sixty-two percent showed no significant abnormality. Q-QS patterns were seen in 6%, twice as frequently in men as in women. ST-T abnormalities were found in 8% of patients, LVH in 9%. Both of these abnormalities were more frequent in women than in men. There was a 1.4% to 2% incidence of conduction defects, such as left bundle branch block (LBBB), right bundle branch block (RBBB), left anterior hemiblock (LAHB) and incomplete RBBB. Atrial fibrillation occurred in 2% of patients under 75 years old, and in 5% over 75 years old. Forty percent of cases showed no codable abnormalities. This frequency decreased sharply to 26% in those over age 75. Twenty-two percent of the patients' records noted minor abnormalities, defined as left axis deviation without LAHB, counterclockwise rotation, clockwise rotation, sinus tachycardia, or sinus bradycardia. Probable LVH was seen in 10% of women over age 75. RVH was seen in only 16 patients, 11 of them men, and all had chronic pulmonary disease. The only arrhythmias commonly observed were frequent ectopic beats and atrial fibrillation. In a companion paper assessing the significance of these findings, Caird et al.[8] studied the 3-year mortality of these 2254 patients. They found that the approximately 1400 patients with no or minor ECG abnormalities had significantly decreased morbidity and mortality compared to those with abnormal ECGs. The average mortality was 2.32 times the expected for Q-QS patterns, probable LVH, major ST-T pattern abnormalities, LBBB, and RBBB. In those patients who died, the percentage of cardiac deaths was 28% in those with no significant ECG abnormalities versus 56% in those with ECG abnormalities.

Mihalick and Fisch[9] studied the ECGs of 671 subjects over 70 years old. Compared to the age group under 70, they found an increase in first degree atrioventricular block; bundle branch block; ST-T wave abnormalities; premature systoles, both atrial and ventricular; left anterior hemiblock; LVH; and atrial fibrillation. In their study the abnormalities that were strongly correlated with cardiac disease were atrial fibrillation, LBBB, and nonspecific intraventricular conduction defect. Q or QS complexes in the precordial leads were not correlated with cardiac disease in their study. ST and T abnormalities in their study were related to digitalis administration rather than cardiac disease. In their study, as in the reports of Campbell et al.[7] and Caird et al.[8] the incidence of left axis deviation increased with age but did not correlate with cardiac disease. Other studies suggest that isolated RBBB is not associated with cardiac disease or increased mortality but that RBBB with LAHB are.

CONGESTIVE HEART FAILURE AND PULMONARY EDEMA

As already stated, congestive heart failure in the elderly patient may have diverse etiologies. The therapy for congestive heart failure is directed toward correcting the salt and water retention and the elevated right- and left-sided filling pressures associated with heart failure. Salt-restricted diets are an invaluable asset in controlling chronic congestive failure. Powerful diuretics, particularly furosemide and ethacrynic acid, are useful in mobilizing refractory edema in severe heart failure, but they and less powerful diuretics are not replacements for salt-restricted diets but are adjuncts to therapy. A careful dietary history should be obtained from the patient with heart failure, and excessive sources of sodium should be eliminated from the diet. Clinical consultation with a dietician who carefully explains the diet to the patient is invaluable. The dietician can also suggest methods of cooking and seasoning to make the salt-restricted diet more palatable. Supplementary diuretics may be of great use as well.[10] Generally in ambulatory patients less powerful diuretics of the thiazide class should be used. Intermittent therapy based on sudden weight gain or edema formation is less likely to produce adverse effects, such as hypokalemia, hyperuricemia, and abnormal glucose tolerance, than daily therapy. Efforts to increase left ventricular performance in the patient with chronic heart failure require careful administration of cardiac glycosides. A proper dose based both on clinical effect and serum level is desired. When both diuretics and digitalis are administered jointly, electrolytes and blood urea nitrogen should be measured periodically, since both hypokalemia and azotemia secondary to diuretic usage may induce digitalis intoxication.

It has been found that quinidine and other antiarrhythmic drugs interfere with digitalis metabolism, probably by decreasing renal clearance. Thus the addition of quinidine and similar drugs will increase serum digoxin levels and may precipitate digitalis intoxication. Such patients should have their digitalis therapy assessed frequently and also have frequent measurements taken of their serum digoxin levels.

It is also true that the therapeutic/toxic ratio of cardiac glycosides decreases with age and the extent of cardiac disease. This ratio is also decreased by severe pulmonary disease.

Severe heart failure requires hospitalization. Beside bed rest and the administration of diuretics and digitalis, other measures that may be useful are anticoagulation and the use of unloading therapy, such as intravenous administration of nitroprusside or nitroglycerin.[3,11] Unloading therapy may also be used in conjunction with potent inotropic agents like dopamine and dobutamine.

The patient with severe heart failure who is on a regimen of bed rest runs a high risk of pulmonary embolization. Furthermore, refractory severe failure can be induced by pulmonary emboli in the presence of preexistent heart disease, thus the rationale for anticoagulation. Nitroprusside or nitroglycerin administered intravenously lowers blood pressure and decreases venous return to the right side of the heart. These effects unload the left ventricle and may result in a dramatic increase in cardiac output and a fall in left and right atrial pressures with a dramatic clearing of refractory failure.[12] Such therapy requires careful monitoring of both blood pressure, pulmonary capillary wedge pressure, and cardiac output and is best done in an intensive care unit.

Pulmonary edema secondary to heart failure occurs when left atrial pressure rises to such levels that pulmonary capillary pressure exceeds that of the oncotic pressure of plasma proteins, and fluid exudes out of the capillaries first into the interstitium of the lung and thence into the alveoli interfering with oxygen transport, thus producing hypoxia and also decreasing lung compliance. Therapy is directed toward correcting hypoxia, reducing the work of ventilation, and lowering pulmonary venous pressure. Useful measures are administration of oxygen; morphine sulfate, in relatively small doses; furosemide, 40 to 80 mg administered intravenously; phlebotomy; tourniquets; or sublingual nitroglycerin. The latter three decrease right-side return and reduce flow to the lungs.

Intravenous nitroglycerin administration also reduces arterial blood pressure and thus helps the left ventricle to empty better with the beneficial result of lowering pulmonary venous pressure. Blood gases should be determined in the patient with pulmonary edema. If the P_{CO_2} is elevated, indicating hypoventilation, and the respiratory rate is greater than 40 times a minute, the patient's larynx and trachea should be intubated and the patient mechanically ventilated to achieve better blood gas values. Usually blood gas determinations in pulmonary edema show hypoxia, with P_{O_2} less than 60 mm Hg and hypocarbia secondary to the hyperventilation caused by hypoxia. The abrupt appearance of pulmonary edema in elderly patients may indicate acute myocardial infarction, and these patients should be admitted to intensive care units and receive careful ECG monitoring.

In the patient with congestive heart failure or in the patient who has recovered from acute pulmonary edema, chronic unloading therapy may be extremely useful in controlling heart failure. Agents like hydralazine hydrochloride, which reduce afterload by decreasing peripheral arterial resistance, will decrease the impedance to left ventricular outflow and increase cardiac output. Oral, sublingual, and topical nitrates that reduce the preload by increasing venous capacitance will lower left ventricular filling pressure and decrease congestion but usually will not increase the cardiac index, although they reduce myocardial work and myocardial oxygen demand. Often combined preload and afterload reduction is desirable. This can be accomplished with administration of nitrates and hydralazine hydrochloride or prazosin hydrochloride, which has both preload and afterload reducing abilities.[1] Another agent with potent unloading abilities is captopril. It may work when other agents have failed but should be used cautiously because of its side effects.

ARTERIOSCLEROTIC HEART DISEASE

Arteriosclerotic heart disease is the most frequently encountered single etiologic cause of heart disease in the patient over 60 years of age. The manifestations of arteriosclerotic heart disease in the elderly are essentially the same as those in younger patients: acute myocardial infarction, angina pectoris, arrhythmias, congestive heart failure, and sudden death.

However, in older patients the presentation of these complications is often atypical. Angina may be perceived as shortness of breath, extreme fatigue, or as faintness or syncope. Acute myocardial infarction is more often silent, particularly in the diabetic, and may appear without pain but with the sudden development of severe heart failure, stroke, and malignant arrhythmias. In some cases the infarction is discovered only by routine electrocardiography. In other cases myocardial infarction may be similar in presentation, clinical features, and therapy to that in the younger patient; however, there is a significantly increased mortality of patients over 60 years of age, a higher incidence of anterior infarction, and complications such as cardiogenic shock, pulmonary edema, and congestive heart failure. Serious arrhythmias, such as complete heart block or bifascicular block also occur with increased frequency. Late mortality, occurring after the first 5 days, from complications of renal failure, sepsis, and both pulmonary and systemic embolization are more common in the elderly. Despite these adverse effects, the majority of patients over 60 years of age who enter the hospital with acute myocardial infarction survive and do well.[13]

Special efforts should be made to prevent sensory deprivation, depression, and deconditioning of reflexes. A bed-chair regimen and the use of bedside commodes or bathroom privileges rather than bedpans improves morale. Most patients can feed themselves, and this helps to avoid unnecessary dependency feelings. The complications of arrhythmias, congestive heart failure, and shock are treated no differently in the elderly patient than in the younger patient with infarction. Age per se does not militate against acute surgical therapy for those complications of acute myocardial infarction that demand prompt surgical intervention, such as papillary muscle rupture and ventricular septal defect with severe failure or hypotension. After discharge from the hospital the patient frequently will be able to resume normal activity. Moderate physical exertion, which does not produce either angina or increase failure or fatigue, is not only permissible but is probably desirable both in terms of morale and overall function. Such therapy may also promote collateral circulation.

Angina pectoris in the patient over 60 years of age is common.[14] Classic angina may either occur before or after acute infarction. Classically the pain or distress will be retrosternal, brought on by exertion, emotional stress, anger, cold, and after meals. The diagnosis should be made with care, since chest discomfort similar to angina can occur with many diverse conditions including hiatal hernia, ulcer, gallbladder disease, esophagitis, and local chest wall pain. An electrocardiogram recorded during pain showing ST depression is useful. Sometimes Holter monitoring can establish that atypical pain is associated with striking changes in the ECG. Carotid sinus massage by reducing blood pressure and heart rate decreases myocardial oxygen demand and thus will often relieve angina. Chest pain abrogated by this maneuver virtually establishes the diagnosis. Finally if clinical history and simple tests fail to establish with certainty the diagnosis of arteriosclerotic heart disease and angina, stress testing, thallium stress testing, and coronary angiography may be performed. Although these tests have an inherent risk, they can be performed with remarkable safety in a geriatric population.

Medical therapy of angina is symptomatic. It is directed at decreasing the myocardial demand for oxygen, which is closely related to heart rate, blood pressure, ventricular size, duration of systolic ejection, and contractility. When angina is provoked by cold, large meals, undue exertion, and emotional upset, general measures such as avoidance of stress, sedation, and multiple small meals rather than large repasts are useful. The most useful single medicine is, of course, nitroglycerin given sublingually. Nitrites lower blood pressure by decreasing arterial resistance and reducing venous tone. By lowering blood pressure, concomitantly decreasing venous return and heart size, and shortening the systolic ejection period nitroglycerin greatly reduces myocardial oxygen demand. Some of this favorable effect, however, may be negated by reflex increases in heart rate and contractility induced by lowered blood pressure. Another possible mechanism by which nitroglycerin may aid in relieving angina is by dilatation of collateral coronary vessels. The patient must be instructed concerning how to take nitroglycerin. It is most effective when taken early in the onset of angina and often can be taken prophylactically before activities that are likely to produce pain in a given patient. Patients should be advised that they may feel a fullness in the head or even a headache after nitroglycerin administration but that this generally will abate with time. It must be emphasized to patients that nitroglycerin is not a dangerous drug and also that if chest pain is not relieved promptly by three nitroglycerin tablets and the pain lasts longer than 15 to 20 minutes, the physician should be called. Long-acting nitrites may be used to supplement basic nitroglycerin therapy. This is still somewhat controversial, since nitrites given orally are often poorly absorbed and their effects are uncertain. Certainly they should never be used alone for the treatment of angina. Sublingual isosorbide dinitrite in 5 mg doses seems to be the most effective long-acting agent. Another long-acting nitrite that has been proved to have therapeutic effects is nitrol ointment; this may be particularly useful in relieving nocturnal pain.

A useful adjunct to medical therapy for angina is propranolol, a beta-adrenergic blocking agent. Propranolol decreases myocardial oxygen demand by reducing contractility, slowing heart rate, and in some cases decreasing blood pressure. On the other hand, it tends to increase ventricular size and prolongs the duration of systolic ejection. It can readily be seen that propranolol and nitroglycerin have synergistic effects; the increased heart rate and contractility associated with nitrites is blocked by propranolol; conversely the increased ventricular size and duration of systolic ejection elicited by propranolol are blocked by nitrites. When propranolol is given for angina, it should be administered in increasing doses until a resting heart rate near 60 beats a minute or significant reduction in angina is achieved. Unfortunately propranolol may induce severe heart failure by its negative inotropic effect, and particularly in the elderly it may produce severe bradycardia or marked exertional fatigue, even with small doses. When angina is accompanied by congestive heart failure, treatment with digitalis and diuretics often improves the angina. Other beta-blockers such as nadolol may also be used.

The calcium antagonists verapamil and nifedipine are also useful agents in treating both Prinzmetal's angina due to coronary vasospasm and ordinary stress induced angina. They are potent coronary as well as peripheral vasodilators and also reduce cardiac contractility.

Medical therapy for angina is successful in the great majority of cases; however, in those cases in which optimal medical care has failed and angina intolerable to the patient continues, surgical therapy should be considered. It is now clear that revascularization procedures using saphenous vein or internal mammary artery can relieve angina in a high percentage of cases, will improve exercise tolerance and quality of life, and can be performed with an extremely low surgical mortality, less than 1%, even in patients in the geriatric age group if their coronary artery anatomy and ventricular function is suitable and there are no other major illnesses. Whether survival is prolonged with these procedures remains moot.

Recent surgical reports of bypass surgery in the patient over 70 years old show a mortality of less than 1% if left ventricular function is normal.[15] Again this procedure should be reserved for those elderly patients whose symptoms remain unbearable despite optimal medical therapy with nitrates and β blockers. However, in these cases the beneficial results of bypass surgery are often striking.

Another invasive procedure used to relieve angina is transcoronary angioplasty.

HYPERTENSIVE CARDIOVASCULAR DISEASE

As previously noted, a significant number of patients over the age of 60 years have hypertension. It is estimated that as many as 25% of people in this age group have high blood pressure, defined as diastolic pressure greater than 100 mm Hg. However, it must be emphasized that blood pressure levels tend to increase with age and that effects on morbidity and mortality of elevated blood pressure decrease as the age of onset of hypertension increases. Particularly in elderly white women elevated blood pressure is extraordinarily well tolerated. From the practical point of view therapy is probably not desirable, unless the diastolic blood pressure on repeated measurement is greater than 110 mm Hg. Systolic hypertension alone, with blood pressure less than 180 mm Hg, should not be treated, although there is evidence that systolic hypertension is associated with increased risk of cerebrovascular accident. Attempts at reducing systolic blood pressure when diastolic pressure is normal may result in extremely low diastolic pressures and resultant syncope, angina, or decreased renal perfusion. Furthermore, at present there is no good evidence for a beneficial effect of lowering systolic pressure in these patients.

Therapy for significant hypertension in the elderly is basically the same as that for younger patients. For mild to moderate hypertension a thiazide diuretic and sedation will often suffice. Although reserpine has been used with great success, its side effects of depression, appetite increase, nasal stuffiness, and other effects make it a less than desirable agent. More potent antihypertensive agents such as methyldopa (Aldomet) or hydralazine (Apresoline hydrochloride) may be required. The former may induce significant postural hypotension, and the latter by increasing cardiac work may provoke significant angina. Truly potent antihypertensive agents such as guanethidine or other ganglionic blocking agents are rarely necessary in the elderly hypertensive patient and are almost certain to produce significant unpleasant side effects.

Beta-blockers such as propranolol, nadolol, and metaprolol have proved to be successful antihypertensive agents. The mechanism of action is unknown, but these agents do lower renin levels. They may be used jointly with other antihypertensive agents, particularly diuretics. The contraindications for their use are the same as for angina, significant heart failure and/or bronchospasm.

The patient receiving antihypertensive therapy should be seen periodically to determine the effectiveness of blood pressure control, side effects of the drug, and the development of electrolyte imbalance or azotemia secondary to therapy. Again it must be emphasized that benefits of therapy in the aged are more difficult to ascertain than in younger patients, and side effects are more frequent.[16]

VALVULAR DISEASE

The kinds of valvular disease that occur in elderly patients include those that occur in younger patients as well as those that are unique to the geriatric population, such as calcification of the mitral annulus and the aortic cusps or ring and myxomatous degeneration of the mitral valve leaflets. Rheumatic heart disease also occurs in a significant proportion of geriatric patients. All valvular lesions, aortic stenosis, aortic insufficiency, mitral stenosis, mitral insufficiency, and combinations occur in the elderly. By and large the two most important lesions are aortic stenosis and mitral insufficiency. Aortic stenosis in the elderly occurs as the result of calcification of the aortic valve cusps or ring, sometimes as an idiopathic process and sometimes as a result of degeneration and fibrosis in a congenitally abnormal valve or one damaged by rheumatic or hypertensive disease processes. Finegan et al.[17] reported 78 cases of severe aortic stenosis in patients over the age of 60 years who underwent surgery at Stanford University Hospital. There was little to differentiate these patients and younger individuals with aortic stenosis except that the elderly patients tend to have wider pulse pressures than younger patients, although the upstroke time was still delayed. A high percentage of the elderly patients, 91%, had congestive heart failure, 55% had angina, and only 21% had syncope. Calcification of the aortic valve on plain x-ray film was common and usually associated with severe stenosis, but its absence did not preclude severe aortic stenosis. ECGs were uniformly abnormal, the most common abnormality being that of left ventricular hypertrophy. X-ray examination usually showed left ventricular hypertrophy and calcification in the aortic valve. The definitive diagnostic test was, of course, left ventricular catheterization. Operative mortality was 11.5%, and long-term follow-up established a favorable prognosis and improvement in symptoms in the surviving group.

Since Finegan's report there are now increasing reports in the literature that demonstrate even better short- and long-term survival after aortic valve replacement in the elderly.[15]

Severe mitral insufficiency in the geriatric age group can result from mucoid degeneration of the mitral valve, calcification of the annulus, ruptured chordae tendineae, or severe papillary muscle dysfunction. The patient will often have severe right- and left-sided heart failure of rather sudden or subacute onset, evidence of pulmonary hypertension, and a loud apical systolic murmur, which may radiate widely even into the neck and sometimes be confused with an aortic murmur. Echocardiography and left heart catheterization with angiography are the diagnostic measures of greatest utility. When angiography shows reasonable left ventricular performance and massive mitral insufficiency, surgery is indicated. Two notable patients of mine, one a 69-year-old woman with atrial septal defect and the other a 75-year-old man with coronary artery disease, had severe heart failure secondary to ruptured chordae tendineae. Both responded well to mitral valve replacement, the woman to closure of the atrial septal defect, and the man to saphenous vein bypass graft to the left anterior descending coronary artery. In both, previously refractory severe heart failure with pulmonary edema and low cardiac output was now correctable.

CONGENITAL HEART DISEASE

It may seem strange to discuss congenital heart disease in a geriatric population, since most congenital heart disease greatly shortens life or occurs much earlier in life. However, atrial septal defect of the ostium secundum type can occur late in life and often produces a confusing clinical picture. The elderly patient with an atrial septal defect may have severe right-sided congestive heart failure, often with marked ascites. This occurs because with age the compliance of the left ventricle decreases and hence filling pressure of the left atrium is increased. Since in a large atrial septal defect there is in essence a common atrium, the pressure is immediately transmitted to the right side, and severe right-sided failure may occur. Another common presentation is by supraventricular arrhythmias, particularly atrial flutter and atrial fibrillation, with signs of failure. On physical examination there is a systolic ejection murmur along the left sternal border at the third intercostal space, there may be a diastolic rumble of relative tricuspid stenosis, and there is fixed splitting of the second heart sound. The ECG will show an incomplete right bundle branch block with a normal or right axis. Echocardiography shows a large right ventricle and often paradoxical motion of the interventricular septum. Definitive study requires cardiac catheterization. The indications for surgery are the same as those for a younger age group: a left-to-right shunt ratio greater than 2:1 in the absence of severe pulmonary hypertension. Although the risk of operating for an atrial septal defect increases with age over 60 years, the risk is less than 5% and the results of surgical therapy and clinical improvement are better than those for medical treatment.

IDIOPATHIC HYPERTROPHIC SUBAORTIC STENOSIS

Idiopathic hypertrophic subaortic stenosis (IHSS) probably represents a congenital defect of heart development with abnormal hypertrophy and disorganization of septal fibers, producing a thick and extremely akinetic septum. Despite the fact that this entity is congenital, it not infrequently occurs first in the geriatric age group. Over the last 2 years I have seen six elderly women ranging in age from 60 to 74 years with IHSS. The condition was not initially diagnosed correctly in any of them. The clinical symptomatology of IHSS in the elderly is entirely similar to that in younger individuals. The most common complaints are chest pain, anginal in quality, and palpitations. Two of our patients had atrial fibrillation. Other complaints may include syncope and symptoms of failure, breathlessness on exertion without overt failure, and fatigue. The angina-like pain is often long lasting and responds poorly to nitroglycerin.

Whiting et al.[18] reported that approximately one third of patients with IHSS studied at the Massachusetts General Hospital were over 60 years of age. Interestingly, they showed a significant increase in the female-male sex ratio in the geriatric patients, whereas in patients under the age of 60 years, sex ratios were equal. Although over 50% of patients with IHSS had a correct diagnosis made before cardiac catheterization, this was true for only one third of the geriatric patients. Unlike the younger patients, the older patients sometimes had diastolic blowing murmurs and also occasionally had calcification of the aortic valve. Clinical clues to the diagnosis included a variable ejection murmur, usually loudest at the apex and lower left sternal border, an S-4 gallop when the heart was in sinus rhythm, a brisk initial carotid upstroke, a carotid pulse with double contour, as well as a prominent and often duplicated apical impulse. The murmur classically will increase when standing, during the Valsalva maneuver, and after inhalation of amyl nitrite. Electrocardiographically there is often significant left ventricular hypertrophy. Whenever a patient over 60 years of age, especially if female, has a variable murmur, ejection in quality, increased by amyl nitrite inhalation, unexplained left ventricular hypertrophy that can be observed either electrocardiographically or radiographically, and palpitations, dyspnea, chest pain, or heart failure, the diagnosis of IHSS must be strongly considered. The most definitive noninvasive test to establish the diagnosis is cross-sectional echocardiography. When positive, a thick akinetic septum much thicker than the left ventricular posterior wall will be seen, as well as systolic narrowing of the outflow tract by a significant systolic bulging of the anterior leaflet of the mitral valve toward the thickened septum.[19] The left ventricular chamber is small with an increased ejection fraction. Echocardiography has reduced the necessity of invasive cardiac catheterization procedures in these patients, although the exact gradient across the functional obstruction below the aortic valve can only be measured by left ventricular catheterization. The most frequent misdiagnosis of IHSS in the elderly is coronary artery disease, but sometimes the possibility of mitral insufficiency or valvular aortic stenosis is entertained.

It is important to diagnose this condition correctly, since functional aortic obstruction is worsened by any agent that increases contractility, decreases ventricular size, or reduces arterial pressure. Digitalis and nitroglycerin, which are often administered erroneously to these patients, will of course worsen the gradient and often produce adverse clinical effects. The most effective medical therapy is propranolol, usually in sizable doses of 160 to 200 mg daily, which decreases contractility, slows the heart rate, and increases ventricular size. There is some evidence that propranolol also improves compliance of the left ventricle. The compliance of these thick hypertrophied ventricles is invariably reduced. Because of the diminished compliance, atrial systole plays an important role in filling the left ventricle. When these patients develop atrial fibrillation, their hemodynamic status may rapidly deteriorate, and they may develop severe heart failure, chest pain, and hypotension. Prompt cardioversion is probably the therapy of choice. Most patients with IHSS do well and have a good prognosis, although chest pain, syncope, and palpitations may be troublesome and there is occasional sudden death. Most conditions are managed well by propranolol therapy, and only the most severe cases require surgical intervention. This is especially uncommon in the elderly patient.

BACTERIAL ENDOCARDITIS

Bacterial endocarditis in the elderly presents a significant problem in diagnosis and therapy. In a review by Thell[20] of endocarditis in patients over 60 years of age the following features were pointed out. The clinical diagnosis of endocarditis was made in only 38% of patients. The lack of clinical suspicion occurred because of the paucity of clinical findings other than fever. Only about two thirds of the patients had significant murmurs. Embolic phenomena, large spleens, and splinter hemorrhages occurred rarely until late in the disease. Almost 40% of the patients had no significant murmurs. About one third of the patients did not have evidence of preexisting valvular disease. Left-sided endocarditis predominated, with the aortic valve the most commonly involved valve. Right-sided endocarditis involved the tricuspid valve. Preexisting conditions included rheumatic valvulitis, calcific aortic valvular disease, and biscuspid aortic valve. Infectious organisms were diverse with a high incidence of staphylococcus and fungal infections. Prolonged fever, signs of neurologic dysfunction, associated with sudden congestive heart failure with or without heart murmur should alert the physician to the possibility of bacterial endocarditis in the aged. With right-sided involvement the clinical course is usually characterized by fever and recurrent multiple pulmonary infiltrates. Even when diagnosed correctly and treated with appropriate antibiotic therapy, the prognosis is poor. Without correct diagnosis the course is almost invariably fatal, although rare self-cures have been noted.

SENILE CARDIAC AMYLOIDOSIS

Senile cardiac amyloidosis seems to be an important cause of heart failure in the elderly. In a study by Pomerance,[21] 10% of patients over the age of 80 years had detectable amyloid deposits in the heart. Microscopically this could be recognized by nodules of amyloid in the atrial endocardium. Nearly 50% of patients over the age of 90 years showed amyloid deposits. One half of the patients at autopsy had a history of congestive heart failure. The clinical diagnosis is difficult to make, since the amyloid deposits are localized to the heart but may be suspected whenever an elderly patient develops congestive failure with no clear-cut cardiac disorder. The heart is usually only moderately enlarged. There are frequently both atrial and ventricular arrhythmias. The ECG is nonspecific, but several authors have noted the increased incidence of low voltage tracings. Patients with senile cardiac amyloidosis are exquisitely sensitive to cardiac glycosides and should not be treated with them. Congestive heart failure is best treated in these patients with salt-restricted diets and diuretics. Echocardiography is useful in diagnosing this condition. It shows a small left ventricular chamber with thick walls. The right ventricle may also be thick. Contractility of the heart may be normal or reduced.

ARRHYTHMIAS

Tachyarrhythmias and extrasystoles increase with age. Their therapy is essentially the same as that in younger age groups; however, a few comments may be made. Tachyarrhythmias such as ventricular tachycardia, atrial fibrillation, atrial flutter, and some supraventricular tachycardias that produce life-threatening cardiac dysfunction should be promptly terminated by cardioversion. Ventricular tachycardia that is established and in which the heart rate is greater than 125 beats a minute but is well tolerated by the patient can be treated with intravenous lidocaine, but if the tachycardia fails to revert, cardioversion should be done. Paroxysmal ventricular tachycardia in the elderly patient is most often caused by coronary artery disease, often with ventricular aneurysm. Surgical removal of the ventricular aneurysm will sometimes abrogate the episodes of ventricular tachycardia.

Ventricular extrasystoles in the elderly, unless the patient is symptomatic, should probably be left alone, since effective antiarrhythmic therapy is difficult to maintain and the present antiarrhythmic agents frequently produce adverse side effects. Procaine amide may cause gastrointestinal upset and lupuslike syndrome; quinidine may cause cinchonism, syncope, rarely thrombocytopenia, or sudden death; phenytoin may give rise to lethargy, confusion, ataxia, blood dyscrasias, and other adverse reactions. When, however, it is decided to use any of these three drugs for symptomatic extrasystoles, serum levels should be measured to ensure that the use of the drug is rational and that drug levels remain in the therapeutic range. Procaine amide, for example, is primarily excreted renally, and it is easy to produce toxic levels of this agent in elderly patients with some renal impairment. New antiarrhythmic agents such as disopyramide are now available, and other agents are under investigation.

Atrial extrasystoles, again if not symptomatic, are best left untreated. When the condition is symptomatic, cardiac glycosides, quinidine, or propranolol alone or in combination are useful. Unless atrial fibrillation in the elderly patient is life threatening or associated with refractory failure, reversion to normal sinus rhythm should not be attempted, since maintenance of normal sinus rhythm in geriatric patients is generally disappointing. Rather, these patients should receive digitalization therapy to control ventricular response. Particularly in the elderly patient with long-standing atrial fibrillation or with a controlled ventricular response no attempt should be made to revert to sinus rhythm.

Atrial flutter on the other hand, which is difficult to control with digitalization and often produces a rapid ventricular response, should be reverted to sinus rhythm if possible. If, despite reversion, it recurs, a combination of propranolol and digitalis therapy will often succeed in controlling ventricular response. Acute atrial fibrillation or flutter with rapid ventricular response in which the patient is only moderately symptomatic can often be treated effectively and reverted to sinus rhythm by infusion of 1 to 3 mg of propranolol over 3 to 10 minutes. The blood pressure and electrocardiogram should be carefully monitored during this therapy. Alternatively, digoxin may be given orally or intravenously with the endpoint being control of ventricular response.

Lastly, when an elderly patient develops a paroxysmal supraventricular tachycardia, the patient should have appropriate tests to determine the presence of occult pulmonary embolization, masked hyperthyroidism, or silent mitral stenosis, since these are frequently unrecognized causes of paroxysmal atrial tachyarrhythmias in the elderly patient.

CONDUCTION DISTURBANCES

Conduction disturbances in the aged are frequent occurrences. The conducting system diseases may manifest themselves either in the proximal portions of the conducting system (proximal to the bundle of His) more distally or diffusely throughout the conducting system. When a disturbance in conduction produces excessive bradycardia or results in rapid escape rhythms, such as ventricular tachycardia or transient ventricular fibrillation, symptoms will occur. These most frequently consist of transient weakness or fainting spells, but actual seizure or strokelike episodes may occur—classic Adams-Stokes attacks. The most frequent cause of high-grade atrioventricular block in adults is so-called Lenègre's disease, idiopathic fibrosis, and sclerosis of the conducting system. Another common cause of chronic heart block, particularly in patients over the age of 70 years, is so-called Lev's disease, which consists of calcification of either the mitral or aortic valve with extension of the calcium into the conducting system. Acute and sometimes chronic heart block may also be secondary to arteriosclerotic heart disease, particularly with acute infarction.

Pathophysiologically, most often high-grade atrioventricular block in geriatric patients is caused by a conduction disturbance distal to the bundle of His. Thus, even when the heart is in normal sinus rhythm, that is, when the complete heart block is intermittent or when AV block is present but not complete, the conducted beats are likely to show intraventricular conduction defect, such as right bundle-branch block, left bundle-branch block, or left anterior or posterior hemiblock associated with right bundle-branch block. When less than complete AV block is present, it is invariably a Mobitz type 2 block, in which there is no Wenckebach phenomenon and all conducted beats have the same P-R interval often with QRS patterns showing intraventricular conduction defect. Adams-Stokes attacks are often misdiagnosed as simple syncope, transient ischemic attacks, or seizures. Whenever an elderly patient's clinical picture is compatible with these diagnoses, particularly if the ECG shows either intraventricular or atrioventricular block, efforts to exclude the diagnosis of Adams-Stokes attacks must be made. Useful tests beside the standard ECG include long-term Holter monitoring, which records 10- and 24-hour periods on the ECG and is likely to demonstrate atrioventricular block if present intermittently, response to exercise, and carotid sinus massage. The prognosis for untreated Adams-Stokes attacks secondary to high degree atrioventricular block is poor, with close to 50% mortality in 3 years. This mortality is greatly reduced by implantation of a permanent pacemaker. The permanent transvenous pacemaker can be inserted in even very old patients with remarkably low morbidity and virtually no mortality. It would be my recommendation to insert a permanent pacemaker in any patient with complete or Mobitz type 2 heart block, even if the patient is asymptomatic, since the risk of fatal cardiac arrest with high-degree heart block far exceeds that of pacemaker implantation.

"SICK SINUS SYNDROME"

"Sick sinus syndrome," or sinoatrial dysfunction,[22-24] in elderly patients is an important cause of fainting, transient dizzy spells, light-headedness, and even seizures. This syndrome, originally described by Lown after cardioversion of patients with long-standing atrial fibrillation, has now been found to occur spontaneously secondary to numerous diseases including arteriosclerotic heart disease and rheumatic and hypertensive cardiac disease or as an idiopathic disorder. It may be characterized by inappropriate sinus bradycardia that is unresponsive to drugs or exercise, periods of sinus arrest with intermittent junctional escape rhythm, frequent atrial premature contractions, and sinoatrial block. In approximately two thirds of cases there is episodic rapid rhythm with intermittent atrial fibrillation, flutter, and atrial tachycardia often with rapid ventricular response. These cases represent the tachycardia-bradycardia syndrome. Beside the fainting episodes or equivalents, which are usually associated with the pauses or extreme bradycardia, the patients may also complain of angina, have symptoms of congestive heart failure, and have extreme palpitations—particularly those patients with the tachycardia-bradycardia syndrome. In some reports of this syndrome systemic embolization has been frequent, although in my experience this has not been the case. The course of this disorder is long; sudden death is rare, unlike the situation in complete heart block.

However, when this syndrome is associated with frequent syncopal attacks or when there are frequent episodes of tachycardia, permanent pacemaker implantation is the treatment of choice. It prevents the symptoms secondary to excessively slow heart rates and allows the treatment of the tachycardic episodes with drugs like digitalis glycosides or propranolol without danger of producing excessive bradycardia. I prefer ventricular pacing because approximately one third of these patients show evidence of either atrioventricular block or conduction defects distal to the bundle of His. Another factor in this decision is that permanent demand ventricular pacing is usually more reliable and easier to achieve than permanent atrial pacing.

The diagnostic procedures most helpful in establishing the presence of sick sinus syndrome include noting periods of inappropriate sinus bradycardia, Holter monitoring which is helpful both in detecting bradycardic and tachycardic episodes, and establishing that symptoms are correlated with arrhythmia. Carotid sinus massage is helpful, since many of the patients show abnormal responses to this maneuver with episodes of sinus standstill or high-degree atrioventricular block. Indeed there is an intermixture of sick sinus syndrome with carotid sinus syncope; the latter occurs often in the geriatric patient frequently with bradycardia at rest. Carotid sinus massage should be done routinely on any elderly patient with episodic fainting or equivalent episode. The procedure can be done safely as long as carotid pulses are normal and the patient has no carotid bruits. To ensure maximum safety the patient should be monitored electrocardiographically. Atropine should be available, 0.5 mg to be given intravenously if excessive bradycardia develops. The carotid arteries should be massaged vigorously with an up-and-down motion for no more than 5 seconds, first on the right side and then the left. If atrioventricular block occurs or standstill greater than 3 seconds is recorded, an abnormal response is present. The diagnosis is even more certain if the massage reproduces the symptoms.

Again the therapy of choice of carotid sinus syncope with or without associated sick sinus syndrome is permanent pacemaking. Another useful test for sick sinus syndrome is atrial pacing. With atrial pacing at rates greater than 100 beats a minute for 2 minutes or longer, followed by sudden cessation of pacing there is an abnormally long period before the sinus node fires again. Usually the pause induced by pacing is the normal sinus cycle length plus a period longer than 540 msec; indeed, 3- to 5-second periods of standstill may occur. Atrial pacing probably represents the most sensitive test for sick sinus syndrome but is only infrequently necessary to make the diagnosis, since long-term ECG monitoring, response to carotid sinus massage, and stress testing will often firmly establish the diagnosis.

DIGITALIS THERAPY

Digitalis, which increases the inotropic force of contraction, is one of the mainstays of therapy for congestive heart failure, a common condition in the elderly. Cardiac glycosides also play an important role in both the acute and prophylactic therapy of supraventricular arrhythmias, such as paroxysmal atrial tachycardia, atrial flutter, and atrial fibrillation; its beneficial effect is mainly exerted through slowing conduction in the atrioventricular node.

Digitalis agents are, however, a two-edged sword. The therapeutic-toxic ratio is extremely low for a widely used agent. It has been estimated that 10% to 25% of patients receiving digitalis manifest toxicity. Toxic manifestations may be either cardiac or noncardiac. Toxicity occurs more frequently with decreased renal function, advanced pulmonary disease, severe cardiac disease with increased heart size, conjoint diuretic therapy, particularly if hypokalemia results, and in the presence of multiple pulmonary emboli. All of these conditions occur more frequently with age, and furthermore, there is some evidence that age itself is a factor in the development of digitalis toxicity. The noncardiac manifestations of digitalis intoxication may be subtle, but any elderly patient receiving digitalis therapy who develops lethargy, muscular weakness, weight loss, and psychic changes ranging from depression and stupor to paranoia and delirium should be considered as possibly digitalis intoxicated. Even when there is no clear-cut history of digitialis administration, the patient may be receiving cardiac glycosides in diet pills or in general tonics. The cardiac manifestations of digitalis toxicity result from an increase in automaticity and slowing of conduction in junctional tissues. Virtually any arrhythmia may be produced by cardiac glycosides, but the most important in frequency are ventricular extrasystoles, accelerated idiojunctional rhythm with atrioventricular dissociation, paroxysmal atrial tachycardia with block, and atrioventricular block, usually Mobitz type 1. Sinoatrial block and extreme sinus bradycardia also occur, particularly in elderly patients. When cardiac arrhythmias are believed to be secondary to intoxication; digitalis administration must be immediately stopped, since the patient may have been given a nearly lethal dose. When increased automaticity represented by premature ventricular contractions, or rapid rhythms, such as paroxysmal atrial trachycardia with block, or nonparoxysmal junctional tachycardia occurs, the patient may be treated with potassium or phenytoin. When bradycardia secondary to atrioventricular block or sinoatrial block occurs, potassium should not be given, since it may further increase the block. If the slow rate produces symptoms, atropine therapy or even temporary pacemaking may be necessary.

The best therapy, however, for digitalis intoxication is prevention. The old dictum of loading a patient to toxicity should be proscribed. Conjoint use of powerful diuretics such as ethacrynic acid or furosemide together with large loading doses of cardiac glycosides are rarely necessary and should be avoided. Electrolyte levels should be determined, since hypokalemia predisposes to toxicity. Serum levels of cardiac glycosides can be determined now by widely available radioimmunoassay techniques. For digoxin, therapeutic serum levels are between 1 and 2 ng/ml; for digitoxin, between 10 and 20 ng/ml. Above these levels toxicity is likely to occur. Elderly patients should have their glycoside levels checked periodically to ensure proper dosage levels. Renal function should be determined by serum creatinine and blood urea nitrogen levels, since cardiac glycosides are mainly excreted by way of the kidney. Digitoxin also has an active hepatic metabolism, but since some of it is converted to digoxin, renal function is still an important determinant of clearance. Although some digitalis intoxication, particularly in the elderly patient, is inevitable secondary to the inherent properties of the drug, much toxicity can be avoided by remembering the aforementioned measures.

SURGERY FOR GERIATRIC HEART DISEASE

As noted in earlier sections of this chapter, age itself is not a barrier to major open heart surgery. Quinlan[25] from the Peter Bent Brigham Hospital, reported open heart surgery in 73 patients over the age of 65 years. There were 33 patients with aortic valve replacement, seven mitral valve replacements, 11 double valve replacements, four aortic dissections, and one closure of an atrial septal defect. The surgical mortality was 12% in elective cases but nearly 50% in emergencies, an experience similar to that of other groups and a potent stimulus for operating early on a patient with severe cardiac disease despite age, rather than waiting until the patient is near death. In this group of 73 patients there were no in-hospital deaths from either elective double valve replacements or from coronary artery bypass procedures. The overall late mortality was 10%, which was mostly related to complications of coronary artery disease. Ninety-eight percent of survivors were in functional class 1 or 2 after operation. This report, as well as experience elsewhere, documents the efficiency and safety of major cardiac surgery for a geriatric population when that surgery is indicated.

REFERENCES

1. Lewis, K.B.: Heart disease in the elderly, Hosp. Pract. **11**(2):99, 1976.
2. Feigenbaum, H.: The value of echocardiography in older patients, Geriatrics, **30**(6):106, 1975.
3. Loten, E.G.: Heart disease at 70, N. Z. Med. J. **88:**336-338, 1978.
4. Burch, G.: Interesting aspects of geriatric cardiology, Am. Heart J. **88:**99, 1975.
5. Pomerance, A.: Pathology of the heart with and without cardiac failure in the aged, Br. Heart J. **27:**697, 1965.
6. Sugiura, M., Hiraoka, K., Ohkawa, S., and Shimada, H.: A clinicopathological study on the heart diseases in the aged, Jpn. Heart H. **16**(5):526-537, 1975.
7. Campbell, A., Caird, F.I., and Jackson, T.F.M.: Prevalence of abnormalities of electrocardiogram in old people, Br. Heart J. **36:**1005-1011, 1974.
8. Caird, F.I., Campbell, A., and Jackson, T.F.M.: Significance of abnormalities of electrocardiogram in old people, Br. Heart J. **36:**1012-1018, 1974.
9. Mihalick, M.J., and Fisch, C.: Should ECG criteria be modified for geriatric patients? Geriatrics **32**(2):65-72, 1977.
10. Frohlich, E.D.: Use and abuse of diuretics, Am. Heart J. **89:**1, 1975.
11. Miller, R., et al. Clinical use of sodium nitroprusside in chronic ischemic heart disease, Circulation **51:**328, 1975.
12. Cohn, J.R.: Vasodilator therapy for heart failure: the influence of impedance on left ventricular performance, Circulation **48:**5, 1973.
13. Kleiger, R.E., Martin, T.F., Miller, J.P., Oliver, G.C.: Mortality of myocardial infarction treated in the CCU, BCL Monograph No. 250, July, 1974.
14. Kleiger, R.E., and Martin, T.F.: The patient with angina: medical management plus sympathetic, continuous care, Geriatrics **28**(3):74, 1973.
15. Shanahan, M., Windsor, H., and Golding, L.: Open heart surgery in the elderly, Aust. N.Z. J. Surg. **42**(2):107-112, 1972.
16. Laragh, J.H., editor: Hypertension manual, New York, 1973, Yorke Medical Books.
17. Finegan, R.E., Gianelly, R.E., and Harrison, D.C.: Aortic stenosis in the elderly: relevance of age to diagnosis and treatment, N. Engl. J. Med. **281:**1261, 1969.
18. Whiting, R.B., Powell, W.J., Jr., and Dinsmore, R.E.: Idiopathic hypertrophic subaortic stenosis in the elderly, N. Engl. J. Med. **285:**196, 1971.
19. Henry, W.C., Clark, C.E., and Epstein, S.E.: Asymmetric septal hypertrophy (ASH): the unifying link in the IHSS disease spectrum. Observations regarding its pathogenesis, pathophysiology and course, Circulation **47:**827, 1973.
20. Thell, R.: Bacterial endocarditis in subjects 60 years of age and older, Circulation **50:**174, 1975.
21. Pomerance, A.: Senile cardiac amyloidosis, Br. Heart J. **27:**711, 1965.
22. Rubenstein, J.J., Schulman, C.L., and Yurchak, R.M.: Clinical spectrum of the sick sinus syndrome, Circulation **46:**5, 1972.
23. Ferrer, M.: The sick sinus syndrome, Circulation **47:**635, 1973.
24. Narula, O.S., Samet, P., and Javier, R.P.: Significance of the sinus-node recovery time, Circulation **45:**140, 1972.
25. Quinlan, R.M., Cohn, L.H., and Collins, J.J., Jr.: Determinants of survival following cardiovascular operations in patients over age of 65, Chest (abst. 333) **66:**3, 1974.

CHAPTER 7 · RESPIRATORY DISEASES

Thomas L. Petty

Emphasis is placed on identification and clinical management of *chronic* obstructive pulmonary disease (COPD), which refers to the emphysema and chronic bronchitis complex, the continuing problem of chronic pulmonary tuberculosis, and the perplexing problem of lung cancer. Common pneumonias and pulmonary embolus, which frequently complicate chronic respiratory diseases, are discussed in this chapter. Practical considerations are stressed throughout.

CHRONIC OBSTRUCTIVE PULMONARY DISEASE

Definitions, identifications, and pathophysiology

Emphysema. Technically emphysema is the loss of alveolar walls, but this is a pathologic diagnosis often only made with confidence at postmortem examination.[1,2]

From autopsy studies it has been demonstrated that the incidence of emphysema increases with age, and by the age of 90 years nearly all individuals have some degree of emphysema pathology. The mean age of patients entering three prospective studies of the course and prognosis of emphysema and chronic bronchitis ranged from 58 to 61 years.[3]

A useful clinical definition of emphysema is the following: chronic dyspnea on exertion usually with a prior cough with progressive disability due to unrelenting dyspnea. Chronic bronchitis may or may not also be present. Other chronic chest diseases such as pulmonary fibrosis and bronchiectasis must be excluded for certainty in diagnosis.

Physiologically, expiratory obstruction is found in severe emphysema, judged primarily by ventilatory function tests—forced expiratory volume in 1 second (FEV_1), maximum midexpiratory flow (MMEF), and maximum voluntary ventilation (MVV). In addition, lung volumes are usually large because of pulmonary overdistention, residual volume is increased because of expiratory trapping, and gas transport is somewhat impaired because of departitioning of the lung. The volume of ventilation per minute is relatively large because of rather profound respiratory drives in the pure form of disease.[4] Because of the respiratory drive, dyspnea is often much more profound in emphysema than in chronic bronchitis. Distribution between ventilation and perfusion is relatively well maintained in emphysema; thus excessive right-to left shunting is minimized.[5] This, coupled with increased volume of ventilation per minute, results in fairly normal levels of blood gases in the compensated state. Therefore hypoxemia and carbon dioxide retention are not observed until the disease is terminal or unless there is intercurrent illness.

Chronic bronchitis. Arbitrarily, chronic bronchitis is defined in clinical terms. This makes things a bit confusing because emphysema is primarily defined in morphologic terms, although the clinical diagnosis for it previously defined has been useful. Chronic bronchitis refers to chronic cough and expectoration that have continued for at least 3 months or for at least 2 years when there is no other cause such as neoplasm or tuberculosis. It is almost always found in smokers, and usually the cough is unrelenting and nonseasonal. Dyspnea usually follows 10 to 20 years of prior chronic cough. The spirogram, no matter how useful, does not separate chronic bronchitis from emphysema.* Re-

*Symptomatic chronic bronchitis patients have ventilatory function abnormalities similar in degree to those of emphysema patients. Hypoxemia (oxygen pressure less than 70 mm Hg) is also often present.

sidual volume is also increased in chronic bronchitis because of air trapping, but the total lung capacity is not greatly increased.[5-7] The diffusion test results may be low or nearly normal.[5,8]

The most important physiologic abnormality in chronic bronchitis is hypoxemia and carbon dioxide retention once the disease is fully established. The hypoxemia is out of proportion to the degree of underventilation, which is due both to the work of breathing and to the relative lack of respiratory drive in this form of COPD, which is itself largely based on hereditary factors.[4] The hypoxemia is largely the result of ventilation-perfusion abnormalities in which there is considerable inequality between the distribution of ventilation and circulation. This is primarily due to localized airway plugging and shunting through these areas of little or no ventilation.

The morphologic counterpart of chronic bronchitis is mucous gland hyperplasia.[9] Also, particularly in exacerbations of disease, acute bronchiolitis with severe inflammation, edema, and plugging of the airways occur and further confound the ventilation-perfusion abnormalities.[9]

Many of the manifestations of chronic bronchitis are a result of hypoxemia. These manifestations include reactive pulmonary hypertension and cor pulmonale with associated congestive heart failure. The heart failure is probably worsened by impaired myocardial contractility due to oxygen lack as well as by impaired renal plasma flow and impaired salt and water clearance. Also secondary polycythemia is a response to the hypoxemic state.

Clinical spectrum. Although emphysema and chronic bronchitis have just been described separately, it must be stressed that these diseases are not commonly found in such pure forms. As a matter of fact, these diseases probably coexist about as often as they exist separately; thus the two basic processes represent a spectrum.

For this reason there is no absolute, typical picture of a patient with emphysema. The so-called barrel chest deformity is not a regular accompaniment of disease, and indeed, question has arisen as to whether the anterior-posterior chest diameter is increased at all in emphysema.[10] Although one thinks of the bronchitic person as "blue and bloated" and the emphysematous patient as "pink and puffing," these important historic phrases also represent an overly simplistic and often inaccurate concept.[6]

One should view each patient as having in his disease an airway component—bronchitis, bronchiolitis, edema, and secretions—and a mechanical component—the collapsing airway and increased work of breathing. The collapsing airway is probably flow limiting, and it is a matter of great debate as to *which segment* of the conducting airway is flow limiting. It is likely that expiratory collapse along both the central and peripheral conducting airways can occur in a variety of places. Factors promoting collapse are bronchial atrophy, loss of radial traction forces, and increased transpulmonary pressure.[11] The mechanical problem of the collapsing airways has implications for breathing retraining.

In addition to the airway problem, the mechanical ventilatory problem, and the blood gas abnormalities, all of which have therapeutic implications, the physician also faces the patient's response to his chronic illness and associated personality change including depression. Therefore the management of patients with COPD involves identification of the underlying treatable features of disease as well as an understanding of the pathologic and physiologic abnormalities involved and of problems of anxiety, depression, and despair.

Management*

Patient education. In the case of any chronic disease, effective therapy largely depends on thorough patient indoctrination. This has been known by diabetic specialists for years and certainly is the backbone of therapy for other chronic diseases such as renal failure requiring dialysis. Patients need a simple but thorough review of anatomy, physiology, work of breathing, and control of respiration and an understanding of their psychologic response to dyspnea, depression, anxiety, and frustration. Simple instruction classes are highly useful. They often can be conducted by a nurse or therapist who has time to provide small group sessions. Instructions are given in generalities concerning COPD, and the therapy prescribed by the physician is then amplified and explained. Simple

*The details of management are based on a 16-year comprehensive care study for COPD,[12] supported by U.S. Public Health Service contract No. 108-66-227, Chronic Respiratory Diseases Control Program.

handbooks with illustrative drawings have been found useful in patient indoctrination and instruction.[13]

Bronchial hygiene. One of the most important aspects in the ambulatory care of patients with COPD is care of the airway. This has been termed *bronchial hygiene*.[13] In brief, this involves measures to improve airway clearance and to prevent further irritation. Certainly smoking must be curtailed, and in areas of high levels of air pollution, room precipitators and air conditioners may be of value. Moving away from a highly contaminated environment may be of benefit.

Beyond these fundamental measures, the concept of bronchial hygiene includes the inhalation of bronchodilator aerosol and then inhalation of moisture followed by expulsive coughing maneuvers. The bronchodilator aerosol found most useful is Bronkosol, containing isoetharine, a selective beta$_2$-stimulator. Isoproterenol (Isuprel) is a short-acting beta-stimulator. Newer bronchodilator drugs that have fewer side effects and longer duration of action will soon be available. Metaproterenol in a metered dose device has recently been introduced (Metaprel, Alupent). The bronchodilator aerosol is inhaled in a regular, controlled fashion by a variety of means. A simple hand bulb nebulizer is suitable for many patients at home, particularly if the degree of airway obstruction is not great (forced expiratory volume in 1 second greater than 1 liter). If patients cannot use a simple hand bulb nebulizer because of lack of strength or coordination, pump-driven devices may be employed. Industry has provided for relatively inexpensive compression-driven devices that are highly useful (Fig. 7-1). If patients require pressure breathing because of severe obstruction, they can use simple home intermittent positive pressure breathing (IPPB) devices. A discussion of the advantages and disadvantages of IPPB therapy in COPD is beyond the scope of this chapter. Today IPPB remains controversial in COPD and is under study in comparison with pump-powered bronchodilator delivery.[14]

In practice at home, patients are generally instructed to place 10 drops of bronchodilator into their nebulizer and dilute with an equal amount of water. This is a simple starting point, and it is stressed that the proper use of bronchodilator drugs must become an art and that judgments on effectiveness, side effects, and dose adjustments must follow a careful assessment by the trained patient and physician together. One generally begins therapy with 10 deep breaths of aerosolized bronchodilator, but later, if side effects such as anxiety and palpations are not observed, nebulizer therapy for 10 or 15 minutes is allowed in certain cases. Often, however, 10 deep breaths suffice.

After the original nebulization period, de-

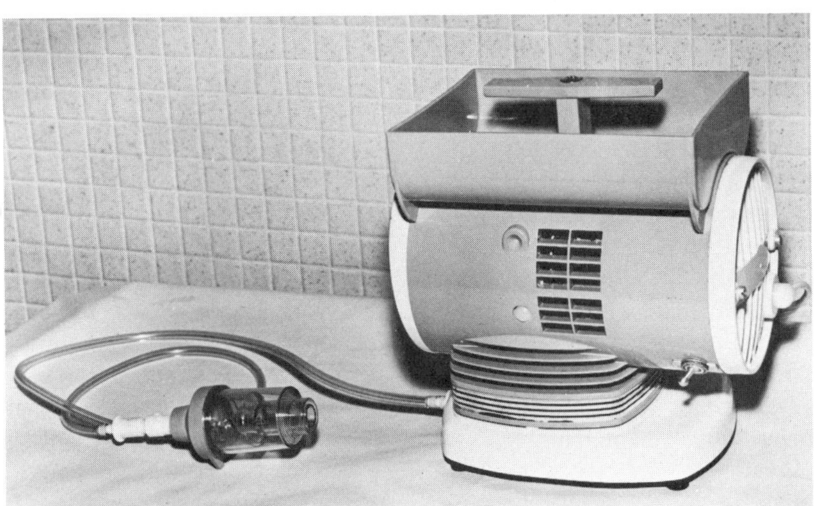

Fig. 7-1. Inexpensive pump-powered nebulizer for home use. (The nebulizer shown is a Maxi-Myst made by Mead Johnson Co., Evansville, Ind.)

signed to reduce airway resistance by reducing muscular bronchospasm and combating mucosal edema and probably also by stimulating mucociliary clearance, patients inhale moisture in the form of steam or nebulized water for approximately 10 minutes. Here, again, a variety of devices are useful. Most commonly a simple baby-bottle warmer with steam attachment is used, which provides large particles and humidified air. This inexpensive device is extremely popular with patients. More complicated devices such as heated nebulizers or ultrasonic nebulizers may be used from time to time in particularly difficult situations.

After the moisture inhalation period expulsive coughing or simple postural drainage maneuvers over pillows in bed or both are useful in helping clear the mobilized secretions. Most patients can clear their lungs by controlled expulsive coughing, which should be encouraged as part of the bronchial hygiene regimen. Useless cough, that is, spasmodic cough, which does not produce secretions, should be discouraged. Most patients cannot tolerate the traditional over-the-bed–head-on-the-floor postural drainage maneuver, which really makes little anatomic sense. Simple positions over pillows in bed are most useful and generally two positions are used each morning and each evening.

The bronchial hygiene program is employed morning and evening, with the recognition that some individuals will feel congestion and dyspnea at midday or other times and thus require further nebulization therapy. The practice of excessive nebulization should be discouraged because of irritation, paradoxical response, and the phenomenon of bronchospasm after nebulization, which is observed in some patients who use too much medication.

Breathing retraining. After a satisfactory bronchial hygiene program is established, breathing retraining is the next step in ambulatory care. Most individuals with severe airway obstruction breathe in a rapid, discoordinated fashion. This breathing favors dead-space ventilation, requires a great degree of effort, and is highly inefficient from the standpoint of gas exchange. Slow breathing favors oxygen transport; therefore patients are taught to relax their abdomen during inspiration and to contract their abdomen during expiration, thus facilitating pulmonary emptying. Numerous studies have been reported, showing the effectiveness of this procedure. In addition, patients are instructed to exhale against pursed lips. The exact mechanism of effectiveness of the pursed-lip maneuver is not entirely known; however, the amount of air that needs to be breathed for a unit of oxygen to be consumed is reduced, and the gas transport at the alveolar level also improves. It is possible that slow exhalation against resistance minimizes expiratory airway collapse. Many patients have spontaneously learned abdominal-diaphragmatic pursed-lip breathing and have called this maneuver to the attention of their physicians. Therefore this must be an adaptive phenomenon. It is a simple technique that provides great relief for many patients and should be taught all patients who can understand the technique and may experience relief from its use.[15]

Physical reconditioning. Simple graded exercises stressing normal walking have been demonstrated to improve the mobility of many patients with COPD.[12,15] Actually, dyspnea on exertion and lack of mobility are the most disabling features of this disease spectrum. Numerous reports have now established the fact that patients with severe COPD can perform greater degrees of exercise after daily exercise training in spite of the fact that their physiologic abnormalities may be irreversible. Nonetheless, increased exercise tolerance can be translated into increased daily activity and increased productivity as well as decreased symptoms. Improved mobility, productivity, and relief—these are what the patient seeks.

Generally patients are taught to exercise in appropriate situations around the home and with a definite goal to be increased each day. Both morning and evening exercises are encouraged. Specific research studies have established the fact that patients' exercise tolerance may be increased 100% or more during training, with this improved activity level being sustained for up to 2 years. Therefore this exercising is important for emphysema patients who must train, not to perform athletic events but to be able to participate more actively in life's normal and pleasurable pursuits.

Oxygen therapy. Continuous oxygen administration is valuable for extremely hypoxemic individuals who exhibit the ravages of impaired oxygenation in terms of severe disability usually with accompanying cor pulmonale and failure of the right side of the heart.[16,17] Oxygen therapy has now been established as practical for home care for COPD and is particularly valuable for the hypoxemic bronchitis patient. Oxygen reverses pulmonary hypertension, controls secondary polycythemia, and greatly improves exercise tolerance.[17] Oxygen administration has been useful and safe without apparent complications for periods of up to 13 years.[16]

New advances in oxygen delivery systems are noteworthy. Oxygen concentrators, employing either a molecular "sieve" or a semipermeable membrane, are used in pump-driven devices that concentrate oxygen from the air. These machines take advantage of the different molecular sizes of oxygen and nitrogen and thereby concentrate the oxygen percentage up to 92% from molecular sieve devices and 40% to 44% with semipermeable membrane units. Thus a stationary source for oxygen delivery is provided to replace conventional tanks, which are cumbersome and inconvenient. For patients requiring continuous oxygen, a backup compressed gas system is still required, however. These devices do not allow for oxygen delivery during exercise but whether or not 24-hour oxygen delivery is really needed in all patients with advanced COPD and hypoxemia is the subject of a current study. It is possible that less than 24-hour oxygen delivery will provide some of the same benefit that continuous oxygen systems including the liquid Linde system and compressed transfilling systems are able to provide. A commercially available molecular sieve-type oxygen concentrator is shown in Fig. 7-2.

Advances in the transfilling Linde liquid system include "walker" devices of two sizes, that is, providing either 5 or 9 hours oxygen supply at 2 liters. The lighter weight device in use is shown in Fig. 7-3, and Fig. 7-4 shows a simple transfilling oxygen tank, representing one of many devices that can be filled from conventional tank sources allowing 30 minutes to 4 hours ambulatory oxygen. Transfilling systems have been proven safe in widespread use over more than 20 years.

Drug therapy. Antibiotics should be used when there are deep chest infections, which are identified by increased production of sputum, which is often yellow or green and which patients learn to recognize by virtue of instruction. Self-administration of antibiotics is certainly advisable and safe, particularly when patients are well taught. The usual infectious organisms are *Haemophilus influenzae* and *Streptococcus pneumoniae;* thus the empiric use of tetracycline, 2 gm daily for the first 2 days followed by 1 gm daily for a total of 5 to 7 days, seems rational. An alternative is ampicillin, 4 gm for the first 2 days, followed by 2 gm daily; this is the required dose for COPD. In addition, for occasional patients who are allergic or refractory to these two antibiotics, chloramphenicol, which has great penetration into pulmonary tissue, is useful. Generally 4 gm daily are used for the first 2 days, followed by 2 gm every 24 hours for a total of 5 days. Chloramphenicol is a highly effective antibiotic, particularly against *H. influenzae*. It is also useful against several gram-negative rods that infect COPD patients.

Trimethoprim with sulfamethoxazole (Bactrim, Septra) is also highly effective against common bacteria associated with episodes of purulent bronchitis.

Cardiac glycosides and the increasing number of effective diuretic drugs are useful in controlling congestive heart failure but are of most value for the patient who is also receiving oxygen for control of reactive pulmonary hypertension. Both digitalis and diuretics are considered dangerous in the face of hypoxemia; thus these two drugs should be considered as adjuncts to the management of patients with cor pulmonale with failure, but only with adequate oxygenation of the myocardium.

Corticosteroid drugs require special mention in any discussion of COPD. Certain patients with apparently irreversible disease may have objective improvement and considerable symptomatic benefit coincident with corticosteroid therapy.[18] In brief, improved patients are mostly those with the bronchitic type of condition and often have superimposed exacerbations of wheezing or choking spells. It is entirely possible that these individuals may really have occult asthma, but clinically the asthma may be indistinguishable from the manifestations of COPD. Identification becomes doubly important because considerable reversibility may be possible. Steroids should be given after patients have received a meticulous bronchial hygiene program. Thereafter steroids can be "tried" with laboratory guidance. Generally, the equivalent of 30 mg of prednisone daily are given for

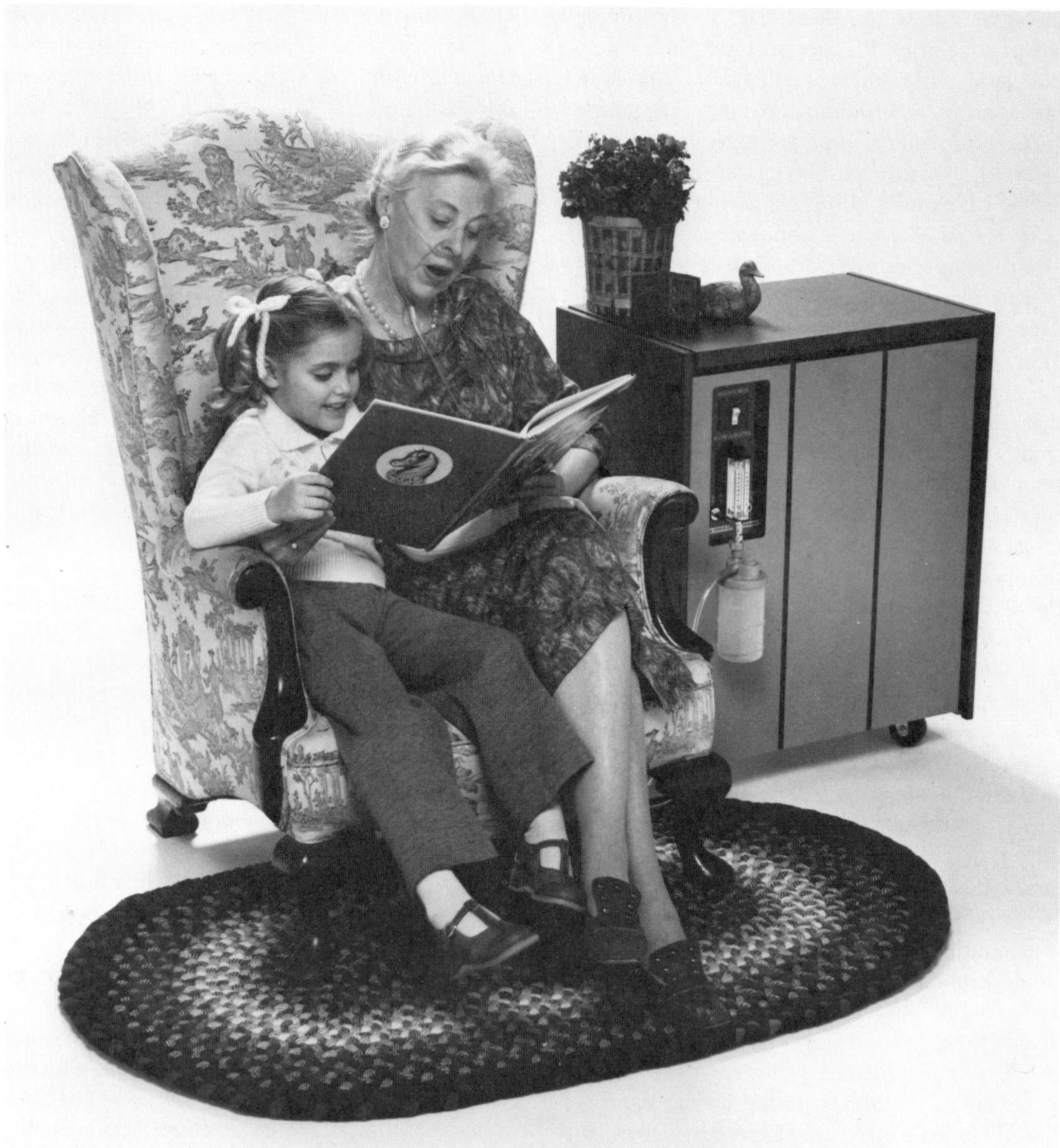

Fig. 7-2. Home oxygen concentrator using molecular sieve principle. Device produces oxygen from air by absorbing nitrogen and releasing the oxygen at approximately 92% concentration at 2 to 4 liters per minute. (Courtesy Briox Corporation.))

approximately 2 weeks, and laboratory function tests, particularly spirometric tests and tests of resting blood gas levels, are repeated. If both symptomatic and objective functional improvement are noted, the steroid dose can be reduced to 15 mg every 24 hours for the next 2 weeks, followed by a low maintenance dose averaging 5 to 10 mg every 24 hours. Alternate day therapy may also produce fewer side effects.

Oral bronchodilators, although popular, are not very effective. Nonetheless, metaproterenol or terbutaline may bring some symptomatic relief. Soluble xanthine drugs such as oxtriphylline (Choledyl) and anhydrous theophylline (Bronkodyl, Elixophyllin, Quibron) are useful oral bronchodilating methylxanthines.

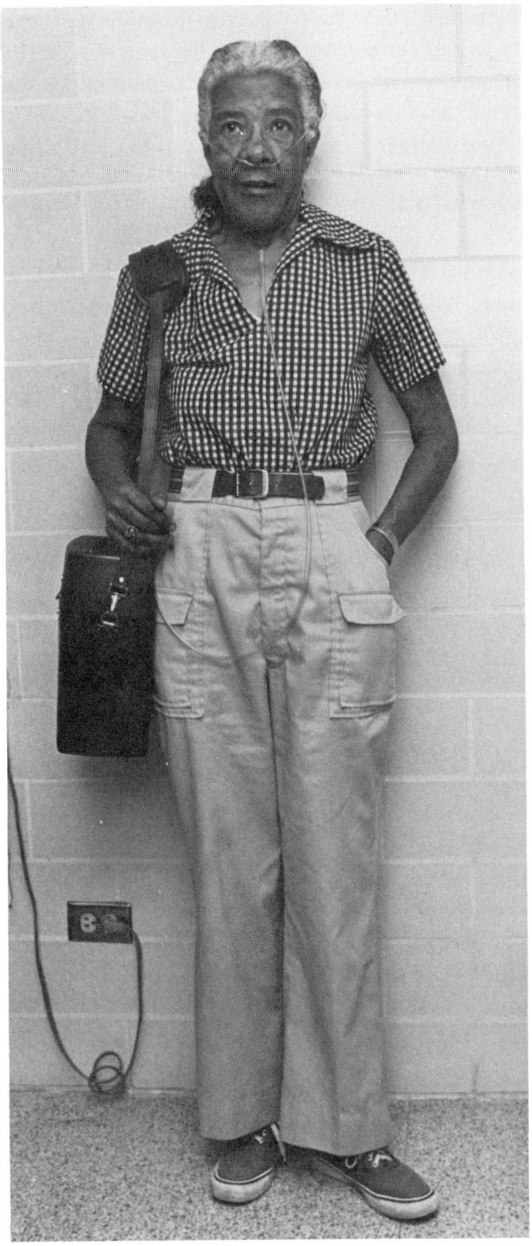

Fig. 7-3. New lightweight Linde transfilling portable liquid system. Device carries an oxygen supply of approximately 5 hours and weighs 6.5 lb. A larger device with a supply of approximately 9 hours is also available. Other manufacturers have similar devices.

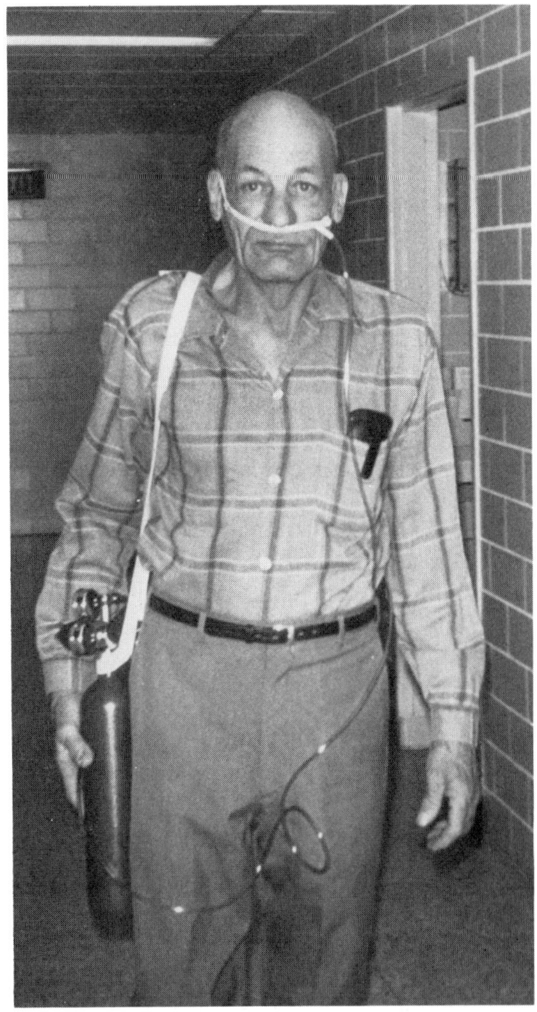

Fig. 7-4. Portable cylinder, which can be transfilled from large H or K cylinder. This offers 1½ to 3½ hours supply, depending on size of tank. Newer tanks are made of aluminum. Transfilling is practical and safe.

So-called expectorants, such as saturated solution potassium iodide (SSKI) and the popular so-called expectorant glyceryl guaiacolate, present in many formulations, have never been proved by critical study to provide significant benefit. Nonetheless, they may be of use for short periods and help to stimulate serous bronchorrhea in some people. So-called respiratory stimulants taken orally are ineffectual. In short, oral pharmacologic therapy with any drugs other than antibiotics, steroids, diuretics, and cardiotonic drugs is of little proved value.

Polyvalent influenza virus vaccine should be given each fall for whatever protection it affords. The vaccine is most useful during specific epidemics. However, influenza remains endemic in certain areas nearly every year; thus there is support for the current belief that influenza virus vaccine should be used on a fairly routine basis each fall for patients with COPD. Polyvalent pneumococcal vaccine (Pneumovax) should be used in all patients with COPD.

Psychologic support. In the management of patients with severe COPD, psychologic support and family counseling are needed. Patients with this disease spectrum are anxious, demanding, and frightened; suffer loss of self-image; and often realize they have an endless and frequently progressive disease. This often leads to profound personality change. Often effective breathing retraining and physical reconditioning along with the other measures just defined provide great relief of anxiety and emotional upset. Also, the educational techniques help make the patient much more independent and capable of coping with problems. It is important for the practitioner to recognize why emphysema patients are the way they are. It is equally important for an excellent physician-patient relationship to be established to help relieve the burdens of disease.

At times the judicious use of psychoenergizing drugs such as imipramine (Tofranil) and amitriptyline (Elavil) helps to combat depression. Most authorities fear the use of any tranquilizing or sedative drugs in view of their ability to depress respiration. Nonetheless, small amounts of tranquilizing agents are required at times, and sometimes diazepam (Valium) and chlordiazepoxide (Librium) are useful and reasonably safe in low dosage. It should be stressed that patients with even moderate degrees of carbon dioxide retention or with exacerbations of disease should not receive a sedative at any time because of the likelihood of further respiratory failure.

• • •

Any discussion of COPD care would be incomplete without brief mention of acute respiratory failure. Acute respiratory failure commonly punctuates the course of the COPD in a patient but represents a medical emergency that today frequently can be identified. Modern respiratory support, with employment of methods of physiologically oriented care in an organized respiratory care unit, has saved the lives of many patients.[19]

In brief, acute respiratory failure is present when the arterial oxygen tension rapidly drops to less than 50 mm Hg, when the carbon dioxide tension is elevated to greater than 50 mm Hg, or when both take place. The urgency of the situation will be inversely proportional to the time for development of these blood gas level abnormalities. Some patients can tolerate these degrees of blood gas level abnormalities if they have occurred over a prolonged period of time.

The details of intensive care management are beyond the scope of this chapter. However, many patients can survive with the controlled administration of oxygen at a low flow, to correct profound degrees of hypoxemia, in conjunction with aggressive nursing care, bronchial hygiene, and liberal use of inhaled moisture in an intensive respiratory care unit. Some individuals with profound respiratory insufficiency require nasotracheal or orotracheal intubation or tracheostomy with assisted or controlled ventilation by an automatic ventilator. Even if such emergencies occur, the physician should approach the care of these patients with enthusiasm, since experience has shown that as many as 75% of patients suffering from acute respiratory failure and requiring ventilatory assistance can recover and return home and, in many cases, lead useful and productive lives.*

The salvage rate of older patients is surprisingly good. Fifty-one percent of patients over the age of 70 years who required mechanical ventilation for acute respiratory failure with chronic obstructive pulmonary disease recovered and left the hospital.[20] It is particularly important to maintain adequate nutrition and muscle tone in older patients. Getting the patient up in a chair as early as possible and encouraging ambulation with assistance are valuable aids in management (Fig. 7-5).

Except in the case of acute respiratory failure, when lives often are saved, one cannot help but wonder whether the natural course of disease is altered by the therapeutic measures previously described. There is no question, however, that patients derive great symptomatic benefit from the therapeutic measures and increased exercise tolerance; at times they return to gainful employment; and a marked reduction in hospital needs has also been documented.[21] A limited number of patients with apparently irreversible COPD *in fact* demonstrate a measure of objec-

*From 10-year consecutive experience, all patients, Respiratory Care Unit, University of Colorado Medical Center, Denver.

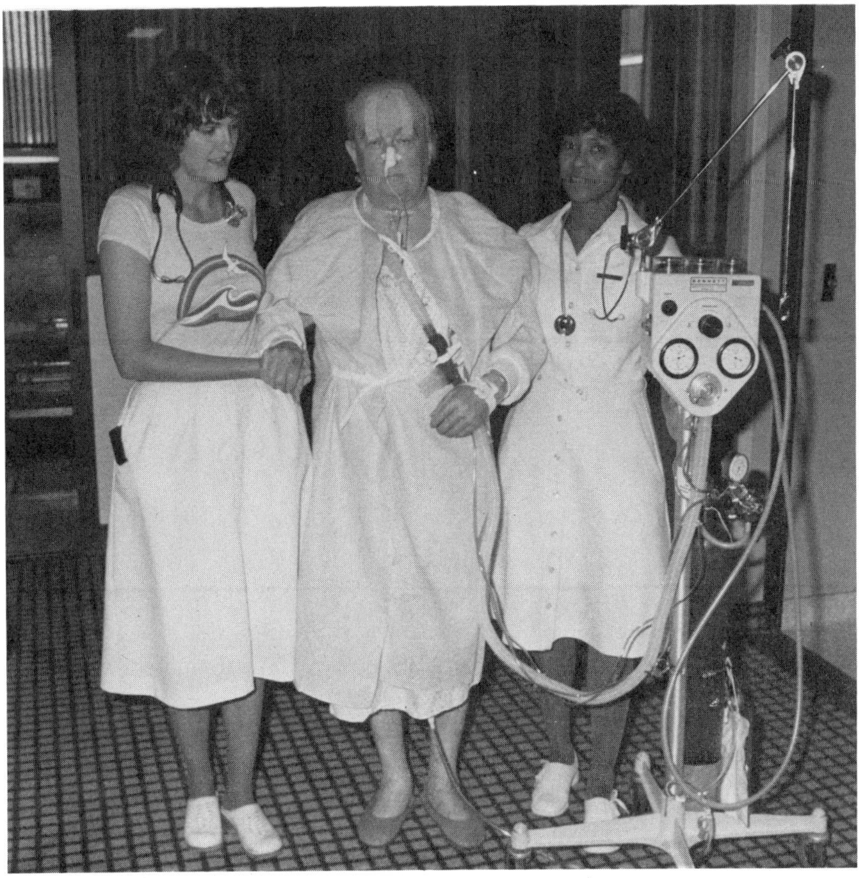

Fig. 7-5. Method of ambulating patients still requiring ventilatory assistance, using pressure-cycled TR1 Bennett ventilator powered by small oxygen E cylinder. The 82-year-old patient has COPD and requires hospitalization for myasthenia gravis.

tive functional improvement with the application of systematic care methods. Occasionally the return of function may be considerable and unexpected.[18]

PULMONARY TUBERCULOSIS

Pulmonary tuberculosis remains this nation's most important infectious disease, since it is a chronic respiratory disease and plagues the elderly population. Today some 20 million tuberculin test reactors—individuals infected with *viable* tuberculosis bacilli—some 25,000 new cases each year, and probably 4000 deaths at least, related to tuberculosis are reported. The natural history of tuberculosis in the United States is primary infection by inhalation of droplet nuclei at any time in life. The tuberculosis bacillus frequently remains dormant after it has initially infected a person, and only at times of impaired host response, which may be in old age, will the clinically overt disease become manifest.[22] Thus, today, tuberculosis is becoming a disease of the elderly, a fact that is apparent to those who still have the opportunity to visit the remaining tuberculosis units in this country.

The tuberculin skin tests have now been well standardized, and the intermediate strength purified protein derivative with Tween additive (PPD-T) should be used, given by intradermal injection. Most experts agree that a reaction of greater than 10 mm of induration in roughly 48 hours is indicative of clinical infection.[22] This does not mean, however, that the tuberculosis *disease* is present; it only identifies the presence of viable organisms. In the elderly population, however, relative degrees of tuberculin anergy are not uncommon, and therefore less reliance is placed on the skin test in this age group.

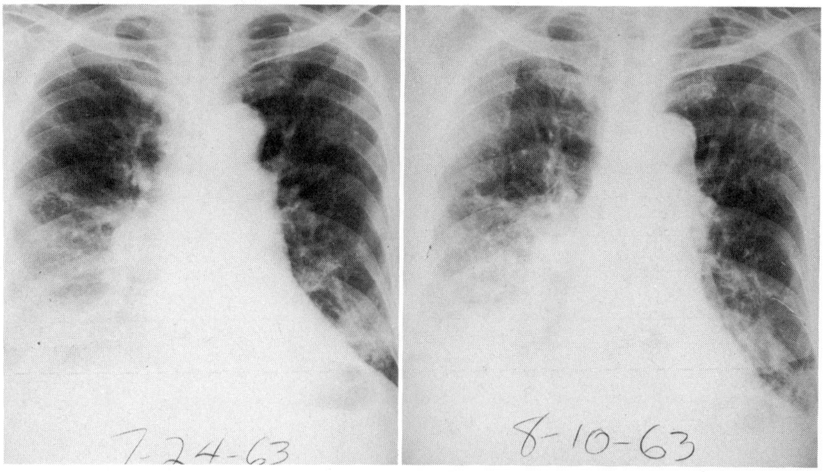

Fig. 7-6. Progressive bilateral lower lobe infiltrates ultimately proved by biopsy to be typical tuberculosis.

It should be stressed that the typical apical cavitation, which is the classic x-ray picture well known to students of tuberculosis, is not always the actual roentgenographic finding. Although suspicion is heightened when this x-ray abnormality is found, it should be stressed that lower lobe infiltrates (Fig. 7-6) and pleural effusion may be manifestations of disease in the elderly.

The final diagnosis of tuberculosis is made by bacteriologic examination. The time-honored acid-fast stain is highly useful for very infectious patients, and in some cases this has been replaced by fluorescent staining, which has the advantage of being somewhat more rapid than the classic Ziehl-Neelsen technique. The diagnosis of tuberculosis, however, must be made by culture, since other organisms such as the so-called atypical mycobacteria[23] also cause pulmonary disease that requires therapy with drugs different from the usual drugs for pulmonary tuberculosis. These are the atypical mycobacteria that Runyon[23] classified into four groups (*Mycobacterium kansasii* and *Mycobacterium battei* cause diseases that are uncommon and will not be considered in this chapter). Culture techniques allow the alert laboratory to identify the presence of atypical acid-fast organisms and to separate these microbes from those that cause human tuberculosis.

Management of the active case

Pulmonary tuberculosis management has undergone a tremendous revolution in the past 30 years, and many cases are now properly managed by the nonpulmonary physician.[24] Almost all cases can be successfully managed by chemotherapy, and no less than 11 effective drugs represent a tremendous armamentarium in the battle against the disease. At the same time the need for sanitarium care has been eliminated, and most states have closed all their chronic care facilities. The infectious phase of tuberculosis often can be brought under control in a matter of a few weeks.

Short course chemotherapy, employing isoniazid (INH) and rifampin has now reduced effective chemotherapy to as little as 9 months. INH, 300 mg per day, and rifampin, 600 mg per day, are at least as effective as three drug regimens, including injectables, which were standard treatments in the past.[25]

Surgery for pulmonary tuberculosis is rarely required and ordinarily reserved for mechanical complications such as bronchial stenosis, empyema, and in some cases destruction of large lung zones. In most cases, chemotherapy is entirely adequate in controlling the infectious state and rendering the patient clinically well.

Prevention

There is growing interest in preventing tuberculosis. High-risk patients are given empiric, so-called preventive therapy, and this generally involves the administration of INH in a single dose of 300 mg. High risk patients include those who have uncontrolled diabetes, require corticosteroid therapy for more than 2 weeks, have conglomerate silicosis, have had gastrectomy, and have impaired immune responses either induced or as part of an underlying disease. Immune processes are known to be impaired when lymphomas, leukemia, Hodgkin's disease, or the uremic state exist. In all cases repeated sputum cultures should be made in the search for active disease, which would require the use of two drugs. The widespread and uncontrolled use of INH prophylaxis for all tuberculin test reactors is advocated by some but is believed by most experts to be a rather inappropriate use of this drug. This attitude at the present time, however, is a subject of current study and remains debatable.

LUNG CANCER

Lung cancer is a *major* disease of the elderly. Although seldom considered a chronic disease, the magnitude of the problem and the fact that lung cancer often coexists with chronic obstructive pulmonary disease (COPD) warrants a consideration of the problem in this chapter.

Lung cancer is truly a disease of the elderly. In a large prospective study more than half the men with lung cancer were 65 years of age or older.[26] The number of patients with surgically resectable lesions was only 24% in this age group, and there were no 5-year survivors. The low percentage of surgically resectable cases and the poor overall prognosis was at least partly due to coexisting pulmonary insufficiency from COPD. So far no form of chemotherapy has clearly been shown to alter the natural course of lung cancer, except in oat cell carcinoma.[27,28] Aggressive chemotherapy employing multiple drugs combined with supervoltage radiotherapy has provided complete remissions and improved survival in selected patients recently.[28]

In view of the overall dismal picture, the only rational approach to the control of lung cancer is prevention. Epidemiologic studies have clearly related lung cancer to cigarette smoking, and evidence has been offered that the cessation of smoking substantially reduces the risk of lung cancer.[29] Reducing the amount of smoking and switching to filtered cigarettes with lower tar content may also reduce lung cancer risk.[29]

The operative risk in elderly patients is at least 10%, and the likelihood of cure is so low that surgery is rarely helpful in elderly individuals with lung cancer. This statement does not apply, of course, to all patients, and particularly vigorous men with good pulmonary function and peripheral solitary nodules may be good surgical candidates.

OTHER CHRONIC RESPIRATORY DISEASES

Chronic bronchial asthma

Bronchial asthma represents a problem in the adult population and often coexists with chronic obstructive pulmonary disease (COPD). The mangement of chronic asthma is similar to that of COPD; it includes the use of bronchial hygiene measures. A more liberal use of corticosteroid drugs is sometimes also required. Corticosteroids in doses equivalent to 10 to 15 mg prednisone are remarkably well tolerated in most most elderly men with otherwise refractory asthma.

Common bacterial pneumonias

Common bacterial pneumonias frequently complicate the treatment of patients with the chronic respiratory diseases described in this chapter and are particularly prevalent in patients with COPD and interstitial diseases. The most common organisms are *Streptococcus pneumoniae, Hemophilus influenzae,* and *Staphylococcus aureus*. Classically *S. pneumoniae* begins with a single chill and is usually associated with high fever. However, the chill and febrile response may be subtle or absent in the elderly. Lobar consolidation is common. Penicillin G remains the therapy of choice. Erythromycin is an alternative for those allergic to penicillin.

H. influenzae pneumonia is most common in patients with underlying COPD. X-ray manifestations may include patchy unilateral or bilateral infiltrates. Therapy with ampicillin or chloramphenicol is effective, but the outcome is largely dependent on the native resistance of the underlying host. Staphylococcal pneumonia frequently follows bouts of acute influenza in the elderly. A florid x-ray infiltrate may be present, including cavitation. Therapy with a semisynthetic penicillin or cephalosporin is required.

Recently pneumonia due to *Legionnella pneumophilia* has received appropriate attention. These pneumonias are commonly present in the late summer or early fall, occur in clusters, and attack the debilitated host. Therapy with erythromycin or rifampin is effective in many patients.[30] Finally, aspiration pneumonia is a common problem and involves anaerobic bacteria and other common enteric organisms.[31]

Pulmonary thromboembolism

Pulmonary embolism with or without infarction also commonly complicates the course of chronic lung diseases. It is most prevalent in patients confined to bed, the obese, those with underlying malignancy, and those with congestive heart failure. The diagnosis, treatment, and prevention has been summarized many times, and the prevalence of this disease has been emphasized. A high index of suspicion and appropriate use of perfusion and ventilation scans provide a presumptive diagnosis in many clinical situations. In the presence of underlying COPD, however, interpretation of both ventilation and perfusion scans is difficult, due to focal abnormalities of both ventilation and perfusion inherent in these clinical conditions, particularly in emphysema. Serial studies improve diagnostic accuracy. Today the "gold standard" in diagnosis is pulmonary arteriography, which is impractical or not available in many cases. Thus the diagnosis remains largely presumptive and the therapy empiric, with heparin used to treat an acute embolic event in the absence of overwhelming bleeding considerations.

Interstitial fibrosis and chronic pneumonitis

Interstitial fibrosis and chronic pneumonitis also are illnesses that represent a spectrum. Most commonly included are diffuse interstitial fibrosis associated with collagen disease and more newly described entities such as fibrosing alveolitis or desquamative interstitial pneumonitis. The importance of the diagnoses of these diseases, only made with certainty by lung biopsy, is the fact that corticosteroid drugs may be beneficial.

Bronchiectasis

Bronchiectasis is a chronic disease that has almost vanished from the American scene, probably because of the early use of antimicrobial agents for episodes of acute bronchitis and pneumonia. Bronchiectasis management is similar to management of chronic bronchitis; it includes the employment of bronchial hygiene and postural drainage. Each patient with bronchiectasis should be treated vigorously with antimicrobial agents in the event of specific deep chest infections.

Suppurative lung diseases

So-called nonspecific lung abscess may require prolonged chemotherapy. Generally, nonspecific lung abscess is managed by penicillin, and for prolonged cases oral penicillin in doses of roughly 2.4 million units every 24 hours is usually effective. Occasionally a resection is required for a remaining cavity, particularly if it is involved with recurrent infection from fungi, such as aspergillosis.

SUMMARY

Chronic obstructive pulmonary disease (COPD) has replaced tuberculosis as the major important pulmonary disease spectrum affecting the adult population. COPD is not a hopeless entity but rather a clinical-pathologic state, which is now recognized and understood better than ever before and for which effective therapy is available. Management is based on patient education, bronchial hygiene, breathing retraining, physical reconditioning, oxygen therapy in some cases, and the judicious use of antibiotics, cardiotonic drugs, and corticosteroids.

Tuberculosis remains the most important chronic infectious disease of adults. Specific chemotherapy, which now includes 11 drugs, has revolutionized management. The sanitarium is disappearing from the American scene. The practitioner and general hospitals now assume more important roles than ever before in tuberculosis management, control, and prevention. Lung cancer is a *major* disease of the elderly. The likelihood of a surgical cure is small, in part because of coexisting pulmonary insufficiency from COPD. Radical radiotherapy or chemotherapy may be helpful in oat cell carcinoma.

REFERENCES

1. Heard, B.E.: Pathology of pulmonary emphysema, Am. Rev. Resp. Dis. **82**:792, 1960.
2. Mitchell, R.S., et al.: Clinical morphological correlations in chronic airway obstruction, Am. Rev. Resp. Dis. **97**:54, 1968.
3. Petty, T.L., Hudson, L.D., and Neff, T.A.: Methods of ambulatory care, Med. Clin. North Am. **57**:751, 1973.
4. Mountain, R., Zwillich, C.W., and Weil, J.: Hypoventilation in obstructive lung disease, N. Engl. J. Med. **298**:521, 1978.

5. Filley, G.F., Beckwitt, H.J., Reeves, J.T., and Mitchell, R.S.: Chronic obstructive bronchopulmonary disease. II. Oxygen transport in two clinical types, Am. J. Med. **44**:26, 1968.
6. Thurlbeck, W.M.: Aspects of chronic airflow obstruction, Chest **72**:341, 1977.
7. Mitchell, R.S., Vincent, T.N., Ryan, S.F., and Filley, G.F.: Chronic obstructive bronchopulmonary disease. IV. The clinical and physiological differentiation of chronic bronchitis and emphysema, Am. J. Med. Sci. **247**:513, 1964.
8. Jones, N.L., Burrows, B., and Fletcher, C.M.: Serial studies of 100 patients with chronic airways obstruction in London and Chicago, Thorax **22**:327, 1967.
9. Mitchell, R.S., Ryan, S.F., Petty, T.L., and Filley, G.F.: The significance of morphologic chronic hyperplastic bronchitis, Am. Rev. Resp. Dis. **93**:720, 1966.
10. Kilburn, K.H., and Asmundsson, T.: Anterior-posterior chest diameter in emphysema, Arch. Intern. Med. **123**:379, 1969.
11. Maisel, J.C., Silvers, G.W., Mitchell, R.S., and Petty, T.L.: Bronchial atrophy and dynamic expiratory collapse, Am. Rev. Resp. Dis. **98**:988, 1968.
12. Petty, T.L., and Nett, L.M.: Pulmonary rehabilitation, Continuing Education **8**:491, 1978.
13. Petty, T.L., and Nett, L.M.: For those who live and breathe with emphysema and chronic bronchitis, ed. 2, Springfield, Ill., 1974, Charles C Thomas, Publisher.
14. Conference on the Scientific Basis of Respiratory Therapy, Am. Rev. Resp. Dis. **110**:13, 1974.
15. Mueller, R.E., Petty, T.L., and Filley, G.F.: Ventilation and blood gas changes induced by pursed lips breathing, J. Appl. Physiol. **28**:784, 1970.
16. Petty, T.L., et al.: Outpatient oxygen therapy in chronic obstructive pulmonary disease (a review of 13 years' experience and an evaluation of modes of therapy), Arch. Intern. Med. **139**:28, 1979.
17. Levine, B.E., et al.: The role of long term continuous oxgyen administration in patients with chronic airway obstruction with hypoxemia, Ann. Intern. Med. **66**:369, 1967.
18. Petty, T.L., Brink, G.A., and Corsello, P.R.: Objective functional improvement in chronic airway obstruction, Chest **57**:216, 1970.
19. Petty, T.L., et al.: Intensive respiratory care unit (review of ten years' experience), J.A.M.A. **233**:34, 1975.
20. Pierson, D.J., Neff, T.A., and Petty, T.L.: Ventilatory management of the elderly, Geriatrics **28**:86, 1973.
21. Hudson, L.H., Tyler, M.L., and Petty, T.L.: Hospitalization needs during an outpatient rehabilitation program for chronic airway obstruction, Chest **70**:606, 1976.
22. Stead, W.W.: Pathogenesis of the sporadic case of tuberculosis, N. Engl. J. Med. **277**:1008, 1967.
23. Runyon, E.H.: Anonymous mycobacteria in pulmonary disease, Med. Clin. North Am. **43**:273, 1959.
24. Byrd, R.B., et al.: Treatment of tuberculosis by the nonpulmonary physician, Ann. Intern. Med. **86**:799, 1977.
25. Dutt, A.K., Jones, J., and Stead, W.W.: Short course chemotherapy for tuberculosis with largely twice-weekly isoniazid-rifampin, Chest **75**:441, 1979.
26. Weiss, W.: Survivorship among men with bronchogenic carcinoma, Arch. Environ. **22**:168, 1971.
27. Carbone, P.O., et al.: Lung cancer: perspectives and prospects, Ann. Intern. Med. **73**:1003, 1970.
28. Greco, F.A., et al.: Small cell carcinoma (complete remission and improved survival), Am. J. Med. **66**:625, 1979.
29. Wyander, E.L., Mabuchi, K., and Beattie, E.J., Jr.: The epidemiology of lung cancer, J.A.M.A. **213**:2221, 1970.
30. Kirby, B.D., Snyder, K.M., Meyer, R.D., and Finegold, S.M.: Legionnaires' disease: clinical features of 24 cases, Ann. Intern. Med. **89**:297, 1978.
31. Lorber, B., and Swenson, R.M.: Bacteriology of aspiration pneumonia (a prospective study of community- and hospital-acquired cases, Ann. Intern. Med. **81**:329, 1974.
32. Hirsh, J.: Venous thromboembolism: diagnosis, treatment, prevention, Hosp. Pract., Aug., 1975, p. 53.

CHAPTER 8 · GASTROINTESTINAL PROBLEMS

Phillip M. Berman
Joseph B. Kirsner

Gastrointestinal disease in the elderly is a major health problem, not only in the United States but throughout the world. This chapter reviews some of the more important digestive problems encountered in this group.

The effects of aging on the human gastrointestinal tract may involve an alteration in a characteristic function of the organ, as in the disorganized motility of the "aged" esophagus (presbyesophagus) or the lowered acid secretion of the "aged" stomach; the effect of age also may involve a change in anatomic structure, as in gastric atrophy and diminished tonus of bowel musculature.[1] More often the digestive problems of the elderly reflect the presence of concomitant diseases that impair general health, limit physical activity, and disturb emotional balance. Also, the increased use of various drugs (e.g., aspirin, nonsteroidal antiinflammatory agents, and laxatives), a common practice among the elderly, results in significant digestive disorders. In general, however, the concept of an "aged" gastrointestinal tract with seriously limited anatomic and physiologic capacities and therefore vulnerable to a spectrum of disorders unique to aging is incorrect, except possibly for cancer of the gastrointestinal tract, whose incidence increases with age. Actually, the anatomic and physiologic integrity of the gastrointestinal tract usually is maintained at least into the eighties, nineties, and older.

ESOPHAGUS

The function of the esophagus is to facilitate the passage of food from the oral cavity to the stomach. In most instances this activity is preserved completely. In some elderly people cineradiography and esophageal motility studies demonstrate an increased number of dysrhythmic, tertiary contractions. Peristaltic contractions may be absent throughout the entire length of the esophagus, or the esophagus is dilated. *Presbyesophagus* designates the clinical syndrome of disorganized and inefficient motor function of the esophagus of the elderly, a situation resembling diffuse esophageal spasm.[2,3]

Achalasia

Achalasia refers to an inability of the lower esophageal sphincter to relax with swallowing, associated with decreased peristaltic activity throughout the length of the esophagus. It ranks second to carcinoma as a cause of esophageal obstruction. The principal manifestations are dysphagia and weight loss, at times so pronounced as to suggest carcinoma. The typical symptom is difficulty in swallowing, at first solid foods and later also liquids. The course initially is intermittent with intervals of freedom from symptoms. Often the disability is progressive; the esophagus is characteristically dilated, and the patient may reach a stage wherein little can be swallowed without therapeutic intervention. Later the patient may relate that after a certain amount of food has been ingested, the esophagus seems consciously to empty because of the accumulation of sufficient pressure from the food and gravity to overcome the resistance at the lower esophageal sphincter, allowing the esophageal contents to pass into the stomach. This sequence is in distinct contrast to a mechanical esophageal obstruction, as in stricture or carcinoma, which cannot be overcome by the pressure of food. Tracheobronchial aspiration of food and secretions from the functionally obstructed, dilated esophagus causes coughing, wheezing, shortness of breath, and recurrent pneumonitis or pneumonia. In severe instances a lung abscess may develop. Radiographically, the esophagus is dilated proximal to a smooth, symmetric, and well-defined narrowing at the lower end of the esophagus, immediately above the gastroesophageal junction. The disorder is characterized physiologically by decreased vagal and augmented sympathetic nervous influences. Histologically, the esophagus is characterized by a decrease or loss of ganglion cells, especially in its lower third. Esophageal motility tests demonstrate decreased amplitude of contractions in the body of the esophagus, disorganized peristalsis, and failure of the lower esophageal sphincter to relax with swallowing, as under normal circumstances.

Because of the impaired postganglionic innervation of the esophagus in achalasia, the intramuscular administration of 2 mg acetyl betamethylcholine (Mecholyl) evokes an exaggerated response of painful, forceful contractions of the lower esophagus, readily observed with fluoroscopy or esophageal manometry. Esophagoscopy and biopsy should be performed to exclude mechanical obstructions such as peptic ulcer or carcinoma. In elderly patients the passage of mercury-filled Hurst dilators may provide temporary relief of the dysphagia by stretching the lower esophageal muscle fibers. Pneumatic dilatation of the distal esophageal sphincter is more effective but carries a higher risk of tearing and perforation of the esophagus. Surgical myotomy of the distal esophagus (Heller operation) relieves the esophageal obstruction when nonoperative dilatation is ineffective, but the procedure may be complicated by esophageal reflux.

Hiatus hernia

The incidence of hiatus hernia in those under the age of 40 years is 9% compared with 69% among persons over 70 years.[4] However, the ability to demonstrate a hiatus hernia radiographically frequently reflects the intensity of the diagnostic effort as well as the aging process. The development of hiatus hernia usually is ascribed to muscle weakness around the diaphragmatic hiatus associated with old age or chronic illness, straining at stool, the wearing of tight belts and garments and kyphoscoliosis of the spine—conditions that presumably increase intraabdominal pressure.[5,6] This pressure then is directed to the stomach and esophagus, forcing these organs upward against the diaphragm. Although most hiatus hernias are asymptomatic or are associated with only minor symptoms, complications may include esophagitis, esophageal stricture, bleeding and ulceration of the esophagus, and tracheobronchial aspiration. Reflux esophagitis also can occur without a demonstrable hiatus hernia. Most patients with hiatus hernia respond to a regimen of weight reduction in the overweight patient; small bland meals; avoidance of tight garments, bedtime snacks, highly sweetened liquids; and not reclining after meals. The regular use of antacids or H_2-receptor blockers serves the dual purpose of neutralizing gastric acid and stimulating the production of the hormone gastrin, which has been shown to increase the lower esophageal sphincter pressure, thereby decreasing gastroesophageal reflux.[7] Anticholinergic medications are contraindicated, since they enhance esophageal reflux by delaying gastric emptying and diminishing lower esophageal sphincter pressure.

Esophagoscopy is helpful in confirming the presence of a gastric protrusion above the level of the diaphragm. The endoscopic findings of esophagitis are erythema, edema, friability, and superficial ulceration. Direct-vision brushing cytology and biopsies are highly accurate diagnostic procedures and are essential in excluding malignancy associated with an esophageal stricture. Benign structures respond to gradual dilatation with bougies after the esophagitis has subsided. The use of mild irradiation (1600 rads) to the gastric fundus may decrease acid output from the stomach and thereby relieve the symptoms of acid-peptic esophagitis, especially in patients who are poor surgical risks because of cardiac, pulmonary, hepatic, or renal disease.[8] Surgical correction of the hernia is required infrequently for disabling symptoms or for complications.

Carcinoma

Carcinoma is the most common cause of obstruction of the esophagus in the aged. The incidence is higher in association with achalasia, alcoholism, acid-peptic stenosis of the esophagus, lye strictures, the Plummer-Vinson syndrome, and perhaps after gastric resection for peptic ulcer.[9-12] Cytology specimens obtained by direct-vision brushing at the time of esophagoscopy now provide almost 100% diagnostic accuracy at the University of Chicago.[13] Nevertheless, the prognosis is poor.

Surgical resection of localized lesions with interposition of the stomach or colon occasionally is feasible. Preoperative irradiation may reduce the size of the lesion and facilitate surgical removal. Postoperative irradiation also may help contain local spread of the tumor. Chemotherapy has little to offer in the treatment of squamous cell carcinoma of the esophagus. If the tumor involving the esophagus is an adenocarcinoma extending from its primary site in the gastric fundus, radiation therapy and 5-fluorouracil administration may be useful, at least temporarily. Palliation for obstruction includes mechanical dilatation and occasionally the insertion of a polyethylene tube by way of a bougie guide and gastrostomy.[14]

STOMACH

Of all the gastrointestinal organs the stomach is the most accessible for study and therefore is most often found in elderly individuals to be altered anatomically and physiologically. Gastric motility allegedly decreases with age, and hunger contractions apparently may be reduced.[15,16] However, the rate of gastric emptying in one study was within normal limits. In all probability gastric motor activity among the elderly is not altered significantly.

Atrophic gastritis

Atrophic gastritis, or gastric atrophy, is perhaps the most common manifestation of the "aged" stomach.[17] The histologic features include decreased thickness of the gastric wall caused by atrophy of the mucosa and muscularis mucosae, infiltration with leukocytes and lymphoid aggregates, "intestinalization," and pyloric gland metaplasia. Because uncomplicated chronic atrophic gastritis is asymptomatic and endoscopy is not a routine diagnostic procedure, its true clinical frequency is unknown. Biopsy studies have shown an incidence of 3.8% in the age group from 21 to 30 years compared with an incidence of 16.2% in a population age group over 70 years.[17] Atrophic gastritis is of interest chiefly because of a potential predisposition to pernicious anemia and to gastric carcinoma.

The secretion of hydrochloric acid by the "aged" stomach is reduced both in volume and concentration, and achlorhydria may develop, although newer stimulants (pentagastrin) demonstrate a much lower incidence of achlorhydria than had been assumed.[18-20] The consequences of true achlorhydria include decreased absorption of iron and vitamin B_{12} as well as a possible predisposition to gastric carcinoma. The concept of gastrogenous diarrhea as a result of achlorhydria has long been abandoned. However, in the absence of hydrochloric acid the bacterial flora within the alimentary tract tends to rise higher than usual, and bacterial overgrowth may be a factor in some instances. Such bacteriologic and metabolic abnormalities are detectable by "breath tests." When glycine-1-^{14}C-cholate is administered orally to patients with bacterial overgrowth, there is an increase in the level of $^{14}CO_2$ in the expired air caused by the increased deconjugation of the bile salt.[21] Peptic activity apparently is diminished in the elderly, paralleling the lower levels of acid secretion, but again this observation is not established conclusively. With aging the usual sex differences in gastric secretion become less pronounced, and acid and pepsin outputs in the elderly female tend to approximate those of the elderly male. In patients without gastrointestinal disease the plasma gastrin level increases with age; however, this elevation correlates better with the presence of antibodies to parietal cells than with age.[22,23]

Peptic ulcer

Peptic ulcer is a common problem among older people.[24] In a recent study 15% of patients hospitalized for peptic ulcer disease were 60 years of age or older.[25] The more common use of potentially ulcerogenic drugs such as aspirin, reserpine, phenylbutazone, steroids, and indomethacin by the elderly contributes to the development of gastric ulceration or erosive gastritis with massive bleeding. The alleged relationship between atherosclerosis of the gastric arteries and gastric ulceration is unproved.[26,27] Gastric ulcer seems to be more common among the elderly than duodenal ulcer. Giant benign gastric ulcer (diameter of 3 cm or more) also appears to occur more frequently among the elderly, with a peak incidence during the decade from 60 to 70 years of age, 5 to 10 years later than the usual age distribution of gastric ulcer.[28] Coexistent duodenal ulcer also may be present.

Approximately 50% of elderly patients with ulcers are admitted for acute gastrointestinal bleeding, and mortality exceeds 30%. Gastric retention may result from distortion of the stomach as a consequence of contraction of the lesser curvature and alteration of the normal anatomic relationships of the antrum pylorus and duodenum, a problem seen less frequently now than previously.

Medical management is effective in approximately 50% of patients. The recurrence rate of gastric ulcer is high, especially in association with a previous duodenal ulcer or with chronic obstructive lung disease. Complications including hemorrhage, perforation, pyloric obstruction, and failure of the gastric ulcer to heal are more common among elderly patients than among younger patients. The diagnosis of ulcer perforation is more difficult in the elderly patient because the manifestation of pain tends to be less typical and is poorly localized.

The incidence of bleeding from peptic ulcer does not increase with age, but the severity of the bleeding is increased. The mortality in a group of patients in their fifties with bleeding gastric ulcer was 25%, whereas the mortality rose to 65% among octagenerians.[29] There also is a rise in mortality in bleeding duodenal ulcers from 12% to 50% among the older patients. These figures suggest that earlier surgical intervention would be appropriate in older patients with bleeding that is definitely attributable to peptic ulcer.

Peptic ulcer with an onset after the age of 65 years generally is less responsive to treatment. The medical program involves several important considerations. A strict bed rest regimen should not be prolonged to reduce the hazard of pulmonary infections, thrombophlebitis, and pulmonary embolism. Antacids containing calcium or magnesium must be prescribed with care for patients with renal impairment; calcium carbonate, a highly effective antacid, may produce severe constipation as well as hypercalcemia. Its use also may be contraindicated because of its tendency to stimulate gastrin production and consequent hypersecretion of hydrochloric acid.

Cimetidine is the first of a new class of drugs known as histamine H_2-receptor antagonists. By blocking the action of histamine on the parietal cell, gastric acid secretion to such stimuli as food, gastrin, acetylcholine, pentagastrin, caffeine, and histamine is suppressed substantially for the period of administration of the drug. The initial dosage varies but usually approximates 300 mg four times daily with a subsequent decrease to maintenance levels (administration once or twice daily usually at night). Cimetidine appears to accelerate the healing of duodenal ulcers via the acid suppression mechanism. Patient compliance with this drug program seems to be the greatest advantage over the use of antacid therapy. When administration of the drug is stopped, gastric secretory patterns return to pretreatment levels, and recurrence of the duodenal ulcer is common. Although continued maintenance with a single bedtime dose of cimetidine reduces the recurrence rate, relapses can occur with administration of less than the full dose.[30]

The incidence of side effects with cimetidine has been low, but there have been reports of central nervous system (CNS) effects. Confusion is the most common CNS symptom, although slurred speech, delirium, hallucinations, and other signs of brain dysfunction have been reported.[31,32] Cimetidine side effects, including renal impairment, seem to be more common at higher doses and in older patients. Other reported side effects are fever, diarrhea, skin rash, and gynecomastia with breast soreness.

The role of cimetidine in other acid-peptic disorders is less certain than with duodenal ulcer. The use of cimetidine in peptic esophagitis results in symptomatic improvement and decreased antacid consumption, often without endoscopic or histologic change.[33]

Cimetidine is used for the treatment of gastric ulcer on the assumption that reduced gastric acid secretion may speed healing. As with the use of antacids for gastric ulcer, the benefit of cimetidine is not readily apparent in controlled studies. The Zollinger-Ellison syndrome, rarely seen in the elderly, can be treated successfully with prolonged administration of cimetidine, thereby avoiding the need for total gastrectomy.

Other pharmacologic effects of cimetidine not reported in the initial studies are now being described, and very likely other mechanisms of action of cimetidine will be elucidated in the near future.[34,35]

Anticholinergic compounds are more likely to precipitate glaucoma and gastric or urinary retention in elderly individuals than in younger patients. Excessive or overly rapid transfusions of blood in the management of bleeding peptic ulcer may induce congestive heart failure, and posttransfusion hepatitis is especially severe among the elderly. The use of washed packed red blood cells from hepatitis-associated antigen-negative volunteer donors may help to reduce the incidence of post-transfusion hepatitis. This condition often is related to cytomegalic virus as well as to non-A, non-B hepatitis virus. Commerically available gamma globulin unfortunately seems to be ineffective in preventing posttransfusion hepatitis.[36,37]

Mild gastric irradiation (1600 rads in divided doses of 160 rads daily) of the gastric fundus (over fluoroscopically outlined anterior and posterior portals) may reduce gastric secretion significantly in patients with peptic ulcer disease and thereby decrease the recurrence rate.[38] This adjunctive therapy is especially valuable in the elderly ulcer patient who is a poor surgical risk. Whether the availability of cimetidine will eliminate the need for this therapy remains to be determined.

Early endoscopy may help to identify a bleeding site and also provides a histologic diagnosis of the lesion by means of direct-vision cytology and biopsy. Celiac arteriography has been helpful in identifying the source of upper gastrointestinal bleeding. With selective catheterization of the bleeding artery, which is identified by the extravascular extravasation of radiopaque dye, infusion of vasoconstrictors or vasopressin (Pitressin), which lowers mesenteric blood flow, may allow nonsurgical control of the bleeding. The endoscopic control of upper gastrointestinal bleeding is being studied.[39]

Postgastrectomy syndromes

A variety of postgastrectomy syndromes may follow gastric resection, with greater incapacity to the elderly individual than to the younger patient. The symptoms of satiety and epigastric fullness and discomfort associated with a generous subtotal gastrectomy tend to improve with time. The dumping syndrome results from the rapid entry of gastric content into the jejunum distended by hypertonic fluid. Vasoactive serotonin and bradykinin have been implicated as mediators of the symptoms of flushing, lightheadedness, headache, sweating, and hyperperistalsis.[40,41] Treatment of the dumping syndrome includes small frequent meals, rest after eating, and separation of fluids from the intake of solid food. Sedatives and anticholinergic medication may be helpful. In a poorly constructed gastroenterostomy, sharp angulation of the gastrojejunal anastomosis, an excessively long afferent loop, or extrinsic adhesive bands may cause incomplete, recurrent upper gastrointestinal obstruction. Stasis associated with bacterial overgrowth of intestinal organisms in the afferent loop can induce deconjugation of bile salts with resultant bile salt steatorrhea, as well as megaloblastic anemia caused by folic acid deficiency. Surgery for peptic ulcer disease also may uncover a latent adult celiac disease.[42] Metabolic bone disease associated with vitamin D deficiency and the decreased absorption of calcium also may follow gastric surgery after long periods.[43] Iron-deficiency anemia can result from decreased iron absorption after gastric resection.[44] Patients who have undergone gastrectomy, resulting in a general decrease of resistance to disease, apparently are more susceptible also to pulmonary tuberculosis and to salmonella infections.[45,46] The more common use of vagotomy and pyloroplasty vagotomy and antral resection or the selective vagotomy procedures available today should reduce the frequency of these problems.

Gastric carcinoma

Although the prevalence of gastric carcinoma has decreased from 2.8 per 100,000 persons in 1930 to 1.1 per 100,000 persons in 1965, approximately 20,000 deaths from cancer of the stomach occur each year in the United States.[47] Intestinal metaplasia associated with chronic atrophic gastritis, especially in association with pernicious anemia, is considered a premalignant state.[48] Gastric adenomas with a tendency to neoplasia often contain the histologic changes of intestinal metaplasia. Consequently, gastric polyps larger than 2 cm require the most thorough scrutiny and surgical removal if carcinoma cannot be excluded completely. Endoscopic polypectomy now can be readily performed through the fiberoptic gastroscope, thereby avoiding a laparotomy and the need for a general anesthetic.[49]

Carcinoma of the postoperative gastric stump is significantly more common than in nonsurgically treated stomachs, especially at the area of anastomosis where polypoid, atrophic, and dysplastic changes occur.[50,51] In general, elderly patients remain more vulnerable to neoplasia of the digestive tract than young individuals. Fortunately, newer diagnostic procedures, including improved double contrast radiologic techniques and fiberoptic endoscopy combined with direct-vision cytology and biopsy, now permit an almost 100% diagnostic accuracy of these neoplasms through the digestive tract.[52]

Lymphoma

Lymphoma of the stomach is rare, but because of therapeutic considerations, lymphoma must be carefully differentiated from adenocarcinoma or the benign condition pseudolymphoma of the stomach.

Patients with lymphoma experience constant upper abdominal pain, weight loss, fever, and anemia most often the result of bleeding. A palpable abdominal mass may be present. Radiographic studies reveal ulcerated polypoid masses and thickened folds caused by submucosal infiltration. Peristalsis usually is preserved. At gastroscopy irregular masses are seen. Cytologic examination reveals large cells with prominent large nuclei that are distinguishable from adenocarcinoma cells. Biopsy may be less useful because the tumor tends to be submucosal in location. During surgical exploration a large gastric resection is performed, and follow-up treatment with radiation and chemotherapy is more successful than in adenocarcinoma.

Pseudolymphoma

Pseudolymphoma of the stomach is a benign inflammatory lesion often associated with large, multiple ulcers. The mucosa and submucosa are infiltrated with mature lymphocytes. The clinical symptoms and signs, as well as the radiographic findings, are difficult to differentiate from a malignant lymphoma. Gastroscopy and biopsy may be misleading so that surgical exploration with generous gastric biopsy is required to establish the diagnosis. Radiation therapy and chemotherapy are not indicated in the treatment of pseudolymphoma.

SMALL INTESTINE

The functional capacity of the small intestine may be altered by advancing age, as reflected in the decreased absorption of D-xylose and vitamins B_1, B_{12}, A, carotene, and folic acid.[53-58] The absorption of vitamin C apparently is not altered.[59] The absorption of fat also may be diminished in the elderly.[60,61]

The lowered intestinal absorption may be attributed to the effects of aging on the small bowel mucosa, with altered function of the mucosal cells as a result of decreased enzyme activity and reduced numbers of epithelial cells. The use of oral or systemic antibiotics in the elderly, as for acute respiratory illness, may disturb the ecology of the gut, allowing pathogenic bacteria or fungi to flourish and subsequently induce alterations in the structure of the small bowel mucosa.

Malabsorption

Malabsorption in the elderly can be caused by a variety of mechanisms. Steatorrhea, that is, more than 7 grams of fecal fat per 24 hours on a daily intake of 100 grams of fat is a common manifestation of malabsorption, regardless of the underlying pathologic condition. The absorption of fat requires the initial intraluminal preparation of dietary fats, which are split by pancreatic lipase in the presence of bicarbonate into monoglycerides and free fatty acids. The monoglycerides are combined with bile acids to form micelles. The micelles are absorbed by the villi of the small intestine and transported by the lymphatics into the portal vein. Steatorrhea can develop if there is an abnormality of the intraluminal phase of digestion, an abnormality of the bowel wall or villi, or obstruction to the lymphatic flow from the intestine.

Intraluminal factors—chronic pancreatitis or obstruction of the pancreatic duct by stones or tumor—will decrease the amount of lipase available within the small intestine to split dietary fats. Hepatobiliary disease can result in either decreased synthesis or an obstruction to the flow of bile acids to the duodenum. Diseases of the terminal ileum, such as regional enteritis or lymphoma, or resection of the terminal ileum may interfere with the enterohepatic circulation of bile acids, decreasing the quantity of bile salts returning to the liver. Although the liver attempts to compensate for this decrease, it cannot accomplish this completely, and usually the bile acid pool available for the formation of micelles in the proximal small intestine is diminished.

Treatment consists of the oral administration

of pancreatic enzymes containing lipase. Replacement therapy for decreased conjugated bile salts currently is not available. Bacterial overgrowth occurs in areas of stasis such as blind intestinal loop, small intestinal (jejunal) diverticula, visceral neuropathy usually associated with diabetes mellitus and scleroderma, and partial small bowel obstruction, which are associated with a deconjugation of bile salts within the bowel. Broad-spectrum antibiotics such as tetracyclines are helpful in reducing bacterial overgrowth and correcting the deconjugation process, at least partially.

Atrophy of the intestinal mucosa by conditions such as celiac disease, tropical sprue, dermatitis herpetiformis, and neoplasms including lymphoma and, rarely, carcinoma of the lung results in a malabsorption syndrome.[62-64]

Infiltration of the small intestinal wall as in scleroderma, amyloidosis, Whipple's disease, and lymphoma also may result in malabsorption.[65] These conditions can be diagnosed best by small bowel biopsy. Celiac disease responds to a gluten-free diet. Although this specific diet therapy is successful, it is expensive and inconvenient for most elderly patients. The diagnosis should be confirmed by small bowel biopsy before gluten is eliminated, and improvement of the villous atrophy should be documented by a repeat small bowel biopsy 3 months after the diet has been maintained.

Tropical sprue, rarely seen in elderly patients, responds to tetracycline and folic acid administration. Whipple's disease currently is classified as an infectious disease that responds to adequate tetracycline therapy. Although most infiltrative small bowel diseases cannot be adequately treated, the concomitant bacterial overgrowth can be managed with antibiotics.

Circulatory disturbances, either ischemic or venous stasis caused by congestive heart failure, also must be considered in evaluating patients with malabsorption.[66-67] Obstruction of mesenteric lymph nodes by Whipple's disease, constrictive pericarditis, congestive heart failure, tuberculosis, or malignant infiltration of the mesentery and its nodes may result in a malabsorption syndrome. Since medium chain triglycerides do not require bile acids for their absorption and are absorbed directly into the bloodstream, thus bypassing the lymphatic channels, they are of value in patients with obstructed lymphatics or with diminished conjugated bile salts.

Regional enteritis

Ten percent of patients with regional enteritis, or Crohn's disease of the terminal ileum, are over the age of 50 years at onset.[68] In Crohn's colitis, 27% of patients are over the age of 50 years.[69]

Crohn's disease of the terminal ileum is a transmural inflammation of the bowel wall associated with thickening of the bowel wall, linear or irregular ulcerations, a chronic inflammatory cellular infiltration, and granuloma formation. Skip areas of inflammation occur in other parts of the large or small intestine and, less often, in the duodenum, stomach, or esophagus. Complications include obstruction, confined perforation, abscess, fistulization, and bleeding. The typical patient has lower abdominal cramping pain, nonbloody diarrhea, weight loss, fatigue, and low-grade fever. The physical findings include right lower quadrant tenderness, peritoneal signs, and an ill-defined mass. Laboratory studies reveal anemia, occult blood in the stool, an elevated sedimentation rate, and hypoproteinemia. Electrolyte abnormalities such as hypokalemia and hypomagnesemia may be present if diarrhea has been severe. Abnormal liver function tests suggest systemic liver involvement such as fatty infiltration or pericholangitis. Vitamin B_{12} malabsorption and steatorrhea may result from terminal ileal disease or follow resection of this portion of the small bowel. Radiographically the terminal ileum is narrowed, irregular, and often fixed in situ by the associated inflammatory reaction. Fistulas from the terminal ileum to other intraabdominal organs such as other loops of small intestine, colon, bladder, or vagina may occur. Skip areas of intestinal inflammation are common.

The etiology of regional enteritis is unknown. Therefore the treatment is nonspecific and largely symptomatic. Dietary management consists of eliminating those foods that might excessively stimulate the bowel and promote diarrhea, such as raw fruits, juices, and raw vegetables. Large amounts of high-residue foods might be impeded by partial obstruction of the bowel lumen, although some observers actually have suggested the use of a high-fiber diet despite the presence of intestinal narrowing.

Milk is poorly tolerated by patients with an associated lactase deficiency. Sulfonamides such as sulfathalidine and salicylazosulfapyridine (sulfasalazine) are helpful in the medical management of Crohn's disease, although not as beneficial as in ulcerative colitis. Anticholinergic medication may be useful in controlling intestinal hypermotility and cramping.

Corticosteroids reduce inflammation and tissue reaction to infection. Their use is contraindicated in the presence of abscess formation, in perforation, and perhaps in fistula formation. Parenteral hyperalimentation is an important adjunct to maintain the nutrition of patients when prolonged bowel rest is indicated. Amino acid food supplements provide an easily absorbed, low-residue source of protein precursors helpful in patients with extrinsic disease. Because of their low residue and high nutritive value, amino acid food supplements provide an oral hyperalimentation alternative to the more expensive and more complicated parenteral hyperalimentation. The use of antibiotics may help to control a confined perforation or small abscess.

Surgery for Crohn's disease is limited to patients with complications such as obstruction, fistula, recurrent bleeding, and continued malnutrition. Surgical intervention does not necessarily cure Crohn's disease, and recurrence rates are high.

Crohn's disease rarely first appears in the geriatric age group, but patients with long-standing disease may be encountered. These individuals present special management problems. Over one half of the patients with Crohn's disease in the older age group will have undergone a surgical resection in the past. If the ileocecal valve has been resected, the patient may experience diarrhea as a result of the anatomic modifications. In addition, the resection of the terminal ileum may produce malabsorption of both vitamin B_{12} and bile salts. If bile salts enter the colon in concentrated amounts, they may irritate the colonic mucosa with loss of fluid and electrolytes, intensifying the diarrhea. The oral administration of psyllium powder (Metamucil) or the resin cholestyramine binds bile salts and renders them less irritating to the colon. The parenteral administration of vitamin B_{12} prevents megaloblastic anemia and the neurologic changes associated with vitamin B_{12} deficiency.

Primary ulcers

Primary ulcers of the small intestine beyond the duodenum are rare. They usually are located in the distal portion of the small intestine and may be complicated by bleeding, obstruction, or perforation. Although the etiology of small bowel ulceration is unknown, the oral ingestion of enteric-coated compounds containing potassium has been implicated in some instances.[70,71]

Intestinal lymphosarcoma, esophageal or gastric cancer, and bronchogenic carcinoma can be associated with partial villous atrophy and steatorrhea. The small bowel biopsy of patients with extragastrointestinal neoplasms may reveal blunted villi, increased lymphocytic infiltration of the lamina propria, and other changes.

Small intestinal obstruction

Obstruction of the small intestine can be either mechanical or adynamic, that is, paralysis or atony of the bowel musculature. The most common cause of mechanical small bowel obstruction in the elderly is intraabdominal adhesions from previous surgery or inflammation. Incarcerated inguinal hernia is another common cause. Symptoms include abdominal pain and distention, nausea, and vomiting followed by obstipation. Peristalsis often is visible through a thin abdominal wall. Bowel sounds are active and occur in rushes in the early stages; intestinal muscular paralysis may occur after prolonged obstruction. Plain abdominal x-ray films demonstrate distended bowel proximal to the obstruction and fluid levels, with a lack of air in the bowel distal to the obstruction. Adenomatous polyps, foreign bodies, lymphoma, and adenocarcinoma are rare causes of small intestinal obstruction.

Paralytic ileus can be caused by drugs such as narcotics, anticholinergics, and ganglionic blocking agents prescribed for hypertension and other disorders. Intraabdominal sepsis such as peritonitis or abscess, ischemia, electrolyte imbalance, and the late stages of mechanical obstruction also may result in paralytic ileus. Patients with adynamic ileus do not have colicky abdominal pain, even though the abdomen is distended. Nausea and vomiting are not as severe as in mechanical obstruction. Bowel sounds are greatly diminished or absent. Plain abdominal x-ray films reveal dilatation of the small intestine and often of the colon as well. Treatment is directed to the underlying cause of the "paralysis."

Malignant tumors

Malignant tumors of the small intestine are rare, consisting of three types—adenocarcinoma, lymphoma, and carcinoid tumor.[72-75]

Adenocarcinoma. Adenocarcinoma tends to develop in the more proximal small intestine and may appear as an obstruction, hemorrhage, a palpable mass, or as perforation of the bowel. Tumors of the duodenum most often are diagnosed on upper gastrointestinal barium examinations. Hypotonic duodenography confirms the presence of a mass. Fiberoptic duodenoscopy allows direct visualization and direct cytologic examination and biopsy of the lesion. Tumors in the jejunum are more difficult to detect by barium study but are discovered usually when celiac arteriography is used to study patients with gastrointestinal bleeding. The improved radiologic technique of controlled enteroclysis may be more beneficial diagnostically.

Lymphoma. Lymphoma occurs in the more distal portion of the small intestine. The patient may have a high temperature, weight loss, and a palpable abdominal mass. Carcinoma of the terminal ileum often causes symptoms and signs suggesting regional enteritis. The radiographic signs of obstruction, perforation, and abscess make differentiation difficult. Surgical exploration and biopsy often are necessary to establish the diagnosis. Radiation and chemotherapy have been of therapeutic value occasionally.

Carcinoid tumors. Carcinoid tumors progress slowly and tend to have a better prognosis than other small bowel malignancies. Appendiceal carcinoid tumors obstruct the appendix and appear as acute appendicitis. Carcinoid tumors of the small intestine tend to metastasize to the liver and are associated with the "carcinoid syndrome." The carcinoid syndrome of flushing, diarrhea, wheezing, and heart murmurs is allegedly mediated by serotonin and bradykinins produced by the tumor cells.[76,77] The diarrhea can be controlled with parachlorophenylalanine, which blocks the hydroxylation of tryptophan to 3-hydroxytryptophan, the precursor of 5-hydroxytryptamine.[78,79] The flush component of the syndrome is associated with excessive bradykinin production and is unaffected by parachlorophenylalanine. The same histologic type of carcinoid tumor is found in the rectum and tends to be less malignant, only locally invasive, and rarely associated with the carcinoid syndrome. Local resection of a carcinoid tumor of the rectum is curative.

APPENDIX

With aging the appendix undergoes true involution, as reflected in the decreased lymphoid tissue and in the obliteration of its lumen.

Acute appendicitis

Acute appendicitis in the elderly person has an increased mortality because of several factors: (1) the symptoms and the localization of pain are often atypical and (2) the inflammation tends to progress rapidly to gangrene and perforation (32% in an elderly group of patients as opposed to 6% in younger patients).[80,81] The lymphoid atrophy and decreased local blood supply may predispose the patient to gangrene, the rapid spread of infection, and bacteremia. The postoperative complications of pneumonia, wound infection, and delayed wound healing contribute to morbidity and mortality. In one series, because of complications, only 16% of elderly patients undergoing appendectomy were discharged from the hospital within the usual 5 postoperative days.

COLON

The familiar notion that the colon atrophies and its musculature becomes thin and atonic with age, causing constipation, is incorrect. Actually, in elderly patients with diverticulosis of the colon there may be pronounced thickening of the circular and longitudinal muscle layers. The high incidence of constipation in the elderly has led to the belief that bowel motor activity decreases with advancing age. Although the gastrointestinal tract motor function in advanced age has not been studied extensively, our clinical experience does not support this view. The tendency to constipation rather is attributable to decreased physical activity and a diminished intake of food fiber and fluids.

Melanosis coli

Melanosis coli is a streaked yellow-brown pigmentation of the bowel surface caused by the deposition of melanin in the submucosa of the colon, attributable to the prolonged use of laxatives containing cascara. This situation causes no physiologic disturbance and no clinical symptoms and is of no clinical significance other than revealing the prolonged overuse of laxatives.

Dolichocolon

Dolichocolon, a condition found predominantly in the very old, is characterized by enormous elongation and dilatation of a portion of or the entire colon. The atonic colon develops after prolonged disregard of the urge to defecate. It is most common in psychotic patients and in patients with Parkinson's disease,[82] as a result of either the disease itself or the overuse of anticholinergic drugs; it reflects loss of tone of the colonic musculature.

Intestinal obstruction

In the elderly the most common cause of mechanical obstruction of the colon is carcinoma. The usual symptoms of carcinoma such as abdominal cramps, change in bowel habits, or blood in the stool may be so mild as to go unnoticed until the patient has complete bowel obstruction, manifested by obstipation, distention, nausea, and vomiting. Digital and proctosigmoidoscopic examinations may reveal an obstructing lesion in the rectum. Barium enema examination also should be performed.

Other causes of mechanical obstruction of the colon include large adenomatous polyps or foreign bodies such as undigested fibers or gallstones. Fecal impactions and barium retained after earlier x-ray examinations also may result in an obstruction. Colonic strictures may follow ischemic colitis, Crohn's colitis, and radiation proctocolitis. Unlike small intestinal obstruction, inguinal hernia and adhesions rarely are causes of colonic obstruction. Extrinsic masses such as abscess formation associated with diverticulitis of the colon and an intraabdominal tumor such as may originate in the ovaries or uterus also may account for bowel obstruction.

Sigmoid volvulus refers to a twisting of the sigmoid colon around its mesentery, resulting in either a complete or partial obstruction. The sigmoid colon often is redundant and may wrap itself around intraabdominal adhesions. Ischemia caused by a compromised mesenteric blood flow may result in gangrene and perforation of the bowel. The patient describes sudden lower abdominal pain, initially colicky, but then steady in nature. This is followed by obstipation, general malaise, and signs of "toxicity." The nonsurgical treatment of sigmoid volvulus includes careful proctosigmoidoscopy or barium enema procedures, which per se may untwist the bowel. If these measures are unsuccessful or if bowel infarction or perforation is suspected, surgical treatment is required.

Irritable colon (functional bowel disease)

The irritable colon is the most common cause of symptoms referable to the gastrointestinal tract among the aged. This diagnosis is best made after a careful evaluation of the patient, including a thorough medical history and physical examination that includes the following: complete gastrointestinal radiologic examinations; proctosigmoidoscopy; examination of the stools for occult blood, pathogenic bacteria, and undigested muscle fiber and fat; and laboratory studies, including complete blood cell counts, urinalysis, sedimentation rate, and liver and pancreatic function tests.

The symptoms of irritable colon include constipation, diarrhea, gaseous distention, cramping abdominal pain, and excessive mucus in the bowel movements. A variety of other symptoms also may be present, including "heartburn," nausea, a sense of abdominal fullness, fatigue, and general malaise. Physical fatigue, dietary indiscretions, the use of laxatives or enemas, and especially emotional difficulties contribute to or aggravate the development of the syndrome. Important roles are played by emotional problems (depression, boredom, isolation, neglect, and a sense of inadequacy and uselessness); fear of disease, particularly cancer; and a lowered standard of living necessitated by the fiscal limitations of retirement.

The therapeutic approach to the patient with an irritable gastrointestinal tract should be positive and encouraging. After a complete evaluation the patient should be assured as to the absence of organic disease. It often is helpful to review some of the x-ray films with the patient during the course of a simple physiologic explanation of the disorder. The patient should be reassured that the symptoms are genuine and that they have a physiologic basis. With proper diet, rest, and appropriate medication (sedatives, anticholinergics, or antidepressants) the patient can be restored to an active and satisfactory life. Patience, understanding, and reassurance by an interested physician are the important components of therapy for this common condition among the aged.

Constipation

Constipation occurs in at least 25% of elderly patients.[83] The contributing factors include (1) lack of sufficient bulk in the diet to stimulate peristalsis, (2) the abuse of laxatives, (3) decreased fluid intake, (4) decreased muscle tone and motor function of the bowel, (5) blunting or loss of the defecation reflex as a consequence of neglect of the urge to defecate, (6) poor dentition (decreasing the intake of food), (7) anorectal lesions inducing spasm of the anal sphincter, tumors, and prolonged immobilization associated with fractures or paralyses, and (8) the use of medications such as sedatives or tranquilizers, antihypertensive and ganglionic blocking agents, narcotics, and calcium carbonate antacid.[84] Although there is no consistent alteration of bowel frequency with advancing age, the ingestion of laxatives increases significantly with aging; in one series people over 70 years of age used laxatives twice as frequently as those in the age group from 40 to 50 years.

Rectal prolapse

Rectal prolapse is more common in women and results in incontinence, soiling, and rectal bleeding. This condition is related to atony of the external and internal anal sphincters as a result of poor sensory appreciation of the urge to defecate.[85] Surgical resuspension of the rectum utilizing a Teflon sling may be helpful in selected instances of severe disability.

Fecal incontinence

Fecal incontinence develops in elderly patients with neurologic problems or mental confusion. The rectum of the incontinent patient is more easily stimulated and empties when a smaller than usual volume accumulates. The sensation to balloon distention of the rectum and anal sphincter tone both are decreased. Fecal impactions are not unusual in elderly patients, and fecal incontinence may involve the passage of semiliquid stool around the fecal obstruction.

Diverticulosis of the colon

Diverticulosis of the colon occurs in 40% of people over 70 years of age.[86] This condition has been recognized for a long time, but understanding of its pathogenesis is recent.[87] Clinically there is a close association between the symptoms of the irritable colon syndrome and the presence of diverticulosis.[88] Radiographically, the changes in the sigmoid colon of patients with an irritable bowel may be indistinguishable from early diverticulosis. Early in the formation of diverticula there is thickening of both the circular and longitudinal muscle layers because of prolonged spasm and shortening of muscle fibers. The thickened muscle layers cause segmentation of the bowel, and increased intraluminal pressure develops within each segment. As the pressure increases, the mucosa herniates through the weakest points in the bowel wall, that is, where it is penetrated by the small straight arteries.

Diverticulosis usually is asymptomatic. The consumption of a nutritious, high-residue diet; the treatment of constipation by diet, fluids, and bulk agents; the avoidance of bowel irritants; and the occasional use of mild sedatives and antispasmodic agents such as phenobarbital and belladonna help to relieve the associated symptoms of an irritable bowel syndrome.

Diverticulitis results from localized perforation of a single diverticulum, with subsequent peridiverticular or pericolonic inflammation.[87,89] Symptoms of diverticulitis consist of discomfort and tenderness in the left lower abdominal quadrant, constipation or diarrhea, fever, occult blood in the stool, and leukocytosis. A palpable mass representing a pericolonic abscess often is present. Barium enema and colonoscopy are contraindicated in acute diverticulitis. Proctosigmoidoscopy is helpful in excluding other conditions, such as carcinoma, ulcerative colitis, or proctitis, but is rarely useful in confirming diverticulitis. The medical management of mild diverticulitis consists of rest, liquid diet, absorbable antibiotics, and mild antispasmodic medication. Severe cases should be treated in the hospital with a regimen of nothing by mouth, intravenous fluids, and antibiotics. Meperidine (Demerol) should be given for pain, since morphine increases intraluminal colonic pressure. Nonabsorbable antibiotics are not helpful in either the treatment or prophylaxis of diverticulitis. Surgical treatment is reserved for patients who develop complications of diverticulitis such as obstruction, hemorrhage, free perforation, unresolved abscess, or frequent recurrence.

Morbidity and mortality associated with surgery for urgent complications are high; consequently, where indicated, resection of areas of diverticulitis before the onset of urgent complications is desirable. The mortality for surgery during acute complications of diverticulitis varies from 14.7% at the Massachusetts General Hospital to 23.3% in England.[90] Associated purulent or fecal peritonitis raises the mortality. The mortality for elective colonic resection approximates 1.5%[91,92]

There are no certain guidelines to indicate which patients will experience one episode of acute diverticulitis and recover without further recurrence and those who will develop frequent episodes of diverticultis or other complications. Approximately 50% of patients with diverticulosis experience one episode of diverticulitis without further recurrence.[93] The complications of diverticulitis—obstruction, hemorrhage, perforation, and fistula formation—occur in one half the patients with colon diverticulitis.

Patients who might most benefit from bowel resection are those who have (1) recurrent attacks of acute inflammation associated with fever and leukocytosis, (2) a persistent tender mass, (3) radiographic narrowing or severe deformity of a colonic segment, (4) dysuria associated with diverticulosis, (5) rapid progression of symptoms, (6) a young patient, (7) clinical or x-ray signs of cancer, and (8) persistent blood in the stools.[87]

Many surgical procedures have been recommended for diverticulitis of the colon. Not infrequently the involved portion of the sigmoid colon can be resected and a direct anastomosis accomplished in one operation. The multistage procedure for diverticulitis with perforation and abscess formation consists of a colostomy to divert the fecal stream and drainage of the abscess during the first stage. Subsequently, the involved segment of colon is resected and a direct anastomosis is accomplished with the colostomy maintained to protect the new suture line. When the anastomosis is healed, the colostomy is closed. Although this sequence requires three separate operations and general anesthesia, it may be safer than trying to accomplish a resection and reanastomosis when the bowel is greatly dilated because of an obstruction, when a large abscess is present, when the bowel has not been well prepared preoperatively, or when the patient is critically ill. A single-stage resection and reanastomosis can be performed electively if the patient is well prepared and the diverticulitis is localized. Myotomy of the circular muscle layer or antimesenteric longitudinal teniae has been advocated in England as a means of preventing increased intracolonic pressure in patients with diverticulitis.[94] Its ultimate value is not yet established. The use of bran as a bulk agent postoperatively has been recommended to decrease the likelihood of recurrent diverticular formation.

Ischemia of the gastrointestinal tract

Ischemia of the gastrointestinal tract may result from either vascular occlusion, caused by atherosclerosis, embolism, or surgical vascular ligation, or by decreased perfusion associated with congestive heart failure, hypotension, or hypovolemia. An extensive network of anastomoses joins the middle colic branch of the superior mesenteric artery, branches of the inferior mesenteric artery, and branches of the inferior mesenteric artery, and branches of the superior hemorrhoidal artery, forming a collateral circulation to the colon. Because of the lack of such collaterals, infarction of the small bowel is more common. Thrombosis of the superior mesenteric artery is more frequent than occlusion of the inferior mesenteric artery. Acute obstruction of the superior mesenteric artery is characterized by colicky periumbilical abdominal pain. Other clinical findings are hypotension, tachycardia, mental confusion and agitation, hemoconcentration, and leukocytosis out of proportion to the overtly minimal abdominal findings. Adynamic ileus, hematemesis, and bloody bowel movements rapidly ensue. Therapy for acute ischemia of the small intestine is surgical. If detected early before gangrene of the intestine has developed, an embolectomy may be possible. If gangrene has already developed, massive small bowel resection in the distribution of the obstructed artery is required; however, the mortality is high, and the patient is often left a nutritional cripple because of the short bowel syndrome.

Intestinal angina

Intestinal angina results from chronic vascular insufficiency of the gastrointestinal tract in elderly patients with other evidence of general atherosclerosis. Two or three major blood vessels usually are involved to produce the clinical picture of cramping periumbilical pain, which occasionally radiates to the back, commonly occurring 20 to 30 minutes after meals and lasting for 2 to 4 hours. The pain induces a fear of eating, which results in considerable weight loss, intensified occasionally by an associated malabsorption. The diagnosis of chronic ischemia is confirmed by celiac arteriography. Therapy is limited to small frequent meals to avoid excessive vascular demands on gut circulation. Surgical endarterectomy or bypass graft of the occluded vessel is the treatment of choice for severe obstructive vascular disease of the bowel.

Colonic ischemia

Colonic ischemia may produce at least three clinical patterns.[95-97] Necrosis, sloughing, and rapid death from peritonitis may occur, associated with bacteremia caused by *Clostridium*. The second pattern includes acute bloody diarrhea and abdominal pain. A limited infarction occurs, usually at the splenic flexure where the arterial supply is most precarious, resulting in a segmental stricture. An elective resection with primary anastomosis can be undertaken after the acute episode subsides and the extent of infarction is determined. The third pattern also includes bloody diarrhea and abdominal pain. Barium enema examination demonstrates a characteristic "thumbprint" pattern. The abnormality may disappear or a smooth stricture may develop. These patients require only symptomatic therapy such as stool softeners and mild antispasmodic medication. Resection of the bowel is unnecessary.

Ulcerative colitis

Ulcerative colitis occurs in approximately 10% of patients over 65 years of age.[98,99] The etiology of this inflammatory lesion of the mucosa of the rectum and/or colon remains unknown. Although infectious agents have been sought for many years, none has been identified as the cause. Altered immunity to endogenous antigens in the colonic epithelium or to exogenous antigens such as fecal bacteria has been an attractive etiologic concept, stimulating much investigation of the immunologic capacities of the small intestine and the colon. Vascular factors that lead to ischemia of the colon may play an etiologic role. Although ulcerative colitis most often appears as a chronic illness associated with bloody diarrhea, weight loss, abdominal cramps, and low-grade fever, a disproportionate number of older patients develop a more acute fulminating illness complicated by hemorrhage, toxic dilatation of the colon, and perforation of the bowel. Proctoscopic examination is helpful in the diagnosis of ulcerative colitis because the rectum is involved in 95% of cases. In the early stages the mucosa is edematous, and the vascular pattern of the mucosa is lost. More severe inflammation is associated with friability of the mucosa, hemorrhage, and purulent exudate. Long-standing disease is characterized by extensive tissue alterations, including pseudopolyposis.

Barium enema should not be performed in acutely ill patients because the examination may predispose the patient to toxic dilatation or perforation of the colon. The typical barium enema in ulcerative colitis demonstrates shortening of the colon, with loss of haustrations, narrowing, and an irregular mucosal pattern indicative of ulcerations. Advanced cases may show destruction of the mucosal pattern. The involvement usually begins in the rectum and includes a portion or all of the colon in a continuous pattern. Carcinoma of the colon and rectum is more common, especially in patients with total involvement of the colon, severe disease, and duration of the colitis for 10 years or longer. These tumors may be rapidly progressive, often are multifocal in origin, and may be difficult to detect early.

The medical treatment of ulcerative colitis consists of the elimination of potential dietary irritants such as raw fruits and vegetables, alcohol, and possibly milk if the patient is lactase deficient or intolerant of milk. Antispasmodics and antidiarrheal agents are helpful in relieving symptoms, but care must be taken to avoid paralysis of the bowel or gastric or urinary retention because of the pharmacologic overresponsiveness of these patients to antispasmodic and anticholinergic agents. Antibacterial agents such as sulfathalidine and salicylazosulfapyridine are helpful in treating the acute episode and in maintaining a remission. Immunosuppressive agents such as corticosteroids have been found to be helpful in controlling inflammation and in improving appetite and sense of well-being. The use of steroid enemas is particularly helpful when the inflammation is limited to the rectosigmoid area.

Surgery is reserved for those patients who fail to respond to comprehensive medical management, for uncontrolled hemorrhage, for perforation, for toxic dilatation, and for suspected colonic malignancy.

Pseudomembranous colitis

Pseudomembranous colitis often is a serious and occasionally fatal inflammation of the colon characterized by elevated white membranous plaques of exudate on the mucosa and leukocytic infiltration of the lamina propria of the colon on light microscopic examination of biopsies. The clinical picture is that of diarrhea, often watery, that contains occult blood and polymorphonuclear leukocytes on fecal smears; abdominal pain; and fever.[100] The onset of diarrhea occurs hours to days after the ingestion or infusion of a variety of antibiotics. Pseudomembranous colitis has occurred in patients receiving clindamycin, lincomycin, tetracycline, semisynthetic penicillins, chloramphenicol, sulfamethoxazole and trimethoprim, cephalosporins, and other antibiotics.[101,102]

The etiology of pseudomembranous colitis, previously attributed to overgrowth of staphylococci, now is recognized as attributable to a cytotoxin produced by *Clostridium difficile*, which is neutralized by *Clostridium sordellii* antitoxin.[103] The organism is resistant to the antibiotic used for therapy and is allowed to proliferate to a high concentration in the colonic flora.[104]

The use of oral cholestyramine resin, an insoluble quaternary anion exchange resin that binds the cytopathic toxin produced by *C. difficile*, provides a convenient and inexpensive treatment for mild cases of pseudomembranous colitis.[102] Vancomycin is active against *C. difficile*, and its oral administration in doses of 500 mg to 2 gm daily in divided doses for 5 to 21 days provides colonic levels of high inhibitory concentrations. Occasionally a relapse occurs after vancomycin therapy because of the inability of the antibiotic to eradicate the spore forms of the organism.[105] Readministration of vancomycin usually is successful.

Adenomatous polyps

Benign adenomatous polyps of the colon increase in frequency and number with age. Most adenomas are asymptomatic, but they may be responsible for both occult and gross blood in the stool. The relationship of adenomas of the colon to adenocarcinoma of the colon is unsettled, although carcinoma is much more common in patients with adenomas than in the general population of the same age.[106-109] Polyps and cancers occur in the same area of the colon, and the peak incidence of colonic cancer occurs a few years after the peak incidence of adenomas. However, a 5-year clinical follow-up has not demonstrated a significant difference in the incidence of carcinoma developing among those whose polyps had been excised when compared with a nonsurgically treated group.[110] The controversy concerns the question whether a single polyp is malignant from origin or whether a benign polyp undergoes malignant degeneration.[111] The histologic features of malignancy such as anaplasia, metaplasia, and cellular atypia but without invasion of the muscularis mucosae do not necessarily signify the presence of invasive cancer. These polyps are adequately treated by complete polypectomy.

Rectal bleeding

Rectal bleeding is an important symptom that must be evaluated completely to determine the source. Hemorrhoids and colonic diverticula in the elderly are so common that their presence cannot be assumed automatically to be the source of bleeding, especially if bleeding, either gross or occult, is persistent. When caused by diverticulosis, bleeding may be massive. Streaking of the stool with red blood more commonly is caused by a polyp or carcinoma. If proctosigmoidoscopy and a barium enema do not disclose a lesion other than diverticulosis, and the bleeding persists after a few days, fiberoptic colonoscopy should be performed. This procedure, in experienced hands, allows examination of the entire colon and also direct-vision brushing for cytology and biopsy of suspicious areas.

At the time of colonoscopy, snare polypectomy can be performed safely and easily by experienced colonoscopists.[112] Recent experience has shown that lesions smaller than 1 cm in diameter, even with a pedicle, may contain carcinoma in situ without invasion of the stalk of invasive carcinoma. It no longer is necessary to continue "to follow" with a barium enema those polyps that can be removed by colonoscopy.

Villous adenomas are more common in the

elderly. This benign polyp is of special interest because of its occasional association with excessive electrolyte secretion, causing depletion of the extracellular fluid volume, its tendency to recur locally, and its increased malignant potential in comparison with other adenomas. Patients have rectal bleeding accompanied by acidosis, and less commonly mucoid diarrhea associated with depletion of sodium, potassium, and chloride. In severe electrolyte depletion the patient may develop hypovolemic shock. The diagnosis often is made by digital examination of the rectum, demonstrating the bulky, velvety, sessile tumor. Proctoscopy and biopsy confirm the diagnosis. This lesion often is sessile and frequently contains areas of malignant alteration. Villous adenomas in the sigmoid colon most often are removed by local bowel resection. Rectal lesions may be treated satisfactorily by snare resection and electrocautery because of the relatively low malignant potential of many of these adenomas.

Cancer screening

The gastrointestinal tract is the site of the most common fatal malignancies. The best opportunity for cure of gastrointestinal cancer lies in the early diagnosis of a localized lesion in an asymptomatic patient. The anatomic distribution of colonic cancers has changed over the years. In the past, about one third of large bowel cancers were within reach of a digital examination; now only about 10% are felt on rectal examination. More tumors are located in the descending and sigmoid colon. As a routine large-scale screening procedure, rigid proctoscopy is expensive and resource consuming and is particularly difficult to perform in the elderly. The examination often is limited to the distal 15 cm of the bowel and is somewhat uncomfortable and requires adequate preparation. Nevertheless, all older patients with signs or symptoms referable to the distal colon should undergo this examination.

A flexible sigmoidoscope, approximately 65 cm long, that allows examination of the rectum and sigmoid and descending colon is now available. Although it is expensive, this instrument allows a much higher frequency of recognition of lesions than the rigid sigmoidoscope and probably will be used more often in the years ahead.[113]

Most proliferative colonic epithelial lesions bleed, at least intermittently. Guaiac-impregnated paper slides have been developed and allow the patient to obtain a stool specimen in the privacy of the home and to return the slides by mail for occult blood testing. In addition to cancer, other lesions associated with occult rectal bleeding are sought in patients with positive tests.

Routine screening with Hemoccult slides should be a regular part of the physical examination of all older patients, regardless of the presence or absence of symptoms. Rigid proctosigmoidoscopy or, if available, flexible colonoscopy should be undertaken in all patients with consistently positive tests, unless there are compelling contraindications such as severe cardiopulmonary disease.

Adenocarcinoma of the colon

Adenocarcinoma of the colon represents approximately 25% of all cancers of the gastrointestinal tract.[114-116] Elderly patients tend to have a better prognosis than younger patients with carcinoma of the colon. However, in our experience, despite an increased incidence of colon carcinoma with aging, the biologic behavior of the tumor in terms of invasiveness and survival rate is not changed significantly in relation to age.[117] Fulguration of adenocarcinomas of the rectum, deemed inoperable because of the patient's general debility, metastases, or other serious associated disease, can reduce the obstruction, bleeding, and rectal discharge.[118] Radiation therapy with high doses of supervoltage irradiation may provide long-term palliation in inoperable primary or recurrent carcinoma of the rectum.[119]

Carcinoembryonic antigen (CEA) is a glycoprotein that can be detected by radioimmunoassay in many patients with colonic cancer.[120-122] Although initially thought to be specific for colorectal cancer, elevated levels of CEA have been reported in patients with malignancies of the stomach, esophagus, pancreas, bile duct, and metastatic carcinoid to the liver, lungs, breast, ovary, urinary bladder, and prostate. Elevated levels also have been reported with neuroblastoma, multiple myeloma, and osteogenic sarcoma. Benign conditions associated with elevated levels of CEA include chronic renal disease, alcoholic liver and pancreatic disease, ulcerative colitis and Crohn's disease, diabetes, diverticulitis, and heavy cigarette smoking.[121]

Higher levels of CEA are usually, but not always, associated with more advanced disease, thus limiting its usefulness as a general screening procedure for early cancer.

Although the lack of specificity of the CEA determination limits its usefulness, an elevated level should support the need to continue the investigation for malignancy. The most valuable application of the CEA determination at this time is to follow the condition of patients with carcinoma of the colon and rectum whose elevated CEA levels fall to normal with tumor resection. A subsequent rise in the CEA level suggests recurrent malignancy.

Anal lesions

Pruritus ani. Pruritus ani is an itching of the anal area caused by irritation or inflammation of the perianal area by anal leakage and poor hygiene or as a result of excessive sweating from prolonged sitting such as occurs in older patients with cerebral vascular accidents who are confined to wheelchairs. Infections such as moniliasis in diabetic patients and pinworms should be sought and treated specifically. The presence of anal fissures or fistula must be excluded.

The treatment consists of improved local hygiene with avoidance of irritating toilet paper, using cotton instead. Drying creams or pastes with or without hydrocortisone are helpful. A straw pad or inflatable ring is helpful for people who must sit for prolonged periods.

Anal fissure. An anal fissure is a linear tear in the anal mucosa caused by stretching of the anus around a large hard stool or foreign body. Sharp pain and burning are associated with bowel movements. Bright red blood streaks the stool. An anoscopic examination often is diagnostic. Warm baths, stool softeners, and soothing anal suppositories or ointments provide symptomatic relief. Surgery is required for chronic fissures.

Hemorrhoids. Hemorrhoids are varicosities of the internal or external hemorrhoidal veins. They result from prolonged standing and particularly straining at stool. Portal hypertension also may be associated with hemorrhoids. The dilated veins protrude from the anus, bleed either chronically or acutely, and may become thrombosed or infected. Treatment includes the regulation of bowel habits and rectal evacuation. The patient must be instructed to avoid prolonged periods of sitting on the toilet and straining at stool. Acute inflammation can be relieved by warm baths and suppositories or ointments. Thrombosed hemorrhoids are acutely painful and distended with blood. Surgical removal of the blood clot gives prompt relief. Rubber band ligation of symptomatic internal hemorrhoids can often replace surgery.

Anorectal fistula. An anorectal fistula is an abnormal communication between the rectal mucosa and the perianal skin. It usually begins as a local anorectal infection; regional enteritis or Crohn's disease among the elderly is a rare associated disorder. Surgical excision of the fistulous tract after the abscess has been treated with hot applications and antibiotics usually is successful.

Epidermal carcinoma. Epidermal carcinoma of the anus is a squamous cell carcinoma that fortunately is rare. The lesion often ulcerates, invades locally, and is extended by way of lymphatic spread. Treatment includes surgery and irradiation.

PANCREAS

In the pancreas of the aged, solid masses of proliferating cells of the intralobular ducts may destroy the lobular architecture. Other changes include increased deposition of adipose tissue, decreased basophilia of the cytoplasm, nuclear degeneration, and focal areas of atrophy. Postmortem retrograde pancreatography has shown dilatation and ectasia of pancreatic ducts in the elderly even without obstruction. However, the volume of pancreatic secretion, the concentration of bicarbonate, and the enzyme content do not decline significantly with age.[123,124]

Pancreatitis

Pancreatitis in the older age group most often is secondary to other digestive disorders. Acute cholecystitis often associated with abscess or empyema can cause inflammation of the head of the pancreas. A posterior wall gastric or duodenal ulcer can penetrate into the pancreas, causing a secondary pancreatitis. These patients complain of pain radiating from the epigastrium straight through to the midback. This pain can be relieved by the patient sitting forward, thereby decreasing pressure on the pancreas. The pancreatitis associated with a penetrating peptic ulcer usually responds to adequate treatment of the peptic ulcer. The hypercalcemia of hyperparathyroidism is associated with pancreatitis. Pancreatic calculi may be responsible for distal obstruction of the pancreatic ducts and consequent inflammation.

Diabetes mellitus is associated with a higher incidence and a more severe form of cholecystitis, which may cause a secondary pancreatitis. Atherosclerosis of pancreatic arterioles also may contribute to a higher incidence of pancreatitis among diabetic patients. Hyperlipemia also has been associated with a higher incidence of pancreatitis.

Adenocarcinoma

Adenocarcinoma of the pancreas represents approximately 10% of digestive malignancies, and the incidence of this neoplasm is increasing in the United States.[125] Although found among younger people, pancreatic neoplasms usually occur in persons over 50 years of age. The combination of periumbilical or left epigastric pain, weight loss, and anorexia in elderly persons should alert the physician to this possibility. The rather abrupt onset of painless jaundice also may be the initial manifestation of pancreatic carcinoma among the aged.

The physical examination often is not revealing except for evidence of weight loss and chronic illness. A palpable gallbladder with painless jaundice reflects extrabiliary obstruction. Compression of the splenic artery by tumor produces an epigastric bruit.[126] The "early" diagnosis of pancreatic carcinoma remains difficult. The secretin test has not been helpful for this purpose, but cytologic examination of the fluid is especially helpful, with a diagnostic accuracy approximating 60%.[127] Newer developments, including fiberoptic duodenoscopy with cannulation of the ampulla of Vater for cytology and pancreatograms, celiac angiography, ultrasonographic and computerized axial tomography (CT scans) of the pancreas, and possibly the measurement of circulating carcinoembryonic antigen, may improve the diagnostic accuracy of this elusive carcinoma.[128]

LIVER

Several changes in the liver have been attributed to aging, including decreased weight and reduced hepatic blood flow, but without decisive supporting evidence.[129-130] A nonspecific reactive hepatitis, characterized by proliferation of ductules around the portal tract, surrounded by increased numbers of lymphocytes, leukocytes, histiocytes, and eosinophils has been described in elderly people, but such changes probably reflect the influence of other illnesses and medications rather than the aging process.[131] The blood chemical changes reflecting the status of the liver are nonspecific. Serum glutamic oxaloacetic transaminase, bilirubin, and cholesterol levels usually are normal. Bromsulphalein retention is increased slightly in about 50% of elderly patients.[132]

Malignant obstruction of the common bile duct

Malignant obstruction of the common bile duct is the most common cause of jaundice in the elderly.[133] Usually involved are tumors of the head of the pancreas or the ampulla of Vater, or tumors metastatic to the liver. Other causes of jaundice are viral hepatitis, cirrhosis, cholelithiasis, and intrahepatic cholestasis caused by drugs such as chlorpromazine.

Newer diagnostic procedures have improved the preoperative diagnosis of jaundice in patients with extrahepatic obstruction. Abdominal ultrasonography uses echo waves to visualize the liver, the gallbladder, the intrahepatic and extrahepatic ducts, and the pancreas. This safe, comfortable, noninvasive, and relatively inexpensive study is based on the principle that tissues of different densities absorb or reflect inaudible sound waves in characteristic patterns. If the hepatic ducts are dilated, and extrahepatic obstruction is confirmed, surgery can be undertaken with greater confidence. The size and precise location of the gallbladder can be confirmed. Stones appear as echogenic areas within the gallbladder. A filling defect in the liver caused by tumor, abscess, or cyst can be detected. Similar lesions within the pancreas also can be detected. Suspected ascites can be confirmed by ultrasonography.

CT scans incorporate roentgenograms taken from different angles in remarkably thin "slices" and group them into a composite pattern that provides a two-dimensional view of this area based on different tissue densities. Although this examination is more expensive than ultrasonography and involves irradiation, it is noninvasive, requires little preparation, and can detect lesions of organs relatively inaccessible previously by conventional x-ray examination and nuclear scans.

In the presence of extrahepatic obstruction, the percutaneous cannulation of an intrahepatic duct by a thin or "skinny" needle and the injection of contrast medium into the ductal system will help locate and determine the type of obstruction.

Endoscopic retrograde cholangiopancreatography (ERCP) is performed by orally introducing an endoscope to the level of the ampulla of Vater. When the ampulla is catheterized and contrast medium is injected, the extrahepatic and pancreatic ducts are visualized. In the hands of an expert this procedure can provide information regarding the state of the pancreas. Removal of stones in the common bile duct and other procedures such as endoscopic papillotomy (incision of the ampulla of Vater for stricture) are now possible through the endoscope.

Thin needles can be guided by ultrasonography to aspirate pancreatic and other tumorous cells. Although these needles may puncture or pass through abdominal viscera or vessels, complications are quite rare.[134]

Viral hepatitis

Viral hepatitis can be a serious problem in the elderly because it occurs in circumstances associated with the treatment of other diseases, for example, transfusion of blood and drugs.[135] Acholic stools associated with the intrahepatic obstructive phase of hepatitis may suggest obstructive surgical jaundice. The mortality for viral hepatitis in the elderly approximates 25%.[136] This poor prognosis correlates with subacute hepatic necrosis, poor nutrition, and associated diseases such as cancer or cardiovascular or chronic pulmonary disease. From an epidemiologic standpoint, care must be taken to avoid the fecal-oral spread of both the short-and long-incubation viruses of hepatitis in institutionalized or nursing home patients.[137]

Postnecrotic cirrhosis

Postnecrotic cirrhosis is an insidious disease often discovered coincidentally in the older age group. Symptoms include vague abdominal pain, weakness, anorexia, nausea, and weight loss. Clinical signs may include splenomegaly, jaundice, ascites, or bleeding. The liver varies in size. Anemia, thrombocytopenia, hypoalbuminemia, hyperbilirubinemia, and elevated alkaline phosphatase levels of hepatic origin suggest hepatic disease. Ascites is a late manifestation of postnecrotic cirrhosis and must be distinguished from malignant ascites. A liver scan may show patchy uptake of radioisotope in the liver, as well as increased uptake in the spleen and bone marrow. Percutaneous needle biopsy of the liver is an important diagnostic test. Infection and bleeding complicate cirrhosis and lead to hepatic coma. Superimposed hepatocellular carcinoma should be considered in patients with long-standing postnecrotic cirrhosis who suddenly show evidence of hepatic decompensation. Measurement of the serum alpha fetoprotein level may provide a diagnostically helpful biochemical supplement to the clinical and needle biopsy findings.

GALLBLADDER

Cholelithiasis

Cholelithiasis is common in the elderly, occurring in 38% of patients 70 to 80 years of age who are brought to autopsy.[138] Without ductal obstruction or cholecystitis the presence of gallstones is asymptomatic. The alleged intolerance of fatty foods and flatulence are unreliable symptoms of cholelithiasis.

Chenodeoxycholic acid, a naturally occurring primary bile acid, has been shown to desaturate human bile of cholesterol and to dissolve cholesterol gallstones over a period of months. Clinical studies during recent years have shown chenodeoxycholic to be safe and effective.[139] What influence gallstone dissolution will have on the course of chronic cholecystitis, which is often associated with the presence of gallstones, or the incidence of carcinoma of the gallbladder remains to be determined. It should be noted that gallstones tend to recur over varying periods of time when chenodeoxycholic acid has been discontinued. The clinical trials in progress during the past few years are being reviewed, and further guidelines as to indications, clinical efficacy, and long-term safety should be forthcoming.

Acute cholecystitis

Acute cholecystitis is the most common complication of cholelithiasis in the elderly. The patient experiences right upper abdominal quadrant pain, which gradually increases in intensity, but the pain usually lacks the intermittent quality suggested by the term *biliary colic*. Anorexia, nausea, vomiting, and fever are common but may not be as pronounced in the elderly as in younger patients. On physical examination there is right upper quadrant tenderness and a palpable mass if the cystic duct is blocked, causing a *hydrops* of the gallbladder. Jaundice is mild unless there is obstruction of the common bile duct. Elevation of the serum alkaline phosphatase level suggests partial common bile duct obstruction, even though the serum bilirubin level may be normal or only slightly elevated. *Empyema* or abscess of the gallbladder can occur without dramatic change in the symptoms, signs, or laboratory findings of the elderly patient. The presence of a tender, palpable gallbladder with a rising white blood cell count, fever, and chills suggests this serious complication.

The treatment of acute cholecystitis includes nasogastric suction and administration of intravenous fluids, electrolytes, and antibiotics such as ampicillin, cephalothin, tetracycline, or rarely, chloramphenicol. If the patient does not respond to medical management, surgery may be necessary even thought mortality in the elderly exceeds 10%.[140-142] At surgery a cholecystostomy with drainage of the gallbladder is performed in the critically ill patient rather than the more formidable procedure of cholecystectomy.

A gallstone may erode through the wall of the gallbladder into the intestine and pass to the ileocecal area where it may obstruct the bowel, producing *gallstone ileus*. A helpful diagnostic clue is the discovery on plain abdominal x-ray film of air in the biliary tree caused by the fistulous communication of the biliary system and the bowel. Other conditions that may show air in the biliary tree are choledochoduodenal fistula from chronic duodenal ulcer, and infection in the biliary tree with gas-producing bacteria.

Carcinoma

Carcinoma of the gallbladder rarely is diagnosed before surgery for a nonfunctioning gall bladder or cholelithiasis. Occasionally, persistent jaundice and a palpable mass in the right upper quadrant with severe pain and progressive debility suggest this diagnosis. The prognosis is poor, but because of its infrequency, it is not a major clinical problem. The causal relationship between gallstones and cancer of the gallbladder remains unsettled, although today it is less emphasized than in the past. The presence of gallstones without symptoms is not an indication for elective cholecystectomy among the elderly.

DIET THERAPY

Diet therapy long has been an important part of the art of managing a variety of gastrointestinal disorders. The more scientific the approach to the recommendation of diets the more differences of opinion emerge. There are several categories of conditions for which diet therapy is symptomatically helpful and a third category in which diet therapy has not been shown to be important from either a symptom-controlling or therapeutic standpoint. Traditionally, patients with active peptic ulcer at one time were advised to observe a restricted diet—initially consuming only milk or cream alternating with antacids on an hourly basis, followed by the gradual introduction of a limited number of bland foods. Although the ingestion of bland foods seemed to relieve the symptoms of most patients with peptic ulcer, their use has not been shown to enhance the healing of peptic ulcers. If the goal of diet therapy is the neutralization of gastric acidity, frequent small feedings are desirable. Whole milk or cream is no more effective than skimmed milk in neutralizing gastric acid, although the fat content slows gastric emptying; actually, milk and its products today are no longer emphasized in the management of peptic ulcer. Foods containing caffeine and alcohol stimulate gastric secretion without neutralizing the acid produced and are best avoided in patients who develop dyspepsia with these foods. The same limitation applies to the use of tobacco.

Patients with gallbladder, liver, or pancreactic disease may have flatulence, cramps, and nausea, frequently attributed to an intolerance of fatty foods. The ideal treatment of patients with gallstones and fatty food intolerance is cholecystectomy, but if the patient's general condition does not permit surgery, a low-fat diet may decrease stimulation of the gallbladder, thereby reducing symptoms and the hazard of an acute biliary colic. Patients with partial intrahepatic or extrahepatic biliary obstruction and individuals with a diseased or resected terminal ileum may develop fat malabsorption resulting from a decrease in the concentration of intraluminal bile acids, caused by interference with the normal intrahepatic circulation of bile salts.

Chronic pancreatitis also may result in the malabsorption of fat because of a relative deficiency of the pancreatic enzymes lipase, trypsin, and others. The symptoms include persistent diarrhea. abdominal distention, and cramps. The reduction of fat in the diet and, if necessary, the addition of medium chain triglycerides that do not require bile acids for their absorption can be helpful. Dietary supplementation of fat-soluble vitamins A, D, E, and K correct the deficiencies caused by their decreased absorption as a result of fat malasorption. Pancreatic enzyme preparations such as pancreatin (Viokase) containing lipase may improve fat digestion.

The use of high-residue diets containing unrefined grains such as bran, unrefined sugar, whole grain bread, and large quantities of fruits and vegetables have been suggested by Burkitt[143] to prevent gallstones, diverticulosis, and bowel cancer. The etiologic relationship between these conditions and the consumption of a low-residue, refined "western" diet is as yet speculative and improved. However, in African and Asian countries where unrefined grain and sugar are consumed, the incidence of diverticulosis is very low, but as people move to urban areas and adopt a lower residue diet, the incidence of diverticulosis rises. Perhaps factors other than diet, such as the stress and strains of urban life, also play a role in the development of diverticulosis of the colon.[144]

Occasionally, older people will not tolerate milk and milk products because of a deficiency of the enzyme lactase, which splits lactose into glucose and galactose. This situation can be documented by a failure of the blood glucose level to rise more than 20 mg/100 ml above the fasting level after the ingestion of 25 gm of lactose. Even though the blood glucose level may rise enough to indicate enzymatic activity, symptoms of diarrhea, flatulence, and distention may be brought on by the ingestion of the milk sugar.

Hyperalimentation

Total parenteral nutrition is one of the most important advances in the medical or surgical treatment of patients with serious gastrointestinal disease. Adequate bowel rest requires the cessation of oral intake of food. Patients who are rendered catabolic by inflammation, infection, or the stress of surgery develop severe nutritional deficiencies that must be overcome to ensure satisfactory tissue repair and surgical wound healing. In the past, this was difficult if not impossible with the parenteral fluids then available. It is now possible to provide intravenously the necessary calories, carbohydrates, fats, amino acids, vitamins, minerals, electrolytes, and trace metals needed to maintain adequate nutrition, to replace nutritional deficits, and to reestablish an anabolic state.[145] As with other modern techniques, skilled and expert supervision is mandatory for intravenous hyperalimentation and to monitor disease and prevent the significant metabolic and biochemical abnormalities associated with this therapeutic procedure. Many older people have a poor nutritional balance. This is intensified when serious illness occurs or multiple surgical procedures are undergone. Following surgery, the gastrointestinal tract may be unable to function properly because of infection such as abscess, massive resection, draining fistulas, prolonged ileus, and anorexia. Other complications in older people such as pulmonary emboli, pneumonia, and depression may delay the resumption of an adequate oral diet. Hyperalimentation can prepare and support the patient with a treatable malignancy during radiation and/or chemotherapy.

Iatrogenic disease

The chronic use or abuse of medications may produce varied abnormalities of the gastrointestinal tract.[146] The prolonged use of laxatives can cause diarrhea, weight loss, and weakness in the elderly. The earliest radiographic changes of chronic laxative abuse appear in the cecum and ileocecal valve, which becomes more patent. In time the entire colon manifests a loss of haustra; however, the length of the colon and its caliber may remain normal. Irregular contractions are seen fluoroscopically. The use of strong bowel irritants such as senna may damage the myenteric nerve plexuses in human beings and in experimental animals, contributing to a loss of muscle tone with irregular dilatation and redundancy of the colon. The changes sometimes are reversible, with discontinuance of laxatives and the reestablishment of normal bowel habits.

The chronic use of aspirin, indomethacin, phenylbutazone, adrenocorticotropic hormone

(ACTH), and adrenal steroids may result in erosive gastritis with bleeding or gastric ulceration, presumably on the basis of mucosal injury and the back diffusion of hydrochloric acid into the mucosal cell rendered susceptible to injury by an altered mucosal barrier.[147,148] Drugs such as monoamine oxidase inhibitors, antituberculosis agents, phenothiazines, oral androgens, aspirin, and cancer chemotherapy can cause jaundice and hepatitis. General anesthetic agents such as halothane also can cause a sensitivity type of hepatitis with hepatic failure and death.[149] Androgens have been implicated in the etiology of peliosis hepatis, a rare condition wherein the liver is characterized by blood-filled spaces and necrosis of liver cells.[150]

Surgery can be an important cause of iatrogenic gastrointestinal problems in the elderly. The postgastrectomy malabsorption syndromes have been mentioned. Cholecystectomy may be followed by problems as disabling as the condition prompting the initial surgery, including stricture of the common bile duct, retained stones, stenosing papillitis, obstruction at the sphincter of Oddi, or an enlarged cystic duct remnant with recurrent stones or inflammation. Massive resection of the small intestine for vascular occlusion leads to the short-bowel syndrome, with excessively rapid transit time and malabsorption, increased gastric acid secretion, and the excessive outgo of electrolytes and fluids, causing hazardous depletion of the extracellular fluid volume and associated cardiovascular and renal problems.[151]

Irradiation damage to the gastrointestinal tract after the irradiation of pelvic neoplasms can produce a variety of problems. Mild gastric irradiation, as employed in the adjunctive treatment of peptic ulcer, causes atrophic gastritis, but this structural change usually is temporary. There is no significant increase in the incidence of carcinoma of the stomach after this procedure. The slight increase in pancreatic carcinoma reflects the general trend of an increased frequency of this neoplasm in the United States. Carcinoma of the cervix treated with pelvic irradiation is complicated by radiation proctitis.[152] The small bowel is most susceptible to irradiation changes after the irradiation of pelvic and abdominal tumors.[153] The acute changes, including inflammation of the mucosal surface with epithelial atrophy, may occur within hours and generally subside over several days. Ulceration with perforation may occur. Delayed manifestations of radiation proctitis are stricture, fistula formation, and malabsorption.

CONCLUSION

This brief review of some of the more common gastrointestinal problems among elderly patients reemphasizes the general biologic uniformity of the human population. Digestive disorders are more common among elderly patients because more time has provided the opportunity for illness to develop and not necessarily because a fundamental or clinically significant alteration in the anatomic or the physiologic capacities of the alimentary canal has occurred. Thus the elderly patient is not subject to a "specific" age-related gastrointestinal disease. On the other hand, disease of other systems directly and indirectly influence the management of digestive illness among the elderly. In this context the understanding of gastrointestinal function and gastrointestinal illness, including the role of the emotional stresses and the contribution of environmental, economic, and sociocultural influences upon the health homeostasis of the elderly patient, represent a distinct "specialty" of practical medical importance.

The problems associated with gastrointestinal disorders among aged patients more often reflect the limited interest of the physician and other health personnel, inadequate attention, and insufficient study rather than a fundamental nonresponsiveness to treatment. The elderly patient who remains active and involved in life's affairs often is as "normal," as healthy, and certainly as productive and as useful or more so in human society as many "younger" individuals.

REFERENCES

1. Berman, P.M., and Kirsner, J.B.: The aging gut, Geriatrics **27**(3):84, 1972.
2. Soergel, K.H., Zboralske, F.F., and Amberg, J.R.: Presbyesophagus: esophageal motility in nonagenarians, J. Clin. Invest. **43**:1472, 1964.
3. Zboralske, F.F., Amberg, J.R., and Soergel, K.H.: Presbyesophagus: cineradiographic manifestations, Radiology **82**:463, 1964.
4. Pridie, R.B.: Incidence and coincidence of hiatus hernia, Gut **7**:188, 1966.
5. McKeown, F.: Pathology of the aged, London, 1964, Butterworth & Co. (Publishers) Ltd., p. 125.
6. Kassem, N.Y., Groen, J.J., and Fraenkel, M.: Spinal deformities and oesophageal hiatus hernia, Lancet **1**:887, 1965.

7. Castell, D.O., and Harris, L.D: Hormonal control of gastroesophageal sphincter strength, N. Engl. J. Med. **282**:886, 1970.
8. Cooper, J.N., Gelzayd, E.A., and Kirsner, J.B.: Mild gastric fundal irradiation in the treatment of peptic esophagitis, Gastrointest. Endosc. **14**:222, 1968.
9. Mosbech, J., and Videbaek, A.: On the etiology of esophageal carcinoma, J. Natl. Cancer Inst. **15**:1665, 1955.
10. Joske, R.A., and Benedict, E.B.: The role of benign esophageal obstruction in the development of carcinoma of the esophagus, Gastroenterology **36**:749, 1959.
11. Spiro, H.M.: Clinical gastroenterology, New York, 1970, The Macmillan Co.
12. Shearman, D.J.C., et al.: Carcinoma of the oesophagus after gastric surgery, Lancet **1**:581, 1970.
13. Kobayashi, S., Prolla, J.C., and Kirsner, J.B.: Brushing cytology of the esophagus and stomach under direct-vision by fiberscopes, Acta Cytol. **14**:219, 1970.
14. Carter, R., and Hinshaw, D.B.: Use of the Celestin indwelling plastic tube for inoperable carcinoma of esophagus and cardia, Surg. Gynecol. Obstet. **117**:641, 1963.
15. Lansing, A.L., editor: Cowdry's problems of aging, Baltimore, 1952, The Williams & Wilkins Co., pp. 481-526.
16. Van Liere, E.J., and Northrup, D.W.: The emptying time of the normal human stomach in the young adult, Am. J. Physiol. **134**:719, 1941.
17. Joske, R.A., Finckh, E.S., and Wood, I.J.: Gastric biopsy: study of 1,000 consecutive successful gastric biopsies, Q. J. Med. **24**:269, 1955.
18. Grossman, M.I., Kirsner, J.B., and Gillespie, I.E.: Basal and Histalog-stimulated gastric secretion in control subjects and patients with peptic ulcer or gastric cancer, Gastroenterology **45**:14, 1963.
19. Fikry, M.E.: Gastric secretory functions in the aged, Gerontol. Clin. **7**:216, 1965.
20. Blackman, A.H., et al.: Computed normal values for peak acid output based on age, sex and body weight, Am. J. Dig. Dis. **15**:783, 1970.
21. Sherr, H.P., et al.: Detection of bacterial deconjugation of bile salts by a convenient breath analysis technique, N. Engl. J. Med. **285**:656, 1971.
22. McGuigan, J.E., and Trudeau, W.L.: Serum gastrin concentrations in pernicious anemia, N. Engl. J. Med. **282**:358, 1970.
23. Ganguli, P.C., Cullen, D.R., and Irvine, W.J.: Radioimmunoassay of plasmagastrin in pernicious anaemia, achlorhydria without pernicious anaemia, hypochlorhydria, and in controls, Lancet **1**:155, 1971.
24. Levrat, M., et al.: Peptic ulcer in patients over 60, Am. J. Dig. Dis. **11**:279, 1966.
25. Cutler, C.W., Jr.: Clinical patterns of peptic ulcer after sixty, Surg. Gynecol. Obstet. **107**:23, 1958.
26. Elkeles, A.: On the pathogenesis of gastic ulcer in the aged and on the antagonism between calcified atherosclerosis and gastric carcinoma: a radiological study, J. Am. Geriatr. Soc. **18**:450, 1970.
27. Larsen, E., Johansen, A., and Anderson, D.: Gastric atherosclerosis in elderly people, Scand. J. Gastroenterol. **4**:384, 1969.
28. Strange, S.L.: Giant innocent gastric ulcer in the elderly, Gerontol. Clin. **5**:171, 1963.
29. Schuster, M.M.: Disorders of the aging GI system, Hosp. Pract. **11**(9):95, 1976.
30. Cimetidine forever (and ever and ever...?) (editorial), Br. Med. J. **1**:1435, 1978.
31. Schentag, J.J., et al.: Pharmokinetic and clinical studies in patients with cimetidine-associated mental confusion, Lancet **1**:177, 1979.
32. Cimetidine (Tagamet): update on adverse effects, Med. Let. **20**:77, 1978.
33. Behar, J., et al.: Cimetidine in the treatment of symptomatic gastroesophageal reflux, Gastroenterology **74**:441, 1978.
34. Puurunen, J., and Pelkonen, O.: Cimetidine inhibits microsomal drug metabolism in the rat, Eur. J. Pharmacol. **55**:335, 1979.
35. Klotz, U., and Reimann, I.: Delayed clearance of diazepam due to cimetidine, N. Engl. J. Med. **302**:1012, 1980.
36. Spellberg, M.A., and Berman, P.M.: The incidence of post-transfusion hepatitis and the lack of efficacy of gamma globulin in its prevention, Am. J. Gastroenterol. **55**:564, 1971.
37. Grady, G.F., et al.: Cooperative study: prevention of posttransfusion hepatitis by gamma globulin, J.A.M.A. **214**:140, 1970.
38. Levin, E., et al.: Observation on the value of gastric irradiation in the treatment of duodenal ulcer, Gastroenterology **32**:42, 1957.
39. Baum, S., and Nusbaum, M.: The control of gastrointestinal hemorrhage by selective mesenteric arterial infusion of vasopressin, Radiology **98**:497, 1971.
40. Peskin, G.W., and Miller, L.D.: The role of serotonin in the "dumping syndrome," Arch. Surg. **85**:701, 1962.
41. Zeitlin, I.J., and Smith, A.N.: 5-Hydroxylindoles and kinins in the carcinoid and dumping syndromes, Lancet **2**:986, 1966.
42. Hedberg, C.A., Melnyk, C.S., and Johnson, C.F.: Gluten enteropathy appearing after gastric surgery, Gastroenterology **50**:796, 1966.
43. Thompson, G.R., et al.: Detection of vitamin D deficiency after partial gastrectomy, Lancet **1**:623, 1966.
44. Baird, I.M., and Wilson, G.M.: The pathogenesis of anemia after partial gastrectomy. II. Iron absorption after partial gastrectomy, Q. J. Med. **28**:35, 1959.
45. Chofnas, I., and Love, R.W.: Postgastrectomy state and tuberculosis, Arch. Surg. **92**:704, 1966.
46. Black, P.H., Kunz, L.J., and Swartz, M.N.: Salmonellosis—a review of some unusual aspects, N. Engl. J. Med. **262**:811, 1960.
47. Pack, G.T.: Tumors of the stomach, Geriatrics **20**(9):699, 1965.
48. Morson, B.C.: Precancerous lesions of the upper gastrointestinal tract, J.A.M.A. **179**:311, 1962.
49. Seifert, E., and Elster, K.: Endoscopic polypectomy in the stomach: indications, technic and results, Dtsch. Med. Wochenschr. **97**:1199, 1972.
50. Hilbe, G., et al.: The risk of carcinoma in the resected stomach, Langenbecks Arch. Klin. Chir. **323**:142, 1968.
51. Kobayashi, S., Prolla, J.C., and Kirsner, J.B.: Late

gastric carcinoma developing after surgery for benign conditions, Am. J. Dig. Dis. **15**:905, 1970.
52. Prolla, J.C.: On the diagnosis of gastric cancer, Gastroenterology **58**:124, 1970.
53. Fowler, D., and Cooke, W.T.: Diagnostic significance of D-xylose excretion test, Gut **1**:67, 1960.
54. Guth, P.H.: Physiologic alterations in small bowel function with age: the absorption of D-xylose, Am. J. Dig. Dis. **13**:565, 1968.
55. Rafsky, H.A., and Newman, B.: Vitamin B excretion in the aged, Gastroenterology **1**:737, 1943.
56. Chernish, S.M., et al.: The effect of intrinsic factor on the absorption of vitamin B_{12} in older people, Am. J. Clin. Nutr. **5**:651, 1957.
57. Rafsky, H.A., and Newman, B.: A study of vitamin A and carotene tolerance tests in the aged, Gastroenterology **10**:1001, 1948.
58. Hurdle, A.D.F., and Williams, T.C.P.: Folic acid deficiency in elderly patients admitted to hospital, Br. Med. J. **2**:202, 1966.
59. Chieffie, M., and Kirk, J.E.: The ascorbic acid excretion in the stool in elderly subjects, J. Nutr. **59**:273, 1956.
60. Ryder, J.B.: Steatorrhoea in the elderly, Gerontol. Clin. **5**:30, 1963.
61. Becker, G.H., Meyer, J., and Necheles, H.: Fat absorption in young and old age, Gastroenterology **14**:80, 1950.
62. Rosa, L., et al.: Functional aspects of the small intestine in the aged, Rev. Gastroenterol. **17**:385, 1965.
63. Fikry, M.E., and Aboul-Wafa, M.H.: Intestinal absorption in the old, Gerontol. Clin. **7**:171, 1965.
64. Sleisenger, M.H.: Malabsorption syndrome, N. Engl. J. Med. **281**:1111, 1969.
65. Levinson, J.D., and Kirsner, J.B.: Infiltrative disease of the small bowel and malabsorption, Am. J. Dig. Dis. **15**:741, 1970.
66. Shaw, R.S., and Maynard, E.P., III: Acute and chronic thrombosis of mesenteric arteries associated with malabsorption: report of two cases successfully treated with thromboendarterectomy, N. Engl. J. Med. **258**:874, 1958.
67. Joske, R.A., Shamma'a, M.H., and Drummey, G.D.: Intestinal malabsorption following temporary occlusion of the superior mesenteric artery, Am. J. Med. **25**:449, 1958.
68. Crohn, B.B., and Yarnis, H.: Regional enteritis, New York, 1958, Grune & Stratton, Inc.
69. Fahrlander, H., and Baerlocher, C.H.: Clinical features and epidemiological data in the Basel area. In Engel, A., and Larson, T., editors: Regional enteritis Crohn's disease, Skandia International Symposia, Stockholm, 1971, Nordiska Bokhandeln Forlag.
70. Baker, D.R., Schrader, W.H., and Hitchcock, C.R.: Small bowel ulceration apparently associated with thiazide and potassium therapy, J.A.M.A. **190**:586, 1964.
71. Brown, C.H., and Akin, N.: Stenosing small intestinal ulcers: report of eleven cases, Cleve. Clin. Q. **33**:85, 1966.
72. Botsford, T.W., Crowe, P., and Crocker, D.W.: Tumors of the small intestine: a review of experience with 115 cases including a report of a rare malignant hemangio-epithelioma, Am. J. Surg. **103**:358, 1962.
73. Bruno, M.S., and Fein, H.D.: Primary malignant and benign tumors of the duodenum, Arch. Intern. Med. **125**:670, 1970.
74. Weber, H.M., and Kirklin, B.R.: Roentgenologic manifestation of tumor of the small intestine, Am. J. Roentgenol. Radium Ther. Nucl. Med. **47**:243, 1942.
75. Moertel, C.G., et al.: Life history of the carcinoid tumor of the small intestine, Cancer **14**:901, 1961.
76. Adicoff, A., Alexander, C.S., and Davis, R.B.: Malignant carcinoid syndrome: serotonin concentrates and hemodynamic studies, Arch. Intern. Med. **117**:250, 1966.
77. Oates, J.A., Melmon, K., and Sjoerdsma, A.: Release of a kinin peptide in the carcinoid syndrome, Lancet **1**:514, 1964.
78. Satterlee, W.G., Serpick, A., and Bianchine, J.R.: The carcinoid syndrome: chronic treatment with para-chlorophenylalanine, Ann. Intern. Med. **72**:919, 1970.
79. Koe, B.K., and Weissman, A.: *p*-Chlorophenylalanine: a specific depletor of brain serotonin, J. Pharmacol. Exp. Ther. **154**:499, 1966.
80. Peltokallio, P., and Jauhiainen, K.: Acute appendicitis in the aged patient, Arch. Surg. **100**:140, 1970.
81. Hangos, G., and Thurzó, R.: Appendicitis in the aged, Gerontol. Clin. **3**(Suppl.):55, 1961.
82. Lewitan, A., Nathanson, L., and Slade, W., Jr.: Megacolon and dilatation of the small bowel in parkinsonism, Gastroenterology **17**:367, 1951.
83. Connell, A.M., et al.: Variation in bowel habits in two population samples, Br. Med. J. **2**:1095, 1965.
84. Hootnick, H.L.: Constipation in elderly patients due to drug therapy, J. Am. Geriatr. Soc. **4**:1021, 1956.
85. Swinton, H.W., and Scherer, W.P.: Complete rectal prolapse or procidentia, Geriatrics **23**(11):113, 1968.
86. Manousos, O.N., Truelove, S.C., and Lumsden, K.: Prevalence of colonic diverticulosis in general population of Oxford area, Br. Med. J. **3**:762, 1967.
87. Berman, P.M., and Kirsner, J.B.: Current knowledge of diverticular disease of the colon, Am. J. Dig. Dis. **17**:741, 1972.
88. Fleischner, F.G., and Ming, S.C.: Revised concepts on diverticular disease of the colon, Radiology **84**:599, 1965.
89. Berman, L.G., et al.: A critical reappraisal of sigmoid peridiverticulitis, Surg. Gynecol. Obstet. **127**:481, 1968.
90. Hartley, R.C.: Dangers of diverticulitis coli, Br. J. Surg. **51**:45, 1964.
91. Marshall, S.F.: Earlier section in one stage for diverticulitis of the colon, Am. Surg. **29**:337, 1963.
92. Colcock, B.P.: Surgical treatment of diverticulitis, Am. J. Surg. **115**:264, 1968.
93. Boles, R.S., Jr., and Jordan, S.M.: The clinical significance of diverticulosis, Gastroenterology **35**:579, 1958.
94. Reilly, M.: Sigmoid myotomy, Proc. R. Soc. Med. **57**:556, 1964.
95. Fagin, R.R., and Kirsner, J.B.: Ischemic disease of the colon, Adv. Intern. Med. **17**:343, 1971.
96. Marston, A., et al.: Ischaemic colitis, Gut **7**:1, 1966.
97. Irwin, A.: Partial infarction of the colon due to reversible vascular occlusion, Clin. Radiol. **16**:265, 1965.
98. Law, D.H., Steinberg, H., and Sleisenger, M.H.: Ul-

cerative colitis with onset after the age of fifty, Gastroenterology **41**:457, 1961.
99. Banks, B.M., and Klayman, M.I.: Idiopathic ulcerative colitis beginning after the age of fifty, N. Engl. J. Med. **249**:91, 1953.
100. Tedesco, F.J., Stanley, R.J., and Alpers, D.H.: Diagnostic features of clindamycin-associated pseudomembranous colitis, N. Engl. J. Med. **290**:841, 1974.
101. Dowell, V.R., Jr.: Antibiotic associated colitis, Hosp. Pract. **14**(4):75, 1979.
102. Tedesco, F.J., et al.: Therapy of antibiotic-associated pseudomembranous colitis, J. Clin. Gastroenterol. **1**:51, 1979.
103. Bartlett, J.G.: Antibiotic associated pseudomembranous colitis, Rev. Infect. Dis. **1**:530, 1979.
104. Bartlett, J.G., et al.: Antibiotic associated pseudomembranous colitis due to toxin-producing Clostridia, N. Engl. J. Med. **298**:531, 1978.
105. Bartlett, J.G., et al.: Symptomatic relapse after oral vancomycin therapy in antibiotic-associated pseudomembranous colitis, Gastroenterology **78**:431, 1980.
106. Terrel, R.: Adenoma and cancer of the rectum and colon: advances and retreats, Surg. Clin. North Am. **39**:1291, 1959.
107. Rider, J.A., et al.: Polyps of colon and rectum: their incidence and relationship to carcinoma, Am. J. Med. **16**:555, 1954.
108. Castleman, B., and Krickstein, H.: Current approach to the polyp-cancer controversy, Gastroenterology **51**:108, 1966.
109. Ortmayer, M.: Carcinoma in small polyps of the distal colon: a sigmoidoscopic and histologic study, Gastroenterology **31**:404, 1956.
110. Colvert, J.R., and Brown, C.H.: Rectal polyps: diagnosis, five-year follow-up and relation to carcinoma of the colon, Am. J. Med. Sci. **215**:24, 1948.
111. Jackman, R.J., and Mayo, C.W.: The adenoma-carcinoma sequence in cancer of the colon, Surg. Gynecol. Obstet. **93**:327, 1951.
112. Wolff, W.I., and Shinya, H.: Polypectomy via the fiberoptic colonoscope: removal of neoplasms beyond reach of the sigmoidoscope, N. Engl. J. Med. **288**:329, 1973.
113. Winnan, G., et al.: Superiority of the flexible to the rigid sigmoidoscope in routine proctosigmoidoscopy, N. Engl. J. Med. **302**:1011, 1980.
114. Sunderland, D.A., and Brinkley, G.E.: Papillary adenomas of the large intestine, Cancer **1**:184, 1948.
115. Swinton, N.W., and Counts, R.L.: Cancer of the colon and rectum: statistical study with end results, J.A.M.A. **161**:1139, 1956.
116. Welch, C.E., and Burke, J.F.: Carcinoma of the colon and rectum, N. Engl. J. Med. **266**:211, 1962.
117. Roth-Moyo, L.A., Devitt, I.E., and Brown, F.N.: The effect of age on the behavior of carcinoma of the colon and rectum, Dis. Colon Rectum **11**:420, 1968.
118. Ramsey, W.H.: Treatment of inoperable cancer of the rectum by fulguration, Dis. Colon Rectum **6**:114, 1963.
119. Wang, C.C., and Schulz, M.D.: Role of radiation therapy in movement of carcinoma of sigmoid, rectosigmoid and rectum, Radiology **79**:1, 1962.
120. Gold, P., and Freedman, S.O.: Specified carcinoembryonic antigen of the human digestive system, J. Exp. Med. **122**:467, 1965.
121. Stillman, A., and Zamcheck, N.: Recent advances in immunologic diagnosis of digestive tract cancer, Am. J. Dig. Dis. **15**:1003, 1970.
122. Thompson, D.M.P., et al.: The radioimmunoassay of circulating carcinoembryonic antigen of the human digestive system, Proc. Natl. Acad. Sci. USA **64**:161, 1969.
123. Kreel, L., and Sandin, B.: Changes in pancreatic morphology associated with aging, Gut **14**:962, 1973.
124. Rosenberg, I.R., et al.: The effect of age and sex upon human pancreatic secretion of fluid and bicarbonate, Gastroenterology **50**:191, 1966.
125. Moldow, R.E., and Connelly, R.R.: Epidemiology of pancreatic cancer in Connecticut, Gastroenterology **55**:677, 1968.
126. Serebro, H.: A diagnostic sign of carcinoma of the body of the pancreas, Lancet **1**:85, 1965.
127. Prolla, J., and Kirsner, J.B.: Handbook and atlas of gastrointestinal exfoliative cytology, Chicago, 1972, University of Chicago Press.
128. Moore, T.L., et al.: Carcinoembryonic antigen assay in cancer of the colon and pancreas and other digestive tract disorders, Am. J. Dig. Dis. **16**:1, 1971.
129. Boyd, E.: Normal variability in weight of the adult human liver and spleen, Arch. Pathol. **16**:350, 1933.
130. Wiener, E., and Rabinovici, N.: Liver haemodynamics and age, Proc. Soc. Exp. Biol. Med. **108**:752, 1961.
131. Schaffner, F., and Popper, H.: Nonspecific reactive hepatitis in aged and infirmed people, Am. J. Dig. Dis. **4**:389, 1959.
132. Smolyansky, B.L., and Kolmakov, V.N.: Functional state of the liver in connection with aging, Klin. Med. **44**:53, 1966.
133. Huete-Armijo, A., and Exton-Smith, A.N.: Causes and diagnosis of jaundice in the elderly, Br. Med. J. **1**:1113, 1962.
134. Yamanaka, T., and Kimura, K.: Differential diagnosis of pancreatic mass lesion with percutaneous fine-needle aspiration biopsy under ultrasonic guidance, Dig. Dis. Sci. **24**:694, 1979.
135. Fenster, L.F.: Viral hepatitis in the elderly, Gastroenterology **49**:262, 1965.
136. Kishko, A.M.: Peculiarities of infectious hepatitis in the aged, Ter. Arkh. **38**:29, 1966.
137. Giles, J.P., et al.: Viral hepatitis: relation of Australian/SH antigen to the Willowbrook MS2 strain, N. Engl. J. Med. **281**:119, 1969.
138. Newman, H.F., and Northup, J.D.: The autopsy incidence of gallstones, Int. Surg. **109**:1, 1959.
139. Thistle, J.L., Hofmann, A.F., Ott, B.J., Stephens, D.H.: Chenotherapy for gallstone dissolution. I. Efficacy and safety, J.A.M.A. **239**:1041, 1978.
140. Glenn, F.: Indications for operation in biliary tract disease among the elderly, Geriatrics **24**:98, 1969.
141. Amberg, J.R., and Zboralske, F.F.: Gallstones after 70, Geriatrics **20**(7):539, 1965.
142. Glenn, F., and Hays, D.: The age factor in mortality rate of patients undergoing surgery of the biliary tract, Surg. Gynecol. Obstet. **100**:11, 1955.

143. Burkitt, D.P., Walker, A.R.P., and Painter, N.S.: Dietary fiber and disease, J.A.M.A. **229:**1068, 1974.
144. Berman, P.M., and Kirsner, J.R.: Diverticular disease of the colon—the possible role of "roughage" in both food and life (editorial), Am. J. Dig. Dis. **18:**506, 1973.
145. Wilmore, D.W., and Dudrick, S.J.: Growth and development of an infant receiving all nutrients by vein, J.A.M.A. **203:**860, 1968.
146. Berman, P.M., and Kirsner, J.B.: Recognizing and avoiding adverse gastrointestinal effects of drugs, Geriatrics **29**(6):59, 1974.
147. Menguy, R.: Pathophysiology of peptic ulcer, Am. J. Surg. **120:**282, 1970.
148. Davenport, H.W.: Salicylate damage to the gastric mucosal barrier, N. Engl. J. Med. **276:**1307, 1967.
149. Davidson, C.S., Babior, Z., and Popper, H.: Concerning hepatotoxicity of halothane, N. Engl. J. Med. **275:**1497, 1966.
150. Gordon, B.S., et al.: Peliosis hepatis and cholestasis following administration of norethandrolone, Am. J. Clin. Pathol. **33:**156, 1960.
151. Reul, G.J., and Ellison, E.H.: Effect of 75 per cent distal small bowel resection on gastric secretion, Am. J. Surg. **111:**772, 1966.
152. Gelfand, M.D., et al.: Acute irradiation proctitis in man: development of eosinophilic crypt abscesses, Gastroenterology **54:**401, 1968.
153. Trier, J.S., and Browning, T.H.: Morphological response of the mucosa of the human small intestine to x-ray exposure, J. Clin. Invest. **45:**194, 1966.

CHAPTER 9 · AGING, BONE, AND OSTEOPOROSIS

Louis V. Avioli

Osteoporosis is not unique to modern humans, having been documented in prehistoric humans living within the third millenium B.C. or circa 2500 to 2000 B.C.[1,2] *Osteoporosis* is a generic term used currently to define a specific form of generalized *osteopenia*, a term initially introduced by Bauer[3] as equal to "too little calcified bone" but herein redefined as signifying a reduction in bone mass below that which normally characterizes the skeleton for the age, sex, and race of an individual. As such, it is a description of a state not a disease.

Histologically, osteoporosis represents a state of decreased bone mass with normal mineralization of the remnant skeletal tissue. Osteoporosis therefore must be differentiated from osteomalacia, wherein the bone is poorly mineralized although total bone mass (i.e., osteoid plus mineral) may be normal, decreased, or even increased. In most instances (i.e., in the absence of pseudofractures) the distinction between osteoporosis and osteomalacia is only established with certainty by bone biopsy, usually of the rib or iliac crest, and by inspection of appropriately stained, undemineralized, histologic sections.[4,5] The characteristic histologic features of osteomalacia are wide osteoid (i.e., poorly mineralized collagen) seams and an increased number of surface seams per unit of bone. In addition to these changes one classically finds a decreased rate of osteoid mineralization or so-called "appositional rate" at the calcification front employing either special staining (i.e., Solochrome) or tetracycline labeling techniques. These combined histologic criteria are essential to the diagnosis of osteomalacia per se, since other pathologic osteopenic disorders characterized by elevated appositional rates (i.e., hyperthyroidism, Paget's disease, or primary hyperparathyroidism) may also lead to an increase in the surface area occupied by osteoid seams, despite ample evidence of osteoid mineralization. Histologic confirmation of osteoporosis as the primary underlying form of osteopenia is considered most essential for the institution of appropriate therapy. Without appropriate bone biopsy documentation therefore, a variety of proposed therapeutic "cures" for osteoporosis may, in fact, represent a remineralization of an associated osteomalacic process. In fact, sometimes osteoporosis and osteomalacia occur in the same individuals, despite the lack of clinical suggestion of osteomalacia in their clinical histories and normal laboratory data and radiographs.[6]

PHYSIOLOGY

In adults, after epiphyseal closure and after longitudinal growth have ceased, the skeletal turnover rate is approximately 2% to 4% a year. During adult life, skeletal growth does not entirely cease, since there is both continuing subperiosteal bone formation and a continuation of the later adolescent shift to endosteal bone formation or apposition. At this time the skeletal maintenance requires the deposition of approximately 100 gm of calcium a year, or 19% of the total skeletal content. The skeleton is in a relatively steady state, since bone formation equals bone resorption with no net change in skeletal mass. Epidemiologic surveys in varied populations with wide ranges in calcium intake demonstrate a shift in this equilibrium between the third and fourth decades with bone resorption dominating; this results in a loss of skeletal mass, especially in the vertebrae and long bones.[7,8] When judged by relatively insensitive radiologic criteria alone, the incidence of osteoporosis of the spine of women between the ages of 45 and 79 years has been estimated as 29%,[9] whereas only 18% of ambulating elderly men are similarly affected.[10] Despite attempts to refine radiographic techniques, this x-ray diagnosis may be somewhat crude and misleading, since a loss of over 30% of bone mineral is necessary (possibly up to 50% to 60%) before the trained radiologist is certain of abnormal demineralization.[11-13] Radiologic criteria such as ballooning of the vertebral discs have been shown to be of little value in assessing the amount of bone loss.[14] The age-related bone loss most probably affects the entire skeleton, although it is far from uniform, proceeding at different rates in different parts.[8,15] Thus the amount of cancellous trabecular bone of the vertebral bodies begins to decrease by the age of 25 to 30 years, whereas the loss of cortical bone occurs much later in time. Furthermore, the rates of bone resorption in various cancellous bones are also different, since vertebral bodies atrophy sooner than the calcaneum.[16] Age-related decreases in mandibular alveolar bone also lead to diminution of tooth support, fenestration of the roots, and ultimate loss of teeth.[17]

There are certain other characteristics of this universal loss of skeletal mass with age: the rate of bone loss does not increase with age in that there appears to be a steady fall in the average amount of bones in persons which begins at 30 to 40 years of age. This is approximately 8% per decade in women and 3% per decade in men. Among young adults the skeletal mass is greater in males than females and greater in blacks than whites. The rate of bone loss is similar in whites and in blacks, and the loss begins earlier in females than in males. Taller individuals of both sexes lose bone less rapidly, and although the onset of loss in the females antedates the menopause, the ratio of skeletal loss in the female is distinctly accelerated after menopause. Thus, since the maximum skeletal maturity is less for the white female than for the white male or the black male or female and because the loss begins earlier in the female and proceeds at a more rapid rate after menopause, net skeletal mass is lowest in the postmenopausal white female.

Genetic and epidemiologic factors all appear to play important roles in determining the total bone mass of adult populations. It seems appropriate therefore to reserve the term *osteoporosis* for disorders with a histologically documented reduction in bone volume and in which the reduction in skeletal mass is characterized by a normal degree of osteoid mineralization and is greater than that anticipated for the age, race, and sex of the individual. The critical level of skeletal mass at which osteoporosis becomes radiologically or symptomatically manifested will be reached much earlier in the individual who failed to acquire the full complement of bone in adolescence. The individual with relatively lower skeletal mass at the time of maturity will not only be more susceptible to the ravages of physiologic osteopenia at an earlier age but also to the symptomatic manifestations of so-called "postmenopausal," "crush-fracture," or "senile" osteoporosis.

DIAGNOSIS

Radiology

Since bone mass is normally gradually decreasing with age in all adults, before osteoporosis is attributed to some other cause the degree of osteopenia must be shown to be inappropriate for the age and sex of the individual. This distinction is often difficult, since estimates of the amount of mineral that must be lost to be evident even to the trained radiologic eye have ranged from 20% to 60%.[11,13,18] Various radioisotopic absorptiometric methods utilizing monoenergetic radiation sources and more sensitive columnated detection devices have led to more precise determinations and the detection of mineral losses of substantially less than 8%.[19] Regional bone mass measurements (radius, spine, and humerus) utilizing photon absorption densitometric techniques have also been shown to correlate well with total bone mineral mass and presently show promise for accurately predicting total body mineral content.[20,21] However, even when lack of mineral can be clearly determined, it may be impossible to differentiate osteoporosis from osteomalacia until certain distinguishing features become apparent.[22]

Fortunately, one need not depend on uncertain estimates of diminished density because there are several "geographic" changes in bone radiographs that, although detectable only when a significant amount of bone has been lost, are suggestive of osteoporosis. In the vertebrae, generally corresponding to the severity of the disorder, accentuation of end plate shadows, preservation and perhaps intensification of vertical trabeculae, and biconcave compressions, localized to one or two vertebrae, usually with expansion of the intervertebral discs are seen. In most forms of osteoporosis the vertebral cortex is thin and uninterrupted and gives the false impression of increased density because of the loss of trabeculae in the main body. Erosion of the cortex is rare and should lead the physician to suspect malignant disease. As the disease progresses, the trabecular structure assumes patterns in vertebrae and femoral necks according to the structural lines of stress.[23,24] Further progression of the osteoporotic process may result in biconcave compression of the end plates by the pressure of the intervertebral discs on the hypomineralized vertebrae, resulting in "codfish" vertebrae and "ballooned" intervertebral discs. Localized herniations of the nucleus pulposus into the vertebral body, producing a concave mushroom-shaped defect in the upper or lower surface of the involved vertebrae or "Schmorl's nodes," may also be observed, although there is no association between Schmorl's nodes and the incidence of osteoporosis.[25] Progressive vertebrae demineralization subsequently leads to wedge or compression fracture. In osteoporosis the apex of the wedge fracture is typically anterior. Posterior wedging strongly suggests a different underlying disease process such as Paget's disease, trauma, or metastatic malignancy.

The osteoporotic spine with irregularly spaced biconcave vertebral bodies containing Schmorl's nodes can often be distinguished from osteomalacia, the latter characteristically leading to biconcavity of most vertebrae with expansion of the intravertebral spaces without Schmorl's nodes. These differences, although often subtle, may be useful for distinguishing osteoporosis and osteomalacia changes in the vertebral column with the following exceptions: the vertebrae of osteoporotic children reveal the regular shape changes described as characteristic for osteomalacia; and when osteoporosis and osteomalacia coexist in the same individual, the appearance of the spine may be classically that of osteoporosis. The presence of vertebral fractures in osteoporosis is highly correlated with the coexistence of other radiographic indications of osteoporosis, the association being particularly strong for the white female.[25] The female with a vertebral fracture (most commonly the twelfth thoracic and first three lumbar vertebrae) has a 98% likelihood of having coexistent generalized osteoporosis as opposed to the male, in whom the coexistence is approximately 70%. Fractures above the sixth thoracic vertebra without concomitant disease below this level are rarely due to osteoporosis. Spontaneous fractures above the fourth thoracic vertebra should suggest metastatic cancer or septic spondylitis. Black individuals with vertebral fractures of the lower spine always should be considered to have generalized osteopenia until otherwise determined.[25]

Radiographic changes, when apparent in peripheral skeletal sites, include cortical thinning of the long bones with irregularities of endosteal surfaces and diffuse demineralization as well as thinning of the tables of the calvaria. Occasionally the demineralization in the skull is spotty, resembling multiple myeloma or metastatic carcinoma. These changes are often associated with decreased density of the floor and dorsum of the sella turcica. Pelvic and femoral involvement are characterized by a thin rim of well-mineralized cortex and a decreased amount of trabecular or cancellous bone. The remaining trabecular pattern in the pelvis and femoral necks reflect the lines of stress applied to the skeleton and may actually appear more dense. In this regard some authors have advocated simple radiographic quantitation of trabecular content in the femoral heads as a reliable method of categorizing various degrees of osteoporosis.[26] An estimate of the severity of the osteoporotic process can also be obtained by measurements of cortical thickness of the femur and metatarsal, metacarpal, and phalangeal bones in relation to the total width of the shaft.[27,28] Related radiographic features of limited diagnostic value are the absence of less than usual amount of osteophytosis or spur formation along the vertebrae, a process that normally accompanies the aging process,[29] and a relative increase in the calcification of the aorta compared with that expected for the age of the patient.[30]

Clinical characteristics

Most patients with osteoporosis are asymptomatic without back pain, despite the presence of one or more vertebral fractures. When present, the back pain is usually localized and of two types. Coincidentally with a vertebral fracture the patient may experience a sudden onset of sharp severe pain, aggravated by motion and located directly over a vertebral process. The pain may be spasmodic and characteristically radiates anteriorly around the flank into various portions of the abdomen, legs, or pelvis. In contrast to osteomalacia, generalized skeletal pain is uncommon, and between episodic bouts of vertebral fracture the patient is usually completely free of pain. Nerve-root and spinal cord compressions are also exceedingly rare complications of spinal osteoporosis, despite the presence of severe spinal deformities. With rest and with slight hyperextension of the back if necessary, the pain gradually subsides within 2 or 4 weeks regardless of any other treatment. The other, more commonly observed pain is dull and aching, of long duration, and located several centimeters to one or both sides of the midline in the lower thoracic or lumbar region. These symptoms are often attributed to "rheumatism" or "lumbago." Careful palpation usually detects associated spasm of the paravertebral muscles. The pain is likely to be exacerbated by sitting or standing for some time and by the Valsalva maneuver, and it is usually relieved by lying down.

The patient's history may also reveal a gradual loss of height over a period of years or sometimes only months. The loss of height that occurs in osteoporosis is due to vertebral compression, greatest in the lumbar vertebrae, although it is also seen in the thoracic vertebrae. Clinically, the loss of height can be shown to be above the pubis by demonstrating that the distance from pubis to heel minus the distance from crown to pubis is greater than 2 inches, whereas the pubis-to-heel dimension is still one half the span from fingertip to fingertip. The resultant lower dorsal kyphosis (commonly referred to as the "dowager's" or "widow's hump") and stepwise decline in height are most reliable clinical signs of progression of osteoporotic process. This progressive deforming process usually leads to downward angulation of the ribs and a narrowing of the normal gap between the lower ribs and the iliac crest, which may become so severe that patients complain of a rubbing together of the iliac crest and lower ribs. Measurable reduction in height ceases when the costal margins come to rest on the iliac crests. For this reason linear height changes as a reflection of therapeutic responsiveness should be interpreted with caution.[31,32] Prominent horizontal skin creases are also seen across the abdomen resulting from an accordian-like folding of the torso. In severe forms of the disease the loss of the anterior lumbar curve may produce a posterior pelvic tilt, hamstring contractures, a shuffling, unsteady gait, and a broad stance. Common sites of fracture other than vertebrae are the border of the radii (i.e., Colles' fracture) and the neck of the femur. At these sites the fracture incidence is closely related to age and diminished bone density as seen radiographically.

Laboratory and biochemical tests

Calcium and inorganic phosphate in the plasma are characteristically normal for the age of the patient, and elevated phosphate values are usually seen in the prepubertal age in both sexes and in the postmenopausal female.[33] Diagnostic significance has been attributed to the serum phosphate level in postmenopausal forms of osteoporosis, and a direct correlation has been observed between circulating phosphate values and bone-resorbing surfaces quantitated micrographically.[34] The serum alkaline phosphatase level is usually normal and if elevated, suggests associated osteomalacia or healing fractures.[35] Immunoreactive parathyroid hormone (iPTH) levels have also been reported as high in certain individuals with the postmenopausal variant of osteoporosis.[36,37] The urinary calcium level is usually normal in elderly patients with osteoporosis and no demonstrable endocrinopathy. In selected instances hypercalciuria with histologic documentation of osteoporosis has been associated in the middle-aged female with an occult form of acquired distal renal tubular acidosis. This diagnosis can only be established with certainty by recording urinary pH for 2 to 3 consecutive days and by determining the response to ammonium chloride (0.1 gm/kg body weight). Normally, the urine pH should fall below 5.3 during this maneuver. The urine hydroxyproline, an indirect measurement of bone collagen turnover, is also normal in osteoporotic patients.[38,39] It must be emphasized, however, that a "normal hydroxyproline" may, in fact, reflect accelerated bone resorption in individuals with reduced skeletal mass.

INCIDENCE

Although a variety of diseases characterized by metabolic or hormonal imbalances result in osteoporosis, the majority of patients thus afflicted are postmenopausal women. It has been estimated that of the approximately 1 million fractures experienced each year by women 45 years of age or older in the United States, about 700,000 are incurred by women with osteoporosis.[40] In 1968, falls were the leading cause of nontransport accidental deaths in all persons and the leading cause of all accidental deaths in elderly white women in the United States. Approximately three fourths of all deaths from falls occur in patients 65 years of age and over, with a female:male fracture incidence ratio of 8:1.[41] The rate (per 1000 population per year) of hip fractures in white women due to minimal trauma increases from two at 50 to 64 years of age to five at 65 to 74 years of age to ten at greater than 75 years of age.[42]

PATHOGENESIS

Since the gradual decrease in bone mass that accompanies aging in both sexes necessarily distorts the structural integrity of strategic weight-bearing skeletal foci such as the neck of the femur or vertebral bodies, the increased fracture rate that attends senescence should be anticipated. Why then is the postmenopausal woman particularly at risk in this regard? Although there are reports that negate a direct causative relationship between accelerated bone loss and the menopause,[43-45] there is evidence that cessation of ovarian function results in an acceleration of the age-related bone loss phenomenon in some individuals.[46-49]

Most data collected to date defining age-related changes in bone mass and the effect of either natural or artificially induced cessation of normal ovarian function[50] thereon have been obtained by quantitating cortical bone content of peripheral tubular bones from radiographs of trabecular content of distal sites of the forearm (i.e., radius) densitometrically. Although changes in the appendicular skeleton appear to reflect the mineral content of the axial skeleton adequately, definitive conclusions regarding the effect of age and the menopause on vertebral mineral content await the development of more sensitive and reproducible techniques applicable to the vertebral column. In one study utilizing photon absorptiometric measurements of bone mineral content in the proximal end of the shaft of the radius, women between 45 and 70 years of age were losing bone at a rate of 10% to 15% a decade, the rate decreasing to 5% a decade thereafter. In contrast, the rate of bone loss in men from 50 to 80 years of age was constant at 5% a decade.[51] The bone density of men with symptomatic osteoporosis is abnormally low when compared with either unaffected age-related men or older men.[51]

One must also account for the fact that the rate of cortical and trabecular bone loss in a population of symptomatic postmenopausal osteoporotic women with vertebral fractures is equal to that of age-matched asymptomatic women without vertebral fractures, although at any age the trabecular bone density is less in the women with symptomatic fractures.[20] Postmenopausal women who develop symptomatic "osteopenia," which is often the correct diagnosis since histologic confirmation of "osteoporosis" is rarely obtained in the majority of patients, may simply represent those selected individuals who approach the menopause with the smaller skeletal mass in the normally distributed population at 45 to 60 years of age. Of note in this regard is the observation that the density of the ulna of clinically normal women over 45 years of age follows a binominal distribution pattern, with 37% of women demonstrating bone densities in the preosteoporotic range.[52] As a consequence of the accelerated bone mineral loss that attends the postmenopausal years in all women, those with lower bone densities should become susceptible to fractures earlier.[20]

Documented seasonal variations in bone mineral content after menopause with increments from winter to summer and decrements from summer to winter should also be considered.[53] Not only does the surface area of osteoid tissue in bones increase with age in women after the fourth decade,[54] but serum vitamin D activity in some postmenopausal women is higher in the summer than in the winter.[55] The possibility that subclinical vitamin D deficiency and resultant osteomalacia might be another contributing factor to the increased fracture ratio incidence in some women with postmenopausal osteoporosis should be entertained, since the combination of both histologic defects in over 30% of postmenopausal osteopenic females has been well documented.[6,56]

The pathogenesis of the accelerated bone loss observed in the postmenopausal state is still conjectural at best. Morphometric analysis of biopsied specimens reveal that bone resorption is increased in this form of osteoporosis, whereas bone formation is in general, but not invariably, reduced.[57-60] Evidence advanced in favor of the hypothesis that inadequate ovarian function is the major determinant in relation to bone mineral loss of the postmenopausal woman primarily stems from reports of salutary effects of estrogens on "well-being" and in preventing height loss as well as improving mineral balance and peripheral bone density.[31,32,50,61-63] In contrast to these reports isolated studies defining therapeutic trials with randomized codes fail to demonstrate any additional beneficial effects of estrogens when added to a regimen containing vitamin D and/or calcium supplements.[63,64] Moreover, when compared to age-matched white women, the bone density of both American-born and Asiatic-born Chinese and Japanese women is strikingly low,[65] although the estrogen profiles of Oriental women outside Asia are substantially lower than those of Oriental women in Asia.[66] Finally, the "estrogen-lack" theory is incompatible with the observation that circulating levels of estradiol and estrone are comparable in postmenopausal women with or without vertebral compression fractures and symptomatic osteoporosis.[67]

Epidemiologic and retrospective dietary analytic studies reveal that calcium deficiency may contribute to the symptomatic osteoporosis seen in postmenopausal and elderly individuals. Some reports reveal no significant difference in the incidence of "osteoporosis" between patients receiving diets containing less than 500 mg of calcium per day and those with intakes greater than 1500 mg per day,[68-70] whereas other reports demonstrate a lower calcium intake in "osteoporotic" individuals than in age-matched normal control individuals.[71-78] Epidemiologic and dietary survey studies may ultimately prove misleading regardless of the conclusions derived, unless more specific emphasis is placed on dietary and alcoholic intake habits, lactase intolerance, the degree of mobilization, the daily intake of minerals other than calcium, the dietary intake of protein and vitamin D, and the extent of sunlight exposure.[73,79-83] Modern acid ash diets, which are characteristically rich in animal proteins and phosphorus, may prove deleterious to bone, since diets that contain excessive amounts of these ingredients promote hypercalciuria and stimulate the release of parathyroid hormone. Immobilization, or the relative inactivity that often attends the infirmities of age, also promotes skeletal demineralization; peculiar dietary habits may also lead to increased urinary calcium loss and a negative calcium balance, despite an adequate intake. Moreover, when dietary phosphorus is ingested in the form of phytin, as may be the case in diets high in unpolished rice or wheatmeal, calcium absorption from the intestine is impaired. Since elderly populations with adequate calcium intakes may have limited sunlight exposure and may be deficient in vitamin D, epidemiologic studies designed to correlate calcium intake with results obtained from radiologic determinants of "osteoporosis" may yield misleading and less than adequate conclusions. In fact, osteomalacia resulting from vitamin D deficiency may prove to be the predominant skeletal histologic lesion.

THERAPY

Data accumulated to date consistently demonstrate that the primary effect of short-term (i.e., 2 to 4 months) estrogen therapy is to decrease the levels of bone resorption if they are in fact increased prior to therapy. This initial short-lived favorable effect is ultimately negated after longer treatment intervals (i.e., 9 to 15 months) by a secondary decrease in bone formation.[84] Although the cause for this biphasic skeletal response to estrogen therapy is still uncertain, it may result from the elevations in circulating parathyroid hormone[36] and free cortisol observed in estrogen-treated individuals.[85] Estrogen therapy may ultimately prove to be prophylactic for the young castrated female and perimenopausal women.[61-63] Long-term therapy in aged women should be considered inappropriate until controlled, prospective, long-term therapeutic trials are conducted in this population. The risk of developing endometrial carcinoma during long-term conjugated estrogen therapy should be considered in this regard.

The calcium requirement for normal adults is still a debatable issue, although it is generally placed between 600 and 1000 mg per day.[73,77,86] The majority of young and middle-aged adults are capable of maintaining a positive calcium balance when receiving this intake,[86,87] although higher intakes may be essential to maintain mineral and skeletal homeostasis in elderly individuals, especially those exposed to stressful environments.[73,77,87-89] The age-related needs for additional dietary calcium may result in part from the observations that absorption as well as the adaptive efficiency of the intestine fluctuations in calcium intake decrease with age.[90-91] Negative calcium balances observed in osteoporotic patients receiving low but seemingly adequate calcium intakes may be a result of a slow and noncompensatory adaptation to low calcium intakes,[92] defective renal adaptation and relative hypercalciuria,[93] and/or lactose intolerance resulting from intestinal lactase deficiency.[82] These observations are consistent with the conclusions that the accepted "normal" adult calcium intake of 400 mg per day may ultimately prove inadequate to compensate for the accelerated mineral defects that accompany the senescent postmenopausal state.[73,77]

Therapeutic claims of high dose or intravenous calcium therapy[94-98] for osteoporosis have been refuted,[68,70,99-101] since the documented reductions in bone resorption results in a parallel suppression of bone formation with no apparent gain for the patient and a potential for renal calculi with intravenous therapy. Those objections to "oral" supplemental, calcium therapeutic regimens are premature and should not be misinterpreted. The reported lack of correlation between calcium intake and incidence of osteoporosis[68,71] is based primarily on retrospective analyses and has not been confirmed by others.[71-77]

The intestinal adaptation to low calcium diets in humans not only varies considerably but is dependent on vitamin D intake and exercise and most probably a host of additional unknown factors. Variations in adaptive absorption efficiencies may explain why certain races and ethnic groups develop osteoporosis when receiving high calcium intakes, whereas others do not despite a calcium intake of less than 500 mg per day. Chronic restrictive calcium intakes, combined with inadequate urinary retention and high phosphate intakes, the latter so characteristic of modern-day high protein diets, may ultimately lead to compensated parathyroid overactivity, osteoclastosis, and increased bone resorption. As such, it seems more than appropriate to ensure that the nutritional status of the symptomatic osteoporotic patient is adequate with specific emphasis on calcium intakes of 1000 to 1500 mg per day until more appropriately designed, long-term prospective studies of high calcium supplementation become available for scrutiny. The exact nature of the osteopenic process should be documented by either appropriate biochemical measurements of vitamin D and/or its biologically active metabolites 25-hydroxycholecalciferol[102] and 1,25-dihydroxycholecalciferol[103] or by localized needle bone biopsy of the iliac crest. Vitamin D supplementation although appropriate treatment for those "osteoporotic" patients with osteomalacia, should not be administered indiscriminately, since hypercalciuria and hypercalcemia and the attendant sequelae may prove hazardous.[104]

Reports of decreased incidence of osteoporosis and collapsed vertebrae in individuals living in the areas where the fluoride content of the water supply was high (i.e., >4 p.p.m.)[105,106] and other reports citing the potential benefit of sodium fluoride therapy in doses varying from 10 to 175 mg per day[107-110] are consistent with the hypothesis that long-term sodium fluoride therapy may prove therapeutic for symptomatic osteoporosis. This form of therapy must still be regarded as experimental, however, and its use tempered by the realization that the chronic ingestion of sodium fluoride leads to osteomalacia and secondary hyperparathyroidism,[109-113] unless calcium intake and absorption are well controlled. Moreover, optic neuritis, arthritis, and chronic gastroenteritis ulceration may complicate the treatment.[114,115] The optimum dose of sodium fluoride for therapeutic effectiveness is reportedly 40 to 45 mg every 24 hours with larger doses (greater than 60 mg every 24 hours) producing morphologically abnormal bone.[107] Any enthusiasm for fluoride therapy in osteoporotic patients must be conditioned by reports that document increased fracture incidence and abnormal bone marrow cytology in patients receiving as little as 16 mg every 24 hours of sodium fluoride for prolonged periods[115,116] and by other reports demonstrating decreased mechanical strength of bones of fluoride-treated animals wherein the bone fluoride content approximated that of humans receiving fluoride, vitamin D, and calcium combinations.[117] Rigorous long-term assessment of the effects of prolonged and continuous fluoride administration on the structural integrity of bone, fracture incidence, and extra-skeletal tissue metabolism and organ function is essential before an adequate appraisal can be made of therapeutic effectiveness in postmenopausal osteoporotic women.

The therapeutic effects reported with calcitonin administration in Paget's disease of the bone have also resulted in limited trials with this agent in patients with senile or postmenopausal osteoporosis. Calcitonin, a peptide hormone normally secreted by the parafollicular or "C" cells of the thyroid gland, functions primarily to suppress bone resorption. Favorable therapeutic responses to porcine calcitonin for periods ranging from 1 to 29 months have been reported, with suppression of bone resorption documented both biochemically and histologically.[118-121] Although a likely candidate for suppressing the bone resorption of osteoporotic patients, calcitonin therapy must presently be considered experimental until more appropriate, double-blind, placebo study protocols are developed with detailed evaluation of the incidence of fracture rates and the development of secondary hyperparathyroidism and antibodies to nonhuman calcitonin preparations.[120,122]

REFERENCES

1. Perzigian, A.J.: The antiquity of age-associated bone demineralization in man, J. Am. Geriatr. Soc. **21**:100, 1973.
2. Moseley, J.E.: The paleopathologic riddle of "symmetrical osteoporosis," Am. J. Roentgenol. Radium Ther. Nucl. Med. **95**:135, 1965.
3. Bauer, G.C.H.: Kinetics of calcium and strontium metabolism in man. In Rodahl, K., Nicholson, J.T., and Brown, E.M., Jr., editors: Bone as a tissue, New York, 1960, McGraw-Hill Book Co.
4. Lemay, M., and Blunt, J.W., Jr.: A factor determining the location of pseudofractures in osteomalacia, J. Clin. Invest. **28**:521, 1949.
5. Steinbach, H.L., Kolb, F.O., and Crane, J.T.: Unusual roentgen manifestations of osteomalacia, Am. J. Roentgenol. Radium Ther. Nucl. Med. **82**:875, 1959.
6. Johnson, K.A., Riggs, B.L., Kelly, P.J., and Jowsey, J.: Osteoid tissue in normal and osteoporotic individuals, J. Clin. Endocrinol. Metab. **33**:745, 1971.
7. Arnold, J.S.: The quantitation of bone mineralization as an organ and tissue in osteoporosis. In Pearson, O.H., and Joplin, J.F., editors: Dynamic studies of metabolic bone disease, Oxford, 1964, Blackwell Scientific Publications.
8. Morgan, D.B., and Newton-John, H.F.: Bone loss and senescence, Gerontologia **15**:140, 1969.
9. Smith, R.W., Jr., Eyler, W.R., and Mellinger, R.C.: On the incidence of senile osteoporosis, Ann. Intern. Med. **52**:773, 1960.
10. Urist, M.R.: Observation bearing on the problems of osteoporosis. In Rodahl, K., Nicholson, J.T., and Brown, E.M. Jr., editors: Bone as a tissue, New York, 1960, McGraw-Hill Book Co.
11. Lachman, E.: Osteoporosis: the potentialities and limitations of its roentgenologic diagnosis, Am. J. Roentgenol. Radium Ther. Nucl. Med. **74**:712, 1955.
12. Wray, J.B., Sugarman, E.D., and Schneider, A.J.: Bone composition in senile osteoporosis, J.A.M.A. **182**:118, 1963.
13. Lachman, E., and Whilan, M.: Roentgen diagnosis of osteoporosis and its limitations, Radiology **26**:165, 1936.
14. Doyle, F.H., Gutteridge, D.H., Joplin, G.F., and Fraser, R.: An assessment of radiological criteria used in the study of spinal osteoporosis, Br. J. Radiol. **40**:241, 1967.
15. Adams, P., Davies, G.R., and Sweetnam, P.: Osteoporosis and the effects of aging on bone mass in elderly men and women, Q. J. Med. **39**:601, 1970.
16. Weaver, J.K., and Chalmers, J.: Cancellous bone: its strength and changes with ageing and an evaluation of some methods for measuring its mineral content, J. Bone Joint Surg. [Am.]**48**:289, 1966.
17. Israel, H.: Loss of bone and remodeling-redistribution in the cranio-facial skeleton with age, Fed. Proc. **26**:1723, 1967.
18. McFarland, W.: Evaluation of bone density from roentgenograms, Science **119**:810, 1954.
19. Cameron, J.R., Mazess, R.B., and Sorenson, J.A.: Precision and accuracy of bone mineral determination by direct photon absorptiometry, Invest. Radiol. **3**:141, 1968.
20. Riggs, B.L., et al.: Differential changes in bone mineral density of the appendicular and axial skeleton with aging, J. Clin. Invest. **67**:328, 1981.
21. Cameron, J.R., and Sorenson, J.: Measurement of bone mineral *in vivo:* an improved method, Science **42**:5, 1963.
22. Rose, G.A.: The radiological diagnosis of osteoporosis, osteomalacia and hyperthyroidism, Clin. Radiol. **15**:75, 1964.
23. Vernon-Roberts, B., and Pirie, C.J.: Healing trabecular microfractures in the bodies of lumbar vertebrae, Ann. Rheum. Dis. **32**:406, 1973.
24. Atkinson, P.J.: Variation in trabecular structure of vertebrae with age, Calcif. Tissue Res. **1**:24, 1967.
25. Boukhris, R., and Becker, K.L.: Schmorl's nodes and osteoporosis, Clin. Orthop. **104**:279, 1974.
26. Singh, M., Nagrath, A.R., and Maini, R.S.: Changes in trabecular pattern of the upper end of the femur as an index of osteoporosis, J. Bone Joint Surg. [Am.] **52**:457, 1970.
27. Exton-Smith, A.N., Millard, P.H., Payne, P.R., and Wheeler, E.F.: Pattern of development and loss of bone with age, Lancet **2**:1154, 1969.
28. Gryfe, C.I., Exton-Smith, A.N., Payne, P.R., and Wheeler, E.F.: Pattern of development of bone in childhood and adolescence, Lancet **1**:523, 1971.
29. Smith, R.W., Jr., and Rizek, J.: Epidemiologic studies of osteoporosis in women of Puerto Rico and southeastern Michigan with special reference to age, race, national origin and to other related or associated findings, Clin. Orthop. **45**:31, 1966.

30. Boukhris, R., and Becker, K.L.: Calcification of the aorta and osteoporosis: a radiographic study, J.A.M.A. **219:**1307, 1972.
31. Henneman, P.H., and Wallach, S.: The use of androgens and estrogens and their metabolic effects: a review of prolonged use of estrogens and androgens in postmenopausal and senile osteoporosis, Arch. Intern. Med. **100:**715, 1957.
32. Herberg, C.A.: Treatment of post-menopausal osteoporosis with estrogens and androgens, Acta Endocrinol. **34:**51, 1960.
33. Keating, F.R., Jr., Jones, J.D., Elveback, L.R., and Randall, R.V.: The relation of age and sex to distribution of values in healthy adults of serum calcium, inorganic calcium, inorganic phosphate, magnesium alkaline phosphatase, total protein, albumin and blood urea, J. Lab. Clin. Med. **73:**825, 1969.
34. Kelly, P.J., Jowsey, J., Riggs, B.L., and Elveback, L.R.: Relationship between serum phosphate concentration and bone resorption in osteoporosis, J. Lab. Clin. Med. **69:**110, 1967.
35. Nilsson, B.E., and Westlin, N.E.: The plasma concentration of alkaline phosphatase, phosphorus and calcium following femoral neck fracture, Acta Orthop. Scand. **43:**504, 1972.
36. Riggs, B.L., et al.: A syndrome of osteoporosis, increased serum immunoreactive parathyroid hormone and inappropriately low serum 1,25-dihydroxyvitamin D, Mayo Clin. Proc. **53:**701, 1978.
37. Fujita, T., et al.: Radioimmunoassay of serum parathyroid hormone in postmenopausal osteoporosis, Endocrinol. Jap. **19:**571, 1972.
38. Guggenheim, K., et al.: An epidemiological study of osteoporosis in Israel, Arch. Environ. Health **22:**259, 1971.
39. Moskowitz, R.W., Kelin, L., and Katz, D.: Urinary hydroxyproline levels in an aged population: a study of non-osteoporotic and osteoporotic patients, Arthritis Rheum. **8:**61, 1965.
40. Iskrant, A.P., and Smith, R.W., Jr.: Osteoporosis in women 45 years and over related to subsequent fractures, Public Health Rep. **84:**33, 1969.
41. Iskrant, A.P.: The etiology of fractured hips in females: a study of suspected relationships between osteoporosis and fractures from falls, Am. J. Public Health **58:**485, 1968.
42. Bollet, A.J., Engh, G., and Parson, W.: Epidemiology of osteoporosis, Arch. Intern. Med. **116:**191, 1965.
43. Saville, P.D.: Symptomatic osteoporosis and the menopause, Clin. Orthop. **55:**43, 1967.
44. Ruikka, I., Gronroos, M., Bourander, L.B., and Virtama, P.: Bone demineralization and estrogen activity after menopause, Geriatrics **23:**165, 1968.
45. Newton-John, H.F., and Morgan, D.B.: Osteoporosis: disease or senescence, Lancet **1:**232, 1968.
46. Nordin, B.E.C.: Clinical significance and pathogenesis of osteoporosis, Br. Med. J. **1:**571, 1971.
47. Aitken, J.M., et al.: Osteoporosis after oophorectomy for nonmalignant disease in premenopausal women, Br. Med. J. **1:**325, 1973.
48. Meema, H.E.: Menopausal and aging changes in muscle mass and bone mineral content, J. Bone Joint Surg. [Am.] **48:**1138, 1966.
49. Meema, H.E., and Meema, S.: Prevention of postmenopausal osteoporosis by hormone treatment of the menopause, Can. Med. Assoc. J. **99:**248, 1968.
50. Donaldson, I.A., and Nassim, J.R.: The artificial menopause, Br. Med. J. **1:**1228, 1954.
51. Mazess, R.B., and Cameron, J.R.: Bone mineral content in normal U.S. whites, International Conference on Bone Mineral Measurement, U.S. Department of Health, Education and Welfare, Pub. No. NIH 75-683, p. 228, 1973.
52. Selle, W.A., and Jurist, J.M.: The onset of postmenopausal osteoporosis as studied by a new technique. J. Am. Geriatr. Soc. **14:**930, 1966.
53. Aitken, J.M., Anderson, J.B., and Horton, P.W.: Seasonal variations in bone mineral content after the menopause, Nature **241:**59, 1973.
54. Frost, H.M.: Human osteoid seams, J. Clin. Endocrinol. Metab. **22:**631, 1962.
55. Smith, R.W., Jr., Rizek, J., and Frame, B.: Determinants of serum antirachitic activity: special reference to involuntional osteoporosis, Am. J. Clin. Nutr. **14:**98, 1964.
56. Aaron, J.E., et al: Frequency of osteomalacia and osteoporosis in fractures of the proximal femur, Lancet **1:**229, 1974.
57. Jowsey, J.: Age changes in human bone, Clin. Orthop. **17:**210, 1960.
58. Frost, H.M.: Postmenopausal osteoporosis: a disturbance in osteoclasia, J. Am. Geriatr. Soc. **9:**1078, 1961.
59. Villanueva, A.R., et al.: Cortical bone dynamics measured by means of tetracycline labeling in 21 cases of osteoporosis, J. Lab. Clin. Med. **68:**599, 1966.
60. Wu, K., Jett, S., and Frost, H.M.: Bone resorption rates in rib in physiological, senile and postmenopausal osteoporosis, J. Lab. Clin. Med. **69:**810, 1967.
61. Weiss, N.S., et al.: Decreased risk of fractures of the hip and lower forearm with post-menopausal use of estrogen, N. Engl. J. Med. **303:**1195, 1980.
62. Hutchinson, T.A., Polansky, S.M., and Feinstein, A.R.: Post-menopausal oestrogens protect against fractures of hip and distal radius, Lancet **2:**705, 1979.
63. Recker, R.R., Saville, P.D., and Heaney, R.P.: Effect of estrogens and calcium carbonate on bone loss in post-menopausal women, Ann. Intern. Med. **87:**649, 1977.
64. Miller, R.G.: The treatment of osteoporosis—a report of a double blind therapeutic trial, Gerontol. Clin. **11:**244, 1969.
65. Garn, S.M., Pao, E.M., and Rihl, M.E.: Compact bone in Chinese and Japanese, Science **143:**1439, 1964.
66. Dickinson, L.E., MacMahon, B., Cole P., and Brown, J.B.: Estrogen profiles of Oriental and Caucasian women in Hawaii, N. Engl. J. Med. **291:**1211, 1974.
67. Riggs, B.L., et al.: Serum concentrations of estrogen, testosterone and gonadotropins in osteoporotic and nonosteoporotic postmenopausal women, J. Clin. Endocrinol. Metab. **36:**1097, 1973.
68. Smith, R.W., Jr., and Frame, B.: Concurrent axial and appendicular osteoporosis, N. Engl. J. Med. **273:**73, 1965.
69. Garn, S.M., Rohmann, C.A., and Wagner, B.: Bone loss as a general phenomenon in man, Fed. Proc. **26:**1729, 1967.

70. Garn, S.M.: Calcium requirements for bone building and skeletal maintenance, Am. J. Clin. Nutr. **23:**1149, 1970.
71. Riggs, B.L., et al.: Calcium deficiency and osteoporosis: observations in 1966 patients and critical review of the literature, J. Bone Joint Surg. [Am.] **29:**915, 1967.
72. Hurxthal, L.M., and Vose, G.P.: The relationship of dietary calcium intake to radiographic bone density in normal and osteoporotic persons, Calcif. Tissue Res. **4:**245, 1969.
73. Avioli, L.V.: Postmenopausal osteoporosis prevention versus cure, Fed. Proc. **40:**82, 1981.
74. Vinther-Paulsen, N.: Calcium and phosphorus intake in senile osteoporosis, Geriatrics **8:**76, 1953.
75. Smith, D.A., and Nordin, B.E.C.: The relation between calcium balance and hydroxyproline excretion in osteoporosis, Proc. R. Soc. Med. **57:**868, 1964.
76. Matkovic, V., et al.: Bone status and fracture rates in two regions of Yugoslavia, Am. J. Clin. Nutr. **32:**540, 1979.
77. Nordin, B.E.C., et al.: Calcium requirements and calcium therapy, Clin. Orthop. Rel. Res. **140:**216, 1979.
78. Krook, L., et al.: Human periodontal disease: morphology and response to calcium therapy, Cornell Vet. **62:**32, 1972.
79. Wachman, A., and Bernstein, D.S.: Diet and osteoporosis, Lancet **1:**958, 1968.
80. Anand, C.R., and Linkswiler, H.M.: Effect of protein intake on calcium balance of young men given 500 mg calcium daily, J. Nutr. **104:**695, 1974.
81. Nilsson, B.E., and Westlin, N.E.: Changes in bone mass in alcoholics, Clin. Orthop. **90:**229, 1973.
82. Birge, S.J., Jr., Keutmann, H.T., Cuatrecasas, P., and Whedon, G.D.: Osteoporosis, intestinal lactase deficiency and low dietary calcium intake, N. Engl. J. Med. **276:**445, 1967.
83. Mazess, R.B.: Bone mineral content in Wainwright Eskimos: preliminary report, Arctic Anthropol. **7:**114, 1970.
84. Heaney, R.P.: Estrogen effects on the skeleton. In Salhanick, H.A., Kipnis, D.M., and VandeWiele, R.L., editors: Metabolic effects of gonad hormones and contraceptive steroids, New York, 1969, Plenum Publishing Corp.
85. Aitken, J.M., Hall, P.E., Rao, L.G.S., Hart, D.M., and Lindsay, R.: Hypercortisolaemia and lack of skeletal response to oestrogen in postmenopausal women, Clin. Endocrinol. **3:**167, 1974.
86. Irwin, M.I., and Kienholz, E.W.: A conspectus on research on calcium requirements of man, J. Nutr. **103:**1019, 1973.
87. Malm, O.J.: Calcium requirements and adaptation in adult man, J. Clin. Lab. Invest. **10**(Suppl):1, 1958.
88. Roberts, P.H., Kerr, C.H., and Ohlson, A.: Nutritional studies of older women: nitrogen, calcium, phosphorus retention on nine women, J. Am. Diet. Assoc. **24:**292, 1948.
89. Malm, O.J.: Adaptation to alterations in calcium intake. In Wasserman, R.H., editor: The transfer of calcium and strontium acress biological membranes, London, 1963, Academic Press, Inc.
90. Avioli, L.V., McDonald, J.E., and Lee, S.W.: The influence of age on the intestinal absorption of ^{47}Ca in women and its relation to ^{47}Ca absorption in postmenopausal osteoporosis, J. Clin. Invest. **44:**1960, 1965.
91. Bullamore, J.R., Wilkinson, R., Gallagher, J.C., Nordin, B.E.C., and Marshall, D.H.: Effect of age on calcium absorption, Lancet **2:**535, 1970.
92. Ireland, P., and Fordtran, J.S.: Effect of dietary calcium and age on jejunal calcium absorption in humans studied by intestinal perfusion, J. Clin. Invest. **52:**2672, 1973.
93. Bhandarkar, S.D., and Nordin, B.E.C.: Effect of low calcium diet on urinary calcium in osteoporosis, Br. Med. J. **1:**145, 1962.
94. Epstein, S., Meighem, W.V., Sagel, J., and Jackson, W.P.U.: Effect of single large doses of oral calcium on serum calcium levels in the young and the elderly, Metabolism **22:**1163, 1973.
95. Pak, C.Y.C., et al.: The treatment of osteoporosis with calcium infusions: clinical studies, Am. J. Med. **47:**7, 1969.
96. Cohn, S.H., Dombrowski, C.S., Hauser, W., and Atkins, H.L.: High calcium diet and the parameters of calcium metabolism in osteoporosis, Am. J. Clin. Nutr. **21:**1246, 1968.
97. Whedon, G.D.: Effects of high calcium intakes on bones, blood and soft tissue: relationship of calcium intake to balance in osteoporosis, Fed. Proc. **18:**1112, 1959.
98. Shafar, J.: Calcium infusions in spinal osteoporosis, Br. J. Clin. Pract. **27:**405, 1973.
99. Schwartz, E., Panariello, V.A., and Saeli, J.: Radioactive calcium kinetics during high calcium intake in osteoporosis, J. Clin. Invest. **44:**1547, 1965.
100. Dudl, R.J., et al.: Evaluation of intravenous calcium as therapy for osteoporosis, Am. J. Med. **55:**631, 1973.
101. Jensen, H., Christiansen, C., Munck, O., and Toft, H.: Treatment of osteoporosis with calcium infusions, Scand. J. Clin. Lab. Invest. **32:**93, 1973.
102. Lawoyin, S., Zerwekh, J.E., Glass, K., and Pak, C.Y.C.: Ability of 25-hydroxyvitamin D therapy to augment serum 1,25- and 24,25-dihydroxyvitamin D in postmenopausal osteoporosis, J. Clin. Endocrinol. Metab. **50:**593, 1980.
103. Gallagher, J.C., et al.: Intestinal calcium absorption and serum vitamin D metabolites in normal subjects and osteoporotic patients, J. Clin. Invest. **64:**729, 1979.
104. Gwinup, G.: Hypercalcemia as a complication of vitamin D therapy in postmenopausal osteoporosis, J. Clin. Endocrinol. Metab. **21:**101, 1961.
105. Bernstein, D.S., et al.: Prevalence of osteoporosis in high and low fluoride areas in North Dakota, J.A.M.A. **198:**499, 1966.
106. Alffram, P.A., Hernborg, J., and Nilsson, B.E.R.: The influence of a high fluoride content in the drinking water on the bone mineral mass in man, Acta Orthop. Scand. **40:**137, 1969.
107. Cohen, M.B., and Rubini, M.E.: The treatment of osteoporosis with sodium fluoride, Clin. Orthop. **40:**147, 1965.
108. Bernstein, D.S., and Cohen, P.: Use of sodium fluoride

in the treatment of osteoporosis, J. Clin. Endocrinol. Metab. **27**:197, 1967.

109. Jowsey, J., Riggs, B., Kelly, P.J., and Hoffman, D.L.: Effect of combined therapy with sodium fluoride, vitamin D and calcium in osteoporosis, Am. J. Med. **54**:43, 1972.
110. Franke, J., Rempel, H., and Franke, M.: Three years' experience with sodium fluoride therapy of osteoporosis, Acta Orthop. Scand. **45**:1, 1974.
111. Baylink, D.J., and Bernstein, D.S.: The effects of fluoride therapy on metabolic bone disease, Clin. Orthop. **55**:51, 1967.
112. Kuhlencordt, F., Druse, H.P., Lozano-Tonkin, C., and Eckermeier, L.: The treatment of osteoporosis with sodium fluoride: a morphological study of bone changes in eight cases, Dtsch. Med. Wochenschr. **94**:1730, 1969.
113. Teotia, S.P.S., and Teotia, M.: Secondary hyperparathyroidism in patients with endemic skeletal fluorosis, Br. Med. J. **1**:637, 1973.
114. Geall, M.G., and Beilin, L.J.: Sodium fluoride and poptic neuritis, Br. Med. J. **2**:255, 1964.
115. Riggs, B.L., et al.: Treatment of primary osteoporosis with fluoride and calcium. Clinical tolerance and fracture occurrence, J.A.M.A. **243**:446, 1980.
116. Duffey, P.H., Tretbar, H.C., and Jarkowski, T.L.: Giant cells in bone marrow of patients on high dose fluoride treatment, Ann. Intern. Med. **75**:745, 1971.
117. Riggins, R.S., Zeman, F., and Moon, D.: The effects of sodium fluoride on bone breaking stength, Calcif. Tissue Res. **14**:283, 1974.
118. Cohn, S.H., et al.: Effects of porcine calcitonin on calcium metabolism in osteoporosis, J. Clin. Endocrinol. Metab. **33**:719, 1971.
119. Caniggia, A., et al.: Calcium metabolism and ^{47}calcium kinetics before and after long-term thyrocalcitonin treatment in senile osteoporosis, Clin. Sci. **38**:397, 1970.
120. Rasmussen, H., et al.: Effect of combined therapy with phosphate and calcitonin on bone volume in osteoporosis, Metab. Bone Dis. Rel. Res. **2**:107, 1980.
121. Bloch-Michel, H., et al.: Traitement au long cours de l'ostéoporose par la thyrocalcitonine, Rev. Rhum. Mal. Osteoartic. **37**:629, 1970.
122. Sluys Veer, J.V.D., Bijvoet, O.L.M., and Smeenk, D.: Effects of long-term porcine calcitonin administration in patients with Paget's disease or osteoporosis, Calcif. Tissue Res. **4**:88, 1970.

CHAPTER 10 · DIABETES MELLITUS

Marvin E. Levin

The incidence of diabetes in the United States has been variously estimated to be between 2% and 5% of the total population. Recent estimates suggest that the incidence is closer to 5%. This means that 5% of the population is now diabetic or will develop diabetes at some point in their lifetime. Furthermore, it is estimated that the number of diabetics is increasing at a rate of 6% per year, doubling the diabetic population every 15 years.[1] Part of this increase is apparent and part is real. Diabetes detection drives and hospital screening programs, using a routine admission chemical profile, have discovered many diabetic patients whose disease was so mild that it would otherwise have gone undetected. An absolute increase is also occurring because diabetics today live longer than they did three to four decades ago.

Most of this increase in longevity is the result of the use of antibiotics, which now prevent previously fatal infections. Before the advent of sulfonamide drugs in 1930 and subsequently of other antibiotics, in-hospital mortality after amputation in diabetic patients was 50%.[2] The availability of antibiotics reduced this rate to between 10% and 20% at the present time. The number of diabetic patients today would probably be even greater if it were not for the problem of cardiovascular disease, which still causes a significant excess risk of death at a relatively early age in these patients. Nevertheless, the number of elderly diabetic patients is continuing to increase at a significant rate. The incidence of diabetes in the various age groups is shown in Table 10-1.[3] Based on these figures it can be observed that the vast majority of patients are over 55 years of age.

Table 10-1. Rates of known diabetes, 1978*

	Age				
	All	*Under 20*	*20-44*	*45-64*	*65+*
Male	20.0	2.0	9.8	47.4	69.1
Female	27.1	2.1	11.1	57.4	88.8
White	23.3	2.1	10.5	49.8	75.7
All other	26.3	1.7	10.4	76.8	129.1
Black	(29.1)	(1.8)	(12.1)	(83.4)	(134.4)

*From Health interview survey, National Commission on Health Services, 1978.

The incidence of age and diabetes can also depend on race. For example, the Pima Indians, a tribe of almost 3000 Indians residing mainly on the Gila River Reservation in South Central Arizona, were studied with glucose tolerance tests. In terms of age and specific prevalence of diabetes, 40% of the males between 65 and 74 years of age had diabetes and 69% of the females between 55 and 64 years of age had diabetes. The overall prevalence of diabetes in the Pima Indians at 35 years of age or over was 50%. This is the highest recorded incidence of diabetes of all ethnic groups reported.[4]

Another explanation for the apparent or real increase in diabetes in the elderly is the impairment of glucose tolerance with aging. As early as 1921, Spence[5] noted variations in glucose tolerance at different ages and observed a decreased glucose tolerance in healthy elderly men. Although glucose tolerance deteriorates with age, the question still remains whether this decreased tolerance makes a diagnosis of diabetes or whether it is simply part of the normal aging process. Furthermore, if it is diagnostic of diabetes, at what level of glucose abnormality can the test be called positive for diabetes in the elderly? The exact incidence of diabetes in the

Table 10-2. Criteria for the interpretation of oral glucose tolerance tests in use in the United States

	Fasting	*1 hour*	*1½ hours*	*2 hours*	*3 hours*
*University of Michigan**†					
Glucose values (mg/100 ml)					
Whole blood	—	160	140	120	—
Plasma or serum		185	160	140	—
Diagnostic criteria			All levels at or above		
Wilkerson point system‡§					
Glucose values (mg/100 ml)					
Whole blood	110 or above	170 or above	—	120 or above	110 or above
Plasma or serum	130 or above	195 or above	—	140 or above	125 or above
Points	1	½		½	1
Diagnostic criteria			Total of 2 points or more		
University group diabetes program‖¶					
Glucose values (mg/100 ml)					
Whole blood			500 or above		
Plasma or serum			600 or above		
Diagnostic criteria			Sum of Fasting, 1-, 2-, 3-hour glucose values		

*Data from Fajans and Conn, 1954[7] and 1959.[8]
†Glucose load 1.75 mg/kg ideal body weight.
‡Data from Wilkerson, 1964.[9]
§Glucose load 100 mg.
‖Data from Report of the Committee on Statistics of the American Diabetes Association, 1969.[6]
¶Glucose load 30 gm/m^2 of body surface.

older age group has been made even more difficult because of the great number of variables involved in glucose tolerance testing. Many of these variables have been outlined by the Committee on Statistics of the American Diabetes Association.[6] Some of the most important variables are the glucose loading doses and the different criteria used in the interpretations of the tests. The most commonly used glucose tolerance tests are outlined in Table 10-2.[6-9] The method of Fajans and Conn[7,8] refers only to those patients under 50 years of age. In addition, standards for the glucose tolerance tests are performed on nonhospitalized healthy people. One must take into consideration the fact that patients who are hospitalized may be under stress or bedridden and may have eaten poorly, all factors that could influence the results of the glucose tolerance test.

Recently there has been an adjustment made in the criteria for diagnosing glucose intolerance and diabetes mellitus in the patient without intercurrent illness. A diagnosis of diabetes can be made if the fasting plasma glucose level is over 140 mg/100 ml; this must be confirmed by at least one additional determination to exclude laboratory error or patient failure to fast. In Table 10-3 is shown the National Institutes of Health (NIH) International Workgroup criteria for making a diagnosis of overt diabetes or what might be termed *impaired glucose tolerance*. The loading dose for this glucose tolerance test is 75 or 100 gm of glucose or 1.7 gm/kg of body weight if the patient is small.

In the interpretation of any of these tests it is important to be familiar with the analytic method used in the particular laboratory. Thus values comparing whole blood and plasma cannot be done unless a conversion is carried out. Conversion of whole blood values to plasma values is done by multiplying the whole blood values by 1.15 and adding 6 mg/100 ml. The values are usually rounded to the nearest 5 mg/100 ml. If capillary blood is used, diagnostic values are slightly higher. The interpretation of glucose tolerance tests also depends on the type of dietary preparation. Although there is not total agreement, the patient should have been receiving a carbohydrate intake of 150 to 300 gm per day for 3 days before the test. Other variables include the route of administration of the glucose load, the time of day that the test was performed, whether the test was fasting or postprandial, whether the source of the blood was venous or capillary, and the analytic procedure used—plasma, serum, or whole blood. In addition, diuretics, estrogens, and levodopa,[10] which may raise the blood glucose level, are drugs commonly used in the older age group and must be taken into consideration in evaluating test results.

Table 10-3. NIH criteria for diagnosis of diabetes mellitus

Minutes	*Overt diabetes*	*Impaired glucose tolerance*
30, 60, 90	1 value: >200 mg/100 ml	1 value: >200 mg/100 ml
	+	+
120	>200 mg/100 ml	>140 and <200 mg/100 ml

A comparison of several health surveys used to evaluate the effect of aging on glucose tolerance is recorded in Table 10-4.[11-16] It is seen from this table that there have been a wide variety of populations studied, various glucose loads used, and blood glucose levels measured at 1 hour and in some studies at 2 hours. In still others, values were reported at both 1- and 2-hour intervals. The mean increase in blood glucose per decade was determined by comparing the blood glucose values obtained in patients in their second decade of life with those obtained in patients in their eighth decade of life. It is seen from this table that despite the various populations studied and techniques used, there was a definite increase in blood glucose level in the older age group. Depending on which studies are used, there is an average increase in 1-hour values that varied anywhere from 6 to 14 mg/100 ml per decade and in 2-hour values from 6 to 11 mg/100 ml per decade. These values then would be in general accord with a mnemonic of adding 10 mg/100 ml to each decade over 50 years of age.[11]

Another method for adjusting glucose toler-

Table 10-4. Selected studies evaluating the influence of aging on glucose tolerance

	Number of subjects	*Glucose load*	*Time of sample after glucose load (hr)*	*Mean blood glucose increase per decade of life (mg/100 ml)*
Dallas* 1957	152	100 gm	2	11
National Health Survey† 1960-1962	111,000	50 gm	1	14
Tecumseh, Michigan, Community Study‡ 1966	4000	100 gm	1	13
London Community Study§ 1966	570	50 gm	1,2	14,7
Australian Community Study‖ 1969	1770	50 gm	1	10
Gerontology Research Center¶ 1971	713	1.75 gm/kg body weight	1,2	6,6

*Data from Unger, 1957.[14]
†Data from U.S. National Center for Health Statistics, 1964.[15]
‡Data from Hayner et al., 1965.[13]
§Data from Butterfield, 1966.[12]
‖Data from Welborn et al., 1969.[16]
¶Data from Andres, 1971.[11]

ance with age is that suggested by Jackson and Vinik.[17] They have studied glucose tolerances with a 50 gm glucose load in clinically normal individuals in different decades of life (Fig. 10-1).[17] It is seen that the curve for each successive decade fits above the preceding one, the shaded zone being "diabetic" by the authors' criteria. Thus patients of varying ages could have dissimilar fasting and 1-hour and 2-hour blood glucose values, and all of these would be within the normal range.

Still another way of evaluating blood glucose values in the aged is by the use of the nomogram suggested by Andres (Fig. 10-2).[11] By this technique each individual's performance is judged against those of the same age. For example, a line extending from the individual's age through the 2-hour blood glucose concentration will intersect the percentile line. Thus a 55-year-old individual with a 2-hour glucose level of 180 mg/100 ml has a percentile rank of 8%; 92% of the individuals of that age will outperform him, and 8% will have an even lower tolerance. This technique cannot designate in which percentile rank one should consider a patient to be diabetic and which percentile rank simply represents the ef-

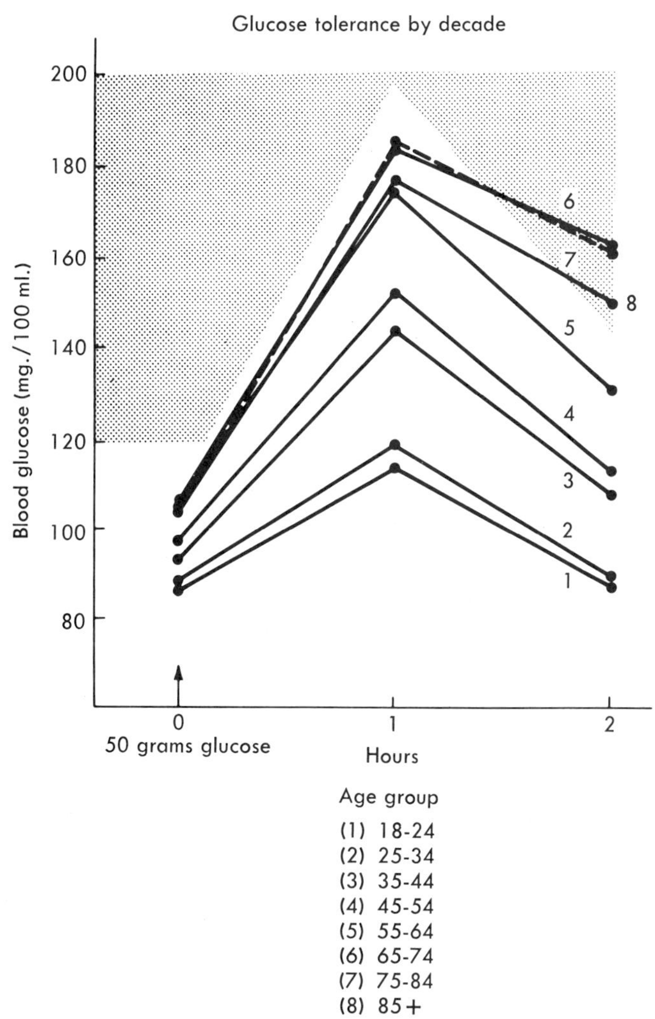

Fig. 10-1. Diminishing glucose tolerance with age. Shaded zone is considered "diabetic." (From Jackson, W.P.U., and Vinik, A.I.: Hyperglycemia and diabetes in the elderly. In Ellenberg, M., and Rifkin, H., editors: Diabetes mellitus, theory and practice. Copyright 1970 by McGraw-Hill Book Co. Used with permission of the publisher.)

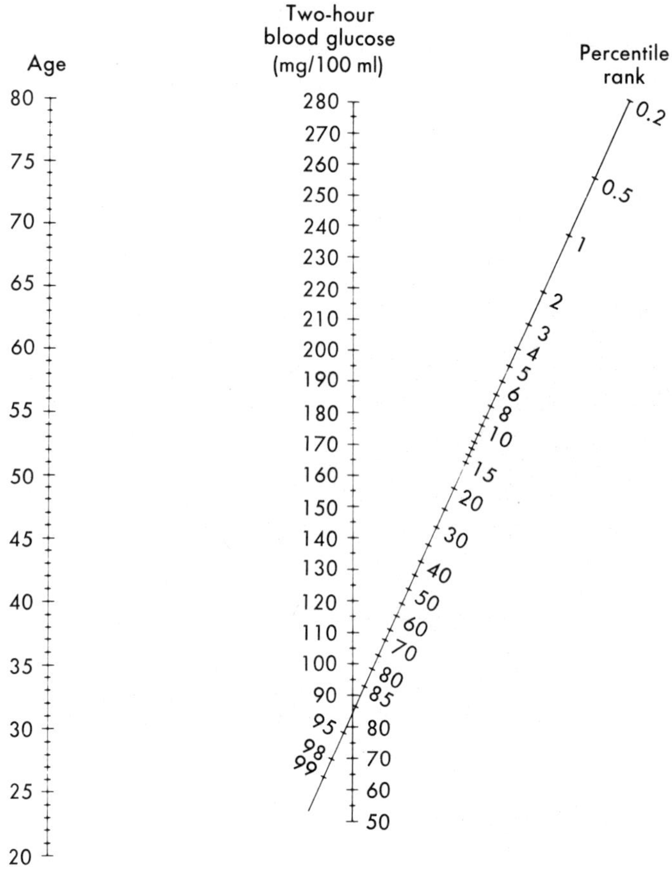

Fig. 10-2. Nomogram for evaluating oral glucose tolerance tests. (From Andres, R.: Med. Clin. North Am. **55:**835, 1971.)

fect of aging on glucose tolerance. However, it does provide a good concept of how any individual ranks compared with a large number of tested individuals of similar age.

Additional means of studying glucose tolerance involve the use of the cortisone glucose tolerance test, intravenous glucose tolerance test, and intravenous tolbutamide response test. These tests also involve additional variables and are used primarily in special situations. There are only extremely limited data available indicating how well these tests can distinguish glucose tolerance associated with aging from that of true diabetes. Therefore these tests have no particular value over the oral glucose tolerance test in testing for diabetes in the aging population. A review of these types of glucose tolerance tests in the aging population has been made by Andres.[11]

One would hope that with all of these multiple studies there would be a standard procedure for evaluating glucose tolerances in the aged. Obviously such standards are not available. The report of the World Health Organization (WHO) recommends diagnostic standards only up to the age of 45 years.[18] The American Diabetes Association Committee on Statistics,[6] although listing multiple factors that influence glucose tolerance and procedures for performing glucose tolerance testing, has not given a definitive answer in this regard. Although the committee recognizes that glucose tolerance deteriorates with age in persons who do not become symptomatic diabetic patients, it has not given a unified opinion on how to evaluate the deterioration in glucose tolerance with aging, as opposed to the intolerance that occurs in true diabetes.

Obviously not all diabeticians agree with these various adjustments of glucose tolerance tests with age, since all elderly people do not have impaired glucose tolerance. Therefore these diabeticians are more likely to make a diagnosis of diabetes at any age if there is a significant abnormality in the curve.

Jackson and Vinik[17] have suggested that the elderly hyperglycemic patient may represent a double population. One group is truly diabetic and more susceptible to the complications of diabetes; the other group, although having an abnormality in glucose tolerance, is not diabetic and is simply unable to handle an unnatural glucose load such as is given in a glucose tolerance test. A final point suggesting the importance of an abnormal glucose tolerance test in the older patient is inheritance. Thus an abnormal glucose tolerance curve in the elderly patient may ultimately prove to be significant in terms of inheritance for other family members.

Perhaps with current information an exact distinction between the carbohydrate abnormalities seen in aging and those of true diabetes is an impossible task, but these various studies do provide guidelines and help the physician to avoid making a false positive diagnosis of diabetes in the elderly patient simply on the basis of an abnormal glucose tolerance test. Once given this diagnosis, patients must live the remainder of their lives with this label. In some cases it can result in loss of employment and can cause unnecessary medical expenses for blood glucose determinations and for the more frequent medical evaluations required for the known diabetic patient. Statistically the life-span of the diabetic individual is shorter than that of the nondiabetic individual. Burdened with this knowledge, diabetics may be forced to change their life-styles completely on the basis of a false diagnosis. One of the most distressing things that happens to individuals who have been diagnosed as diabetic is the change in diet. They are requested to give up sugar-containing foods and to change a lifelong way of eating. If they have the disease, this is a necessity, but if, in fact, they do not have diabetes, requesting this change in diet does them a gastronomic injustice.

In summary, once the diagnosis of diabetes is made, the patient takes on new anxieties, a new way of eating, a change in life-style, and additional expenses. Therefore, in the elderly patient the diagnosis of diabetes on the basis of a glucose tolerance test must take into consideration all the previously noted variables that can influence the test.

Table 10-5. Death rate per 100,000 population for diabetic patients in United States, 1974*

Age group	*Incidence*
25-34	1.9
34-44	4.3
45-54	11.4
55-64	31.7
65-74	81.6
75-84	172.0
85-Plus	248.4

*Data from National Center for Health Statistics: Advance report final mortality statistics, 1974. Monthly vital statistics report, vol. 24, no. 11, DHEW Pub. no. (HRA) 76-1120. Report of National Commission on Diabetes, vol. 3, part 1, DHEW Pub. no. (NIH) 76-1021, Washington, D.C., U.S. Government Printing Office.

MORTALITY

The frequency and relatively early age of death in the adult diabetic patient is largely the result of stroke and myocardial infarction (Table 10-5). Silent or painless myocardial infarctions have been reported to be more common in the elderly diabetic patient. Bradley and Schonfeld[20] reported that 42% of myocardial infarctions in diabetic patients were essentially painless. The frequency of death, mainly the result of vascular disease, increases approximately 20 times from 40 to 70 years of age, compared with only a tenfold increase in the nondiabetic individual in the same age span.[21]

Insurance studies have confirmed the diabetic to be a heavily substandard risk with a mortality ratio far in excess of normal. In a 20-year mortality study of over 10,000 diabetics, Goodkin[22] found the following: (1) The age of onset is the most significant factor in mortality, with the highest mortality ratio in those with diabetes before age 14. The juvenile insulin dependent diabetic is therefore a poor insurance risk. (2) Mortality increases with duration until the fourteenth year of the disease, when it tends to flatten out. (3) Poor control appears to be associated with about two and one half times the mortality of the well-controlled group. (4) Diabetics treated by diet alone or by diet and oral medication show lower mortality ratios than those who are insulin dependent. It must be kept in mind that a diabetic who can be controlled by diet alone or by diet and oral medication tends to be a milder diabetic and is usually of the adult non-insulin requiring type. (5) Underweight diabetics have a higher mortality than overweight diabetics. This would further confirm the conclusion that the thin or insulin dependent diabetic is a greater mortality risk than the milder adult onset diabetic who tends to be obese. (6) Obesity alone is not a significantly adverse prognostic factor in diabetes. (7) The mortality risk of hypertension is multiplied in the diabetic as compared to the nondiabetic, especially at ages under 40. (8) The finding of albuminuria is an extremely unfavorable prognostic sign. (9) Coronary heart disease represented the most common cause of death among diabetics. Of all deaths, 62% were attributed to cardiovascular and renal disease.[22]

The age of onset is especially important in predicting longevity. Goodkin[22] found the mortality ratios of diabetics versus nondiabetics to be the greatest in those under age 15. Table 10-6 compares the life expectancy and mortality ratios of diabetics diagnosed at various ages compared with the overall life expectancy of the standard nondiabetic. It is seen that the diabetic with an onset at age 15 has a life expectancy of another 32 years as compared to 59 plus years for the nondiabetic at the same age, a difference of 27 years. A diabetic diagnosed between ages 30 and 39 would be expected to live another 28 years, whereas the nondiabetic of the same age could expect another 39 years of life, a difference of 11 years. The difference in length of life decreases progressively until age 65. Diagnosis at this age has only a 5-year difference in life expectancy between diabetic and nondiabetic, indicating that a diagnosis of diabetes in the older or geriatric patient carries a better outlook than for the patient who develops diabetes at a younger age.[22]

ACCELERATED AGING IN THE DIABETIC

The diabetic patient's age is generally accepted as being 10 years or more than his chronological years. For example, the islet cells of the diabetic pancreas at age 50 may look like those of a nondiabetic 100 years or older.[23] This accelerated aging process or premature senescence is evidenced not only by changes in the islet cells but also by the early development of cataracts, macular degeneration, and by a decrease in bone mass. The decrease in bone mass is comparable to that in much older patients, suggesting premature osteoporosis.[24] By far the most impressive and important change resulting from accelerated aging is atherosclerosis, which leads to premature heart attacks, stroke, and peripheral vascular disease (PVD).

There are several experimental lines of evidence that demonstrate premature aging in diabetics. One of the most important is the collagen study. Evidence has accumulated that cross-linking of collagen and connective tissue is accelerated in diabetics. This results in generalized stiffness with age, senile cataracts, and some of the stiffness in blood vessel walls. Collagen studies can be used to estimate with considerable precision the chronological age of individuals.[25] In an attempt to determine the apparent rates of aging in persons with diabetes, Hamlin et al.[26] analyzed specimens of collagen taken shortly after death from the central tendon of the diaphragm of three subjects with juvenile onset diabetes and compared these specimens

Table 10-6. Diabetic mortality study: expectation of life among all diabetic insurance applicants compared with standard lives by age of onset

	Mortality ratios (%)		*Expectation of life (in years)*	
Age of onset	*Diabetics*	*Standard lives*	*Diabetics*	*Standard lives*
Under 15	1127	100	32	59
15-19	926	100	33	56
20-29	443	100	33	49
30-39	344	100	28	39
40-49	301	100	20	30
50-59	213	100	17	23
60-70	234	100	11	16

with those taken from 14 nondiabetics. They found remarkable agreement between the true ages of the nondiabetic patient and the estimated age as determined from the collagen specimen but vast discrepancies in the actual and estimated ages of the diabetic patients. Among the diabetics there was a 51- to 65-year differential between the subject's actual and estimated ages. The three diabetic patients had died at ages 31, 41, and 44 years, but their respective estimated ages by collagen analysis were 84 years in one patient and 106 years in the other two.[26] Since collagen is a major component of blood vessel walls and basement membranes, it is most likely that changes in the collagen structure are involved in many of the diseases and disabilities of aging. Thickening of the capillary basement membrane (CBM), of which collagen is a major component, normally occurs with advancing age; however, this process is accelerated in the diabetic.[27] Further evidence of very early senescence in the blood vessels of diabetics is seen in the study by Pillsbury et al.[28] In a comparison study of 39 diabetic children and 27 normal children, the diabetic children showed changes in pulse wave velocity that could be associated with increased wall stiffness similar to that seen with aging, suggesting that the large arteries and the brachial and carotid arteries of diabetic children may exhibit acceleration of the aging process.

Finally, aging may also be related to antibody formation against the islet cell. Ohneda[29] has proposed that antibody formation against the islet cell is intrinsic with aging. This may be another cause for the aging changes seen in the diabetic's islet cells.

CONTROL VERSUS GENETICS IN AGING

Whether diabetic control is or is not critical in preventing complications and accelerated aging is an important question that continues to be asked. A substantial amount of evidence suggests that genetic factors play an important role and that elevated blood sugar levels alone cannot be the sole explanation for accelerated aging. In Pillsbury's study,[28] the severity of the changes in pulse wave velocity bore no direct correlation with the degree of carbohydrate tolerance as judged by insulin requirement. In the study of Levin et al.[24] relating to a decrease in bone mass in diabetics, a greater than 10% loss of bone mass in 50% of both the juvenile and adult onset diabetics was found to be present at the time of initial diagnosis. While it is difficult to ascertain the exact onset of diabetes in the adult onset diabetic and therefore its duration, the juvenile diabetic has a relatively abrupt onset, and the exact date of onset and duration are readily determined. However, the duration of diabetes in both adult and juvenile onset diabetic patients failed to show an acceleration of bone mass loss,[24] suggesting a genetic factor in determining bone structure and mass.

There is also some evidence that CBM thickening may have, at least in part, a genetic factor. If CBM thickening were purely an environmental or hyperglycemic effect, one might expect the thickening to be uniform throughout the capillary, but in fact the width may differ in a single tissue and capillary.[30] There is also no correlation between severity of retinopathy and muscle CBM thickening.[31,32] Further evidence for a genetic factor is documented by Camerini-Davlos et al.[33] On the basis of age adjusted 95%-tolerance limit, 23% of their 30 patients with genetic prediabetes (the offspring of diabetic parents) had CBM thickening compared with only 5% of their 40 control patients. This figure is similar to the 29% seen in the Pima study.[34]

Additional evidence of a genetic factor in premature aging of the diabetic is established by the observations of Goldstein et al.[35] on fibroblasts. Skin fibroblasts in the diabetic had a decreased growth capacity similar to that seen with the aging process, and it was felt that the fibroblasts had a diabetic genotype. While detrimental effects of the diabetic gene on cell growth were more pronounced in the overt diabetic patient than in those genetically predisposed, the effects of decreased fibroblast growth were seen in some juvenile diabetic and prediabetic patients, suggesting that the aging process in diabetics is at least in part inherited and not a factor totally related to hyperglycemia.[35]

AGING FACTORS INFLUENCING CARBOHYDRATE METABOLISM

Insulin

The causes of decreased carbohydrate tolerance with aging are multifactorial. The first factor to consider is the effect of age on insulin levels, insulin release, decreased peripheral effectiveness of insulin, or a combination of these. O'Sullivan et al.[36] have found that with advancing age blood glucose and immunoreactive insulin (IRI) levels tend to rise. However, insulin release required a higher blood glucose level in the older group, suggesting the primary disorder in the insulin release mechanism occurring with age is the need for a higher blood glucose level to produce an equivalent insulin level.[36] There is also evidence of delayed insulin release with aging. In a group of healthy men, young and old, Dudl and Ensinck[37] found that with advancing age the basal glucose level rose from 80 to 100 mg/100 ml although basal insulin levels were unaltered. After a glucose load there was a decreased rate of glucose disappearance with age, and the acute insulin response measured by the percent of change in the mean 3 to 5 minute levels also declined. Thus the rise of glucose levels with age may be explained by inappropriately low levels of insulin in the fasting state and a delayed insulin response.

A decreased peripheral responsiveness to insulin is another explanation for glucose intolerance with age. This may begin as early as 20 years of age.[38,39] Elsas et al.[39] found that the muscle of 50-day-old rats compared with that of younger rats loses its responsiveness to insulin, as measured by the amino acid uptake by the rat diaphragm. In the older rat the preparation relies completely on indirect stimulation through new protein synthesis. This observation suggests that with increasing age the muscle membrane loses direct responsiveness to insulin. Dobrzanski[40] has also shown decreased peripheral adipose tissue sensitivity to insulin with age. He found adipose tissue of older rats to be less sensitive to insulin and to have a decreased uptake of glucose compared with that of younger rats. Recent evidence confirms that glucose intolerance with aging is related to a decrease in peripheral insulin sensitivity. Defronzo,[41] employing intravenous glucose and/or insulin administration at set levels, found impaired tissue sensitivity to insulin to be the primary factor responsible for the decrease in glucose tolerance observed with advancing age. He felt that this insulin resistance resided primarily in peripheral tissue and not in the liver. However, Freeman[42] and Olefsky[43] have shown that the insulin receptors on liver cell membranes as well as those on fat cells decreased with age. Runyan et al.,[44] in studying the effect of age on insulin degrading activity in rat tissue, found that in animals over 1 year old insulin degrading activity in muscle, the liver, and the kidney was significantly less than the activity in either 4- or 7-week-old animals. Insulin degradation has been shown by Terris et al.[45] to occur as part of the hormone's interaction with its receptor, and it has been suggested that degradation of the insulin molecule might be required for part of the action of insulin.[46]

Finally obesity and age must be taken into account as major factors in peripheral insulin resistance beyond that related to a decrease in binding sites.[47] Adipose tissue disposes of less than 3% to 5% of an administered glucose load.[48,49] Therefore peripheral utilization depends largely on muscle mass. With aging there is a decrease in tissue (muscle) available to metabolize a glucose load and an increase in tissue (fat) with a low rate of glucose metabolism.

Proinsulin

An additional factor involving insulin release from the pancreas is increased levels of proinsulin in the elderly. Proinsulin has less biologic activity than insulin. Duckworth and Kitabchi[50] have shown that normal individuals 40 to 60 years of age had significantly higher levels of plasma immunoreactive proinsulin-like material compared with insulin than did normal individuals who were 20 to 40 years of age.

Glucagon

Another hormonal substance affecting glucose tolerance with aging is glucagon. In a group of healthy young men, Dudl and Ensinck[37] demonstrated normal basal levels of glucagon, but elevated levels in older men after a glucose load. Unger et al.[51] have suggested that with advancing age or a long duration of diabetes glucagon secretion is not readily suppressed by hyperglycemia. More recently Berger et al.[52] confirmed an effect of age on blood glucagon levels. They demonstrated a rise in the plasma glucagon level occurring primarily in the third and fourth decade of life; but the level of plasma glucagon failed to increase thereafter.

Lipids

By acting as an insulin inhibitor, hyperlipemia may cause hyperglycemia. With aging there is a tendency toward prolonged alimentary hyperlipemia. These high values for serum lipids may be the result of a decrease in postheparin lipase activity. Brodows and Campbell[53] have found the postheparin lipase activity to be one half as great in elderly men after administration of a dose of heparin of 10 mg/kg body weight as in a control group of young men.

It is well established that diabetics have a higher incidence of atherosclerosis than do nondiabetics. This correlates with the fact that these patients have elevated levels of cholesterol and triglycerides.[54] High density lipoproteins (HDL cholesterol) seem to have a coronary protective effect and are known to be inversely related to the risk of coronary artery disease and correlate positively to life expectancy. There is some evidence that the diabetic may have a lower level of HDL cholesterol than the nondiabetic. However, there is some debate as to whether or not lowering serum lipid and cholesterol values will have a positive effect in reducing the atherosclerotic process. Nikkila and Hormila[55] have concluded that the average serum lipid and lipoprotein pattern of insulin treated diabetics is not more atherogenic than that of the diabetic of similar age and sex. They also found elevated HDL cholesterol levels in the insulin treated diabetics that should make these diabetic individuals less liable to develop coronary artery disease. It was their feeling that the excessive cardiovascular disease associated with insulin dependent diabetes should be credited to factors other than lipid abnormalities.

TREATMENT OF DIABETES

Diet

Diet is the cornerstone of all diabetic therapy. This is especially true in the adult onset diabetic whose disease usually is mild and in most instances controllable by diet alone. Therefore the greatest therapeutic effort should be directed toward proper diet. However, the ideal diet for the elderly diabetic patient may be difficult to achieve for many reasons. Patients in the older age group frequently are financially unable to purchase the proper foods, and their diet may be unusually high in fats and disproportionally low in the more expensive protein containing foods. Understanding the diet may also be difficult for the elderly patient, and dietary instruction therefore must be especially designed for these patients. Social factors are also important. Frequently the elderly diabetic lives alone, with no one to cook for and no one to share the meal; the incentive to eat properly is lost. They frequently eat their meals out and are not always able to obtain a totally proper diet. Those who live in nursing homes, an ever increasing problem, do not always receive a correctly calculated diabetic diet. Faulty dentures or absent teeth are also common problems in the elderly and must be taken into consideration in the preparation of the diet. Many of these patients require a soft or mechanically soft diet. In addition, the diet must be realistic in terms of the patient's socioeconomic and ethnic background. Any dietary instruction that fails to take all of these factors into consideration is doomed to failure.

The diet should be calorically adjusted according to the individual patient's activity. Since most of these patients are over age 65 and are sedentary, a diet consisting of 20 to 25 calories/kg of ideal body weight is a useful guideline. The diet should contain 50% to 55% carbohydrates, 15% to 20% protein, and 20% to 25% fat. Diets high in fiber should also be used. Concern over saturated fats and cholesterol in the diet may not be as important in the elderly diabetic as in the younger diabetic patient. It is doubtful that additional severe restrictions in dietary cholesterol and fats would have any long-range effect in preventing atherosclerosis in this age group. However, whenever possible, polyunsaturated fats should be prescribed.

Insulin

Although most elderly diabetic patients can be controlled by diet alone, a significant number will require insulin. The indications for the use of insulin in the geriatric diabetic are no different than in the younger diabetic patient. If blood sugar levels and symptoms cannot be controlled by diet alone or the patient is prone to ketoacidosis, insulin administration is indicated. Geriatric patients with infections or surgical stress may require insulin even though under normal conditions their diabetes is controllable by diet alone. While there is evidence that strict diabetic control may prevent complications, tight control of the geriatric patient can carry some risks. Hypoglycemia with its concomitant release of catecholamines may lead to cardiac dysrhythmia and even death in the elderly patient. Furthermore, the older patient with cerebral atherosclerosis may have more profound central nervous system (CNS) symptoms associated with hypoglycemia. It is not unusual for the older patient with hypoglycemia to exhibit CNS symptoms rather than those related to catecholamine release. Because these patients are more vulnerable to the effects of hypoglycemia, rigid control in the elderly diabetic may be inadvisable. These patients should maintain fasting blood sugar levels in the range of 140 mg/100 ml and 2-hour postprandial sugar levels of 150 to 175 mg/100 ml. Keeping blood sugar levels in these ranges minimizes the risk of hypoglycemia.

Many elderly diabetic patients are blind. It is my feeling that automatic insulin measuring devices carry significant risks because of the possibility of drawing up too much or too little insulin. If these patients are living with their families, their insulin should be measured by a family member. If the patient is blind and living alone, a family member or friend can draw up a week's supply of insulin syringes and leave them in the refrigerator for the patient to use each day. The patient should be cautioned, however, to shake and rotate the syringe to make sure that the precipitate is equally distributed. If a family member or friend is not available, the Visiting Nurses Association can provide a nurse to perform this service at weekly intervals.

In the 1980s new, highly purified, monocomponent insulins were introduced. These insulins appear to decrease the incidence of local and generalized skin reactions and lipoatrophy. To date, prevention of diabetic complications has not been demonstrated with these insulins. These newer insulins will be more expensive than the single peak, slightly less purified insulins previously used. In the patient requiring a large insulin dose, gradual reduction may be necessary, as it has been estimated that patients who are switched to the newer insulins may require 15% less insulin.

Oral hypoglycemic agents

Oral hypoglycemic drugs are frequently prescribed for the adult onset diabetic patient whose disease is relatively mild. These drugs are being used primarily in the treatment of the older patient, since adult onset diabetes usually occurs after the age of 40 to 50 years. It is estimated that from 1 to 1.5 million Americans are taking these medications. How necessary are these drugs in controlling diabetes? Recent clinical research has shown that of a large number of patients who discontinued these drugs one third were totally unaffected, that is, the drugs used were having no effect and were not needed; one third required more rigid dietary management but could be controlled without medication; and one third required insulin or oral hypoglycemic drugs.[56,57]

There is also evidence of increased cardiovascular mortality associated with the use of oral hypoglycemic agents. In 1970 the University Group Diabetes Program (UGDP) reported an increase in cardiovascular deaths in patients taking tolbutamide,[58] and in 1971 a similar finding of increased cardiovascular mortality was reported in patients taking phenformin.[59] Phenformin has since been removed from the market because of the increased incidence of lactic acidosis associated with its use. Since the UGDP report there has been a great deal of controversy over whether or not there is a cardiovascular risk associated with the use of the sulfonylureas, although it should be pointed out that only tolbutamide was used in the study. While some studies have confirmed the UGDP findings, others have not. In both a retrospective and prospective study, Hadden et al.[60] found that diabetic patients receiving a flexible dose of oral hypoglycemic agents had almost twice as many myocardial infarctions and twice as high a death rate as those using diet alone or diet and insulin to control their disease. A study by Soler et al.[61] of diabetic patients treated and monitored in a coronary care unit found the incidence of ventricular fibrillation, a highly lethal event, in 12% of the patients receiving oral agents, compared with 7% in those using diet alone and 3% in those receiving insulin. Additional evidence supporting the hypothesis that the use of these drugs may result in increased mortality from cardiovascular disease has come from recent surveys in England[62] and Wales for the WHO.[63] Using age-adjusted mortality figures, these surveys have shown an increased rate of death from cardiovascular disease, beginning around 1960, that correlates with increased usage of the oral hypoglycemic agents. At the same time the death rate for juvenile onset diabetic patients receiving insulin had fallen.

The manner in which sulfonylureic agents might precipitate increasing mortality has not been conclusively demonstrated. However, there is increasing experimental evidence both in animals[64] and humans[65] that these agents have positive inotropic effects on the heart and may therefore cause increased ventricular irritability and death in patients with preexisting myocardial disease.

Confirmation of the UGDP findings has been made by the Biometric Society[66] and by the Food and Drug Administration (FDA).[67] However, controversy still remains regarding the reliability of the UGDP data. The most vigorous opponents of the UGDP are Kilo et al.[68] In their recent review of the UGDP data they make the point that in patients over 53 years of age, especially women, there is an increased cardiovascular death rate in those who have fasting blood sugar levels over 200 mg/100 ml and are taking tolbutamide.[68] The adult onset diabetic tends to be obese and has difficulty following a prescribed diet; one would be naive and unrealistic to believe that the majority of these patients can be consistently controlled with blood sugar levels below 200 mg/100 ml. Therefore Kilo et al. are in fact warning of cardiovascular risk with the use of oral agents in this large group of patients.

If oral hypoglycemic agents are used, it must be kept in mind that severe hypoglycemia can result. The hypoglycemic effect of these drugs may be potentiated by decreased food intake and the use of ethanol, salicylates, monoamine oxidase inhibitors, sulfonamides, bishydroxycoumarin, and phenylbutazone.[69-72] Oral hypoglycemic agents must be used with great caution in patients who have renal or hepatic disease. Most of these agents are excreted by the kidneys in an active form. For example, chlorpropamide (Diabinese) is excreted unchanged. Acetohexamide (Dymelor) is metabolized by the liver into several active compounds that are also excreted by the kidneys. Therefore in the face of liver disease these compounds may not be metabolized and in the presence of renal disease they can accumulate and produce severe prolonged hypoglycemia that lasts for several days.[73] In addition, elderly patients living alone may be skipping meals, thus decreasing glycogen stores and predisposing themselves to hypoglycemia. Severe hypoglycemia in the elderly patient can mimic a cerebral vascular accident. Therefore any patient taking insulin or a hypoglycemic agent who has a cerebral vascular accident-like picture must be evaluated for the possibility of hypoglycemia.

It should be noted that chlorpropamide has a tendency to cause fluid retention, which may lead to mild to moderate congestive heart failure, particularly in the diabetic predisposed to arteriosclerotic heart disease. The fluid retaining property of chlorpropamide also accounts for some cases of hyponatremia on a dilutional basis.

Exercise

Celsus, around the time of Christ, first advocated exercise as a component of diabetes management.[74] The importance of exercise in diabetes care was rediscovered in 1926 when Lawrence[75] again pointed out that exercise potentiates the effect of insulin in lowering the concentration of blood glucose. Lutwak and Whedon[76] have observed an abnormal glucose tolerance test level in normal persons after a regimen of 1 to 3 weeks of bed rest. Lipman et al.[77] have also shown a significant reduction of peripheral glucose uptake as early as 72 hours after the onset of absolute bed rest. In addition, they found that individuals on a regimen of bed rest tend to be somewhat resistant to exogenously administered insulin with a smaller fall in their glucose level after insulin administration compared with active control subjects. It has also been shown that physical activity can produce an insulin-like effect. Goldstein[78] demonstrated a circulating humoral factor that was released from exercising muscle. This substance appeared to have a significant hypoglycemic effect in resting parabiotic animals. More recently Felig[79] showed that insulin mediated blood glucose uptake increased by 30% after physical training. Felig felt that insulin sensitivity improved in proportion to physical fitness and that it was probably attributable, at least in part, to increased insulin binding at the receptor sites.

Exercise may also influence clotting factors and thrombi formation. The adhesion of platelets to endothelium followed by aggregation of platelets is an important contributing factor to atheromatous changes in blood vessels. This process tends to be acclerated in the diabetic. A significant difference in platelet adherence before and after exercise has been demonstrated.[79] Before exercise a normal subject has a 40% adherence rate and 36% after exercise. In a diabetic subject the percentage of adherence was 74% before exercise and 53% afterwards. This decrease in adherence of platelets was maintained for 9 hours after exercise in one subject and 24 hours after exercise in another subject.[79]

A detailed symposium on diabetes and exercise can be found in a recent review on this subject.[74]

With increasing age individuals tend to decrease physical activity, thus decreasing the opportunity for peripheral utilization of glucose. In addition, with increasing age muscle mass decreases to a proportionally greater degree than does fat mass, even though the total body weight may remain the same, further decreasing the muscle tissue available for utilization of glucose. It is therefore extremely important for the diabetic patient to have a definite exercise program. This should be worked out by the physician and programed to the age of the patient and his cardiovascular status. The minimum daily activity should be walking.

DIABETIC COMPLICATIONS

Vascular disease

The complications of vascular disease are the most common and serious disorders affecting the diabetic patient, both in morbidity and mortality. Vascular disease can be divided into two major categories, macrovascular disease that comprises the larger vessels, and microvascular disease that includes arteries smaller than 115 μm in diameter, arterioles, and capillaries.

Microvascular disease involving the capillary is characterized by CBM thickening and is the hallmark of vascular disease in the diabetic patient. An example of CBM thickening in the elderly nondiabetic individual is depicted in Fig. 10-3. By contrast, the greatly thickened CBM in an 83-year-old man with diabetes of 26 years' duration is shown in Fig. 10-4. A highly significant degree of thickening of muscle CBM as an aging phenomenon both in the diabetic and the nondiabetic individual is seen in Fig. 10-5.[27] This age related CBM thickening is significant in both sexes; however, the rate of thickening is not the same in normal males and females. In males the CBM width increases throughout life, but at a decreasing rate. In females the CBM width parallels that of males up to approximately 25 years of age and then plateaus until approximately 10 to 15 years after menopause, at which time it increases rapidly to catch up with that of the males. CBM thickening increases with age even more dramatically in the diabetic than in normal individuals and is thicker in the diabetic at all

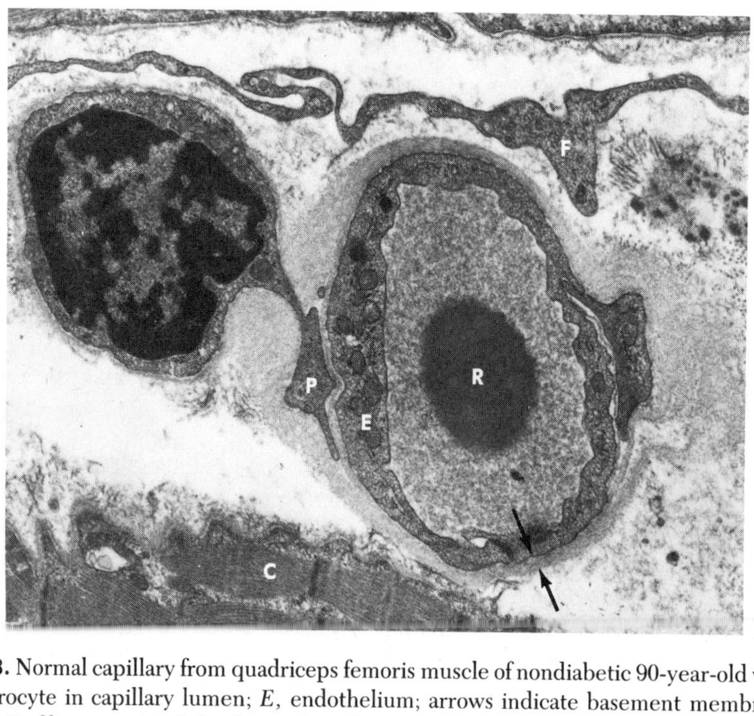

Fig. 10-3. Normal capillary from quadriceps femoris muscle of nondiabetic 90-year-old woman. *R*, erythrocyte in capillary lumen; *E*, endothelium; arrows indicate basement membrane; *P*, pericyte; *F*, fibrocyte; *C*, skeletal muscle cell. (×14,600.) (From Williamson, J.R., Kilo, C., and Crespin, S.R.: Vascular disease. In Levin, M., and O'Neal, L., editors: The diabetic foot, ed. 3, St. Louis, 1982, The C.V. Mosby Co.)

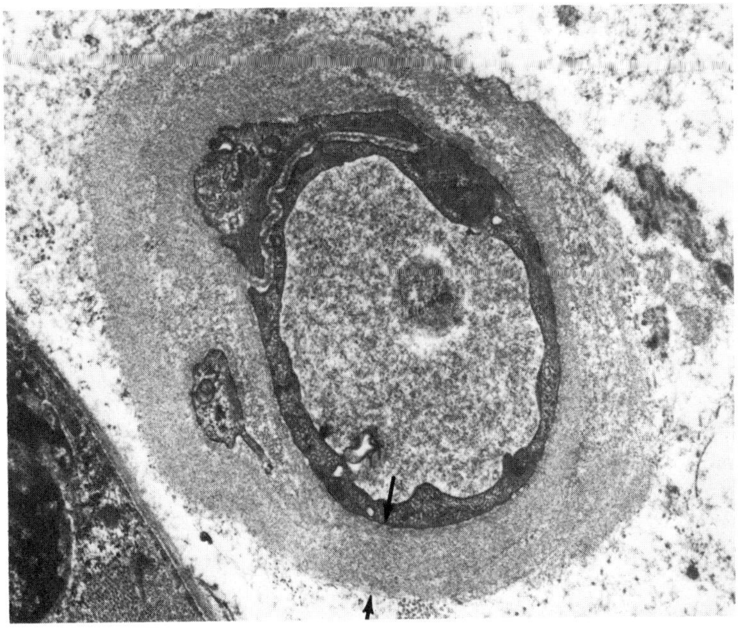

Fig. 10-4. Capillary from quadriceps femoris muscle of 83-year-old man with diabetes of 26 years' known duration. Basement membrane (arrows) is greatly thickened around the entire circumference of vessel. (×18,200.) (From Williamson, J.R., Kilo, C., and Crespin, S.R.: Vascular disease. In Levin, M., and O'Neal, L., editors: The diabetic foot, ed. 3, St. Louis, 1982, The C.V. Mosby Co.)

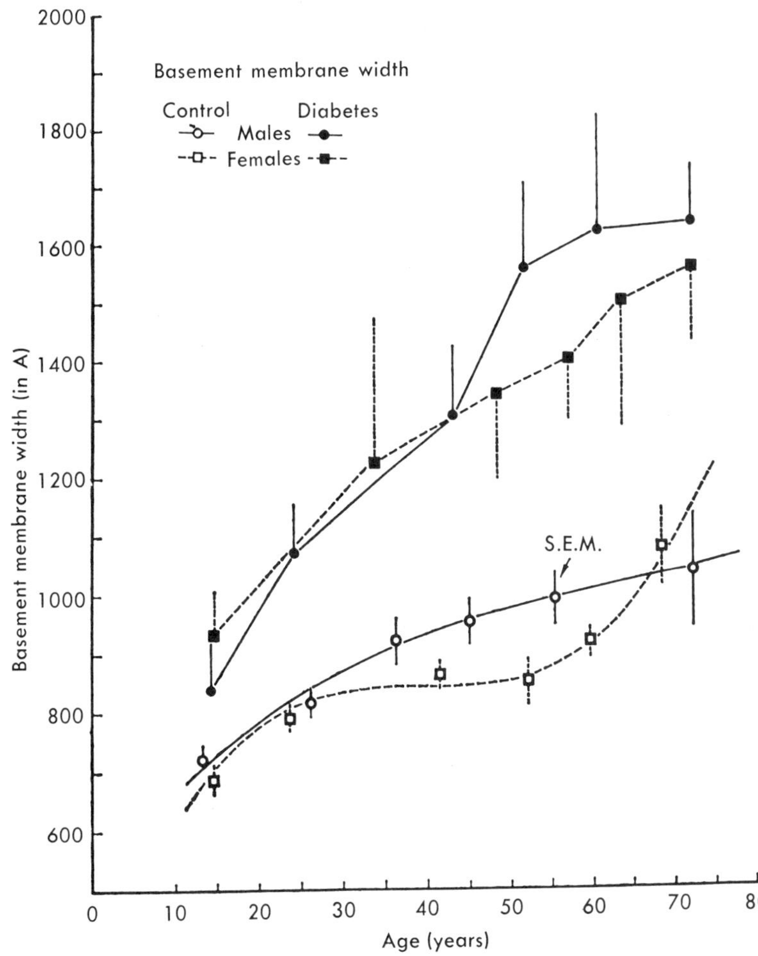

Fig. 10-5. Basement membrane width in controls and diabetics. *S.E.M.*, Standard error of the mean. (From Kilo, C., Vogler, N., and Williamson, J.R.: Diabetes **21:**881, 1972.)

ages. However, the difference is minimal in younger individuals and increases with age (Fig. 10-5).

The clinical significance of CBM thickening remains unknown. Theoretically, the CBM might act as a barrier to the egress of intravascular nutrients into the interstitial space. This concept is given some support by Ismail et al.,[80] who observed a decrease in microvascular permeability of intravenously injected radioactive iodinated albumin in diabetic patients. However, more recently Alpert et al.[81] have shown the converse effect by demonstrating that diabetic patients with microvascular disease may actually have an abnormally increased permeability of the capillary wall to ions and albumin. An important factor of the thickened CBM is its potential effect in infection. It has been postulated that leukocytes may have difficulty in transversing a thickened CBM and thus be unable to reach an infection in the interstitial space.[82] Microvascular disease leads to major diabetic complications such as retinopathy and nephropathy, which will be discussed in-depth in special sections of this chapter.

Macrovascular disease leads to myocardial infarction, stroke, and PVD and is common in the diabetic. Butterfield[83] reported that 43.3% of the hyperglycemic patients studied had vascular disease, while only 27.9% of the normoglycemic patients of similar age were affected. The pathogenesis of vascular disease in large vessels, macrovascular disease, when compared with the nondiabetic is not significantly different in the diabetic. The changes in the vessel wall both in the media and intima, consisting of deposits of lipid and cholesterol, are qualitatively the same in both groups although quantitatively greater in the diabetic patient. However, the atherosclerotic process is more common in the diabetic patient than in the nondiabetic individual; it appears at a younger age, advances more rapidly, and is more common in women than in men.

Stroke has now become a major public health problem. The common factors contributing to development of strokes and transient ischemic attacks (TIA) are hypertension, diabetes mellitus, hyperlipidemia, and the use of oral contraceptives. Hypertension is perhaps the most important risk factor. Diabetes mellitus, while somewhat less significant as a risk factor, is frequently a concomitant disease in stroke cases. Diabetes associated with stroke has been reported to have occurred in 5% to 30% of these patients. In a study of 1522 new stroke cases, Lavy[84] found that 20% had overt diabetes, with the same percentage in both sexes. When compared with the prevalence of diabetes in the general population, Lavy found diabetes to be associated with stroke four times as often as in the nondiabetic population.

In a review by Palumbo et al.[85] of a community based, maturity onset, diabetic population, they found the frequency of TIA and stroke to be increased when compared with the general population. The median age for occurrence of TIA and/or stroke was 74 years of age in the diabetic, not significantly different from the nondiabetic. Diabetic patients with hypertension at the time of diagnosis had increased frequency of TIA and/or stroke, but with control of their hypertension and/or diabetes mellitus, the frequency decreased. Obesity, clinical coronary heart disease, and an abnormal electrocardiogram (ECG) at the time of diagnosis of diabetes were not associated with a significantly increased frequency of TIA and/or stroke.[85]

Age is a critically important factor in the occurrence of TIA and stroke. When diabetes is coupled with advancing age, there is marked predisposition to stroke. This is probably secondary to the contribution of diabetes to atherogenesis in the cerebral and extracerebral vessels. This is evidenced by the effect of diabetes and advancing age on cerebral blood flow. This has been well documented in the study by Baker and Iannone.[86] They found a diffuse and progressive reduction of gray matter, blood flow, and brain weight as well as an increase in cerebral vascular resistance with advancing age. This was partially the result of cerebral arteriosclerosis. These vascular changes were most evident in the middle cerebral artery distribution and were enhanced by associated hypertension, diabetes, and hyperlipidemia. These studies are in accord with necropsy studies that show a predilection of cerebral vascular arteriosclerosis in the carotid and middle cerebral arteries. The anterior and posterior cerebral arteries, as well as branches of the vertebrobasilar arterial system appeared to be less frequently involved. Small cerebral arteries and arterioles measuring 50 to 500 μm in diameter are known to regulate cerebral vascular resistance. This is in keeping with the fact that diabetes has a marked propensity to cause atherosclerotic changes and microthrombi in the small arteries and arterioles. CNS disturbances resembling stroke can also be produced by hypoglycemia. These localizing neurologic disturbances are resolved after correction of the hypoglycemia; however, in the older patient syncope, coma, and neurologic signs caused by hypoglycemia may take several days to be resolved completely.

Arteriosclerotic heart disease (ASHD) has an earlier onset in the diabetic than in the nondiabetic. Furthermore, the frequency of ASHD tends to be equal in both sexes of diabetics as compared to a greater frequency of ASHD in the nondiabetic male than in the nondiabetic female. The tendency for painless heart attacks in diabetics has already been noted.[20] The management of heart disease is reviewed in chapter 6 and is no different for the diabetic than for the nondiabetic. Whether or not tight control of the blood sugar level will delay the atherosclerotic process remains a question of great controversy. Treatment with oral hypoglycemic agents has alread been reviewed in this chapter. Their use in patients with known ASHD should be undertaken with caution.[58] This is especially true if these patients tend to have fasting blood sugar levels over 200 mg/100 ml.[68]

Because renal shutdown can occur after an injection of radiocontrast material, especially in diabetics, the diabetic patient undergoing coronary or peripheral angiography, as well as intravenous pyelography or gallbladder studies with contrast material should have special precautions taken before injection of contrast medium and a careful postinjection follow-up. This is discussed in more detail later in this chapter.

Diabetes is one of the leading causes of PVD. Bell[87] found that vascular changes leading to gangrene occur 53 times more often in diabetic men and 71 times more often in diabetic women than in nondiabetic individuals. He also reported that gangrene is 156 times more common in the diabetic than in the nondiabetic in the fifth decade of life, 85 times more common in the sixth decade, and 53 times more common in the seventh decade. PVD is so common in the diabetic that of the nontraumatic amputations in the United States as high as 70% of them are performed on diabetics.[88] Despite the large number of amputations, only 3% of the diabetic population are amputees at any given time. This is the result of the early death of these patients from heart attack and stroke. PVD has become more prevalent in the diabetic because of the number of older diabetics; the majority are over age 50. While large vessel disease is less common in the diabetic than in the nondiabetic, it is still significant. PVD in the diabetic is characterized primarily by involvement of the small arteries and arterioles, resulting in patchy areas of gangrene of the foot and toes and atrophic skin changes with loss of subcutaneous fatty tissue.

Risk factors for PVD vary from series to series. In the Framingham study[89] the strongest risk factor for intermittent claudication was smoking. This was followed by hyperglycemia, hypercholesterolemia, and hypertension. Hyperlipoproteinemia has been high in most clinical studies of diabetic PVD. A number of animal and human studies have suggested a direct relationship between the presence of hyperglycemia and diabetic complications of retinopathy and nephropathy. Evidence that hyperglycemia is critical in the development of PVD is less convincing and must take into consideration the duration of diabetes; the presence or absence of lipid abnormalities; and the patient's age, sex, and, to a degree, genetic and racial factors. Duration is extremely important as a factor in development of PVD. Nilsson et al.[90] found severe calcification in 4.8% of the nondiabetic controls, in 8.7% of the short duration diabetics, and in 17.9% of the long duration diabetics.

Treatment of PVD. Avoidance of risk factors, especially smoking, is the first line of therapy in treating PVD. As noted, hyperglycemia does not appear to be as important a factor in development of PVD as it does in the development of retinopathy and/or nephropathy. Because poor diabetic control can lead to hypertriglyceridemia, which may affect the endothelium and lead to atherosclerotic changes, it is important to control the blood sugar level as well as is possible. Unfortunately, proper control of hyperglycemia and adherence to diet do not always prevent PVD. Therefore vascular surgery must be considered for the diabetic patient. The procedure required could be endarterectomy, an arterial bypass, or percutaneous transluminal angioplasty. Angiography is required to establish correctable obstructive vascular lesions. Indications for angiography are the occurrence of rest pain or night pain, not caused by neuropathy; a blood pressure (Doppler method) reading above the ankle that is 50% or less than that in the upper extremity; ulcerations that do not heal despite vigorous care; and early or insidious gangrene. Angiography carries some risk and should not be undertaken without prior consultation with a vascular surgeon. Thrombus formation can occur following injection of the contrast medium, with hematoma and bleeding at the site of injection. The patient should not be receiving anticoagulation therapy, and blood clotting studies should be obtained before the procedure is performed.

Renal shutdown caused by an injection of radiocontrast medium has been reported following intravenous urography, angiography, oral cholecystography and cholangiography.[91] Harkonen and Kjellstrand[92] felt that patients with renal insufficiency caused by diseases other than diabetes and myeloma did not have as great a risk of sustaining renal shutdown from the injection of radiocontrast medium. In Harkonen and Kjellstrand's series 76% of the diabetic patients with creatinine levels of more than 2 mg/100 ml had exacerbation of renal failure following intravenous pyelography. In nine patients this was irreversible. Particularly at risk are patients with early onset diabetes and creatinine levels over 5 mg/100 ml. Of these patients 93% had problems after intravenous pyelography and 56% had irreversible deterioration. It was their feeling that the injection of contrast medium is particularly dangerous in patients with juvenile onset diabetes who have creatinine levels of more than 5 mg/100ml. Most cases of renal failure are reversible. In Harkonen and Kjellstrand's review of the literature, permanent renal damage was observed in only 17% of the patients. The higher percentage of irreversibility in this series may be related to the fact that these patients had serious renal disease before the injection of radiocontrast medium.[92]

Factors that may predispose an individual to renal failure after injection of radiocontrast medium are as follows: (1) dehydration, which seems to be an important factor, although all investigators are not convinced of this; (2) precipitation of proteinaceous casts in the tubule that may occur; (3) changes in renal hemodynamics; (4) direct tubule toxicity; (5) changes in red blood cells; (6) hyperuricemia and oxaluria that appear to follow the injection of contrast medium, causing uric acid and oxalate crystal formation.[92]

Another predisposing factor may be the amount of contrast material used.[93] This is particularly important in patients undergoing angiography in which the dose of contrast medium injected may be two to three times the amount in pyelography. Preinjection precautions consist of good hydration, correction of hyperuricemia, the use of as small a dose of contrast medium as possible, and avoidance of multiple contrast procedures in close temporal proximity.

As noted, most episodes or renal shutdown are reversible, particularly if the baseline creatinine level is 4.5 mg/100 ml or less.[92] Any diabetic patient undergoing renal angiography should be followed closely after the procedure with blood urea nitrogen (BUN) and/or creatinine level determinations, with close attention to urinary output and daily weight to check for fluid retention. Should renal shutdown occur, proper adjustment of fluid intake must be made. In some cases dialysis may become necessary. Renal shutdown is usually reversed within 1 week. Close attention to the diuretic phase must be maintained and when necessary, treated with appropriate fluids and electrolytes.

Vasodilators are widely advertised for treatment of PVD. Although these drugs have been shown to increase blood flow in experimental animals and in some normal human subjects, their use in PVD remains questionable.[94] This is especially true in the diabetic patient when vascular narrowing is primarily due to plaque formation because of the atherosclerotic process rather than vasospastic disease.

Sympathectomy rarely has any therapeutic value when vascular insufficiency is primarily the result of atherosclerotic narrowing of the vessels and not of vasospastic disease. In addition, because of involvement of the autonomic nervous system, many of these patients have already had "autosympathectomy."[95]

Retinopathy

The exact incidence of diabetic retinopathy is difficult to ascertain since many studies are not in complete agreement. A good estimate, based on 17,000 diabetic patients, is an incidence of 23.5%[96] Most of these patients had simple or background retinopathy; proliferative retinopathy was less common.[97,98] However, with approximately 10 million diabetic patients in the United States, proliferative retinopathy is responsible for a significant number of blind diabetics. Today diabetes is the leading cause of new blindness in the United States. This was true as early as 1969 for the 41 to 60 years of age group.[99] It is estimated that in the next 20 years approximately 500,000 to 600,000 diabetics will become blind, and a considerable number of these will be in the older age group. If the high incidence of senile macular degeneration, cataract, and glaucoma is added to these figures, it is evident that the elderly diabetic patient's eye is vulnerable in at least three categories besides diabetes. In the older diabetic there is an accumulation of lipid material, particulary in the macula. This causes a loss of central vision, which makes reading and driving impossible, and results in legal blindness. In the older patient, the changes of diabetic retinopathy are frequently superimposed on somewhat compromised blood vessel trees. Some of the changes associated with diabetic retinopathy have an earlier onset in the older diabetic than in the juvenile diabetic. This may be more apparent than real since the exact date of maturity onset diabetes is uncertain because the disease may have existed for a considerable length of time before being diagnosed. In contrast, the onset of juvenile diabetes is frequently more dramatic and the date of onset more readily determined.

Diabetic retinopathy occurs in three stages. The first is background retinopathy, characterized by microaneurysms, retinal edema, hard exudates, retinal hemorrhages, cotton wool patches, intraretinal microvascular abnormalities, and sclerosis of the retinal arterioles. The second is the proliferative stage, which occurs when there is neovascularization in response to retinal tissue hypoxia.[100] This stage consists of a formation of new blood vessels that are fragile and have a tendency to hemorrhage. These hemorrhages may occur spontaneously or may result from an increase in pressure caused by straining, lifting, coughing, or a head down position. The third stage is vitreous contraction. This is characterized by fibrous proliferation, preretinal and vitreous hemorrhage, and finally retinal detachment.[101] The duration of diabetes is an important clinical factor and can influence the appearance and progression of retinopathy. Juvenile diabetics in whom the date of onset is fairly definite, show simple retinopathy after 10 to 15 years and proliferative retinopathy a few years later. In this group, after 20 to 25 years of the disease, approximately 80% have either simple or proliferative retinopathy.[102] In adult onset diabetic patients the course is not typical, and retinopathy may sometimes be found at the time of diagnosis or soon thereafter.[103,104] Caird et al.[105] have also reported the effects of a long duration of diabetes and age on retinopathy and vision. They followed two different age groups of individuals with early retinopathy and good vision in both eyes for 5 years. In the group under 60 years of age, impaired vision developed in 13.6% of the patients and blindness in 3%. By contrast, of the group over 60 years of age, 31.5% developed impaired vision and 20% developed blindness in 5 years. Thus with early retinopathy there is a risk of visual impairment and blindness after 5 years in 10% to 30% of the diabetics, the course being more rapid in the older patient.

The presence of retinopathy serves as a prognostic factor for longevity. The interval between discovery of retinopathy to blindness is 17.4 years, and when one eye is blind, there is a 60% possibility of the remaining eye becoming blind in 1 year. The interval between blindness and death in these patients is 9 to 10 years.[106] Approximately 65% of the diabetic patients with proliferative retinopathy and less than 50% of the newly blind survive more than 5 years.[105] The chief causes of death are renal failure and cardiovascular disease. These data emphasize the close relationship between retinopathy and other vascular complications of diabetes.

Despite these frightening statistics and the high incidence of diabetic retinopathy, a variety of treatments are available to delay the ultimate end-point of blindness. The first line of therapy is prevention of diabetic retinopathy whenever possible. Today there is good evidence that microangiopathy affecting the retina and glomeruli can be prevented or delayed and perhaps even improved by good diabetic control.[107,108] Hypertension may be an important factor leading to retinopathy; therefore diabetic and hypertensive control should be a sustained effort at any age. This can result in preservation of vision and avoidance of tremendous inconvenience, discomfort, and expense.

The effects of diabetic control on complications of the disease are difficult to assess. Some investigators believe that early control of diabetes is the most important factor in preventing complications,[109-112] while others feel that both early and late control are very important. One interpretation of this difference is that early control may influence the fundamental process that leads to the initiation of diabetic complications but with good control later in the disease it might be possible to modify the complications. This could explain in part the difficulty in evaluating the degrees of control of retinopathy in the adult onset diabetic, since the date of onset is unknown and in all probability the disease had been present for a number of years before being diagnosed. This is substantiated by the UGDP study,[58] in which 16% of the patients had retinopathy at the time of diagnosis.

When proliferative changes or hemorrhage occurs, a variety of treatments are available. These include photocoagulation, xenon[113] or argon[114,115] laser beam therapy, scleral buckling in some cases, and in highly selective cases, pituitary ablation. In addition, when hemorrhage fills the vitreous, vitrectomy and combined approaches are available. Each technique has its advantage. At the Washington University School of Medicine the xenon photocoagulator is the preferred method.[106] While this technique necessitates the use of retrobulbar injections or local anesthetic, it does allow the entire treatment to be performed at one time as opposed to the argon laser technique. There is evidence from the national collaborative diabetic retinopathy study that the long-term effects of argon laser photocoagulation may not be as good as those of the xenon photocoagulator.[116]

Retinal detachment is another complication of diabetic retinopathy. It is characteristically a traction type complication that can progress slowly or rapidly. The treatment of choice is scleral buckling. Using this technique, Okun and Fung[117] found a 65% anatomic reattachment rate with 50% of this group of patients achieving visual acuity of 20/400 or better. Many of these eyes had been considered inoperable.

Eyes totally full of blood and fibrous tissue had previously been considered inoperable. However, with the advent of vitrectomy, vision was restored to 75% of these patients.[118] Vitrectomy is accomplished with the use of a motorized sucking and cutting device that maintains a constant volume in the eyeball with saline solution. Using this technique, the blood in the eye can be removed. This procedure is not without risks and complications such as iris neovascularization with secondary glaucoma; retinal hole or detachment may result. Until diabetic retinopathy can be prevented, a close association of ophthalmologists, internists, and family practitioners is important; patients must be seen frequently and funduscopic examinations performed so that proliferative retinopathy can be detected early and treated appropriately.

Nephropathy

It is estimated that by 1980 there were 70 new end-stage renal patients for each million in the population of the United States. At least half, 35 million, would have had terminal renal failure because of diabetes.[106] Part of this influx of patients will be the result of the excellent management of juvenile onset diabetics who are now living long enough to develop terminal renal failure. This anticipated increase of patients with end-stage diabetic nephropathy will place a significant burden on renal disease programs in this country, both in terms of cost, available dialysis machines, and available kidneys for transplantation; the result will be numerous moral, ethical, and economic issues that will be raised with regard to how these patients will be managed.

Diabetic glomerulosclerosis occurs in both young and elderly diabetic patients but is more common in younger patients. When renal failure occurs in the patient over 50 years of age, causes other than diabetic glomerulosclerosis must be considered. For example, nephrosclerosis is a common finding in the elderly diabetic and may be the primary cause of renal failure in this group. In addition, pyelonephritis leading to renal impairment is common in diabetics. Renal failure can also result from obstructive nephropathy and the possibility of kidney stone must always be ruled out. Red blood cells in the urine are most likely to be found in association with ureteral calculi and rarely occur as part of the diabetic picture. Prostatic enlargement in the elderly male may cause hydronephrosis and must always be considered as a possible source of renal failure. In the diabetic a neuropathic bladder can cause obstructive nephropathy. The incidence of vesical dysfunction in diabetes is much higher than the clinical picture would suggest. Buck et al.[119] showed that 32 out of 40 randomly selected diabetic patients had abnormal urodynamic studies, but only 11 had urinary symptoms. The bladder in these individuals can become greatly distended (Fig. 10-6). Incompetence of the ureteral orifices occurs, resulting in ureteral reflux, and hydronephrosis can be demonstrated by injection of contrast material.[120] Keeping in mind the possible risks of using contrast material in these patients, the presence of hydronephrosis can be detected by ultrasound without having to resort to pyelography.

Decreased renal function in the elderly diabetic patient may also result from congestive heart failure. In addition, overzealous use of diuretics for treatment of hypertension and edema in these elderly patients may lead to dehydration and prerenal azotemia.

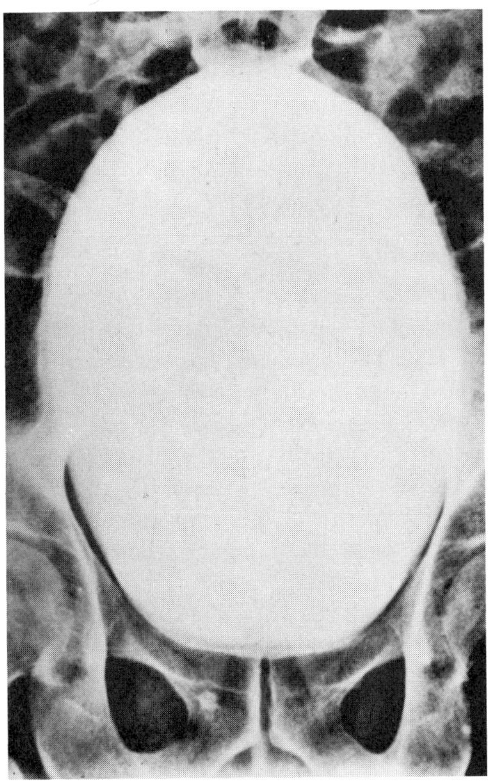

Fig. 10-6. Cystogram showing enormously enlarged, dilated bladder in a diabetic patient with neurogenic vesical paralysis. (From Ellenberg, M.: Diabetes neuropathy. In Ellenberg, M., and Rifkin, H., editors: Diabetes mellitus, theory and practice. Copyright 1970 by McGraw-Hill Book Co. Used with permission of the publisher.)

Nephropathy also influences the various types of therapy for the diabetic patient. Once there is a decrease in renal mass and function, the degradation and excretion of insulin is decreased and the insulin requirement frequently will decrease. As previously noted, the oral hypoglycemic agents are excreted primarily through the kidney, usually in an active form. In the face of renal failure those compounds may accumulate, leading to severe and prolonged hypoglycemia. They must therefore be used with great caution in patients with decreased renal function.

Once the diabetic patient has developed the signs and symptoms of renal failure, the clinical course generally leads to death in a relatively short period of time. Kussman et al.[121] in a retrospective study of juvenile diabetic patients found that the mean duration of the disease to renal failure with serum creatinine levels over 5 mg/100 ml was 21.6 years, plus or minus 6.3 years. The duration of life after development of severe renal disease was 7 months. Therefore those patients who develop severe diabetic nephropathy rarely live to an old age.

As with diabetic retinopathy, the first line of defense for prevention, stabilization, or improvement of diabetic glomerulosclerosis is control of diabetes. Although agreement on this form of therapy for prevention or improvement of diabetic nephropathy is not universal, it is the only therapy available to us at this time. Animal studies have suggested that tight control can play an important therapeutic role.[112,122] Evidence to date suggests that this improvement occurs more often in the younger diabetic than in the older diabetic whose renal disease can be and frequently is complicated by atherosclerosis of the renal vessels. Large vessel atherosclerotic disease such as in the retinal arteries is probably less influenced by diabetic control as compared with the effect of blood sugar control on the smaller vessels.

Until recently, there was no specific treatment for the diabetic patient dying of renal disease. Even hemodialysis, a long accepted procedure, was, until a few years ago, denied to most diabetic patients. Now although increasing numbers of diabetics are being accepted for hemodialysis, they do not tolerate the procedure as well as nondiabetic patients. This is particularly true of the elderly diabetic who often has severe and generalized vascular disease and is susceptible to infection. Renal transplantation is now becoming the accepted form of treatment for end-stage renal disease in the diabetic. The first human renal allograft was done in 1950. However, it was not until 1970 that this treatment became clinically practical. The Kidney Transplant Registry report indicates that the 3-year patient survival and kidney function survival rates for cadaver donor transplants are 57% and 26%, respectively. However, for living, related donors, the 3-year survival rates are 74% and 58%, respectively. The 15% to 30% difference between patient survival and kidney survival is the result of unsuccessfully transplanted patients returning to chronic dialysis.[123-125] Because patients on chronic dialysis do worse than those with transplantation, the preferred method of treatment is renal transplantation, preferably with a close matching HL-A family member or, failing that, from a well-matched cadaver kidney.

The postoperative management of the diabetic transplant patient is generally recognized to be more difficult than that of the nondiabetic. Mortality following transplantation is 33% for diabetics and approximately 20% for nondiabetics. This is the result of the higher incidence of cardiovascular deaths in the diabetic population than in the nondiabetic. Superficial wound infection and bladder leaks are twice as common in the diabetic. Diabetic transplant patients tend to have an acceleration of the atherosclerotic process following transplantation, with 25% to 30% having had some form of amputation of either fingers, toes, or legs.[106] A problem unique to diabetic transplant patients is pseudo-rejection which is manifested by 0.5 mg/100 ml rise in serum creatinine levels, for every 100 mg/100 ml increase in the serum glucose level.[126] This has been attributed to intracellular dehydration and subsequent renal malfunction. Control of hyperglycemia results in a lowered serum creatinine level.

Biopsy of the kidney transplant functioning in a diabetic for at least 2 to 5 years shows evidence of diabetic nephropathy; all biopsies after 5 years have changes consistent with diabetic nephropathy.[122] However, most of these kidneys show no evidence of deterioration in renal function despite the histologic findings. This is in keeping with the fact that it takes the juvenile diabetic an average of 17 years before evidence of glomerulosclerosis develops as evidenced by proteinuria .

A serum creatinine level of 8 mg/100 ml is an indication that death will probably occur from renal failure in less than 1 year and probably closer to 6 months. Renal transplantation should be carried out before this stage of failure occurs. After renal transplantation, peripheral neuropathy and visual acuity stabilize or improve in about 75% of these patients. Most centers therefore prefer to electively transplant diabetics before they require long-term hemodialysis.[127] Although renal transplantation is the preferred method for treating end-stage renal disease in juvenile onset diabetics, the older diabetic has not been refused this form of therapy. In a study by Kjellstrand et al.[128] of 69 patients over age 50, kidney transplants from related donors had essentially the same high rate of success as in the younger patient. Over 80% of these diabetic patients who received kidneys from related donors were surviving 5 years, in contrast to 52% of those who had to settle for cadaver kidneys. Infection posed the most serious hazard after surgery in the older patient group.[128]

The Washington University Medical Center has transplanted kidneys into seven patients over age 50. The survival rate in this small group is 41% at 6 to 42 months.[129]

Neuropathy

The true incidence of diabetic neuropathy, like other diabetic complications, is difficult to ascertain. The incidence has been reported to be anywhere from 13% to 62%.[130] The average age of the patient with neuropathy often exceeds 50 years. Neuropathy in the diabetic nerve is associated with degeneration of the myelin sheath. A decrease in nerve myelin with age has been demonstrated in human studies and in the sciatic nerve of aging rabbits. This decrease was greater in diabetic animals than in nondiabetic animals.[131] An age related drop in myelin from the human peripheral nerve as been shown to occur fairly abruptly in the sixth and seventh decades of life.[132]

The average duration of diabetes before there is evidence of neuropathy is usually 5 years or more, but this may be the presenting sign or symptom of the disease. In other cases neuropathy may not develop until diabetes has been present for over 30 years. The most serious complication of neuropathy in the elderly diabetic patient is that affecting the lower extremities.

Although hyperesthesia and paresthesia are the most distressing symptoms to the patient, hypoesthesia is the neuropathic complication that most often leads to serious trouble. With loss of sensation, the diabetic's feet become extremely vulnerable. For example, because of poor circulation that results in cold feet, the patients frequently use heating pads or hot water bottles to warm their feet. Because of the loss of sensation to temperature, this can result in a severe burn, followed by ulceration, infection, gangrene, and finally, amputation. The use of chemical agents to remove corns and calluses also can result in undetected chemical burns to the feet. Because the diabetic patient has greatly decreased or absent sensation to pain, he tends to cut his toenails or calluses too deeply, and infection frequently develops in these areas. The classic plantar ulcer is the result of the loss of pain sensation. These ulcers can become extensive without the patient being aware of their presence. They become infected, and the infection leads to gangrenous changes and ultimately to amputation. A detailed discussion of these problems involving the diabetic foot has been presented by Levin.[95]

Diabetic neuropathy, with increasing age and duration of the disease can lead to impotence and retrograde ejaculation in the male and decreased orgasms in the female.[133]

Treatment of neuropathy. Treatment of diabetic neuropathy consists of two approaches. The first is diabetic control. There is ample evidence that excessive blood sugar levels lead to accumulation, through the polyol pathway, of sorbital and fructose within the myelin sheath. These substances result in an increase in osmotic pressure, causing swelling and degeneration of the myelin sheath. However, even in the well-controlled diabetic, signs and symptoms of neuropathy can develop. A multitude of approaches have been recommended for treatment of painful neuropathy. Among these have been the use of a variety of vitamins, including thiamin, B_{12} injections, and large doses of vitamin E. None of these have proven to be of consistent value. Phenytoin (Dilantin) has been reported to be effective in some of these patients and has been used for many years. It has also been reported to be more effective in relieving the discomfort of diabetic neuropathy in women than in men.[134] Despite its many recommendations, I have not found this drug to be particularly effective. Carbamazepine (Tegretol) has been helpful in many patients with painful neuropathy. However, this drug must be used with caution because of the high frequency of side effects. In the study by Rull et al.[135] side effects occurred in 28 out of 30 patients.

A form of therapy recommended by Davis et al.[136] which I have also found to be most effective in treating neuropathic paresthesia and pain, is a combination of amitriptyline and fluphenazine hydrochloride. When this combination is effective, the pain is diminished and sometimes totally relieved within only a few days, suggesting that the effects of these medications are not due to psychiatric effects, which take much longer. Because these drugs may cause cardiac problems, especially in the elderly patient, they must be used with caution.

Diabetic neuropathy causes insensitivity in the foot. Therefore the most important approach to saving the diabetic foot is patient education. The boxed list details the instructions I give my patients. It is important to recognize that simply handing a sheet of instructions to a patient is not sufficient; each precaution must be explained thoroughly. This should be done at the first visit and repeated periodically on follow-up visits. It is critical to remove the shoes and stockings of these patients at each visit to inspect the feet, particularly between the toes as painless interdigital ulceration and/or infection is not uncommon.

Miscellaneous complications

A variety of other complications associated with diabetes occur in the elderly patient. Cataracts have been reported to be more common and to occur at a somewhat earlier age in the diabetic than in the nondiabetic.[137] Dupuytren's contracture is also more common in the elderly diabetic than in the elderly nondiabetic.[138] Itching is frequently generalized and tends to be more common in the elderly diabetic.[139-141] Amyotrophy is a primary neuromuscular disorder characterized by proximal muscle weakness and atrophy. This tends to affect elderly diabetic men in particular.[142] Hypertension is also more common in the diabetic patient, caused in part by the increased incidence of nephrosclerosis[143] and pyelonephritis. Sourander[144] found urinary tract infection to be present in 48% of a series of elderly diabetic patients as opposed to an incidence of only 20% in the elderly nondiabetic population. Osteoporosis, particularly in the older age group, has been suggested as a complication of diabetes, as early as 1948 by Albright and Reifenstein.[145] They found an increased incidence of osteoporosis in a series of poorly controlled diabetic patients. A more recent report from Israel also suggested an increased incidence of osteoporosis in the diabetic patient. In this study the authors found a 22% higher incidence of proximal hip fractures in diabetic patients who tended to be younger than the nondiabetic control group with hip fractures.[146]

Nonketotic hyperosmolar coma is a serious and potentially lethal diabetic syndrome, occurring most often in the elderly diabetic patient. This complication, although uncommon, is not rare. Arieff and Carroll[147] noted that the syndrome occurs with equal frequency in both men and women. With the exception of three young diabetic patients, the ages in their series ranged from 41 to 88 years. Only five patients were insulin dependent. The initiating event in many of these cases is usually a severe or concurrent illness such as chronic renal insufficiency or infection. Nonketotic hyperosmolar coma may also be precipitated by diuretic therapy, which is commonly used in the elderly patient. Lavender and McGill[148] reported a case of nonketotic hyperosmolar coma after furosemide therapy; nonketotic hyperosmolar coma has also been reported in patients receiving thiazide and/or chlorthalidone therapy.[149,150] Diuretic therapy may contribute to the hyperosmolar state by causing excessive salt and water diuresis, resulting in dehydration. Thiazides and furosemides are also known to aggravate diabetes and in some instances actually to convert latent diabetes into clinical diabetes. The postoperative diabetic patient must have periodic blood glucose determinations performed to detect possible severe hyperglycemia that may occur without ketosis. The metabolic derangement in this

Patient instructions for the care of the diabetic foot

1. Do not smoke.
2. Inspect toes and between toes daily for blisters, cuts, and scratches. The use of a mirror can aid in seeing the bottom of the feet.
3. Wash feet daily, dry carefully, especially between the toes.
4. Avoid extremes of temperatures. Test water before bathing.
5. If feet feel cold at night, wear socks; do not apply hot water bottles or heating pads.
6. Do not use chemical agents for the removal of corns and calluses.
7. Inspect inside of shoes daily for foreign objects, nail points, and torn linings.
8. Wear properly fitted stockings; do not wear mended stockings; avoid stockings with seams; change stockings daily.
9. Do not wear garters.
10. Shoes should be comfortable at the time of purchase. Do not depend on them to "stretch out".
11. Do not wear shoes without stockings.
12. Do not wear sandals with thongs between the toes.
13. Do not walk barefooted, and never on hot surfaces such as sandy beaches or around swimming pools.
14. Cut nails straight across.
15. Do not cut corns and calluses: follow special instructions from your physician or podiatrist.
16. See your physician regularly and be sure your feet are examined at each visit.
17. If your vision is impaired, have a family member inspect feet daily, trim nails and buff down calluses.
18. Be sure to inform your podiatrist that you are diabetic.

Levin, M.E., and O'Neal, L., editors: The diabetic foot, ed. 3, St. Louis, 1982, The C.V. Mosby Co.

syndrome can be successfully corrected in most of these patients by fluid intake, electrolyte replacement, and moderate doses of insulin.

SUMMARY

Diabetes effects a significant number of the adult population. However, caution must be used in making this diagnosis merely on the basis of an abnormal glucose tolerance test, since there is a normal decrease in glucose tolerance with aging. Reasons for this have been discussed in detail in this chapter. The elderly diabetic is prone to develop vascular disease of both the macrovascular and microvascular systems. Areas that are particularly affected in elderly diabetic patients are the eye; the heart, with a significant increase in myocardial deaths compared with the nondiabetic population, and the peripheral vascular system, which along with neuropathy contributes to a significant number of diabetic foot problems. Patient education in foot care is critical to saving the diabetic foot.

Diet is the mainstay of therapy for the elderly diabetic patient. This must be carefully tailored to the individual and his socioeconomic status. Oral hypoglycemic agents are being used to excess in this age group; the possibility of increased cardiovascular risks associated with their use should be kept in mind.

Photocoagulation and vitrectomy are beneficial in maintaining or improving vision in the diabetic. Renal transplantation, even in the older diabetic with end-stage renal disease, offers the possibility of increased life span with quality.

REFERENCES

1. Crofford, O.B.: Report of the National Commission on Diabetes to the Congress of the United States, Department of Health, Education, and Welfare Pub. No. (NIH) 67-1018, Washington, D.C., 1975, U.S. Government Printing Office.
2. Rosenberg, N., Aniarte, E., Bujdoso, L.V., and Backwinkel, K.D.: Mortality factors in major limb amputations for vascular disease: a study of 176 procedures, Surgery **67**:437, 1970.
3. U.S. Department of Health, Education and Welfare: Diabetes source book, P.H.S. Pub. No. 1168, rev. ed. Washington, D.C., 1968, U.S. Government Printing Office, p. 9.
4. Bennett, P.H., Burch, T.A., and Miller, M.: Diabetes mellitus in American (Pima) Indians, Lancet **2**:125, 1971.
5. Spence, J.C.: Some observations on sugar tolerance with special reference to variations found at different ages, Q.J. Med. **14**:314, 1921.
6. Standardization of oral glucose tolerance test, Report of the Committee on Statistics of the American Diabetes Association, June 14, 1968, Diabetes **18**:299, 1969.
7. Fajans, S.S., and Conn, J.W.: The approach to the prediction of diabetes mellitus by modification of the glucose tolerance test with cortisone, Diabetes **3**:296, 1954.
8. Fajans, S.S., and Conn, J.W.: The early recognition of diabetes mellitus, Ann. N.Y. Acad. Sci. **82**:298, 1959.
9. Wilkerson, H.L.: Diagnosis, oral glucose tolerance tests. In Danowski, T.S., editor: Diabetes mellitus: diagnosis and treatment, New York, 1964, American Diabetes Association, p. 31.
10. Sirtori, C.R., Bolme, P., and Azarnoff, D.L.: Metabolic responses to acute and chronic L-dopa administration in patients with parkinsonism, N. Engl. J. Med. **287**:729, 1972.
11. Andres, R.: Aging and diabetes, Med. Clin. North Am. **55**:835, 1971.
12. Butterfield, W.J.H.: Bedford Diabetic Survey and its related studies. In Duncan, L.J.P., editor: Diabetes mellitus, Edinburgh, 1966, Edinburgh University Press.
13. Hayner, H.S., Kjelsberg, M.O., Epstein, F.H., and Francis, T., Jr.: Carbohydrate tolerance and diabetes in a total community, Tecumseh, Michigan. I. Effects of age, sex, and test conditions on one-hour glucose tolerance in adults, Diabetes **14**:413, 1965
14. Unger, R.H.: The standard two hour oral glucose tolerance test in the diagnosis of diabetes mellitus in subjects without fasting hyperglycemia, Ann. Intern. Med. **47**:1138, 1957.
15. United States National Center for Health Statistics: Glucose tolerance of adults, United States, 1960-1962: diabetes prevalence and results of a glucose tolerance test, by age and sex, Washington, D.C., 1964, United States Department of Health, Education and Welfare, p. 25.
16. Welborn, T.A., Stenhouse, N.S., and Johnstone, C.G.: Factors determining serum-insulin response in a population sample, Diabetologia **5**:263, 1969.
17. Jackson, W.P.U., and Vinik, A.I.: Hyperglycemia and diabetes in the elderly. In Ellenberg, M., and Rifkin, H., editors: Diabetes mellitus, theory and practice, New York, 1970, McGraw-Hill Book Co.
18. Diabetes mellitus: Report of a WHO Expert Committee, WHO Tech. Rep. Ser. N310, p. 45, 1965.
19. U.S. Department of Health, Education and Welfare: Diabetes mortality in the United States, 1950-67, Vital and Health Statistics Series 20, No. 10, p. 17, July, 1971.
20. Bradley, R.F., and Schonfeld, A.: Diminished pain in diabetic patients with acute myocardial infarction, Geriatrics **17**:322, 1962.
21. U.S. Bureau of Census: Statistical abstract of the United States, ed. 94, Washington, D.C., 1973, U.S. Government Printing Office.
22. Goodkin, G.: Mortality factors in diabetes, J. Occup. Med. **17**:716, 1975.
23. Cahill, G.: Recent developments in diabetes, Today's Clin. **7**:53, 1978.

24. Levin, M.E., Boisseau, V.C., and Avioli, L.V.: Effects of diabetes mellitus on bone mass in juvenile and adult-onset diabetes, N. Engl. J. Med. **294**:241, 1976.
25. Hamlin, C.R., and Kohn, R.R.: Determination of human chronologic age by study of collagen sample, Exp. Gerontol. **7**:377, 1972.
26. Hamlin, C.R., Kohn, R.R., and Luschin, J.H.: Apparent accelerated aging of human collagen in diabetes mellitus, Diabetes **24**:902, 1975.
27. Kilo, C., Vogler, N., and Williamson, J.R.: Muscle capillary basement membrane changes related to aging and diabetes mellitus, Diabetes **21**:881, 1972.
28. Pillsbury, H.C., III, Hung, W., Kyle, M.C., and Freis, E.D.: Arteriole pulse waves in velocity and systolic time intervals in diabetic children, Am. Heart J. **87**:783, 1974.
29. Ohneda, A., et al.: Hypoglycemia due to apparent autoantibodies to insulin. Characterization of insulin-binding protein, Diabetes **23**:41, 1974.
30. Peterson, G.E., and Forsham, P.H.: Variation in thickness of the capillary basement in single muscles of diabetic subjects, Diabetes **28**:548, 1979.
31. Dunn, P.J., et al.: The association between diabetic retinopathy and skeletal muscle capillary basal lamina thickening corrected for the influence of age and duration of diabetes, Diabetes **28**:858, 1979.
32. Deckert, T., et al.: Basement membrane thickness, insulin antibodies and HLA-antigens in long standing insulin dependent diabetes with and without severe retinopathy, Diabetologia **17**:91, 1979.
33. Camerini-Davalos, R.A., et al.: Muscle capillary basement membrane width in genetic prediabetes, J.Clin. Endocrinol. Metab. **48**:251, 1979.
34. Aronoff, S.L., et al.: Muscle capillary basement membrane (MCBM) measurements in prediabetic, diabetic, and normal Pima Indians and normal Caucasians, Clin. Res. **24**:455A, 1976.
35. Goldstein, S., et al.: Diabetes mellitus and genetic prediabetes: decreased replicative capacity of cultured skin fibroblasts, J. Clin. Invest. **63**:358, 1979.
36. O'Sullivan, J.B., Mahan, C.E., Freedlender, A.E., and Williams, R.F.: Effect of age on carbohydrate metabolism, J. Clin. Endocrinol. Metab. **33**:619, 1971.
37. Dudl, R.J., and Ensinck, J.W.: The role of insulin, glucagon, and growth hormone in carbohydrate homeostasis during aging, Diabetes **21**(Suppl. 1):357, 1972.
38. Gries, F.A., and Steinke, J.: Insulin and human adipose tissue in vitro: a brief review, Metabolism **16**:693, 1967.
39. Elsas, L.J., MacDonell, R.C., Jr., and Rosenberg, L.E.: Influence of age on insulin stimulation of aminoacid uptake in rat diaphragm, J. Biol. Chem. **246**:6452, 1971.
40. Dobrzanski, J.: Age effect on insulin action in rat adipose tissue, Diabetes **15**:430, 1966.
41. DeFronzo, R.A.: Glucose intolerance and aging: evidence for tissue insensitivity to insulin, Diabetes **28**:1095, 1979.
42. Freeman, C., Karoly, K., and Adelman, R.C.: Impairments in availability of insulin in vivo and in binding of insulin to purified hepatic plasma membranes during aging, Biochem. Biophys. Res. Commun. **54**:1573, 1973.
43. Olefsky, J.M., and Reaven, G.M.: The effects of age and obesity on ^{125}I insulin binding to isolated rat adipocytes, Endocrinology **96**:1486, 1975.
44. Runyan, K., Duckworth, W.C., Kitabchi, A.E., and Huff, G.: The effect of age on insulin-degrading activity in rat tissue, Diabetes **28**:324, 1979.
45. Terris, S., and Steiner, D.F.: Binding and degradation of ^{125}I insulin by rat hepatocytes, J. Biol. Chem. **251**:8389, 1975.
46. Steiner, D.F.: Insulin today, Diabetes **26**:322, 1977.
47. DeFronzo, R.A., et al.: Insulin binding to monocytes and insulin action in human obesity, starvation, and refeeding, J. Clin. Invest. **62**:204, 1978.
48. Bjorntorp, P., Berchtold, P., and Larson, B.: The glucose uptake of human adipose tissue in obesity, Eur. J. Clin. Invest. **1**:480, 1971.
49. Bjorntorp, P., Krotkjewski, M., Larson, B., and Somlo-Szues, Z.: Effects of feeding states on lipid radioactivity in liver, muscle, and adipose tissue after injection of labeled glucose in the rat, Acta Physiol. Scand. **80**:29, 1970.
50. Duckworth, W.C., and Kitabchi, A.E.: Effect of age, obesity and degree of carbohydrate intolerance on proinsulin response to oral glucose, Diabetes **21**(Suppl. 1):356, 1972.
51. Unger, R.H., Madison, L.L., and Muller, W.A.: Abnormal alpha cell function in diabetic's response to insulin, Diabetes **21**:301, 1972.
52. Berger, D., et al.: Effect of age on fasting plasma levels of pancreatic hormones in man, J. Clin. Endocrinol. Metab. **47**:1183, 1978.
53. Brodows, R.G., and Campbell, R.: Effects of age on post-heparin lipase, N. Engl. J. Med. **287**:969, 1972.
54. Santen, R.J., Willis, P.W., III, and Fajans, S.S.: Atherosclerosis in diabetes mellitus: correlations with serum lipid levels, adiposity, and serum insulin level, Arch. Intern. Med. **130**:833, 1972.
55. Nikkila, E.A., and Hormila, P.: Serum lipids and lipoproteins in insulin-treated diabetes: demonstration of increased high density lipoprotein concentrations, Diabetes **27**:1078, 1978.
56. Davidson, J.K.: Panel on diabetes, in epidemiologic studies and clinical trials in chronic diseases. Symposium, Pan American Health Organization Advisory Committee on Medical Research, Washington, D.C., PAHO Sci. Pub. No. 257, p. 44. 1972.
57. Tomkins, A.M., and Bloom, A.: Assessment of the need for continued oral therapy in diabetics, Br. Med. J. **1**:649, 1972.
58. University Group Diabetes Program: A study of the effects of hypoglycemic agents on vascular complications in patients with adult-onset diabetes. II. Mortality results, Diabetes **19**(Suppl. 2):747, 1970.
59. Knatterud, G.L., et al.: Effects of hypoglycemic agents on vascular complications in patients with adult-onset diabetes. IV. A preliminary report on phenformin results, J.A.M.A. **217**:777, 1971.
60. Hadden, D.R., Montgomery, D.A.D., and Weaver, J.A.: Myocardial infarction in maturity-onset diabetes, Lancet **1**:475, 1974.

61. Soler, N.G., Pentecorst, B.L., and Bennett, M.A.: Coronary care for myocardial infarction in diabetics, Lancet **1**:475, 1974.
62. Reid, D.D., and Evans, J.G.: New drugs and changing mortality from non-infectious disease in England and Wales, Br. Med. Bull.**26**:191, 1970.
63. Abramson, J.H., editor: World health news: apparent rise in mortality from diabetes, Isr. J. Med. Sci. **7**:1209, 1971.
64. Crass, M.F., III, et al.: Tolbutamide-induced inotropic responses in the perfused working heart: effects of albumin, Proc. Soc. Exp. Biol. Med. **142**:861, 1973.
65. Levey, G.S., Lasseter, K.C., and Palmer, R.F.: Sulfonylureas and the heart, Annu. Rev. Med. **25**:69, 1974.
66. Report of the committee for the assessment of biometric aspects of controlled trials of hypoglycemic agents, J.A.M.A. **231**:583, 1975.
67. Audit confirms conclusions of U.G.D.P. study on oral diabetes drugs, FDA Drug Bull. **8**:34, 1978.
68. Kilo, C., Miller, J.P., and Williamson, J.R.: The achilles heel of the University Group Diabetes Program, J.A.M.A. **243**:450, 1980.
69. Field, J.B., et al.: Potentiation of acetohexamide hypoglycemia by phenylbutazone, N. Engl. J. Med. **277**:889, 1967.
70. Goodman, L.S., and Gilman, A.: The pharmacological basis of therapeutics, ed. 6, New York, 1980, The Macmillan Co., p. 1510-1514.
71. Harris, E.L.: Adverse reactions to oral antidiabetic agents, Br. Med. J. **3**:29, 1971.
72. Seltzer, H.S.: Drug induced hypoglycemia: review based on 473 cases, Diabetes **21**:955,1972.
73. Gardner, P., Goodner, C.J., and Dowling, T.J.: Severe hypoglycemia in elderly patients receiving therapeutic doses of tolbutamide, J.A.M.A. **186**:117, 1963.
74. Vranic, M., Horvath, S., and Wahren, J.: Exercise and diabetes: an overview, Diabetes **28**(Suppl. 1):107, 1979.
75. Lawrence, R.D.: The effect of insulin action in diabetes, Br. Med. J. **1**:648, 1926.
76. Lutwak, L., and Whedon, G.D.: The effect of physical conditioning on glucose tolerance, Clin. Res. **7**:143, 1959.
77. Lipman, R.L., et al.: Glucose intolerance during decreased physical activity in man, Diabetes **21**:101, 1972.
78. Goldstein, M.S.: Muscular exercise and subsequent glucose utilization. In Leibel, B.S., and Wrenshall, G.A., editors: On the nature and treatment of diabetes, Amsterdam, 1965, Excerpta Medica Foundation.
79. Felig, P.: Exercise therapy "rediscovered" for diabetes, but what does it do? J.A.M.A. **242**:1591, 1979.
80. Ismail, A.D., Khalifa, K., and Madwar, K.R.: Capillary loss of radioiodinated serum albumin in diabetics, Lancet **2**:1188, 1965.
81. Alpert, J.S., et al.: Capillary permeability and blood flow in skeletal muscle of patients with diabetes mellitus and genetic prediabetes, N. Engl. J. Med. **286**:454, 1972.
82. Siperstein, M.D., Unger, R.H., and Madison, L.L.: Studies of muscle capillary basement membranes in normal subjects, diabetic and prediabetic patients, J. Clin. Invest. **47**:1973, 1968.
83. Butterfield, W.J.H.: Summary of results of the Bedford diabetes survey, Proc. R. Soc. Med. **57**:196, 1962.
84. Lavy, S.: Medical risk factors in stroke, Adv. Neurol. **25**:127, 1979.
85. Palumbo, P., Jr., Elveback, L.R., and Whisnant, J.P.: Neurologic complications of diabetes mellitus: transient ischemic attack, stroke, and peripheral neuropathy, Adv. Neurol. **25**:593, 1979.
86. Baker, A.B., and Iannone, A.: Cerebral vascular disease. III. The intracerebral arterioles, Neurology **9**:441, 1959.
87. Bell, E.T.: Atherosclerotic gangrene of the lower extremities in diabetic and nondiabetic persons, Am. J. Clin. Pathol. **28**:27, 1957.
88. Warren, R., and Kihn, R.B.: A survey of lower extremity amputation for ischemia, Surgery **63**:107, 1968.
89. Gordon, T., and Kannel, W.B.: The Framingham study: predisposition to atherosclerosis in the head, heart and legs, J.A.M.A. **221**:661, 1972.
90. Nilsson, S.E., Nilsson, J.E., and Frostbert, E.: Kristianstad Survey II: studies in a representative adult diabetic population with special references to comparison with adequate control group, Acta Med. Scand. **496**:1, 1967.
91. Ansari, Z., and Baldwin, D.F.: Acute renal failure due to radio-contrast agents, Nephron **17**:28, 1976.
92. Harkonen, S., and Kjellstrand, C.M.: Exacerbation of diabetic renal failure following intravenous pyelography, Am. J. Med. **63**:939, 1977.
93. Weinrauch, L.A., et al.: Coronary angiography and acute renal failure in diabetic azotemic nephropathy, Ann. Intern. Med. **86**:56, 1977.
94. Coffman, J.D.: Vasodilator drugs and peripheral vascular disease, N. Engl. J. Med. **300**:713, 1979.
95. Levin, M.E.: Medical evaluation and treatment. In Levin, M.E., and O'Neal, L., editors: The diabetic foot, ed. 3, St. Louis, 1982, The C.V. Mosby Co.
96. Ashton, N.: Diabetic microangiopathy, Adv. Ophthalmol. **8**:1, 1958.
97. Burditt, A.F., Caird, F.I., and Draper, G.J.: The natural history of diabetic retinopathy, Q.J. Med. **37**:303, 1968.
98. Lundbaek, K.: Ocular manifestations of diabetic angiopathy, J.R. Coll. Surg. Ireland **1**:28, 1963.
99. Welch, R.J.: Causes of blindness in addition to MRA Registers for 1967, Proceedings of the 1969 Conference of Model Reporting Area for Blindness, Washington, D.C., 1970, U.S. Government Printing Office.
100. Davis, M.D., et al.: Clinical observations concerning the pathogenesis of diabetic retinopathy. In Goldberg and Fine, editors: Symposium on the treatment of diabetic retinopathy, Washington, D.C., 1969, U.S. Government Printing Office, p. 47.
101. Davis, M.D.: Vitreous contraction in proliferative diabetic retinopathy, Arch. Ophthalmol. **74**:741, 1965.
102. White, P.: Natural course and prognosis of juvenile diabetes, Diabetes **5**:445, 1956.
103. Oakley, W.G., Pyke, D.A., and Taylor, K.W.: Clinical diabetes and its biochemical basis, Oxford, 1968, Blackwell Scientific Publications, p. 456.
104. Soler, N.G., Fitzgerald, M.G., Malins, J.M., and Summers, R.O.C.: Retinopathy at diagnosis of dia-

betes, with special reference to patients under 40 years of age, Br. Med. J. **3**:567, 1969.
105. Caird, F.I., Pirie, A., and Ramsell, T.G.: Diabetes and the eye, Oxford, 1968, Blackwell Scientific Publications, p. 94.
106. Levin, M.E., Boniuk, I., and Anderson, C.B.: Prevention and treatment of diabetic complications, Arch. Intern. Med. **140**:691, 1980.
107. Job, D., Eschwege, E., Guyot-Argenton, C., and Tschobroutsky, F.: Effect of multiple daily insulin injections on the course of diabetic retinopathy, Diabetes **25**:463, 1976.
108. Eschwege, E., et al.: Delayed progression of diabetic retinopathy by divided insulin administration: a further followup, Diabetologia **16**:13, 1978.
109. Burditt, A.F., Caird, F.I., and Draper, G.J.: The natural history of diabetic retinopathy, Q.J. Med. **37**:303, 1968.
110. Caird, F.I.: Control of diabetes and diabetic retinopathy. In Goldberg, M.P., and Fine, S.L., editors: Symposium on the treatment of diabetic retinopathy, Washington, D.C., 1969, U.S. Government Printing Office, p. 107.
111. Constam, G.R.: Zur Spätprognose des Diabetes mellitus, Helv. Med. Acta **32**:287, 1965.
112. Pirart, J.: Diabetes mellitus and its degenerative complications: a prospective study of 4400 patients observed between 1947 and 1973, Diabetes Care **1**:168, 252, 1978.
113. Okun, E.: The effectiveness of photocoagulation in the therapy of proliferative diabetic retinopathy (PDR) (a controlled study in 50 patients), Trans. Am. Acad. Ophthalmol. Otolaryngol. **72**:246, 1968.
114. L'Esperance, F.A., Jr.: Argon laser photocoagulations, Trans. Am. Acad. Ophthalmol. Otolaryngol. **73**:1077, 1969.
115. Zweng, N.C., editor: Recent advances in photocoagulation, Int. Ophthalmol. Clin. **16**(4):79, 1976.
116. Diabetic retinopathy study research group: preliminary report on effects of photocoagulation therapy, Am.J.Ophthalmol. **81**:383, 1976.
117. Okun, E., Fung, W.E.: Therapy of diabetic retinal detachment. In Symposium on retina and retinal surgery, Transactions of the New Orleans Academy of Ophthalmology, St. Louis, 1969, The C.V. Mosby Co.
118. Okun, E., and Burgess, D.: Pars plana lensectomy and vitrectomy with the Douvas roto-extractor in diabetic retinopathy. In Irvine, A., and O'Malley, C., editors: Advances in vitreous surgery, Springfield, Ill., 1976, Charles C Thomas, Publisher, pp. 555-560.
119. Buck, A.C., et al.: The diabetic bladder, Proc. R. Soc. Med. **67**:81, 1974.
120. Friedenberg, R.M., and Ney, C.: Radiographic findings in neurogenic bladder, Radiology **76**:795, 1961.
121. Kussman, M.J., Goldstein, H.H., and Gleason, R.E.: Clinical course of diabetic nephropathy, Diabetes **23**:337, 1974.
122. Mauer, S.M., et al.: Development of diabetic vascular lesions in normal kidneys transplanted into patients with diabetes mellitus, N. Engl. J. Med. **295**:915, 1976.
123. Advisory Committee to the Renal Transplantation Registry: The Thirteenth report of the Human Renal Transplant Registry, Transplant Proc. **9**:9, 1977.
124. Najarian, J.S., et al.: Kidney transplantation for the uremic diabetic patient, Surg. Gynecol. Obstet. **144**:682, 1977.
125. Zincke, H.: Renal transplantation in patients with insulin-dependent diabetes mellitus, J.A.M.A. **237**: 1101, 1977.
126. Matas, A.J., et al.: Hyperglycemic pseudo-rejection in the diabetic transplant patient, Surgery **79**:132, 1976.
127. Kussman, M.J., Goldstein, H.H., and Gleason, R.E.: The clinical course of diabetic nephropathy, J.A.M.A. **236**:1861, 1976.
128. Kjellstrand, C.M., et al.: Kidney transplants in patients over 50, Geriatrics **31**:65, Sept., 1976.
129. Anderson, C.: Transplantation in older patients. Personal communication.
130. Prockop, L.D.: Diabetic neuropathy in diabetes mellitus. In Fajans, S.S., and Sussman, K.E., editors: Diabetes mellitus: diagnosis and treatment, vol. 3, New York, 1971, American Diabetes Association, p. 337.
131. Spritz, N., Singh, H., and Marinan, B.: Decrease in myelin content of rabbit sciatic nerve with aging and diabetes, Diabetes **24**:680, 1975.
132. Spritz, N., Singh, H., and Geyer, B.: Myelin from human peripheral nerves. Quantitative and qualitative studies in two age groups, J. Clin. Invest. **52**:520, 1973.
133. Kolodny, R.C.: Sexual dysfunction in diabetic females, Diabetes **20**:557, 1971.
134. Ellenberg, M.: Treatment of diabetic neuropathy with diphenylhydantoin, N.Y. State J. Med. **68**:2653, 1968.
135. Rull, J.A., Quibrera, H., Gonzales-Millan, H., and Castaneda, O.L.: Symptomatic treatment of peripheral diabetic neuropathy with carbamazepine (Tegretol): double blind crossover trial, Diabetologia **5**:215, 1969.
136. Davis, J.L., et al.: Peripheral diabetic neuropathy treated with amitriptyline and fluphenazine, J.A.M.A. **238**:2291, 1977.
137. Beckett, A.G., and Hobbs, H.E.: Cataract extraction and diabetes, Br. Med. J. **2**:1605, 1961.
138. Schneider, T.: Late manifestations of diabetes mellitus, S. Afr. Med. J. **27**:466, 1953.
139. Hellier, F.F.: Itching and diabetes, Br. Med. J. **2**:628, 1964.
140. Murray, I.: Itching and diabetes, Br. Med. J. **2**:877, 1964.
141. Oakley, W.G.: Itching and diabetes, Br. Med. J. **2**:818, 1964.
142. Locke, S., Lawrence, D.G., and Legg, M.A.: Diabetic amyotrophy, Am. J. Med. **34**:775, 1963.
143. Pell, S., and d'Alonzo, C.A.: Some aspects of hypertension in diabetes mellitus, J.A.M.A. **202**:10, 1967.
144. Sourander, L.B.: Urinary tract infection in the aged: an epidemiological study, Ann. Med. Intern. Fenn. **55**(Suppl.45):1, 1966.
145. Albright, F., and Reifenstein, E.C.: Parathyroid glands and metabolic bone disease, Baltimore, 1948, The Williams & Wilkins Co.
146. Menczel, M.M., Robin, G., Jaye, I., and Naor, E.: Prevalence of diabetes mellitus in Jerusalem: its as-

sociation with presenile osteoporosis, Isr. J. Med. Sci. **8**:918, 1972.

147. Arieff, A.I., and Carroll, H.J.: Nonketotic hyperosmolar coma with hyperglycemia: clinical features, pathophysiology, renal function, acid-base balance, plasma-cerebrospinal fluid equilibria and the effects of therapy in 37 cases, Medicine **51**:73, 1972.
148. Lavender, S., and McGill, R.J.: Case report: nonketotic hyperosmolar coma and furosemide therapy, Diabetes **23**:247, 1974.
149. Curtis, J., et al.: Chlorthalidone-induced hyperosmolar hyperglycemic nonketotic coma, J.A.M.A. **220**: 1592, 1972.
150. Solvsteen, P., Olsen, F., and Hansen, E.L.: Diabetic coma without ketoacidosis, Acta Med. Scand. **184**:83, 1968.

CHAPTER 11 · HEMATOLOGIC DISORDERS OF THE ELDERLY

John R. Walsh

A selective approach is a primary requisite for an overview of hematologic disorders in the elderly. The objective of this survey is to discuss common conditions and to update students and physicians on contemporary approaches and management of hematologic problems.

Active, healthy elderly people develop hematologic problems similar to young adults and respond analogously to treatment. Some older people may have altered responses to blood problems because of lower reserves and poor health. Furthermore, multiple disorders characteristic of elderly patients modify and confuse the clinical presentation. Multiple drug therapy increases the risk of drug-induced hematologic disorders. Nutritional deficiencies of the elderly related to underlying disease, dementia, depression, alcohol, drugs, lowered income, living alone, or residing in nursing homes are prominent causes of hematologic problems. Finally, some hematologic disorders, such as chronic lymphocytic leukemia and pernicious anemia, are more common in aged persons than in younger individuals.

ANEMIA

Anemia is characterized by a reduced hemoglobin concentration. Clinical manifestations depend on reduced oxygen transport of blood; the effects of reduced oxygen transport are reflected by tissue hypoxia. There is no such entity as anemia of the aged. There is some disagreement about normal hemoglobin levels in the elderly, with some observers indicating that there is no change from normal adult values while others report a 1 to 2 gm/100 ml reduction, especially in men, presumably due to diminished androgen. Clearly, many of the differences in studies reflect population sampling, and further studies are needed to separate active, healthy elderly men and women from sedentary, disabled nursing home residents. Recent studies of apparently healthy institutionalized residents have described hemoglobin and hematocrit levels below accepted normal values.[1,2] Further iron and bone marrow studies are indicated before accepting these values as normal. Elderly people with even mild anemia deserve the same consideration for diagnostic studies as younger adults. It is risky to assume that anemia in the elderly is due to aging.

The clinical manifestations of anemia include fatigue, dyspnea, pallor, and tachycardia, which are similar at any age. Signs and symptoms of anemia may appear at higher hemoglobin levels in the elderly and may be more difficult to evaluate because of coexisting diseases. Fatigue is more difficult to assess in the frail elderly. Exertional dyspnea may be due to anemia or concomitant chronic pulmonary or cardiac disease, each of which impair oxygen transport. Anemia may produce confusional states or worsen existing dementia. Elderly patients with coronary artery disease may develop ischemic chest pain or congestive heart failure with mild to moderate decreases in hemoglobin levels.

Anemia itself is not a diagnosis but must be considered a sign of disease. Successful management of anemia is dependent on an accurate diagnosis. Classifying anemia as hypochromic or macrocytic narrows the differential diagnosis within each group. On the other hand, normochromic anemias include a large variety of disorders. The reticulocyte count further classifies the mechanism of anemia: reticulocytopenia reflects a decreased marrow erythrocyte production while an elevated reticulocyte count suggests an increased marrow response to the anemia and implies that the anemia is due to hemolysis or acute blood loss.

Iron deficiency

Hemoglobin consists of two components, heme and globin, and defective formation of either moiety can lead to defective hemoglobin formation. In iron deficiency and in the anemia of chronic disease, there is failure to form heme due to lack of available iron to combine with protoporphyrin. In thalassemia syndromes, globin production is impaired and in sideroblastic anemia production of porphyrin is impaired. Although the reason for impaired hemoglobin formation is different in each of the four disorders, they are all characterized by the production of hypochromic anemia. Iron deficiency is the most common cause of defective hemoglobin synthesis resulting in poorly hemoglobinized red blood cells. Iron deficiency anemia and the anemia of chronic disease are the two most common types of anemia in old people.

Symptoms of iron deficiency anemia are related to diminished oxygen transfer to tissues due to a decreased quantity of hemoglobin and to iron deficiency itself.[3,4] This is further substantiated by treatment with iron, which produces significant improvement in physical activity prior to an increase in hemoglobin concentration.[3,4] Furthermore, the clinician is often surprised by unexpected improvement with iron therapy in patients who have minimal decreases in hemoglobin concentration.

The usual sequence of events in iron deficiency is an initial loss of reticuloendothelial cell iron, which can be detected by a low serum ferritin level, followed by a low serum iron level, an increase in total iron-binding capacity (TIBC), and, finally, the appearance of hypochromic microcytic red cells typical of iron deficiency anemia. However, with mild degrees of iron deficiency, erythrocyte morphology and indices may be normal. In this situation, a low serum iron level associated with an elevated TIBC (greater than 350 μg/100 ml) and resulting in a low iron saturation of transferrin (less than 16%) indicates iron deficiency. However, almost one third of iron deficient patients have a low normal or even a decreased TIBC level related to the underlying cause of their anemia or to other associated disorders. In this circumstance, a low serum ferritin level establishes the diagnosis. Since serum ferritin level is ordinarily a good indicator of the amount of stored iron, it can be substituted for bone marrow assessment of iron stores.[5,6] This test is now becoming universally available and may eventually replace serum iron and TIBC, since it is a reliable and sensitive indicator of iron deficiency. Serum ferritin level reflects decreasing iron stores before characteristic changes occur in serum iron and TIBC. In patients with iron deficiency anemia, serum ferritin values are below 12 μg/liter. When iron deficiency and inflammatory disease coexist, the serum ferritin is disproportionately high. Therefore, serum ferritin must be interpreted with knowledge of the clinical condition, that is, values will not be as low with coexistent inflammatory, renal, liver, or Hodgkin's diseases, as with an uncomplicated iron deficiency anemia.

The management of a patient with iron deficiency anemia involves two important steps: (1) identification and correction of any abnormality causing iron deficiency and (2) treatment of iron deficiency. Dietary deficiency is seldom the sole cause. Nonetheless, we should be alert to poor nutrition as a contributing cause of iron deficiency. The average daily diet normally contains 15 to 20 mg of food iron of which 5% to 10% is absorbed (0.5 to 1.5 mg per day). The amount of dietary iron is closely related to caloric intake, which is usually about 6 mg of elemental iron per 1000 calories. Iron from animal tissue is better absorbed than iron in vegetables. Vegetable sources may be high in iron content, but the iron is poorly absorbed because of inhibitors to iron absorption such as phosphates and phytates. Therefore, although spinach may contain ample iron, it is not recommended as a dietary source because of its poor absorption. Tea has been shown to be an inhibitor of iron absorption.[7] Some elderly people drink enormous amounts of tea daily, which may be a factor in producing iron deficiency, especially in those whose diet consists mainly of vegetables. Nonetheless, the explanation that iron deficiency anemia in an elderly person is due to poor diet should never be accepted until investigation for a bleeding lesion has been completed. On the other hand, bleeding from a gastrointestinal lesion superimposed on iron stores depleted by poor diet is not uncommon. Testing for occult blood in the stool is an essential part of the examination of every patient. More often, iron deficiency in the elderly is due to chronic blood loss, especially bleeding from gastrointestinal lesions. Bleeding may be intermittent and, therefore, if the test for occult blood is negative, a search for a gastrointestinal lesion is still warranted. Major gastrointestinal bleeding induced by drugs is a serious and relatively common event in the elderly. Aspirin is a prominent cause of gastrointestinal bleeding. Phenylbutazone, indomethacin, steroids, and alcohol have been implicated, and, recently, gastrointestinal bleeding has been observed in patients receiving intravenous ethacrynic acid.[8] It is, however, unwise to attribute gastrointestinal bleeding to drugs unless other causes, especially gastrointestinal lesions, are excluded.

Treatment consists of the oral administration of ferrous sulfate 3 or 4 times daily. This provides approximatley 180 to 240 mg elemental iron, which, assuming a 20% absorption, supplies approximately 35 to 50 mg of iron to bone marrow. A rise in hemoglobin concentration usually occurs after 10 days of treatment, and it becomes normal within 6 weeks. The daily hemoglobin production averages about 0.25 gm/100 ml in severe anemia. It has been observed that there is no difference in iron absorption in young or old patients with iron deficiency.[9] After correction of anemia, the amount of iron absorbed diminishes and therapy must be continued for an additional 4 months to replenish bone marrow iron stores; this provides a buffer against future losses.

Parenteral iron therapy with iron-dextran (Imferon) is reserved for patients who do not comply with oral therapy, do not tolerate side effects, or are unable to absorb orally administered iron because of gastrointestinal disease or surgery. Iron-dextran can be given intramuscularly or intravenously. A test dose of 0.25 ml is injected the first day, followed by 2.5 ml in each buttock intramuscularly until the calculated dose has been given. In patients with small muscle mass or hemorrhagic disorders, the entire calculated dose diluted in 100 ml of normal saline for each 5 ml of iron-dextran, is infused intravenously over a period of 30 to 60 minutes.

Sideroblastic anemias

In the elderly, impaired erythropoiesis due to defective heme synthesis produces a hypochromic anemia associated with tissue iron overload. Impairment of porphyrin synthesis prevents combination of iron with protoporphyrin to form heme, and iron accumulates within the mitochondria of nucleated red cells. Ringed sideroblasts, which are bone marrow nucleated red cells with a ring of Prussian-blue staining mitochondrial iron around the nucleus, are diagnostic. An elderly patient with hypochromia who is not iron deficient and who does not have evidence of chronic disease is likely to have sideroblastic anemia. The peripheral blood smear shows hypochromic cells which are small or normal-sized, in addition to macrocytes. The serum iron is increased along with an iron saturation of transferrin greater than 50% and often close to 100%. Elevated serum ferritin levels are common.

It is reasonable to treat patients with sideroblastic anemia with 200 mg of pyridoxine per day, although it is seldom effective. A rare response to intramuscular injections of pyridoxal phosphate suggests a defect in the conversion of pyridoxine to pyridoxal. Sideroblastic changes occurring with megaloblastic anemia disappear with appropriate folic acid or vitamin B_{12} treatment. The most common secondary cause of sideroblastic anemia is alcohol. The erythropoietic disorder disappears usually within 10 days after alcohol consumption ceases. Anemia may be severe enough in primary acquired sideroblastic anemia to require transfusions over long periods of time. In some elderly patients, sideroblastic anemia represents a preleukemic syndrome, which precedes acute nonlymphocytic leukemia.

Anemia of chronic disease (ACD)

An anemia is frequently seen in elderly patients who have chronic inflammatory states such as rheumatoid arthritis or hepatitis, infections such as tuberculosis or osteomyelitis, or neoplastic disease. It is often confused with iron deficiency, and the patient sometimes mistakenly receives long-term iron therapy. The anemia is usually not severe with hematocrit values ranging from 27% to 35%. Although there is some shortening of the red cell life span, the major problem is a diminished compensatory bone marrow response, indicating a marrow production defect. Bone marrow iron stores are sufficient, but a block in the release of iron from reticuloendothelial cells results in low plasma iron levels. The increased iron in reticuloendothelial cells is reflected by a rise in serum ferritin levels.

The laboratory findings for ACD may be similar to those for iron deficiency anemia.[6,10] In both normochromic or hypochromic anemia with low reticulocyte indices and low serum iron and elevated erythrocyte protoporphyrin levels may be present. However, in contrast to iron deficiency anemia, the low serum iron level is accompanied by a low normal or low TIBC, and the serum ferritin value is high-normal or elevated. Until serum ferritin determinations became available, bone marrow examination showing absent iron with iron deficiency and adequate iron in reticuloendothelial cells with ACD usually distinguished these conditions. The serum ferritin determination is presently a simple and inexpensive method of making this distinction.

Management consists of finding and treating the underlying disorder. Iron therapy is not beneficial and androgens are not helpful.

Vitamin B_{12} and folate deficiencies

A detailed dietary history is important in establishing a diagnosis. Vitamin B_{12} is found in all foods of animal origin including meat, poultry, fish, eggs, and dairy products, but it is not found in plant sources. Most normal diets contain 5 to 30 μg vitamin B_{12} with an absorption fo 1 to 5 μg per day. Preliminary binding with gastric intrinsic factor is necessary for the absorption of vitamin B_{12}, which occurs through specific intrinsic factor (IF)-B_{12} receptors in the terminal ileum. In the stomach, R-proteins have a greater avidity for vitamin B_{12} than intrinsic factor, but R-protein–vitamin B_{12} complexes are not absorbed by ileal receptors, which have specificity for IF-vitamin B_{12} complexes.[11] Pancreatic enzymes (trypsin and chymotrypsin) degrade R-proteins in the small intestine, releasing vitamin B_{12} and making it available for subsequent binding with intrinsic factor.[11] It requires 8 to 10 hours for vitamin B_{12} to reach peak plasma activity because of transit time in the gastrointestinal tract and processing of IF-B_{12} complex in the ileal mucosa.

A storage pool of 3000 to 5000 μg of vitamin B_{12} is present in adults, of which 1000 to 3000 μg is stored in the liver. Since the daily requirement of vitamin B_{12} is approximately 2 to 5 μg per day, it is estimated that it would take 2 to 5 years to exhaust body stores if no vitamin B_{12} was present in the diet or if none was absorbed. A patient must be on a strict vegetarian diet to produce a vitamin B_{12} deficiency on a dietary basis. Obviously, vitamin B_{12} deficiency occurs with pernicious anemia or after total gastrectomy due to absent gastric intrinsic factor. More subtle forms of vitamin B_{12} deficiency occur, even in the presence of adequate intrinsic factor, due to insufficient gastric secretions, which are needed to liberate vitamin B_{12} from food.[12] This may occur in several situations such as a patient with partial gastrectomy, vagotomy with gastroenterostomy, or chronic gastritis with achlorhydria or hypochlorhydria. Under these circumstances, orally administered radioactive vitamin B_{12}, as given with the Schilling test, would be normally absorbed, thereby resulting in a normal test. In patients with severe pancreatic insufficiency, vitamin B_{12} is not released from R-protein in the absence of pancreatic enzymes (trypsin and chymotrypsin), although this rarely produces a clinical problem. Obviously, removal of ileal receptors for vitamin B_{12} in the terminal ileum by either surgical resection or disease such as regional ileitis results in malabsorption of vitamin B_{12}.

Nutritional folate deficiency is more common than vitamin B_{12} deficiency in the elderly as a consequence of poor dietary intake. This is more common in persons living alone and in alcoholics. Megaloblastic anemia occurs almost exclusively in alcoholics who have been eating poorly. It occurs more frequently with wine and whiskey drinkers rather than with beer drinkers, since the former contain practically no folate whereas there is ample folate in beer.[13] The addition of folic acid to alcoholic beverages has even been recommended to prevent deficiency in alcoholics.[14] Folic acid is soluble in alcoholic beverages and does not alter its taste. The amount of folate in the normal daily diet is 200 to 500 μg, with the daily requirement being 100 to 200 μg. Folates are found in nearly all raw foods such as green vegetables, liver, kidney, and dairy products; but excessive cooking readily destroys folates. Elderly persons whose daily diet does not include fresh or fresh-frozen uncooked fruit, fruit juice, or fresh, lightly cooked vegetables are at risk to develop folate deficiency. Most dietary folates are polyglutamates, which are less well absorbed than monoglutamates. An intestinal enzyme (conjugase) hydrolyzes the glutamyl peptide bonds, thereby reducing the chain length and facilitating absorption. Folate is absorbed in the small intestine. The liver is the most important storage organ for folates, normally containing approximately 10 mg.

Abnormalities of the blood and bone marrow are similar for vitamin B_{12} or folate deficiency. Following are the laboratory features common to vitamin B_{12} and folate deficiencies:

1. Mean corpuscular volume (MCV) greater than 100 μm^3
2. Macro-ovalocytes
3. "Hypersegmented polys"
4. Thrombocytopenia
5. Megaloblastic marrow
6. Increased serum lactate dehydrogenase (SLDH)
7. Increased serum bilirubin level

Megaloblastic anemia in either deficiency is characterized in the peripheral blood by macro-ovalocytes, fishtail red blood cells, and hypersegmented neutrophils, which is the most helpful clue to making the diagnosis. The mean corpuscular volume (MCV) is greater than 100 μm^3, and a value greater than 115 μm^3 would be highly suggestive of megaloblastic anemia, since it is unusual for a normoblastic macrocytic anemia to be present with an MCV of this magnitude. There is often a leukopenia and a thrombocytopenia. Bone marrow examination shows characteristic erythroid and myeloid megaloblastosis. Early death of erythroid cells within the bone marrow, intramedullary hemolysis, results in a decreased number of normal cells delivered to the peripheral circulation. This is called *ineffective erythropoiesis;* consequences of this are an increased serum iron and an increased number of sideroblasts, producing a picture that resembles iron overload. The blood chemistry findings that reflect hemolysis are an increased serum lactate dehydrogenase level and a modestly elevated serum bilirubin level. A low or low normal serum iron level, especially if associated with an elevated total iron-binding capacity in a patient with megaloblastic anemia, is most likely the result of a coexistent iron deficiency.

Clinical findings are helpful in separating folate from vitamin B_{12} deficiency. A symmetrical peripheral neuropathy occurs with vitamin B_{12}; this originates in peripheral nerves and progresses to the posterior and lateral columns of the spinal cord and is associated with symmetrical paresthesias and a loss of proprioception and vibratory sensation. A family history of pernicious anemia or of thyroid disease and early graying of the hair suggest a diagnosis of pernicious anemia. On the other hand, a diet lacking fresh vegetables and fruit, especially in an alcoholic individual, points to folate deficiency. Measurement of serum levels of vitamin B_{12} and folate distinguishes these deficiencies. A serum vitamin B_{12} level below 120 pg/ml establishes vitamin B_{12} deficiency; patients with folate deficiency have a low serum folate level of less than 3 ng/ml. A bone marrow examination is not always essential for the patient with macro-ovalocytes and hypersegmented polys who, in addition, has a low serum vitamin B_{12} or a low folate level. The Schilling test is helpful in confirming clinically significant vitamin B_{12} deficiency or ascertaining the cause of the vitamin B_{12} deficiency (Table 11-1). Radioactive vitamin B_{12} absorption test performed by either measuring radioactivity in the urine (Schilling test) or plasma uptake of radioactivity is especially useful in confirming clinically significant vitamin B_{12} deficiency whether or not the patient has been receiving vitamin B_{12} therapy. An abnormal Schilling test corrected by the addition of intrinsic factor provides evidence of intrinsic factor deficiency characteristic of pernicious anemia or occurring after gastric resection. Misleading results can be avoided if it is remembered that vitamin B_{12} deficiency may produce a "megaloblastic gut"[12] and, consequently, impaired ileal absorption of vitamin B_{12}. This produces low uptake of radioactive vitamin B_{12} with intrinsic factor in the

Table 11-1. Clinical results of radioactive vitamin B_{12} absorption tests

Cause	*Without intrinsic factor*	*With intrinsic factor*	*With antibiotics*
Deficient diet	Normal	—	—
Absent intrinsic factor	Low	Normal	—
Ileal lesion	Low	Low	—
Bacteria	Low	Low	Normal

Schilling test, but this absorptive defect is transient and reversible, usually within a few weeks. Obviously, a Schilling test is dispensable in a patient with an extensive gastric resection, ileal resection, or a regional enteritis with an associated vitamin B_{12} deficiency.

Specific replacement therapy should be started after determination of the specific deficiency. A correct diagnosis is essential prior to treatment with folic acid, which produces a hematologic remission in patients with vitamin B_{12} deficiency and eventually an irreversible neuropathy. The objectives of therapy are to correct the anemia, replenish body stores of vitamin B_{12} or folate, eliminate the underlying cause, and assure long-term maintenance therapy. Vitamin B_{12} deficiency is treated with either cyanocobalamin or hydroxocobalamin. Both preparations produce similar results, although the latter is preferable because it is retained in the body better than cyanocobalamin. Initial therapy with hydroxocobalamin consists of 1000 μg intramuscularly every 2 to 3 days for a total of six injections. This is followed by maintenance therapy of 500 to 1000 μg intramuscularly every 3 months.[15] If cyanocobalamin is used, initial therapy is similar with the administration of 1000 μg intramuscularly for a total of six injections; but maintenance therapy is given more frequently because of greater urinary excretion of cyanocobalamin than hydroxocobalamin. Usually 500 to 1000 μg intramuscularly is administered once a month. While minimal doses of 30 μg per month may be adequate, vitamin B_{12} is not expensive and not harmful; therefore a larger dose provides better assurance. Prompt therapy is indicated in patients who bleed because of a low platelet count or who have infection associated with neutropenia due to either deficiency. Occasionally, immediate therapy is indicated prior to establishing the specific deficiency responsible. A blood sample should be drawn for serum assays, and both folate and vitamin B_{12} therapy should be initiated, with the appropriate therapy subsequently continued as indicated by the results of the serum assay. Patients who have had a total gastrectomy or an ileal resection should receive hydroxocobalamin, 1000 μg every 3 months, as preventive therapy. In patients with severe anemia causing symptoms such as dyspnea or angina, cautious transfusions of packed cells are indicated. Transfusions may cause congestive heart failure, and it may be necessary to remove 100 ml of blood from the other arm or to administer a diuretic. It is important that the patient with vitamin B_{12} deficiency be educated about the disorder, its treatment, and the necessity for lifetime therapy. When a physician considers withdrawal of vitamin B_{12} therapy on the assumption of a misdiagnosis, a complete review of the data on which the diagnosis is based is mandatory.

Therapy for folate deficiency is effective with 1 mg folic acid orally per day. The length of therapy depends on the underlying cause but is usually 4 months. The underlying cause must be corrected and attention given to improve the diet with foods containing folate, such as fresh vegetables, fruits, nuts, liver, and dairy products.

The response to either vitamin B_{12} or folate therapy is evident by a reticulocytosis and an increased neutrophil and platelet count in 5 to 10 days. Bone marrow converts from a megaloblastic to a normoblastic morphology in 48 to 72 hours. Serum iron decreases to a low value in 4 to 5 days and, subsequently, rises to normal over a period of a few weeks. Serum bilirubin and the serum lactate dehydrogenase return to normal in 1 to 3 weeks. A rare complication of therapy is hypokalemia, and there have been reports of sudden unexplained deaths due to this phenomenon.

ALCOHOL-RELATED BLOOD DISORDERS

Alcohol abuse has been associated with various hematologic disorders including anemia, thrombocytopenia, and leukopenia. It is often difficult to separate alcohol-induced anemia from that due to underlying liver disease. Alcohol produces vacuolization in erythroid precursors, especially proerythroblasts, but there is little evidence of marrow suppression. Several types of anemia are associated with alcohol intake including folate deficiency, blood loss, sideroblastic anemia, hypersplenism, and hemolytic anemia. Folate deficiency is due mainly to decreased dietary folate and an antifolate action of ethanol, and often it produces thrombocytopenia and leukopenia in addition to macrocytic anemia. A round cell macrocytosis associated with erythrocyte membrane lipid changes is recognized in liver disease, but macrocytosis (MCV greater than 100 to 110) without neutrophil hypersegmentation is present in greater than 40% of alcoholics who have neither folate deficiency nor overt liver disease.[16]

Alcohol abuse is a common cause of sideroblastic changes in the marrow. It is usually associated with megaloblastic changes in the marrow due to folate deficiency.[17] Upper gastrointestinal hemorrhage results from esophagitis and gastritis in acute alochol ingestion and from esophageal varices in long-term liver disease. Bleeding may be complicated by coagulation abnormalities and thrombocytopenia. ACD may occur in hepatic cirrhosis and is characterized by a diminished marrow response to mild hemolysis. Several types of hemolytic disease are recognized with alcoholism or liver disease.[16] Hypophosphatemia is associated with alcoholism and accompanied by low levels of erythrocyte adenosine triphosphate (ATP) and spherocytic hemolytic anemia.[18] The serum phosphorus and ATP levels return to normal within 3 to 14 days after cessation of alcohol ingestion, with or without phosphate supplementation. Hemolysis frequently ensues with alcoholic liver disease due to splenic sequestration, spur cells, stomatocytosis, Zieve syndrome, and hypophosphatemia. Zieve syndrome consists of alcoholic fatty liver, hyperlipemia, lactescent serum, and an acute hemolytic anemia.

Platelet abnormalities in alcoholism are related to alcohol itself, hepatic cirrhosis, or folate deficiency. Alcohol-related thrombocytopenia with platelet counts less than 100,000/mm^3 occurs in 3% of nonacutely ill chronic alcoholics and 25% of acutely ill alcoholics with acute intoxication, alcoholic withdrawal, or complications of alcoholism.[19] Platelet counts as low as 10,000/mm^3 have been observed. Folate deficiency may also cause thrombocytopenia, but alcoholic-related thrombocytopenia occurs independently. Platelet counts return to normal after cessation of alcohol ingestion. The platelet count begins to rise 2 to 3 days after interdicting alcohol, with a rapid increase at a rate of 20,000 to 60,000/mm^3 each day. Maximum elevation is seen in 5 to 21 days. In approximately one third of patients, an elevated count (greater than 450,000/mm^3) is observed, which gradually declines to the normal range within 1 to 3 weeks. Rebound thrombocytosis has been responsible for thromboembolic episodes.[20] Both qualitative and quantitative abnormalities appear with alcohol-related thrombocytopenia. There is an increased rate of platelet destruction in addition to a productive defect leading to ineffective thrombopoiesis.

Alcoholics have an increased incidence of infection due to impaired host defense mechanisms, which is at least partly due to abnormalities in number and functions of granulocytes and lymphocytes. Granulocytopenia is sometimes due to folate deficiency or hypersplenism. In the absence of infection, folate or vitamin B_{12} deficiency, or hypersplenism, an acute episode of excessive alcohol intake may cause granulocytopenia, which disappears within a week after alcohol withdrawal.[16] The bone marrow is usually hypocellular, and the functional marrow granulocyte reserve is reduced. But granulocytopenia is also seen in alcoholics with infection, usually pneumococcal pneumonia. The granulocytopenia is evanescent and lasts only 2 to 4 days. Because granulocyte marrow reserve is low, the infection is usually protracted. Alcohol also causes functional impairment of granulocytes, macrophages, and lymphocytes.

PRELEUKEMIA SYNDROME (HEMOPOIETIC DYSPLASIA, MYELODYSPLASTIC SYNDROME)

The term *preleukemia* has been criticized because some patients have this disorder for years and never develop leukemia. Notwithstanding the terminology, a recognizable clinical syndrome often precedes the development of acute nonlymphocytic (granulocytic) leukemia.[21,22] This syndrome is observed mainly in patients over 50 years of age and occurs in approximately 30% of elderly patients who develop acute granulocytic leukemia. Abnormalities of all marrow elements (erythrocytic, granulocytic, and megakaryocytic cells) are invariably present. Peripheral blood cytopenias are prevalent, and patients have symptoms and signs of fatigue, weakness, bleeding, and infection.

The bone marrow is always abnormal, exhibiting erythroid hyperplasia with prominent megaloblastic features and multinucleated forms. Ringed sideroblasts are frequently observed. Atypical megakaryocytes are prominent despite peripheral thrombocytopenia. Monocytosis or monocytoid granulocytic cells may be seen. There is insufficient evidence to support a diagnosis of leukemia. The peripheral blood smear shows variable-sized erythrocytes with prominent macro-ovalocytes and sometimes circulating nucleated red cells. The hematologic picture is often suggestive of vitamin B_{12} or folate deficiency, but serum vitamin B_{12} and folate levels are normal and treatment with these medications are ineffective. It is critical to recognize a treatable vitamin B_{12} or folate deficiency and to avoid inadvertently attributing an atypical megaloblastic picture to the preleukemic syndrome.

A preleukemic syndrome usually persists for 6 to 24 months prior to the development of overt leukemia. However, it has occasionally lasted as long as 5 to 10 years. There is no specific or effective treatment for the preleukemic syndrome. Red cell transfusions are appropriate for symptomatic anemia. Severe thrombocytopenia may require intermittent platelet transfusions. Rarely, patients have responded to pyridoxine (150 mg per day for 2 to 3 months). A few patients have responded to a 3- to 4-week trial of prednisone at doses of 60 to 80 per day. In vitro marrow culture studies may indicate which patients will likely achieve success with corticosteroids.[23] Cytotoxic drugs have not been effective in the therapy of preleukemia and should only be tried when the patient is symptomatic from thrombocytopenia or neutropenia.

ACUTE LEUKEMIA

Acute leukemia in adults is predominantly acute nonlymphocytic leukemia (myeloblastic). Impressive advances in treatment of this leukemia have been made. Acute nonlymphocytic leukemia is primarily a disease of the elderly; 70% of patients are over 50 years of age. Until recently, acute leukemia in the elderly was associated with an unfavorable prognosis. Patients over 60 years of age were considered not only to be refractory to chemotherapy, but also to poorly tolerate bone marrow aplasia from therapy, resulting in an early death. Recent studies, however, indicate that elderly patients do achieve complete remissions followed by long survivals similar to young adults.[24,25] Furthermore, they are apparently not exposed to a higher risk of death due to treatment than younger adults.[24]

In contrast to the abrupt onset of acute leukemia in younger patients, approximately 30% of elderly patients have a preleukemic phase. Elderly patients present with nonspecific complaints such as malaise; anorexia; weight loss, weakness, and fatigue due to anemia; bleeding and bruising due to thrombocytopenia or disseminated intravascular coagulation (DIC); and fever due to infections associated with granulocytopenia. In addition, bone and joint pain, lymphadenopathy, hepatosplenomegaly, and neurologic symptoms from leukemic infiltrates may be present. Initial laboratory studies usually reveal anemia, thrombocytopenia, and granulocytopenia with myeloblasts, monoblasts, or both in the peripheral blood. The marrow is usually hypercellular with myeloblasts, monocytoid features of the granulocytic cells, and, not infrequently, megaloblastic changes of erythroid cells and atypical megakaryocytes. If untreated, the median duration from the onset of symptoms to death is less than 6 months due to infection or hemorrhage.

The decision to treat should be made only after discussion with the patient and family of benefits and hazards likely to result from treatment. Current chemotherapeutic regimens produce profound bone marrow hypoplasia, sometimes lasting for weeks and requiring supportive care. Therapy, nonetheless, can be offered optimistically, since the introduction of cytarabine and daunorubicin has produced remission rates of up to 60% in patients over 50 years of age. Complete remissions have even been induced in several patients in the ninth decade of life.[26] The median duration of remission is approximately 10 to 12 months. However, approximately 20% to 25% of patients achieving complete remission have remained in continued remission for 5 years or longer. Because of these encouraging results, aggressive therapy should be made available to all patients regardless of age. The management of acute leukemia requires considerable expertise and extensive support facilities so that once the diagnosis is made, patients should be referred to an appropriate center. A few elderly patients have "smoldering leukemia," which is characterized by mildly elevated white blood cell counts with relatively few myeloblasts, mild anemia, and a tendency to infection or hemorrhage. The leukemia has an indolent course for several years and requires no chemotherapy. In our experience, however, these patients usually progress to the point where a specific antileukemic therapy is indicated.

Granulocyte (blast) counts greater than 100,000 per mm^3 and infection worsen initial prognosis. With the former, large numbers of leukemic cells involve small blood vessels in the brain and produce leukemic perivascular infiltration, which results in intracranial hemorrhage and death. Infection is a common complication and the major cause of death due to the combined effects of the leukemia and antileukemic therapy, which inevitably produces profound neutropenia. Neutropenia caused by leukemia or its treatment is the most important factor contributing to susceptibility to infection. In any patient with less than 1000 neutrophils/mm^3, the presence of an unexplained temperature over 101° F calls for emergency measures. Immediate cultures (of blood, urine, pharynx, and sputum) for bacteria and fungi should be obtained, and potential sites of infection, such as the perianal area and lungs, should be carefully examined. Because of granulocytopenia, the usual signs of infection, such as swelling and purulent discharge, are absent and only mild erythema and local tenderness may be present. Pneumonia is a common infection that occurs without the usual clinical signs or symptoms. Therefore, a chest x-ray film is essential. After obtaining appropriate cultures, empiric antibiotic therapy must be started without waiting for identification of organisms. Antibiotic combinations with nafcillin or a cephalosporin, carbenicillin, and gentamicin have been effective. These antibiotics should be continued for 7 to 10 days after the patient becomes afebrile and until granulocytopenia has resolved. Granulocyte transfusions have been effective in severely granulocytopenic patients with a serious infection.[27] Granulocyte transfusions are usually recommended in patients with a granulocyte count less than 500/mm^3 who remain febrile after 48 to 72 hours of broad spectrum antibiotic therapy or earlier if an overwhelming infection is present with shock, pneumonia, or a rigid abdomen.

The use of platelet transfusions to combat severe thrombocytopenia has decreased the incidence of death from bleeding. Platelets are usually maintained above 15 to 20,000/mm^3. A single platelet transfusion consisting of eight units of platelets will increase the platelet count to a level of approximately 80,000, with the count remaining above 20,000 for several days. The use of platelet transfusions from random donors results eventually in immunologic refractoriness to treatment, and in such circumstances HLA-matched donor transfusions may be effective. The patient may need transfusions of packed red cells for symptoms due to anemia. Packed red cells keep fluid load to a minimum and lessen antigen load with removal of plasma proteins and other cellular elements.

CHRONIC LYMPHOCYTIC LEUKEMIA (CLL)

This is the leukemia most frequently seen in the elderly, with the greatest incidence in persons over 60 years of age. Eighty percent of new diagnoses are made in patients over 50. It is an extremely variable disease and can no longer be viewed as an indolent disease afflicting the elderly. Its discovery may be an accidental finding on a routine blood count or on examination of a peripheral blood smear. Enlarged lymph nodes or splenomegaly may be palpated during an examination for another problem. Usually, however, protean symptoms correlate with adenopathy, splenomegaly, and high lymphocyte counts.

CLL is a lymphoproliferative disorder characterized by excessive lymphocytes in the bone marrow accompanied by lymphocytosis in peripheral blood. Early in the disease, the marrow may show only mild lymphocytosis, but eventually lymphocytes replace normal marrow, thereby producing anemia, thrombocytopenia, and neutropenia. The white cell count ranges from 20,000/mm^3 to 200,000/mm^3 with 70% to 90% mature lymphocytes. Many smudged cells are seen.

Most elderly patients with CLL have a variable course, but it is not unusual to follow some patients for 10 to 15 years. Unfortunately, the disease in some patients follows a more aggressive course. Rai has suggested a staging system that correlates clinical findings with survival (Table 11-2).[28] This provides a logical approach to prognosis rather than establishing a single median survival for a disease with such a varied course.

Clinical and laboratory manifestations of CLL can be attributed to immunologic deficiencies and cytopenias associated with CLL. Susceptibility to infection is related to hypogammaglobulinemia, poor cellular immune response, and granulocytopenia. Anemia and thrombocyto-

Table 11-2. Clinical staging and prognosis of chronic lymphocytic leukemia

Stage	*Clinical criteria*	*Median survival (months)*
0	Lymphocytosis	150
I	Lymphocytosis + lymphadenopathy	101
II	Lymphocytosis + splenomegaly and/or hepatomegaly	71
III	Lymphocytosis + anemia	19
IV	Lymphocytosis + thrombocytopenia	19

Data from Rai, K.R., et al.: Blood **46**:219, 1975.

penia result from bone marrow replacement with leukemic cells, chemotherapy, or hypersplenism. Approximately 20% of patients will develop a Coombs' positive autoimmune anemia and, less frequently, an autoimmune thrombocytopenia, both of which may respond dramatically to corticosteroid therapy.

With the benign form of CLL, the patient often dies from an unrelated cause. However, with aggressive disease, the terminal event is generally bleeding due to thrombocytopenia or infection due to granulocytopenia and immunologic deficiency. Additionally, chemotherapeutic agents may produce granulocytopenia and thrombocytopenia, and alkylating agents or glucocorticoids inhibit immune function, thereby increasing susceptibility to bacterial, viral, or fungal infection. It follows, therefore, that therapy is not indicated for the asymptomatic patient. Alkylating agents such as chlorambucil or cyclophosphamide are effective in returning blood counts to normal and reducing lymphadenopathy, splenomegaly, and hepatomegaly. Chlorambucil is the agent most commonly used. Alkylating agents are often given alone, but prednisone along with the alkylating agent is beneficial for cytopenias due to lymphocytic bone marrow infiltration, autoimmune hemolysis or thrombocytopenia, or hypersplenism. Initially, corticosteroids may produce a transient rise in peripheral blood lymphocytes, but this is soon followed by a decrease in lymph node size and in the peripheral blood lymphocyte count. Therapy results in substantial cell destruction and liberation of excessive uric acid, which may lead to deposition in renal tubules and subsequent renal failure. Uric acid stones and nephropathy can be prevented by the administration of allopurinol and by sustaining good hydration.

Radiation therapy is particularly useful for bulky adenopathy or localized lymphocytic infiltration, which cause blockage of ureters, bile ducts, or bronchi. Splenic radiation is of no proven benefit for hypersplenic manifestations of CLL. Splenectomy has been helpful in a few patients with prednisone resistant hypersplenism with severe cytopenia.

Leukapheresis removes a significant number of lymphocytes in patients with CLL and is especially suitable for the management of patients with significant anemia and thrombocytopenia.[29] Recovery of marrow production with elevation of both hemoglobin and platelet values occurs concomitantly with reduction of lymphoid cells.

MULTIPLE MYELOMA

The incidence of myeloma is increasing, apparently because of the increasing number of elderly persons and better methods for diagnosis. It usually appears in persons over 50 years old with the greater incidence in persons over 60 years old. Only 2% of patients in one series were younger than 40 years of age. Plasma cell (multiple) myeloma is a malignant disease of plasma cells that typically involves bone marrow but often other tissues as well. Myeloma results from a selective proliferation of a single clone of lymphocytes (B cells), producing a specific immunoglobulin. This monoclonal protein serves as a tumor marker, indicating the size of the myeloma cell mass.[30,31] The growth of plasma cells is slow, as evidenced by a doubling time of 3 months for IgG myeloma. A monoclonal spike on serum protein electrophoresis is seen when the tumor size reaches 10^{11} cells. Symptoms usually correlate with a cellular mass of approximately 0.5×10^{12} cells, and death ordinarily occurs when the tumor mass reaches 5×10^{12} myeloma cells. The frequency of the types of protein abnormalities found in patients with myeloma are IgG, 61%; light chain, 19.5%; IgA, 17%; IgD, 1.5%; and IgE, less than 1%.[32]

The major features of myeloma are plasma cell infiltration of bone marrow greater than 10%, monoclonal gammopathy of serum or urine greater than 1 gm/100 ml, osteolytic lesions or osteoporosis, hypercalcemia, anemia, and azotemia. The most prominent symptom is bone pain due to myeloma cells in the marrow cavity, causing osteolytic lesions or osteoporosis. Osteoporosis may be the only bone lesion in 25% of cases. Pathologic fractures often occur with minimal or no trauma. An osteoclastic activating factor in plasma cells of patients with myeloma is responsible for bone resorption, which causes skeletal destruction and leads to hypercalcemia.[33] Marrow involvement with myeloma cells accounts for anemia and its associated symptoms of weakness and fatigue. Myeloma should be suspected in any elderly patient with bone pain, especially with unexplained anemia associated with rouleaux formation on the peripheral blood smear. Routine urinalysis and "dip-stick" methods will not detect Bence Jones protein, but sulfosalicylic acid and *p*-toluene sulfuric acid are good screening methods. The diagnosis of monoclonal light chain excretion should always be confirmed by electrophoresis and immunoelectrophoresis of concentrated urine. A diagnosis of myeloma should not be made solely on the basis of a monoclonal spike. Approximately 1% to 3% of elderly individuals have monoclonal gammopathy (M spike) but do not develop myeloma. These are designated "benign" idiopathic monoclonal gammopathy and are characterized by monoclonal spikes seldom greater than 1 gm/100 ml but always less than 3.0 gm/100 ml, less than 20% marrow plasma cells, absence of Bence Jones proteinuria, and no apparent bone destruction.

Acute and chronic renal failure (see list below) occur in myeloma:

1. Myeloma kidney
2. Hypercalcemia
3. Hyperuricemia
4. Amyloidosis
5. Plasma cell infiltration of kidneys
6. Pyelonephritis

Renal disease is the presenting problem in 10% to 20% of patients and is found in 50% during the course of the disease. Renal failure is a serious prognostic sign and is second only to infection as a cause of death. Myeloma should be suspected in an elderly patient with nonhypertensive azotemia. Tubular dysfunction secondary to light chain proteinuria (Bence Jones proteins) produces the typical "myeloma kidney." Renal disease is especially common in light chain myeloma and IgD myeloma. Hypercalcemia is a treatable cause of renal failure. About 50% of patients with myeloma have elevated serum calcium levels. Hyperuricemia occurs, especially after initiating treatment, and should be managed prophylactically with adequate hydration and allopurinol to avoid complications produced by urate precipitation in renal tubules or ureters causing ureteral colic, azotemia, and oliguria. Acute renal failure occurs with intravenous pyelography, hypercalcemia, dehydration, antibiotics, and sepsis. Hence intravenous pyelography should be performed only if absolutely necessary and in a well-hydrated patient. Nephrotoxic antibiotics should be used only as a last resort. Urinary tract instrumentation should be minimal or avoided.

Infection is a common complication and major cause of death in patients with plasma cell myeloma. Recurrent infection, especially pneumonia and urinary tract infections, are common and should be promptly diagnosed and treated. A decrease in normal immunoglobulin levels or granulocytopenia is responsible for increased susceptibility to infections.

Several risk factors have been identified that correlate with a poorer response to treatment and shorter survival. These factors include azotemia, hypercalcemia, infection, anemia, leukopenia or thrombocytopenia, hypoalbuminemia, hyperuricemia, and non–light chain urinary protein excretion. It has been observed that several of these prognostic indicators correlate with tumor load.[34]

Plasma cell myeloma pursues a relentless downhill course with a mean survival of 7 months from the time of diagnosis. However, supportive therapy along with reduction of the tumor mass with chemotherapy, has resulted in a median survival time of 23 to 40 months. Alkylating agents, either melphalan (Alkeran) or cyclophosphamide (Cytoxan) with prednisone, reduces myeloma gammopathy reflecting shrinkage of the myeloma cell mass. Patients who fail to respond may improve with agents or combinations such as doxorubicin (Adriamycin) and lomustine (CeeNU). The addition of vincristine to other chemotherapeutic agents for the management of patients with high tumor mass, that is, the group with the worst prognosis, results in significantly higher response rates and length of survival.[35] Radiation therapy is effective for the relief of localized pain caused by myelomatous lesions and for localized tumors composed of plasma cell (plasmacytoma). However, so-called "solitary" plasmacytomas usually progress to generalized disease with marrow plasmacytosis, osteolytic lesions, and monoclonal gammopathy despite resection or radiation therapy.

Spinal cord compression is an emergency requiring prompt diagnosis and treatment.[36] Tumor compression of the spinal cord can be due to an extramedullary plasmacytoma or to a pathologic fracture of a vertebral body. Lumbar puncture should be done in conjunction with a myelogram because the neurologic symptoms worsen after the tap in 8% of patients. Laminectomy followed by radiation therapy is indicated for rapidly progressing neurologic symptoms. Radiation therapy alone may suffice in patients with minimal or slowly progressing neurologic symptoms. Dexamethasone, 4 mg every 6 hours, is sometimes given prior to radiation therapy.

Asymptomatic patients with monoclonal gammopathy should be followed closely but not treated. Many of the complications of myeloma such as infection, hypercalcemia, hyperuricemia, anemia, hyperviscosity, and pathologic fracture can be anticipated and therefore prevented or minimized by appropriate therapy. Adequate hydration and physical activity are encouraged to decrease the hazards of hyperuricemia, hypercalcemia, and renal failure due to Bence Jones proteinuria. Hypercalcemia may be managed by adequate hydration and encouraging activity, but other measures are usually required. The combination of saline and furosemide, administered intravenously, is one of the more effective therapies. Prednisone decreases mobilization of calcium from the bone in myeloma and reverses hypercalcemia in the majority of patients. Therapy with orally administered phosphate may be helpful in some patients who do not have renal failure. Calcitonin is a rapidly acting, powerful inhibitor of bone absorption whose use has been disappointing because of its transient activity. However, the combination of calcitonin with glucocorticoids produces a rapid fall in serum calcium levels toward the normal range, an effect that is maintained for 4 days.[37] Mithramycin produces a rapid but transient decrease in calcium but causes acute hepatotoxicity and a unique coagulopathy associated with depressed coagulation factors II, V, VII, and X and sometimes thrombocytopenia.

Waldenström's macroglobulinemia is a disease of the elderly characterized by a high concentration of monoclonal IgM macroglobulins which cause a hyperviscosity syndrome with sludging and consequent dilatation of retinal veins, loss of vision, loss of hearing, bleeding, congestive heart failure, headache, dizziness, and coma. The bone marrow is infiltrated with cells having characteristics of both plasma cells and lymphocytes. Plasmapheresis reverses the clinical manifestations when used as emergency treatment of the hyperviscosity syndrome. Chemotherapy inhibits further production of immunoglobulin.

MYELOPROLIFERATIVE DISORDERS

Erythroleukemia, polycythemia vera, essential thrombocythemia, agnogenic myeloid metaplasia, and chronic granulocytic leukemia are classified as the myeloproliferative disorders. Chronic granulocytic leukemia is the only one that occurs most commonly in middle age and infrequently in older patients. The myeloproliferative disorders are characterized by proliferation of erythroid, myeloid, or megakaryocytic cells as well as fibrocytes or reticulum cells of the bone marrow. This proliferation may also occur in extramedullary sites such as the spleen, liver, or lymph nodes.

Agnogenic myeloid metaplasia

The characteristic feature is extramedullary hematopoiesis due to the development of a clone of cells, which proliferate in the spleen, liver, and lymph nodes. Abnormal peripheral blood findings, splenomegaly, or both, are critical diagnostic features of this disorder. The peripheral blood smear shows teardrop-shaped red cells, nucleated red cells, immature granulocytes, and abnormal platelets. The white blood cell count is frequently elevated and may suggest chronic granulocytic leukemia; however, it is usually not as high in agnogenic myeloid metaplasia, usually less than 30,000/mm^3 and rarely reaching 100,000/mm^3. Leukocyte alkaline phosphatase scores are elevated or normal. Platelet counts may be low, normal, or high. A prominent feature is a thrombocytosis with large, bizarre platelets on the peripheral blood smear. Bone marrow is usually difficult to obtain, and dry tap often results. Bone marrow biopsy reveals fibrosis and, in some cases, new bone formation or osteosclerosis. The presence of myelofibrosis strongly supports the diagnosis of agnogenic myeloid metaplasia, but its absence does not rule out the condition. The spleen is enlarged, usually hard and irregular. Initial symptoms may be related to anemia, thrombocytopenia, or pain over the splenic infarcts. Gout may occur from an increase in uric acid secondary to increased cell turnover.

The mean life span after diagnosis is approximately 4 to 5 years. Patients usually die of complications of infection, hemorrhage, thrombosis, or portal hypertension. In approximately 10% of patients leukopenia develops with the appearance of sufficient blast forms indicating transition to acute leukemia. Agnogenic myeloid metaplasia must be distinguished from chronic granulocytic leukemia, and the bone marrow must be examined carefully for evidence of metastatic disease, which may produce a similar leukoerythroblastic blood picture.

Elderly patients with agnogenic myeloid metaplasia may be severely symptomatic and require blood transfusions to treat anemia. Androgens have not shown significant benefits. Pyridoxine, 250 mg daily, has been used to increase hemoglobin. Folic acid is given for patients who develop megaloblastic changes associated with low folic acid levels.

Thrombocytosis has been associated with either bleeding or thrombosis, especially with platelet counts greater than 1,000,000/mm^3. Aspirin and other antiplatelet agents are useful therapy for the hypercoagulable state due to thrombocytosis.[38] Chemotherapy with alkylating agents such as busulfan, chlorambucil, or cyclophosphamide decreases platelets and often reduces splenic size. Hydroxyurea has been effective in reducing platelets.

Splenectomy is indicated for severe thrombocytopenia, hemolytic anemia unresponsive to medical therapy, symptoms due to massive splenomegaly, splenic infarcts, and portal hypertension with bleeding.[39] Since extramedullary hematopoiesis in the spleen is ineffective and does not contribute greatly to the peripheral blood count, removal of the spleen is not considered harmful. Early splenectomy to prevent complications is not advocated at this time.

Polycythemia vera

Polycythemia vera is regarded as a clonal proliferation of the pluripotential stem cell[40] and is distinguished by hyperplasia of the bone marrow with increased numbers of circulating erythrocytes, granulocytes, and platelets. Although the term *polycythemia* is popularly used in reference to an excessive number of red cells regardless of cause, *erythrocytosis* is a more appropriate term for such a condition, with the term *polycythemia* thereby reserved specifically for polycythemia vera. Patients with either polycythemia vera or secondary erythrocytosis have absolute erythrocytosis with an increase in red cell volume. In relative or spurious erythrocytosis, the hematocrit level is elevated but the red cell volume is normal. These people have a decreased plasma volume, often associated with cigarette smoking, obesity, and hypertension. Management is, therefore, aimed at controlling hypertension, encouraging the patient to stop smoking, and correcting the obesity. It is crucial to recognize this condition because it is frequently mistaken for polycythemia vera and therapy to reduce the red cell volume for spurious erythrocytosis is unwarranted. The red cell volume is measured with ^{51}Cr-labelled red cells. Values of greater than 36 ml/kg of body weight for men and greater than 32 ml/kg for women indicate absolute erythrocytosis. When absolute erythrocytosis has been established, the two major possibilities are polycythemia vera and erythropoietin-producing disorders (secondary) (Fig. 11-1).[41] The latter, which are several times more common than polycythemia vera, involve only erythropoiesis. This is in contrast to polycythemia vera, which involves all hematopoietic cells. However, even in polycythemia vera, erythrocytosis may be the sole finding, especially in the early stages. The erythrocytosis of polycythemia vera is autonomous and not dependent on erythropoietin (levels are low to absent). Tissue hypoxia, because of diminished blood oxygen saturation secondary to pulmonary or cardiac disorders, commonly causes secondary erythrocytosis. Cigarette smoking increases red cell volume apart from its effect in reducing plasma volume; therefore, a thorough history of cigarette smoking should be obtained before embarking on an extensive diagnostic evaluation for an increased hematocrit level. Smoking more than 1.5 packages of cigarettes per day may

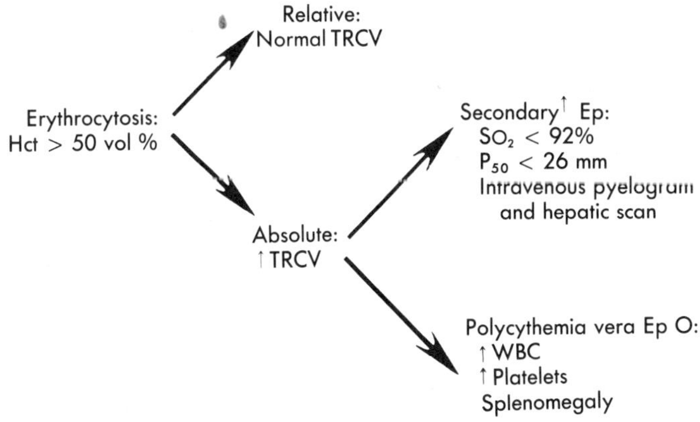

Fig. 11-1. Evaluation of erythrocytosis. *TRCV*, Total red cell volume; *EP*, Erythropoietin; SO_2, arterial blood oxygen saturation; P_{50}, partial pressure of oxygen at which hemoglobin is 50% saturated. (From Walsh, J.R.: Geriatrics **33**:61, 1978. Reprinted with permission.)

cause hematocrit elevations that return to normal with cessation of smoking. Cigarette smokers with long-term lung disease have the added effect of carboxyhemoglobin superimposed on respiratory failure for production of secondary erythrocytosis. Carboxyhemoglobin from cigarette smoking does not bind oxygen and, consequently, causes hypoxemia, which accounts for tissue hypoxia with the elaboration of erythropoietin and ultimately erythrocytosis. Less commonly, secondary erythrocytosis is due to an inappropriate increase of erythropoietin associated with renal tumors, cysts, hydronephrosis, renal parenchymal disease, and tumors of the liver (hepatoma), ovary, adrenal gland, and cerebellum.

In patients with an elevated red cell volume, secondary causes of erythrocytosis must be differentiated from polycythemia vera. Erythropoietin assays are not routinely available and, therefore, other clinical and laboratory features are substituted to make a diagnosis. Measurement of arterial oxygen saturation (SO_2) is the first logical step in evaluating erythrocytosis. Measurement of $P_{50}O_2$ (the partial pressure of oxygen at which hemoglobin is 50% saturated) is used to exclude hemoglobinopathies in which there is an increase in hemoglobin affinity for oxygen. When hypoxia has been excluded, intravenous pyelography and hepatic scans are obtained to exclude renal or hepatic lesions. A diagnosis of polycythemia vera is facilitated if the erythrocytosis is accompanied by leukocytosis, thrombocytosis, and/or the presence of splenomegaly. A leukocyte alkaline phosphatase score of greater than 100, a serum B_{12} of 900 pg/ml or unbound B_{12}-binding capacity greater than 2200 pg/ml are helpful clues in establishing a diagnosis of polycythemia vera. When erythrocytosis alone is present, the diagnosis of polycythemia vera is largely made by excluding other secondary causes of an increased red cell volume.

Phlebotomy, ^{32}P, and chemotherapy are the major modalities used for therapy of polycythemia vera. Treatment should be instituted only after a definitive diagnosis is established. Reduced cerebral blood flow with its attendant risk of thromboembolism exists with hematocrit levels above 45 volumes percent. Phlebotomy should be initiated early to reduce the hematocrit level to 45%, which accordingly increases cerebral blood flow and reduces whole blood viscosity.[42] This can be accomplished by removal of 300 to 500 ml of blood two to three times a week. Frequent phlebotomies result in iron deficiency, which suppresses red cell production; however, iron deficiency may become symptomatic and require iron replacement. For patients who undergo frequent phlebotomy or who have advanced disease or thrombocytosis, ^{32}P is the treatment of choice. After a single intravenous administration of ^{32}P, most patients have a normal blood picture in 1 to 2 months, and it remains normal for months or years. If a remission is not achieved in 3 months, the patient is retreated.

Chemotherapy with alkylating agents have been effective in treating polycythemia vera. Busulfan (Myleran), chlorambucil (Leukeran), or melphalan (Alkeran) have been used. Busulfan should be used cautiously, since it induces persistent thrombocytopenia and leukopenia, skin pigmentation, and pulmonary fibrosis. Chlorambucil is the alkylating agent that, until recently, had been recommended as the drug of choice. However, the polycythemia vera study group has reported that the incidence of acute leukemia in the chlorambucil-treated group has been higher than the phlebotomy or ^{32}P therapy.[43] It would seem, therefore, that ^{32}P is the treatment of choice for patients who cannot be controlled by phlebotomy alone. Hyperuricemia and clinical gout is treated with allopurinol, 300 to 400 mg orally per day. With control of the disease, uric acid metabolism usually returns to normal and allopurinol need not be given indefinitely.

Treatment unquestionably prolongs life, and the average life span of patients after diagnosis is approximately 10 to 12 years. Acute leukemia is a terminal complication in 10% to 15% of patients with polycythemia vera. The incidence of acute leukemia with phlebotomy is 0.7, with chlorambucil 10.6, and with ^{32}P 3.8%.[43] Patients who develop acute leukemia have an indolent preleukemic phase characterized by an evolving pancytopenia over a period of several months. This leukemia is more difficult to treat than that developing spontaneously in adult patients. Postpolycythemia myeloid metaplasia occurs as a late complication in 15% to 20% of patients with polycythemia vera.[44] It is characterized by increasing splenomegaly, a peripheral blood smear showing leukoerythroblastic features, teardrop erythrocytes, and bone marrow fibrosis. The clinical picture, course, and treatment are similar to agnogenic myeloid metaplasia.

HEMORRHAGIC DISORDERS

Thrombocytopenia

Thrombocytopenia is caused by decreased marrow platelet production or excessive platelet destruction. Reduced production occurs with marrow aplasia, leukemia, multiple myeloma, myelofibrosis, carcinoma, lymphoma, toxins, chemotherapy, ethanol, irradiation, drugs, and vitamin B_{12} or folic acid deficiencies. Increased platelet utilization or consumption occurs with disseminated intravascular coagulation. Splenic pooling associated with an enlarged spleen may cause thrombocytopenia. On the other hand, excessive platelet destruction may be on either an immune or nonimmune basis.

Immune thrombocytopenia is most commonly due to drugs, particularly thiazide diuretics, quinine, quinidine, sulfonamides, aspirin, heparin, oral hypoglycemic agents, and sedatives.[45] A careful drug history, which includes over-the-counter drugs, borrowed drugs, and home remedies, may uncover the cause of thrombocytopenia. Ingestion of gin and tonic which contains quinine should be considered. Quinine and quinidine are rapidly excreted and bleeding symptoms disappear over a period of 3 to 4 days. Idiopathic thrombocytopenia purpura (ITP) in the adult is usually a long-term disorder that initially must be differentiated from drug-induced thrombocytopenia. The latter patients quickly improve within a few weeks after medication is discontinued. ITP in the elderly may require splenectomy if glucocorticoids are ineffective.

Bleeding is rare with platelet counts above 100,000/mm^3. Hemorrhage with thrombocytopenia progressively increases as the platelet count falls below 40,000/mm^3. At levels of 10,000/mm^3 or less, bleeding is a constant threat. Platelet concentrates are administered for support of bleeding patients, but many clinicians routinely administer platelets when the platelet count falls below 20,000/mm^3.

Disseminated intravascular coagulation (DIC)

An imbalance beween blood procoagulant factors and inhibitors may result in activation of coagulation mechanisms leading to diffuse intravascular fibrin deposition with consumption of platelets and clotting factors. If fibrinolytic enzymes do not clear fibrin promptly, formation of thrombi in the microcirculation leads to ischemia of organs such as skin, kidney, and adrenal glands. Generalized bleeding is a sequela of consumption of platelets, fibrinogen, and other coagulation factors utilized in the formation of thrombi. The bleeding is usually purpuric. Among the causes of DIC in the elderly are infections, acute nonlymphocytic leukemia, hemolytic reactions, metastatic carcinoma, chemotherapy, heat stroke, and hepatic disease.

Laboratory values are conspicuously abnormal in severe DIC.[46] The most important initiating event of DIC is the conversion of prothrombin to thrombin. Thrombin activity causes consumption of fibrinogen, factors V and VIII. As a result, hypofibrinogenemia and prolonged prothrombin and partial thromboplastin times are usually seen.[46] Fibrin monomer resulting from the action of thrombin on fibrinogen produces positive protamine sulfate and ethanol gel tests.[47] Fibrinolysis leads to soluble fibrin degradation products and in 50% of cases, a prolonged thrombin time. Thrombocytopenia of varying degrees accompany coagulation defects. Fragmentation of red blood cells by fibrin strands in the microcirculation produces schistocytes or helmet cells seen on the peripheral blood smear.

Management of the underlying condition determines outcome in most cases, and the use of anticoagulants such as heparin to control the coagulopathy is often ineffective and may even increase bleeding. Treatment of the cause of DIC is, therefore, crucial. In circumstances where it is impossible to rapidly control the underlying disease, the clinician must consider replacing platelets and clotting factors by administering platelet concentrates, cryoprecipitate (to supply fibrinogen and factor VIII) and fresh frozen plasma to provide factor V.[48] Heparin should be reserved for selected patients, especially those with uncontrolled intravascular thrombosis involving the kidney or leading to cutaneous gangrene.[46] Oliguria and a rising serum creatinine level suggest the former, and heparin should be used concomitantly with replacement of depleted clotting factors and platelet infusions.[49]

REFERENCES

1. Vogel, J.M.: Hematologic problems of the aged. Mt. Sinai J. Med. **47:**150, 1980.
2. Shaver, H.J., Loper J.A., and Lutes R.A.: Nutritional status of nursing home patients, J. Parenteral Enteral. Nutr. **4:**367, 1980.
3. Finch, C.A., et al.: Iron deficiency in the rat. Physiological and biochemical studies of muscle dysfunction, J. Clin. Invest. **58:**447, 1976.
4. Ohira, Y., et al.: Work capacity, heart rate and blood lactate responses to iron therapy. Br. J. Haematol. **41:**365, 1979.
5. Lipschitz, D.A., Cook, J.D., and Finch, C.A.: A clinical evaluation of serum ferritin as an index of iron stores, N. Engl. J. Med. **290:**1212, 1974.
6. Walsh, J.R., and Fredrickson, M.: Serum ferritin; free erythrocyte protoporphyrin and urinary iron excretion in patients with iron disorders, Am. J. Med. Sci. **273:**293, 1977.
7. Disler, P.B., et al.: The effect of tea on iron absorption, Gut **16:**193, 1975.
8. Jick, H., and Porter, J.: Drug-induced gastrointestinal bleeding, Lancet **2:**87, 1978
9. Marx, J.J.M.: Normal iron absorption and decreased red cell iron uptake in the aged, Blood **53:**204, 1979.
10. Walsh, J.R., Cassel, C.K., and Madler, J.J.: Iron deficiency in the elderly: it's often nondietary, Geriatrics **36**(3):121, 1981.
11. Allen, R.H., Seetharam, B., Podell, E., and Alpers, D.H.: Effect of proteolytic enzymes on the binding of cobalamin to R protein and intrinsic factor, J. Clin. Invest. **61:**47, 1978.
12. Lindenbaum, J.: Aspects of vitamin B12 and folate metabolism in malabsorption syndromes, Am. J. Med. **67:**1037, 1979.
13. Lindenbaum, J.: Folate and vitamin B12 deficiencies in alcoholism, Semin. Hematol. **17:**119, 1980.
14. Kaunitz, J.D., and Lindenbaum, J.: The bioavailability of folic acid added to wine, Ann. Intern. Med. **87:**542, 1977.
15. Hoffbrand, A.V.: Restoring color in megaloblastic anemia, Drug Ther. **1:**167, 1975.
16. Colman, N., and Herbert, V.: Hematologic complications of alcoholism: overview, Semin. Hematol. **17:**164, 1980.
17. Hines, J.D.: Reversible megaloblastic and sideroblastic marrow abnormalities in alcoholic patients, Br. J. Haemotol. **16:**87, 1969.
18. Territo, M.C., and Tanaka, K.R.: Hypophosphatemia in chronic alcoholism, Arch. Intern. Med. **134:**445, 1974.
19. Cowan, D.H.: Effect of alcoholism on hemostasis, Semin. Hematol. **17:**137, 1980.
20. Haselager, E.M., and Vreeken, J.: Rebound thrombocytosis after alcohol abuse: a possible factor in the pathogenesis of thromboembolic disease, Lancet **1:**774, 1977.
21. Linman, J.W., and Bagby, G.C.: The preleukemic syndrome (hemopoietic dysplasia), Cancer **42:**854, 1978.
22. Koeffler, H.P., and Goldie, D.W.: Human preleukemia, Ann. Intern. Med. **93:**347, 1980.
23. Bagby, G.C., Gabourel, J.D., and Linman, J.W.: Glucocorticoid therapy in the preleukemic syndrome (hemopoietic dysplasia), Ann. Intern. Med. **92:**55, 1980.
24. Reiffers, J., Raynal, F., and Boustet, A.: Acute myeloblastic leukemia in elderly patients. Treatment and prognostic factors, Cancer **45:**2816, 1980.
25. Bloomfield, C.A.: Treatment of adult acute nonlymphocytic leukemia—1980, Ann. Intern. Med. **93:**133, 1980.
26. Richert-Boe, K.E., and Bagby, G.C.: Treating acute nonlymphocytic leukemia, Geriatrics **33**(2):50, 1978.
27. Higby, D.J., and Burnett, D.: Granulocyte transfusion: current status, Blood **55:**2, 1980.
28. Rai, K.R., et al.: Clinical staging of chronic lymphocytic leukemia, Blood **46:**219, 1975.
29. Cooper I.A., et al.: Intensive leukapheresis in the management of cytopenias in patients with chronic lymphocytic leukemia (CLL) and lymphocytic lymphoma, Am. J. Hematol. **6:**387, 1979.

30. Hobbs, J.R.: Immunocytoma O' mice an' men. Br. Med. J. **2**:67, 1971.
31. Salmon, S.E.: Expansion of growth fraction in multiple myeloma with alkylating agents, Blood **45**:119, 1975.
32. Mass, R.E.: Brief review: diagnosing and managing plasma cell (multiple) myeloma, Geriatrics **33**(7):53, 1978.
33. Mundy, G.R., et al.: Evidence for secretion of an osteoclastic stimulating factor in myeloma, N. Engl. J. Med. **291**:1041, 1974.
34. Durie, B.G., and Salmon, S.E.: A clinical staging system for multiple myeloma, Cancer **36**:842, 1975.
35. Paredes, J.M., and Mitchel, B.S.: Multiple myeloma. Current concepts in diagnosis and management, Med. Clin. North Am. **64**:729, 1980.
36. Bruckman, J.E., and Bloomer, W.D.: Management of spinal cord compression, Semin. Oncol. **5**:135, 1978.
37. Binstock, M.L., and Mundy, G.R.: Effect of calcitonin and glucocorticoids in combination on the hypercalcemia of malignancy, Ann. Intern. Med. **93**:269, 1980.
38. Wu, J.K.: Platelet hyperaggregability and thrombosis in patients with thrombocythemia, Ann. Intern. Med. **88**:7, 1978.
39. Silverstein, M.N., and Remine, W.H.: Splenectomy in myeloid metaplasia, Blood **53**:515, 1979.
40. Golde, D.W., and Cline, M.J.: Pathogenesis of polycythemia vera—new concepts, Am. J. Hematol. **1**:351, 1976.
41. Walsh, J.R.: Polycythemia vera: diagnosis, treatment and relationship to leukemia, Geriatrics **33**(5):61, 1978.
42. Pearson, T.C., and Wetherley-Mein, G.: Vascular occlusive episodes and venous hematocrit in primary proliferative polycythemia, Lancet **2**:1219, 1978.
43. Silverstein, M.N., et al.: The incidence of acute leukemia in a randomized clinical trial for polycythemia vera. Blood **54**(1):209a, 1979.
44. Silverstein, M.N.: The evolution into the treatment of late stage polycythemia vera, Semin. Hematol. **13**:79, 1976.
45. Ungaro, P.C.: Intravascular coagulation in fibrinolysis. In Hematologic diseases: new directions in therapy, ed. 2, New York, 1979, Medical Examination Publishing Co., Inc.
46. Goodnight, S.H.: Hemostatic complications in leukemic patients, Geriatrics **33**(3):53, 1978.
47. Kidder, W.R., Logan, L.J., and Rapaport, S.E.: The plasma protamine paracoagulation test: clinical and laboratory evaluation, Am. J. Clin. Pathol. **58**:675, 1972.
48. Goodnight, S.H., Kenoyer, G., and Rapaport, S.E.: Defibrination after brain-tissue destruction: a serious complication of head injury, N. Engl. J. Med. **290**:1043, 1974.
49. Penner, J.A.: Hypercoagulation and thrombosis, Med. Clin. North Am. **64**:743, 1980.

CHAPTER 12 · DERMATOLOGIC DISORDERS

Arnold W. Gurevitch

Advancing years place special and ever-increasing burdens on the skin. With the passage of time, the skin reacts in a relatively predictable fashion.[1-3] The skin surface often becomes dry and develops fine cracks and scale. In addition, the color of the skin changes, with the occurrence of mottled erythema and hyperpigmentation. The epidermis becomes thinner, and the dermis not only thins but also has less turgor and elasticity, resulting in the fine wrinkling of aged skin.[4] The subcutaneous fatty layer also decreases in thickness. This combination of dermal and subcutaneous changes causes a more flaccid and superfluous skin, which lies in coarse folds over the underlying muscular and bony structures. The result is the typical changes in facial contour that we associate with age. Other common age-related changes include hyperpigmentation and hypopigmentation of the skin, especially on sun-exposed areas. Coarse hairs become more prominent on the face, especially on areas such as the nose, ears, upper lip, chin, and eyebrows. Sebaceous gland function declines in elderly women, while remaining quite high in men. However, in both men and women apocrine glands atrophy and eccrine sweating also declines.

To a great extent, society's perception of a person's age depends on the changes in skin appearance outlined above. However, the onset of these aging changes is somewhat unpredictable. Therefore, certain individuals may look significantly older, or younger, than their true years. There are two major interrelated factors involved in the aging of the skin:

1. *Environmental factors*. Of these, sunlight is by far the most significant. The sun exposed skin of our faces and forearms "ages" vastly more rapidly than does the skin of the buttocks. Other environmental conditions, such as chronic exposure to wind, may also play a role.
2. *Heredity*. The most important hereditary factor is skin color and response to sunlight. However, even on non–sun exposed skin, there are familial aging patterns.

The aging of skin, in addition to its cosmetic and psychologic significance, is also related to a variety of pathologic states. The incidence of skin disease is directly related to age, with prevalence rates for skin disease as a whole being lowest for children and reaching a maximum in the 65 to 74-year-old age group. The elderly patient can have an amazing number of dermatologic ills, many of which, however, occur equally or even more frequently in other age groups. This chapter will deal specifically only with those problems that have their greatest incidence in the elderly or that present special and significant problems in this age group.

PRURITUS AND DRY SKIN

Itching is the most common dermatologic complaint of the elderly. In the absence of a primary skin disease, itching is usually felt to be due to dry skin (asteatosis, xerosis).[5] This type of itching may be localized, especially to the legs, but it is often widespread and intense. The thinned horny layer in aged skin is able to retain less water. In addition there may be less sebaceous secretion and less sweat, resulting in dry, scaly skin that reacts with an itch response to a variety of often minor stimuli. Environmental factors, especially low relative humidity and cool air, contribute to dehydration of the horny layer.[6] Examples of important environmental situations of this type are the overheated cold dry air found in the northern United States in the

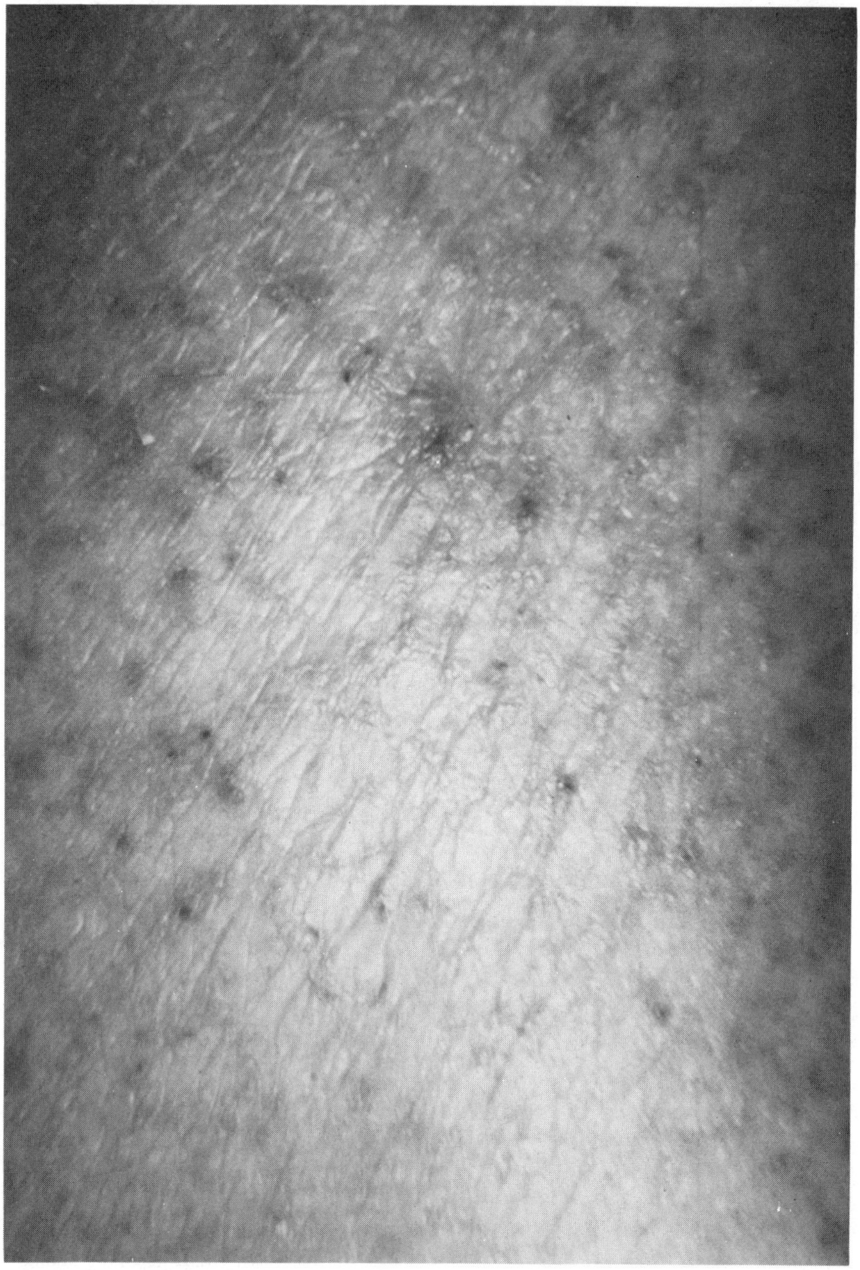

Fig. 12-1. Typical superficially fissured dry skin of asteatotic eczema (eczema craquelé).

winter; dry, cold, windy environments; and air-conditioned summer desert air. Asteatotic pruritus is so prevalent where there are dry, cold winters that it is commonly called "winter itch." An additional major factor in overdrying the skin is excessive bathing, especially with hot water and strong, drying soaps. Furthermore, some patients use various drying topical preparations, such as rubbing alcohol, for minor cutaneous problems. In this over-dried skin, itching may be triggered by such a minimal stimulus as undressing, possibly via a sudden temperature change or the passage of cool air across the roughened, dehydrated horny layer.

Pruritus of this sort may show itself only as excoriations on a background of dry skin. However, after an extended period of itching, scratching, rubbing, and more itching, a dermatitis may develop. Poorly defined areas of scaly erythema often occur on the lateral aspect of the legs and less commonly on the arms. At times there is a characteristic superficial cracking through the stratum corneum, which gives a netlike arrangement of erythematous or hemorrhagic fissures (eczema craquelé, asteatotic eczema) (Fig. 12-1).

Although pruritus in the elderly is usually due to dry skin, it also may occur in its absence. In essential or primary pruritus, with no diagnostic underlying skin disorder, certain systemic diseases must be considered. Hyperthyroidism, hepatobiliary disease, renal disease, lymphomas, drug allergy, and parasitic infestations have all been associated with generalized pruritus. However, some elderly patients have severe pruritus and no other related conditions, either cutaneous or systemic. This entity has been termed *senile pruritus*. Psychologic factors may be operative, but the true pathophysiology of senile pruritus remains unknown.[1] These patients usually do not respond to the regimen utilized for asteatosis, nor are they well controlled by systemic antihistamines.

Localized pruritus, with a resulting dermatitis, is also a relatively common problem. In addition to the lower legs, the most comon sites for this disturbing situation are the genital and perianal areas.[3,5] A variety of factors may be operative in pruritus ani, scroti, or vulvae. Excessive dryness of the skin may play a role in some cases. In others, poor hygiene, increased secretions from anal crypts, hemorrhoidal tags that trap stool and anal discharge, an incompetent sphincter, or vaginal infection or discharge may be important. Burning and itching can even develop in the anal canal from strong food seasoning present in the feces. Other exacerbating factors include the use of rough toilet paper, frequent enemas or excesive use of laxatives, and the wearing of tight-fitting, nonabsorbent undergarments.

The most important aspect of the treatment of dry, itchy skin is to decrease the frequency and duration of bathing and to avoid hot water and strong soaps. Patients are advised to take short, lukewarm baths or showers, no more than once daily. In more severe cases, even fewer baths are advisable. The use of a mild soap, such as Dove, is recommended. A bath oil can be used in the tub, but if the patient is elderly and infirm it is advisable that there be another person present to assist in order to prevent slipping. If the patient prefers showers, the bath oil can be applied with a damp wash cloth immediately after showering, following which the skin is patted dry. Emollient creams or lotions may be used during the day or night, but irritating or sensitizing topical preparations should not be applied. The patient is also advised to wear loose, permeable clothing and to avoid direct contact with wool. If possible, the temperature and humidity should both be in the moderate range. A systemic antipruritic agent, such as hydroxyzine, is often helpful along with the aforementioned program. Occasionally, mood elevators may bring relief. Reassurance and psychologic support are valuable additional measures, especially if anxiety or depression seems to be a factor. For local itching, a cool compress or ice bag may be useful. If the dry skin has become eczematized (asteatotic eczema), a mild topical corticosteroid, such as 1% hydrocortisone cream, is beneficial. Hydrocortisone cream may also be used for pruritus ani or vulvae.

DERMATITIS

Nummular dermatitis

In nummular dermatitis, discrete erythematous, coin-shaped eczematous patches occur, especially on the legs, but also on the arms, dorsum of the hands, and trunk[7] (Fig. 12-2). In lesions that have recently appeared, there are often tiny vesicles on the surface of an edematous, crusted patch. Later the lesions are more scaly and become thickened. These pruritic lesions occur more often in men and have a peak incidence in the 55 to 65-year-old age group. Some patients have only one or at most a very few such patches, although extensive nummular eruptions may also occur. Lesions usually come and go spontaneously, but they tend to be a chronic and recurrent problem. Although the etiology of nummular dermatitis is not known, many patients do have an associated dry skin. Exacerbations are more common in winter and can be brought on by wool clothing, strong soaps, and excessive bathing. The management of patients with this problem, in addition to therapy directed at the associated dry skin, includes the use of a topical steroid cream or ointment, usually applied three times a day. A systemic antihistaminic agent is also helpful to control the

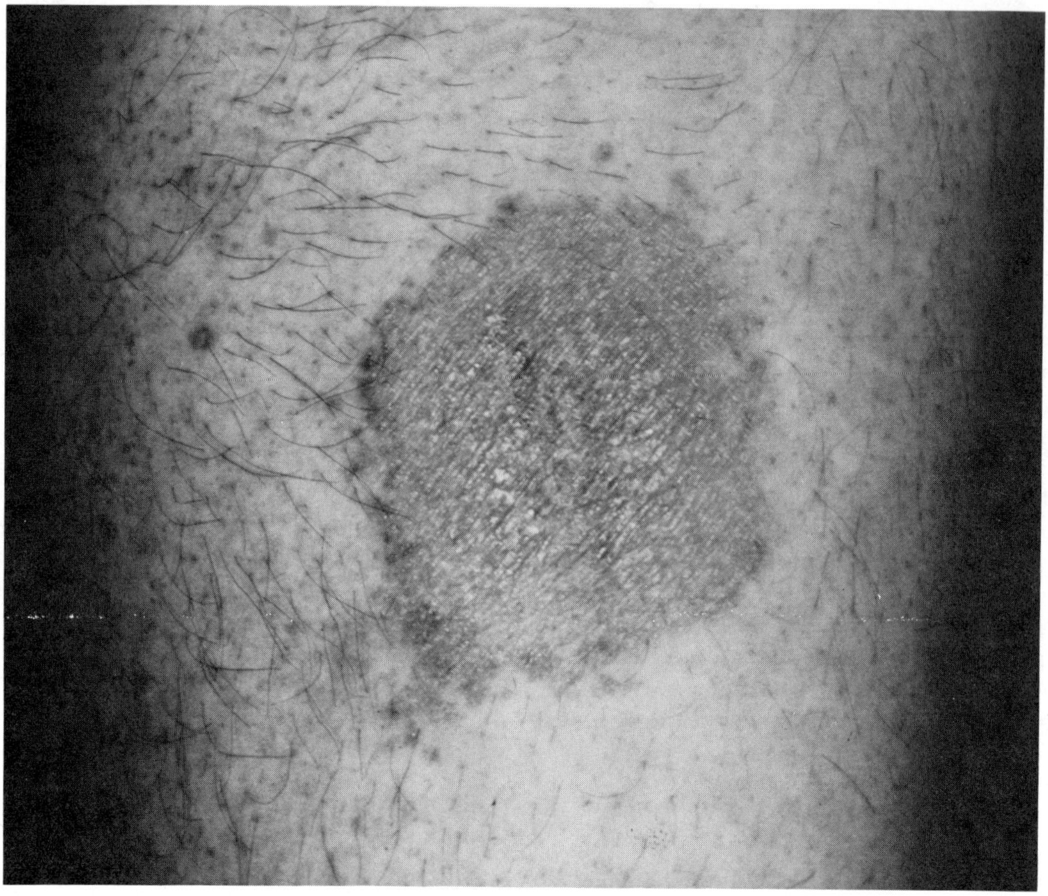

Fig. 12-2. Round erythematous scaly patch of nummular dermatitis.

pruritus. In cases with severe, extensive involvement, use of a systemic corticosteroid agent may be necessary for initial control. Prednisone, in a dosage of 30 to 40 mg per day for 1 to 3 weeks, is often effective, although sometimes only temporarily.

Stasis dermatitis

Stasis dermatitis occurs on the lower legs and ankles and is secondary to the edema of chronic peripheral venous disease.[3] Varicose veins are usually evident, and there is often a history of thrombophlebitis. The eruption begins as an erythematous, scaly, sometimes weeping patch, most often above the medial malleolus. It can spread around the entire lower leg and may be unilateral or bilateral (Fig. 12-3). With time, secondary pigmentation occurs in the involved area and a stasis ulcer may even result. Treatment is directed chiefly toward reduction of the edema by such measures as elevation of the leg, supportive elastic bandages or hose, gelocast dressing or Jobst stockings. In the initial stages, rest and elevation of the leg are of critical importance, whereas the various forms of pressure stockings or dressings are more useful in preventing recurrence. At times the dermatitis is markedly exudative, in which case wet compresses or soaks are helpful. A topical steroid will help decrease the pruritus and inflammation.

Intertrigo

Intertrigo is a dermatitis of an intertriginous area due to local factors such as heat, moisture, and rubbing of skin surfaces.[3] It occurs in the groin, axillae, intergluteal cleft, and inframammary area and in the abdominal skin folds of the obese patient. Initially, the involved skin becomes red and macerated and may ultimately become superficially eroded. In these circumstances, the local bacterial and fungal flora can

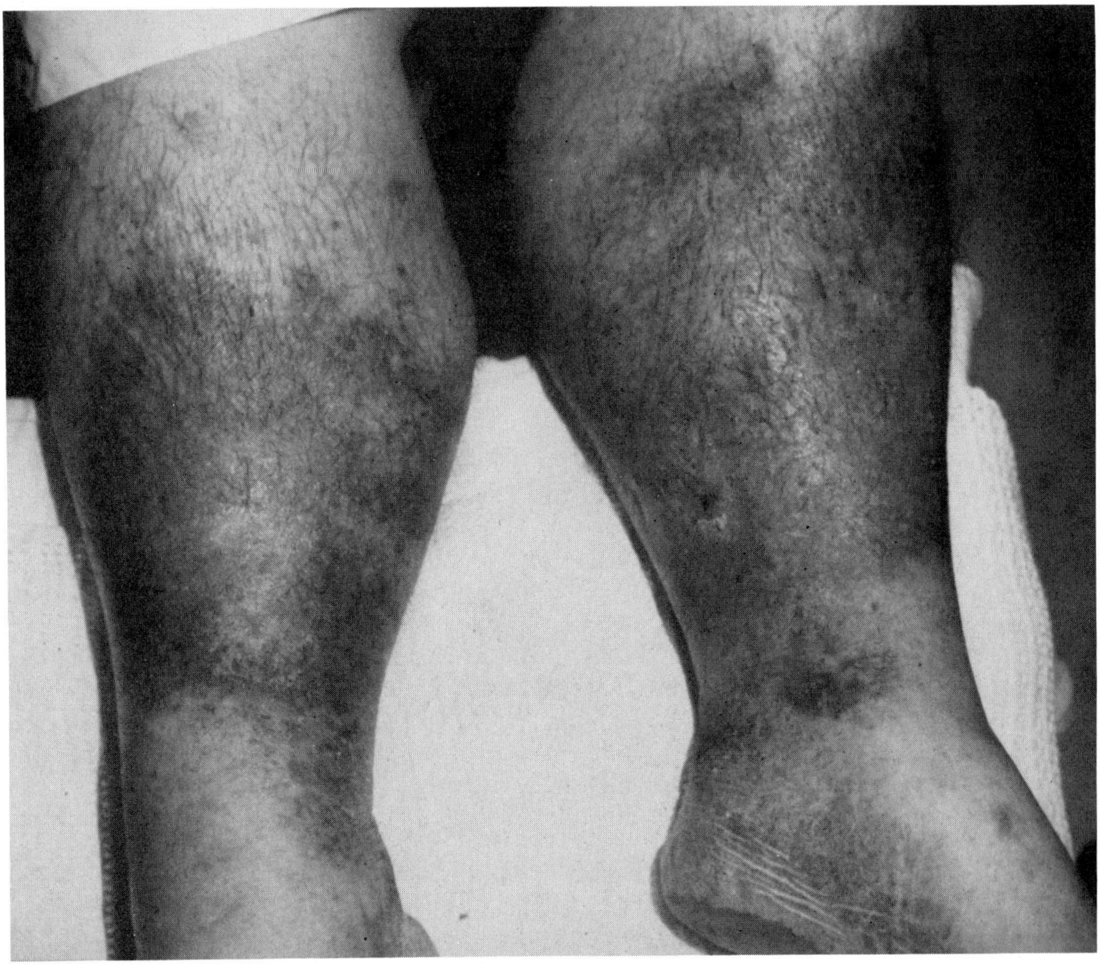

Fig. 12-3. Stasis dermatitis, demonstrating erythema, hyperpigmentation, scaling, and crusting involving the lower legs.

grow luxuriantly, and secondary infection is common, especially with *Candida albicans*. Thorough cleansing and drying of the involved areas at least once or twice a day are essential in treatment. The skin folds should be kept separated as much as possible, and a cool environment and loose fitting clothing may also be helpful. One percent hydrocortisone cream, applied 2 to 3 times per day, reduces the inflammation and pruritus. Since *C. albicans*, as well as various bacteria, is often present, a cream containing a combination of 1% hydrocortisone with 3% iodochlorhydroxyquin (Vioform) may be even more effective. After rubbing the cream in thoroughly, the patient is instructed to liberally apply a topical powder to coat the opposing surfaces and absorb excess moisture and thus to prevent maceration.

Angular cheilitis

Angular cheilitis, or perlèche, is essentially an intertrigo at the corners of the mouth. There is redness and maceration, which usually leads to fissuring and occasionally to ulceration. The skin is involved, but usually not the buccal mucosa. Secondary infection, chiefly from *C. albicans*, is quite common.[1] Although certain vitamin deficiencies can cause angular cheilitis, most cases are not due to hypovitaminosis. The basic cause is an anatomic change involving the face and the mouth. With age, the skin becomes more lax and folded, with a deepening furrow at the angles of the mouth. In patients who have worn down teeth or ill-fitting dentures, or who are edentulous, the upper lip tends to override the lower, thus accentuating the furrow. Saliva and food collect and an intertrigo develops.[5] Drooling at night and licking the area are aggravating factors. Mild cases can often be managed by faithful use of Mycolog ointment or 1% hydrocortisone with 3% iodochlorhydroxyquin (Vioform) cream. The patient is also advised to avoid licking the area. In severe or recurrent cases, cure will depend on correction of the dental problem and return of the facial contours to normal.

Generalized exfoliative dermatitis

By definition, this is a dermatitis that involves all, or nearly all, of the skin surface. There are varying degrees of erythema and scaling, often with crusting and oozing. Elderly persons are especially prone to develop this problem, which can evolve from a variety of preexisting dermatoses.[1] Although atopic dermatitis, psoriasis, seborrheic dermatitis, stasis dermatitis, and contact dermatitis can eventuate into a generalized eruption, a great many of these cases, especially in the elderly population, are idiopathic. However, approximately 10% of patients with this disorder have an underlying malignancy, usually in the leukemia or lymphoma group. In addition to the problems associated with the extensive dermatitis itself, these patients are susceptible to secondary bacterial infection of the involved skin. Other secondary problems include loss of protein from the skin, fluid and electrolyte imbalance, chills, weakness, and alopecia. In patients with preexisting cardiac disease, cardiac failure may rarely occur.

Treatment is basically the same as for other eczematous eruptions. Daily baths, especially with a bath oil, are usually beneficial, as is persistent use of a topical corticosteroid cream. Systemic antihistamines help control the accompanying pruritus. In addition, fluid and electrolyte levels should be monitored carefully and the patient maintained in an environment of both moderate temperature and humidity. The physician must be alert to the development of a secondary bacterial infection of the skin and treat it rapidly. If the above measures fail to give adequate improvement, or if the case is very severe, systemic steroids in a dosage of 30 to 60 mg of prednisone per day may be necessary.

BENIGN TUMORS

Skin tags

Skin tags, which are also known as *acrochordons* or *fibroepithelial polyps*, are small (1 to 5 mm) soft, pedunculated papules. The surface may be either smooth or irregular, and their color varies from skin-colored to brown. Skin tags are asymptomatic unless the pedicle twists and infarction occurs. They appear very commonly after middle life, especially in women. Sites of predilection are the neck, axillae, eyelids, and upper trunk.[1] Some patients want them removed because of their appearance. They can easily be snipped off with a curved iris scissors. In some cases, multiple lesions may be removed by liquid nitrogen application or electrodesiccation.

Seborrheic keratosis

Seborrheic keratoses usually begin in middle life on both exposed and unexposed areas of skin. Classically, they present as irregularly round or oval, flat-topped, well-demarcated plaques, which look as though they have been "stuck on" the skin[2] (Fig. 12-4). The surface is usually verrucous, but some are smooth, and the color can vary from skin-colored to tan, brown, or even black. Often there are many such lesions, most commonly on the upper part of the trunk or on the face. Large, dark seborrheic keratoses, especially those on visible areas, may be of concern to patients. If the diagnosis is in doubt, a shave biopsy followed by electrodesiccation will be curative. If the patient wishes one or a few lesions removed, a simple technique is electrodesiccation following injection of a local anesthetic. The desiccated material is then easily curetted off. An alternate approach, especially useful for multiple lesions, is cryotherapy utilizing liquid nitrogen.

Sebaceous hyperplasia

These are small (2 to 5 mm) slightly yellowish papules, which often have a central depression from which sebum may be expressed (Fig. 12-5). They are most common after about 40 years of age and occur especially on the forehead and cheeks. Lesions may be single or multiple and represent a cluster of enlarged sebaceous glands around a central duct. Occasionally a large lesion of sebaceous hyperplasia resembles early basal cell carcinoma, and biopsy must be undertaken for exact diagnosis.[2] Otherwise, removal of these lesions is for cosmetic reasons only. Shave excision followed by light electrodesiccation, or liquid nitrogen cryotherapy, is the most common procedure.

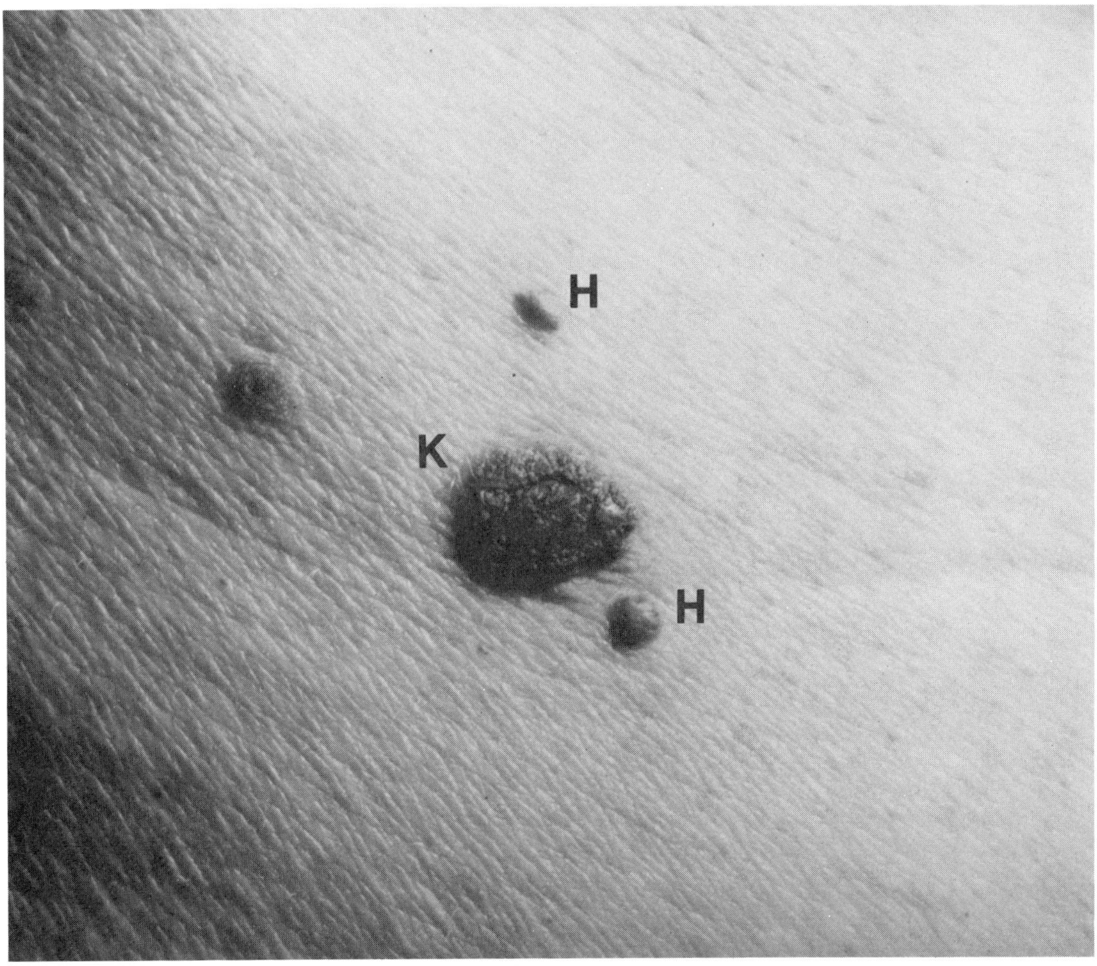

Fig. 12-4. A markedly hyperpigmented, verrucous, "stuck-on" appearing seborrheic keratosis (*K*). Nearby are two small cherry hemangiomas (*H*).

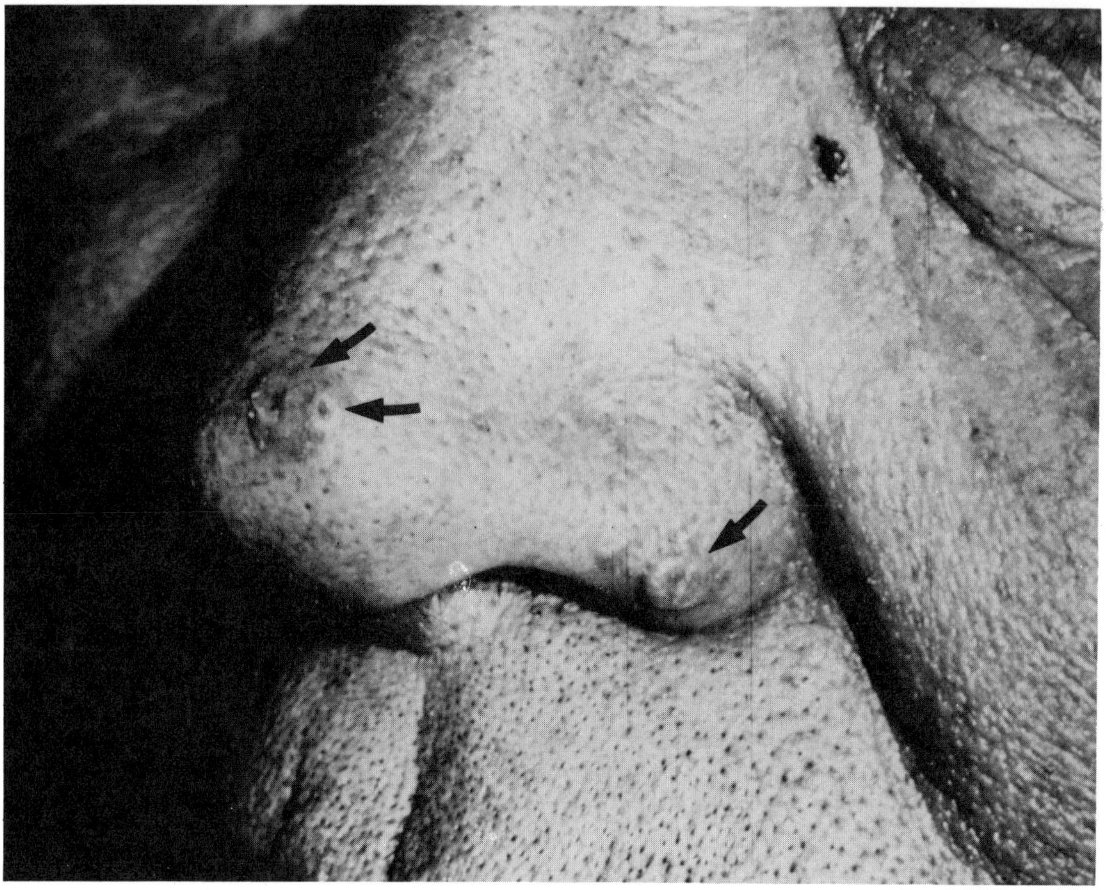

Fig. 12-5. Three umbilicated papules of sebaceous hyperplasia (arrows).

VASCULAR LESIONS

Cherry hemangioma

These small bright red papules are also called *senile angiomas, cherry spots*, or *De Morgan's spots*[3] (Fig. 12-4). They vary from one to several millimeters in size and are often numerous, especially on the upper trunk and forehead. Although occasionally found on young adults, they tend to increase in number and size with advancing age. Treatment is not necessary, but for cosmetic reasons they may be removed by electrodesiccation or freezing with liquid nitrogen.

Venous lake

A venous lake, or varix, is a dark blue vascular nodule that may be emptied with pressure. It is usually small and irregularly shaped, often seen on the face and ears, and may resemble a blood blister. Occasionally such a lesion will thrombose and involute spontaneously but most persist indefinitely. Treatment is not usually indicated, although small lesions can be removed by electrosurgery.[3]

Angiokeratoma of Fordyce

Angiokeratomas of Fordyce are small red to purple keratotic papules that occur on the scrotum and less often on the vulva. They are quite common in elderly men, although they may arise during middle age. Occasionally such lesions can also be seen on the penile shaft, lower abdomen, and inner thighs. These angiokeratomas are asymptomatic and removal is not required.

INFECTIONS AND INFESTATIONS

Herpes zoster

This viral infection consists of grouped vesicles on an erythematous base occuring in a unilateral dermatomal distribution. The vesicular eruption is often preceded for up to 1 week by a tingling, stinging, or painful sensation in the area. The eruption itself can progress for about 1 week, with new groups of vesicles occurring in crops. The vesicles will often become pustular within a few days of development and then heal during a 1- to 2-week period. The involved area of skin remains hyperesthetic during the active stage of the infection, and this may be a helpful clinical sign if the diagnosis is not clear-cut. C_2 and L_2 are the most commonly involved dermatomes, but infection in the areas of the fifth and seventh cranial nerves also are frequent. Any dermatome may be involved.

Although herpes zoster can occur from childhood through old age, its incidence rises with age and it presents special problems in the elderly. Generally the skin lesions tend to be more necrotic in the elderly, resulting in greater scarring. Even more important, the eruption itself is more painful in older patients, and this pain can persist for weeks to months after the healing of the skin lesions.[1] Postherpetic neuralgia occurs chiefly in persons over the age of 50, with an attack rate of almost 20% in the 50- to 59-year old age group and of almost 50% in patients above the age of 70.

The vesicular stage of herpes zoster may be treated with cool compresses, using Burow's solution for its drying and debriding effect. If the eruption is severely crusted or secondarily infected, a topical antibiotic ointment may be used. Analgesics should be given as needed for control of pain. In patients above the age of 55, it may be worthwhile to attempt to prevent the development of postherpetic neuralgia by a relatively short course of systemic corticosteroids. Sixty milligrams of prednisone is given daily for 5 to 7 days, followed by 30 mg daily for 5 to 7 days, and then 15 mg daily for the third such period. To be effective, this treatment program must be initiated within 5 days of onset of the eruption. It will have no effect on the healing time of the zoster lesions and does not cause an increased incidence of disseminated zoster. If postherpetic neuralgia does develop, there are reports of successful treatment using intralesional or subcutaneous injections of triamcinolone, oral tricyclic antidepressants in combination with either perphenazine (Trilafon) or thioridazine (Mellaril), or chlorprothixene (Taractan) given either intramuscularly or orally. However, in some patients the pain persists and requires surgical or chemical destruction of the nerve.

Pediculosis corporis

Body lice most commonly occur on persons living in crowded unhygienic conditions or in those with poor personal hygiene habits. It is often called *vagabonds' disease* because it is so often seen in single men, often elderly, who have no permanent residence and inhabit "skid row" areas of the city. Currently, most cases are seen in public hospitals. Both the adult body lice and the nits may be found on the seams of clothing, epecially around the collar, waistline, and armpits. Transmission occurs through infested clothing or bedding. Clinically, the initial lesion is a hemorrhagic or erythematous macule or papule at the site of the bite. Because of severe pruritus, many linear excoriations are soon seen, and they may become crusted and secondarily infected. With persistence, hyperpigmentation often occurs. Therapy includes a cleansing bath and a change to clean clothing and bedding. Lice are rarely found on the body, so treatment of the skin may not be necessary. However, one application of gamma benzene hexachloride lotion to the entire cutaneous surface, followed in 12 hours by another bath, is often recommended. Infested clothing should be laundered, boiled, or dry cleaned. If the patient's skin is markedly eczematized, a topical corticosteroid may be used as in the eczematous dermatoses, together with a systemic antihistaminic for control of pruritus.

Scabies

Among the elderly, scabies is most often seen in patients confined to nursing homes. The causative mite is usually transmitted by close person-to-person contact. However, in a nursing home, contaminated bedding is probably the major factor. In these patients the lesions, which can vary from few to hundreds, are usually on areas in contact with the sheets. The initial lesion is a tiny blister on an erythematous base, adjacent to which a short, wavy line, the burrow, may occasionally be seen. Pruritus is severe, usually worse at night, and the vesicles are often scratched rapidly, appearing as small crusted papules. Secondary eczematization and bacterial infection may occur. Diagnosis is suggested when a typical eruption occurs in a living environment in which there are other cases. One should attempt to prove the diagnosis by identifying the mite on direct skin scrapings from lesions. Treatment involves application of a scabicide, commonly gamma benzene hexachloride lotion, to the entire trunk and extremities from the neck down. This medication is left on for 12 hours and then washed off in a bath. One application is usually adequate, although a second treatment after 1 week is often recommended. Fresh clothing and bedding should be used after the first application. All persons who have had contact with the patient's skin or bedding should probably be treated at the same time. Oral antipruritic agents may be helpful, and severely eczematized skin may be treated with topical corticosteroids following completion of the first course of scabicidal therapy.

SUN-RELATED DERMATOSES AND TUMORS

Those visible skin changes that are popularly associated with aging are, in fact, more closely related to sun exposure. How old we look has more to do with a combination of our genetically determined skin color plus total sun exposure than it does with age in years alone. As a result, darker skinned people tend to look younger than fair-skinned Caucasians of the same chronological age. Some cutaneous changes, such as laxity, wrinkling, and yellowing, can occur from aging itself. However, these changes are highly exaggerated and hastened on areas of skin exposed to excessive sunshine. Other alterations, such as the mottled and irregular pigmentation of sun-exposed skin, do not occur on unexposed sites.

Solar elastosis

Solar elastosis is seen histologically as degeneration of the collagen fibers in the upper dermis. Clinically, sun-damaged skin is leathery, lax, and wrinkled, with an increase in skin markings.[2] These changes tend to be most striking on the back of the neck. The term "farmer's and sailor's skin" has been used to describe severe solar changes occurring in fair skinned persons. These alterations can probably be prevented by avoidance of the sun and routine use of a sunscreen beginning at a relatively early age. However, once solar elastosis occurs, it will remain. In very severe cases, a dermabrasion may be indicated to remove most of the damaged dermis, along with the accompanying epidermal changes. This is usually done to help prevent the development of premalignant and malignant skin lesions, which almost always occur on a background of solar elastosis. In some individuals, especially elderly men, the sun-damaged skin of the face may develop a yellowish irregularly nodular thickening with many comedones and small cysts. This is known as *senile comedones*, or nodular elastosis with cysts and comedones (Favre-Racouchot syndrome), and occurs most commonly in the periorbital areas. Removal of these unsightly lesions is best accomplished by a combination of topical retinoic acid plus incision and expression of the comedones.

Another common clinical problem related to solar elastosis is *senile purpura* (solar or Bateman's purpura). Irregular areas of ecchymosis occur on the backs of the hands and forearms after minimal trauma.[3] Hyperpigmentation usually develops when the ecchymoses resolve. In some people with senile purpura, there are also white, irregular scarlike lesions on the backs of the arms. Often these white areas are stellate or linear and have been termed *spontaneous stellate pseudoscars*.[8] Basically, both senile purpura and spontaneous stellate pseudoscars are due to sun-induced fragility of the skin. In the latter condition, superficial well-marginated ulcerations occur first after mild trauma. The ulcerations heal leaving the characteristic white scars.

Solar lentigo (senile lentigo, liver spots)

These sharply circumscribed, light brown flat spots occcur on sun-exposed areas in over one half of light-skinned persons above the age of 45 years. Most are seen on the backs of the hands and arms and also on the forehead and cheeks (Figs. 12-6 and 12-7). The color is uniform and can vary from light tan to very dark brown. These lesions do not fade when no longer exposed to the sun. The average solar lentigo is about 0.5 cm in diameter, but occasionally they can reach several cm. These are benign lesions of cosmetic significance only. If removal is desired, a light or gentle freezing with liquid nitrogen is the easiest method. Bleaching creams are of no benefit.

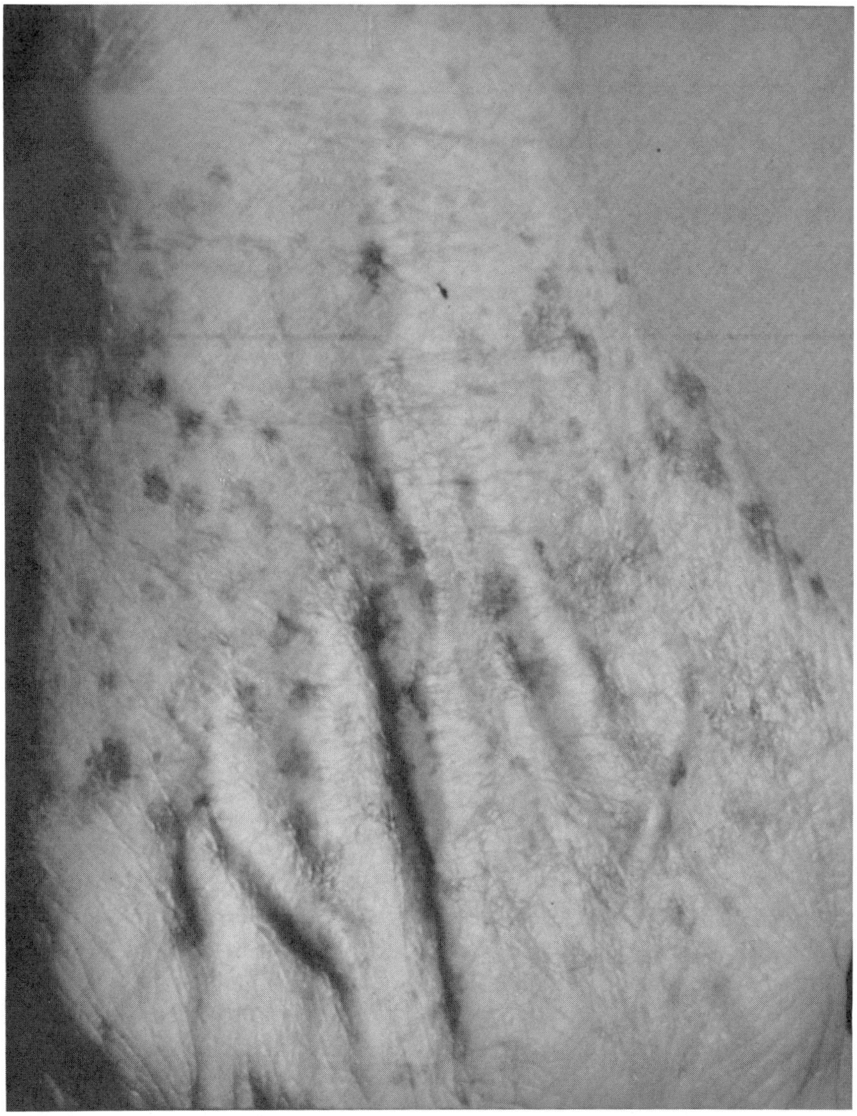

Fig. 12-6. Multiple flat brown solar lentigines on sun-damaged skin of the back of the hand.

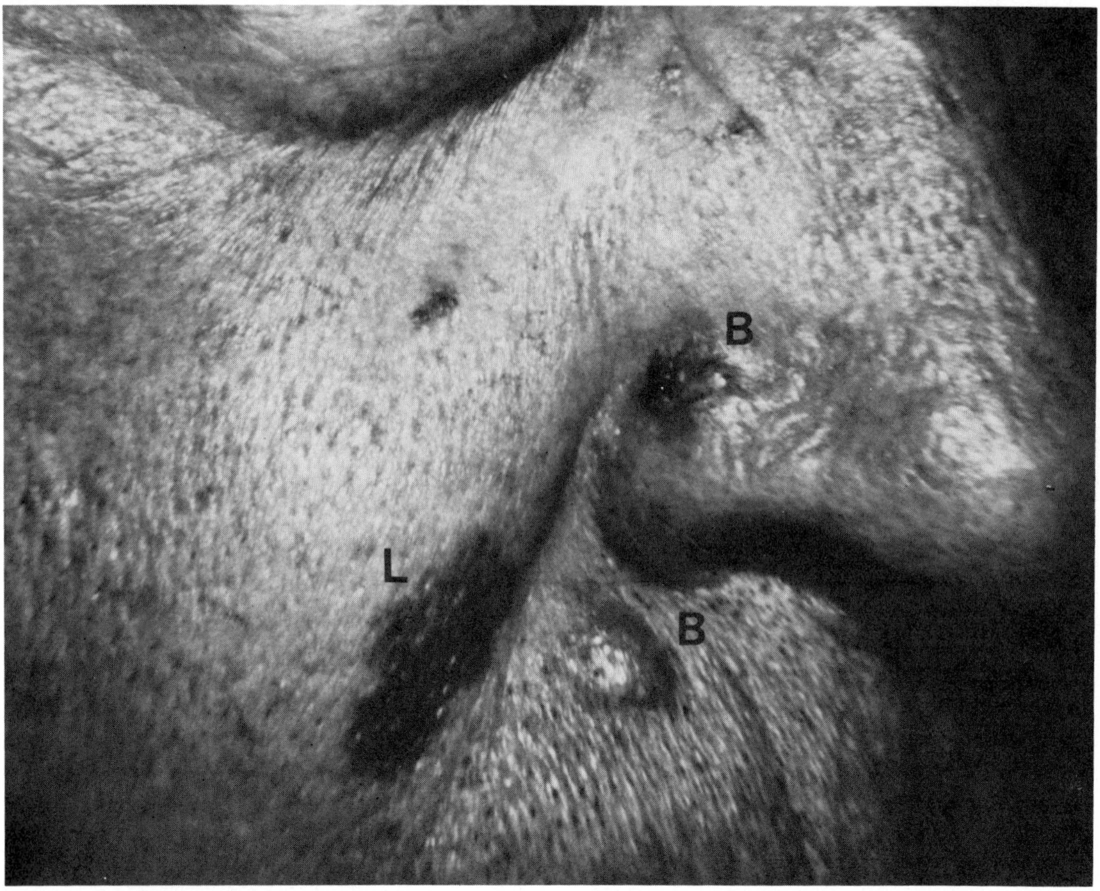

Fig. 12-7. Two basal cell carcinomas (*B*), the upper of which is crusted. At the lower left is a solar lentigo (*L*).

Lentigo maligna

Lentigo maligna is essentially a form of in situ (intraepidermal) melanoma. If it invades into the dermis, it becomes a lentigo maligna melanoma. Lentigo maligna itself somewhat resembles a routine solar lentigo. It is also a flat hyperpigmented spot primarily on the sun-exposed skin of elderly people. It begins as a small, flat, tan, frecklelike spot, which then enlarges. As it enlarges it develops variations in color, chiefly gradations of tan to dark brown, often with speckling or stippling (Fig. 12-8). There may be reticulated dark areas in a tan background. This variability in color helps distinguish the lentigo maligna clinically from the more uniformly pigmented solar lentigo. Definitive diagnosis, however, requires a biopsy. A lentigo maligna should be removed by simple excision.

Lentigo maligna melanoma

When a lentigo maligna develops irregular thickening or nodularity, it usually signifies progression to an invasive melanoma. The flat areas of a lentigo maligna melanoma can vary in color from tan to brown or black, and at times there are blue or gray and white areas intermingled.[9] The nodular areas are usually dark brown to black. The lesions are often quite large, up to 3 to 6 cm in diameter. Treatment is basically surgical, dependent to a great extent on the depth of invasion of the tumor. Level II lesions, which extend down into the papillary dermis, may be excised with a 1-cm margin beyond the clinically visible edge of the lesion. Tumors that invade more deeply are excised more radically, with margins from 2 to 3 cm when possible.

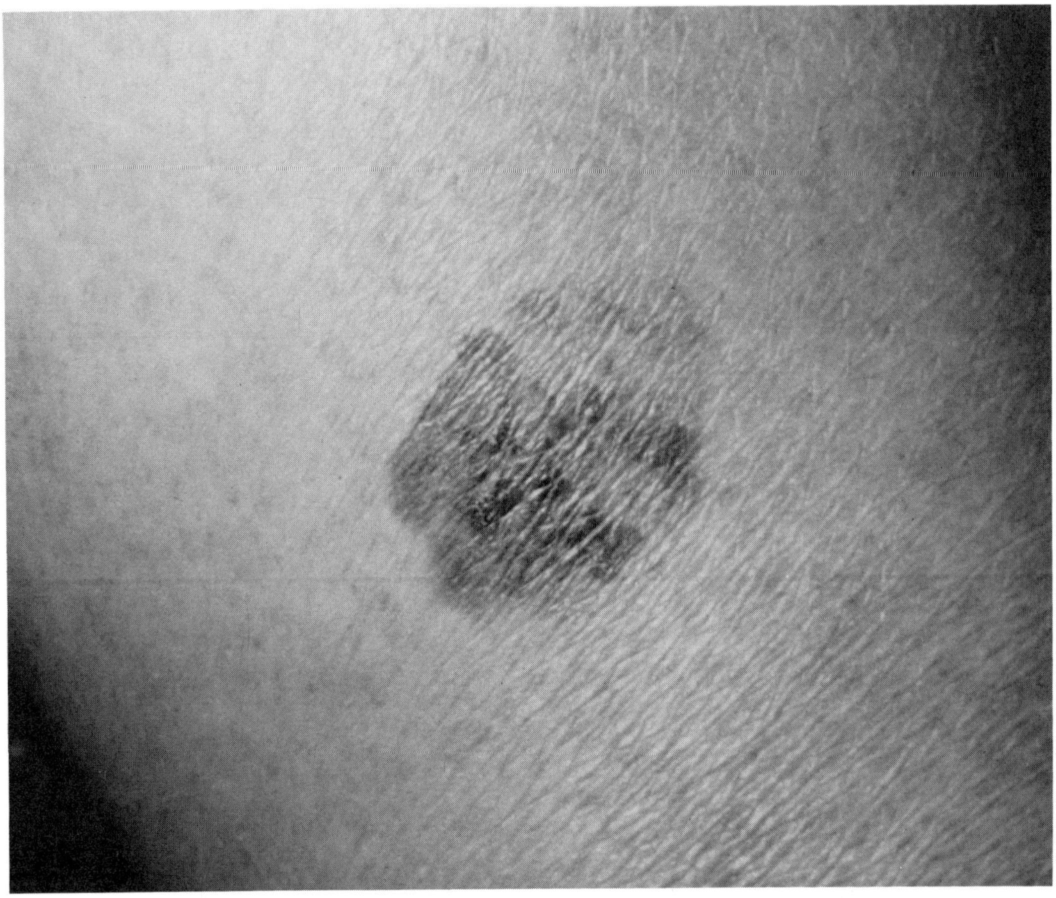

Fig. 12-8. A flat, irregularly pigmented, well-demarcated lentigo maligna with a notched border.

Solar keratosis

Solar (senile, actinic) keratoses are the most common premalignant lesion of the skin.[10] Most can be found on the dorsum of the hands and arms, rims of the ears, neck, and face. Occasionally there is a single lesion, but more often they are multiple. Clinically, the solar keratosis is a flat to slightly raised erythematous lesion, usually less than 1 cm in diameter (Fig. 12-9), with an irregular roughened keratotic surface. Sometimes they are more easily felt than seen. Occasionally they can be skin-colored or even tan. The surrounding skin usually shows the previously described features of chronic sun damage. A solar keratosis can usually be diagnosed clinically, but, if it is large or atypical, a biopsy should be done. Thickening of the base below the keratotic surface suggests progression into a skin cancer, which will occur in approximately 20% of persons with solar keratoses.

Solar keratoses may be removed by any one of a number of techniques involving superficial destruction of the skin. The most popular form of therapy, especially for multiple lesions, is cryotherapy using liquid nitrogen. Similar results can be achieved by the application of trichloroacetic acid, 50% concentration or greater, or by shave excision or curettage, followed by light electrodesiccation. Topical 5-fluorouracil (5-FU) is quite helpful for multiple lesions, especially on the face. 5-FU is generally applied as a 1% or 2% solution or cream to the face and in a 5% concentration to the arms and hands twice daily until a brisk inflammatory reaction occurs at the sites of lesions. Treatment time for the face is usually 2 to 3 weeks, whereas 3 to 6

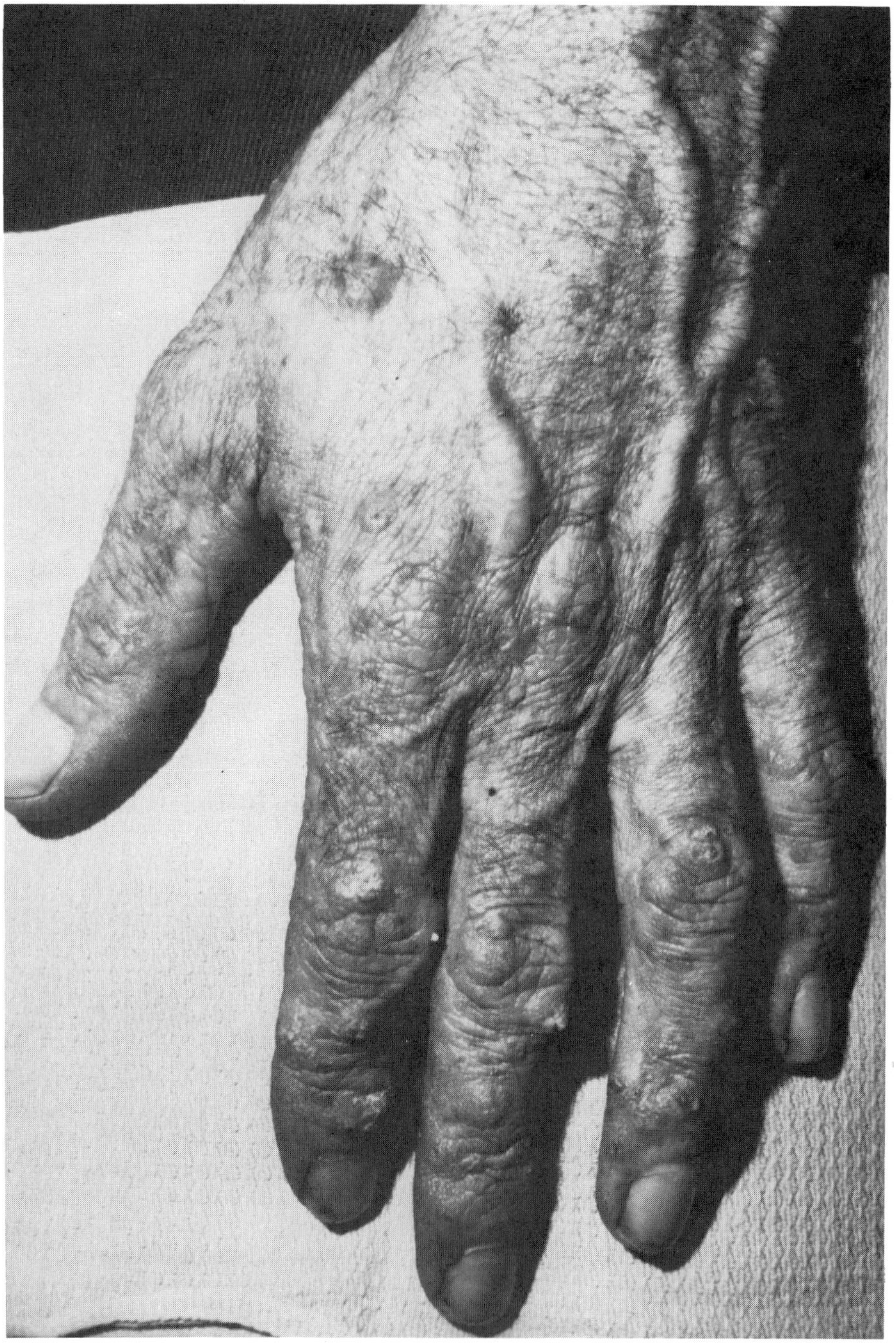

Fig. 12-9. Multiple solar keratoses on the dorsum of the hand.

weeks are required for the hands and arms. In patients with severely sun-damaged skin and multiple actinic keratoses of the face, a dermabrasion may be indicated. Topical 5-FU and dermabrasion not only remove the visible keratoses but also decrease the number of new lesions to develop in the treated area. Patients with solar keratoses should also be advised to avoid the sun, especially between the hours of 10:00 AM and 4:00 PM, to wear protective clothing, and to use an effective sunscreen.

Basal cell carcinoma

Basal cell carcinomas (epitheliomas) are far and away the most common form of skin cancer. Usually one lesion occurs at a time and most often on the face. Other areas of hair-bearing skin that are chronically exposed to sunlight may also develop these tumors. The basal cell carcinoma is slow growing and locally invasive with little tendency to metastasize. Clinically, the most common type of basal cell carcinoma begins as a small, smooth, rounded, pearly or waxy-looking papule with telangiectatic vessels on its surface[10] (Fig. 12-7). A central depression, surrounded by a pearly, rolled border, usually develops. These tumors tend to bleed easily with minimal trauma due to their marked friability. When the central area ulcerates, a typical "rodent ulcer" is produced.

Although a typical basal cell carcinoma can often be recognized clinically, a biopsy is necessary for definitive diagnosis. These tumors may be treated by curettage and electrodesiccation, surgical excision, or irradiation.[11] Each lesion and each patient should be treated individually with respect to age, physical condition, previous treatment, location, size, depth, and type of tumor. With proper patient selection and competent performance of therapy, a cure rate of 95% or better is anticipated.

Squamous cell carcinoma

Cutaneous squamous cell carcinomas usually arise on the chronically sun-damaged skin of the backs of the hands, arms, ears, neck, and face. Those squamous cell carcinomas that arise in sun-damaged skin have a low metastatic potential, whereas tumors that arise from mucosal surfaces, burn scars, chronic radiodermatitis, and chronic ulcerative conditions of the skin will metastasize more frequently. This tumor usually begins as an erythematous papule, which develops a shallow ulceration surrounded by a wide indurated border as it enlarges[10] (Fig. 12-10). Occasionally, however, the tumor may be exophytic or warty. A biopsy is necessary for diagnosis, following which it may be treated in a manner similar to basal cell carcinoma. However, except for very small lesions, curettage and electrodesiccation are less desirable than is surgical excision.

Keratoacanthoma

Clinically, the keratoacanthoma may resemble a squamous cell carcinoma. However, it grows much more rapidly and tends to have a characteristic volcano-like shape.[10] The tumor is a dome-shaped erythematous nodule with a cup-like keratin-filled center (Fig. 12-11). These lesions are thought to be benign, and they often regress spontaneously after several months. Keratoacanthomas develop twice as often in men than in women and most often occur in the 60- to 65-year-old age range. Sites of predilection are the face and dorsum of the hands, and exposure to sunlight may be a predisposing factor. Although the tumor may have a very characteristic clinical appearance and growth rate, a biopsy is often necessary for definitive diagnosis. Some keratoacanthomas are removed for cosmetic reasons alone. In other cases, it is advisable to remove the lesion before it enlarges further, even though spontaneous involution may be expected. The scar from surgical removal is usually more acceptable than that from spontaneous resolution. A simple method of removal consists of shaving the elevated part of the tumor flush with the surrounding skin, followed by curettage of the remainder of the lesion. However, if the diagnosis is in doubt, a complete surgical excision is recommended.

Bowen's disease

Bowen's disease is not truly a sun-induced lesion. It is an intraepidermal squamous cell carcinoma that can occur on either sun-exposed or non–sun-exposed sites. Most commonly there is one lesion, but occasionally a few lesions may occur. Bowen's disease begins as a reddish patch with a sharp but irregular outline and a scaly surface.[10] It slowly enlarges and may reach a diameter of several centimeters. In some lesions, brownish pigmentation may occur, and in

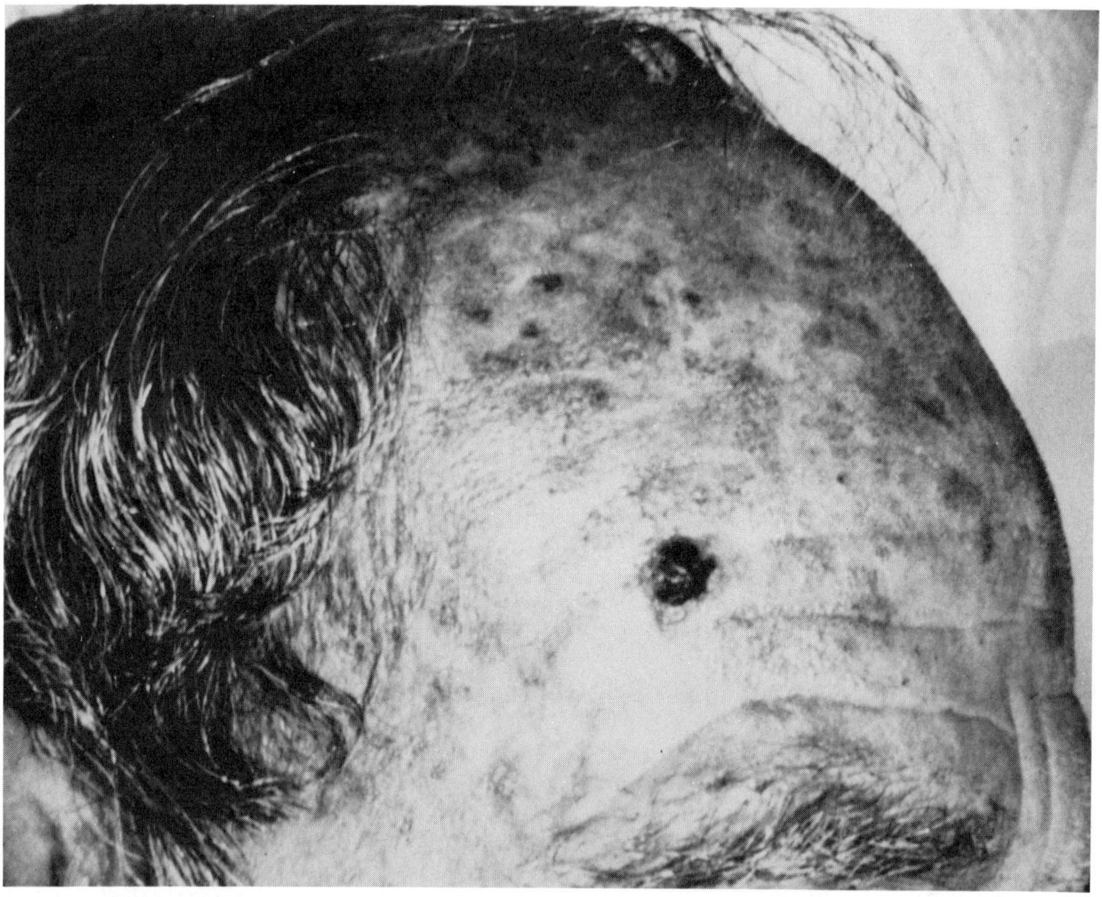

Fig. 12-10. Squamous cell carcinoma of the forehead, presenting as a shallow crusted ulcer with a raised erythematous border. The forehead demonstrates the blotchy pigmentary changes of excessive sun exposure.

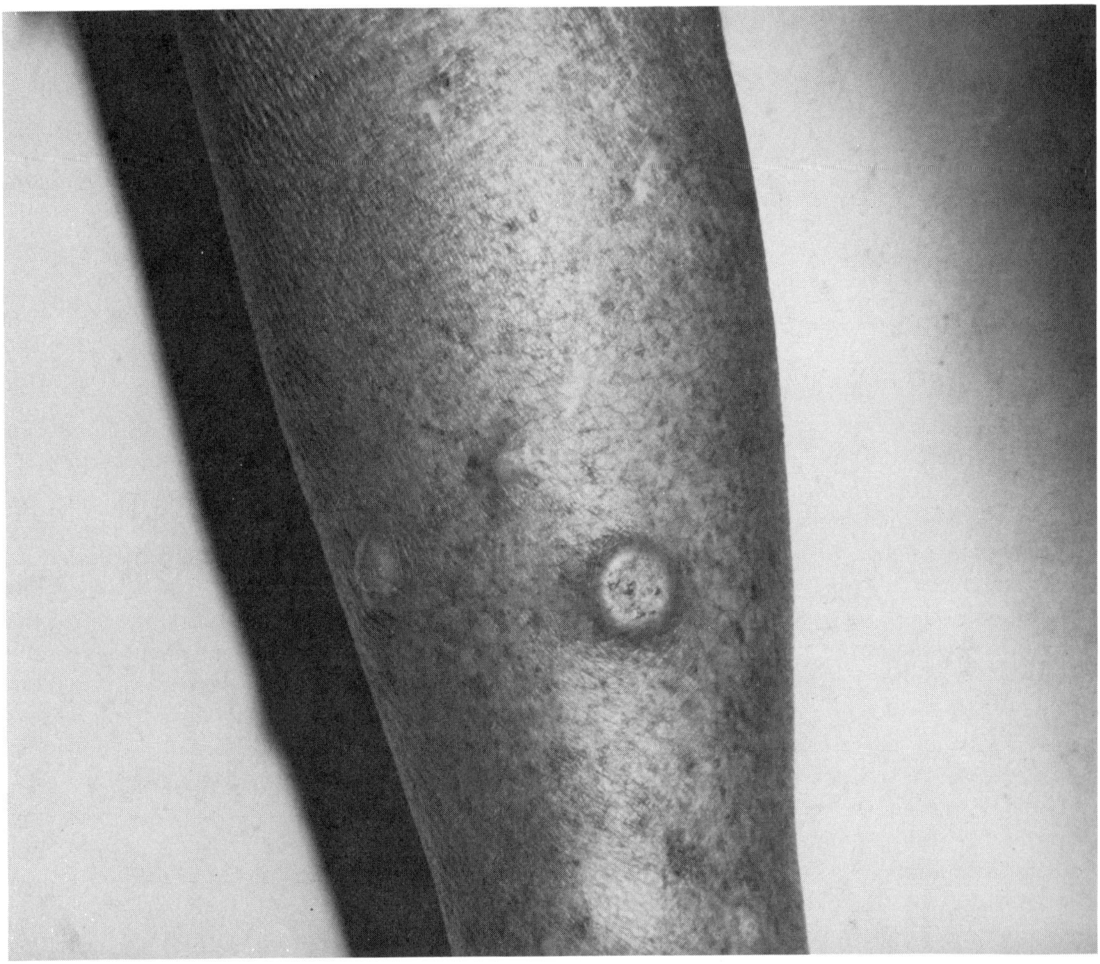

Fig. 12-11. Two dome-shaped keratoacanthomas on the leg.

cerated. These tumors tend to remain intraepidermal for a few to several years, but ultimately some develop marked induration, usually signifying the occurrence of dermal invasion. Bowen's disease may be mistaken for psoriasis, lichen simplex chronicus, tinea corporis, nummular dermatitis, or superficial basal cell carcinoma. Therefore a biopsy is required for diagnosis. Once the diagnosis is established, the lesion should be removed by simple surgical excision.

REFERENCES

1. Halpern, L.K.: Skin disease in the aged. Unit 4-42. In Demis, D.J., et al., editors: Clinical dermatology. New York, 1980, Harper and Row, Publishers Inc.
2. Selmanowitz, V.J.: Cutaneous changes associated with aging, J. Dermatol. Surg. Oncol. **3:**628, 1977.
3. Verbov, J.: Skin diseases in the elderly, Philadelphia, 1974, J.B. Lippincott Co.
4. Spoor, H.J.: Wrinkles, Cutis **17:**236, 1976.
5. Waisman, M.: A clinical look at the aging skin, Postgrad. Med.**66:**87, 1979.
6. Johnson, S.A.M.: Relieving itching in the geriatric patient, Postgrad. Med.**58:**105, 1975.
7. Chenowith, B.R.: Nummular eczema. Unit 13-9. In Demis, D.J., et al., editors: Clinical dermatology, New York, 1980, Harper & Row, Publishers Inc.
8. Björnberg, A., and Mobacken, H.: "Spontaneous stellate pseudoscars" of the arms caused by increased skin fragility, Acta Derm. Venereol. (Stockh.) **52:**151, 1972.
9. Kopf, A.W., Bart, R.S., and Rodríguez-Sains, R.S.: Malignant melanoma: a review, J. Dermatol. Surg. Oncol. **3:**41, 1977.
10. Knox, J.M., and Freeman, R.G.: Detection and diagnosis of skin cancer, CA **15:**216, 1965.
11. Knox, J.M.: Skin cancer: appropriate therapy, Cutis **16:**848, 1975.

CHAPTER 13 · NUTRITION

Vernon R. Young

The foods we eat fulfill various functions. They serve as a source of water, energy, and the essential nutrients required to maintain normal functioning of body tissues and various physiologic processes necessary to maintain good health and resistance to disease. In addition, foods play important roles in cultural and social behavior, and these roles must be considered in the comprehensive evaluation of nutrition and the health of adults. The focus of the discussion in this chapter will be on physiologic and metabolic aspects of diet, the nutrients it contains, nutritional status, and well-being of older adults.

In the first part of this discussion the nutrients required by healthy adults will be considered, followed by a summary account of the nutritional characteristics of the elderly individual. The consequences of an inadequate diet on the health of adults will be reviewed briefly. The purpose will be to convey to those responsible for the care of elderly patients an indication of the importance of including nutrition as a critical component in the comprehensive medical management of individuals.

It would be a difficult task to present in a single chapter all of the details that would be useful to the reader who is genuinely concerned about the food and nutrition needs and problems of the elderly individual, healthy or sick. Thus it is necessary to be selective with respect to the topics chosen for discussion and the depth to which each is treated. There are a number of books[1-4] and review articles[5-8] concerned with various aspects of nutrition in relation to the aging adult that may serve as sources of more extensive information. Furthermore, additional consideration of nutritionally related problems, such as osteoporosis, diabetes mellitus, and arteriosclerotic heart disease, are presented elsewhere in this book (Chapters 6, 9, and 10).

ESSENTIAL NUTRIENTS

In older adults nutrients are required for maintenance of cells and organs, for tissue repair, and for resisting disease. Foods provide these nutrients, some supplying only a few and others supplying many; no single food provides all of the nutrients in amounts and proportions necessary for adequate health. However, if the total diet supplies all essential nutrients, the cells and body organs can synthesize many thousands of physiologically significant compounds needed to maintain health, to resist infection, and to promote recovery from minor or catastrophic injuries such as a leg fracture or extensive body burn.

In a brief consideration of essential nutrients, it is convenient to classify them into six general classes: carbohydrates, fats, proteins, vitamins, minerals, and water.

Carbohydrates, fats, and proteins serve as major sources of food energy, with alcohol sometimes accounting for sizeable proportions of total energy intake. However, the primary need for protein is to supply substrate (indispensable amino acids and a utilizable source of nitrogen) for protein synthesis. The proteins of cells commonly consist of about 20 amino acids, but only half of these can be made by the body. The remaining amino acids, the essential or indispensable amino acids, must be provided by protein foods, otherwise amino acid deficiency will develop. Some food protein sources, such as eggs, milk, meat, and other animal protein foods, contain high concentrations of these essential amino acids, while some vegetable or plant protein sources, such as cereal grains and legumes, may contain lower concentrations of one or more of these amino acids.[9] A suitable mixture of plant protein sources can supply the essential amino acids in amounts and propor-

Table 13-1. Structural features of the components of dietary fiber

Major groups	*Principal structural types*	*Main variations*
Structural		
Noncellulosic polysaccharides	Galacturonans	Methoxy groups; side chains
	Arabinoxylans; glucuronoxylans	Branched and linear xylan chain; number and distribution of side chains
	Glucosmannans; galactomannans	Number and distribution of side chains
	Arabino galactans	Branching and side chains
Cellulose	β-D-glucan	Degree of polymerization
Lignins	Aromatic polymer	Type of polymer; functional groups
Unstructural		
Pectin	Galacturonans	Methoxy group; side chains
Gums, mucilages	Great variety including arabinoxylans, glucomannans, and galactomannans	Branching; side chains
Algal polysaccharides	Sulphated galactans; guluronomannuronans	Variations in composition of backbone chain
Modified celluloses	Esters; ethers	Cross-linking

Adapted from Southgate, D.A.T.: Br. Med. Bull. **37**:65, 1981.

tions that adequately meet nutritional requirements. Thus expensive animal protein foods are not nutritionally essential. Nevertheless, animal and dairy products serve as palatable sources of quality dietary protein and contain sources of other essential vitamins and minerals that make them a desirable component of a balanced diet for elderly individuals.[10]

Fats or lipids are concentrated sources of dietary energy and are also carriers of fat-soluble vitamins. Furthermore, dietary fats are the source of *essential fatty acids*, linoleic and archidonic, which are intimately involved in the maintenance of normal membrane structure and function. These fatty acids cannot be made by the body but are a constituent part of the unsaturated fats in the diet and account for a relatively large part of some vegetable oils. They are parent substances for the formation of prostaglandins and prostacyclins that play multiple roles, including maintenance of the normal function of blood platelets, smooth muscle metabolism, and nervous system activity.[11] Thus an adequate intake of these fatty acids is necessary to maintain good blood circulation and to assure adequate heart function.

Although dietary fats do play an important part in the maintenance of normal metabolism and health, excessive dietary intakes can lead to or promote disease. Numerous epidemiologic studies indicate that high intakes of fats are correlated with coronary heart disease[12] and other degenerative diseases, including various cancers.[13] There is, however, considerable debate concerning the etiologic significance of these associations and the extent to which these diseases are caused or promoted by dietary and environmental factors.

Dietary carbohydrates are also important sources of energy intake; the nutritionally important carbohydrates are as follows: (1) monosaccharides, such as glucose and fructose; (2) disaccharides such as sucrose and lactose; and (3) polysaccharides, such as starch and glycogen. In human nutrition the celluloses and other plant polysaccharides are not used to meet energy requirements because they are not hydrolyzed by secretions of the human digestive tract, although some digestion may take place through the action of intestinal microflora.[14] However, they comprise the *dietary fiber* (unavailable plant polysaccharides and lignin) of foods, which may play an important role in the maintenance of normal gastrointestinal function, metabolism, and health (Table 13-1).[15] The decrease in the intake of dietary fiber by populations in the United States and western Europe during the past quarter century has been thought by some investigators[16,17] to be a major reason for the increase in digestive diseases in our society, although this remains speculative.[18] Alternatively, dietary fiber may reduce the absorption and availability of some trace nutrients. If the latter are already in low amounts in the diet, there

Table 13-2. Generic descriptors and trivial names for vitamins and related compounds in human nutrition (IUNS Committee on nomenclature)

Vitamin	*Generic use (compounds with same qualitative biologic activity)*
Fat-soluble vitamins and related compounds	
Vitamin A	β-ionone derivatives with retinol activity
Provitamin A carotenoids	Carotenoids with β-carotene activity
Vitamin D	Steroids with cholecalciferol activity
Vitamin E	Tocol and Tocotrienol derivatives with activity of α-tocopherol
Vitamin K	2-methyl-1,4 naphthoquinone and derivatives with phylloquinone activity
Water-soluble vitamins and related compounds	
Folacin	Folic acid and compounds with folic acid activity (e.g., THFA)
Niacin	Pyridine 3-carboxylic acid and derivatives with nicotinamide activity
Riboflavin (B_2)	
Thiamine (B_1)	
Vitamin B_6	2-methylpyridine and derivatives with pyridoxine activity
Vitamin B_{12}	Corrinoids exhibiting cyanocobalamin activity
Vitamin C	Compounds with ascorbic acid activity
Pantothenic acid	
Biotin	
Choline	

Adapted from International Union of Nutritional Sciences Committee on Nomenclature: Nutr. Abstr. Rev. **40**:395, 1970.

may be untoward health effects;[19] but the inclusion of fruits, vegetables, and whole grains in the diet makes it possible to obtain sufficient fiber, and there is little reason to resort to the use of fiber supplements to ensure adequate intake.

Available carbohydrates, such as sucrose, lactose, and starch, are not specifically required as far as is known. However, they contribute about 40% of energy intake, with sucrose consumption ranging from 15% to 20% of the total energy intake in the American diet.[20]

The vitamins are another class of essential nutrients, 13 of which are necessary dietary constituents for human health (Table 13-2).[21] Their metabolic functions are diverse: thiamine, pyridoxine, riboflavin, and niacin act as coenzymes; and a low dietary intake causes reduced activities of enzymes associated with reactions involved in energy metabolism and the efficient use of amino acids.

Vitamins A, D, E, and K have attracted considerable research interest in recent years, and significant advances have been made in unravelling their metabolism and mechanism(s) of action. Thus the recent discovery of a retinol-phosphate-mannose-glycolipid intermediate suggests that vitamin A may play a primary role in glycoprotein synthesis.[22] Vitamin K now appears to be required for the conversion of a precursor to prothrombin in a vitamin K-dependent step involving the α-carboxylation of glutamic acid residues.[23] Finally, the identification of 1α, 25- $(OH)_2$-D_3(1,25-dihydroxyvitamin-D_3) as the *active* form of vitamin D[24] and the discovery of its exclusive formation in the kidney are examples of this new knowledge. Indeed, the recent work concerned with vitamin D and, possibly, vitamin A metabolism and action leads to the conclusion that these nutrients may be more appropriately defined as hormones. Furthermore, research developments in the metabolism of vitamin D have led to the successful therapeutic application of vitamin D metabolites and analogs in the treatment of various disorders of calcium metabolism.

The mineral elements constitute the final class of essential nutrients that should be mentioned. The so-called macroinorganic elements (sodium, potassium, chlorine, calcium, magnesium, phosphorus) are present in the body in significant quantities, their combined mass being about 3 kg in adult men. The microelements, or trace minerals, on the other hand, are required in smaller amounts in the diet, usually less than 30 mg per day, and their total body content is about 30 gm.

The major mineral elements, such as sodium, potassium, calcium, magnesium, and chloride, fulfill electrochemical functions. Calcium, potassium, magnesium, copper, and zinc participate as catalysts in enzyme systems, and some minerals, for example, calcium, phosphorus, and fluorine, play a role in maintaining the structure of the bony tissues, skeleton, and teeth. Other essential mineral elements include io-

Table 13-3. Classification of the essential trace elements

Element	Function	Deficiency signs: Animals	Deficiency signs: Humans	Imbalances in humans
Fluorine	Structure of teeth, possibly of bones; possibly growth effect	Caries; possibly growth depression	Increased incidence of caries; possibly risk factor of osteoporosis	Deficiency and excess known
Silicon	Calcification; possibly function in connective tissue	Growth depression; bone deformities	Not known	Not known
Vanadium	Not known	Growth depression; change of lipid metabolism; impairment of reproduction	Not known	Not known
Chromium	Potentiation of insulin	Relative insulin resistance	Relative insulin resistance; impaired glucose tolerance; elevated serum lipids	Deficiency known in malnutrition; aging; total parenteral alimentation
Manganese	Mucopolysaccharides metabolism; superoxide dismutase	Growth depression; bone deformities; β-cell degeneration	Not known	Deficiency not known; toxicity by inhalation
Iron	Oxygen, electron transport	Anemia; growth retardation	Anemia	Deficiencies widespread; excesses dangerous in hemochromatosis; acute poisoning
Cobalt	As part of vitamin B_{12}	Anemia; growth retardation in ruminant species	Only as vitamin B_{12} deficiency	Inability to absorb Vitamin B_{12}; low B_{12} intake in vegetarian diets
Nickel	Interaction with iron absorption	Growth depression; anemia; ultra-structural changes in liver; impaired reproduction	Not known	Not known
Copper	Oxidative enzymes; interaction with iron; cross-linking of elastin	Anemia; rupture of large vessels; disturbances of ossification	Anemia; changes of ossification; possibly elevated serum cholesterol	Deficiencies in malnutrition; total parenteral alimentation
Zinc	Numerous enzymes involved in energy metabolism and in transcription and translation	Failure to eat; severe growth depression; skin lesions; sexual immaturity	Growth depression; sexual immaturity; skin lesions; depression of immunocompetence; change of taste acuity	Deficiencies in Iran, Egypt, in total parenteral nutrition; genetic diseases; traumatic stress
Arsenic	Not known	Impairment of growth, reproduction; sudden heart death in third generation lactating goats	Not known	Not known
Selenium	Glutathione peroxidase; interaction with heavy metals	Different, depending on species; muscle degeneration (ruminants); pancreas atrophy (chicken)	Endemic cardiomyopathy (Keshan disease) conditioned by selenium deficiency	Deficiency and excess in areas of China; one case resulting from total parenteral alimentation
Molybdenum	Xanthine; aldehyde oxidases	Difficult to produce; growth depression	Not known	Excessive exposure in parts of Soviet Union associated with gout-like syndrome
Iodine	Constituent of thyroid hormones	Goiter, depression of thyroid function	Goiter; depression of thyroid function; cretinism	Deficiencies widespread; excessive intakes may lead to thyrotoxicosis

From Mertz, W.: Science **213**:1332, 1981. Copyright 1981 by the American Association for the Advancement of Science.

dine, used for formation of thyroid hormones, and iron, required for the formation of hemoglobin, which serves as an oxygen carrier to tissues and organs. Dietary iron inadequacy, therefore, leads to low blood levels of hemoglobin muscular weakness and a reduced capacity to carry out physical work (Table 13-3).

Improved methods for the chemical analysis of the elements present in small amounts in body fluids and tissues and the development of refined systems for rearing experimental animals in "clean" environments have also led to the identification of a number of newer essential minerals[25,26]—nickel, tin, vanadium, and silicon. Not many years ago these minerals were considered only health hazards. They are widely distributed in foods, and a primary dietary deficiency appears unlikely. Nevertheless, changes in the balance among them and among the other mineral elements in diets may have health consequences. For example, it has been claimed that imbalances among the mineral elements might be contributing factors to the development of diseases such as atherosclerosis[27,28] or even cancer.[29] Again, however, this is an area that is characterized by much speculation.[29] Much careful, additional study will be necessary before the causal associations, if any, between the intake and balance of the mineral elements and chronic disease states are adequately defined.

ESTIMATES OF NUTRITIONAL REQUIREMENTS

Approaches

The problems involved with estimating the quantitative requirements of essential nutrients in human subjects are difficult, and current knowledge in this area, particularly in relation to elderly individuals, is generally unsatisfactory. Choosing the appropriate criterion for assessing the requirement level for a given nutrient is a complex task.[30]

Much of the current knowledge of the quantitative requirement for the various essential nutrients in human nutrition is based on the concept of the development of clinically evident nutritional disease. Fig. 13-1 depicts the stages of development of nutritional disease, leading to appearance of clinical symptoms that may be nonspecific.[31] The sequence begins with an inadequate supply of a nutrient to cells and body tissues. This may arise through a primary dietary deficiency or from a number of factors that result in reduced absorption and retention of the nutrient. Examples of some of these factors[32] are listed below.*

Delivery to cells and organs:
- Chemical form in the diet
- Diet constituents and composition
- Absorption–digestion
- Cellular and intracellular transport
- Conversion to metabolically active form

Loss of nutrients:
- Renal clearance
- Intestinal secretion and elimination
- Oxidation and metabolism
- Chemical or drug inactivation

Alterations in cellular and organ function:
- Size and activity of organs
- Binding to enzymes

One approach, suggested by the sequence of events shown in Fig. 13-1, that may be used for determining nutrient requirements is to assess the nutrient intake of individuals in populations free of nutritional disease. Comparable information may then be obtained from individuals in populations where the specific nutritional deficiency occurs, giving an estimate of the approximate range of intake that is consistent with maintenance of good health. However, this is not an exact procedure; there are difficulties in determining precisely the nutrient intakes of free-living subjects. Furthermore, the diagnosis of subclinical deficiency is often uncertain.

A more satisfactory approach involves the conduct of metabolic studies in which volunteer subjects receive highly controlled diets. Under these study conditions the level of the test nutrient intake is altered during experimental dietary periods, often for only a short time, to determine the minimum level of intake necessary to meet a given criterion, such as the maintenance of a specific biochemical function. In the case of thiamine this might be erythrocyte transketolase,[33,34] or it might be albumin in the case of studies concerned with estimation of protein needs.

Although this approach is a more precise method than the dietary method mentioned above, metabolic studies with humans are laborious, time-consuming, and expensive. Furthermore, these studies may involve the use of monotonous experimental diets and pose strict

*Adapted from Brown, R.R.: J. Agric. Food Chem. **20**:498, 1972.

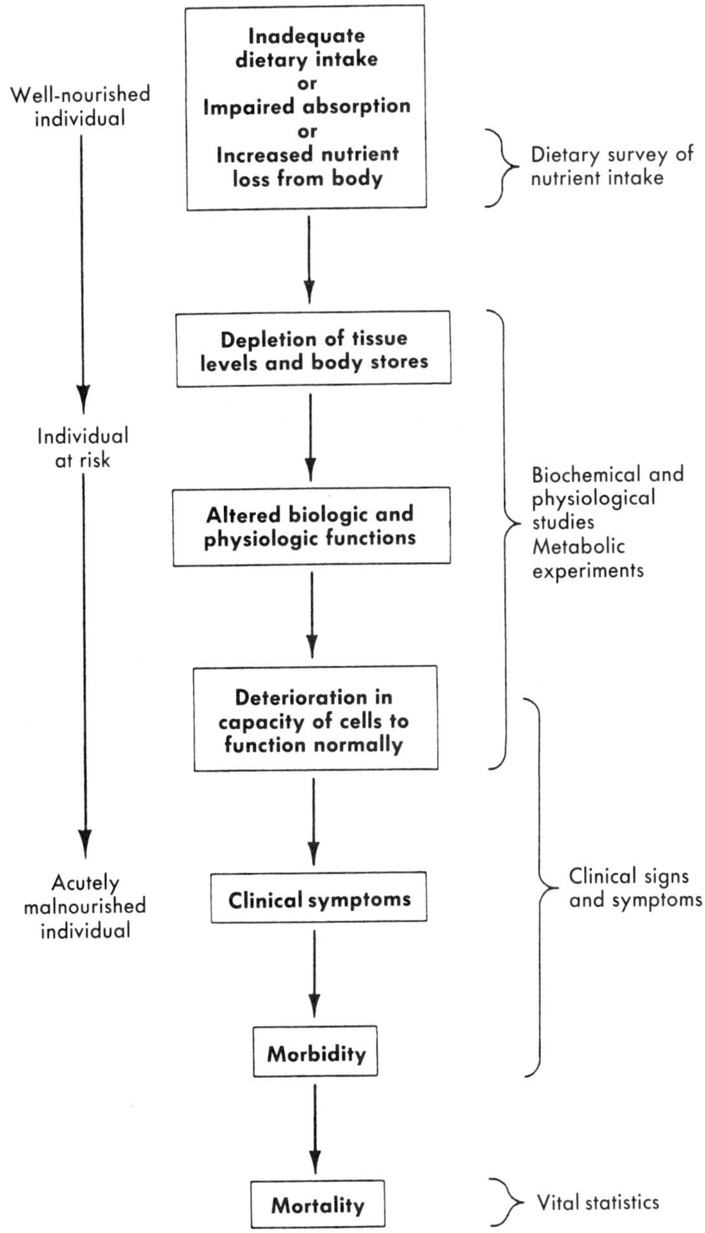

Fig. 13-1. Major stages in development of nutritional deficiency disease. Nutritional deficiency begins with inadequate supply of a nutrient to body cells and organs. This inadequacy may be the result of various factors, including low dietary intakes or relatively high rates of loss from the body. Subsequently biochemical deterioration occurs with the appearance of clinical symptoms. Knowledge of these stages provides a means for evaluating, by various approaches, human nutrient requirements. (Adapted from Beaton, G.H., and Patwardhan, V.N.: Physiological and practical considerations of nutrient function and requirements. In Beaton, G.H., and Bengoa, J.M., editors: Nutrition in preventive medicine, Geneva, 1976, World Health Organization.)

requirements, including complete collection of urine and feces over many days, making it difficult to use many volunteer subjects. For this reason such studies are frequently of short duration and include only a few volunteer subjects. Thus the data obtained will be quite limited in terms of application to populations. Nevertheless, this technique, or modifications of it, has been used extensively in the determination of human nutrient requirements.

For some of the essential nutrients, it has not been possible to use these or other satisfactory approaches. We must rely, therefore, on cautious extrapolation of data obtained in animal experiments or on dietary and epidemiologic information to approximate dietary intakes that might be considered adequate for human health.

It should be emphasized, however, that very few studies have been directly carried out with elderly subjects; most of the current information applies strictly to studies in young adults.

Factors that affect nutritional requirements

In addition to the specific issue of approaches and methods applied for the determination of nutrient requirements it should also be recognized that these requirements are influenced by numerous factors, which are listed below, according to host, environmental, and agent (dietary) factors. The variable importance of these requirements for different individuals further complicates a definition of the quantitative nutrient requirements in the elderly.

Agent (dietary) factors:
- Chemical form of nutrient
- Energy intake
- Food processing and preparation (may increase or decrease dietary needs)
- Effect of other dietary constituents

Host factors:
- Progressive old age
- Sex
- Genetic makeup
- Pathologic states
- Drugs
- Infection
- Physical trauma
- Chronic disease, cancer
- Psychologic states

Environmental factors:
- Physical (unsuitable housing, inadequate heating)
- Biologic (poor sanitary conditions)
- Socioeconomic (poverty, dietary habits, food choices, physical activity)

Nutrient requirements differ among individuals. A fundamental component of this variation is that introduced by genetic differences, although the importance of this factor is difficult to judge for the population as a whole.

Dietary factors affect nutrient requirements. A few examples are given here. In the case of iron, its chemical form, the type of diet, and composition of individual meals affect the use of iron. These factors will determine, in part, the intake of the element necessary to maintain an adequate iron supply in the individual.[35] It is now well-established that meat improves overall iron absorption. Because the degree of absorption of dietary iron is a major factor in determining the minimum intake necessary to meet physiologic needs, a better understanding of the factors that affect iron absorption and utilization in the elderly is required to define the basis and extent of variation in iron requirements for this age group.

Another example concerning the effects of dietary factors on estimated nutrient requirements relates to the question of protein needs in elderly subjects. It has long been recognized that the level of energy intake influences the efficiency of use of dietary protein[36,37] and that relatively small reductions in energy intake are associated with higher protein requirements. The characteristic decline in total energy intake in adults as they grow older[38] may have, therefore, an important impact on the metabolism of and requirement for dietary protein, although the extent to which the requirement might be affected remains to be studied. This does emphasize, however, the need to determine protein and amino acid requirements directly in elderly individuals rather than to rely on information obtained in younger adults.

Of particular importance in considering nutrient needs in the elderly population is the effect of stressful stimuli, such as those arising from infection or physical trauma or even those of psychologic origin. It is known that early in the infectious episode there is an increased rate of synthesis of immunoglobulins and of other proteins characteristic of the initial metabolic response to the infectious agent.

Nutritional aspects of the catabolic response to infection*

1. Most prominent metabolic response to a generalized febrile infection of any cause
2. Caused by increased metabolic requirements of

*Adapted from Beisel, W.R.: Infectious diseases. In Schneider, H., et al.: Nutritional support of medical practice, New York, 1977, Harper and Row, Publishers, Inc., p. 350.

body tissues in the presence of a generally inadequate dietary intake

3. Modulated by complex hormonal influences
4. Consistent features include:
   a. Onset time following that of fever
   b. Muscle wasting and weight loss
   c. Negative balances of nitrogen and other nitrocellular elements
   d. Persistence into convalescence
5. Minimized by effective control of illness
6. Magnified during severe, uncontrolled, complicated, or recurrent illness
7. Followed by wasting and malnutrition if infection becomes chronic

This is followed by a net catabolic response that results in increased losses of body nitrogen and of some vitamins and minerals and in decreases in blood levels of these nutrients.[39,40] Furthermore, absorption of nutrients may be interfered with if there is a significant pathologic condition of the gastrointestinal tract. The net result of these responses is depletion of body nutrients followed by an increase in the physiologic need for nutrients during convalescence to promote recovery and compensate for earlier losses. Although acute and chronic infections and other stressful stimuli, including anxiety, pain, and physical trauma, generally increase the requirement for many essential nutrients, there are inadequate quantitative data to help determine how much nutrient intake should be increased under these circumstances. However, by way of an example, an approximation of the changes in protein needs in some major disease states is presented in the following outline. As shown here the requirement may be altered by different circumstances.[41]

Protein needs in specific diseases*

1. Normal adults
   a. For N equilibrium: 0.75 gm/kg of good quality, highly digestible protein; 0.8 to 0.9 gm/kg for proteins of low digestibility
   b. Customary intake: 1 to 2 gm/kg
2. Metabolic response to severe burn injury and trauma
   a. Acute phase: 2 to 4 gm/kg plus energy
   b. Convalescence: 2 gm/kg or more
3. Malabsorption of GI diseases
   a. Malabsorption syndrome: 1 gm/kg
   b. Ulcerative colitis*: 1 to 1.4 gm/kg
   c. Ileocecostomy†: 1 to 1.4 gm/kg
4. Liver disease
   a. Acute hepatic encephalopathy*: very low
   b. Recovered encephalopathy: 1 to 1.5 gm/kg
   c. Chronic encephalopathy*: 0.5 gm/kg
5. Renal disease
   a. Uremia*: 0.5 gm/kg (ketoanalogs)
   b. Nephrosis†: 1 to 1.4 gm/kg
6. Malignant disease
   a. Increased protein and energy

*Adapted from Munro, H.N., and Young, V.R.: Protein metabolism and requirements. In Exton-Smith, A.N., and Caird, F.I., editors: Metabolic and nutritional disorders in the elderly, Bristol, England, 1980, John Wright & Sons, Ltd., p. 13.

*Intake restricted on clinical grounds.

†In each condition, losses of protein can double minimal requirement.

Finally it should be mentioned that drugs may have profound effects on nutrient requirements by decreasing nutrient absorption or by altering the utilization of the nutrients by tissues.[42] The effects of drugs on nutrient requirements will depend on the dose, period, and frequency of administration. The multiple administration of drugs may have synergistic effects, altering nutritional status and the requirements for nutrients. Reduced appetite may be a consequence of drug therapy and further compromises the individual's nutritional status, particularly if the diet is marginally adequate to begin with.

The quantitative effects of these various factors on the requirements for individual nutrients have not been established, but this information is necessary if rational dietary allowances are to be developed for the elderly segment of the population. In spite of this lack of knowledge there is a continuing need for estimates of nutrient intakes that are sufficient to maintain health in population groups. These estimates are embodied in the Recommended Dietary Allowances (RDA); in the following section a brief account of RDA will be given.

Recommended dietary allowances (RDA) for elderly individuals

The RDA are intakes considered sufficient to meet the nutritional needs of practically all *healthy* persons within a particular population group.[43] They are higher than the average minimum requirement for a given nutrient, because they incorporate an estimation of the variation in nutrient requirements within a group of apparently similar individuals. This variation is as-

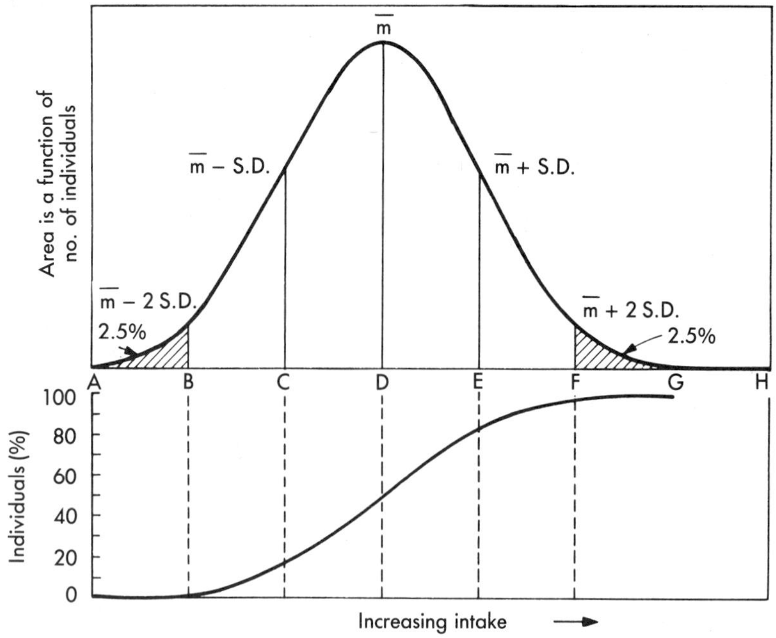

Fig. 13-2. Schematic distribution of nutrient requirements of any population. Nutrient requirements of individuals within a given population group, for example, healthy elderly people, vary around the mean requirement for the population according to distribution curve shown in the top panel. To cover nutrient needs of practically all individuals it is necessary to determine range of variation. The objective of this approach is to set recommended intakes at a level equal to the mean requirement *plus* two standard deviations (S.D.) so that the requirements of 97.5% of the population will be met. This point is emphasized by the curve in the lower panel, indicating that dietary intakes at recommended levels meet requirements of nearly all individuals. The allowance for dietary energy is based on an estimate of the mean requirement for the population.

sumed to be normally distributed (Fig. 13-2). Provided that the mean or average requirement for the nutrient is known and an estimate is available for the distribution in requirements about this mean, an RDA can be developed. Because it is not practical to formulate recommendations sufficient to cover *all* members of a population group, since a few normal individuals in the population may require considerably more of a given nutrient than most others, the usual convention is to take the mean requirement plus two standard deviations above the mean as a reasonable basis for establishing RDA. Thus an intake that equals the RDA should be sufficient to cover the requirements of about 97.5% of the population.

For energy requirements the situation is different because allowances for energy are based on the average requirement for the population. Intakes of either well above or well below an individual's requirement would, of course, result in a deterioration of health. It is assumed, therefore, that most individuals select diets providing energy intakes that either meet or closely approximate actual needs. Thus the average energy requirement is often given as a guideline for establishing levels of dietary energy.

Table 13-4 summarizes the RDA for adults as proposed by the U.S. Food and Nutrition Board. It should be noted that not all of the essential nutrients are listed in this table because available information is insufficient for making a reliable recommendation as to dietary allowances. However, the U.S. Food and Nutrition Board discusses these other nutrients in the text of their report. For some of these nutrients an adequate and safe intake has been established, as shown in Table 13-5, as a step toward eventually setting RDA as further information becomes available.

Before terminating a discussion of RDA, it

Table 13-4. Recommended dietary allowances for young and older adults

Nutrient	Young adult (19-22 yr.)		Older adult (51+ yr.)	
	Male	Female	Male	Female
Energy (kcal/day)	2500-3300	1700-2500	2000 2800	1400-2200
Protein (gm/day)	56	44	56	44
Vitamins				
A (μgRE)	1000	800	1000	800
D (μg)	7.5	7.5	5	5
E (mg α-tocopherol)	10	8	10	8
C (mg)	60	60	60	60
Thiamine (mg)	1.5	1.1	1.2	1.0
Riboflavin (mg)	1.7	1.3	1.4	1.2
Niacin (mg)	19	14	16	13
B_6 (mg)	2.2	2.0	2.2	2.0
Folacin (μg)	400	400	400	400
B_{12} (μg)	3	3	3	3
Minerals				
Ca (mg)	800	800	800	800
P (mg)	800	800	800	800
Mg (mg)	350	300	350	300
Fe (mg)	10	18	10	10
Zn (mg)	15	15	15	15
I (μg)	150	150	150	150

From National Research Council/National Academy of Sciences: Recommended dietary allowances, rev. ed. 9, Washington, D.C., 1980, National Academy of Sciences.

Table 13-5. Estimated safe and adequate daily intake for adults of selected vitamins and minerals

Nutrient	Safe and adequate intake
Vitamins	
K	70-140 μg
Biotin	100-200 μg
Pantothenic acid	4-7 mg
Electrolytes	
Sodium	1100-3300 mg
Potassium	1875-5625 mg
Chloride	1700-5100 mg
Iron elements	
Copper	2.0-3.0 mg
Manganese	2.5-5.0 mg
Fluoride	1.5-4.0 mg
Chromium	0.05-0.2 mg
Selenium	0.05-0.2 mg
Molybdenum	0.15-0.5 mg

From National Research Council/National Academy of Sciences: Recommended dietary allowances, rev. ed. 9, Washington, D.C., 1980, National Academy of Sciences.

must be made clear that they represent intakes considered *sufficient for the maintenance of health in nearly all adults*. These recommendations focus on *health maintenance* and are not intended to be sufficient for therapeutic purposes. Therefore, they may not be adequate to meet the additional requirements that may occur during and following recovery from infection or as a consequence of malabsorption, trauma, metabolic disease, or other significant stress. It is also worth pointing out that the RDA refer to intakes with reasonable daily variation persisting over a period of time and do not mandate that the daily intake should be at this level to minimize risk of nutritional deficiency.

VULNERABLE STATE OF NUTRITION IN THE ELDERLY

Although there are no good indications that old age per se substantially changes nutrient requirements, providing the individual is physically and mentally healthy, there are a broad range of conditions that accompany progressive old age that may have important effects on the nutritional requirements and status of the elderly. Important factors, especially those experienced frequently in elderly persons, include the following:

- Psychological problems; apathy; loneliness
- Physical disability: immobility at home; poor vision; arthritis; etc.
- Disease: infection; cancer; other chronic illnesses
- Malabsorption; gastrointesintal disorders and discomfort
- Poverty
- Mental deterioration
- Inadequate knowledge of dietetic principles; food fads; poor dietary habits
- Alcoholism
- Drugs
- Alterations in metabolism of and requirements for nutrients
- Unsuitable housing situation

Physical and mental disabilities affect the mode of living and may lead to changes in dietary patterns and a deterioration of nutritional status. Underlying medical problems, emotional disturbance, loneliness, and poverty are all factors that diminish appetite and the ability to maintain an adequate diet. Risk of nutritional deficiencies will increase under these circumstances. Furthermore, because energy requirements and intake are reduced, as stated earlier, even in healthy groups[38] this means that adequate intakes of essential nutrients may require a change in the dietary choices towards foods with higher nutrient density. These factors are further compounded by changes in taste and in the deteriorating health of oral tissues.

NUTRITIONAL STATUS OF THE ELDERLY

A large number of surveys have been conducted to assess the nutritional status of institutionalized or noninstitutionalized populations of elderly subjects. Because many of these studies have been reviewed,[44-47] little purpose is served in presenting an extensive account of various findings. However, few surveys have been sufficiently comprehensive to provide a definitive assessment of the extent to which the health and function of subjects have actually been affected by a change in their nutritional status. Although many of the studies suggest that there is an increased risk of vitamin and mineral deficiences, for example, in the elderly groups examined, overt manifestations of nutritional deficiency disease are generally uncommon. For example, low levels of leukocyte ascorbic acid (LAA) have been reported by several observers, which indicates reduced body stores of this vitamin.[48,49] However, it is unclear in many cases whether the diminished blood levels of vitamins or changes in blood parameters that are indicative of nutritional status are caused by inadequate intake of foods that contain particular nutrients in question or to the processing and cooking of foods. Thus in the study of Burr et al.[49] the consumption of fresh fruits appeared to be a major but not the only factor in determining LAA levels.

In relation to vitamins, considerable interest has focused on the folate status of older people, and Herbert[50] has suggested that folate deficiency is a common nutritional problem. A number of surveys suggest that possibility, based on biochemical evidence, that a folate inadequacy may be widespread in elderly subjects.[7,44] For other B vitamins, including thiamine, riboflavin, and B_{12}, studies suggest that there may be significant numbers of elderly people who do not have adequate sources of calories, iron, thiamine, and niacin in their diets. Sugars, sweets, and fats add appreciably to energy intake but make little contribution to protein, mineral, and B-complex vitamin intakes. Milk and dairy products make important contributions to meeting protein, calcium, and riboflavin requirements but are poor sources of vitamins A and C. The meat group and beans, peas, nuts, poultry, and fish are good sources of protein and also of many vitamins and minerals. Thus for planning a healthy diet, foods should be selected from among each group, although it is not essential that every food group be represented. Some diets contain little or no meat, but when planned carefully they can be nutritionally adequate.

Successful meal planning depends on many other factors in addition to consideration of physiologic requirements for nutrients. These factors include family composition, food habits, cultural influences, food costs, and time for food preparation. All of these factors caution against rigid recommendations about use of specific foods for the elderly. However, the important point is that there is considerable flexibility possible in designing diets that are nutritionally adequate and acceptable. It is not profitable to consider any food as being a detriment to health unless there are specific clinical indications for doing so. In the final analysis a balanced intake of a variety of foods is the best guarantee of an adequate diet in elderly individuals.

Of course, the normal oral ingestion of foods may not be possible for various reasons,[52] as shown in the following list.* In this case it may be necessary to resort to use of special nutritional formulations intended for oral or intravenous use to prevent nutritional deficiencies and to promote recovery from earlier depletion, although it is beyond the scope of this short chapter to consider.

- Obstruction, partial or total
- Impairment of swallowing mechanisms
- Ileus
- Fistulas, especially of upper tract
- Coma
- Symptomatic exacerbation of disease with oral intake
- Severe malabsorption and/or diarrhea
- Severe vomiting

FOOD CHOICES AND HEALTH

Identification of the essential nutrients and of the amounts required for health maintenance provides a rational basis for food and menu planning and for assessment of the nutritional adequacy of food sources and diets.

As stated earlier, requirements for the essential nutrients are met via the various foods eaten. The principal foods are as follows: (1) cereals; (2) starchy roots; (3) sugars and syrups; (4) pulses, nuts, and seeds; (5) vegetables; (6) fruits; (7) meat, fish, and eggs; (8) milk and milk products; (9) oils and fats; and (10) beverages. Some of these foods serve as a dietary staple, such as wheat, and therefore can have an important impact on nutritional health. Other foods may be used in lesser amounts, perhaps for flavoring or for other culinary purposes. All foods supply some nutrients, but no single natural food is complete.

Where medical, economic, or social factors are not constraints, it is possible to select a diet based on a wide variety of foods that guarantee the requirements for energy and the essential nutrients can readily be met. Indeed when there is ample availability of many foods nutritional deficiencies do not usually arise, although problems associated with excess intakes may be of importance. An adequate diet would be based on the above; various categories of foods and many basic plans could be constructed to meet individual needs, taking into account not only physiologic requirements but also psychologic, emotional, social, and economic factors. The wide variety of foods allows consideration of individual preferences while selecting a nutritionally balanced diet.

To explore this further, we know that cereals provide significant nutrition. It is pertinent that in the study by Harrill and Cervone,[51] individuals who received vitamin supplements were apparently at a lower risk of nutritional deficiency.

In this regard, however, Exton-Smith[44] has pointed out that vitamin D deficiency, leading to osteomalacia in older persons, is often multifactorial in origin; a low dietary intake of vitamin D, limited exposure to sunlight, inadequate absorption, or impaired conversion of 25-hydroxycholecalciferol to the active 1,25-dihydroxycholecalciferol because of a decline in renal function in old age, alone or in combination can contribute to development of vitamin D deficiency in elderly people.

For these various reasons it is recommended that where a deficiency of a particular nutrient or number of nutrients is suspected a careful and thorough assessment of dietary intake and biochemical and clinical evaluations of the problem be undertaken. Only on this basis can an appropriate diagnosis of a possible nutritional problem be made. It is recognized, however, that the taking of low-potency multivitamin or vitamin-trace mineral capsules by many older individuals may represent a reasonable means for ensuring against the consequences of poor dietary choices and for covering brief periods associated with increased needs for these nutrients.

However, groups of elderly people who are at particular risk of a nutritional inadequacy must be identified and the means developed for improving their nutrient intakes. Only a small percentage of the total elderly population might be affected; of course, many elderly individuals will never experience nutritional deficiencies. However, adequate nutrition for the increasing numbers of elderly persons in our society represents a medical, nutritional, and public health problem that cannot be ignored.

*From Shils, M.: Cancer Res. **37**:2432, 1977.

A few points might be made in regard to special diets or approaches to the nutritional support of sick patients, particularly with respect to the cancer patient, by way of example.

As stated earlier, disease alters the nutritional characteristics of the host. In the context of our example, patients with cancer may experience profound changes in their intake of nutrients, their metabolism, and their nutritional status. Cachexia is a frequent consequence of the presence and growth of tumors, and anorexia or diminished food intake is a major contributor to the overall morbidity of the cancer patient.[53] The degree of cachexia, however, does not appear simply related to food intake, tumor burden, or anatomic site of involvement but as the result of various factors that interact in complex ways, including changes in metabolism, altered food intake and absorption of nutrients, and anatomic changes.[53] Because of the fundamental role of the gastrointestinal tract in the ingestion and use of nutrients, the occurrence of cancer in this system is likely to have significant effects on the nutritional status of the patient. Furthermore, surgical procedures, for example, as in the case of resection of the organs of the gastrointestinal tract, together with administration of chemotherapeutic and immunotherapeutic agents and curative doses of radiotherapy, all have important nutritional consequences.[54]

Hence the cancer itself as well as the treatment modalities can affect the nutritional needs and status of the cancer patient. It is essential, therefore, that particular attention be given to the matter of nutritional support as an important aspect of the comprehensive approach to the treatment of elderly cancer patients.

Wretlind[55] has proposed a series of guidelines or postulates that should be followed and considered in approaches to maintain an adequate nutritional status in hospitalized patients. Some of these guidelines and postulates include the following*:

1. Good nutritional status—prerequisite for optimal resistance to infection and optimal response from medical treatment
2. Daily supply of nutrients in adequate amounts
3. Easier to maintain good nutrition status than to treat malnutrition
4. Oral or tube feedings first choice; intravenous feeding second choice
5. Many preparations available for nutritional support of patients

These guidelines apply equally to the elderly cancer patient. Of course the preferred approach of assuring an adequate intake of nutrients is by voluntary ingestion of a well-balanced diet. However, anorexia may necessitate tube feeding or there may be contraindications to feeding by mouth as discussed by Shils.[52] In this case the alternative involves some form of parenteral nutrition. The indications and possible benefits gained by use of this means of nutritional support in the cancer patient have been discussed.[56]

The specific indications for use of nutritional support via the parenteral route are still under investigation. The evaluation will depend in part on improved methods for assessment of nutritional status, an area that requires particular attention in reference to the elderly patient. Indeed there is a critical need to develop appropriate guidelines for interpretation of anthropometric, biochemical, and functional indices (such as measures of immune function) of nutritional status as applied in elderly individuals.

In spite of the lack of information concerning the role of nutrition and the type of nutritional support in the optimum treatment of elderly patients with cancers, there is little doubt that maintenance of an adequate nutritional state or reversal of nutritional deficiencies will aid the patient's chances for recovery and survival. Thus nutrition constitutes a major consideration in the management of hospitalized elderly patients.

CONCLUSION

For the active, healthy, elderly person, the requirements for essential nutrients are the same as those for the younger adult. However, the elderly suffer from increased disease and experience a range of social, cultural, and economic adjustments that increase the risk of nutritional deficiencies in this age group. This emphasizes the importance of considering nutritional factors and diet in preventive medicine and in the comprehensive approach to the management of elderly patients. Eating habits acquired at an earlier age may be modified by changes in life-style and by disabilities. Indeed nutritional problems appear to be largely a consequence of superimposed disease or the result

*Adapted from Wretlind, A.: Nutr. Rev. **39**:257, 1981.

of other factors rather than of any dramatic changes in the physiology of nutrient metabolism and requirements per se. Each older individual represents a specific case, making it difficult to make generalizations that are helpful. However, the principles of nutrition apply equally at all ages. This makes it essential for physicians to recognize the key role of nutrition in the maintenance of health and the relationships between nutrition and disease processes. In this way the significant contribution to be made by nutrition to maintaining health and well-being for a greater proportion of adult life might be achieved.

REFERENCES

1. Winick, M.: Nutrition and aging, New York, 1976, John Wiley & Sons, Inc.
2. Rockstein, M., and Sussman, M.L.: Nutrition, longevity and aging, New York, 1976, Academic Press, Inc.
3. Albanese, A.A.: Nutrition for the elderly, New York, 1980, Alan R. Liss, Inc., p. 332.
4. Exton-Smith, A.N., and Caird, F.I.: Metabolic and nutritional disorders in the elderly, Bristol, England, 1980, John Wright & Sons, Ltd., p. 227.
5. Watkin, D.M.: Nutrition for the aging and aged. In Goodhart, R.S., and Shils, M.E., editors: Modern nutrition in health and disease, Philadelphia, 1978, Lea and Febiger, p. 781.
6. Munro, H.N.: Nutrition and ageing, Br. Med. Bull. **37:**83, 1981.
7. Young, V.R., Gersovitz, M., and Munro, H.N.: Human aging: protein and amino acid metabolism and implications for protein and amino acid requirements. In Moment, G.B., editor: Nutritional approaches to aging research, Boca Raton, Fla., 1981, CRC Press, Inc.
8. Young, V.R.: Vitamins and the aging process. In Platt, D., editor: Handbook of gerontology, Heidelberg, 1981, Springer-Verlag. (In press.)
9. Young, V.R., Scrimshaw, N.S., and Milner, M.: Food from plants, Chemistry Industry **14:**588, 1976.
10. Young, V.R.: Animal foods, past, present and future: a nutritionist's view. In Baldwin, R.L., editor: Animals, feed, food and people, American Association of Advanced Sciences Symposium Series, No. 42, Washington, D.C., 1980, American Association of Advanced Sciences, p. 121.
11. Wills, A.L.: Nutritional and pharmacological factors in eicosanoid biology, Nutr. Rev. **39:**289, 1981.
12. Levy, R.I., Rifkind, B.M., Dennis, B.H., and Ernst, N.D., editors: Nutrition, lipids and coronary heart disease, New York, 1979, Raven Press, p. 566.
13. Doll, R., and Peto, R.: The causes of cancer: quantitative estimates of avoidable risks of cancer in the United States today, J. Natl. Cancer Inst. **66:**1191, 1981.
14. Cummings, J.H.: Dietary fibre, Br. Med. Bull. **37:**65, 1981.
15. Southgate, D.A.T.: Dietary fiber: analysis and food sources, Am. J. Clin. Nutr. **31**(Suppl. 10): S107, 1978.
16. Trowell, H.: Diabetes mellitus and dietary fiber of starchy foods, Am. J. Clin. Nutr. **31**(Suppl. 10): S53, 1978.
17. Burkitt, D.P.: Colo-rectal cancer: fiber and other dietary factors, Am. J. Clin. Nutr. **31**(Suppl. 10):S58, 1978.
18. Spiller, G.A., and Freeman, H.J.: Recent advances in dietary fiber and colorectal diseases, Am. J. Clin. Nutr. **34:**1145, 1981.
19. Kelsay, J.L.: Effect of dietary fiber on bowel function and trace metal balances of human subjects, Cereal Chem. **58:**2, 1981.
20. Lee, V.A.: The nutritional significance of sucrose consumption, 1970-1980, CRC Crit. Rev. Food Sci. Nutr. **14:**1, 1981.
21. International Union of Nutritional Sciences (IUNS) Committee on Nomenclature: Tentative rules for generic descriptors and trivial names of vitamins and related compounds, Nutr. Abstr. Rev. **40:**395, 1970.
22. Wolf, G.: Vitamin A. In Alfin-Slater, R.B., and Kritchevsky, D., editors: Nutrition and the adult: micronutrients, New York, 1980, Plenum Publishing Corp., p. 97.
23. Olson, R.E.: Vitamin K. In Alfin-Slater, R.B., and Kritchevsky, D., editors: Nutrition and the adult: micronutrients, New York, 1980, Plenum Publishing Corp., p. 267.
24. De Luca, H.: Vitamin D. In Alfin-Slater, R.B., and Kritchevsky, D., editors: Nutrition and the adult: micronutrients, New York, 1980, Plenum Publishing Corp., p. 205.
25. Mertz, W.: The essential trace elements, Science **213:**1332, 1981.
26. Carlisle, E.: Silicon, Nutr. Rev. **33:**257, 1975.
27. Masaroni, R.: Trace elements and cardiovascular diseases, Bull. WHO **40:**305, 1969.
28. Schroeder, H.A.: The role of trace elements in cardiovascular diseases, Med. Clin. North Am. **58:**381, 1974.
29. Young, V.R., and Richardson, D.P.: Nutrients, vitamins and minerals in cancer prevention: facts and fallacies, Cancer **43:**2125, 1979.
30. Young, V.R., and Scrimshaw, N.S.: Genetic and biological variability in human nutrient requirements, Am. J. Clin. Nutr. **32:**486, 1979.
31. Beaton, G.H., and Patwardhan, V.N.: Physiological and practical considerations of nutrient function and requirements. In Beaton, G.H., and Bengoa, J.M., editors: Nutrition in preventive medicine, Geneva, 1976, World Health Organization, p. 445.
32. Brown, R.R.: Normal and pathological conditions which may alter the human requirement for Vitamin B_6, J. Agric. Food Chem. **20:**498, 1972.
33. Brin, M.: Erythrocyte as a biopsy tissue for functional evaluation of thiamine adequacy, J.A.M.A. **197:**762, 1964.
34. Sauberlich, H.E., Herman, Y.F., Stevens, C.O., and Herman, R.H.: Thiamin requirement of the adult human, Am. J. Clin. Nutr. **32:**2237, 1979.
35. Hallberg, L.: Bioavailability of dietary iron in man, Annu. Rev. Nutr. **1:**123, 1981.
36. Munro, H.N.: Carbohydrate and fat as factors in protein utilization and metabolism, Physiol. Rev. **31:**449, 1951.
37. Young, V.R., et al.: Protein and energy intake in relation

to protein turnover in man. In Waterlow, J.C., and Stephen, J.M.L., editors: Nitrogen metabolism in man, London, 1981, Applied Science Publishers, Ltd. p.419.

38. Shock, N.W.: Energy metabolism, caloric intake and physical activity of the aging. In Carlson, L.A., editor: Nutrition in old age, Uppsala, 1972, Swedish Nutrition Foundation, p. 12.
39. Beisel, W.R., Sawyer, W.D., Ryll, C.D., and Crozier, D.: Metabolic effects of intracellular infections in man, Ann. Intern. Med. **67**:744, 1967.
40. Beisel, W.R.: Infectious diseases. In Schneider, H., Anderson, C.E., and Coursin, D.B., editors: Nutritional support of medical practice, New York, 1977, Harper & Row, Publishers, Inc., p. 350.
41. Munro, H.N., and Young, V.R.: Protein metabolism and requirements. In Exton-Smith, A.N., and Caird, F.I., editors: Metabolic and nutritional disorders in the elderly, Bristol, England, 1980, John Wright & Sons, Ltd., p. 13.
42. Hathcock, J.N., and Coon, J., editors: Nutrition and drug interrelations, New York, 1978, Academic Press, Inc., p. 927.
43. National Research Council/National Academy of Sciences: Recommended dietary allowances, rev. ed. 9, Washington, D.C., 1980, National Academy of Sciences.
44. Exton-Smith, A.N.: Vitamins. In Exton-Smith, A.N., and Caird, F.I., editors: Metabolic and nutritional disorders in the elderly, Bristol, England, 1980, John Wright & Sons, Ltd., p. 26.
45. Flemming, B.B.: The vitamin status and requirements of the elderly. In Moment, G.B., editor: Nutritional approaches to aging research, Boca Raton, Fla., 1981, CRC Press, Inc. (In press.)
46. Brin, M., and Bauernfeind, J.C.: Vitamin needs of the elderly, Postgrad. Med. **63**:155, 1978.
47. Exton-Smith, A.N.: Nutritional problems of elderly populations. In Hawkins, W.W., editor: Nutrition of the aged, Quebec, 1978, Nutrition Society of Canada, p. 1.
48. Andrews, J., Letcher, M., and Brook, M.: Vitamin C supplementation in the elderly: a 17-months trial in an old persons' home, Br. Med. J. **2**:416, 1969.
49. Burr, M.L., et al.: Plasma and leucocyte ascorbic acid levels in the elderly, Am. J. Clin. Nutr. **27**:144, 1974.
50. Herbert, V.: Biochemical and hematologic lesions in folic acid deficiency, Am. J. Clin. Nutr. **20**:562, 1967.
51. Harrill, I, and Cervone, N.: Vitamin status of older women, Am. J. Clin. Nutr. **30**:431, 1977.
52. Shils, M.: Enteral nutrition by tube, Cancer Res. **37**:2432, 1977.
53. Costa, G.: Cachexia, the metabolic component of neoplastic diseases, Cancer Res. **37**:2327, 1977.
54. Milder, J.W., editor: Conference on nutrition and cancer therapy, Cancer Res. **37**:2321, 1977.
55. Wretlind, A.: Parenteral nutrition, Nutr. Rev. **39**:257, 1981.
56. Brennan, M.F.: Total parenteral nutrition in the management of the cancer patient, Annu. Rev. Med. **32**:233, 1981.

CHAPTER 14 · INFECTIONS IN THE ELDERLY

Ian M. Smith

Man and bacteria coexist sometimes in symbiosis and sometimes in a state of uneasy truce. The body is well protected against bacterial invasion, both by natural barriers such as skin and by a population of normal flora. Knowledge of infectious diseases of the elderly enables one not only to save lives but also to improve the quality of life in the remaining years.[1] A recent study of 190 patients in nursing homes showed that among patients who were actively treated for fever with antibiotics, 9% died whereas among those denied such treatment, 59% died.[2] Some of these patients would have died anyway of other diseases but many of them would not. Infections are eminently treatable, and a proper knowledge of the types that occur in the elderly and their treatment is essential for a geriatrician.

Certain characteristics of elderly populations militate against early specific diagnosis of infection.[3] Elderly patients have multiple conditions, and some of the manifestations of infection duplicate the symptoms and signs of the underlying disease rather than indicate the presence of a new disease.[4] Fever, for example, may be absent. In pneumonia, instead of dyspnea, cough, or chest pain, confusion is frequently present. In other infections the development of congestive cardiac failure may be the only indication of a complicating infection. In a study of 315 patients over the age of 70 who died in an acute care hospital, in males the most common disease was myocardial infarction with its complications, the second most common was pneumonia, and the third septicemia. Females also died most frequently of myocardial infarction; the second most common cause of death was pulmonary embolus; and the third lymphoma-leukemia.[5] Approximately 65% of the elderly die in acute care hospitals. When patients die of infectious disease, approximately half of them die of the direct effects of overwhelming infection. The other half die because the burden of infection strains an underlying system defect to the point of failure, as for example, when the patient dies of renal failure precipitated by infection. Since organ function decreases with age, most elderly people have one or more of their systems functioning at a level with little reserve. These underlying factors of aging are reflected in a diminished ability to respond to stress. The elderly patient sometimes has a poor white blood cell response to infection.[6,7] For example in *Haemophilus influenzae* pneumonia, only 61% of people over age 50 produced a leukocytosis. However, when the differential count was examined, 95% had a shift to the left. Thus, although the total white count was deficient, there still was evidence of a white cell response to infection, which could be found if the clinician realized the importance of a differential count in such patients.[8] Elderly people frequently are unable to increase body temperature in response to infection. An elderly patient with tachycardia should be carefully examined to rule out infection even if there is no fever.

A digression on fever is appropriate at this point. Fever develops in the human body when there is an interaction between the polymorphonuclear leukocyte (PMN) and something it ingested. Phagocytosis causes the PMN to shed endogenous pyrogen, a protein that causes fever. There are three main entities that can be phagocytosed: microorganisms, antibody-antigen complexes, and dead tissue. For this reason, some fevers are caused by drug allergy. Other fevers are due to the mopping up of dead tissue as in myocardial infarction (fever for 1 to 3 days is quite common). Another example is dead tissue produced by an alcoholic bout in cirrhosis. However, the most common cause of fever is interaction between phagocytosing polymorphonuclear cells and bacteria. Healthy people have a higher temperature from 6 to 8 PM and a lower temperature around 2 to 3 AM. The fever of infection is added on to the normal diurnal swing of the body temperature, which varies about 1° F. When temperatures are monitored once a day in the morning, fever can be missed for several days. Single daily temperatures must be taken in the evening. Many elderly people have a low normal temperature and a degree or so of fever can remain undetected if this is not taken into account. It is possible that constant aspirin therapy may mask a fever. Adrenocorticosteroid therapy will certainly mask a fever, and patients receiving steroids must have their pulse rate monitored carefully because tachycardia may be the only sign of a complicating infection such as pneumococcal septicemia. Renal failure, which is quite common in the elderly, causes impairment of febrile responses.

Since fever is an exaggeration of the normal diurnal swing of temperature, patients most often have an evening spike while the morning temperature may be normal or somewhat elevated but not as elevated as in the evening. When a fever responds successfully to antibiotic treatment, the fever will fall like a bouncing ball; that is the 6 to 8 PM temperature will be reduced each evening or at least not elevated over the previous evening if the antibiotic therapy has been properly chosen and is successful. If the temperature fails to fall 2 days in succession after the institution of antibiotic therapy, the antibiotic should be changed. Chills at the onset of fever occur in the elderly but are less common, and one must look for other reactions such as confusion.

There are some definite changes in the immunologic responses in the aged. Elderly persons have a reduced IgM from an average of 179 to 106, an increased native C3 from an average of 25 to 36, and a slightly increased properdin level from 100 to 113.[10] The unitage is not important, but the trend is. There is also evidence of a relationship between changes in delayed hypersensitivity and reaction to disease in the elderly. Roberts-Thomas et al. have shown that if skin tests of five common antigens such as mumps, candida, tuberculosis, trychophyton, and streptokinase-streptodornase are done on people of different age groups, 68% of the population over 80 react to none or only one of these antigens. Of those who react to none or only one antigen, 80% are dead within 2 years, whereas 65% of those who react to two or more antigens are still alive 2 years later.[11] These findings require further investigation, but they do indicate the importance of delayed hypersensitivity in elderly individuals.

Normal flora of the body forms a mantle of protection against the invasion of pathogens. Normal flora may sometimes become pathogenic after an acute viral infection, as this may change bacterial adherence on which ability to invade depends. Flora can also change under adverse circumstances such as immobilization in a crowded health care institution. For example, in normal adults and in active and socially involved elderly people approximately 8% have flora from the bowel in their throats. When the elderly are confined to a chair, this increases to 10% and when confined to a bed to 15%. If they are confined to the nursing home, this becomes 20% and becomes 60% if they are in an acute care unit of a general hospital.[12]

Some infections in the elderly represent an increase in the incidence of diseases that also occur in younger adults. For example, there is a steady increase in pneumococcal pneumonia, gram-negative rod septicemia, and urinary tract infection (particularly in women). There are also infections peculiar to the elderly, such as urinary tract infections following obstruction by benign prostatic hypertrophy or vaginitis following degeneration of the vaginal epithelium associated with endocrine changes of aging. As the incidence of diabetes increases markedly with age, infections of diabetics increase because of defective recruitment of white cells to an infected area, defective phagocytosis of bacteria, and defective ability to kill bacteria once they are phagocytosed.[1]

Bacterial infections in the elderly are frequently polymicrobial and represent invasion of bacterial flora into an area that has been damaged, for example, by a decubitus ulcer or by necrosis following vascular obliteration in diabetes. Loss of the skin barrier increases the likelihood of infection by fecal organisms, many of which are anaerobes. The pathophysiology here is that the aerobes in the inoculum first use up the oxygen and then the anaerobes are able to survive and multiply. In addition, for unknown reasons herpes zoster and reactivation of tuberculosis acquired initially at a younger age become more common as people age.

DIAGNOSTIC SKILLS IN INFECTIOUS DISEASES

There are three essential diagnostic steps in infectious disease: first, one must diagnose the probable presence of infection; second, the location of the infection should be delineated; and third, the specific bacterial or viral agent should be definitively diagnosed. Sometimes while awaiting specific agent identification likely possibilities must be considered to begin treatment. Fever is the most frequent indication of infection. If infection becomes generalized with temporary invasion of the bloodstream (bacteremia) or permanent invasion of the bloodstream (septicemia), shaking chills occur in approximately two thirds of cases. If fever for some reason is suppressed, then tachycardia is usually present and must be regarded with suspicion. The probabilities for various bacteria by region are summarized in Table 14-1. For example, in the urinary tract in women, *Escherichia coli* is by far the most likely organism, whereas in the cerebral spinal fluid in the elderly, *Streptococcus pneumoniae* and *Listeria* are most common. To learn the probabilities of infections in different areas of the body cultures should be taken in all the difficult infections. One learns little by curing an infection with antibiotics if one does not know what one is curing. Taking a culture benefits the patient under treatment and also educates the physician. If the urine is examined, unspun, and many bacteria are seen, this is equivalent to a quantitative urine culture and is much more reliable than seeing pus cells in the urine. If bacteria are seen by gram stain in an exudate from an area of the body where there are no bacteria normally present, infection can be presumed, for example, in the cerebral spinal fluid. This does not work in the throat because of the presence of normal flora that is similar in staining properties to the pathogens.[13]

Gram staining should be viewed as a dyeing procedure. In dyeing one has to use not only a dye but also a mordant that binds the dye to fiber. In the case of bacteria, crystal violet is a dye and the mordant is iodine. If this is not fixed

Table 14-1. Most common bacterial pathogens in designated infectious diseases in the elderly

Disease	*Pathogens*
Burns	*S. aureus*
	P. aeruginosa
	Klebsiella enterobacter
Peritonitis	Bacteroides sp.
	E. coli
	Peptostreptococcus
Endocarditis	*S. viridans*
	S. aureus
	S. epidermidis
Meningitis	*S. pneumoniae*
	Gram-negative rods
	L. monocytogenes
Septicemia	*E. coli*
	S. aureus
Urinary tract infections	
Females	*E. coli*
	E. coli and *P. vulgaris*
	P. vulgaris
Males	*P. vulgaris*
	E. coli
	E. coli and *P. vulgaris*
Diarrhea	Enteropathogenic *E. coli*
	C. difficile
	(Rotaviruses)
Pneumonia	*S. pneumoniae*
	Gram-negative rods
	L. pneumophilia

or bound, then one is able to wash out the dye with acetone-ether mixture and the counterstain, which is red Safranin, makes the gram-negative bacteria pink. A gram stain can be done in 20 minutes by a competent observer. When pus is visible, it is important to make a culture. If the pus is not visible but there is fluctuance, it is important to aspirate material for culture. I carry blood culture bottles with me in my physician's bag and often directly inoculate non-blood specimens into these as a suitable way for transporting them to the laboratory.

Blood cultures are extremely important in the elderly.[14] In the presence of pneumonia, at least one blood culture should be taken in the initial diagnostic workup. It is positive in 25% to 33% of most pneumonias with the exception of Legionnaires disease. A single blood culture should also be taken to diagnose meningitis. If one suspects septicemia, that is, if the patient has shaking chills, three blood cultures should be taken, approximately 2 hours apart. The timing serves to exclude temporary bacteremias, which usually last only an hour. If a heart murmur is also present, five blood cultures should be taken. These procedures will reveal 95% of all possible positive cultures within 3 days if the patient is not taking antibiotics. If something that is labeled "contaminant" is isolated like *Staphylococcus epidermidis*, then a second course of three to five blood cultures should be taken. Aspiration cultures are useful from joints, occasionally from the bladder or the skin, and frequently by transtracheal aspiration.

If an elderly person has a fever of 102° F or higher, which has lasted for 1 to 2 weeks and has been investigated for several days to a week without solution, it is labeled a *fever of unknown origin*. These difficult-to-diagnose fevers need to be studied as completely as possible. About one third of them are caused by infections of the usual sort such as pneumonia, urinary tract infection, or septicemia. Approximately 20% are caused by connective tissue diseases such as rheumatoid arthritis or polyarteritis nodosa. An important group is the 20% of patients with fevers of unknown origin who have cancer. This relates to necrosis occurring in tumors and leading to phagocytosis, production of endogenous pyrogen, and fever. Ten percent to twenty percent of fevers of unknown origin are due to miscellaneous identifiable causes, and about 10% are not diagnosed. Causes of fevers of unknown origin in the elderly are very similar to those in younger adults.[15]

PREVENTION OF INFECTION

The immune system decreases in effectiveness with aging. Vaccination against influenza is recommended for elderly people, pneumococcal pneumonia, and in rural areas against tetanus. There are two primary causes of influenza: influenza A and influenza B. The genetic makeup of influenza B tends to be stable, whereas that of influenza A varies from year to year making a new vaccine necessary each year. Patients with long-term heart disease, long-term lung disease, long-term renal disease, severe anemia such as sickle cell disease, or diabetes mellitus should be vaccinated. A good case can be made for vaccinating all those over 65 against influenza. In addition to protecting the elderly in nursing homes, one must also remember to protect the staff in nursing homes and hospitals. The vaccine is given in a single dose of 0.5 ml subcutaneously. Mild soreness can occur, and the Guillain-Barré syndrome may occur in a ratio of 10 cases for every million people vaccinated. It most frequently resolves without any residual weakness, but approximately 5% of cases are fatal. Amantadine, a simple chemical, has a 70% efficacy in the prevention of influenza A. It is not effective against influenza B. It is particularly useful in people with cardiopulmonary, metabolic, or immunodeficiency diseases. Persons in semiclosed institutional environments, especially older persons who have not received influenza vaccine, should receive amantadine prophylaxis (200 mg daily administered orally) if there is an outbreak of influenza. Influenza vaccine should be given at the same time because amantadine does not suppress the antibody responses to inactivated influenza vaccine. Amantadine can be discontinued 10 days after vaccination unless the patient is immunocompromised. Amantadine is inexpensive, and the rare side effects are mental confusion, tremulousness, and insomnia.

Fourteen antigenic types of pneumococci account for 83% of septicemic pneumococcal infections most commonly encountered in the elderly population. Large scale tests have shown that the vaccine is 80% effective in preventing pneumococcal pneumonia and septicemia. Patients who are under treatment for Hodgkin's disease respond poorly. Transient local discomfort is very common; 35% of recipients develop local erythema, and 3% develop a mild fever. Vaccination consists of a single injection of 0.5 ml subcutaneously or intramuscularly. The main problem is expense; at present it costs approximately $5 per dose. It is recommended primarily for elderly patients with cardiorespiratory, renal, hepatic, neoplastic, or diabetic disease. It can be administered at any time of the year and will produce solid immunity within 1 month or less. Reimmunization requirements for the new vaccine have not yet been determined, but studies suggest that immunity may persist as long as 5 years. It should not be repeated within 3 years as the Arthus reaction with local necrosis is likely to occur.

Infection prevention in the elderly also involves the preservation of natural barriers. Bladder indwelling catheters and bed sores are prime examples of breaches of natural barriers. In paraplegic patients intermittent catheterization has been shown to be safer than indwelling catheters. This procedure needs to be investigated in elderly people. Bed sore prevention means prevention of local pressure and prevention of the exposure of the skin to moisture. Patients with a hemoglobin level of less than 12 gm should be carefully checked for protein malnutrition, which interferes with healing. Every effort should be made to provide proper nourishment for patients. Active and passive movements help prevent decubitus ulcers.

Postoperative infections increase in incidence with age, and prevention involves the use of aseptic techniques. In certain situations antibiotic prophylaxis can be effective, such as when there is a contaminated wound or a probably contaminated wound. In these cases antibiotics can be effective if they are begun approximately 1 hour before the skin is cut and continued for 48 hours. The use of the antibiotic varies with the type of risk, but cephalosporins are commonly used. Excessive doses of antibiotics or the use of too many antibiotics for too long may predispose patients to superinfection because the normal flora has been reduced. Louria and Kaminski studied the development of superinfectious pneumonia in patients initially treated for pneumococcal pneumonia. The results of this investigation are summarized in Table 14-2.

Table 14-2. Superinfection as shown by quantitative sputum culture in patients originally treated for pneumococcal pneumonia

Daily dose of antibiotic in patients with ≥ 10^5 S. pneumoniae per milliliter sputum and with pneumonic infiltrate	*Percent positive culture of new pathogen ≥ 10^5 organism per milliliter sputum*
Penicillin ≤ 2.4 million units	0
Penicillin ≥ 10 million units	29
Penicillin and streptomycin	19
Tetracycline	5
Chloramphenicol	5
Penicillin with tetracycline or chloramphenicol	47

From Louria, D.B., and Kaminski, T.: Am. Rev. Resp. Dis. **85**:649, 1962.

Persons who are traveling to foreign countries should be protected against traveler's diarrhea. Within 3 to 21 days of arrival in a new country the patient develops an acute watery diarrhea. For the elderly traveler, this diarrhea is dangerous because dehydration is a threat to renal and circulatory systems. About one half to two thirds of traveler's diarrhea is due to infection with enterotoxigenic *E. coli*. This can be prevented with tetracycline, 250 mg four times per day for 3 days, taken after the second diarrhea stool. A few cases are due to shigellosis or salmonellas (which usually but not always respond to tetracyclines) or to rotavirus or *Giardia lamblia* (which do not respond to tetracyclines).

REGIONAL AND SYSTEMIC INFECTIONS

Skin infections

The incidence of *wound infections* increases with age.[16] Elderly patients are likely to have operations with the following postoperative wound infection rates: cholecystectomy, 4%; herniorrhaphy, 3%; colon resection, 10%; below knee amputation, 15%; hysterectomy, 3%; total hip replacement, 3%; and total knee replacement, 1%. As mentioned before, there are specific indications for preoperative wound sepsis prophylaxis with antibiotics.

Elderly dependent patients are predisposed to *burns*. In addition, alcoholism or psychiatric disorders increases the risk. Infection of burns and complicating septicemia are responsible for 20% to 30% of all deaths from burns. Dead tissue must be removed and the wound must be covered if possible by grafting. Severe protein calorie malnutrition must be combatted. An isolated controlled environment is needed, and local antibacterial agents such as 0.5% aqueous silver nitrate, mafenide (Sulfamylon), or silver sulfadiazine cream should be applied to the burn area. Systemic antibiotics may be used for short periods of decreased host resistance or in the presence of established infections. Penicillin G is given early in the course of treatment to prevent hemolytic streptococcal infection. Short-term antibiotic prophylaxis is also indicated in periods surrounding anesthesia, surgery, or cardiac shock. Antistaphylococcal antibiotics are also indicated. If the patient's condition deteriorates with the development of either fever or hypothermia, paralytic ileus, leukocytosis, disorientation, tachycardia, or septic shock, it is important to know the specific type of infection. Blood culture and wound culture should be taken often enough to indicate appropriate antibiotics. *E. coli*, Klebsiella, enterobacter, *Staphylococcus aureus* and *Pseudomonas aeruginosa* are the most common lethal invaders.

Staphylococcal infections are common in the elderly. Infection of a single hair follicle produces a boil and of multiple hair follicles a carbuncle. Various host resistance problems such as renal failure, diabetes, and cross-infection in a long-term care institution predispose patients to these infections. *S. aureus* lives in the human nose about as far as the exploring finger can reach and travels by hand contact to the attendant or to the patient's skin. Patients who have recurrent boils, perhaps 10 or more in number lasting 6 months or longer, usually have established carriage in the nose. If the infections are primarily between the waist and the knee, the carriage is likely to be in the perineum between the anus and the scrotum or around the vulva. These areas are not cleared by systemic chemotherapy and require local antibiotic ointment such as bacitracin (500 units/gm).[13]

Skin infections in diabetics are frequent and the consequences are serious. The majority of these patients have poor circulation with 60% having absent dorsalis pedis and 25% no popliteal pulses. The skin is frequently anesthetic. The diabetic elderly often have poor vision and intend to cut a toenail and cut a toe instead. This becomes infected with aerobes, which prepare the way for fecal anaerobes to take over. The most frequent infections are anaerobic streptococcus and anaerobic staphylococcus (peptostreptococcus and peptococcus), *E. coli, Klebsiella* enterobacter species, and bacteroides. About 10% to 20% have gas palpable or visible in the tissues on x-ray films. If not treated with antianaerobic antibiotics, gangrene may develop with a resulting need for amputation. About one third have underlying osteomyelitis. There is a slight preponderance of females, and most of them have had diabetes for 13 years or more. Thirteen percent of the patients who develop these problems are controlled by diet alone; 43% are receiving oral antidiabetic agents and 43% are receiving insulin. The onset of the infection usually leads to an increase in the insulin requirement. About 50% to 60% also have cardiovascular disease, renal disease, retinopathy or cataracts, peripheral vascular disease, or some or all of these in combination. Overt gangrene develops in 40% and ketoacidosis in 3%. Proper antianaerobic chemotherapy decreases the need for amputation below the knee from 10% to 1%.[17,18]

Pressure sores occur in 5% to 10% of hospitalized patients and in 5% to 30% of patients in nursing homes. Patients over 70 years old account for 70% of these bed sores. Patients confined to a chair have more pressure sores than bed-fast patients with similar degrees of helplessness. Elderly patients at home have a similar incidence of bed sores. In a study survey, 1% to 6% of patients under 50, 10% of those aged 50 to 59, and 20% to 25% of those 60 and over had bed sores. Prolonged pressure and moist bed clothes cause bed sores, and disordered metabolic states increase the risk. Infection causes healing problems. Patients with fever attributable to decubitus ulcers are most frequently infected with anaerobic organisms, particularly *Bacteroides fragilis*. Septicemia often develops, and when it does the fatality rate is about 50%. Culture requires proper anaerobic techniques. Surgical debridement is an important part of the treatment. Decubitus ulcers are caused by pressures greater than 44 gm/cm^2 on large sites and for 2 or more continuous hours. Contributing factors are advanced age, immobilization, tranquilizers, cachexia, and lowered arteriolar pressure. Decubitus ulcers in patients in nursing homes are best managed by a team of nurses specially trained in surgical debridement. Enzymatic methods of debridement can also be used. Antipressure padding and water mattresses are extremely helpful.[19,20]

Herpes zoster, most frequently found in the elderly, is caused by varicella zoster virus and is a reactivation of chickenpox. This infection occurs worldwide equally in men and women. If a cohort of 1000 people were to live to be 85, half would have had one attack of zoster, 10 would have had two attacks, and one would have had a third attack. A unilateral painful vesicular eruption develops, which is localized in a dermatome of a specific dorsal root or extramedullary cranial ganglion. Herpes zoster, herpes simplex, or chickenpox lesions have multinucleated giant cells in their bases, which can be shown by a Tzanck test. Using a No. 15 scalpel the top

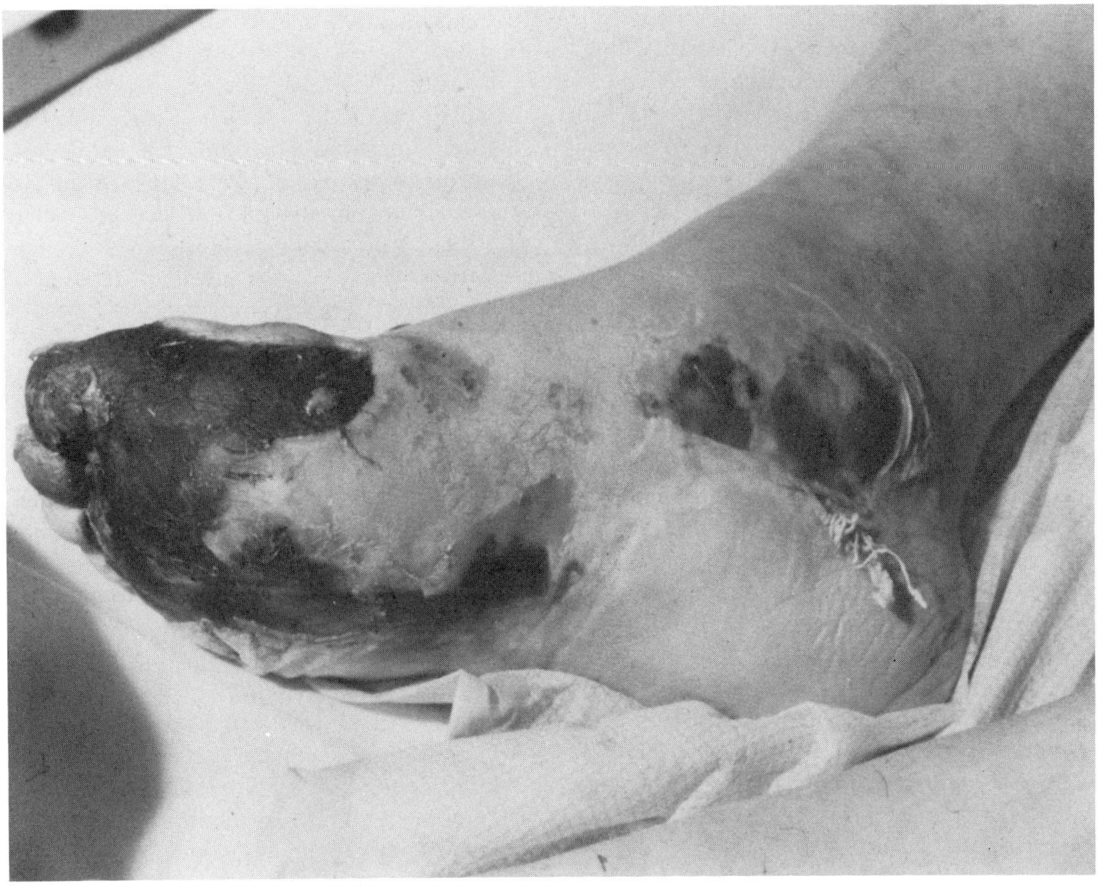

Fig. 14-1. Infected gangrenous ulcer in a diabetic patient. These lesions frequently give rise to septicemia sometimes due to bacteroides alone and at other times multimicrobial in type.

is removed from a vesicle and it is scraped vigorously. When lightly heat fixed and examined with Giemsas, Wright, or Papanicolaou stain, the smear reveals multinucleated giant cells with intranuclear inclusions. Pain and paresthesia occur in the dermatome site 1 to 10 days before the eruption. (Rarely the attack stops here; "zoster sine herpete.") A bandlike pattern of erythematous grouped papules are topped by clear vesicles within 12 to 24 hours and progress to pustules in 72 hours. In 7 to 8 days the pustules begin to dry; crusts occur in 10 to 12 days and fall off in 2 to 3 weeks. Zoster involves the thoracic nerves in over half of the patients, trigeminal and cervical nerves in 10% to 20%, lumbar zoster in 3% to 18%, and sacral zoster in 3% to 5%. Half the patients who have vesicles on the tip of their nose develop ocular complications indicating involvement of the ophthalmic division of the fifth cranial nerve. Sacral zoster is sometimes complicated by neurogenic bladder dysfunction. The incidence of postherpetic neuralgia increases with age. Prednisone has been used in controlled trials to minimize postherpetic neuralgia in patients over 60, 60 mg per day for the first week, 30 mg per day for the second, and 15 mg per day for the third. To be effective this treatment should be started within the first 7 days of illness. Neuralgia occurs in 30% of patients over 60 who are treated with steroids and in 73% of untreated patients. Aspirin or codeine are used to control the pain. For eye involvement referral to an ophthalmologist is necessary.

Respiratory infections

Influenza occurs in epidemics. Epidemics occur at approximately 2-year intervals with pandemics or worldwide outbreaks occurring 10 to 11 years apart. The two main viruses are influenza A and influenza B. Influenza B does not change much, but influenza A shows an antigenic drift and new vaccines have to be produced yearly. When an outbreak occurs, approximately 20% of a family practice clientele will be involved. The outbreak spreads over a 7- to 8-week span. After an incubation period of 1 to 3 days, there is an abrupt onset of fever, approximately 102° F with headache, aches and pains, and a dry cough. Many of the patients start off with an acute rigor (shaking chill) and can time the onset of the disease to the minute. The myalgia involves the long muscles of the back and some aching occurs in the limbs but it is less noticeable. The patient has a raw throat and a dry nonproductive cough, sometimes with substernal aching at the time of coughing. Abnormal findings in the uncomplicated disease are fever, red eyes, and congestive respiratory mucosa. The fever usually lasts 2 to 3 days. After this the patient is very weak or prostrate. Convalescence may last for 1 to 2 weeks. The uncomplicated disease is a nuisance and is severe for only a couple of days. In contrast to this, complications can be lethal.

The disease in the elderly follows the same pattern as in younger patients except that pulmonary involvement is much more common. Pneumonia and bronchitis together occur in approximately 10% of all influenza patients, but this combination occurs in 36% of patients age 60 to 69 and in 73% of patients age 70 and older. The patient with pneumonia is more ill and dyspneic and may be cyanotic. The most important indicator of pneumonia is an increased respiration rate. There may be rales or lobar consolidation. About one third of the pneumonias show discrete consolidation, and there are about an equal number of pneumonias and bronchitis patients. Only 7% of people developing pneumonia have underlying disease, so one must be aware that apparently healthy individuals can develop severe complications. Bacterial pneumonia complicating influenza is most frequently caused by *S. pneumoniae*, then by *S. aureus*, and rarely by *H. influenzae*. Most deaths occur in the elderly. The overall case fatality rate is 5% to 10%, and the case fatality rate in the elderly is 20% to 30%. As usual the fever response in the elderly may be lower than in younger patients. A gram stain of the sputum is useful and if no bacteria are seen, one must suspect a primary influenza virus pneumonia or Legionnaires disease if there is a chest x-ray infiltrate. Bacterial appearance on gram stain can help in the choice of antibiotic. Most frequently this will be penicillin G or an antistaphylococcal penicillin, such as nafcillin.

Pneumonia is the only infectious disease that is one of the 10 most common causes of death. It accounts for 10% of all medical service admissions to acute care hospitals. In adults 70% or more of pneumonia cases are bacterial in origin, whereas in children 50% or less are caused by bacteria. In both age groups, pneumonia of unknown etiology comprises 5% to 15%. Pneumonias are categorized as follows: (1) pneumococcal pneumonia; (2) mycoplasmal pneumonia; (3) Legionnaires pneumonia; (4) gram-negative rod pneumonia; and (5) staphylococcal pneumonia. Pneumococcal, mycoplasmal, and Legionnaires pneumonia are usually acquired in the community, whereas gram-negative rod pneumonia and staphylococcal pneumonia are usually acquired in the hospital.

The disease of most concern in the elderly is pneumococcal pneumonia. This pneumonia occurs in the winter and early spring and affects three males for every two females. It progressively affects more people from the age of 30 on upward in a straight line relationship to age. Patients may first develop a coryzal illness, then abruptly develop a shaking chill (in over 80%) with a rapid rise in temperature to 102° to 104° F. Three-fourths of patients develop sharp stabbing pain on coughing or deep breathing. Dyspnea and cough with pinkish, bloody, or rust-colored sputum develops within a few hours. The respirations are rapid with expiratory grunting and sometimes cyanosis. Early the breath sounds are diminished in a localized area with "just wet" rales. Later signs of consolidation appear, but a diagnosis should be made before this happens. Mild jaundice may occur in 5% to 10%, and the abdomen is often bloated due to a medical ileus. Approximately 10% of this population has a history of a previous attack of pneumonia. One-lobe involvement occurs in 66% and two-lobe involvement in 25%. A pleural effusion is present in 5%. Approximately 40% have serologic evidence of coexisting viral infection.[13,21,22]

The most effective and rapid diagnosis is by

gram stain of a properly obtained sputum specimen. Suitable sputum contains 25 or more PMN and less than 10 mouth epithelial cells per high power field. The presence of easily seen gram-stained bacteria in the sputum differentiates an active infection from a carrier as there have to be 10^5 organisms per milliliter or more present in an infection. It also gives assurance that the patient does not have gram-negative rod pneumonia.

Before antibiotics were available, blood cultures in pneumococcal pneumonia were positive in 25% of persons under age 65, 38% of persons aged 60 to 69, and in 58% of persons aged 70 and over. More recent figures show positive pretreatment blood cultures in 15% to 30%.[23] Six to twenty-five percent of pneumococcal pneumonia diagnoses are made where the sputum is negative but a culture of the blood is positive. Lung puncture cultures are mainly used in children but are beginning to be used more in the compromised host, including the elderly. Transtracheal aspirates were introduced in 1959. They are indicated for the diagnosis of anaerobic infections and in patients who have failed to be diagnosed by the more usual methods, who are unable to cough, or who are critically ill. Contraindications are bleeding disorders and patients unable to cooperate.

Approximately 10% to 20% of the lung is behind the heart shadow, and a lateral as well as an anterior-posterior view is necessary to diagnose pneumonia. Pneumococcal pneumonia in young people and women is typically lobar. In men over age 40 and men over 65 in particular, the appearance is distorted in about 50% by underlying emphysema. Consolidation of pneumococcal pneumonia disappears by 6 weeks in those under age 60. Alcohol and underlying emphysema may lead to delayed resolution. X-ray resolution occurs in 14 weeks in persons over age 50 but in 18 weeks if there is emphysema. I only have the x-ray film repeated if the patient's condition appears to be deteriorating.

The treatment of choice in pneumococcal pneumonia is aqueous (not procaine) penicillin G, 1,200,000 units daily in divided doses until 72 hours after the last sign of illness. Higher doses of penicillin are not helpful except in meningitis or endocarditis. The first dose must be aqueous penicillin injected intramuscularly. Thereafter oral treatment is adequate. Strains of penicillin-resistant pneumococci were reported in 1977 in South Africa and in Minnesota. These strains were also resistant to erythromycin and chloramphenicol. Usually, however, erythromycin is a suitable substitute for penicillin G in patients known to be allergic to penicillin G. The cephalosporins can also be used but have some cross-reaction with penicillin antigens. Tetracyclines fail to kill approximately 20% of pneumococci.

The prognosis in pneumococcal pneumonia illustrates principles applicable to other types of pneumonia.[22] In the 1930s in patients of all ages, pneumococcal pneumonia had a 30% case fatality rate. The case fatality rate in the age group 10 to 20 years was 10% and in those over 60 years was 72%. The overall rate now is 5%, with 1% aged 10 to 20 years and 8% over 60 years. If one lobe is involved with modern treatment there is a 1% fatality rate; if two or more lobes are involved, the rate is 10% or more. Nowadays alcoholics are treatable with a 4% fatality rate compared to a 3% rate in nonalcoholics. Underlying disease such as emphysema leads to an 11% fatality rate compared with 1% when there is no other disease. With bacteremia the fatality rate is 9% and without it the rate is 1%.[22] The elderly frequently have two or more lobes involved. Also they often have underlying pulmonary disease, and bacteremia is common. Various studies show fatality rates of 28% to 35% in elderly persons. Patients who have a PCO_2 of 55 or higher or PO_2 of 55 (acutely) or lower can benefit from mechanical ventilation. This might be thought excessive in the elderly, but it has been shown that of individuals age 70 to 74 treated with a respirator, 57% were saved; at age 75 to 79, 53% and at age 80 to 95, 39% saved after respirator treatment in the intensive care unit. Therefore careful assessment should be made as to whether the patient requires ventilator assistance.

Gram-negative rods cause 5% to 10% of all pneumonias, but estimates of 30% to 40% may be more correct for hospital pneumonias or for those found in long-term care establishments.[23,24] Over 80% are males usually age 50 or older. Serious underlying disease is the rule, and about 25% have had pneumonia previously. Predisposing factors are alcoholism, heart disease, diabetes, and emphysema. The patient usually develops severe dyspnea with fever and one or more chills. Profuse diaphoresis may be present and cough, sputum, and pleuritic chest pain are usual. Hemoptysis can occur with *Klebsiella* enterobacteror or proteus infections. Cardiomegaly or congestive heart failure occur in about one fourth of the patients. Half of the patients are anemic. White blood counts usually lie between 15 and 20 thousand/mm^3. Over 90% have a shift to the left even when the white cell count is normal.[8] Over 80% have abnormal liver function tests and the bilirubin level is elevated in one half of patients. In 85% the lower lobes are involved. Diagnosis follows the same plan as in pneumococcal pneumonia. An aminoglycoside, usually gentamicin, is the treatment of choice. Persons with renal disease should be followed by using gentamicin levels; those over 80 years old can be assumed to have some degree of renal failure.

In adults *staphylococcal pneumonia* is found after influenza or other viral disease and occasionally as a nosocomial infection in geriatric debilitated patients. Approximately one third of postinfluenza pneumonias are staphylococcal; the patients have cough, sputum production, high fever, shaking chills, and often cyanosis. Patients become progressively and rapidly ill. They may be disoriented or in coma or shock. Staphylococci are identified in gram stain of the sputum. The treatment of choice is administration of nafcillin or some other semisynthetic penicillinase-resistant penicillin. In some cases an aminoglycoside can be added with advantage. Lung abscess occurs in 25% and empyema in 10%.

Legionnaires disease can be asymptomatic but is usually an acute pneumonia affecting older men twice as often as women. They usually have underlying lung disease or a history of cigarette smoking. After a 2-day prodromal phase of malaise, myalgia, and headache, there is a relatively sudden onset of fever (102° to 105° F) often with rigor and frequently with bradycardia. A nonproductive cough occurs with pleuritic chest pain. There is often confusion and diarrhea. Confusion occurs in 30% at onset and in 50% during the course of the illness. Rales are heard, most often unilaterally; rarely shock or respiratory failure occurs. Gastrointestinal bleeding or renal failure can be complications. A moderate leukocytosis is common, sometimes with a raised sedimentation rate and moderately abnormal liver function tests. A clue to the diagnosis is a gram stain of the sputum with many pus cells but no visible bacteria. Diagnosis is made by a rising titer of indirect fluorescent antibody, by culture on hemoglobin isovitale x-enriched media under CO_2, or by Dieterle's silver impregnantion stain on biopsy specimens. Chest x-ray films reveal patchy pneumonia, which is often unilateral. Treatment is based on clinical suspicion after the appropriate tests have been taken and is with erythromycin, 2 to 4 gm daily. This pneumonia is acquired from the environment, perhaps from the soil or air-conditioning or water systems. Person-to-person transmission has not been shown, and isolation is not necessary. Hospital outbreaks have occurred.

Aspiration of exogenous material or of gastric contents may cause sudden asphyxia or long-term debilitating pulmonary disease.[25] The severity depends on the type of material aspirated and its pH and volume. An inert aspirate causes no distinctive lesions, whereas a large volume of toxic aspirate produces extensive clinical pneumonia. Unfortunately there is no diagnostic test for unwitnessed aspiration. Although bronchoscopy may yield some clues, diagnosis usually depends on the high index of suspicion and evaluation of the clinical situation with a knowledge of the following predisposing factors: reduced level of consciousness with diminished or absent gag and cough reflexes, esophageal disorders, endotracheal intubation, the use of nasogastric tubes, and tracheostomy. Silent aspiration is reported in 7% to 16% of those cases in which general anesthetics are used. The ideal treatment is prevention. If the aspirate is an admixture of liquid and solid material, for example, stomach contents, vigorous tracheal suction followed immediately by bronchoscopy is essential. The correction of hypoxia is mandatory and blood gases should be monitored. Patients' vital signs, urinary output, electrocardiogram, arterial blood gases, and intraarterial pressures should also be monitored whenever possible.

Aerosolized isoproterenol or a similar bronchodilator should be administered for the relief of bronchospasm. Aminophylline, given intravenously, may also be useful. Purulent sputum and extending infiltrates on chest x-ray films are reliable indicators of pulmonary infection. In contrast, fever and leukocytosis often represent a nonspecific inflammatory response. If the patient appears to have developed pneumonia, penicillin G, administered intravenously in high doses, is useful, and clindamycin or chloramphenicol can be used for those allergic to penicillin G. Short-term steroid therapy with antibiotic coverage is valuable in the management of aspiration pneumonitis if given within the first 12 to 24 hours.

Sixty percent of new patients with *tuberculosis* are 45 years old or older, an age group that comprises 30% of the total population. The tuberculosis case rates in the United States per 100,000 are 6 under age 25; 17 between ages 25 and 44; 28 between 45 and 65; and 38 above 65. Some states have case rates that are approximately one third of these figures, and in these states tuberculosis is becoming a medical rarity, not expected and easily missed until others are exposed. An additional factor in the elderly is ethnic origin; the rate for white females is 20, white males 50; nonwhite females 66 and nonwhite males 170/100,000 population. The vast majority of these cases represent reactivation and not fresh reinfection. It is estimated that 4% of the tuberculin-positive population will reactivate within the next 50 years. Initial infection with tuberculosis means the entry of live tubercle bacilli usually into the lung. A minor Ghon focus is formed and the disease subsides. After this has happened, however, the presence of live tubercle bacilli in the body can be demonstrated by a positive tuberculin test with 10 mm or more of induration. It is very important, therefore, to find out from elderly patients what their exposure to tuberculosis was when they were in their 20s or younger as this is the time of life when their skin reactivity usually changed. Reactivation in the elderly occurs in relation to malnutrition, alcholism, cancer, and possibly because of age alone. This population carries a much higher incidence of positive tuberculin tests.[26,27]

The symptoms of tuberculosis are fever, weight loss, cough, sputum, and debility, all of which are common in other maladies in the elderly. Fever usually occurs in the evening or nightime and is associated with night sweats. Productive cough and particularly hemoptysis are clear indications for a chest x-ray film; the diagnosis becomes obvious with infiltrate or cavities in the apical posterior segments of the upper lobes. Unfortunately, when tuberculosis is diagnosed in elderly persons, 40% of them have advanced disease. This may be due to increased virulence of the organisms, decreased host resistance, or failure to suspect the disease early. An elderly person may have only a vague general decline in health before tuberculosis is eventually diagnosed. In people under age 65 who have positive cultures for tuberculosis, first strength tuberculin is positive in 72%, intermediate in 92%, and second strength in 99.3%. In some studies in the elderly, only 80% to 85% of known tuberculous patients have positive intermediate tuberculin tests. Elderly persons with a previous history of acute tuberculosis who have not received modern chemotherapy should be given 1 year of treatment with isoniazid whether or not their sputum is positive on culture.

Diagnosis is made on the basis of smear and culture of three morning deep cough sputum specimens; 24-hour specimens are no longer used as they easily become contaminated with atypical mycobacteria. Skin tests in the elderly are useful but not necessarily diagnostic. Chest x-ray films are mandatory, and comparison with earlier films is very helpful. The diagnosis of extrapulmonary tuberculosis involves urine culture or biopsy culture of the involved area.

The modern treatment of tuberculosis is very effective except in socially maladjusted people, noncompliant patients, alcoholics, or patients in whom the organisms are drug resistant. One must therefore take a history of a previous treatment for tuberculosis or contact with people who have been treated with modern antituberculosis drug therapy. It is important to be aware that drug resistance is more common in the foreign-born than the native. Before embarking on treatment, one must be aware of decreased organ function in the elderly, particularly decreased renal function. Tuberculosis is treated with any two antituberculous drugs so long as one of them is isoniazid. In advanced disease, infection of the kidney, or tuberculous meningitis, three drugs are indicated. The initial drugs are usually isoniazid INH, 300 mg per day, and ethambutol, 15 mg/kg per day in a single daily dose. Rifampin is a useful third drug. The dose of rifampin is 600 mg orally, and it should be noted that it interacts with warfarin sodium (coumadin). Rifampin can cause red tears and red urine early in the course of therapy, but this usually stops with continued treatment. There is more risk of toxicity when the drug is given erratically. Pyridoxine, 50 mg daily, is necessary in poor nutritional states or if other pyridoxine antagonist drugs such as cycloserine or pyrazinamide are given. Some patients are given streptomycin, 500 to 1000 mg daily, but ototoxicity occurs more easily in the elderly than in the young. Occasionally in the very ill, the concomitant use of steroids is justified. Many patients will benefit by brief hospitalization for tests and education. There is no indication for surgery in tuberculosis. Patients should receive monthly sputum cultures and smears until the cultures are negative for 2 successive months. Once the smear becomes negative, (often 2 weeks after the onset of treatment), the patient is no longer infectious. Treatment is carried on for 9 months if INH and rifampin are used, depending on the compliance of the patient.[26-29]

Gastrointestinal infections

Diarrhea caused *pseudomembranous enterocolitis* can occur after a variety of insults such as antibiotics, surgery, uremia, and myocardial infarction. It is now seen primarily after treatment with antibiotics, particularly after administration of clindamycin. The majority of cases appear to be due to a change in bowel flora with an overgrowth of certain clostridia. Possibly it can also be caused by an overgrowth of *Candida* or staphylococci, but the prime problem is an overgrowth of *Clostridium difficile,* which is resistant to the antibiotics being used. There is usually an abrupt onset of abdominal pain and fever 4 to 10 days after beginning antibiotic treatment, but it can occur after treatment has stopped. The offending antibiotic should be stopped immediately. Oral vancomycin is the treatment of choice, but oral metronidazole may also be effective.

Various diarrheas are caused by food or water. The causes of major *food-borne* diarrheas are *Salmonella,* 22%; *S. aureus,* 20%; *C. botulinum,* 6%; *Shigella,* 3%; *Vibrio parahemolyticus,* 1%; ciguatera, 6%; scombroid, 5%; and mushrooms, 4%. The onset is fairly typical in relation to the clinical picture. Nausea and vomiting occur within 1 to 6 hours of eating due to *S. aureus* in the majority of cases and *Bacillus cereus* in a few. Although most patients have vomiting and diarrhea, fever is uncommon. The illness usually lasts 12 hours or less. Staphylococci are resistant to salt and grow in animal protein foods such as ham and cream dressings or fillings. If abdominal cramps and diarrhea occur 8 to 16 hours after eating, an enterotoxin from *Clostridium perfringens* or *B. cereus* can be suspected. This is also a brief illness. The patient may be nauseated but rarely vomits, and fever is uncommon. Patients with fever, abdominal cramps, and diarrhea beginning 16 to 28 hours after eating usually are infected with *Salmonella,* occasionally with *Shigella* or *V. parahemolyticus, Yersinia enterocolitica,* or invasive *E. coli.* If only abdominal cramps and watery diarrhea occur within 16 to 72 hours, the major causes are enterotoxogenic *E. coli, V. parahemolyticus,* and noncholera vibrios. Nausea, vomiting, diarrhea, and paralysis within 18 to 36 hours strongly suggest food-borne botulism.

Fluid replacement is extremely important in elderly patients who have severe diarrhea. If groups are traveling together, it is helpful to carry foil packages containing 20 gm of glucose, 3.5 gm of salt, 2.5 gm of sodium bicarbonate, and 1.5 gm of potassium chloride; these can be made up by the local pharmacist. When needed, the contents can be dissolved in a liter of water. Patients with five to ten watery stools per day should sip 1 to 1.5 liters daily in divided doses every 6 hours; for more than ten watery stools, 2 liters daily is recommended. Medications such as opiates and diphenoxylate (Lomotil) may prolong some forms of infectious diarrhea and are best avoided. Iodochlorohydroxyquin (Entero-Vioform) sold abroad for diarrhea can cause neurologic damage and should not be used.[13]

Viral hepatitis is caused by three main viruses: hepatitis A (infectious hepatitis, HAV); hepatitis B (serum hepatitis, HBV); and non-A, non-B, intermediate between these two. The clinical picture is very similar for these diseases and is divided into preicteric and icteric phases. In 75% the onset is gradual. Anorexia and weakness occur in 90%; nausea and vomiting and a vague right upper quadrant discomfort or pain is found in a lesser number. These symptoms are predominant for a period of 3 to 10 days. The next phase is that of jaundice and dark urine lasting 1 to 3 weeks. There may also be light stools. The patient usually feels better after the onset of jaundice. Two variants on this general picture are that the disease can be essentially asymptomatic or it can be fulminant with liver failure. Some patients, particularly those with hepatitis B syndrome, have an onset with serum sickness syndrome consisting of fever, urticaria, and arthralgia or arthritis. In the elderly, the clinical picture is frequently less definite, and only 50% are correctly diagnosed initially.[30,31] Delayed appreciation of the problem leads to delayed admission to hospital. These patients frequently have other diseases and in a population in their 80s and 90s this may be as high as 90% of patients. The elderly often lose 8 to 10 kg in weight, and a mistaken diagnosis of cancer may be made. The mood and mentality of the older patient is frequently aberrant even in the absence of hepatic coma. The laboratory findings in this disease are a rise in SGOT to approximately eight times normal and a similar rise in SGPT. The LDH is usually 2 to 3 times normal, and the alkaline phosphatase level is mildly elevated (more elevated in younger patients with hepatitis). The bilirubin usually rises to levels of 8 to 15 mg/100 ml and the direct reacting bilirubin is equal to the indirect. Both SGOT and bilirubin return to normal more slowly in older than younger patients. Antigenemia also persists for a longer time. Leukocyte count and sedimentation rate increase more than in younger patients with hepatitis. Certain diseases can be associated with hepatitis, particularly hepatitis B. These are periarteritis nodosa and polymyalgia rheumatica.

The HB surface antigen is elevated in approximately two thirds of these patients and may remain elevated after treatment. In theory this may be an important trigger of these immunologic diseases in response to infection in the elderly. The general case fatality rates in hepatitis A are approximately 0.1% to 5% and in hepatitis B they are 1% to 2%. In the elderly, fatality rates can be increased five- to ten-fold; fatality rates for hepatitis undifferentiated as A or B have ranged from 15% to 25%. Subacute necrosis has been reported in 40% and a severe course in 46%, compared to 23% in patients age 30 to 39. A prolonged course has been reported in 16%. Fibrotic lesions of the liver are more pronounced in the elderly, and cirrhosis has been reported in 7% to 18%. Other complications are mixed cryoglobulinemia, membranous glomerulonephritis, and possibly hepatocellular cancer and aplastic anemia. Poor prognostic findings are a bilirubin over 20 mg/100 ml and a low blood sugar level. Elderly patients usually spend more time in hospitals than younger patients. The disease has to be distinguished from hepatitis caused by Epstein-Barr virus and liver damage from drugs, toxins, anoxia, or congestive cardiac failure. Hemolysis must also be differentiated from hepatitis. The combination of significant weight loss and cholestatic features may suggest extrahepatic blockage and signal a need for surgery. The fatality rate for operating on elderly people with hepatitis is approximately 50% to 60% and should be avoided at all costs. Drugs likely to damage the liver in this age group are phenothiazines and testosterone. Management is rest and a nutritious diet. Steroids are not beneficial. Outbreaks can occur in homes for the elderly because serum hepatitis can pass in very minute amounts of blood, stool, tears, or saliva. A nail brush used by the group as a whole is a good example. Discharges from decubitus ulcers of patients with hepatitis are infectious. Serum hepatitis occurs in approximately a third of hepatitis cases in the elderly. Physical findings can be disappointingly few and consist of icterus and an enlarged or tender liver. The disease affects both sexes equally. Prophylaxis of hepatitis A is achieved with 0.02 ml/kg of immune serum globulin intramuscularly. With hepatitis B, hepatitis B immune globulin (H-BIG) is given in 3 ml volume.[32] This has been found to reduce the hepatitis attack rate in exposed personnel of hospitals from 7% to 11% to 2% to 3%, a significant reduction. There is suggestive but not certain evidence that specific hepatitis immune globulin protects significantly better against hepatitis B than normal pooled serum globulin.

Appendicitis can occur in the elderly. Vomiting occurs in elderly patients in 33% compared to 72% in younger persons, but chills are twice as frequent in the elderly. Abdominal guarding is less frequent, 61% compared to 77%, and positive rectal examination is less frequent, 45% compared to 51%. A normal white count is found in 30% compared to 14%. Seventy-two hours or more elapse before diagnosis in 18% of geriatric patients compared with 6% in children. Perforation occurs in 46% versus 18% and abscess in 30% versus 10%. Surgical drains are needed in 37% versus 14%. The case fatality rate is 5% to 10% compared to less than 1%. Five percent of all cases of appendicitis occur in persons over age 60. Every third elderly patient has postoperative complications, and only 16% of the patients are discharged from hospitals within the norm of 5 days. The highest risk group consists of patients with so-called latent unrecognized heart failure. In general up to 80% of the elderly patients could be operated on earlier if physicians had a greater suspicion of the possibility of appendicitis.[16,33-35]

Diverticulitis is inflammation of colonic diverticula particularly in the sigmoid colon. The incidence of diverticula increases with age and the numbers of diverticula increase also. In routine barium enemas approximately 5% of adults show diverticula; of these 15% show associated diverticulitis. Of patients with diverticulitis, 15% to 20% require surgery. All these patients are over the age of 35 and 40% are over 70.[36]

Diverticula are often asymptomatic. The average age of presentation with problems is 64 with an equal distribution of sexes. Urinary symptoms associated with it occur rarely. Fifty percent of all patients have a single attack without recurrence. Many of the patients are obese. They complain of pain in the left lower quadrant or, rarely, in the right lower quadrant. Diarrhea may alternate with constipation. Occasionally they have symptoms of colonic obstruction. Lower abdominal tenderness is present and peritoneal irritation with muscle spasm, guarding, rebound tenderness, fever, and leukocytosis. Rectal examination may reveal a tender mass. Occult blood is frequently present in the stool. Seventy-five percent of the patients have their problem in the sigmoid colon and the remainder in the descending colon. A barium enema may not be possible during the acute phase of the disease and when done may be doubtful in 20%. A differential diagnosis has to be made from regional enteritis, appendicitis, and septic gynecologic problems. Once the patient is hospitalized, complications are present in up to 50% and surgery is required in 20%.[37] Eighty percent of patients with complications have no previous history of diverticular disease. Twenty percent have hemorrhage; chronic or acute perforation occurs in 60%. Other complications are pelvic cellulitis, obstruction, and pelvic abscess. Cancer can be found in 5% and polyps in a further 10%. The disease, however, has no direct relationship with cancer, and these are incidental findings.[13,36]

Treatment of diverticulitis is bed rest in the acute phase of the disease and a high fiber diet. Antibiotics required for complications must be carefully chosen. They must not only be directed against anaerobes but also against aerobes. The acute initial phase of the disease is largely aerobic, but if treated only with antiaerobic antibiotics it will be complicated later by anaerobic abscesses. A good choice is a cephalosporin with clindamycin. Frequently this has to be given intravenously initially and intravenous fluids may be required. Patients are usually treated medically for two to three attacks and then if the attacks continue a partial colectomy is performed during a well interval. Patients who do not respond to conservative measures in 48 hours may be considered for surgery.[37] The overall operative fatality rate is 15% to 25%. This high rate is caused by complicating underlying diseases and delayed diagnosis. Increased surgical death rate occurs with increasing age. Septicemia often causes death. The fatality rate with elective surgery is 2% to 3% compared to 15% to 25% with emergency surgery. Surgery procedures other than resection are drainage of abscesses, correction of fistulae, freeing of obstruction, and treating perforation.[38]

Genitourinary infections

Brocklehurst et al. found 20% of women between the ages of 65 and 90 to be infected in the urinary tract; infection was present in 43% of those over 90.[39,40] In men, however, 3% of those aged 65 to 70 were infected and 20% of those over 70. In 1965, Sir Ferguson Anderson found infection in 50% of women averaging 79 years of age in a long-term care facility. Another study of patients admitted to a geriatric assessment unit from their own homes with a wide variety of illnesses, largely unconnected with diseases of the urinary tract, showed 31% infection in males and 34% in females. Urinary incontinence was more common in patients with urinary infection. Other studies of patients in long-term care facilities have found up to 46% with urinary infection.[41,42] This is especially a problem in the demented. In hospitals where nosocomial infections can occur, enterococcal infections were found in 30 out of 34 instrumented patients. It was thought to be secondary to fecal contamination caused by failure to clean the perineum before instrumentation. Proteus species can also spread by nosocomial means and can be typed to show specific spread of some species of organisms. There is a progressive increase in urinary tract infection with increasing disability and patient dependence. The loss of bactericidal activity of the urine associated with a decrease of prostate secretions is a predisposing factor as is the presence of residual urine in the bladder. There is a difference of opinion as to whether bacteriuria alone can cause incontinence in females or if it must be associated with an active infection.[40] In women *E. coli* are the primary pathogens, alone causing 49% of urinary infections. In a study of 425 elderly people who were chronically ill and averaged 72 years of age, 31% were found infected with *E. coli,* 21% with coliform bacteria, 28% with Proteus, and 4% with Pseudomonas, whereas 16% had other bacteria. *E. coli* appeared significantly more frequently in women and *Proteus* in men. Some women are highly susceptible to urinary tract infections. Fecal bacteria are the reservoir for recurrent infection. This is preceded by colonization of the vagina. During trimethoprim-sulfamethoxazole prophylaxis, 9% of monthly vaginal and 27% of monthly fecal cultures grew *E. coli* compared to 36% and 96%, respectively, of those receiving nitrofurantoin. *E. coli* resistance developed in 2% of the patients treated with nitrofurantoin, and in 9% of the women treated with trimethoprim-sulfamethoxazole. Ninety-two episodes of recurrent urinary tract infections occurred in the 12 months before treatment, six during treatment with nitrofurantoin, and none during treatment with trimethoprim-sulfamethoxazole.[43]

Infections with indwelling catheters can be reduced by using good technique and proper catheter care, that is, using the smallest size catheter possible to minimize trauma and monitoring the time of insertion of catheters with cultures at insertion and withdrawal. Of 416 patients successively admitted to geriatric clinics, 21% had indwelling catheters. Ninety percent of those with catheters had urinary tract infection. Removal of the catheter led to urinary retention in only 2% of the women and 12% of the men. In women, 71% had *E. coli*. In men, *Proteus* occurred in 42% and *E. coli* in 17%. The indications for catheterization were hemiplegia, 43%; fractured femur, 12%; benign prostatic hypertrophy, 12%; pressure sores, 7%; and incontinence, 6%. The catheter is usually prescribed by the head nurse. Indwelling catheters should be confined to cases of chronic retention and temporary drainage following urologic surgery. Incontinence and pressure sores should not be indications. With indwelling catheters, the value of a truly closed system of urinary drainage cannot be overemphasized. Proper catheter maintenance is the door to success in patients requiring catheterization, and sterile technique is the key. Twice daily perineal cleansing is essential. The drainage tube must not dip into the collected urine. Continuous irrigation is not useful. All patients should receive a perineal wash prior to instrumentation. In the past a 90% to 100% infection rate has been reported in 3 to 5 days. The risk of acquiring bacteriuria after a single straight catheterization is approximately 3% in women and 0.5% to 1% in men. Another approach is to combine a daily change of catheter with preparation of the external genitals with a polymyxin-bacitracin spray and irrigation of the anterior urethra with a solution containing 1% each of bacitracin (Mycitracin) and neomycin and 0.4% polymyxin. This has been successfully used to keep paraplegic patients free of infections for 10 weeks or more.[43,44]

The diagnosis of urinary tract infection should be made by quantitative urine culture showing 100,000 or more bacteria per cubic milliliter. This should be confirmed in a second specimen. There are many ways to do this with commercially available paddles or similar techniques. In patients difficult to catheterize, suprapubic bladder puncture can be used with little risk and in some cases this has been found superior to the clean catch quantitative urine culture. If two or more organisms are found, contamination is likely.[45]

Urinary tract infection may be asymptomatic (bacteriuria) or symptomatic (cystitis or pyelonephritis). Most postoperative urinary tract infections are related to catheters. This can be reduced by aseptic placement, meticulous catheter care, and early removal.

Patients with infected urine have a variety of symptoms; nocturia is most common. The infections damage the epithelium of the nephron and prevent reabsorption of water. This is most obvious at night. Precipitancy occurs in 30% and incontinence in 20%. Almost half of the incontinence is stress incontinence. Scalding occurs in 11% and frequency in 10%. Precipitancy and difficulty in passing urine relate strongly to infected urine.[40] Urinary tract infection is common in the presence of prostatitis, and it is easiest to diagnose by taking a quantitative culture before a prostatic massage and repeating the quantitative culture afterward. Some investigators believe that chronic bacteriuria may not interfere with renal function, but others have found that silent bacteriuria can lead to a decrease in glomerular filtration rate in 20% of the patients compared to 5% and a decreased renal plasma flow of 17% compared to 3% in controls free of bacteriuria but of the same age and rechecked 22 months later. No difference is found in the prevalence of hypertension in bacteriuric versus nonbacteriuric outpatient subjects, nor is there a difference in prevalence of bacteriuria in hypertensive versus nonhypertensive subjects. However, in hospitalized patients a relationship between hypertension and bacteriuria was statistically significant.[46,47]

Treatment is easier in cystitis of recent onset. Renal biopsy shows that after the third attack it is frequent to find the same serologic type of organism in the kidney substance as in the bladder urine. Treatment can be with sulfonamide, nitrofurantion, or ampicillin. In a trial of ampicillin used for 1 week in a dose of 0.5 gm daily, a 3-month follow-up showed a 45% cure rate and in half of those relapsing, a new organism was present. Two weeks of treatment works as well as 6 weeks of treatment. For cystitis 1 to 2 days of treatment *may* be as good as 2 weeks. Approximately two thirds of those who were incontinent became continent. In general terms, the asymptomatic bacteriuric patients cleared less well than those with symptomatic disease.[39] Cephalexin is well tolerated in the elderly with few side effects. There is a good clinical response in 87% of patients and a good bacteriologic response in 72%. Seven percent have mild reactions such as rashes.[48] In some patients methenamine (Mandelamine) can be used as a suppressant, and up to 70% of bacteriurias can be suppressed with essentially no medical risk.

Trimethoprim-sulfamethoxazole has also been used for long-term suppression. Mild nausea, stomach disorders, and an occasional drug rash were found. The drug has been used for as long as 12 months in the treatment of patients with recurrent urinary tract infections and was tolerated for this period with continuous sterile urine in 65% of the patients compared to only 8% of those treated with nitrofurantoin. A minor rise in serum creatinine was observed in some patients but no other side effects were found.[43]

Outbreaks of resistant organisms have been described in long-term care units, indicating the need for careful nosocomial infection prevention studies. One such outbreak was associated with the carriage of trimethoprim-resistant organisms with many noninfected patients being carriers of the offending organism. Half of the carriers had been exposed to trimethoprim in the past, and the carriers had been in the unit 15 months longer than noncarriers. Carriage was in the rectum. Discontinuation of the agent leads to a decrease and disappearance of resistant organism carriage. Initially this resistant organism only caused mild infections. Eventually, however, two patients developed septicemia and one of them died. This makes clear the importance of infection surveillance in long-term care units.[49]

In prostatitis, if bacteriuria is present, ampicillin, cephalexin, and nitrofurantoin should be given for 2 to 3 days to sterilize the urine; then the urine is cultured before and after prostate massage or ejaculation. An ejaculate should also be cultured. Chronic bacterial prostatitis is difficult to cure and likely to persist and cause relapsing urinary tract infection. Erythromycin and trimethoprim or metronidazole enter the prostate (probably because their basic nature makes them capable of entering the acid milieu and fatty tissue of the prostate gland). Trimethoprim-sulfamethoxazole appears to be the most effective therapy available for chronic bacterial prostatitis.[13]

In general the prognosis of chronic lower urinary tract infection is good from the point of view of serious complications. There is no severe harm to the bladder or urethra nor does it usually cause acute pyelonephritis or septicemia. However, one group of investigators has found that the initially lowered glomerular filtration rate and renal plasma flow in bacteriuric individuals 24 months later are further reduced by 20% in contrast to 4% in controls. When patients with urinary tract infections do develop chronic renal disease or septicemia they often have structural abnormalities or neurologic disease or have been receiving long-term catheterization.

Central nervous system infections

Meningitis is a life-threatening disease with an untreated fatality rate in the aged close to

100%. The incidence has risen from 4 to 6 cases/100,000 in the 1930s to approximately 10 cases/100,000 in the 1980s. In the elderly there has been a greater increase from 5 to 15/100,000. Most larger hospitals have five cases of meningitis per 10,000 admissions per year. The disease is community acquired, and nosocomial infections are found only in neonates. Elderly patients make up from 5% to 15% of large series of meningitis cases.

Neisseria meningitidis, *H. influenzae*, and *S. pneumoniae* are the chief causative organisms except in the elderly where *H. influenzae* is not seen and *N. meningitidis* is rare. *S. aureus* and *S. pneumoniae* each make up 15% to 20%. Bacterial meningitis due to unidentified organisms makes up 20% both in the young and in the elderly. The remainder are caused by a group of unusual organisms such as *Listeria monocytogenes*, gram-negative rods, cryptococcus, and *M. tuberculosis*. These unusual pathogens make up a varying percentage but have been described in as many as 60% of all cases in the elderly.[50]

The symptoms of meningitis in the geriatric patient are severe headache and decrease in mental ability associated with fever, nuchal rigidity, or both. Patients who have urinary tract infection or respiratory disease leading to meningitis frequently show one of the unusual pathogens. Unfortunately, underlying disease may mimic some of the findings of meningitis and may delay the diagnosis and in particular delay the performance of a lumbar puncture. Seventy-five percent of elderly patients with meningitis have chronic underlying disease. Many of them have prolonged fever and go into septic shock. It is also important to rule out the possibility of trauma. If respiratory failure develops, these patients may require mechanical ventilation.[51]

Pneumococcal meningitis is the most common form of meningitis. Coma occurs in 25% of patients, and only 20% to 30% are fully conscious. Fifteen percent have convulsions. Ninety-five percent of patients are febrile. Coma in meningococcal meningitis occurs in only 10% when the diagnosis is made early. Predisposing causes such as cranial fracture, pneumonia, and otitis media should be looked for strenuously.

S. aureus meningitis is often a complication of diagnostic or surgical procedures, particularly those with indwelling foreign bodies. About 20% the patients have this disease as a complication of septicemia or endocarditis, with males predominating. Patients complain of headache, nausea, vomiting, and neck pain. About one fourth are obtunded, stuporous, or in coma. Nuchal rigidity is almost universal but seizures are rare. The peripheral white count in the majority of cases is 12,000 to 20,000 and 25% are over 20,000 per cubic millimeter. Some of the elderly do not have a raised white count, but in almost all cases there is a shift to the left in the differential count.

Listeria meningitis resembles tuberculosis in many ways. The patients usually have a low grade fever and a personality change. There is no clinical way of differentiating this type of meningitis. The organism can often be seen on smear. It is a gram-positive, non–spore-forming aerobic rod, motile at room temperature but not very motile at 37° F. Half of the patients with this meningitis are over 40, and the case fatality rate is about 50%. There is usually a purulent exudate in the cerebral spinal fluid with a protein of 100 to 300 mg/100 ml, but the spinal fluid glucose level is not always low. The focus for this organism is in the soil, dust, water, and sewage and it may occasionally be a nosocomially acquired infection. It occurs in winter and early spring. Patients with cancer or cirrhosis are more likely to get *Listeria* meningitis than those without these diseases.[51] Beware of the label "contaminant"; it may represent unidentified Listerella.

The diagnosis of meningitis is based on a healthy suspicion and lumbar puncture in patients who are febrile and confused. Gram stain shows the pathogen in about 70% of patients. If there has been preceding antibiotic treatment, both the gram stain and the culture may not be positive but the biochemical changes such as protein and sugar will remain as well as the increase in PMN cells. A differential diagnosis without a positive culture is extraordinarily difficult as summarized below:

Conditions that may make diagnosing purulent meningitis in the aged difficult*

Cerebral apoplexy
Subarachnoid hemorrhage
Febrile delirium
Senile confusion

*From Quaade, F.: Geriatrics **18**:860, 1963.

Diabetic coma
Intoxication (barbiturate, alcohol, carbon monoxide, chlorpromazine, bromide)
Cerebral anoxia and hypercapnia (respiratory insufficiency, Stokes-Adams syndrome)
Head injury (cerebral hemorrhage or edema)
Senile psychosis
Cerebral tumor, primary or secondary
Hypertensive encephalopathy
Acute encephalitis
Postepileptic coma
Hypoglycemic coma
Cerebral abscess
Hepatic coma
Uremic coma

The prognosis of meningitis in the elderly is poor. In various large series of meningitis cases, the general fatality rate in recent years has varied from 10% to 15%. The fatality rate for patients over 60 has been 40% to 60% or even higher in the oldest patients. There has been an increase in fatality rate from the 1930s to the 1960s in the elderly from 10% to 60%. This may be due to the different composition of today's population of elderly patients and the larger number of underlying diseases in frail elderly. Morbidity and mortality are higher in males. In pneumococcal meningitis, the fatality rate has varied between 17% and 25%. Poor prognostic findings are an age greater than 60 years old, coma, pneumonia, convulsions, bacteremia, and a cerebral spinal cell count of less than 1000. In one controlled series, the case fatality rate was 27% in controls and 11% in patients who received steroids in addition to penicillin G. In summarizing the fatality rate from pneumococcal meningitis, the two main factors are underlying disease and the severity of the infection as demonstrated by bacteremia, low cerebral spinal fluid glucose level, or poor host resistance in relation to white cells in the cerebral spinal fluid. The severity of the bacterial disease is also indicated by impaired consciousness. Meningitis in the elderly not due to pneumococci or staphylococci has a fatality rate that varies from 25% to 55%.

Bone and joint infections

Pyogenic *septic arthritis* is not rare in the elderly because predisposing factors are common, such as diabetes mellitus, cirrhosis, cancer, rheumatoid arthritis, immunosuppressive treatment, or treatment with steroids. There has been prior antibiotic treatment in approximately 20% of the cases. Usually other concurrent infections are present, particularly of the skin but also of the urinary tract, lungs, or throat. The patient complains of a hot, swollen, red joint. The redness is particularly important. Redness usually occurs only in gout and in infectious arthritis. Twenty-five percent to forty percent of patients with septic arthritis have shaking chills, and 90% are febrile; but in the elderly, particularly in those immunosuppressed or those receiving corticosteroids, fever may not be present. About 60% have a white blood cell count increased to approximately 13,000. The remainder usually have a shift to the left. The joints involved in diminishing frequency are knees, wrists, shoulder, elbow, hips, and ankles. In the young, gonococci are the common infecting organisms, but in the elderly *S. aureus*, *S. hemolyticus*, gram-negative rods, and *S. pneumoniae* are the causes (in order of descending frequency). Diagnosis is based on the aspiration of joint fluid. The joint fluid white cell count may be elevated to 200,000; 85% are PMN. There is a mucin clot and the gram stain is positive in 65%. The glucose is low and culture is mandatory. X-ray changes showing a loss of cartilage usually do not occur for 1 to 2 weeks. Treatment is with the appropriate systemic antibiotics for 2 to 4 weeks; the longer course is particularly necessary for *S. aureus*. Daily arthrocentesis can be done on all joints except the hips. Surgery is indicated for the hips if there is no response to medical treatment. Intraarticular antibiotics are not necessary and lead to chemical arthritis. Oral antibiotics give adequate intraarticular levels. In the presence of gram-negative rods, gentamicin and carbenicillin may be used. Good responses to treatment are found in 70% if the treatment is started less than 7 days from onset and in only 27% if started after that. Older patients do less well than younger ones. The predisposing factors as noted above militate against a good prognosis. Patients with rheumatoid arthritis have to be watched carefully as septic arthritis may only be diagnosed at autopsy. Least favorable results are found in patients receiving dialysis with a 60% fatality rate and in patients with rheumatoid arthritis with a 45% fatality rate.

A particular kind of *osteomyelitis*, pyogenic vertebral osteomyelitis, is common in elderly males, particularly diabetics. These patients complain of neck or back pain over a fairly long period of time. There may also be some chest pain associated with it. The erythrocyte sedimentation rate is always elevated, but only half of the patients have fever or leukocytosis. In about one third of these patients the infection comes from the urinary tract. The lumbar region is more frequently affected than the thoracic region. It is not unusual to see narrowing of the disc spaces with vertebral end-plate involvement on the x-ray film. About 60% of the cases are caused by *S. aureus*. Bed rest and systemic antibiotic therapy, initially parenteral and later oral, are given for 4 weeks. Approximately 5% die, and an equal number have neurologic deficits.

Infections in prosthetic joints.[52] With greater surgical experience the occurrence of 10% has been reduced to about 1%. Artificial joints are inserted to give the patient pain-free mobility. Infection is regarded as a disastrous complication because it may result in less function than before the prosthesis was inserted. The fact that a prosthesis is a foreign body increases the virulence of organisms considerably. In most but not all patients the bacterial inoculum becomes established at the time of surgery. Elaborate isolation precautions can be used to prevent infection at the time of surgery, or moderate precautions can be taken with prophylactic antibiotics. Antibiotics can also be incorporated in the cement. Half of the reported infections become manifest within the first 4 to 6 months. Late infections may appear up to 2 years after surgery. Both early and late infections are caused by *S. aureus*, *S. epidermidis*, or Peptococcus. The diagnosis is not difficult if the infection is in the soft tissues. The patient usually has tenderness, erythema, and fluctuance. However, infection restricted to the bone adjacent to the cement does not have a classic presentation. There is pain in the affected joint and a high erythrocyte sedimentation rate. X-ray films may reveal loss of bone density adjacent to the implant. The joint may be unstable. Such patients should be considered to be infected until it is proven that they are not. The joint should be aspirated for smears and cultures; arthrograms may be helpful. *S. aureus* is sensitive to the cephalosporins and so is *S. epidermidis*, but the latter is resistant to methicillin. It is advisable to begin treatment with a cephalosporin such as cephalothin or cephazolin at 8 to 12 gm per day rather than a penicillinase-resistant penicillin. If gram-negative rods are identified in the aspirate, an aminoglycoside should be added. Laboratory assessment of the sensitivities is mandatory. Patients with a prosthetic joint who develop cystitis, pyelonephritis, or other infections at a remote area should be treated promptly and actively to prevent seeding of the joint. In some severe infections the joint will have to be opened and possibly removed. In some cases treatment is by the placement of a second prosthetic joint.

Tetanus

Persons in the geriatric age group are susceptible to tetanus. The prognosis is also worse in the elderly. The incidence of tetanus is 0.10/100,000 in the neonatal period; less than 0.05/100,000 from age 10 to 30; 0.05 to 0.10/100,000 from age 30 to 60; and from 0.10 to 0.20/100,000 in those over 60. The mortality rate in the neonate is 0.05/100,000 population and 0.025/100,000 in the 20- to 40-year-old age group. There is an increasing fatality rate starting at 0.05 in 60-year-olds, increasing to 0.15 in those over 70. This increase is also shown by the case fatality rate, which is 60% in neonates, 20% to 40% in young adults, and 60% or higher in the 60 years and over age group.[53] The disease may follow a relatively minor wound, and although many occur on the farm or in automobile accidents, many are sustained in the home, particularly involving lawn mower accidents. The toxin may develop from a few bacilli or spores in the original wound. The patient complains of stiffness in the muscles of the head and neck and then of difficulty in swallowing and opening the mouth. This may progress to involve the muscles of the back and can progress to spasms and then generalized convulsions. The spasm of facial muscles produces a characteristic risus sardonicus as shown in Fig. 14-2. The diagnosis is totally clinical. Tetanus bacilli can be isolated from the wound when the patient does not have tetanus or no organisms may be isolated when the patient does have tetanus. When the disease develops within 10 days of the injury it is usually more serious than that developing after 10 days, the comparative case fatality rates being 35% and 60%. The wound should be cleansed and debrided. If there is a history of no tetanus tox-

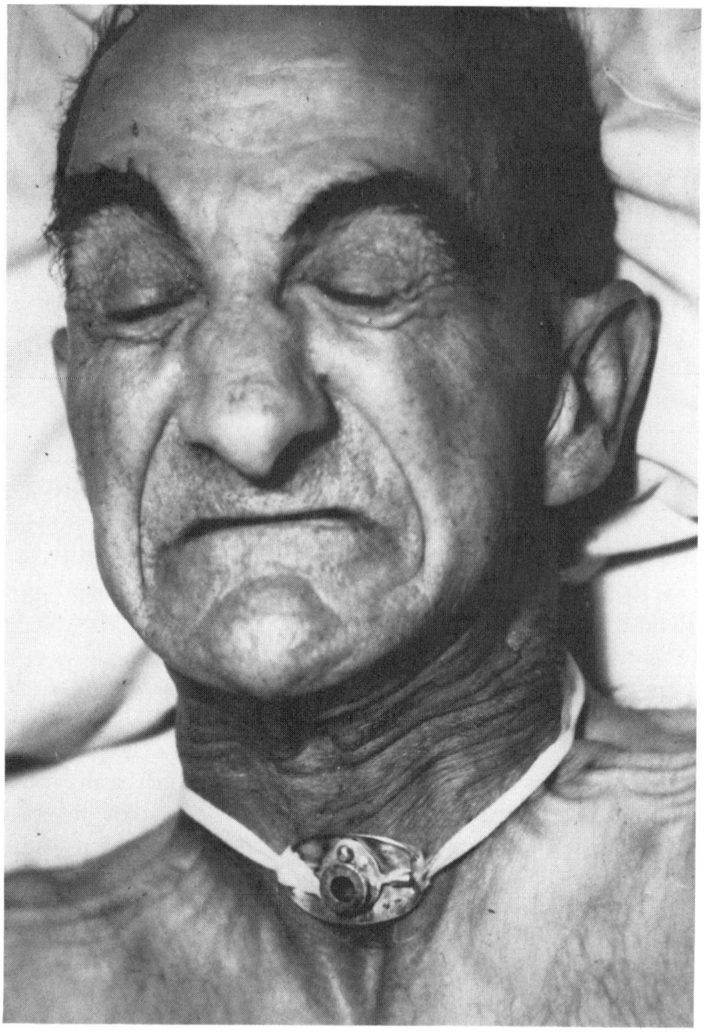

Fig. 14-2. The risus sardonicus of tetanus.

oid or one or two shots, then tetanus toxoid should be given. If there have been three or more shots, it is not necessary provided they have been given within 10 years. When the wound is major, tetanus immune globulin should also be given unless there is a clear history of three tetanus toxoid shots having been given within the past 10 years. If tetanus has already developed, between 3000 and 10,000 units of tetanus immune globulin should be given intramuscularly. Penicillin, 1 million units intravenously, is given every 6 hours for 7 days; in patients allergic to penicillin 500 mg of tetracycline is given orally or intravenously every 6 hours for 7 days. Tracheostomy is recommended early in the treatment. Muscle relaxation by diazepam should be controlled by consultation with the anesthesiologist. The patient should be fed by a nasogastric or gastrostomy tube and should be nursed in a quiet dark room. The patient should be monitored to avoid urine retention, urinary tract infection, and pulmonary infection. The patient will not be immune after the attack of tetanus and should receive three injections of tetanus toxoid.[13]

Infections in diabetics

In diabetics the white cells will not migrate normally to an area of infection, will not phagocytose, and will not kill bacteria if they do happen to phagocytose them. The most important infection in diabetics is gangrene of the feet, often with underlying osteomyelitis. All age groups are involved, but most frequently it is those individuals between ages 40 and 90 who are affected. Any diabetic with a skin infection should have careful aerobic and anaerobic cultures taken. Early and adequate use of antianaerobic antibiotics, such as clindamycin and chloramphenicol, is indicated. These infections are almost always polymicrobial, with two anaerobes and three aerobes isolated in most carefully studied patients. Gas is often found in the tissue without clostridial infection and occurs in approximately 20% of patients with gangrene. However, 2% to 3% can have a clostridial infection. Diabetics have more complications; are often overweight; and often have atherosclerosis, renal disease, and various neuropathies as well. Gangrene occurs 53 times more often in the diabetic man than in the nondiabetic man and 71 times more often in the diabetic woman than in the nondiabetic woman.[17,18]

Such complications were uniformly fatal until the availability of insulin; the fatality rate was recorded at 50% and fell to 33% in the 1950s when insulin became available. In the 1960s 22% to 25% of subjects died in various large series; with the availability of antibiotics, in the 1970s special study units have reduced the fatality rate to 9% to 12%. With the appreciation of the importance of anaerobes and of the use of clindamycin, chloramphenicol or carbenicillin, even better results are expected. The most frequent long-term effect is osteomyelitis, leading to amputation of the affected tissue. Affected individuals become long-term care candidates with major health problems. In various studies 50% to 83% of patients with gangrene have required amputation. More skilled antibiotic therapy may reduce this problem.

Systemic infections

Bacteremia is a temporary presence of bacteria in the bloodstream, and *septicemia* is the established presence of organisms in the bloodstream with signs and symptoms of generalized sepsis. Patients over 60 years old make up 40% to 50% of community-acquired septicemia cases in general hospitals and 50% to 60% of hospital-acquired septicemias. In patients over 60 years old, septicemias in general hospitals have increased from 15% to 50% in community-acquired cases and from 25% to 55% in hospital-acquired cases.[54,55] Limited studies have been done in geriatric facilities. In one study among those thought to merit taking blood cultures, 6% were found to have significant pathogens in the bloodstream. A general increase in gram-negative rod septicemia with age has been noted by a number of investigators. Nosocomial infections increase with age in persons over 40 years old, especially after cardiac surgery. The clinical sources of septicemia have been urinary tract infection in 34%, biliary tract infection in 20%, and lung infection in 13%. Other surveys have shown skin lesions or pyarthrosis and rheumatoid arthritis to be sources of septicemia in the elderly. The findings are frequently nonspecific malaise with fever and sometimes recent onset of confusion. The temperature is usually between 101 and 105° F. Septic shock is common and can be associated with confusion, stupor, delirium, and agitation. Patients with decubitus ulcers frequently develop bacteroides septicemia.[20] Following prostatic surgery, septicemia is common, particularly after prolonged catheterization and drainage. Postprostatectomy studies have shown that many of these patients also have diabetes and arteriosclerosis. The organisms causing the septicemia are *Proteus* and *E. coli*. If the septicemia is associated with biliary tract infection, about one third will have jaundice. Septicemia in the elderly can follow perforated colonic diverticula and a variety of intraabdominal abscesses.[33,36,38] Elderly patients who are neutropenic as a result of hematologic or lymphoreticular malignancies and their treatment are unusually susceptible to septicemia, particularly when the PMN count is less than 500/mm^3.[56]

When septicemia is suspected, three blood cultures should be taken, usually 2 hours apart unless there is pneumonia or fulminant infection. If a heart murmur is present or endocarditis is suspected, five should be taken. In the presence of a urinary tract focus, *E. coli* is the most common organism with *Proteus* species being second. In the presence of biliary tract disease, one should suspect *E. coli* or *Klebsiella* species. Following pneumonia by far the most common is *S. pneumoniae*. If the focus is unknown, *E. coli* or *Bacteroides* are the likely pathogens.[57] If abdominal problems are present, polymicrobic infection is most frequent and in the presence of endocarditis, *S. viridans*, *S. aureus*, or *S.*

epidermidis are prevalent; the latter two are more common after heart surgery. If meningitis is present *S. pneumoniae* is a likely cause.

Twenty-five percent to thirty-five percent of elderly persons die when they have septicemia. In septic shock the fatality rate increases to 61% or higher. Hypothermia, dementia, diabetes mellitus, and cancer all worsen the prognosis. If rapidly fatal underlying disease is present (i.e., disease likely to kill within 1 year such as acute leukemia) the overall fatality rate is approximately 80%. Since 1935, the case fatality rate of septicemia in patients over age 60 has fallen from 91% to 46%. In patients with hospital-acquired septicemia, the case fatality rate has fallen from 84% to 48%.[54,55]

In septicemia with decubitus ulcers, surgical debridement is indicated and in the presence of an abscess, incision and drainage are essential.

An increase in endocarditis in the elderly has been noted, from 12% to 25% of all cases in the 1940s to 21% to 45% in the 1960s. In general the aortic valve is involved more than twice as often in the elderly as in patients of all ages and as would be expected, congenital heart lesions are rare. Recently calcified or otherwise deformed aortic valves have been found in 20%, rheumatic fibrosis in 15%, and a flopping of the mitral valve in 3%. No underlying valvular disease has been found in 37%, and some quote a figure as high as 53%.

In general the findings are the same as in younger patients but less accentuated.[58,59] The symptoms may be overshadowed by the patient's other diseases or by complications precipitated by the endocarditis. Weight loss, coma, confusion, and hemiplegia are common in older patients. Emboli occur in only 11%, congestive cardiac failure and azotemia are more common, and heart enlargement is found in over 50%. Splenomegaly occurs in 53% and hematuria in 61%. There is biochemical evidence of renal damage in 75%, and central nervous system emboli are present in 14%. Males outnumber females approximately 2 to 1. Some patients may have a psychosis or apoplexy. There is a paucity of physical signs. It is usual to find a leukocytosis of 13,000 to 14,000 in streptococcal disease and 15,000 or higher in staphylococcal endocarditis, with the red count averaging 3.2 million and a hemoglobin of approximately 10 gm in staphylococcal disease and 13 gm in streptococcal disease. A correct initial diagnosis is made in 20% to 60% in different series. The underlying multiple pathology of the elderly may confuse and mask this picture; the correct diagnosis being made in 86% under age 50 and in only 20% over 50. The diagnosis should be based on the presence of a cardiac murmur, fever, embolization, and positive blood cultures. Endocarditis has to be differentiated from rheumatic heart disease, renal disease (confused by the presence of hematuria), psychosis, gastrointestinal disease, digitalis toxicity, pyelonephritis, and cerebral-vascular accident. The type of organisms has varied over the years from a predominance of *S. viridans* in the 1940s to the emergence with cardiac surgery of *S. aureus* and *S. epidermidis* in the 1970s and 1980s. *S. aureus* now causes 35% to 45% of cases and *S. viridans* 25% to 30%. Gram-negative rods and fungi are uncommon. The prognosis relates to the organism. Without treatment all patients die. In patients under age 50, fatality rates have varied from 7% to 14%, and those over 50 the fatality rate has varied from 30% to 80%. Although some organisms such as pneumococcus truly cause *acute* bacterial endocarditis, the categorization by organism is much more useful and accurate.

Syphilis

The onset of slowly progressive syphilis of the aorta and central nervous system begins early in latent syphilis. Asymptomatic neurosyphilis is present in patients who have cerebral spinal fluid abnormalities such as pleocytosis, elevated protein, or a positive spinal fluid VDRL; this is found in 25% of untreated syphilis after 2 years. About 20% of these patients will progress in the next 10 years. *Neurosyphilis* is twice as common in men as in women and three times as common in whites as in blacks. There are three kinds of involvement: meningovascular, general paresis, and tabes dorsalis, occurring approximately 7 years, 20 years, and 30 years, respectively, after onset.[60] *Cardiovascualr syphilis* affects the large vessels such as the aorta and produces an aneurysm, anytime from 10 to 40 years after infection. It is more common in men and in blacks.[61] In the 10% that develop cardiovascular syphilis, aortic regurgitation is more common than aneurysms. Gummata, which are painless ulcerating lesions of the skin and other tissues, are rarely seen nowadays with this disease.[61]

The standard nontreponemal test used in the United States is the Venereal Disease Research Laboratory slide test called VDRL. In this test heated serum is tested for its ability to flocculate a suspension of cardiolipin-lecithin antigen. Since the treponemal tests are more sensitive than the nontreponemal test in late syphilis, the FTA-ABS test on serum should be part of the diagnostic workup. When spinal fluid is examined to rule out neurosyphilis, a quantitative VDRL test on the cerebral spinal fluid is the test of choice. In screening elderly patients on occasions such as admissions to nursing homes, the VDRL should be used because of its simplicity and low cost. If this test is positive, a second serum sample should be tested to exclude laboratory or specimen labeling error. Since nontreponemal tests are relatively nonspecific, a second reactive result should be confirmed with the treponemal test. If patients are being treated for syphilis, it is customary to use a quantitative VDRL test and check for its reduction in titer over the next 2 years. Patients with late syphilis, however, may be serofast so that failure to observe a titer fall does not indicate a need for retreatment. The recommended treatment for syphilis of more than 1 year's duration (latent syphilis; indeterminate syphilis of more than 1 year's duration; cardiovascular, late benign, or neurosyphilis) is (1) benzathine penicillin G, 7.2 million units total, that is, 2.4 million units in two intramuscular injections for 3 successive weeks; (2) aqueous procaine penicillin G, 9 million units total, 600,000 units by intramuscular injection daily for 15 days. Patients who are allergic to penicillin should receive (1) tetracycline hydrochloride, 500 mg four times a day orally for 30 days or (2) erythromycin (stearate, succinate, or base), 500 mg four times a day orally for 30 days. There are, however, no published clinical data that adequately document the efficacy of drugs other than penicillin for syphilis of more than 1 year's duration. Cerebral spinal fluid examinations are strongly recommended before therapy with these regimens.

In various series of cardiovascular syphilis, 15% to 25% of patients have been over age 60. It appears that this disease may, like pulmonary tuberculosis, become temporarily a disease of the older age group because of lessened incidence of infection and improved methods of treatment in younger individuals. It has to be pointed out, however, that syphilis is much more prevalent in homosexuals than in heterosexuals, and we may therefore expect to see aging homosexuals with cardiovascular syphilis. Approximately one third of elderly people may have a negative VDRL, although they have underlying syphilis. Syphilitic carditis may present as aortic incompetence or stenosis but frequently it is combined with other diseases. There may be a superimposed bacterial endocarditis or coincident arteriosclerotic or hypertensive heart disease. Furthermore syphilitic aortic disease may be complicated by closure of the coronary ostia, producing acute myocardial involvement. The FTA-ABS test remains positive for life.

TREATMENT OF INFECTIONS[62,63]

General approach to the use of antibiotics

Suitable antibiotic agents are available for almost all infections in normal hosts. Well-trained personnel in an adequately staffed laboratory can find a causative bacterium in most severe infections. The physician must learn to think microbiologically and ask himself such questions as, "Is this a Listeria infection?" He should say, "a staphylococcal carbuncle," not "a carbuncle"; "meningococcal meningitis," not "meningitis"; "pneumococcal pneumonia," not "lobar pneumonia." The microbial etiology indicates which antibiotic to use.

Learning to recognize *P. aeruginosa* septicemia by clinical clues such as blue-green pus is based on seeing this peculiar color and associating it with cultures taken in previous cases.

When confronted with an infection, the physician should ask himself whether the infectious agent will respond to penicillin G (pneumococci, streptococci, gonococci, and meningococci) or whether it is a staphylococcal infection (boils, wound infections, osteomyelitis, etc.) that will require nafcillin or a cephalosporin (vancomycin or erythromycin); a mild gram-negative rod infection (urinary tract infection and some wound infections); a severe gram-negative rod infection (which may require more toxic or expensive medication than would be used in a less serious infection, such as an aminoglycoside (gentamicin, carbenicillin, or co-trimoxazole); or an anaerobic infection that should be treated with penicillin G, chloramphenicol, clindamycin, carbenicillin, rifampin, vancomycin, or metronidazole.[63]

Septic shock

Septic shock results in inadequate tissue perfusion, usually evidenced by confusion or poor urine output. The physician must monitor blood pressure, central venous pressure, urine output, and mental clarity. Abscesses should be drained. Cephalothin and gentamicin or chloramphenicol and gentamicin should be used initially if an anaerobe is not suspected. Clindamycin should be given for an established anaerobe infection. Blood volume must be restored. Patient should not be allowed sodium-containing fluids if carbenicillin, which is sodium-rich, is given. If patients need digitalis, only three fourths of the normal dose should be given as these patients are hypersensitive. Norepinephrine and phentolamine or dopamine are used to support the circulation. Hydrocortisone, 30 to 50 mg/kg of body weight, should be given immediately and for an additional 1 or 2 days if these measures fail. Oxygen by positive end expiratory pressure (PEEP) is used if the oxygen partial pressure is less than 55 on room air.

REFERENCES

1. Smith, I.M.: Infections in the elderly. Cont. Ed. Family Physician **7**:18, 1977.
2. Brown, N.K., and Thompson, D.J.: Nontreatment of fever in extended care facilities, N. Engl. J. Med. **300**:1246, 1979.
3. Gladstone, J.L., and Recco, R.: Host factors and infectious diseases in the elderly, Med. Clin. North Am. **60**:1225, 1976.
4. Howell, T.H.: Some terminal aspects of disease in old age. A clinical study of 300 patients, J. Am. Geriatr. Soc. **17**:1034, 1969.
5. Smith, I.M.: Deaths in the elderly compared and contrasted with deaths in young adults. Analysis of 630 autopsies in an acute care hospital. (In preparation.)
6. Gabbert, W.R., Hutaff, L.W., and Harrell, G.T.: The effect of age on the leukocyte count, Geriatrics **2**:96, 1947.
7. Williams, W.J.: Hematology in the aged. In Williams, W.J., Beutler, E., Erslev, A.J., and Rundles, R.W.: Hematology, ed. 2, New York, 1977, McGraw-Hill Book Co.
8. Everett, E.D., et al.: *Hemophilus influenzae* pneumonia in adults, J.A.M.A. **238**:319, 1977.
9. Fox, R.H., et al.: Body temperatures in the elderly: a national study of physiological, social and environmental conditions, Br. Med. J. **1**:200, 1973.
10. Phair, J.P., et al.: Host defenses in the aged. Evaluation of components of the inflammatory and immune responses, J. Infect. Dis. **138**:67, 1978.
11. Roberts-Thomas, I.C., Whittingham, S., Youngchaiyud, U., and Mackay, I.R.: Ageing, immune response and mortality, Lancet **2**:368, 1974.
12. Valenti, W.M., Trudell, R.G., and Bentley, D.W.: Factors predisposing to oropharyngeal colonization with gram-negative bacilli in the aged, N. Engl. J. Med. **298**:1108, 1978.
13. Mandell, G.L., Douglas, R.G., Jr., and Bennett, J.E.: Principles and practice of infectious disease, New York, 1979, John Wiley & Sons Inc.
14. Denham, M.J., and Goodwin, G.S.: The value of blood cultures in geriatric practice, Age Ageing **6**:85, 1977.
15. Esposito, A.L., and Gleckman, R.A.: Fever of unknown origin in the elderly, J. Am. Geriatr. Soc. **26**:498, 1978.
16. Wenzel, R.P., Hunting, K.J., and Osterman, C.A.: Postoperative wound infection rate, Surg. Gynecol. Obstet. **144**:749, 1977.
17. Bessman, A.N., and Wagner, W.: Nonclostridial gas gangrene: report of 48 cases and review of the literature, J.A.M.A. **233**:958, 1975.
18. Kahn, O., Wagner, W., and Bessman, A.N.: Mortality of diabetic patients treated surgically for lower limb infection and/or gangrene, Diabetes **23**:287, 1974.
19. Barbenel, G.C., Jordan, M.M., Nidid, S.M., and Clark, M.O.: Incidence of pressure sores in the greater Glasgow Health Board Area, Lancet **2**:548, 1977.
20. Golpin, J.E., Chow, A.W., Bager, A.S., and Guze, L.B.: Sepsis associated with decubitus ulcers, Am. J. Med. **61**:346, 1976.
21. Valenti, W.M., Jenger, M., and Bentley, D.W.: Type-specific pneumococcal respiratory disease in the elderly and chronically ill, Am. Rev. Respir. Dis. **117**:233, 1978.
22. Van Meter, T.: Pneumococcal pneumonia treated with antibiotics. Prognostic significance of certain findings, N. Engl. J. Med. **251**:1048, 1954.
23. Ebright, J.R., and Rytel, M.W.: Bacterial pneumonia in the elderly, J. Am. Geriatr. Soc. **28**:220, 1980.
24. Barb, J.L., Brown, R.B., Garb, J.R., and Tuthill, R.W.: Differences in etiology of pneumonias in nursing home and community patients, J.A.M.A. **240**:2169, 1978.
25. Zavala, D.C.: The threat of aspiration pneumonia in the aged, Geriatrics **32**(3):46, 1977.
26. Kasik, J.E., and Schuldt, S.: Why tuberculosis is still a health problem in the aged, Geriatrics **32**(3):62, 1977.
27. Iseman, M.D.: Tuberculosis in the elderly. Treating the white plague, Geriatrics **35**(3):90, 1980.
28. Hermans, P.E., editor: Special series on antimicrobial agnets, Mayo Clin. Proc. **52**:601, 673, 1977.
29. The choice of antimicrobial drugs, Med. Lett. **22**:5, 1980.
30. Bracomer, J.H., and Nordenfeld, T.E.: Serum hepatitis at a home for the aged, Scand. J. Infect. Dis. **4**:279, 1972.
31. Fenster, L.F.: Viral hepatitis in the elderly: an analysis of 23 patients over 65 years of age, Gastroenterology **49**:262, 1965.
32. Iwarsen, S., et al.: Hepatitis B immune globulin in prevention of hepatitis B among hospital staff members, J. Infect. Dis. **135**:473, 1977.
33. Coran, A.G., and Wheeler, H.B.: Early perforation in appendicitis after age 60, J.A.M.A. **197**:745, 1966.
34. Peltoballio, P., and Jauhiainen, K.: Acute appendicitis

in the aged patient. Study of 300 cases after the age of sixty, Arch. Surg. **100:**140, 1970.
35. Yusuf, M.L., and Dunn, E.: Appendicitis in the elderly; learn to discern the untypical picture, Geriatrics **34**(9):73, 1979.
36. Kratzer, G.L., and Sanett, O.N.: Diverticulitis in the elderly, J. Am. Geriatr. Soc. **21:**25, 1973.
37. Tohms, S.H.: Surgical treatment of diverticulitis. Experience at a large municipal hospital, J.A.M.A. **232:**830, 1975.
38. Chaiten, H., and Wienick, L.: Peritonitis in geriatric patients. J. Am. Geriatr. Soc. **18:**834, 1970.
39. Brocklehurst, J.C., Dillane, J.V., Griffiths, L., and Fry, J.: A therapeutic trial in urinary infections in old age, Gerontol. Clin. **10:**345, 1968.
40. Brocklehurst, J.C., Bee, P., and Jones, D.: Bacteriuria in geriatric hospital patients. Its correlates and management, Age Ageing **6:**240, 1977.
41. Lye, M.: Defining and treating urinary tract infections, Geriatrics **33**(3):71, 1978.
42. Mayer, T.R.: Urinary tract infection in the elderly. How to select treatment, Geriatrics **35**(3):67, 1980.
43. Scherwin, J., and Hohn, P.: Long-term treatment with sulfamethoxazole/trimethoprim (Bactrim) and nitrofurantoin in chronic urinary tract infections. A controlled clinical trial, Chemotherapy **23:**282, 1977.
44. Keresteci, A.G., and Leers, W.D.: Indwelling catheter infection, Can. Med. Assoc. J. **109:**711, 1973.
45. Barry, A.L., Smith, P.B., and Turck, M.: Laboratory diagnosis of urinary tract infections, American Society of Microbiology, Washington, D.C., Cumitech **2:**1, 1975.
46. Dontas, A.S., Papanayiotou, P., Marketos, S., and Papanicolaou, N.: The effect of bacteriuria on renal functional patterns in old age, Clin. Sci. **34:**73, 1968.
47. Marketos, S.G., Dontas, A.S., and Papanoyiotou, P.: Bacteriuria and arterial hypertension in old age, Geriatrics **25**(7):136, 1970.
48. Smith, I.M.: Cephalexin. Clinical effectiveness in geriatric patients. Geriatrics **32**(3):91, 1977.
49. Bendall, M.J., and Grueneberg, R.N.: An outbreak of infection caused by trimethoprim-resistant coliform bacilli in a geriatric unit, Age Ageing **8:**231, 1979.
50. Quaade, F.: Meningitis in the aged, Geriatrics **18:**860, 1963.
51. Massanari, R.M.: Purulent meningitis in the elderly: when to suspect an unusual pathogen, Geriatrics **77:**55, 1977.
52. Pesanti, E.: Infections in prosthetic joints, Cont. Educ. Family Phys. 1982. (In press.)
53. Center for Disease Control: Tetanus surveillance, 1977-78; summary, U.S. Department of Health, Education and Welfare, 1978.
54. McGowan, J.E., Jr., Barnes, M.W., and Finland, M.: Bacteremia at Boston City Hospital: occurrence and mortality during 12 selected years (1935-1972) with special reference to hospital acquired cases, J. Infect. Dis. **132:**316, 1975.
55. Setia, U., and Gross, P.A.: Bacteremia in a community hospital, Arch. Intern. Med. **137:**1698, 1977.
56. Singer, C., Caplan, M.H., and Armstrong, D.: Bacteremia and fungemia complicating neoplastic disease. A study of 364 cases, Am. J. Med. **62:**731, 1977.
57. Ellner, P.D., and Wasileuskas, B.L.: Bacteroides septicemia in older patients J. Am. Geriatr. Soc. **19:**296, 1971.
58. Habte-Gabor, E., January, L.E., and Smith, I.M.: Bacterial endocarditis: the need for early diagnosis, Geriatrics **28**(3):164, 1973.
59. Thell, R., Martin, R.H., and Edwards, G.E.: Bacterial endocarditis in subjects 60 years of age and older, Circulation **51:**174, 1975.
60. Luxon, L., Lees, A.J., and Greenwood, R.J.: Neurosyphilis today, Lancet **1:**90, 1979.
61. Zeman, F.D., and Storch, S.: Syphilitic heart disease in the aged. Ann. Intern. Med. **36:**1423, 1952.
62. Triggs, E.J., and Nation, R.L.: Pharmacokinetics in the aged. A review. J. Pharmacokinet. Biopharm. **3:**387, 1975.
63. Smith, I.M., and Habte-Gabr, E.: Life-threatening infections. How to choose the right antibiotics, Geriatrics **32**(3):83, 1977.

CHAPTER 15 · CLINICAL PHARMACOLOGY

Rubin Bressler
Kenneth A. Conrad

The geriatric population has increased in recent years as a result of both an increasing life span and a decreasing birth rate.[1-5] Health care costs rise with the increase in the geriatric population. Although the elderly population constitutes only 12% of the British population, it is responsible for 30% of drug prescription costs.[1,3,4] The elderly population uses more drugs because of its greater incidence of chronic illness.[6-11] Moreover, a number of these illnesses are treated with multiple drug therapy which results in a potential for drug-drug interactions.[12-14] The elderly experience considerably more adverse drug reactions.[4,15,16] Among hospitalized patients, those 70 to 80 years old had twice the number of adverse drug reactions as those in the 40- to 50-years-old group.[4]

In recent years, considerable attention has been focused on the factors influencing drug therapy of geriatric patients. The increased frequency of adverse drug reactions in the elderly has resulted in a substantial literature on the effects of aging on pharmacokinetics (the time course of drug absorption, distribution, metabolism, and excretion), pharmacodynamics (the clinical aspects of drug response), and to a lesser degree, drug sensitivity.[4,6,17-19]

To best use pharmacologic agents in elderly patients, the following factors should be considered: (1) Potential impairment of pharmacokinetic systems that may result in higher blood and tissue levels of active drug. (2) Decreased homeostatic mechanisms that can create difficulty in compensating for drug effects. (3) Sensitivity changes defined as diminished responses to a drug in the absence of changes in blood or tissue concentrations of the drug. This alteration may be the result of decreased drug binding at receptor sites or structural and functional alterations of the responsive tissue;[4,20-22] (4) Compliance to the recommended therapeutic regimen.

Most adverse drug reactions in the elderly are not idiosyncratic but are extensions of the usual effects of the drug. To understand the pathogeneses of the problem the effects of aging on drug pharmacokinetics will be briefly reviewed. The effects of changes in drug absorption, distribution, metabolism, and excretion will be discussed.

DRUG ABSORPTION

There are no data to support a diminished or increased capacity for drug absorption in the gastrointestinal tract in the elderly.[4,17,19]

Despite decreased intestinal blood flow, increased gastric pH and decreased intestinal motility, drug absorption appears to be undiminished in the elderly. There is evidence of a decrease in active transport in the gastrointestinal tract of the elderly (galactose, 3-methylglucose, calcium, iron, thiamine), but most drugs are absorbed by passive diffusion. Studies on the gastrointestinal absorption of sulfamethizole, acetaminophen, and phenylbutazone have not shown any age related changes.[4,17,19,23]

DRUG DISTRIBUTION

There are a number of age related physiologic changes that may have a significant influence on drug distribution. For example, with increasing age there is a decrease in total body water and lean body mass and an increase in body fat.* These factors may contribute to altered distribution of highly water soluble or highly lipid

*References 3, 4, 8, 24-26.

soluble drugs. There is a redistribution of regional blood flow that may influence drug distribution characteristics. Visceral blood flow is decreased while cardiac and cerebral flow are maintained.

The apparent volume of distribution (V_d) of a drug indicates how a drug is distributed in the body. The magnitude of V_d gives an indication of the extent to which a drug is taken up into tissues other than plasma. V_d is large when tissues avidly take up a drug (phenothiazines) and small when most of the drug remains in the plasma (gentamicin).

A study carried out on ethanol elimination in elderly subjects revealed that the higher blood levels found in these subjects were attributable to smaller and to decreased lean body mass.[4,17,27]

Patients aged 51 to 75 averaged 70% higher peak serum morphine levels after intravenous administration of 10 mg/kg than patients aged 23 to 50. This suggests a smaller V_d in the older patients.[28] This alteration in morphine distribution appears to be one of the factors contributing to the increased sensitivity of older patients to narcotics.

PROTEIN BINDING OF DRUGS

Free drug concentration is an important determinant of drug distribution and elimination. Alterations in the binding of drugs to plasma proteins, red blood cells, and other body tissues may be important causes of altered pharmacokinetics in aged patients. Serum albumin is reduced in old age.[29,30] Chronic illness can further reduce plasma protein levels. The resultant reduced drug binding allows more unbound (free) drug to be available for distribution to body tissues, causing enhanced drug effects.[31]

Alterations in the binding of drugs to plasma proteins underlie some adverse effects in the elderly. It is a common clinical finding, for example, that a narcotic dose must be reduced in the elderly patient because of increased sensitivity to the drug's respiratory depressant effects. In a time study of meperidine plasma concentration following intravenous injection in surgical patients and normal patients,[32] the older patients had higher unbound (free) drug fractions. It was found that the diminished warfarin binding capacity in the elderly was proportional to a fall in plasma albumin levels.[33]

REGIONAL BLOOD FLOW

Changes in regional blood flow can significantly change the way drugs are handled by affecting absorption, distribution, metabolism, and excretion. Little is known about how regional blood flow changes with age. It is known that in general peripheral circulation decreases with advancing age and that coronary and cerebral blood flows are better maintained. Certain diseases are known to be associated with increased or decreased regional blood flows, as may be seen in the decreased hepatic blood flow in patients with congestive heart failure and the increased joint blood flow in patients with arthritis. Local blood flow is controlled by a multitude of local and remote elements, including vasoconstrictor and vasodilator nerves, blood flow, excitatory and inhibitory factors, local tissue metabolites, myogenic "pacemaker" cells, and positive feedback from blood pressure stretch receptors.[4,6,17,19]

HEPATIC DRUG METABOLISM

Drugs and other foreign materials are metabolized by the enzyme systems of the liver, kidney, lung, and gastrointestinal tract. These systems convert lipid soluble (nonpolar) compounds into more water soluble (polar) compounds, which may be pharmacologically more or less active but are usually more readily excreted via the kidney or bile.[34] Elderly subjects may have a reduced capacity to metabolize certain drugs.[4,7,8] The liver is around 2.5% of the body weight until middle age and then decreases to around 1.6% of body weight in the aged.[35]

Hepatic blood flow also decreases with age. A fall of 40% to 45% in hepatic blood flow can occur between ages 25 and 65. This is in part the result of decreased cardiac output.[4,36-38]

Studies on the relative rates of drug clearance in young and elderly subjects demonstrated that the mean plasma half-lives were greater in geriatric subjects for both antipyrine (45%) and phenylbutazone (29%). In a number of elderly individuals the metabolism of the two drugs was found to be extremely slow.[39-40] Propranolol clearance is also significantly reduced with aging, particularly in cigarette smokers.[41] The enzyme-inducing effect of smoking appears to decline with age.

Acetaminophen, indomethacin, and sulfamethizole are drugs whose metabolism involves a conjugation step. The study of these drugs in elderly subjects suggested that the elderly subjects had a reduced capacity to form conjugates.[42] Reduced rates of biotransformation in the elderly have been found for aminopyrine, warfarin, and amobarbital.[4]

It has recently been demonstrated that older patients have higher plasma levels and longer plasma half-lives of imipramine or amitriptyline and their active desmethyl metabolites. These effects were not accounted for by smoking (which may increase drug metabolizing enzymes) or the changes in body size associated with aging. Decreased biotransformation may result from a gradual decrease in specific activities of drug metabolizing enzymes as well as a loss of liver mass relative to body size. Because of the increase in the half-lives of tricyclic antidepressants (TCA) from 20 to 35 hours in the general patient population to 40 to 50 hours in the age group over 65 years, steady state drug levels may not be reached for up to 2 weeks. ("Rule of fives": 96% of steady state levels are reached after a period of five half-lives.) Thus in the elderly it is prudent to reduce standard TCA doses by one third to one half.[43]

The pharmacokinetics of benzodiazepines appear to be significantly influenced by age. In a study of adverse reactions to flurazepam (Dalmane) in 2542 hospitalized patients, toxicity (primarily excessive daytime drowsiness or confusion) increased progressively with age (1.9% among those under 60 years old to 7.1% in those over 80 years old). However, a dosage of 15 mg per day or less of flurazepam caused only 2% of those 70 years or older to experience adverse reactions, while 39% of those receiving 30 mg per day had difficulty.[44,67] Higher flurazepam doses produced more reactions regardless of age, but the dose effect is most striking in the elderly. These findings suggest that 15 mg of flurazepam per day can be prescribed safely for most elderly patients. However, toxic accumulation can occur over time at any dose, and patients, especially the elderly, should be monitored for increasing daytime sedation and confusion while taking flurazepam, diazepam, or some other benzodiazepine. While this study does not identify the mechanism of enhanced toxicity, it is probable that the pharmacokinetic properties of flurazepam change with aging, as has been already shown for chlordiazepoxide hydrochloride and diazepam. The clearance of chlordiazepoxide by the liver is reduced significantly in elderly subjects.[45] Although the plasma half-life of diazepam exhibits a striking age dependent increase, with half-life of diazepam at age 20 being about 20 hours and 90 hours[46-48] at age 80, clearance of this drug appears to be lower only in elderly males. Central nervous system (CNS) side effects of diazepam increase significantly from ages 40 to 70 years.[49] Downward adjustment of benzodiazepine dosage is suggested in patients over 65 years old.

It is of interest that nonmicrosomal drug metabolizing pathways such as acetylations and the aldehyde dehydrogenase catalyzed oxidation of ethanol are not affected by aging.[41]

Congestive heart failure is associated with significant decreases in the V_d and clearance rates of several drugs. Recent studies have established that loading doses of lidocaine, procainamide, quinidine, and theophylline should be decreased by at least one third in patients with significant congestive heart failure.[50-52] Furthermore, maintenance doses of these (as well as other drugs eliminated by the liver) need to be reduced in the presence of congestive heart failure because of decreased biotransformation and resultant prolonged half-life caused by decreased blood flow to the liver and impairment of hepatic function.*

RENAL EXCRETION OF DRUGS

Compounds of low lipid solubility are readily excreted by the kidney, and their rate of elimination is primarily dependent on the glomerular filtration rate.[48,54] Highly lipid soluble drugs are reabsorbed by the renal tubule, and their elimination is affected by their conversion to a more water soluble derivative via oxidative metabolism catalyzed by the microsomal drug metabolizing enzymes of the liver and then renal excretion of the metabolite.[55] Renal excretion of drugs can be altered by changes in renal blood flow, glomerular filtration rate, tubular secretion, or reabsorption.

A progressive reduction in the number of functioning nephrons and the decrease in plasma flow to the kidneys that occurs with increasing age have been demonstrated to produce a significant decrease in renal function. From age 20 to 90 years, renal plasma flow is decreased by

*References 4, 17-19, 38, 53.

about 53%, and the glomerular filtration rate (as measured by inulin clearance) is decreased by about 46%.[56-61]

The maximum capacity of the renal tubules for both reabsorption and secretion shows approximately the same percentage change with age, probably reflecting the reduction in absorbing and secreting surface. The general reduction in renal function with age is reflected by a decrease in creatinine clearance; however, it is not reflected by a change in serum creatinine levels. This latter observation is probably a consequence of creatinine production decreasing with age. Many drugs with a primarily renal mode of elimination have been shown to have half-lives progressively prolonged with advancing age. Prominent examples are digoxin, penicillin, tetracycline, streptomycin, gentamicin, and procainamide. The direct influence of age related changes in renal function on the pharmacokinetics of renally eliminated drugs has been clearly demonstrated for a number of drugs. The following table (Table 15-1) taken from a recent review[17] on the influence of age on pharmacokinetics illustrates the effect of age on renal drug elimination.

Digoxin is excreted predominantly by the kidneys. Studies on the pharmacokinetics of tritiated digoxin in groups of young (mean age of 27 years) and old (mean age of 77 years) men showed that the same dose of digoxin resulted in higher blood concentrations and longer blood half-lives in the elderly. The elderly group had creatinine clearances that averaged 56 ml/1.73 M^2 per minute compared to the average in the young men of 122 ml/1.73 M^2 per minute. Digoxin clearances averaged 53 ml/1.73 M^2 per minute in the elderly and 83 in the young. These studies show that the same dose of digoxin given to elderly and young adult subjects results in blood concentrations that are much higher in the elderly and may partially explain the higher incidence of digitalis intoxication in older patients.[62]

Table 15-1. Pharmacokinetic data on drugs eliminated by the kidney

Drug (route)	Findings*		Age groups (yr)	
			Young	*Elderly*
Dihydrostreptomycin (p.o.)	12 hr and 24 hr levels higher in elderly		18-33	63-87
Tetracycline (p.o.)	12 hr levels higher in elderly†			
Benzylpenicillin (IV)	Plasma T½	24 vs 55 hr†	>50 (men)	>70
		21 vs 39 hr†	>30 (women)	>65
Phenobarbitone (p.o.)	Serum T½	70 vs 105 hr	20-40	>70
Digoxin (IV)	Blood T½	51 vs 73 hr	20-30	73-81
	Renal clearance	83 vs 53 ml/ min 1.73 M^2†		
Benzylpenicillin (IM)	Serum levels of both drugs higher in elderly		15-33	71-86
Procaine penicillin (IM)	Plasma T½	0.56 vs 0.66 hr	20-30	60-80
Propicillin (p.o.)	V_d	29.1 vs 18.4L†		
	AUC	28.7 vs 53.0 hr/ units/ml†		
	Percent urinary recovery	53.4% vs 51.4%		
Kanamycin (IV)	Plasma T½	107 vs 282 min	20-50	70-90
Sulphamethizole (p.o.)	Blood T½	105 vs 181 hr†	22-30	73-91
	Blood clearance	167 vs 90 ml/ min 1.73 M^2†		
	V_d	345 vs 338 ml/kg		

From Crooks, et al.: Clin. Pharmacokinet. **1**:280, 1976.

*Values are given in order: young vs old T½, plasma half-life; V_d, apparent volume of distribution; AUC, area under serum concentration time curve.

† Significant difference between values in young and elderly subjects.[17]

A number of antibiotics, several cardiac glycosides, some antidiabetic sulfonylureas, and the active metabolites of acetohexamide (hydroxyhexamide) and allopurinol (hydroxy derivative) undergo renal excretion.

A wide variety of drugs are organic compounds that are actively secreted by the kidney in the renal tubular fluid.[54,55] Such drugs may be present in the plasma bound to proteins. This is the mechanism by which penicillin is removed from the body. The secretory capacity of the renal tubules depends on renal blood flow and the functional state of the secretory process. The effects of a decreased secretory capacity on plasma drug concentration are shown by the pronounced effects of probenecid (a drug that blocks the tubular excretion of certain drugs) in raising plasma levels of penicillin. Studies in humans have shown that the plasma levels of a number of renally excreted antibiotics are higher in elderly patients. Examples from various literature sources are shown in Fig. 15-1.[17,18,60,63]

In using drugs that have a narrow therapeutic index and are eliminated primarily by renal excretion (i.e., digoxin and gentamicin) appropriate reductions in dosage should be made. Nomograms or formulae that predict creatinine clearance for age and weight may be used to estimate dosage, and determination of plasma drug levels should be done to be certain that the appropriate adjustment in dosage has been made.

It has long been known that elderly patients may develop toxic effects when given the usual therapeutic dosages of drugs. Increases in tissue sensitivity in the aged were previously proposed, but recent evidence suggests that impaired renal and hepatic functions explain most adverse responses to drugs in the elderly.

Age decrements are more marked in physiologic adjustments that require the integrated activity of several organ systems than in adjustments involving a single system.[4,58] The impairment of renal, hepatic, cardiac, respiratory, neuromuscular, and endocrine vitality with ag-

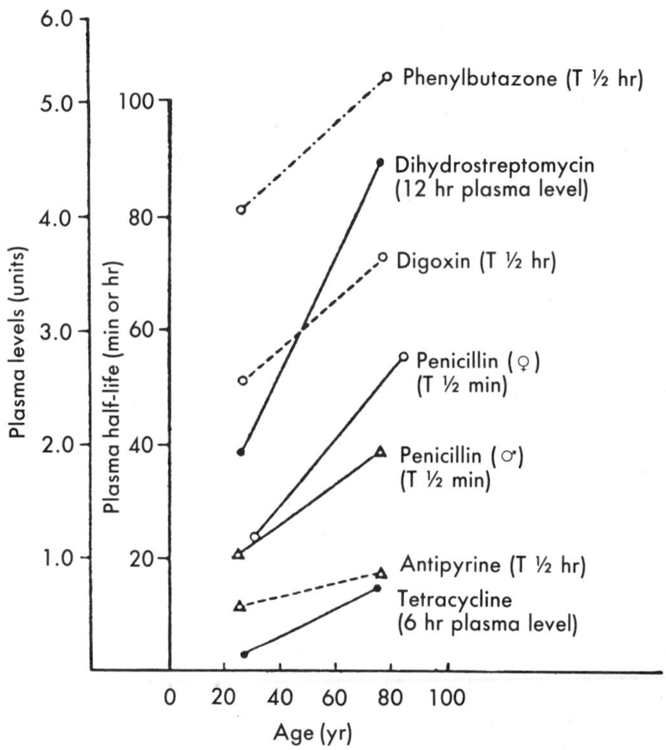

Fig. 15-1. Changes in drug plasma level or plasma half-life in young and old human subjects after parenteral administration of various drugs. (From Bender, A.D.: J. Am. Geriatr. Soc. **22:**296, 1974.)

ing results in a slower rate of recovery following a variety of physiologic displacements.* Aging is characterized by a diminution of the adaptive capacity to a variety of inputs. The reduced homeostatic responses of the elderly may contribute to more frequent adverse drug reactions than would be expected in younger patients. Because of decreased capacity for cardiovascular homeostasis, elderly patients are more prone to postural hypotension secondary to the use of diuretics, sympatholytics, nitrates, phenothiazines, TCA, procainamide, and antihypertensive drugs.[58]

COMPLIANCE TO A SUGGESTED THERAPEUTIC REGIMEN

The success of a program of medical management of illness depends in large measure on the degree to which patients follow their physicians' advice concerning behavior, diet, and the way in which prescribed medications are taken. Poor compliance with drug therapy has been described many times.[65,66] Many factors may contribute to poor compliance of some elderly patients—the cost of medication, poor vision, difficulty opening bottles because of arthritis, impaired memory.

Although some authors believe that the elderly are less likely or less able to follow drug regimens as outpatients,[67,68] others have found no correlation between age per se and compliance.[65,69] For example, compliance with digoxin treatment has been found to be as good in elderly patients as in younger patients when measured by interview and by serum digoxin concentrations.[70]

A general rule of therapeutics is that the correct dosage for every patient must be empirically determined. For the elderly, it is especially important to individualize therapy. When one deals with these patients unusual responses, including hypersensitivity and toxicity, should all be suspected and carefully evaluated if they occur.

EFFECTS OF AGE ON SPECIFIC DRUGS

Some of the more commonly used drugs will be briefly discussed, and the effects of age on drug disposition and adverse responses will be assessed. The drugs to be discussed include the following: (1) digoxin; (2) thiazide diuretics; (3) beta-adrenergic receptor blockers (propranolol); (4) antihypertensive drugs; (5) anticoagulants; (6) theophylline; (7) analgesics; (8) sedative-hypnotic agents; (9) TCA and antipsychotic drugs (neuroleptics); and (10) antiparkinsonian drugs.

Digoxin. Digoxin is widely used in therapy of the elderly and is a major cause of adverse drug reactions. As has been shown earlier, the elderly are probably no more sensitive to the actions of the drug, either therapeutic or toxic, but have a decreased clearance capacity secondary to diminished renal function.[53,62,71] The half-life of digoxin has been found to increase by as much as 40% in the elderly in association with reduced renal function.[62]

Thiazide diuretics. It is known that elderly patients are more susceptible to the adverse effects of thiazide diuretics.[4] These drugs are widely used for therapy of heart failure, edema secondary to cirrhosis and renal disease, and hypertension and are a common cause of adverse drug reactions.[72] These effects include hypokalemia, hypovolemia, hypotension, impaired glucose tolerance with occasional frank diabetes and hyperuricemia, and occasional symptomatic gout. The reason for the adverse effects may lie in the elderly patient's reduced homeostatic capacity with renal, hepatic, cardiac, and peripheral vascular diseases. Because of reduced compensatory mechanisms, drug effects from usual therapeutic dosages are more marked.

Beta-adrenergic receptor blockers (propranolol). Alterations in the autonomic nervous system occur in the elderly.[4] The heart rate response to isoproterenol is less in elderly subjects.[73] Propranolol has been found to reduce the heart rate response to exercise and isoproterenol less in elderly subjects.[73,74] Elderly subjects are often treated with propranolol for angina, hypertension, and cardiac arrhythmias. Elderly subjects attain higher plasma levels of propranolol in response to usual therapeutic dosages than other subjects. Given a single 40 mg oral dose of propranolol elderly subjects attained much higher plasma levels of the drug than younger subjects.[75] This effect is the result of reduced hepatic blood flow resulting in decreased drug clearance.[41,76,77]

Antihypertensive drugs. Elevated blood pressure in subjects over 65 years of age rep-

*References 4, 20-22, 58, 64.

resents a risk factor for cardiovascular disease. The treatment of hypertension in the elderly is, however, more complicated. Impaired baroreceptor responses, decreased venous tone, and diminished cardiovascular and autonomic nervous system functions all dispose the elderly patient to postural hypotension.[58,78-80]

The diminished capacity to compensate for excessive drug actions creates increased sensitivity to the effects of antihypertensive agents in the elderly.[81] Although the central nervous system depressant effects of alpha methyldopa may be troublesome in some elderly patients,[58,82] most tolerate this drug remarkably well.[83] The use of reserpine in the elderly carries the risk of insidious depression in settings where adverse effects may not be detected.

Anticoagulants. Elderly subjects are more sensitive to the effects of both heparin and warfarin.[84,85] The increased risk of bleeding has been attributed to the diminished mechanical homeostatic response of the aging vascular system.[4] No effects of age on warfarin pharmacokinetic parameters have been reported. However, greater inhibition of vitamin K–dependent clotting factor synthesis has been found in the elderly.[86] It has been suggested that reduced dietary vitamin K or reduced gastrointestinal absorption of the vitamin could create a relative deficiency.

Theophylline. Age per se does not affect the clearance of theophylline.[51] Cigarette smoking produces an increase in theophylline clearance in the elderly, in contrast to the lack of effect of smoking on antipyrine and propranolol clearance in older subjects.[41] There is no evidence of any intrinsic increase of sensitivity to theophylline in the elderly, but the presence of congestive heart failure or cirrhosis decreases clearance of the drug and raises plasma levels.[44,87,88] The dangers of elevated plasma levels of theophylline in patients with cerebral and cardiovascular diseases may be considerable (seizures, arrhythmias).[89]

Analgesics. Age has been shown to be the most important variable in determining the degree of pain relief following administration of a potent analgesic.[90] Under double-blind conditions, interviews revealed an age related increase in relief of pain intensity in 712 patients receiving 10 mg of morphine sulfate and 20 mg of pentazocine (Fig. 15-2). There were no differences in the frequency of side effects with age. Available data suggest that this increased responsiveness is most likely the result of age related differences in pain perception. Pharmacokinetic age related differences have been reported following intravenous administration of morphine, 10 mg/70 kg body weight. Serum levels at 2 minutes correlated directly with patient age and averaged 70% higher in the older age group.[90] The serum half-life, however, was independent of age. Plasma binding of meperidine also correlated negatively with age.[91]

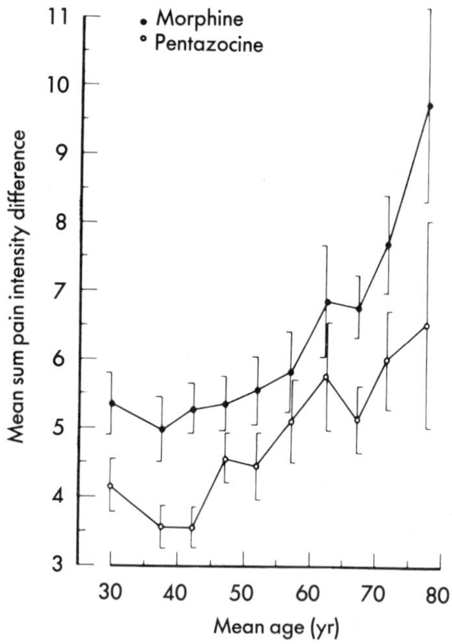

Fig. 15-2. Correlation of estimate of pain relief (mean sum pain intensity differences) with age group after administration of 10 mg morphine (slope = 0.039, $p<0.001$) and 20 mg pentazocine (slope = 0.052, $p<0.001$) administered intramuscularly to 712 patients for acute postoperative pain. (From Bellville, J.W., Forrest, W.H., Miller, E., and Brown, B.W.: J.A.M.A. **217:**1835, 1971.)

Age related changes such as these may contribute to the enhanced effect of analgesics in the elderly. Whether the reduced clearance of acetaminophen in the elderly has clinical importance remains to be determined.[92]

Sedative-hypnotic agents. Sedative-hypnotic drugs are widely used in the elderly. Clinical recountings of increased sensitivity and paradoxical responses to these drugs are well known.[27,93,] The paradoxical excitement in the

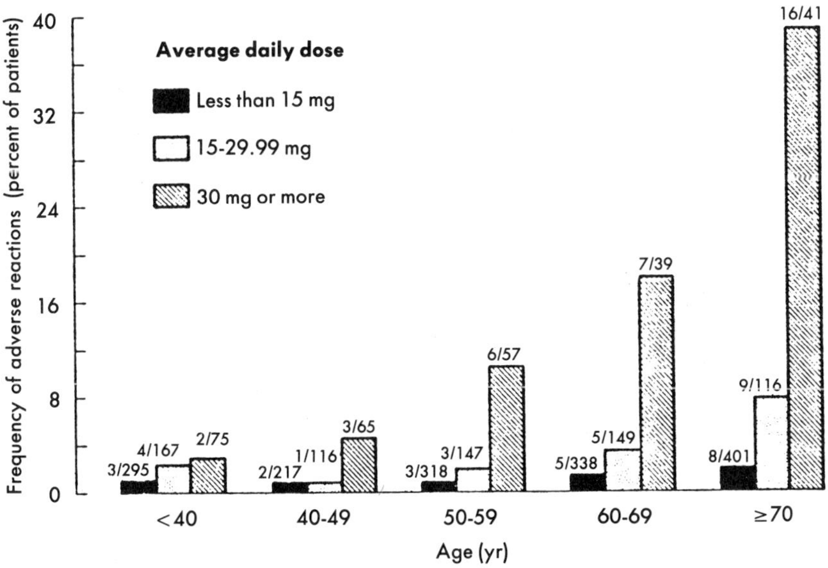

Fig. 15-3. Frequency of adverse reactions of flurazepam in relation to age and average daily dose. (From Greenblatt, D.J., Allen, M.D., and Shader, R.I.: Clin. Pharmacol. Ther. **21**:355, 1977.)

elderly can range from mild restlessness to excitement. The elimination of amobarbital is prolonged in the elderly.[94] The pharmacokinetic differences probably result from decreased drug metabolism as well as reduced renal excretion.[95,96] Clearance of chlordiazepoxide is reduced about 40% in the elderly.[97] An increasing literature is developing on the pharmacology of the benzodiazepines in the elderly.* Clearance of diazepam is reduced in elderly males but not in elderly females. Thus only elderly males would be expected to achieve higher steady-state plasma levels of diazepam. Clearance of desmethyldiazepam, the major active metabolite of diazepam, is not reduced in the elderly.[100] Liver disease is associated with reduced clearance of diazepam.[46] The increased sensitivity of the elderly to the sedative effects of benzodiazepines is a function of age, hepatic activity, and other nonpharmacokinetic factors, which as yet cannot be defined but probably encompass numbers of brain cells, cerebral blood flow, and brain metabolic activity.[47,93,98,99] The relationship between reactions of a series of flurazepam doses and the age of subjects is shown in Fig. 15-3. It is obvious that the frequency of adverse reactions increases with advancing age.[44] The clearance of oxazepam, a shorter acting benzodiazepine, appears to be unaffected by age. The use of this type of preparation may result in "rebound" hypersomnia if used intermittently.[1,101] The greater sensitivity of the elderly to the effects of diazepam, chlordiazepoxide, and flurazepam (excessive drowsiness, impaired psychomotor performance, confusion) may be compounded by the concomitant use of ethanol.[1,93,96]

TCA and antipsychotic drugs. TCA, while not extensively used in elderly patients, have great potential for adverse drug reactions.[1,102] Higher plasma levels of TCA have been reported in older patients being treated with the usual dosages of the drugs.[43] The decreased compensatory mechanisms in elderly patients make them more prone to the hypotensive, sedative, and anticholinergic adverse effects of these agents.

Antipsychotic drugs are more extensively used in the elderly than TCA. They are used in state hospitals and home-care settings over long periods of time. These drugs have prominent cardiovascular, anticholinergic, and sedative effects that can be dangerous in this group of patients.[102] Adverse effects of antipsychotic drugs (phenothiazines and butyrophenones) are more frequent in the elderly probably because of their

*References 44-47, 49, 93, 98, 99.

decreased compensatory mechanisms. The neurologic effects, which include akathisia, parkinsonian syndrome, and choreiform movements, are all increased in elderly patients taking antipsychotic drugs. The combination of decreased homeostasis and chronic illness engenders increased adverse drug reactions.[96]

Antiparkinsonian drugs. The anticholinergic drugs used in the treatment of Parkinson's disease cause classic excess drug effects. Signs of intolerance include mild confusion, nightmares, and increased forgetfulness. It is often the evening dose that precipitates signs of toxicity. Additional anticholinergic side effects such as urinary hesitancy and retention and constipation and obstipation with fecal impaction are also prominent. Behavior alterations may be observed with levodopa. Emotional states may be depressed or elated, and cognitive function may be normal or markedly impaired. Signs of dementia may be aggravated with increased paranoid or agitated behavior.[82,103]

DRUG-DRUG INTERACTIONS

Drug interactions are an important consideration in therapy and are more common in the elderly patient. These interactions occur in a setting of multiple drug therapy used for the many chronic disease states found in an elderly population. Drug interactions can arise from drug effects on the absorption, distribution, biotransformation, or excretion of other drugs. Drug interactions can be and have been used as beneficial contributions to therapy. However, undesirable or unsuspected interactions that are deleterious to the patient must be anticipated in elderly patients receiving a large number of drugs and having impaired homeostatic mechanisms.

Drug-drug interactions are modifications of the effects of a drug when used in association with another drug. These interactions can result in either augmentation or diminution of pharmacologic activity and may account for a significant proportion of all adverse drug reactions. It has been reported that hypersensitivity (the signs and symptoms resulting from an immune response to a standard dose of drug), idiosyncrasy (the inordinate response to a usual dose), and the predictable response (toxicity expected from overdose) account for less than 50% of drug reactions.[12-14,104]

The treatment of a number of pathologic states such as hypertension, arthritis, congestive heart failure, depression, neoplastic disease, infectious disease, and inflammatory disease involves the use of multiple drug therapy. The trend toward simultaneous use of increasing numbers of pharmacologic agents over long periods of time raises new considerations and concerns. Since the efficacy and toxicity of any new pharmacologic agent is ascertained by tests in which the drug is the sole agent used, the testing results may not be valid in the clinical arena of actual drug use. It is unrealistic to assume that drugs do not interact and that a drug will produce the same effect when used with another drug as when used alone.[105-107] Each chemical agent has its separate and distinct side effects that occur with characteristic frequency. The concomitant use of two or more drugs, however, may result in unexpected increases or decreases in potencies of the several drugs being used simultaneously. It has been found that there is a 7% adverse drug reaction rate in patients using 6 to 10 drugs, whereas the reaction rate is 40% in patients using 16 to 20 drugs.[11,15,16]

Tissue levels of physiologically or pharmacologically active substances are limited by their rates of appearance (synthesis or absorption) and their rates of removal (enzymatic inactivation, binding, or excretion). Since drugs may directly or indirectly alter enzymatic activity, binding capacity, and transport processes, it might be expected that the presence of one drug might markedly influence the efficacy of another drug either by affecting the rate of appearance or removal of the drug itself or of an endogenous compound necessary for the action of the second drug. The course of such interactions may enhance drug efficacy, lead to undesirable side effects, or even result in marked toxicity.

PHYSICAL-CHEMICAL PROCESSES

In vitro chemical reactions

The drug-drug interactions that occur before administration usually represent physical-chemical incompatibilities. For example, the delayed hypoglycemia that follows the mixture of regular insulin with protamine zinc insulin is caused by the binding of regular insulin by the excess of protamine present in the sustained action insulin preparation. Other instances of drug inactivation before administration include the diminution of penicillin and semisynthetic penicillin activity caused by carbohydrate solutions with alkaline pH and the decreases in gentamicin activity caused by chemical alteration of aminoglycoside when given in solutions containing carbenicillin or ticarcillin. As this interaction is dependent on a high penicillin concentration it may also occur in vivo, particularly in patients with renal failure who have very high carbenicillin or ticarcillin levels.[108]

Absorption

Clinical responses to orally administered drugs can be modified by changes in the rate of drug absorption or the total quantity of drug absorbed. Since nonionized drugs are better absorbed, acidic drugs are more readily absorbed in the stomach (salicylates, sulfonamides, phenytoin, barbiturates, warfarin) and basic drugs in the small intestines (phenothiazines, TCA, antihistamines, quinidine, erythromycin). However, the small intestine, because of its greater surface area, accounts for the majority of absorption of both acidic and basic drugs.

Drugs that alter gastric and small intestinal motility can affect the rate or quantity of drug absorption. Drugs such as anticholinergics and opiates increase gastric retention time and decrease intestinal motility. This serves to increase transit time in the small intestines where most drug absorption occurs because of the large mucosal absorption surface. Digoxin, a drug whose absorption is normally incomplete, has its plasma levels increased by simultaneously administered anticholinergic agents.[109] This effect presumably occurs as a result of prolonged intestinal transit time. Decreased digoxin absorption would be anticipated with simultaneous use of drugs that shorten intestinal transit time such as cathartics and cholinomimetics (methacholine, neostigmine).

Impairment of drug absorption may result from binding of drugs to other interacting drugs or to foods. This is exemplified by the binding of iron and penicillin to food and the precipitation of tetracyclines as insoluble complexes with magnesium, calcium, and aluminum commonly found in antacid preparations and with iron.

Drug absorption can be affected by the concomitant use of antacid and kaolin products. The large surface area of these preparations favors nonspecific absorption of drugs. Simultaneous use of acidic drugs with antacid preparations may further promote the ionization of the acidic drugs in the small intestines where they are already ionized to some extent. The ionized drug state favors nonspecific drug adsorption to the antacid preparation and decreases and/or delays absorption. The absorption of lincomycin is imparied by ingestion of kaolins. Phenothiazines, which are bound by antacid preparations, lose their effects with chronic use of antacids.

Therapeutic use of these nonspecific surface adsorption phenomena has led to the use of charcoal and kaolin for treatment of drug overdoses. These preparations diminish drug absorption and permit removal of the drug from the gastrointestinal tract.

Cholestyramine and polystyrene sulfonate are insoluble exchange resins that have been used to prevent intestinal absorption and facilitate elimination of certain substances (bile acids, potassium). Cholestyramine is an anion exchanger that has been found to alter the absorption of warfarin and digoxin. Interactions of the exchange resins and acidic and basic drugs is probable, but the extent and clinical significance are not known.[9,48,110,111]

Protein binding

Most drugs are reversibly bound to plasma albumin to varying degrees. The drug-albumin complex serves as a circulating reservoir of drug. Only the unbound form of the drug is active—free to diffuse through capillary walls and reach tissue sites of drug action. The availability of drugs to sites of drug action is directly related to the quantity of free drug present. The quantity of free drug is related to the total concentration of drug, the amount of albumin present, and the binding affinity of the drug for albumin. Albumin is capable of binding anionic and cationic drug species. These ionic interactions are not strong, and other forces play important roles in binding. These include hydrogen bonding, hydrophobic bonding, and van der Waals' forces.

When two or more drugs are simultaneously administered, the binding of one may be affected by the other(s). Displacement of a drug initially results in a greater concentration of free drug and a resultant intensification of pharmacologic action. However, since the free drug is more rapidly eliminated via glomerular filtration and hepatic metabolism, the half-life may be shortened. This shortened half-life would apply when the drug displaced from plasma proteins does not have a high tissue affinity. Displaced drugs with high tissue affinities have increased apparent volumes of distribution, increased plasma half-lives, and little alteration in clearance.[112,113]

Most displacing drugs are acidic. The displacement is more marked with high concentrations of drugs that have high affinities for albumin binding sites relative to the bound drug. A list of highly bound drugs is shown. The bound/free percentage of drug is shown at therapeutic plasma levels.

Diazepam	99-1
Phenylbutazone	99-1
Tolbutamide	99-1
Dicloxicillin	99-1
Indomethacin	97-3
Warfarin	97-3
Chlorpromazine	96-4
Amitriptyline	96-4
Propranolol	94-6
Methotrexate	94-6
Phenytoin	91-9
Clofibrate	90-10
Digitoxin	90-10
Acetylsalicylic acid	84-16

Even a small displacement of a highly bound drug can result in a large increase in the free (active) species.[112] For highly bound drugs, the free form can be doubled by as little as a 1% displacement of the bound drug. A 1% displacement of phenylbutazone doubles the free drug concentration, whereas a 3% displacement will do so for warfarin.

The pharmacologic effects of drug displacement are most marked if the displaced drug is highly bound (greater than 80% at therapeutic plasma levels), has a narrow therapeutic index, and a small apparent V_d. If the V_d of the drug is large, then displacement only results in a small rise in plasma concentration of free drug and the pharmacologic effect will be small. If the V_d is small, then displacement will result in a significant rise in plasma concentration of the free drug, resulting in a more marked pharmacologic effect. Many drugs bound to plasma albumin can be displaced with few discernible clinical effects because they do not fulfill these criteria for intensification of drug action. For example, dicloxicillin has a large therapeutic index and amitriptyline a large V_d.

A number of clinically significant displacement reactions have been reported with oral anticoagulants and tolbutamide. These drugs are displaced from their albumin binding sites by acidic drugs such as sulfonamides, phenylbutazone, ethacrynic acid, nalidixic acid, and acetylsalicylic acid, resulting in bleeding or hypoglycemia.

Displacement can occur both competitively and noncompetitively. Acetylsalicylic acid influences the binding of other drugs to albumin by acetylating a lysine residue of albumin that modifies the binding of anionic drugs.

Hepatic and renal diseases are associated with decreased drug binding to plasma albumin. This is the result of decreased levels of plasma albumin and qualitative changes in the albumin that diminish binding affinity.[29,32,33,112]

Drug interactions at receptor sites and cell membranes

The actions of some drugs and endogenous compounds are associated with their binding to cell surface receptors. Alterations of this binding by other drugs can modify the usual receptor response.

Antagonism is based on inhibition of drug binding to receptors and may be competitive or noncompetitive. These types of inhibitions are the basis of the actions of a number of drugs and include the following: inhibition of the cardiac accelerator actions of norepinephrine by propranolol, a beta-adrenergic receptor blocking agent; reduction of the respiratory depression effects of morphine by naloxone; inhibition of the bradycardic effect of acetylcholine by atropine, a cholinergic receptor blocking agent. These are all examples of competitive inhibitions. Thyroxine has been reported to potentiate the anticoagulant effects of warfarin without altering the warfarin plasma half-life. This probably is a noncompetitive effect.

Drugs may influence the actions of other drugs by blocking their uptake into or facilitating their release from cells. The monoamine oxidase (MAO) inhibitors deter intracellular inactivation of active catecholamines that accumulate in adrenergic neurons. These vasoactive catecholamines can be released from the cell by a number of drugs including amphetamines. A variety of foods contain tyramine, which is normally metabolized in the gastrointestinal tract by MAO. Because of MAO inhibition, the tyramine gains access to the circulation and acts like amphetamines to release the increased stores of catecholamines and causes marked adrenergic effects (tachycardia, hypertension, headache).[104,106,107,114]

TCA inhibit amine uptake and facilitate release of norepinephrine and serotonin in neural tissues. However, TCA also inhibit the uptake of guanethidine, which cannot gain access to its site of action, and its antihypertensive effect is reversed by simultaneous use of TCA.[104,106,107,115]

DRUG DISPOSITION

Drug excretion

Renal clearance of drugs may occur by means of glomerular filtration or tubular secretion. Drug-drug interactions can influence drug clearance by either of these mechanisms.

Nonprotein bound drugs are filtered through the glomerulus. The free drug in the glomerular filtrate is reabsorbed by the renal tubules through passive diffusion. Reabsorption occurs in varying degrees depending in part on the polar nature of the drug and on the pH of the urine. Because less polar (uncharged) drugs are more readily reabsorbed, the pH of the urine can determine the extent of drug clearance. Weakly acidic drugs like salicylic acid and phenylbutazone are rapidly excreted in alkaline urine, whereas weakly basic drugs such as amphetamine and antihistamines are readily excreted in acid urine. Drugs can alter the pH of urine and influence the half-lives of other drugs that are significantly excreted by the kidney (more than 20%). Drugs such as sodium bicarbonate and acetazolamide alkalinize the urine, whereas drugs such as mandelic acid and ascorbic acid acidify urine. These principles are the basis for alkalinization of the urine in the treatment of aspirin and phenobarbital overdoses and for acidification of the urine in amphetamine overdoses.

Drug-drug interactions may occur if a drug that is cleared by the kidney is used in conjuction with a drug that is nephrotoxic. The aminoglycoside antibiotics such as gentamicin and kanamycin may decrease glomerular filtration. Digoxin and chlorpropamide toxicity may occur when these drugs are used in association with gentamicin because they are significantly cleared by glomerular filtration.

Many acidic drugs such as penicillins, thiazides, salicylic acid, and indomethacin are eliminated by renal tubular secretion, an active process. Drug-drug interactions occur when two drugs, which are both cleared by renal tubular secretion, are used simultaneously. The elimination of methotrexate is slowed by acetylsalicylic acid, and phenylbutazone inhibits the elimination of hydroxyhexamide, a potent hypoglycemic metabolite of acetohexamide. The inhibitions result in increased half-lives of active drugs and overdose toxicities. This type of interaction has been used beneficially in the case of simultaneous use of penicillin and probenecid. Probenecid blocks the tubular secretion of penicillin, resulting in higher blood levels for longer periods of time.[13,14,54,55]

Stimulation of drug metabolism

Drugs and other xenobiotics are mainly metabolized in the liver but also to a lesser extent in the kidney, the gastrointestinal tract, and lungs. These compounds undergo a variety of structural modifications that tend to produce products that are more polar and water soluble. The biotransformations in general create drug metabolites that are less capable of permeating cells. The more polar metabolites are in general more readily eliminated by means of renal or biliary excretion.

The enzymes of drug metabolism are both nonpotent and nonspecific. The number of these enzymes is not known; isolation and purification studies are being undertaken. Many but not all of these enzymatic reactions are oxidative and often followed by additional conjugation reactions.

Biotransformation of drugs usually implies loss of pharmacologic activity, but this is not always so. There are instances in which metabolism results in the conversion of an inactive precursor to an active metabolite and in which both the precursor and metabolite are both pharmacologically active. Some examples of these reactions are as follows:

Procainamide (active)	→	N-acetylprocainamide (active)
Propranolol (active)	→	4-hydroxypropranolol (active)
Quinidine (active)	→	2-hydroxyquinidine (active)

Parathion (inactive)	→	paraoxon (active)
Acetohexamide (active)	→	hydroxyhexamide (more active)
Phenylbutazone (active)	→	oxyphenylbutazone (active)
Imipramine (active)	→	Desipramine (active)

The enzymes of drug metabolism are sensitive to a variety of chemical influences that can increase their activity. The increased activity may be engendered by prior in vivo exposure to drugs, insecticides, environmental chemicals, and by smoking cigarettes. The augmentation of drug metabolizing enzyme activity is termed *induction* and is thought to be caused by the synthesis of more enzymes in the liver.[14,34,48,104]

It has been established that induction is a nonspecific phenomenon. For example, phenobarbital and phenytoin are both capable of accelerating the metabolic disposition of a number of other drugs.[105,106,116,117,118]

In general, drugs are capable of inducing the metabolism of other drugs depending on their lipid solubility at physiologic pH, their concentration, and their duration of exposure.

The effects of enzyme induction can be clinically important when a drug is either added to or withdrawn from a therapeutic regimen of multiple drug therapy. In the case of the addition of a second drug there may be an acceleration of metabolic disposition of the first drug resulting in decreased plasma concentrations and diminished therapeutic effect. In the case of withdrawal of a drug from multiple drug therapy regimen the opposite effect may occur. Drug withdrawal results in the concentration of the drug whose metabolism had been accelerated, rising to higher and perhaps toxic blood levels.

Induction of drug metabolizing enzymes by xenobiotics has produced a variety of unexpected clinical responses to drugs. An often cited example is drug metabolizing enzyme stimulation induced by phenobarbital. When phenobarbital is administered both warfarin and bishydroxycoumarin are metabolized more rapidly. When a patient receiving anticoagulants is given a barbiturate that patient will require larger doses of anticoagulants than usual to maintain a suitable state of anticoagulation. On the other hand, if the barbiturate is discontinued and the dose of anticoagulants is not readjusted bleeding may occur. Phenobarbital also stimulates metabolism of corticosteroids.[116] Similar effects have been seen in other conditions of multiple drug usage. Adjustments of drug regimens must be considered when a drug that stimulates drug metabolizing enzymes is instituted or discontinued. A clue to the ocurrence of drug interations caused by altered drug metabolism is the development of unexpected sensitivity to a drug under conditions in which a drug has been discontinued from a therapeutic regimen or drug resistance has developed after the addition of a drug to a therapeutic regimen.[119]

Environmental exposures to chlorinated hydrocarbon insecticides such as lindane and dichlorodiphenyltrichloroethane (DDT) have been found to accelerate the metabolism of antipyrine in subjects chronically exposed to these agents. A loss of the anticoagulant effects of warfarin has also been reported after occupational exposure to insecticides. This exposure required an increase in the warfarin maintenance dose from 7.5 to 17.5 mg a day.[120-122]

An effect of cigarette smoking on the plasma clearance of phenacetin and theophylline has been described. The accelerated disposition of phenacetin and theophylline from the plasma of cigarette smokers was probably caused by increased drug metabolism resulting from induction of drug metabolizing enzymes by xenobiotics contained in the inhaled cigarette smoke.[123-126]

It has been found that long-term therapy of epilepsy with phenobarbital, phenytoin, or both may result in hypocalcemia, osteomalacia, and depressed plasma levels of 25-hydroxycholecalciferol in some patients. It is believed that these drugs accelerate the metabolism of vitamin D_3 (cholecalciferol) to hydroxylated metabolites that are biologically inactive.[127]

Ethanol also may play a role in drug interactions because of its capacity to induce metabolism of other drugs such as tolbutamide and warfarin.[105,107]

Inhibition of drug metabolism

Drug inhibition of drug metabolism is not uncommon and may be clinically more important than stimulation interactions. Because of the nonpotent and nonspecific nature of drug metabolizing enzymes, inhibition of drug metabolism may be nonspecific, and the metabolism of a drug may be inhibited by chemically and pharmacologically unrelated drugs. The inhibition is thought to be caused by saturation of drug metabolizing enzymes. Drug inhibition of drug metabolism usually results in both an intensification of drug action and an increase in its duration. A number of human studies have shown that inhibition of drug metabolism by other drugs increases the half-life of the primary drug and elevates its steady state plasma concentration. Tolbutamide metabolism is inhibited by bishydroxycoumarin, chloramphenicol, probenecid, and sulfaphenazole, which increase the half-life of tolbutamide from a range of 4.5 to 6 hours to 11 to 18 hours. Cimetidine inhibits the metabolism of warfarin,[128] antipyrine, propranolol, theophylline, chlordiazepoxide, and diazepam. The metabolism of phenytoin is inhibited by simultaneous administration of bishydroxycoumarin, phenylbutazone, chloramphenicol, and isoniazid. These inhibitions produce toxic effects at therapeutic doses of the drugs: tolbutamide, hypoglycemia; phenytoin, ataxia; warfarin, bleeding.[52,105,107]

Although inhibition of drug metabolism by other drugs is generally a nonspecific phenomenon, there are interesting exceptions. Simultaneous use of warfarin and metronidazole has resulted in increased steady state plasma levels of warfarin and increased prothrombin times. This is probably caused by metronidazole inhibition of warfarin metabolism.[129] The inhibitory effect was found when either S(−) warfarin or the racemic mixture was used. No inhibition of the metabolism of R(+) warfarin was found. The stereoselective inhibition of S(−) warfarin metabolism by metronidazole could be lessened or avoided by long-term therapy with R(+) warfarin.[129]

A number of drugs exhibit dose-dependent pharmacokinetics. The plasma levels of these drugs decline more slowly after administration of a large dose than after a small dose of drug. This phenomenon has been well studied in the case of bishydroxycoumarin, phenytoin, acetylsalicylic acid, and ethanol. The plasma half-life of bishydroxycoumarin at an oral dose of 2 mg/kg is around 24 hours, whereas at a dose of 4 mg/kg the half-life is 48 hours. Dose-dependent kinetics is a limitation of drug metabolism secondary to saturation of the metabolizing enzymes. It has important implications for therapy of drug overdoses. Larger drug intakes would be expected to lengthen the clearance time of drugs from plasma.[130]

Allopurinol is an inhibitor of xanthine oxidase. Since both azathioprine and mercaptopurine are metabolized to inactive compounds via xanthine oxidase, the inhibition of xanthine oxidase by allopurinol serves to prolong the duration and increase the intensity of action of these two drugs.[131]

L-dihydroxyphenylalanine (levodopa) is converted to dopamine (DA), a CNS transmitter, by the nonspecific L-aromatic amino acid decarboxylase which is ubiquitous in tissues. Normally 90% or more of orally administered levodopa is decarboxylated outside the CNS, and DA does not penetrate into the CNS where it can relieve the signs and symptoms of Parkinson's disease. Because of this, levodopa doses have to be high, in the 4 to 12 gm per day range. These doses of levodopa cause nausea, vomiting, tachycardia, hypotension, and cardiac arrhythmias secondary to the DA formed extracerebrally. Combinations of levodopa and a levodopa decarboxylase inhibitor (dopa hydrazide) that do not penetrate into the CNS have been used. The inhibition of DA formation in extracerebral tissues increases the quantity of levodopa available for decarboxylation to DA in the CNS and reduces the deleterious side effects of peripheral DA. The inhibition of the DOPA decarboxylase is a beneficial one that has permitted a reduction in the quantity of levodopa used in the therapy of Parkinson's disease by two or three times.[132,133]

Ethanol has been found to play a complex role in drug metabolism. Ethanol is a poor substrate for the hepatic drug metabolizing enzyme system, and ethanol metabolism is not significantly influenced by these enzymes (induction or inhibition) because most ethanol metabolism proceeds via the alcohol dehydrogenase-aldehyde dehydrogenase systems. However, ethanol at a blood concentration of 200 to 300 mg/100 ml does influence drug metabolism in spite of its behavior as a poor substrate for these enzymes. Ethanol can induce microsomal enzymes of drug metabolism and can act as a competitive inhibitor of the metabolism of other drugs. In the chronic alcoholic who is acutely intoxicated, ethanol may potentiate the action of other drugs by decreasing their metabolism (competitive inhibition caused by high blood levels). On the other hand, in the sober chronic alcoholic ethanol is an inducer of drug metabolism, and the patient may be less responsive to other drugs (the result of an increased rate of drug metabolism).[107,134,135]

The metabolism of a number of drugs including bishydroxycoumarin, phenytoin, phenobarbital, and meprobamate has been found to be inhibited by ethanol.[105,133]

Hepatic blood flow

Orally administered drugs pass through the liver before entering the systemic circulation. Drugs that are highly extracted by the liver have a low order of bioavailability. This is termed *first pass effect*. Drugs known or suspected of first pass effect pharmacokinetics include lidocaine, nortriptyline, morphine, pentazocine, and propranolol. Lidocaine has been extensively studied in humans because of its intravenous use in cardiac arrhythmias. It undergoes rapid intravenous clearance and has a low oral availability. Its hepatic extraction ratio is approximately 0.7. Pathologic decreases in hepatic blood flow secondary to congestive heart failure or portacaval shunting significantly affect lidocaine's clearance from plasma.

A number of drugs have been shown to alter hepatic blood flow and therefore influence the clearance from plasma of drugs with high hepatic extraction ratios.

Drugs that increase hepatic blood flow include glucagon, isoproterenol, and phenobarbital. Halothane and propranolol decrease hepatic blood flow by 33% and simultaneous administration of lidocaine and propranolol results in a 50% reduction in lidocaine clearance.[38,136] Cimetidine also reduces hepatic blood flow.[137]

Significant reductions in hepatic blood flow have a potential for increasing the activity and duration of the actions of drugs handled by first pass pharmacokinetics. The simultaneous use of drugs that decrease hepatic blood flow and drugs having high hepatic extraction ratios has a potential for adverse effects caused by unexpectedly high levels of bioavailability. Little information is as yet available from human studies in regard to these drug interactions, but there is good probability of their existence.[77]

A number of significant drug interactions have been validated and their mechanisms elucidated. Several of these are presented in Table 15-2. Because of the multiple mechanisms available for drug interactions, these phenomena may be complex, involving more than one mechanism. Such an interaction occurs with simultaneous use of tolbutamide and warfarin. Warfarin inhibits tolbutamide metabolism, causing hypoglycemia, and tolbutamide displaces warfarin from its albumin binding sites, causing bleeding.[77,104,107]

RECOMMENDATIONS FOR PHARMACOLOGIC THERAPY IN THE ELDERLY

Some guidelines and considerations for drug therapy of the elderly patient are as follows:

1. Establish a diagnosis before treating. Drug therapy should ideally be considered for a def-

Table 15-2. Drug interactions

Primary drug	*Interacting drug*	*Adverse effect*	*Mechanism*
Lincomycin	Kaolin-pectin	Decreased lincomycin effect	Decreased absorption
Tetracyclines	Antacids	Decreased tetracycline effect	Decreased absorption
Tolbutamide	Salicylates	Increased hypoglycemic effect	Displacement from binding
Warfarin	Nalidixic acid	Increased anticoagulant effect	Displacement from binding
Chlorpropamide	Salicylates	Increased hypoglycemic effect	Inhibition of renal excretion
Salicylates	Probenecid	Salicylate toxicity	Inhibition of renal excretion
Tolbutamide	Warfarin	Increased hypoglycemic effect	Inhibition of drug metabolism
Phenytoin	Isoniazid	Cerebellar ataxia	Inhibition of drug metabolism
Warfarin	Barbiturates	Decreased anticoagulant effect	Induction of drug metabolism
Tolbutamide	Rifampin	Decreased hypoglycemic effect	Induction of drug metabolism

From Bressler, R.: Adverse drug reactions. In Conrad, K.A., and Bressler, R.: Drug therapy for the elderly, St. Louis, 1982, The C.V. Mosby Co.

inite period of time and for a definite symptomatic or biochemical end point. Treatment should be aimed at altering the natural history of a disease (hypertension, depression, psychosis, diabetes mellitus) and not merely be used as a symptomatic intervention. The gain and risk aspects of drug therapy in the elderly must be considered because of the higher frequency and severity of adverse drug reactions.

2. Review the elderly patient's drug regimen frequently and be alert to the possibility of other physicians prescribing drugs for the patient. The elderly patient with multiple diseases usually is treated with multiple drugs. These include drugs directed against specific diseases as well as nonprescription drugs such as aspirin, antihistamines, caffeine, and anticholinergics. Periodic drug review and compliance evaluation are worthwhile.

3. Minimize the number of drugs used. Review the pharmacologic actions of the drug(s) being used and their mode of inactivation and/ or elimination from the body (i.e., renal excretion, hepatic metabolism). Monitor the patient for both therapeutic and adverse effects until steady state levels have been reached (five half-lives). This may be up to twice the time period for the younger patient. Use the lowest dose that is effective in the individual patient by careful attention and monitoring of the patient during the drug induction period. Adjust the maintenance dose downward if advancing age is associated with impairment of the major mode of drug elimination.

4. When encountering symptoms that mimic stereotypes associated with old age (forgetfulness, weakness, confusion, anorexia, anxiety) suspect a drug reaction as a contributing factor, especially if the patient is receiving a psychotropic drug, sedative-hypnotic agent, or drugs affecting cardiac output or the renal system.

REFERENCES

1. Achong, M.R., Bayne, J.R.D., Gerson, L.W., and Golshan, S.: Prescribing of psychoactive drugs for chronically ill elderly patients, Can. Med. Assoc. J. **118:**1503, 1978.
2. Fottrell, E., et al.: Long-stay patients with long-stay drugs. A case for review: a cause for concern, Lancet **1:**81, 1976.
3. O'Malley, K., Judge, T.G., and Crooks, J.: Geriatric clinical pharmacology and therapeutics. In Avery, G.S., editor: Avery drug treatment, Philadelphia, 1976, Lea & Febiger, p. 123.
4. Vestal, R.E.: Drug use in the elderly: a review of problems and special considerations, Drugs **16:**358, 1978.
5. Wilson, L.A., Lawson, I.R., and Braws, W.: Multiple disorders in the elderly. A clinical and statistical study, Lancet **2:**841, 1962.
6. Bender, A.D.: Pharmacodynamic principles of drug therapy in the aged, J. Am. Geriatr. Soc. **22:**296, 1974.
7. Bender, A.D.: Pharmacologic aspects of aging: a survey of the effect of increasing age on drug activity in adults, J. Am. Geriatr. Soc. **12:**114, 1964.
8. Freeman, J.T., editor: Clinical principles and drugs in aging, Springfield, Ill., 1963, Charles C Thomas, Publisher.
9. Gallo, D.G., Bailey, K.R., and Sheffner, A.L.: The interaction between cholestyramine and drugs, Proc. Soc. Exp. Biol. Med. **120:**60, 1965.
10. Reichel, W.: Complications in the care of 500 elderly hospitalized patients, J. Am. Geriatr. Soc. **13:**973, 1965.
11. Seidl, L.G., et al.: Studies on the epidemiology of adverse drug reactions. III. Reactions in patients on a general medical service. Bull. Johns Hopkins Hosp. **119:**299, 1966.
12. May, F.E., Stewart, R.B., and Cluff, L.E.: Drug interactions and multiple drug administration, Clin. Pharmacol. Ther. **22:**322, 1977.
13. Melmon, K.L.: Preventable drug reactions—causes and cures, N. Engl. J. Med. **284:**1361, 1971.
14. Morrelli, H.F., and Melmon, K.L.: Drug interactions. In Morrelli, H.F., and Melmon, K.L., editors: Clinical pharmacology, New York, 1978, MacMillan, Inc., p. 983.
15. Hurwitz, N.: Predisposing factors in adverse reactions to drugs, Br. Med. J. **1:**536, 1969.
16. Smith, J.W., Seidl, L.G., and Cluff, L.E.: Studies on the epidemiology of adverse drug reactions. V. Clinical factors influencing susceptibility, Ann. Intern. Med. **65:**629, 1966.
17. Crooks, J., O'Malley, K., and Stevenson, I.H.: Pharmacokinetics in the elderly, Clin. Pharmacokinet. **1:**280, 1976.
18. Richev, D.P., and Bender, A.D.: Pharmacokinetic consequences of aging, Annu. Rev. Pharmacol. Toxicol. **17:**49, 1977.
19. Triggs, E.J., and Nation, R.L.: Pharmacokinetics in the aged. A review. J. Pharmacokinet. Biopharm. **3:**387, 1975.
20. Roberts, J., and Goldberg, P.B.: Changes in responsiveness of the heart to drugs during aging, Fed. Proc. **38:**1927, 1979.
21. Roth, G.S.: Hormone receptor changes during adulthood and senescence: significance for aging research, Fed. Proc. **38:**1910, 1979.
22. Snyder, S.H.: Receptors, neurotransmitters and drug responses, N. Engl. J. Med. **300:**465, 1979.
23. Bender, A.D.: Effect of age on intestinal absorption: implications for drug absorption in the elderly, J. Am. Geriatr. Soc. **16:**1331, 1968.
24. Forbes, G.B., and Reina, J.C.: Adult lean body mass declines with age: some longitudinal observations, Metabolism **19:**653, 1970.
25. Norris, A.H., Lundy, T., and Shock, N.W.: Trends in

selected indices of body composition in men between the ages of 30 and 80 years, Ann. N.Y. Acad. Sci. **110**:623, 1963.
26. Novak, L.P.: Aging, total body potassium, fat-free mass and cell mass in males and females between ages 18 and 35 years, J. Gerontol. **27**:438, 1972.
27. Vestal, R.E., et al.: Aging and ethanol metabolism, Clin. Pharmacol. Ther. **21**:343, 1977.
28. Berkowitz, B.A., et al.: The disposition of morphine in surgical patients, Clin. Pharmacol. Ther. **17**:629, 1975.
29. Bender, A.D., et al.: Plasma protein binding as a function of age in adult human subjects, J. Pharm. Sci. **64**:1711, 1975.
30. Cammarata, R.J., Rodnan, G.P., and Fennell, R.H.: Serum antigamma-globulin and anti-nuclear factors in the aged, J.A.M.A. **199**:115, 1967.
31. Koch-Weser, J., and Sellers, E.M.: Binding of drugs to serum albumin, N. Engl. J. Med. **294**:311, 526, 1976.
32. Mather, L.E., et al.: Meperidine kinetics in man: intravenous injection in surgical patients and volunteers, Clin. Pharmacol. Ther. **17**:21, 1975.
33. Hayes, M.J., Langman, M.J.S., and Short, A.H.: Changes in drug metabolism with age. I. Warfarin binding and plasma proteins. Br. J. Clin. Pharmacol. **2**:69, 1975.
34. Gillette, J.R.: Biotransformation of drugs during aging, Fed. Proc. **38**:1900, 1979.
35. Geokas, M.C., and Haverback, B.J.: The aging gastrointestinal tract, Am. J. Surg. **117**:881, 1969.
36. Brandfonbrener, M., Landowne, M., and Shock, N.W.: Changes in cardiac output with age, Circulation **12**:557, 1955.
37. Harris, R.: Cardiac changes with age. In Goldman, R., and Rockstein, M., editors: The physiology and pathology of human aging, New York, 1975, Academic Press, Inc., p. 109.
38. Nies, A.S., Shand, D.B., and Wilkinson, G.R.: Altered hepatic blood flow and drug disposition, Clin. Pharmacokinet. **1**:125, 1976.
39. Liddell, D.E., Williams, F.M., and Briant, R.H.: Phenazone (antipyrine) metabolism and distribution in young and elderly adults, Clin. Exp. Pharmacol. Physiol. **2**:481, 1975.
40. O'Malley, K., Crooks, J., Duke, E., and Stevenson, I.H.: Effect of age and sex on human drug metabolism, Br. Med. J. **3**:607, 1971.
41. Vestal, R.E., et al.: Effect of aging and cigarette smoking on propranolol disposition, Clin. Pharmacol. Ther. **26**:8, 1979.
42. Farah, F., Taylor, W., Rawlins, M.D., and James, O.: Hepatic drug acetylation and oxidation: effects of aging in man, Br. Med. J. **2**:255, 1977.
43. Nies, A., et al.: Relationship between age and tricyclic antidepressant plasma levels, Am. J. Psychiatry **134**:790, 1977.
44. Greenblatt, D.J., Allen, M.D., and Shader, R.I.: Toxicity of high-dose flurazepam in the elderly, Clin. Pharmacol. Ther. **21**:355, 1977.
45. Roberts, R.K., et al.: Effect of age and parenchymal liver disease on the diposition and elimination of chlordiazepoxide (Librium), Gastroenterology **75**:479, 1978.
46. Klotz, U., et al.: The effects of age and liver disease on the disposition and elimination of diazepam in adult man, J. Clin. Invest. **55**:347, 1975.
47. Rowland, M.: Drug administration and regimens: absorption, distribution, excretion, pharmacokinetics. In Melmon, K.L., and Morrelli, H.F., editors: Clinical pharmacology, New York, 1978, MacMillan, Inc., p. 25.
48. Greenblatt, D.J., Allen, M.D., Harmatz, J.S., and Shader, R.I.: Diazepam disposition determinants, Clin. Pharmacol. Ther. **27**:301, 1980.
49. Boston Collaborative Drug Surveillance Program: Clinical depression of the central nervous system due to diazepam and chlordiazepoxide in relation to cigarette smoking and age, N. Engl. J. Med. **288**:277, 1973.
50. Conrad, K.A., Molk, B.L., and Chidsey, C.A.: Pharmacokinetic studies of quinidine in patients with arrhythmias, Circulation **55**:1, 1977.
51. Mitenko, P.A., and Ogilvie, R.I.: Pharmacokinetics of theophylline, Clin. Pharmacol. Ther. **14**:509, 1973.
52. Thomson, P.D., et al.: Lidocaine pharmacokinetics in advanced heart failure, liver disease and renal failure in humans, Ann. Intern. Med. **78**:499, 1973.
53. Thomson, P.D.: Alteration in pharmacologic response induced by cardiovascular disease. In Melmon, K.L., editor: Cardiovascular drug therapy, Philadelphia, 1974, F.A. Davis Co., p. 55.
54. Weiner, I.M.: Excretion of drugs by the kidney. In Brodie, B.B., and Gillette, J.R., editors: Concepts in biochemical pharmacology, vol. 28, New York, 1971, Springer-Verlag New York, Inc., p. 328.
55. Reidenberg, M.: Renal function and drug action, Philadelphia, 1971, W.B. Saunders Co., pp. 5, 33.
56. Lakatta, E.G.: Alterations in the cardiovascular system that occur in advanced aged, Fed. Proc. **38**:163, 1979.
57. McLachlan, M.S.F.: The aging kidney, Lancet **2**:143, 1978.
58. Shock, N.W.: Systems physiology and aging, Fed. Proc. **38**:161, 1979.
59. Rowe, J.W., et al.: Age-adjusted standards for creatinine clearance, Ann. Intern. Med. **84**:567, 1976.
60. Vartia, K.O., and Leikola, E.: Serum levels of antibiotics in young and old subjects following administration of dihydrostreptomycin and tetracycline, J. Gerontol. **15**:392, 1960.
61. Gault, M.H., and Cockcroft, D.W.: Creatinine clearance and age, Lancet **2**:612, 1975.
62. Ewy, G.A., et al.: Digoxin metabolism in the elderly, Circulation **39**:449, 1969.
63. Leikola, E., and Vartia, K.O.: On penicillin levels in young and geriatric subjects, J. Gerontol. **12**:48, 1957.
64. Finch, C.E.: Neuroendocrine mechanisms and aging, Fed. Proc. **38**:178, 1979.
65. Parkin, D.M., Henney, C.R., Quirk, J., and Crooks, J.: Deviation from prescribed drug treatment after discharge from hospital, Br. Med. J. **2**:686, 1976.
66. Sackett, D.Z., and Haynes, R.B., editors: Compliance with therapeutic regimens, Baltimore, 1976, The Johns Hopkins University Press.
67. Gibson, I.I.J.M., and Hare, M.M.: Prescription of drugs for old people at home, Gerontol. Clin. **10**:271, 1968.
68. Schwartz, D., Wang, M., Zeitz, L., and Goss,

M.E.W.: Medication errors made by elderly, chronically ill patients, Am. J. Public Health **52:**2018, 1962.
69. Boyd, J.R., Covington, T.R., Stanaszek, W.F., and Coussons, R.T.: Drug defaulting. I. Determinants of compliance, Am. J. Hosp. Pharm. **31:**362, 1974.
70. Weintraub, M., Au, W.Y.W., and Lasagna, L.: Compliance as a determinant of serum digoxin concentrations, J.A.M.A. **244:**481, 1973.
71. Chamberlain, D.A., White, R.J., Howard, M.R., and Smith, T.W.: Plasma digoxin concentrations in patients with atrial fibrillation, Br. Med. J. **3:**429, 1970.
72. Caranasos, G.J., Stewart, R.B., and Cluff, L.E.: Drug-induced illness leading to hospitalization, J.A.M.A. **28:**713, 1974.
73. Vestal, R.E., Wood, A.J.J., and Shand, D.G.: Reduced β-adrenoceptor sensitivity in the elderly, Clin. Pharmacol. Ther. **26:**181, 1979.
74. Conway, J., Wheeler, R., and Sannerstedt, R.: Sympathetic nervous activity during exercise in relation to age, Cardiovasc. Res. **5:**577, 1971.
75. Castleden, C.M., Kaye, C.M., and Parsons, R.L.: The effect of age on plasma levels of propranolol and practolol in man, Br. J. Clin. Pharmacol. **2:**303, 1975.
76. Shand, D.G., Kornhauser, D.M., and Wilkinson, G.R.: Effects of route of administration and blood flow on hepatic drug elimination, J. Pharmacol. Exp. Ther. **195:**424, 1975.
77. Wilkinson, G.R., and Shand, D.G.: A physiological approach to hepatic drug clearance, Clin. Pharmacol. Ther. **18:**377, 1975.
78. Caird, F.I., Andrews, G.R., and Kennedy, R.D.: Effect of posture on blood pressure in the elderly, Br. Heart J. **35:**527, 1973.
79. Gribbon, B., Pickering, T.G., Sleight, P., and Peto, R.: Effect of age and high blood pressure on baroreflex sensitivity in man, Circ. Res. **29:**424, 1971.
80. Jackson, G., Mahon, W., Pierscianowski, T.A., and Condon, J.: Inappropriate antihypertensive therapy in the elderly, Lancet **2:**1317, 1976.
81. Dollery, C.T., and Harington, J.: Methyldopa in hypertension. Clinical and pharmacological studies, Lancet **1:**759, 1962.
82. Holloway, D.: Drug problems in the geriatric patient, Drug Intell. Clin. Pharm. **8:**632, 1974.
83. Lawson, D.H., Gloss, D., and Jick, H.: Adverse reactions to methyldopa with particular reference to hypotension, Am. Heart J. **96:**572, 1978.
84. Jick, H., Slone, D., Borda, I.T., and Shapiro, S.: Efficacy and toxicity of heparin in relation to age and sex, N. Engl. J. Med. **279:**284, 1968.
85. O'Malley, K., et al.: Determinants of anticoagulant control in patient receiving warfarin, Br. J. Clin. Pharmacol. **4:**309, 1977.
86. Shepherd, A.M., Hewick, D.S., Moreland, T.A., and Stevenson, I.H.: Age as a determinant of sensitivity to warfarin, Br. J. Clin. Pharmacol. **4:**315, 1977.
87. Nielsen-Kudsk, F., Magnussen, I., and Jakobsen, P.: Pharmacokinetics of theophylline in ten elderly patients, Acta Pharmacol. Toxicol. **42:**226, 1978.
88. Piafsky, K.M., Sitar, D.S., Rangno, R.E., and Ogilvie, R.I.: Theophylline kinetics in acute pulmonary edema, Clin. Pharmacol. Ther. **21:**310, 1977.
89. Zwillich, C.W., et al.: Theophylline-induced seizure in adults. Correlation with serum concentrations, Ann. Intern. Med. **82:**784, 1975.
90. Bellville, J.W., Forrest, W.H., Miller, E., and Brown, B.W.: Influence of age on pain relief from analgesics. A study of postoperative patients, J.A.M.A. **217:**1835, 1971.
91. Chan, K., Kendall, M.J., Mitchard, M., and Wells, W.D.E.: The effect of aging on plasma pethidine concentration, Br. J. Clin. Pharmacol. **2:**297, 1975.
92. Briant, R.H., Dorrington, R.E., Cleal, J., and Williams, F.M.: The rate of acetaminophen metabolism in the elderly and the young, J. Am. Geriatr. Soc. **24:**359, 1976.
93. Shader, R.I., and Greenblatt, D.J.: The psychopharmacology treatment of anxiety states. In Shader, R.I., editor: Manual of psychiatric therapeutics, Boston, 1975, Little, Brown and Co., p. 27.
94. Irvine, R.E., Grove, J., Toseland, P.A., and Trounce, J.R.: The effect of age on the hydroxylation of amylobarbitone sodium in man, Br. J. Clin. Pharmacol. **1:**42, 1974.
95. Learoyd, B.M.: Psychotropic drugs and the elderly patient, Med. J. Aust. **1:**1131, 1972.
96. Saltzman, C., Shader, R.I., and Van der Kolk, B.A.: Clinical psychopharmacology and the elderly patient, N.Y. State J. Med. **76:**71, 1976.
97. Shader, R.I., et al.: Absorption and disposition of chlordiazepoxide in young and elderly male volunteers, J. Clin. Pharmacol. **17:**709, 1977.
98. Castleden, C.M., George, C.F., Marcer, D., and Hallett, C.: Increased sensitivity in nitrazepam in old age, Br. Med. J. **1:**10, 1977.
99. Reidenberg, M., et al.: The relationship between diazepam dose, plasma level, age and central nervous system depression in adults, Clin. Pharmacol. Ther. **23:**371, 1978.
100. Allen, M.D., and Greenblatt, D.J.: Desmethyldiazepam kinetics following oral prazepam in the elderly, Clin. Pharmacol. Ther. **29:**244, 1980.
101. Kales, A., Scharf, M.B., Kales, J., and Soldatos, C.R.: Rebound insomnia: a potential hazard following withdrawal of certain benzodiazepines, J.A.M.A. **241:**1692, 1979.
102. Hollister, L.E.: Clinical use of psychotherapeutic drugs, Springfield, Ill., 1973, Charles C Thomas, Publisher, pp. 13, 72.
103. Godwin-Austen, R.B., Frears, C.C., and Bergmann, S.: Incidence of side effects from levodopa during the introduction of treatment, Br. Med. J. **1:**267, 1971.
104. Robinson, D.S.: Pharmacokinetic mechanisms of drug interactions, Postgrad. Med. **57:**55, 1975.
105. Adverse interactions of drugs, Med. Lett. **19:**5, 1977.
106. Cohen, S.N., and Armstrong, M.F.: Drug interactions: a handbook for clinical use, Baltimore, 1974, The Williams & Wilkins Co.
107. Hansen, P.D.: Drug interaction, Philadelphia, 1972, Lea & Febiger.
108. Simberkoff, M.S., et al.: Inactivation of penicillins by carbohydrate solutions at alkaline pH, N. Engl. J. Med. **238:**116, 1970.
109. Koch-Weser, J.: Drug interactions in cardiovascular therapy, Am. Heart J. **90:**93, 1975.
110. Brown, D.D., and Juhl, R.P.: Decreased bioavailabil-

ity of digoxin due to antacids and kaolin-pectin, N. Engl. J. Med. **295**:1034, 1976.

111. Hogben, C.A.M., Tocco, D.J., Brodie, B.V., and Schanker, L.S.: On the mechanism of intestinal absorption of drugs, J. Pharm. Exp. Ther. **125**:275, 1959.
112. Brodie, B.B.: Displacement of one drug by another from carrier or receptor sites, Proc. R. Soc. Med. **58**:946, 1965.
113. Hayes, M.J., and Langman, M.J.S.: An analysis of carbenoxolone binding and clearance in young and elderly people. In Avery, G.S., Jones, A., and Parke, D. V., editors: Fourth symposium on carbenoxolone, London, 1975, Butterworth & Co., p. 107.
114. Sjoqvist, F.: Psychotropic drugs. II. Interaction between monoamine oxidase (MAO) inhibitors and other substances, Proc. R. Soc. Med. **58**:967, 1965.
115. Leishman, A.W.D., Mathews, H.L., and Smith, A.J.: Antagonism of guanethidine by imipramine, Lancet **1**:112, 1963.
116. Brooks, S.M., et al.: Adverse effects of phenobarbital on corticosteroid metabolism in patients with bronchial asthma, N. Engl. J. Med. **286**:1125, 1972.
117. Breckenridge, A., et al.: Increased rates of drug oxidation in man. In Morselli, P.L., Garattini, S., and Cohen, S.N., editors: Drug interactions, New York, 1974, Raven Press, p. 223.
118. Gelehrter, T.D.: Enzyme induction, N. Engl. J. Med. **294**:522, 589, 1976.
119. Koch-Weser, J.: Drug interactions with coumarin anticoagulants, N. Engl. J. Med. **285**:487, 547, 1971.
120. Kolmodin, B., Azarnoff, D.L., and Sjoquist, F.: Effect of environmental factors on drug metabolism: decreased plasma half-life of antipyrine in workers exposed to chlorinated hydrocarbon insecticides, Clin. Pharmacol. Ther. **10**:638, 1969.
121. Kolmodin-Hedman, B.: Decreased plasma half-lives of antipyrine and phenylbutazone in workers occupationally exposed to lindane and DDT. In Morselli, P.L., Garattini, S., and Cohen, S.N., editors: Drug interactions, New York, 1974, Raven Press, p. 249.
122. Jeffery, W.H., Ahlin, T.A., Goren, C., and Hardy, W.R.: Loss of warfarin effect after occupational insecticide exposure, J.A.M.A. **236**:2881, 1976.
123. Hart, P., et al.: Enhanced drug metabolism in cigarette smokers, Br. Med. J. **2**:147, 1976.
124. Hunt, S.N., Jusko, W.J., and Yurchak, A.M.: Effect of smoking on theophylline disposition, Clin. Pharmacol. Ther. **19**:546, 1976.
125. Pantuck, E.J., Kuntzman, R., and Conney, A.H.: Decreased concentration of phenacetin in plasma of cigarette smokers, Science **175**:1248, 1972.
126. Pfeifer, H.J., and Greenblatt, D.J.: Clinical toxicity of theophylline in relation to cigarette smoking, Chest **73**:455, 1978.
127. Hahn, T.J., Hendin, B.A., Scharp, C.R., and Haddad, J.G.: Effect of chronic anticonvulsant therapy on serum 25-hydroxycalciferol levels in adults, N. Engl. J. Med. **287**:900, 1972.
128. Serlin, M.J., et al.: Cimetidine interaction with anticoagulants in man, Lancet **2**:317, 1979.
129. O'Reilly, R.A.: The stereoselective interaction of warfarin and metronidazole in man, N. Engl. J. Med. **295**:354, 1976.
130. Dayton, P.G., and Perel, J.M.: Physiological and physiochemical bases of drug interactions in man, Ann. N.Y. Acad. Sci. **179**:67, 1971.
131. Wyngaarden, J.B., Rundles, R.W., and Metz, E.N.: Allopurinol in the treatment of gout, Ann. Intern. Med. **62**:842, 1965.
132. Selby, G.: Treatment of parkinsonism, Drugs **11**:61, 1976.
133. Yahr, M.D.: Levodopa, Ann. Intern. Med. **83**:677, 1975.
134. Becker, C.E., and Morrelli, H.F.: Alcohol and drug abuse. In Melmon, K.L., and Morrelli, H.F., editors: Clinical pharmacology, ed. 2, New York, 1978, MacMillan, Inc., p. 1008.
135. Rubin, E., Gang, H., Mistra, P., and Lieber, C.S.: Inhibition of drug metabolism by acute ethanol intoxication: a hepatic microsomal mechanism, Am. J. Med. **49**:801, 1970.
136. Ochs, H.R., Carstens, G., and Greenblatt, D.J.: Reduction in lidocaine clearance during continuous infusion and by coadministration of propranolol, N. Engl. J. Med. **303**:373, 1980.
137. Jackson, J.E., et al.: Cimetidine decreases theophylline clearance, Am. Rev. Respir. Dis. **123**:615, 1981.

CHAPTER 16 · ENDOCRINOLOGY

Philip E. Cryer

Clinical endocrinology has been revolutionized by the radioimmunoassay. Virtually all hormones of clinical importance can now be measured, although there are limitations (sensitivity, specificity, and precision) to many individual assays that are relevant to their clinical application.

Typical symptoms and signs are the cornerstone of most endocrinologic diagnoses. Although some endocrinologic disorders can be diagnosed biochemically before they produce a typical clinical picture, the physician must be particularly rigorous in the interpretation of such tests when clinical manifestations are not present. The array of hormonal measurements now available can supplement, but not supplant, thorough assessment of the individual patient.

Most patients with recognized endocrinologic disorders have excessive or deficient secretion of a given hormone or hormones. However, an increasing number of clinical disorders caused by altered hormone action are being recognized. It is likely that major future progress in the field of clinical endocrinology will be in this direction.

This chapter deals with disorders of several of the classic endocrine glands—the pituitary, the thyroid, the adrenal cortices and medullae, the gonads and the parathyroids. Metabolic disorders, such as diabetes mellitus and metabolic bone disease, are covered elsewhere in this book.

A variety of age related alterations of endocrine physiology have been identified. Some, such as diminished pituitary growth hormone secretion in elderly persons, are clinically irrelevant. Several are normally compensated. For example, decreased cortisol clearance is matched by decreased cortisol secretion, and plasma cortisol concentrations remain normal. Other age related endocrine changes are of potential pathophysiologic importance. Diminished renin and aldosterone secretion, coupled with the age related decrease in renal function, may cause a propensity to hyperkalemia. Diminished renal production of 1,25-dihydroxyvitamin D results in decreased intestinal calcium absorption; a compensatory increase in parathyroid hormone secretion results in maintenance of the serum calcium concentration but may accelerate the development of osteopenia. The most dramatic normal age-related change in endocrine function is virtual cessation of ovarian function—the menopause. Advancing age also affects the pathophysiology and clinical expression of endocrine disease. Thus the diagnostic and therapeutic approach to the geriatric patient often differs from that used in younger persons.

PITUITARY GLAND AND HYPOTHALAMUS

Physiology

The anterior pituitary (adenohypophysis) is anatomically distinct from, but functionally tightly linked to, the hypothalamus. The posterior pituitary is an extension of the hypothalamus (neurohypophysis). Its hormones, such as arginine vasopressin (AVP), or antidiuretic hormone, are synthesized in the supraoptic and paraventricular nuclei of the hypothalamus and transported through axons to the posterior pituitary where they are stored and from which they are secreted. Thus adequate AVP secretion can occur in the absence of the posterior pituitary if the hypothalamus remains intact.

Hormones secreted from the anterior pituitary include prolactin (PRL); growth hormone (GH, somatotropin); thyroid stimulating hormone (TSH, thyrotropin); adrenocorticotropic hormone (ACTH, adrenocorticotropin); and the gonadotropins, luteinizing hormone (LH), and follicle stimulating hormone (FSH). The secretion of these hormones is regulated by hypothalamic (hypophysiotropic) hormones released from the median eminence region of the hypothalamus and transported to the anterior pituitary by the hypothalamo-adenohypophyseal portal circulation. The hypophysiotropic hormones are listed in Table 16-1.

Although dual control, by both releasing and inhibiting hypophysiotropic hormones, of the secretion of each of the anterior pituitary hormones has been postulated, the predominant tonic effect of the hypothalamus is to inhibit PRL secretion but to stimulate GH, TSH, ACTH, LH, and FSH secretion. Thus disconnection of the hypothalamus from the pituitary, or destruction of the hypothalamus leaving the pituitary intact, results in excessive PRL secretion but deficient GH, TSH, ACTH, LH, and FSH secretion.

Although the pituitary hormones have been shown to exert a variety of effects under experimental conditions, their physiologically important biologic actions are quite specific: PRL promotes postpartum lactation; GH promotes growth; TSH stimulates the thyroid gland; ACTH stimulates the adrenal cortices; the gonadotropins stimulate the gonads (in general, LH stimulates gonadal hormone synthesis and secretion and FSH stimulates maturation of ova and sperm); and AVP stimulates water reabsorption by the kidneys.

Table 16-1. Hypothalamic regulation of anterior pituitary function

Anterior pituitary hormone	*Hypothalamic control (hypophysiotropic hormones)*
Prolactin	Prolactin inhibiting factor (PIF)—? dopamine
Growth hormone	Growth hormone releasing factor (GH-RF) >somatostatin
Thyrotropin	Thyrotropin releasing hormone (TRH)
Adrenocorticotropin	Corticotropin releasing factor (CRF)
Gonadotropins (luteinizing hormone and follicle stimulating hormone)	Gonadotropin releasing hormone (Gn-RH)

Disorders of adenohypophyseal function

Prolactin. During the last decade it has been found that hyperprolactinemia is a common cause of reproductive dysfunction. In women, it can result in galactorrhea (nonpuerperal lactation), functional hypogonadism with infertility, and amenorrhea and sexual dysfunction or both. However, the most specific sign, galactorrhea, is often absent in hyperprolactinemic women (and some galactorrheic women have normal serum PRL levels). In men, hyperprolactinemia can also result in functional hypogonadism with infertility and diminished libido; galactorrhea is distinctly unusual in hyperprolactinemic men.

The serum PRL concentration should be measured in all patients with any of the symptoms or signs mentioned. Reproducibly elevated serum PRL concentrations are most commonly due to PRL secreting pituitary tumors, prolactinomas. The frequency of the recently documented pituitary prolactin cell hyperplasia as a cause of hyperprolactinemia remains to be determined; it is conceivable, but unproven, that hyperplasia and tumor formation are stages in the evolution of a common pathophysiologic sequence. Other common causes of hyperprolactinemia are hypothyroidism and a variety of drugs commonly used in geriatric patients such as methyldopa, reserpine, phenothiazines, cimetidine, estrogens, and tricyclic antidepressants. Clearly, the possibilities of drug ingestion and hypothyroidism should be carefully considered when hyperprolactinemia is discovered. Hyperprolactinemia has been noted in patients with renal failure and rarely attributed to secretion from nonendocrine tumors (lung and kidney) or to chest wall irritation. Hyperprolactinemia, usually associated with deficient secretion of other pituitary hormones, can accompany hypothalamic disease. Recall that physiologic hyperprolactinemia occurs during pregnancy and that bursts of prolactin secretion are associated with breast-feeding. It has been reported that increments in serum PRL follow manipulation of the breast in nonpuerperal women, although this is not a universal finding. Because of this, some physicians avoid measuring the serum PRL shortly after examination of the breasts.

When other causes of hyperprolactinemia can be excluded on clinical grounds, the probability of prolactinoma is high. In general, the higher the serum PRL, the higher the likelihood of prolactinoma; most patients with serum PRL concentrations greater than 100 ng/ml, and virtually all with PRL levels greater than 300 ng/ml, have prolactinomas. Occasional prolactinomas are large enough to cause headaches and to extend upward into the optic chiasm causing visual field defects. Most alter the radiographic contour of the sella turcica although polytomography may be required to demonstrate this. Undue weight should not, however, be given to subtle alterations noted on polytomography, since recent evidence indicates that these have sometimes been overinterpreted. Many prolactinomas are too small to distort the sella. These microadenomas can generally be seen with modern, high resolution computed tomographic (CT) scans.

Surgical, radiotherapeutic, and medical approaches to the treatment of prolactinoma are available. Transsphenoidal pituitary microsurgery with selective adenomectomy offers the potential for cure with preservation of normal pituitary function and is perhaps the most widely used treatment in the United States. External pituitary irradiation is effective in some patients, although the published experience with it is not great; maximal therapeutic effects may take years. There is considerable interest in medical therapy with bromocriptine, or similar dopaminergic agonists, which reduces hyperprolactinemia in most patients regardless of its etiology. At this writing bromocriptine is recommended by the U.S. Food and Drug Administration only for the short-term treatment of galactorrhea in patients who do not have a demonstrable pituitary tumor and who are willing to avoid conception during therapy. However, the drug has been used sucessfully to restore fertility and sexual function, largely in Europe, and broader recommended uses can reasonably be expected in this country. Recently, bromocriptine has been shown to reduce the size, as well as PRL secretion, of some large prolactinomas. It should be emphasized that this drug does not cure the disease; recurrent hyperprolactinemia follows discontinuation of the drug.

The decision to treat a patient with a prolactinoma should not be made reflexively. Hyperprolactinemia is not known to shorten survival. Symptoms caused by hyperprolactinemia may or may not be sufficiently bothersome to warrant therapy. Large tumors should be treated because of their potential for compressing the normal pituitary or adjacent structures such as the optic chiasm, the base of the brain, or both. Admittedly, all large tumors were at one time small tumors, and one could argue that small tumors should be removed to prevent later mass lesions; further, cure rates are better with small tumors. However, the natural history of pituitary microadenomas is not known. It cannot be assumed that all microadenomas will become macroadenomas. In those that do, the time interval required is not known; it may be years or even decades. Thus it may be reasonable to follow selected asymptomatic or minimally symptomatic patients with PRL secreting microadenomas, especially those in the older age group, without therapy.

Growth hormone. Chronic excessive GH secretion is uncommon. If it occurs prior to puberty, gigantism results. If it begins after puberty, the long bones cannot become longer because of epiphyseal fusion, but tissue overgrowth occurs resulting in the clinical picture of acromegaly. Fully developed acromegaly is easily recognized by enlargement of the hands and feet (due to thickening of soft tissues and an increase in the diameter of the bones), coarsening of facial features (due to thickening of the skin and bony overgrowth often including enlargement of the mandible with spacing of the lower teeth and protrusion of the jaw, prognathism), and generalized tissue overgrowth including thickening of the skin and an increase in soft tissue bulk.

Although the vast majority of patients with acromegaly have GH secreting pituitary tumors, relatively few have symptoms, such as headaches or visual field defects, referable to mass effects of the tumor.

Once suspected on clinical grounds, the diagnosis of acromegaly is usually easily confirmed by the finding of a markedly elevated serum GH level. In some patients, however, serum GH elevations are not striking. In such cases, multiple serum GH measurements or GH measurements during the first hour of an oral glucose tolerance test (GH levels generally fall to undetectable levels during hyperglycemia) may be helpful. However, measurement of the serum somatomedin level is more direct. The growth promoting effects of GH are not direct but are mediated through promotion of secretion of other hormones, the somatomedins, from the liver and perhaps other sites. Serum somatomedin levels are elevated in patients with acromegaly.

Long-standing chronic GH excess is associated with considerable morbidity, including hypertension, heart disease, cerebral vascular disease, and degenerative joint disease among others, in addition to the cosmetic deformity. Further, it shortens life. Thus patients with acromegaly should generally be treated when the diagnosis is made. The choice between pituitary surgery (usually via the transsphenoidal route) and external pituitary irradiation is a matter of debate. My practice is to recommend surgery initially and reserve radiotherapy for those patients not cured by surgery. The maximal GH lowering effect of radiation may require several years.

Effective therapy (normal serum GH and somatomedin levels) can be expected to result in regression of the soft tissue changes of acromegaly in most patients. Bony enlargement does not change.

Although most patients with acromegaly should be treated, some patients are recognized late in life and do not appear too troubled by their acromegaly. It may be reasonable to follow such patients without therapy.

GH deficiency is responsible for roughly 10% of short stature in childhood. It is treatable, by human GH injections, only when detected prior to puberty. In later life, its major importance is that it is a diagnostic clue to the possible presence of other pituitary hormone deficiencies. Since normal serum GH concentrations are often below the limit of detectability of commonly used GH radioimmunoassays, failure of the serum GH concentration to rise in response to a provocative stimulus is required to document deficient GH secretion. Commonly used provocative stimuli include the ingestion of L-dopa (which may cause nausea), a 30-minute infusion of arginine hydrochloride (which is well tolerated, although it may cause hyperkalemia in patients with renal failure), and the production of hypoglycemia by the intravenous injection of regular insulin. The latter can be unpleasant for the patient, requires continuous physician attendance so that symptoms can be treated with intravenous glucose if necessary, and has been reported to precipitate cardiac arrhythmias in patients with heart disease. Thus it is not recommended for older patients. Further, one could question the utility of GH testing in older patients, since as many as 30% of apparently normal persons over the age of 50 years fail to have a GH response to a given provocative stimulus. It is my pratice to measure a random serum GH level (a normal value indicates intact GH secretion even though a low value does not indicate deficient GH secretion) and the serum somatomedin level to assess GH secretion in older patients suspected of having deficient pituitary function.

Thyrotropin. TSH hypersecretion is appropriate in patients with primary hypothyroidism (see later discussion). TSH secreting pituitary tumors have occurred in some patients with long-standing, untreated primary hypothyroidism. Rarely TSH secreting pituitary adenomas develop in the absence of antecedent hypothyroidism and cause hyperthyroidism.

Deficient TSH production can be the result of disease of the anterior pituitary or the hypothalamus causing secondary or tertiary (TRH deficient) hypothyroidism, respectively. A hypothyroid patient with a low plasma TSH level that does not increase after intravenous TRH has pituitary (secondary) hypothyroidism, whereas a hypothyroid patient with a low plasma TSH level that increases after intravenous TRH has hypothalamic (tertiary) hypothyroidism. Although TRH testing may help to localize the lesion in difficult cases, its practical utility is open to question. Such information seldom alters the therapeutic approach.

Adrenocorticotropin (ACTH). ACTH hypersecretion is appropriate in patients with primary adrenocortical insufficiency (Addison's disease; see later discussion). A primary abnormality in the regulation of pituitary ACTH secretion resulting in ACTH hypersecretion causes Cushing's disease (see later discussion). The majority of such patients have ACTH secreting pituitary microadenomas. These infrequently become macroadenomas except following bilateral adrenalectomy when ACTH secreting pituitary tumors may grow rapidly and be associated with intense hyperpigmentation (Nelson's syndrome). ACTH-like peptides are commonly released from nonendocrine tumors, such as carcinoma of the lung, and can cause Cushing's syndrome.

Deficient ACTH secretion causes secondary adrenocortical insufficiency (see later discussion). Since synthetic corticotropin releasing factor is not available, a functional distinction between pituitary and hypothalamic causes cannot be made.

Gonadotropins. Gonadotropin hypersecretion is appropriate in patients with primary hypogonadism (see later discussion). In general, clear-cut elevations in plasma FSH are associated with azoospermia in men and the absence of ova in women, whereas elevations in plasma LH are associated with deficient gonadal sex steroid production. As with TSH secreting adenomas, gonadotropin secreting pituitary tumors have occurred in patients with long standing, untreated primary hypogonadism, and primary gonadotropin secreting pituitary tumors have been recognized rarely.

Deficient gonadotropin secretion causes secondary hypogonadism. Acute testing of the plasma gonadotropin response to Gn-RH does not reliably separate hypothalamic from pituitary causes; reduced plasma LH and FSH responses are the rule. Gn-RH testing after 7 to 10 days of priming with Gn-RH may, however, reveal gonadotropin responses in patients with hypothalamic hypogonadism. Gn-RH testing of this magnitude is hardly practical; again, its relevance to patient management is questionable.

Disorders of neurohypophyseal function

Excessive AVP secretion from the neurohypophysis, or the ectopic secretion of AVP-like peptides from nonendocrine tumors, causes the syndrome of inappropriate antidiuretic hormone secretion (SIADH). At least on medical services, hyponatremia is more commonly due to SIADH and consequent water retention than to total body sodium depletion. Patients are commonly asymptomatic until the serum sodium concentration is quite low (115 to 120 mEq/liter) when nonspecific symptoms such as headache, malaise, and impaired mentation may occur. More profound hyponatremia can cause seizures.

The possibility of SIADH should be considered in aged patients who have become confused and whose serum sodium concentrations is low.

The diagnosis of SIADH is suspected when hyponatremia is discovered in a patient with no clinical evidence of intravascular volume contraction—skin turgor is normal, the mucous membranes are not dry, the heart rate is not increased and does not rise disproportionately when the patient stands, and the blood pressure is well maintained in both the supine and standing positions. Edema is not a feature of the syndrome. Diagnostic clues can be gleaned from routine laboratory data. For example, the serum urea nitrogen is disproportionately low in SIADH because plasma (and total body) water is increased, whereas the urea nitrogen is generally increased in patients with hyponatremia due to sodium depletion.

SIADH is best diagnosed by measurement of plasma AVP concentrations. The primary determinant of normal AVP secretion is the tonicity of the serum. As serum tonicity rises, AVP is secreted; water is therefore reabsorbed from the distal renal tubules and collecting ducts and serum tonicity is reduced to normal. Conversely, as serum tonicity falls, AVP secretion normally decreases, resulting in water diuresis and a rise in serum tonicity. In SIADH, on the other hand, the plasma AVP level is inappropriately high in the presence of hypotonicity of the serum.

Since plasma AVP results will not be immediately available, indirect criteria are used to make a provisional diagnosis of SIADH to guide initial therapy. These include (1) serum hypotonicity (hyponatremia) with urine that is less than maximally dilute in the absence of renal failure, implying the presence of AVP at the renal tubules; and (2) absence of intravascular volume contraction on clinical and laboratory grounds, including continued urinary sodium excretion appropriate to sodium intake. Volume contraction is, in itself, a stimulus to AVP secretion. Therefore the secretion of AVP is not "inappropriate" in a volume-contracted patient even in the presence of serum hypotonicity. Thus the necessary measurements are of serum sodium, creatinine, and osmolality (if unavailable, the serum osmolality can be estimated from the serum sodium concentration) and, in a "spot" urine sample, the urine sodium and osmolality (if unavailable, the urine specific gravity can be used). Some would add additional exclusions, including the absence of hypothyroidism and adrenocortical insufficiency. The hyponatremia that occasionally occurs in patients with hypothyroidism or secondary (ACTH deficient) adrenocortical insufficiency resembles that of SIADH and may indeed be AVP mediated. Thus, it may be an example of SIADH.

Common causes of SIADH include (1) ectopic

AVP secretion from nonendocrine tumors, especially carcinoma of the lung but also from many other tumors; (2) virtually any disorder of the brain (vascular disease, tumor, trauma, infection, subarachnoid hemorrhage, etc.); (3) pneumonias, including pulmonary tuberculosis; and (4) drug ingestion (chlorpropamide, clofibrate, diuretics, narcotics, barbiturates, cyclophosphamide, vincristine, etc.). Clearly many of these disorders are more common in the geriatric population.

Treatment of SIADH includes restriction of fluid intake, initially limited to 500 to 600 ml per day. Since thirst is not a feature of the disorder, this can usually be accomplished. The administration of hypertonic (3%) sodium chloride solution intravenously is seldom necessary and is of only temporary benefit, since the administered sodium is promptly excreted in the urine, but may be required in patients with severe and symptomatic hyponatremia. Indeed, a prompt and sustained increase in the serum sodium concentration after sodium chloride administration should be cause to carefully reconsider the provisional diagnosis of SIADH, since such an increase is more typical of patients with sodium depletion. Obviously, correction of the cause of the SIADH is in order, if possible. The SIADH is sometimes transient. Some drugs, such as demeclocycline, have been empirically observed to be helpful in patients with chronic SIADH in whom long-term fluid restriction has not proved to be practical.

Deficient AVP secretion causes diabetes insipidus (DI), sometimes referred to as *central diabetes insipidus* to distinguish it from the syndrome of nephrogenic diabetes insipidus due to resistance of the kidneys to the action of AVP. The diagnosis of central DI implies hypothalamic disease. As mentioned earlier, adequate AVP secretion can be maintained in the absence of the posterior pituitary if the hypothalamus is intact. Although DI is often idiopathic (and may be familial) in children, the diagnosis should prompt thorough evaluation for a structural hypothalamic lesion in adults.

Patients with DI typically have striking polyuria and polydipsia. Daily urine volumes of 5 to 10 liters are not unusual. They awake frequently at night to void. When they do, they also drink large amounts of water, an important historical point since patients with more common causes of nocturia generally do not do so. As long as thirst mechanisms are intact, the patient is alert enough to respond to thirst, and there is free access to water, patients with DI are able to maintain water balance. However, they are at risk for severe dehydration if the ability to drink large amounts of water is in any way compromised.

In fully developed DI, the diagnosis is rather obvious and easily confirmed. It may be more difficult in patients with partial AVP deficiency. Clearly, more common causes of polyuria—diabetes mellitus and various renal diseases, including those caused by hypercalcemia or hypokalemia—should be considered initially. Also the possibility of primary polydipsia due to psychiatric or other central nervous system disorders need to be considered. Obviously, the clinical distinction between true polyuria and urinary frequency due to bladder neck obstruction or urinary tract infection is of fundamental importance. DI is not a common disorder.

Once the presence of unexplained polyuria is established, the diagnosis of DI is best made by measurement of the plasma AVP concentration. Because of the limited sensitivity of available AVP radioimmunoassays, the diagnosis of DI cannot be made by a random plasma AVP measurement in a compensated patient, that is, a patient who is maintaining water balance and normal serum tonicity by a high water intake. Thus the diagnostic finding is that of a plasma AVP level that is disproportionately low when it should normally be elevated, that is, when the water balance is negative and serum hypertonicity is present. This usually requires short-term deprivation.

Plasma AVP measurements can thus be combined with less direct data derived from a water deprivation test and used to make a provisional diagnosis of DI pending the plasma AVP results. One approach is to withhold water in the morning and measure body weight, serum osmolality (or sodium), and urine volume, osmolality, and specific gravity at hourly intervals. Plasma AVP levels are measured before the test and when the urinary osmolality (or specific gravity) reaches plateau. At that point aqueous vasopressin (Pitressin) is given subcutaneously, and the standard serum and urine measurements repeated 1 hour later. Patients with DI will lose weight (loss of more than 3% of body weight is dangerous), serum hypertonicity will develop, and they will not concentrate their urine substantially until after vasopressin is injected. Further, their plasma AVP levels will not rise as their serum becomes hypertonic.

Replacement therapy for DI has been greatly advanced by the development of long-acting AVP analogs, such as desmopressin acetate (DDAVP), which can be administered by nasal insufflation.

Hypopituitarism

Hypopituitarism can involve deficient secretion of one or more pituitary hormones with intact secretion of other pituitary hormones (fractional hypopituitarism) or deficient secretion of all pituitary hormones (panhypopituitarism). It can be due to (1) primary disease of the pituitary gland or (2) disease directly involving the hypothalamus or that which disrupts the hypothalamo-adenohypophyseal portal circulation. Causes of hypopituitarism are outlined in Table 16-2.

Table 16-2. Hypopituitarism

Pituitary cause	*Hypothalamic cause*
1. Primary (rarely secondary) tumor 2. Infarction (including postpartum infarction, Sheehan's syndrome) 3. Ablation (surgery, irradiation) 4. Idiopathic pituitary fibrosis 5. Others a. Infiltrative/granulomatous disease (hemochromatosis, sarcoidosis, histiocytosis, etc.) b. Infections (tuberculosis, syphilis, brucellosis, mycoses, etc.)	1. Tumor (craniopharyngioma, optic glioma, meningioma, epidermoid cyst, etc.) 2. Trauma (including surgery as well as penetrating or closed head trauma) 3. Idiopathic (especially with isolated hormone deficiency) 4. Others a. Infiltrative/granulomatous disease (sarcoidosis, histiocytosis, etc.) b. Infections (postmeningitis, tuberculosis, etc.)

Assessment of the older patient with suspected hypopituitarism should include an evaluation of pituitary function and an attempt to determine the etiology of any pituitary deficiency state documented. The functional assessment should include search for historical and physical evidence relevant to PRL and GH secretion and measurements of the basal serum PRL, GH, and somatomedin concentrations, as discussed earlier, as well as an evaluation of TSH, ACTH, and gonadotropin secretion. The clinical aspects of deficient secretion of the latter hormones will be discussed later. Laboratory measurements should include those of serum thyroxine, TSH, cortisol, LH, FSH, and testosterone (men) or estradiol (women) at a minimum. Provocative tests of ACTH secretion (discussed later) and measurement of the TSH response to intravenous TRH (discussed earlier) may also be of value. The finding of a morning urinary specific gravity of 1.020 or greater is good evidence against the presence of diabetes insipidus. More definitive testing (discussed earlier) is in order if the history suggests this diagnosis and the morning urinary specific gravity is low.

Features favoring a hypothalamic, rather than primary pituitary, cause for hypopituitarism include (1) the presence of diabetes insipidus; (2) documented hypothalamic hypothyroidism (hypothyroidism with a plasma TSH that is not elevated but rises after TRH injection); and (3) hyperprolactinemia associated with deficient secretion of other pituitary hormones. Other evidence of hypothalamic dysfunction, such as disordered body temperature or appetite regulation, is suggestive. In general, isolated deficiencies of pituitary hormone secretion are thought to be more likely due to hypothalamic than primary pituitary disease.

The etiology of hypopituitarism is often obvious from the history. If not, diagnostic evaluation is generally limited to a search for pituitary or hypothalamic mass lesions, most definitively with CT scans.

Patients with hypopituitarism not due to a lethal disease can be expected to feel well and live a normal life span with appropriate replacement therapy. GH replacement is unnecessary (in adults) as is PRL replacement. Thyroid hormone replacement with thyroxine (generally 0.1 to 0.2 mg daily) is straightforward. Cortisol replacement with cortisone (generally 25 mg in the morning and 12.5 mg in the late afternoon) or prednisone (5 mg and 2.5 mg) is effective. Increased glucocorticoid doses are critical during stress. Since the clearance of thyroxine and glucocorticoids declines with advanced age, lower replacement doses may be appropriate in elderly patients. Replacement of gonadal hormones (testosterone or an estrogen preparation) can be done if clinically indicated.

Evaluation of a patient with an enlarged sella turcica

Enlargement of the sella turcica is a not uncommon serendipitous finding on skull radiographs obtained because of head trauma, headaches, and so on. In such patients, three questions need to be answered. First, is there clinical or laboratory evidence of excessive pituitary hormone secretion? GH hypersecretion (and that of TSH or ACTH) can generally be excluded on clinical grounds. PRL hypersecretion cannot; thus the serum PRL must be measured. Second, is there clinical or laboratory evidence of deficient secretion of one or more pituitary hormones? The appropriate evaluation was discussed previously. Third, what is the intrasellar and parasellar anatomy? Particularly in patients with an enlarged sella but with entirely normal pituitary function, the important distinction is between an asymptomatic intrasellar mass (usually a pituitary adenoma but sometimes a suprasellar mass extending into the sella or rarely a carotid artery aneurysm) and the so-called "empty sella syndrome."

The empty sella syndrome (ESS) is due to herniation of the subarachnoid space into the sella. The sella is not empty but rather contains cerebral spinal fluid. Although often associated with obesity, hypertension, or both, it may be the result of a congenital defect in the diaphragm sella. Remarkably, although the pituitary gland is compressed, it typically functions normally. Thus the ESS is a generally benign condition.

The distinction between an intrasellar mass and the ESS is being made more frequently with modern, high resolution CT scans. However, CT scans after the intrathecal injection of a contrast agent may be required.

THYROID GLAND

Physiology

Thyroidal synthesis and secretion of thyroid hormones are regulated by pituitary TSH, the secretion of which is modulated by hypothalamic TRH. The principal secretory product of the thyroid gland is thyroxine (tetraiodothyronine [T_4]), although some triiodothyronine (T_3) is secreted. Approximately 80% of the T_3 in the circulation is the product of extrathyroidal (in the liver and other tissues) conversion of T_4 to T_3. T_3 is more potent in accelerating metabolic activities than T_4. Thus some have taken the position that T_4 is primarily a precursor and T_3 is the primary metabolically active thyroid hormone.

Thyroid hormones circulate bound to serum proteins, primarily thyroxine binding globulin (TBG). It is the unbound, or free, component that enters the tissues to produce biologic actions (including negative feedback on pituitary TSH secretion). The free T_4 and T_3 concentrations are only a small fraction (roughly 0.04% and 0.4%, respectively) of the serum total T_4 and T_3.

Thyroid function tests

The major thyroid function tests are listed below. These include radioimmunoassay measurements of serum total T_4, total T_3, and TSH; the T_3 uptake test; and, in special circumstances, measurement of the serum free T_4. The latter commonly involves measuring, by equilibrium dialysis, the proportion of added radioactively labelled thyroxine that does not bind to serum proteins (the free component) and then calculating the free thyroxine concentration from this value and the total serum T_4 concentration. The free T_4 measurement should not be confused with the various "free thyroxine indices," which are estimated from the total T_4 and T_3 uptake values.

Major thyroid function tests

Serum thyroxine (T_4): measures total thyroxine and, therefore, largely reflects protein-bound thyroxine

Serum T_3 uptake test (T_3U): used to estimate the number of available binding sites on the serum proteins; does *not* measure T_3

Serum triiodothyronine (T_3): measures total triiodothyronine and, therefore, largely reflects protein-bound triiodothyronine

Plasma thyrotropin (TSH): provides a biologic index of the adequacy of the tissue supply of thyroid hormones in that plasma TSH levels are increased when tissue thyroid hormone levels are low as the result of disease extrinsic to the hypothalamic-pituitary axis; can be interpreted to indicate excessive tissue thyroid hormone levels if TSH levels are low and unresponsive to TRH

Serum free thyroxine (free T_4): measures unbound thyroxine and is, therefore, unaffected by changes in the levels of binding proteins

Variations in TBG levels are common. Since these result in corresponding changes in the serum total T_4 and T_3 concentrations, they are a potential source of diagnostic confusion. Increments in TBG are commonly caused by estrogen therapy (or pregnancy); other causes include acute hepatitis, long-term narcotic use, or familial TBG elevation. Decrements in TBG result from androgen therapy, chronic liver disease, and other hypoproteinemic states or familial TBG deficiency. In practice, abnormalities in the serum binding capacity for thyroid hormones, which are not readily explained, also occur.

Because of the frequency of binding abnormalities and the resultant distortion of total thyroid hormone concentrations, it is best to couple an estimate of the number of available binding sites, the T_3 uptake test, with the initial T_4 or T_3 measurement in a given patient. The T_3 uptake test is performed by mixing radioactively labelled T_3 with the patient's serum and determining the proportion of radioactive T_3 that does not bind to the serum proteins. If TBG is elevated or if the number of unoccupied binding sites is increased due to decreased thyroid hormone production (hypothyroidism), more labelled material will distribute to the binding proteins and the T_3 uptake result will be low; the serum total T_4 (and T_3) will be increased in the former circumstance and decreased in the latter. If TBG decreases or the number of unoccupied binding sites is decreased due to increased thyroid hormone production (hyperthyroidism), less labelled material will distribute to the binding proteins and the T_3 uptake result will be high; the serum T_4 (and T_3) will be decreased in the former circumstance and increased in the latter. Thus the serum thyroid hormone concentrations and the T_3 uptake value change in the same direction in hyperthyroidism (both increased) and in hypothyroidism (both decreased).

Divergent changes in the thyroid hormone level and the T_3 uptake test are indicative of a binding abnormality. In my judgment, mathematical adjustments, the "free thyroxine index," or similar indices, are not sufficiently reliable to permit the diagnosis of hyperthyroidism or hypothyroidism when a binding abnormality is apparent from the discrepant thyroid hormone and T_3 uptake results. Specific measurement of the free thyroxine concentration is indicated.

The routine availability of assays for TSH in plasma is a useful advance. Elevated TSH levels are a sensitive indicator of primary hypothyroidism, and their suppression to normal can be used to assess the adequacy of replacement therapy. Plasma TSH levels are suppressed in hyperthyroidism (except in the rare patient with hyperthyroidism due to a TSH secreting pituitary tumor), but basal measurements are not diagnostically useful since many euthyroid persons have plasma TSH concentrations below the level of detectability of most available immunoassays. The plasma TSH response to intravenous TRH is suppressed even in mild hyperthyroidism. I seldom use this test, however, since hyperthyroidism is usually more easily diagnosed by thyroid hormone measurements. I am reluctant to treat a patient with hyperthyroidism that is so biochemically subtle as to be manifested only by an absent TSH response to TRH, especially since some euthyroid persons have very small TSH increments after TRH injection.

The ^{131}I thyroid uptake is an overused test. It is not a sensitive test for hyperthyroidism and is even worse for hypothyroidism because of a wide normal range and substantial overlap in states of abnormal thyroid function. Its use has been limited to estimation of the dose of ^{131}I to be used to treat hyperthyroidism. There has, however, been renewed interest in ^{131}I uptakes with the increasing recognition of transient hyperthyroidism, during which the ^{131}I uptake is low due to subacute thyroiditis or painless thyroiditis (discussed later). However, similar information can be obtained in patients with that condition with a ^{99m}technetium thyroid scan. This scan is quicker and delivers a much lower radiation dose to the thyroid gland. Because of the latter advantage ^{99m}technetium thyroid scans have largely replaced ^{131}I scans. However, in general, thyroid scans are perhaps the most overused thyroid test; their main use is to assess thyroid nodules.

The only age related change in the commonly used thyroid function tests is a decline in the serum total T_3 concentration. This is attributable to diminished T_3 formation from T_4. Despite diminished T_4 clearance, correspondingly decreased T_4 secretion results in normal serum total T_4 concentrations; TSH levels are not increased. Basal metabolic rates are often slightly reduced, but appropriate to lean body mass.

Hyperthyroidism

Thyroid hormone excess is characterized clinically by manifestations of a generalized increase in metabolic activity. Accelerated oxidation of metabolic fuels results in increased heat generation, causing the common symptom of heat intolerance, and in weight loss. Although some younger patients increase their caloric consumption sufficiently to maintain their body weight, older patients rarely do so. Accelerated proteolysis causes muscular weakness. The skin becomes noticeably soft and the hair fine. A fine tremor, brisk reflexes, a moderate increase in heart rate, and retraction of the upper lid, which may reflect a thyroid hormone-induced increase in sensitivity to sympathoadrenal catecholamines, are common findings. Although the presence of a goiter is the rule, it has been reported that as many as one third of hyperthyroid patients over the age of 60 years do not have a goiter.

It has been suggested that older patients often have more subtle clinical evidence of hyperthyroidism than do younger patients. They may exhibit less generalized hyperkinesis and fewer typical symptoms and signs and may not have a goiter. Although it is my view that these differences have been overemphasized, I would agree that unexplained weight loss or the recent onset of tachyarrhythmias, particularly atrial fibrillation, are an indication for biochemical assessment of thyroid function even in the absence of overt clinical thyrotoxicosis.

Common causes of hyperthyroidism include diffuse thyroid hyperfunction caused by the elaboration of thyroid stimulating immunoglobulins (Graves' disease) and autonomous thyroid nodules that may be multiple (Plummer's disease) or single (toxic adenoma). Iatrogenic hyperthyroidism or that due to the surreptitious ingestion of thyroid hormones occurs not uncommonly. Hyperthyroidism due to a TSH secreting pituitary tumor, caused by ectopic thyroid hormone secretion (as in struma ovarii) or secondary to massive overproduction of chorionic gonadotropin (as a molar pregnancy), is rare.

Although it can occur at any age, Graves' disease is typically a disorder of young adults, especially women. Infiltrative ophthalmopathy (conjunctival injection and edema, proptosis, fibrosis of the extraocular muscles causing diplopia, or, rarely, optic neuritis with visual loss) and infiltrative dermopathy (pretibial myxedema) are features of Graves' disease not attributable to thyroid hormone excess. Their presence permits a confident diagnosis of Graves' disease in a thyrotoxic patient, although the disorder is commonly assumed in their absence when hyperthyroidism is associated with diffuse thyroid enlargement.

In older hyperthyroid patients the frequency of Graves' disease declines and that of toxic nodular (usually multinodular) goiter increases. This distinction is made by careful physical examination; thyroid scans are not required.

The diagnosis of hyperthyroidism is generally not difficult. The clinical picture is highly suggestive, or unequivocal, and the serum T_4 and T_3 uptake values are clearly elevated. Occasional patients have T_4 levels within the normal range but elevated serum T_3 levels (T_3-toxicosis). Rare causes of normal or low T_4 levels in hyperthyroid patients include TBG deficiency (suggested by a high T_3 uptake value) and hyperthyroidism due to T_3 ingestion.

In contrast to the forms of persistent hyperthyroidism mentioned before, transient hyperthyroidism is being recognized with increasing frequency. This may occur in the early phase of subacute thyroiditis, which is characterized by a painful, tender goiter often associated with nonspecific symptoms suggestive of a viral illness and believed to be the result of viral infection. The hyperthyroidism of subacute thyroiditis is the result of inflammatory disruption of the gland (which is characterized histologically by granulomas and acute inflammatory cells). Circulating thyroid hormone levels are high but, if measured, the thyroid uptake of ^{131}I is very low. The presence of a tender goiter permits clinical recognition of this form of transient hyperthyroidism. Treatment of the hyperthyroidism of subacute thyroiditis may not be necessary although a beta-adrenergic antagonist such as propranolol can be used to minimize thyrotoxic symptoms. Steroids are commonly prescribed to ameliorate the inflammatory symptoms.

A more difficult diagnostic problem is transient hyperthyroidism in the absence of thyroid pain or tenderness, so-called *painless thyroiditis*. Although a short history of thyrotoxic symptoms should raise this possibility, it is often difficult to distinguish hyperthyroidism due to painless thyroiditis from that due to Graves' disease without infiltrative ophthalmopathy or pretibial myxedema. If it is the physician's practice to treat Graves' thyrotoxicosis with ^{131}I, a serious error will not be made because the ^{131}I uptake, performed to calculate the ^{131}I therapeutic dose, will be found to be quite low, making the diagnosis of painless thyroiditis apparent. If, on the other hand, one plans to treat presumed Graves' thyrotoxicosis with thionamide drugs, thyroidectomy, or both, the possibility of painless thyroiditis could be used to defend routine performance of an ^{131}I uptake before beginning drug therapy. Alternatively, one could perform a thyroid scan, since the gland will be poorly visualized, if at all, in painless thyroiditis.

The therapeutic options for Graves' thyrotoxicosis include long-term thionamide drug therapy, thyroidectomy, or ^{131}I therapy. The thionamide drugs—propylthiouracil (PTU) and methimazole (Tapazole)—act to block thyroid hormone synthesis; PTU also impairs T_4 conversion to T_3. The premise of long-term (1 to 2 years) treatment with a thionamide is that the thyrotoxicosis may remit spontaneously during the course of treatment. However, relapse rates average 70%. This, plus the occurrence of side effects (even though life-threatening side effects such as agranulocytosis or hepatic necrosis are uncommon), makes me reluctant to use these drugs. Thyroidectomy is an effective form of therapy. The standard approach is to treat with a thionamide until the patient is euthyroid (on average about 2 to 3 months) and then perform surgery. More recently, preparation for thyroidectomy over a few days with propranolol has been shown to be generally safe. The disadvantages of thyroidectomy include the surgical risks (potential complications include hypoparathyroidism and section of the recurrent laryngeal nerve, although these occur rarely when surgery is performed by an experienced thyroid surgeon), discomfort, the need for hospitalization, and costs. Persistent or recurrent hyperthyroidism is surprisingly infrequent; postoperative hypothyroidism does occur, although perhaps less frequently than after ^{131}I therapy.

Because of the disadvantages of thionamide therapy and of thyroidectomy and the relative ease and safety record of ^{131}I therapy, an increasing proportion of patients are being treated with ^{131}I. Hypothyroidism is a very real, albeit easily treated, complication of ^{131}I therapy. It occurs in 40% to 50% of patients; some would argue that it will occur in virtually all patients if they are followed long enough. Theoretical concerns about carcinogenesis (leukemia, thyroid carcinoma) have not been supported in a now large experience. Hypothetical concern that ^{131}I therapy might cause genetic damage have not been supported; first generation offspring of women treated with ^{131}I (for hyperthyroidism or with ten-fold larger doses for thyroid carcinoma) have not had an increased frequency of congenital abnormalities, although the experience is not large enough to exclude a small effect. Further, the gonadal radiation dose is now recognized to be comparable to that of commonly performed diagnostic x-rays. Clearly, this argument is moot in patients beyond the childbearing age.

^{131}I therapy is also used to treat patients with hyperthyroidism caused by autonomous thyroid nodules, although larger doses are generally required.

Hypothyroidism

Thyroid hormone deficiency results in generalized slowing of metabolic activities. Diminished oxidation of metabolic fuels results in diminished heat production, with the common complaint of cold intolerance, and results in weight gain. The latter is seldom more than 10 to 20 pounds; hypothyroidism does not cause massive obesity. Lethargy, an increased sleep requirement and impaired mentation are common symptoms of fully developed hypothyroidism (myxedema) as are constipation and deepening of the voice. Typical physical findings include dry, coarse skin and hair and dermal infiltration most noticeable in puffiness around the eyes, although fullness of the hands and feet and even the extremities in general may occur. Relative or absolute bradycardia, ptosis, and a delayed relaxation phase of the reflexes may be a reflection of decreased sensitivity to sympathoadrenal catecholamines. A goiter may or may not be present.

The extreme expression of the hypothyroid state is myxedema coma characterized by central nervous system depression with hypoventilation, hypothermia, and stupor proceeding to coma.

Hypothyroidism is a common endocrine disorder, especially in women. The vast majority of hypothyroid patients have primary disease of the thyroid gland—primary hypothyroidism. A small minority have hypothyroidism due to deficient TSH secretion because of disease of the pituitary gland (secondary hypothyroidism) or hypothalamus (tertiary or hypothalamic hypothyroidism).

Chronic (Hashimoto's) thyroiditis is a common cause of primary hypothyroidism. Typically, the patient has a long-standing goiter and hypothyroidism develops insidiously. The gland is usually diffusely enlarged, although the surface may be irregular, and asymmetric enlargement is not uncommon. The histologic picture is that of chronic inflammation often with the pattern of "germinal centers." Serum antithyroid antibodies (antimicrosomal, antithyroglobulin) are often present in high titer; the disease is believed to be the result of an autoimmune process. There is a recognized association between primary hypothyroidism due to chronic thyroiditis and Addison's disease (Schmidt's syndrome).

Many patients have primary hypothyroidism without goiter; the gland is atrophic although chronic inflammatory cells can be seen histologically. It may be that this is the end-stage of chronic thyroiditis. Occasionally, hypothyroidism with goiter is precipitated by iodine or lithium administration; such patients are presumed to have underlying thyroid disease, perhaps chronic thyroiditis, since the majority of patients so treated do not become hypothyroid. Other forms of iatrogenic primary hypothyroidism—those due to thyroidectomy, ^{131}I therapy, or thionamide therapy—occur rather commonly. Defined defects in thyroid hormone biosynthesis, resulting in goitrous hypothyroidism that is typically congenital, are rare. Dietary iodine deficiency is still common in some parts of the world but is rarely, if ever, the cause of goiter and hypothyroidism in the United States today.

The diagnosis of full blown clinical hypothyroidism is not difficult. In general, the serum T_4, the T_3 uptake test, and the plasma TSH should be measured. Both the T_4 and the T_3 uptake values are low; since the vast majority of patients have primary hypothyroidism, the plasma TSH is usually elevated. Since the presence of a goiter is direct evidence of primary thyroid disease, the TSH measurement could reasonably be omitted in goitrous hypothyroidism. Clearly, the uncommon finding of hypothyroidism without an elevated plasma TSH dictates thorough assessment of hypothalamic and pituitary function as discussed earlier.

More subtle clinical hypothyroidism may be more difficult to document on the basis of the serum T_4 concentration. TSH secretion is very sensitive to diminished tissue levels of thyroid hormones, and plasma TSH elevation is reasonably considered diagnostic of hypothyroidism, theoretical arguments notwithstanding. The diagnosis is generally rejected if the plasma TSH is not elevated, an acknowledgment of the rarity of TSH deficient hypothyroidism.

The serum T_3 should not be measured when hypothyroidism is suspected. Some hypothyroid patients have serum T_3 levels within the normal range, presumably reflecting enhanced fractional conversion from thyroxine. More importantly, many persons believed to be euthyroid not infrequently have depressed serum T_3 levels. It is now recognized that many patients with acute or chronic extrathyroidal diseases exhibit diminished T_4 to T_3 conversion, with low serum T_3 levels, but are euthyroid. This has been called the *euthyroid sick syndrome*. Serum free T_4 concentrations are typically elevated, explaining the maintenance of euthyroidism. Whether T_4 acts directly or after conversion to T_3 in the target tissues, this clinical observation indicates that T_4 is a biologically important thyroid hormone and not exclusively a T_3 precursor.

Replacement therapy for hypothyroidism is straightforward. Replacement with thyroxine, in a daily dose of 0.1 to 0.2 mg, results in resolution of the clinical syndrome, elevation of the serum T_4, and suppression of plasma TSH in 3 to 6 weeks. Thyroxine is the drug of choice. It is the hormone normally secreted by the thyroid, is inexpensive, can be taken once a day, and is safe when given in the appropriate dose. As mentioned earlier, the lower doses may be sufficient in elderly patients.

Many physicians start therapy with small

doses of thyroxine (0.025 to 0.050 mg daily) in patients with known ischemic heart disease or in older patients in general because of the fear that a rapid increment in oxygen demand will precipitate myocardial ischemia. Most who have treated large numbers of hypothyroid patients have had a patient who suffered a myocardial infarction a few days after the initiation of thyroid hormone therapy. Although a cause-and-effect relationship remains speculative in such anecdotal observations, it is not unreasonable. Since approximately 5 weeks of daily thyroxine ingestion is required to achieve steady state thyroid hormone levels, dosage increments should be made at intervals of no less than 6 weeks. Thus the potential benefit of low dose initial therapy must be balanced against the realization that the duration of hypothyroidism will be appreciably prolonged.

Goiter

Thyroid enlargement can be due to one or more of three general mechanisms: (1) hyperplasia, (2) inflammation, and (3) tumor. Thyroid hyperplasia in the euthyroid or hypothyroid patient is due to limited thyroid hormone production, caused by any of the primary thyroid diseases discussed earlier, and the consequent compensatory increase in TSH production. In hyperthyroid patients it is commonly due to the thyroid stimulating immunoglobulins of Graves' disease and rarely due to a TSH secreting pituitary tumor. Inflammatory infiltration of the thyroid gland is the result of thyroiditis as exemplified by chronic thyroiditis. Such patients may have both inflammatory and hyperplastic components to the pathogenesis of their goiter. In contrast to diffuse goiters resulting from hyperplasia, inflammation, or both, nodular goiter can be viewed as the result of tumor, using the term in its broad sense. Thyroid nodules may be cysts, benign adenomas, or, as discussed below, carcinomas.

Nodular goiters become increasingly common in older populations. Their pathogenesis is unknown. Evidence that growth of nodules is dependent on TSH has been sought but not convincingly demonstrated. In my experience, nodular goiters seldom regress dramatically during thyroid hormone therapy. This is in contrast to diffuse goiters caused by chronic thyroiditis, which often become substantially smaller during thyroid hormone administration. If one elects to attempt to reduce the size of a multinodular goiter by administering thyroxine, one must recognize the possibility of autonomous thyroid hormone secretion by one or more of the nodules and follow the patient carefully to be certain that the usual thyroxine doses do not produce iatrogenic thyrotoxicosis.

Thyroid carcinoma

Thyroid carcinomas can be classified as papillary, follicular, medullary, or anaplastic. Well-differentiated carcinomas (especially papillary but also follicular) are generally very slow growing. Survival is measured in decades, especially when the diagnosis is made before the age of 40 years. Although these carcinomas tend to be somewhat more aggressive when diagnosed later in life, death from metastatic carcinomas is the exception rather than the rule. Differentiated thyroid carcinomas are usually treated by subtotal thyroidectomy, with removal of only clinically involved cervical lymph nodes (not radical neck dissection), plus lifelong thyroid hormone therapy. The latter is based on the fact that at least some of these tumors are TSH dependent. Bad prognostic signs may dictate more aggressive therapy with large doses of ^{131}I, external irradiation or chemotherapy. Papillary carcinomas that penetrate the thyroid capsule directly are somewhat more aggressive than those that are limited to the thyroid gland (with or without cervical lymph node metastases). Follicular carcinomas tend to metastasize hematogenously; vascular invasion histologically and, of course, distant metastases to lung, liver, or bone make the prognosis poorer but far from dismal.

At the other end of the spectrum, anaplastic carcinoma of the thyroid gland is an aggressive malignancy with survival measured in months, regardless of therapy.

Medullary carcinoma of the thyroid gland has an intermediate prognosis. It is the form of thyroid carcinoma that is a component of the multiple endocrine neoplasia, type 2 syndrome (primary hyperparathyroidism, medullary carcinoma of the thyroid gland, and pheochromocytoma), which is often a familial, autosomal dominant disorder. Medullary carcinomas commonly secrete calcitonin, and serum calcitonin measurements (especially after provocative stimuli such as pentagastrin or calcium) have been used to identify occult medullary carcinoma in members of an affected family. Indeed, prospective testing of family members has permitted identification of a premalignant lesion, C-cell hyperplasia. In general, the older the patient at diagnosis, the greater the likelihood that he or she has a sporadic rather than a familial disorder. Nonetheless, serious consideration should be given to the possibility of pheochromocytoma before thyroid surgery is performed in a patient with medullary carcinoma of the thyroid gland.

Thyroid nodules are common, particularly in an older population. Clinically important thyroid cancer, on the other hand, is not common. The challenge, incompletely met with current techniques, is to select those patients with thyroid cancer for thyroidectomy from the larger group with benign thyroid nodules. Factors that increase the probability that a given thyroid nodule is malignant include the following:

1. Prior history of low dose irradiation (for acne, enlarged tonsils, and many other indications then thought appropriate) that included the neck; more than 10% of exposed patients will have carcinoma of the thyroid gland, typically well differentiated, at some time in their life.
2. Failure of the nodule to take up radionuclide on thyroid scan. Although the majority of benign thyroid nodules are also "cold" on scan, nodules that take up the radionuclide are almost invariably benign.
3. A solitary nodule or, in a multinodular gland, a dominant nodule.
4. Youth (under 40 years of age) and the male sex.
5. An unusually hard or irregular nodule.
6. Progressive enlargement of the nodule over weeks and months (acute enlargement is often due to hemorrhage into a cyst).
7. Stippled calcifications (psammoma bodies in papillary carcinoma) on films of the neck.

Obviously the finding of palpably enlarged cervical lymph nodes or of distant metastases make the diagnosis of thyroid carcinoma likely.

What should one do with an older patient who has a definite thyroid nodule that does not concentrate radionuclide on scan and who does not have a history of neck irradiation or clinical evidence of cancer? Only 10% to 20% of such patients have cancer. One approach would be to remove all such nodules surgically on the premise that one cannot categorically exclude carcinoma without histologic examination of the entire nodule. Clearly many benign nodules would be found, and therefore much unnecessary surgery would have been performed. At the other extreme one could follow all such patients on the premises that most of the lesions are benign, most of the carcinomas are low grade malignancies, and there is little evidence that therapy affects the course of the high grade thyroid malignancy. Since neither of these approaches is acceptable, there have been considerable efforts to develop more decisive ways to distinguish malignant from benign thyroid nodules. Although serum thyroglobulin levels correlate with thyroid tumor burden and can be used to follow patients with known thyroid cancer, thyroglobulin measurements are not a sensitive way to diagnose carcinoma of the thyroid gland. Thyroid nodules that are solid by ultrasonography are more likely to be malignant than those that are cystic. However, many solid lesions will be benign, and the distinction between solid and cystic lesions cannot always be made with confidence. Recently there has been renewed interest in aspiration biopsy, using fine needles, of thyroid nodules. This is said to be reasonably simple and safe, but it requires an experienced cytopathologist for accurate interpretation. Occasionally, the contents of a cyst can be entirely aspirated resulting in disappearance of the nodule. The preliminary data with this approach are promising. If conservatively interpreted (for example, the distinction between follicular adenoma and follicular carcinoma cannot be made by aspiration biopsy), this technique may well reduce the frequency of surgery for benign lesions without a corresponding increase in untreated thyroid carcinoma.

ADRENAL CORTEX

Physiology

The adrenal cortex produces three categories of hormones: (1) glucocorticoids (chiefly cortisol), (2) mineralocorticoids (chiefly aldosterone), and (3) sex steroid precursors (chiefly androstenedione). Glucocorticoids are critical to survival. Among their various effects are the stimulation of glucose production (hence the name) and protein catabolism, immunosuppressive and antiinflammatory effects (the reason for their widespread therapeutic use), sensitization of vascular tissues to vasoconstrictors, and central nervous system stimulation. The mineralocorticoids promote sodium conservation and potassium excretion and are therefore critical to maintenance of sodium and potassium balance.

Although aldosterone is the physiologic mineralocorticoid, other steroids such as 11-deoxycorticosterone and even cortisol exert mineralocorticoid effects when they are produced in excess. Gender-appropriate sex steroids are predominantly derived from the gonads, testosterone from the testes and estradiol from the ovaries. However, estrogens in men and androgens in women are in part derived from the adrenal cortex, largely by peripheral conversion from adrenal androstenedione.

The adrenocortical secretion of cortisol is ACTH dependent; cortisol exerts negative feedback on pituitary ACTH secretion. Androstenedione secretion and 11-deoxycorticosterone secretion are also ACTH dependent, but they do not exert feedback on ACTH secretion. In contrast, aldosterone secretion is largely controlled by the renin-angiotensin system; it is also a direct function of the serum potassium concentration. Although ACTH stimulates aldosterone secretion acutely, this effect is not sustained. Further, essentially normal aldosterone secretion continues in the absence of ACTH.

Like the thyroid hormones, cortisol circulates bound to serum proteins, principally corticosteroid binding globulin (CBG). The unbound or free component is the biologically active one. It enters the tissues to produce biologic effects (including negative feedback); it also enters the urine. Like that of TBG, CBG production is increased by estrogen therapy (or pregnancy) and decreased by androgen therapy or chronic liver disease. These changes in CBG result in parallel changes in the serum total cortisol. Similar changes occur in the serum aldosterone and sex steroid binding proteins.

As a group, elderly persons have decreased cortisol clearance rates and secretion rates resulting in plasma cortisol levels similar to those of younger individuals. However, an approximate 30% reduction in the plasma aldosterone concentration in older persons has been reported, attributable to a similar reduction in plasma renin activity. This, coupled with the age related decrease in renal function, may make them more susceptible to hyperkalemia.

Disorders of glucocorticoid secretion

Excessive cortisol secretion is the hallmark of Cushing's syndrome. Endogenous Cushing's syndrome can be caused by the following:

1. Excessive pituitary ACTH secretion, usually from a pituitary microadenoma (pituitary ACTH dependent Cushing's syndrome is by convention referred to as *Cushing's disease*).
2. Autonomous hormone hypersecretion from an adrenocortical tumor (adenoma or carcinoma) or tumors (micronodular hyperplasia).
3. Ectopic secretion of ACTH-like peptides from nonendocrine tumors, carcinoma of the lung among others.
4. Rarely, ectopic secretion of peptides with corticotropin releasing factor activity from nonendocrine tumors resulting in excessive pituitary ACTH hypersecretion and the resultant Cushing's syndrome.

None of these is common. The common form of Cushing's syndrome is that caused by the administration of glucocorticoids such as prednisone in the treatment of nonendocrine diseases. The latter pure glucocorticoid excess syndrome will not be discussed further here.

Although cortisol excess is the constant and diagnostically the central feature of Cushing's syndrome, excessive production of sex steroids, the ACTH dependent mineralocorticoid 11-deoxycorticosterone, or both occurs not infrequently in patients with endogenous Cushing's syndrome. Clinical features reasonably attributed to cortisol excess include obesity (sometimes more striking in the trunk and face), thinning of the skin with striae and ecchymoses, muscle wasting, osteopenia resulting in fractures, glucose intolerance, and perhaps psychiatric changes. Although hypertension may be the result of cortisol excess, increased 11-deoxycorticosterone production with hypokalemia occurs in some patients, particularly in those with ectopic ACTH syndrome. Adrenal androgen over production may result in hirsutism, acne, and amenorrhea in women with Cushing's syndrome.

The clinical picture of the ectopic ACTH syndrome differs from that of other forms of Cushing's syndrome. The patients are generally older, and the malignant disease is usually, although not invariably, clinically apparent. Weight loss is more common than weight gain, typical skin changes are absent or minimal, but hyperpigmentation is common, weakness can be profound, and hypokalemia is a common finding.

Obesity, weakness, back pain, hypertension, and glucose intolerance are common. They are rarely due to Cushing's syndrome. Thus the problem is to select the patient who has a high probability of Cushing's syndrome from the large group who have a suggestive constellation of symptoms and signs but who do not have Cushing's syndrome. This can be accomplished with the overnight dexamethasone suppression test—the morning plasma cortisol concentration after dexamethasone, 1.0 mg, is administered orally at 11:00 to 12:00 PM the preceding evening. Normals have suppressed ACTH secretion and morning plasma cortisol levels of less than 5.0 μg/100 ml. If the cortisol is greater than 5.0 μg/100 ml, the screening test is positive and definitive testing is indicated. False positives do occur, due to massive obesity, estrogen treatment, stress, or failure to take the dexamethasone among other possibilities. However, since false negatives cannot be tolerated with a screening test—an important diagnosis would be erroneously rejected—the possibility of false positives must be accepted.

Definitive diagnosis of Cushing's syndrome requires the demonstration of reproducibly elevated urinary cortisol excretion in a patient with a compatible clinical picture. Since only free cortisol is normally filtered and excreted in the urine, the urinary cortisol measurement provides an index of the serum free cortisol. Dissection of the mechanism of established Cushing's syndrome require (1) measurement of the morning plasma ACTH concentration—markedly elevated in the ectopic ACTH syndrome and suppressed in patients with adrenocortical tumors; and (2) measurement of the urinary cortisol response to oral dexamethasone (0.5 mg every 6 hours for 48 hours and 2.0 mg every 6 hours for 48 hours)—partially suppressed with low dose dexamethasone, suppressed to less than 50% of baseline with high dose dexamethasone in Cushing's disease, and not suppressed at all in the other forms of Cushing's syndrome. If these data suggest an autonomous lesion and not the ectopic ACTH syndrome, CT scans of the adrenal glands will generally demonstrate a tumor. If they suggest Cushing's disease, anatomic assessment of the pituitary gland, including CT scans, is in order.

Cushing's disease is most commonly treated by transsphenoidal pituitary adenomectomy and Cushing's syndrome due to an adrenal tumor by resection of the tumor. Resection of ACTH secreting tumors causing Cushing's syndrome is curative but seldom possible because the tumors are commonly metastatic. Bilateral adrenalectomy may be required if the Cushing's syndrome is intense and there is a reasonable possibility of some comfortable life before the primary malignant process is fatal. Chemotherapy, the use of inhibitors of adrenal steroidogenesis, or both can be tried.

Adrenocortical insufficiency can be primary—due to disease of the adrenal cortices per se (Addison's disease)—or secondary to deficient ACTH secretion. Addison's disease results in decreased secretion of all categories of adrenocortical hormones causing clinical manifestations of glucocorticoid, mineralocorticoid, and, in women, androgen insufficiency. In contrast, aldosterone secretion is maintained in ACTH deficient patients; the renin-angiotensin system is still operative. Thus these patients have clinical manifestations of glucocorticoid and, if they are women, androgen insufficiency.

The symptoms of glucocorticoid deficiency are nonspecific—weakness, fatigue, anorexia (often with nausea and vomiting), and weight loss. Patients with primary adrenocortical insufficiency have increased ACTH secretion resulting in hyperpigmentation. They also have aldosterone deficiency with hyponatremia and hyperkalemia often with hypotension and some degree of azotemia. Adrenal androgen insufficiency can result in loss of axillary and pubic hair in women.

Addison's disease is most often idiopathic and believed to be the result of an autoimmune process. Infectious destruction of the adrenal cortices, by tuberculosis for example, is less common. Uncommon causes include bilateral adrenalectomy, hemorrhage into the adrenal glands (during therapy with anticoagulants; as the result of sepsis or of trauma), amyloidosis, and bilateral metastases. Deficient ACTH secretion can be the result of any of the hypothalamic or pituitary diseases discussed earlier.

More commonly it is the result of withdrawal of prolonged steroid therapy for nonendocrine disorders.

The diagnosis of adrenocortical insufficiency is started with measurement of the morning plasma cortisol and ACTH concentrations. A low cortisol level with a high plasma ACTH indicates primary adrenocortical insufficiency. The plasma cortisol concentration will not rise after the injection of ACTH. A frankly low morning plasma cortisol concentration coupled with an ACTH level that is not elevated suggests secondary adrenocortical insufficiency and is diagnostically sufficient if the clinical picture is clear-cut. A reduced plasma cortisol response to an ACTH mediated provocative stimulus, such as hypoglycemia, is confirmatory. In some patients the morning plasma cortisol concentration is not clearly low, and the diagnosis is considered possible but not likely. Measurement of plasma 11-deoxycortisol (compound S), the precursor to cortisol, after administration of metyrapone (Metopirone), an inhibitor of the last step in cortisol synthesis, is then appropriate. A fall in the morning plasma cortisol concentration without a rise in the morning plasma 11-deoxycortisol concentration after metyropone is indicative of ACTH deficiency (assuming primary adrenocortical insufficiency has been excluded).

Glucocorticoid replacement therapy is commonly accomplished with cortisone acetate (25 mg in the morning and 12.5 mg in the evening) or prednisone (5 mg in the morning and 2.5 mg in the evening). As mentioned earlier, doses one-third lower may be sufficient for older patients. Larger doses are needed during times of stress. Patients with primary adrenocortical insufficiency also require mineralocorticoid replacement with fluorohydrocortisone (Florinef), usually 0.05 to 0.1 mg daily along with a liberal dietary sodium intake.

Disorders of mineralocorticoid secretion

Primary mineralocorticoid overproduction causes hypertension typically with hypokalemia. Mineralocorticoid overproduction in Cushing's syndrome was discussed before. Rarely, 11-deoxycorticosterone overproduction is the result of enzymatic defects in steroid biosynthesis—C_{17}-hydroxylase deficiency resulting in deficient sex steroid secretion or C_{11}-hydroxylase deficiency resulting in excessive androgen production. It has been speculated that overproduction of an as yet unidentified mineralocorticoid is the basis of "low renin" essential hypertension.

Primary aldosteronism (Conn's syndrome) is recognized in a small percentage, perhaps 1% to 2%, of patients with hypertension. However, because hypertension is so common, primary aldosteronism is not a rare disease. Primary aldosteronism is characterized by hypertension, spontaneous hypokalemia with urinary potassium wasting, elevated aldosterone levels, and suppressed plasma renin activity (PRA). A hypertensive patient with spontaneous hypokalemia and urinary potassium excretion of greater than 30 mEq every 24 hours deserves biochemical assessment for primary aldosteronism. In my practice this includes the following:

1. Measurement of the overnight fasted, supine plasma aldosterone concentration after a liberal sodium intake and no antihypertensive therapy for at least 1 week
2. Measurement of the supine plasma aldosterone concentration after the intravenous infusion of 2 liters of saline over 4 hours
3. Measurement of the morning plasma aldosterone concentration before and after 4 hours of upright activity
4. Measurement of PRA after sodium depletion and 4 hours of upright activity

Primary aldosteronism can be caused by an aldosterone producing adenoma (APA) or idiopathic hyperplasia of the adrenal cortex. Surgical removal of an APA will cure hypertension in approximately 50% of patients; hypertension will be improved in an additional 30%. In contrast hypertension in patients with idiopathic hyperplasia is not amenable to surgical therapy and is best treated medically, with a regimen including the aldosterone antagonist spironolactone (Aldactone).

In patients with primary aldosteronism, findings favoring APA include marked biochemical abnormalities and failure of the plasma aldosterone concentration to rise after upright activity. More definitive information comes from lateralizing evidence. This can often be accomplished by CT scans of the adrenal glands, which may demonstrate a tumor. If not, adrenal vein catheterization to demonstrate an aldosterone gradient on one side but not on the other may be required.

Aldosterone deficiency as a component of Addison's disease was discussed earlier. Isolated hypoaldosteronism, often secondary to deficient renin production, also occurs. It is usually recognized because of hyperkalemia, less often because of frank sodium depletion.

Disorders of sex steroid production

Androgen or estrogen excess can result from adrenal or gonadal abnormalities. Androgen excess is difficult to recognize clinically in an adult man, although it could suppress gonadotropin secretion resulting in testicular atrophy. Similarly, estrogen excess in an adult woman is difficult to recognize, although it could result in dysfunction or postmenopausal uterine bleeding.

Gynecomastia is the result of absolute estrogen excess in men or more commonly estrogen excess relative to androgen levels. When sought it is a common physical finding especially in the older age group. Indeed, some have suggested that gynecomastia is a physiologic feature of aging. It is my view that the differential diagnosis of gynecomastia should be carefully considered before gynecomastia is attributed to old age per se (see outline below).

Differential diagnosis of gynecomastia in adult men

1. Drugs—estrogens, digitalis, spironolactone, heroin, marijuana, cimetidine, etc.
2. Hypergonadotropic states
   a. Primary hypogonadism
   b. Ectopic gonadotropin secretion—testicular tumors, nonendocrine tumors
3. Increased estrogen formation (aromatization)
   a. Chronic liver disease
   b. Thyrotoxicosis
   c. Malnutrition → refeeding
4. Estrogen hypersecretion—testicular or adrenocortical tumor
5. Androgen resistance
6. Aging (?)

Androgen excess in women, causing hirsutism, acne, and amenorrhea, is most commonly due to the polycystic ovary syndrome, less commonly due to ovarian hyperthecosis, and occasionally due to adrenocortical androgen overproduction. Androgen secreting adrenocortical or ovarian tumors are rare but may cause frank virilization with clitoromegaly, an increase in muscle mass, male pattern balding, and deepening of the voice.

The typical patient with androgen excess due to the polycystic ovary syndrome has a moderately elevated free serum testosterone concentration (the serum total testosterone concentration may be within the normal range because of androgenic supression of the sex steroid binding globulin level) and an elevated plasma LH to FSH ratio. Distinct elevation of the plasma dehydroepiandrosterone sulfate (DHA-sulfate) level dictates further evaluation of the adrenal glands, since secretion of this compound is unique to the adrenal cortex. Therapy with an estrogen preparation may suppress androgen secretion in patients with the polycystic ovary syndrome. Therapy with clomiphene often restores fertility.

Androgen excess caused by the common nontumor disorders usually becomes apparent during young adult life. Thus the onset of clinical evidence of androgen excess in middle or late life should raise the possibility of an ovarian or an adrenocortical tumor. Clearly, marked serum testosterone elevations and clinical virilization increase the likelihood of tumor. When tumor is suspected, a careful pelvic examination and ultrasonography of the pelvic structures are in order. If these are negative, adrenal CT scans should be obtained. Occasionally, a virilizing ovarian tumor is so small that it is found only when the ovary is bisected at laparotomy.

Deficient androgen or estrogen formation from adrenocortical precursors is not clinically recognizable in men with normal testes. Similarly, deficient estrogen formation from adrenocortical precursors is not recognizable in adult women with normal ovaries. Deficient adrenocortical estrogens could worsen the symptoms of estrogen deficiency in postmenopausal women. As noted earlier, loss of androgens from adrenocortical precursors can result in loss of axillary and pubic hair in women.

ADRENAL MEDULLA

Physiology

Epinephrine is the hormone secreted by the adrenal medullae. They also release norepinephrine, although most circulating norepinephrine represents that released from sympathetic postganglionic neurons throughout the body. Since neural norepinephrine is largely dissipated locally—by axonal reuptake, metabolic modification, or both—norepinephrine in plasma represents only a fraction of that released from nerves (plus that released from the adrenal medullae). Epinephrine functions as a classic hormone; norepinephrine functions primarily as a neurotransmitter. Substantial increments in plasma norepinephrine are required to produce "hormonal" biologic effects.

Epinephrine is approximately 10 times more potent than norepinephrine with respect to most biologic actions of these catecholamines. The hemodynamic patterns of response differ. In physiologic concentrations epinephrine produces net vasodilation and cardiac inotropic and chronotropic effects; heart rate and systolic blood pressure increase and pulse pressure widens. Norepinephrine release causes vasoconstriction with a rise in systolic and diastolic blood pressures; it also has cardiac inotropic and chronotropic effects, but the latter is masked by reflex slowing of heart rate secondary to the elevated blood pressure. Metabolic effects of the catecholamines include hyperglycemia among others.

Catecholamines are metabolized to the metanephrines and 3-methoxy-4-hydroxymandelic acid, the latter better known as vanillylmandelic acid (VMA), which are excreted in the urine.

Disorders of adrenomedullary function

The role of the catecholamines in human metabolic physiology and pathophysiology is only beginning to emerge. The only well-established disorder of the adrenal medullae is the overproduction of catecholamines from a pheochromocytoma.

Pheochromocytomas are tumors that arise from chromaffin cells. Since the adrenal medullae are the major clusters of chromaffin cells that persist during postnatal life, 90% of pheochromocytomas arise there. The remaining 10% arise from extraadrenal chromaffin cells, generally in relation to the sympathetic ganglia. Although pheochromocytomas have been found in sites ranging from the carotid body to the pelvic floor, roughly 99% are in the abdomen and most of the rest are in the posterior mediastinum. Multiple pheochromocytomas occur, especially in familial disease where bilateral adrenomedullary pheochromocytomas are the rule.

Norepinephrine is the predominant secretory product of most pheochromocytomas. Thus hypertension is the common result. Pheochromocytoma is an uncommon cause of hypertension; fewer than one in 200 hypertensive patients harbors a pheochromocytoma. It is, however, an important diagnosis. Pheochromocytoma is a generally curable cause of hypertension, and patients with pheochromocytomas are at continuous risk for a lethal hypertensive paroxysm. Further, there is an incidence, probably less than 5%, of malignant pheochromocytoma. Last, the presence of a pheochromocytoma is a diagnostic clue to the presence of associated, and often familial, disorders (neurofibromatosis, von Hippel-Lindau disease, or multiple endocrine neoplasia with pheochromocytoma, medullary carcinoma of the thyroid gland, and hyperparathyroidism).

Because of episodic, often stress associated, increments in catecholamine release, a pheochromocytoma can produce hypertension that is truly episodic. More often, affected patients have sustained hypertension but the blood pressure is highly variable. The most common paroxysmal symptoms are headache, diaphoresis, and palpitations. If these occur episodically, and especially if they can be shown to be associated with a marked increase in blood pressure, diagnostic evaluation for pheochromocytoma is indicated.

Occasional pheochromocytomas release epinephrine predominantly. Clinical features may include episodes of hypotension, tachycardia, or serious tachyarrhythmias and noncardiac pulmonary edema.

The biochemical diagnosis of pheochromocytoma is commonly made by the finding of increased urinary excretion of catecholamines or their matabolites, such as total metanephrines or VMA. Recently, sensitive radioenzymatic methods used to measure catecholamines in plasma have been effectively applied to the diagnosis of pheochromocytoma. In most affected patients these biochemical measurements are markedly elevated. In an occasional patient with truly paroxysmal or limited catecholamine release from the pheochromocytoma, repeated measurements are required. Once the diagnosis is established biochemically, anatomic localization of the tumor can generally be established by CT scans.

Pheochromocytomas are treated by surgical excision following medical preparation of the patient, usually with a long acting alpha-adrenergic antagonist such as phenoxybenzamine (Dibenzyline).

GONADS
Physiology

The gonads serve two basic functions: the secretion of sex steroids (predominantly testosterone from the testes and estradiol and progesterone from the ovaries) and the production of gametes (sperm and ova). In general, sex steroid production from the gonads is driven by pituitary LH whereas gamete development is driven by FSH, although there are important interactions between the actions of the gonadotropins and between sex steroid production and gametogenesis. Further, negative feedback relationships primarily relate LH to sex steroid secretion and FSH to gametogenesis.

The regulation of ovarian function is more complex than that of the testes. Cyclic gonadotropin secretion, including a midcycle surge in LH and FSH secretion with a resultant burst of estrogen secretion that stimulates ovulation, is critical to normal ovarian function. Ovarian estrogen and progesterone secretion in the postovulation (luteal) phase prepares the uterine endometrium for implantation of the fertilized ovum. If fertilization does not occur, the late luteal decline in ovarian hormone secretion allows the endometrium to slough resulting in menstrual bleeding.

Cross-sectional data indicate that a gradual decline in testicular function, with decrements in serum testosterone and increments in gonadotropin levels, occurs in some men beyond the age of 50 years. Since this is not a universal phenomenon, it is not known whether this is the result of age per se or of unrecognized disease. In contrast, virtual cessation of ovarian function, the menopause, is normal in women.

It should be emphasized that total estrogen deficiency does not occur in the postmenopausal state. Estrogens, principally estrone, are derived from adrenocortical precursors.

Like the thyroid hormones and the adrenocortical steroids, sex steroids circulate bound to serum proteins. Testosterone and estradiol bind to sex steroid binding globulin (SSBG, also known as testosterone-estradiol binding globulin) whereas progesterone binds to corticosteroid binding globulin. Again, binding protein increments produced by estrogen excess, including prescribed estrogens and pregnancy, result in increments in serum total sex steroid concentrations; binding protein decrements produced by androgen excess, chronic liver disease, and so on result in decrements in serum total sex steroid concentrations.

Sex steroids are responsible for the establishment and maintenance of secondary sex characteristics. In men, testosterone promotes growth of sexual hair, including the beard, and an increased muscle mass as well as a deepened voice. In women, maintenance of breast development is a prominent example of estrogen action. Maintenance of vaginal lubrication and effects on the endometrium mentioned earlier are additional functions.

Disorders of gonadal function

Hypogonadism can be primary—the result of gonadal disease—or secondary to hypothalamic-pituitary dysfunction. Patients with primary hypogonadism have low circulating sex steroid levels (testosterone in men, estradiol in women) and elevated gonadotropin levels (hypergonadotropic hypogonadism). Gonadotropin levels are not increased in patients with secondary hypogonadism (hypogonadotropic hypogonadism).

Loss of testicular testosterone secretion results in loss of sexual hair, including diminished beard growth. Muscle mass may decrease. Diminished libido is common. Infertility can result from decreased testosterone production per se. A decrease in testicular size implies loss of seminiferous tubules, which comprise 90% of testicular volume. Gynecomastia (discussed earlier) occurs more commonly in hypergonadotropic hypogonadism.

Primary hypogonadism in men can be the result of congenital disorders, most commonly Klinefelter's syndrome. Acquired gonadal disorders include those caused by infections (mumps, gonorrhea), trauma, irradiation, and chemotherapy. Patients with chronic renal failure and advanced hepatic cirrhosis commonly exhibit primary hypogonadism. With respect to the latter, it should be emphasized that alcoholism per se can result in suppressed testicular function that is sometimes reversible with cessation of alcohol consumption. Primary hypogonadism can also be idiopathic, perhaps the result of an autoimmune process. The causes of secondary hypogonadism were discussed earlier (Disorders of adenohypophyseal function). The recently recognized role of hyperprolactinemia deserves reemphasis.

Treatment of hypogonadal men involves correction of the etiologic mechanism when possible or testosterone replacement. Restoration of fertility is not possible in patients with primary testicular disease; it has occasionally been accomplished by gonadotropin administration in patients with hypogonadotropic hypogonadism.

Loss of ovarian estrogen secretion can result in atrophy of the breasts, diminished vaginal lubrication, hot flashes, and accelerated osteopenia. Infertility and amenorrhea also result. Primary hypogonadism in women can be congenital—most commonly due to Turner's syndrome—or due to the acquired disorders that were mentioned before as causes of primary or secondary hypogonadism in men. Hyperprolactinemia and excessive androgen secretion are common causes. Clearly, pregnancy and in middle life the menopause are common causes of amenorrhea.

Many physicians limit estrogen replacement to patients with symtoms referable to estrogen deficiency. Some urge routine postmenopausal estrogen replacement to prevent clinically important osteopenia. Because of the possibility of estrogen-stimulated endometrial carcinoma, use of an estrogen-progestin combination and cyclic administration are often recommended.

Excessive production of sex steroids was discussed earlier (Disorders of the adrenal cortex).

PARATHYROID GLANDS

Physiology

Parathyroid hormone (PTH) promotes calcium and phosphate mobilization from bone, calcium reabsorption and phosphate excretion by the kidneys, and, indirectly, calcium and phosphate absorption from the gastrointestinal tract. It functions in concert with vitamin D. Dietary vitamin D and that formed in the skin are converted to 25-hydroxyvitamin D (25-OHD) in the liver. 25-OHD is converted to 1,25-dihydroxyvitamin D (1,25-$(OH)_2D$) in the kidney. 1,25-$(OH)_2D$ is the most potent form of vitamin D. It promotes calcium and phosphate absorption from the gastrointestinal tract and favors their deposition in bone.

Parathyroid hormone secretion is primarily regulated by the serum calcium concentration in a negative feedback fashion. Elevated PTH levels (and serum phosphate levels) favor 1,25-$(OH)_2D$ formation.

Roughly half of circulating calcium is bound to serum proteins such as albumin. Thus the total serum calcium concentration varies directly with the serum albumin concentration. Disorders causing changes in serum albumin do not, however, result in changes in the regulated, biologically important serum free ("ionized") calcium concentration.

Perhaps as the result of diminished renal 1,25-$(OH)_2D$ formation and the resulting diminution in intestinal calcium (and phosphate) absorption, the serum free calcium concentration is slightly lower and the PTH level is slightly higher in elderly individuals.

Disorders of parathyroid function

Primary hyperparathyroidism causes hypercalcemia, typically with hypophosphatemia, and can result in urinary tract stones due to hypercalciuria or in osteopenia (osteitis fibrosa). Major hypercalcemia per se causes nonspecific symptoms such as anorexia, nausea and vomiting, and polyuria. A change in mental status is particularly common in older patients with hypercalcemia and can occur with less marked hypercalcemia than that required to produce mental changes in younger individuals.

The differential diagnosis of hypercalcemia is outlined below.

Differential diagnosis of hypercalcemia

1. Malignant disease
   a. Direct bone involvement
      (1) Primary bone tumors (including multiple myeloma)
      (2) Secondary (metastatic) bone tumors
   b. Indirect bone involvement—tumors (especially carcinomas of the lung, kidney, or female reproductive tract) that produce hypercalcemic humoral factors (PTH, prostaglandins, others)
2. Primary hyperparathyroidism
3. Others
   a. Thyrotoxicosis
   b. Vitamin D (or A) intoxication

c. Milk-alkali syndrome
d. Sarcoidosis
e. Addison's disease

In older patients, hypercalcemia is often the result of malignant disease that either directly or indirectly accelerates calcium mobilization from bone. In general, the older the patient and the higher the serum calcium concentration, the greater the likelihood of malignant hypercalcemia. Primary hyperparathyroidism due to PTH hypersecretion from a parathyroid adenoma (rarely, a carcinoma) occurs, however, at all ages. Although its frequency is a matter of debate, parathyroid hyperplasia appears to be primarily a disorder of younger patients.

The diagnosis of primary hyperparathyroidism is based on the findings of hypercalcemia and hypophosphatemia and an elevated serum PTH concentration. Since occasional cancers elaborate a PTH-like material, the diagnosis of malignant hypercalcemia must be considered even when this classic triad is present. Elevated serum 1,25-$(OH)_2D$ levels have recently been found to characterize primary hyperparathyroidism but not malignant hypercalcemia. Nonetheless, this distinction often involves clinical judgment.

Primary hyperparathyroidism is treated by subtotal parathyroidectomy. Whether or not all patients with mild, asymptomatic primary hyperparathyroidism require therapy remains to be established. It is my practice to recommend surgery to all younger patients. Some older patients who have totally asymptomatic disease and no evidence of renal dysfunction or osteopenia disproportionate to their age are followed carefully without surgery.

Secondary hyperparathyroidism is caused by chronic hypocalcemic states and can result in osteitis. A common example is chronic renal failure in which both deficient 1,25-$(OH)_2D$ production and secondary hyperparathyroidism play a pathogenic role in renal osteodystrophy.

Primary hypoparathyroidism, resulting in hypocalcemia and hyperphosphatemia, is an uncommon disorder. In children it is most often idiopathic; in adults it is most often due to parathyroid damage at the time of thyroid or parathyroid surgery. Rarely, hypoparathyroidism is due to massive iron overload, ^{131}I therapy for hyperthyroidism, or thyroid carcinoma or metastases to the parathyroid glands.

A decreased serum total calcium concentration is most commonly the result of decreased serum proteins. Measurement of the serum free calcium concentration is required to confirm this artifact. True hypocalcemia of sufficient degree causes overt tetany with paresthesias and muscle cramps most noticeable as carpopedal spasm. Signs, such as Chvostek's sign and Trousseau's sign, may be present in the absence of overt tetany.

Hypocalcemia can be due to mechanisms other than hypoparathyroidism. These include a number of disorders that result in deficient 1,25-$(OH)_2D$ production. Magnesium depletion can result in functional hypoparathyroidism; hypocalcemia is not responsive to calcium administration, but PTH secretion resumes and the serum calcium rises promptly with magnesium replacement. Rarely, hypocalcemia is the result of resistance to the biologic actions of PTH (pseudohypoparathyroidism).

Aside from hypocalcemia caused by magnesium depletion or vitamin D deficiency, chronic hypocalcemia generally requires therapy with pharmacologic doses of calcium and vitamin D or 1,25-$(OH)_2D$.

REFERENCES

1. Cryer, P.E.: Diagnostic endocrinology, ed. 2, New York, 1979, Oxford University Press.
2. DeGroot, L.J., et al.: Endocrinology, New York, 1979, Grune & Stratton, Inc.
3. Felig, P., Baxter, J., Broadus, A., and Frohman, L., editors: Endocrinology and metabolism, New York, 1981, McGraw-Hill Book Co.

PART II SURGICAL CARE

CHAPTER 17 · GENERAL SURGERY

James H. Mason
Fred C. Gau
Mitchel P. Byrne

The first edition of this text was published in 1958. Since that time there have been significant changes in the age structure of the population of the United States. The portions of our population undergoing the most dramatic changes have been the young adult (18 to 34 years old) and older adult populations (65 years and older). This latter group now comprises 11.2% of the population and has increased 23.5% since 1970 (20.0 million to 24.7 million). The greatest increase has occurred in the female segment of the population (26.2% versus 19.7%) and as a result, the ratio of men to women has dropped.[1] A projection of the population of the United States by age is shown in Fig. 17-1.[2] Current trends and these projections clearly indicate that geriatric surgery will be a rapidly expanding field and must be included in all hospital expansion plans and postgraduate education programs.

PREOPERATIVE EVALUATION

Surgical risk

In the preoperative evaluation of the geriatric patient for elective surgery one question is usually paramount in the physician's mind. How much greater is the risk assumed by the aged patient than that usually accepted for a given procedure? The consensus expressed in the literature on this subject and a recent review of the Professional Activity Studies mortality data (Table 17-1) suggest that the risk for a less traumatic procedure is not significantly different from that expected in younger patients. For emergency procedures however, the mortality is found to be greater in the aged than in younger individuals.

Much of this increased risk is caused by compromise of secondary physiologic systems not specifically related to the problem that brings the patient to the hospital.[3] For example, both emphysema and uremia are found much more frequently in the elderly patient but may be well compensated under ordinary circumstances. Anesthesia and a prolonged abdominal procedure that possibly requires transfusion usually result in fluid shifts, restriction of diaphragmatic movement, and a myriad of other more subtle changes that rapidly upset the tenuous balance that exists between the host and the kidneys or lungs. Recognition of the degree of impairment in the diseased backup system can lead to plans for support with *simple measures*, such as preoperative education in coughing, stopping smoking, antibiotic therapy to clear existing bronchitis and to decrease secretions, intermittent positive-pressure breathing, and intravenous hydration; *intermittent measures*, such as plans for postoperative respirator support or diuretic therapy; or *severe measures*, such as hemodialysis or insertion of a pacemaker.

Recognizing the degree of impairment is an emerging science that has moved pulmonary and renal physiology out of the medical school laboratory and into the intensive care unit. The development of effective, reliable, relatively simple respirators and dialysis machines has stimulated surgeons to use them in an increasing number and variety of clinical problems.

When evaluating the 80-year-old patient, it is frequently necessary to remind everyone concerned that the patient has not necessarily reached his full life expectancy. Indeed, they have survived those years when heart disease, cancer, and accidents take their greatest toll.

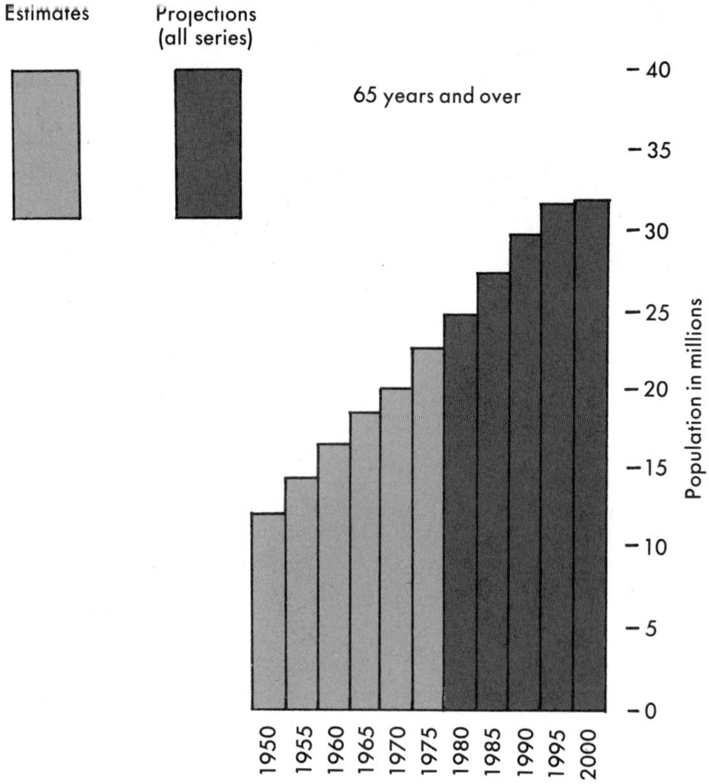

Fig. 17-1. A projection of the population of the United States by age. (From Population estimates and projection series, P25, No. 704, Washington, D.C., July, 1977, U.S. Government Printing Office, p. 13.)

Table 17-1. Mortality for geriatric patients, January to December, 1972*

Surgical procedure	*Mortality rate*			
	Less than 60 years		*Greater than 60 years*	
Cholecystectomy	0.09%	(1053)†	2.4%	(411)†
Acute cholecystitis or cholangitis with cholecystectomy	0%	(84)	6.1%	(49)
Partial gastrectomy	1.5%	(132)	9.9%	(81)
Inguinal herniorrhaphy (not recurrent)	0.09%	(1090)	0.84%	(358)
Transurethral prostatectomy	2.8%	(145)	1.5%	(670)
Segmental resection of colon	6%	(116)	9.7%	(148)
Complete lobectomy	0%	(32)	5.8%	(17)

Surgical procedure	*Mortality rate*					
	60 to 69 years		*70 to 79 years*		*80 to 89 years*	
Cholecystectomy	1.8%	(226)†	2.7%	(146)†	5.1%	(39)†
Acute cholecystitis or cholangitis with cholecystectomy	0	(20)	10.5%	(21)	11.1%	(19)
Partial gastrectomy	11.1%	(15)	0	(20)	30%	(10)
Inguinal hernia (not recurrent)	0	(214)	1.7%	(119)	4.0%	(25)
Transurethral prostatectomy	0	(277)	1.8%	(284)	3.7%	(109)
Segmental resection of colon	4.1%	(73)	12.5%	(56)	25.0%	(16)
Complete lobectomy	0	(12)	20%	(5)		

*Sample includes every forty-second patient discharged from all large (15,000+ discharges per year) hospitals in 1972. Basic data used in Table 17-1 were supplied by the Commission on Professional and Hospital Activities. In these data the identities of the individual hospitals were not revealed in any way.

†Actual number of patients in each category.

Table 17-2. Estimated 5-year survival by age and sex 1980-1985

Age (yr)	*Female (%)*	*Male (%)*
Up to 5	98.7	98.4
20-24	99.7	99.1
40-44	98.7	97.7
60-64	93.5	86.2
70-74	84.2	72.5
80 and over	53.0	44.4

Fifty percent of the 80-year-old population will live another 5 years (Table 17-2). In contrast to the earlier years, the elderly black individual has a better life expectancy than his white counterpart.

In all age groups emergency surgery carries a greater risk than the elective planned procedure. In the elderly this is especially true (Table 17-3). Therefore an indicated procedure should be recommended when the patient is "well" and all compromised systems are compensated. The difference in mortality between an individual with a strangulated and a simple hernia or between an individual with a ruptured and an unruptured abdominal aortic aneurysm are well known, and yet many patients are discharged from hospitals every year with these diagnosed conditions untreated primarily on the basis of age. Cole,[8] using U.S. vital statistics information, emphasizes how poorly emergency conditions are tolerated by the elderly. During 1964 there were 884 deaths in the United States from appendicitis in persons 65 years of age or older. This represented one half the deaths from appendicitis in all age groups. This is especially significant, since appendicitis is relatively uncommon past the age of 65 years.

DISCHARGE PLANNING AND TREATMENT GOALS

About 40% of the elderly patients under general hospital care are admitted for surgical treatment.[9] A recent study of posthospital discharge plans involving 545 patients at New York Hospital indicates that 91.8% of hospital discharges returned home and did not require treatment in an extended care facility. Of the patients entering extended care facilities in the New York Hospital study, 82% had a diagnosis involving malignant neoplasms, diseases of the circulatory system, and diseases involving the nerve or sense organs.[10] Posthospitalization plans for geriatric patients also involve nursing home care far less frequently than most physicians realize. Only 5% of geriatric patients need a protective setting at the point of discharge from a hospital.[11]

Table 17-3. Mortality of aged in emergency operations compared with elective operations[4-7]

	Mortality (%)		
Author	*Emergency operations*	*Elective operations*	*Age of patients*
Estes	16.4	5.0	Over 60
Haug and Dale	21.9	5.7	Over 60
Bosch et al.	17.4	8.8	Over 60
Average	19.7	5.9	
Cohn et al.	23.0	4.0	Over 70

It is most appropriate to begin discharge planning on the day the patient is admitted to the hospital, whether or not he is going to an extended care facility. The medical social worker has been a great help in assessing, with appropriate input from the physician, the patient's medical and nonmedical needs so that plans can be implemented to meet these needs. Community services will vary, but they can be coordinated to aid in adjustment to activities of daily living such as colostomy care or amputation until rehabilitation is indicated.

When are the skilled services of a nursing home or shelter care facility appropriate for the patient, or when do they provide simply a convenient discharge plan for the family? Is the family taking over decision making for the patient and treating that patient like a dependent child? Geriatric patients often desire to and are capable of making their own decisions. The medical social worker can investigate and support the proper plan for each patient. Definition of goals of treatment are extremely valuable and place all aspects of a patient management problem in better perspective. Unfortunately the patient may occasionally be treated as a decubitus ulcer rather than as a whole person.

Repeated attempts to secure healing may entail many weeks of hospitalization, after which the patient is returned to the same setting and circumstances that produced the problem originally. It is especially important in the very aged patient for physicians to ask what would they like to accomplish in order to cure or improve the quality of remaining life.

Treatment goals must be carefully communicated to the family, since they are often unaware that the contemplated procedure can be carried out with reasonable safety. Family members frequently are much more receptive to the plan if they can see a design for improving the quality of the patient's remaining life, and they can be of great help in the management of such things as postoperative delirium if counseled about it preoperatively.

HIGH-RISK PATIENT RECOGNITION

It is well recognized that a recent myocardial infarction dramatically increases the risk of surgery. Skinner and Pierce[12] reported their experience with 857 cardiac patients, most of whom were in the geriatric age group. The mortality for individuals who had surgery within 3 months of an acute myocardial infarction was 40%, whereas it was only 14% for those with a healed infarct. At the Mayo Clinic, patients who were operated on within 3 months of infarction had a 37% reinfarction rate. This rate decreased to 16% between 3 and 6 months and remained at 4% to 5% when infarction had occurred more than 6 months before.[13]

An additional group at high risk about whom there are less available data are those patients with an unstable arrhythmia. Every attempt should be made to stabilize the arrhythmia preoperatively. Consultation with the cardiologist and anesthesiologist, together with continuous intraoperative and postoperative cardiac monitoring are essential features of the successful management of this whole group of problems.

Patients with long standing obstructive jaundice frequently deteriorate rapidly following decompressive surgery. Recently preoperative external biliary decompression using percutaneous catheterization of a major biliary radicle has improved the picture. Using this technique, the bilirubin can be lowered preoperatively.

Severe malnutrition associated with hypoalbuminemia is a frequently overlooked high-risk factor, especially in the patient with abdominal neoplasia. Cole[8] states that approximately one half of the patients over 65 years of age requiring surgery for a serious disease will have sustained recent weight loss varying from 5 to 50 pounds. It is his opinion and that of most others that the incidence of complications can be decreased if some of this weight loss can be regained. Oral intake is the most reliable means of achieving weight gain. A carefully planned diet with between-meal feedings after consultation with the dietician is ideal. Often the patient is anorexic, and supplementation of oral intake with tube feedings will be required. Tube feedings should always be initiated as a diluted solution, gradually increasing them to full strength over 3 to 5 days. This will decrease the incidence of diarrhea. All feedings commercially available contain about 1 kcal/ml. Higher caloric concentrations result in unacceptable diarrhea because of hyperosmolarity of the solution. The amount of protein can be varied according to the degree of depletion. In general, those products with the highest protein content are less palatable and must be given by tube. Tube feedings should be administered between meals and at night to avoid interference with oral intake. The rate of administration should be as slow as possible, consistent with infusion of the desired volume. The head of the bed should be elevated. These last precautions are important so as to avoid aspiration, particularly in the debilitated patient. In patients with preoperative or postoperative gastric outlet obstruction placement of a tube in the duodenum for feeding using the gastroscope has been very helpful.

If hypoproteinemia is severe, daily administration of intravenous albumin may be indicated. If the patient is also receiving blood, care must be taken not to overload the circulatory system. It may be prudent in many patients to insert a central venous catheter at this time to monitor central venous pressure. Those patients who cannot be fed because of intestinal obstruction or intestinal fistula today may be repleted by hyperalimentation. Dudrick and Douglas[14] have shown that hyperosmotic solutions (1000 kcal/liter) may be given through catheters placed in the superior vena cava by way of cephalic, subclavian, or external jugular veins. As many as 3000 calories per day derived from hypertonic glucose and amino acid solutions supplemented with sodium, potassium, vitamins, and trace elements can be given. These solutions are commercially available or may be prepared in the hospital pharmacy. Weight gain has been consistently observed, and because of the high blood flow rates in the vena cava, chemical phlebitis usually does not occur. Complications associated with this form of therapy most frequently noted are infection, inability to tolerate the feedings, and rarely hyperosmolar coma.

The nutritionally depleted patient represents one of the clearest indications for retention sutures, especially in the geriatric age group. We use them routinely and especially when the operation is for the treatment of cancer, jaundice, a thoracoabdominal problem, or in a patient taking steroids.

Pulmonary insufficiency is more capable of being evaluated and treated today than ever before. If there is evidence of pulmonary disease by history, physical examination, or roentgenography, pulmonary function studies complemented by blood gas determinations are obtained so that appropriate plans for postoperative pulmonary support can be made. We no longer have any hesitation in keeping an endotracheal tube in place postoperatively for up to 5 days. It is removed only when we are satisfied that the patient can maintain his Po_2 and Pco_2 in a reasonable range without excessive effort. This will be discussed in more detail under postperative care.

Preoperative evidence of impaired liver function is an especially ominous finding when the proposed operation will not provide the liver with some mechanical advantage. Little can usually be done preoperatively to improve liver function other than to correct hypoprothrombinemia by the administration of vitamin K or to delay the procedure while awaiting spontaneous improvement from general supportive measures. Because of the possible implication of the halogenated hydrocarbons in some cases of postoperative hepatitis, our anesthesiologists are using an increasing amount of nitrous-narcotic anesthesia. It is used routinely for all patients with preexisting liver disease or for those who have had a recent anesthetic with halothane. (See Chapter 18.)

The importance of assessing renal function preoperatively has already been mentioned. The blood urea nitrogen (BUN) and creatinine levels are primarily used in this evaluation. It has been our experience that blood in the gastrointestinal tract alone seldom elevates the BUN above 50 mg/100 ml (prerenal azotemia). Urea levels above 50 mg/100 ml in the bleeding patient usually indicate intrinsic renal disease. In the elective setting when uremia is present, attempts to return the BUN to normal by hyperhydration are carried out. Even when these chemistries are normal, *all* elderly patients are given 1 liter of 5% dextrose and Ringer's lactate solution between midnight and their *early* morning operation so as to avoid arrival in the operating room in a dehydrated state. Patients who in the past have been considered categorically inoperable with BUN levels in excess of 100 mg/100 ml have now been operated on successfully after consultation with the nephrologist and either peritoneal dialysis or hemodialysis have been done. Although peritoneal dialysis may be carried out after intraabdominal surgery, we prefer hemodialysis, especially in the presence of a draining fistula, colostomy, or anastomosis of any type.

Although some medical centers have recommended the use of prophylactic anticoagulation in all patients undergoing major surgery, we have restricted this therapeutic modality to the high-risk patient. This group would include, for example, the patient with a prior history of pulmonary embolism or thrombophlebitis; patients who will either require prolonged bed rest or who are no longer ambulatory; patients undergoing major lower extremity surgery (e.g., hip fracture); the extremely obese patient; and patients undergoing major cancer surgery. From this list, it is obvious that a high proportion of the geriatric population will have prophylactic heparin administration in their preoperative plan. Heparin is usually administered in 5000-unit doses every 12 hours (subcutaneously). Heparin administration is begun 2 hours preoperatively and continued until the patient is about ready for discharge.[15]

Although we have not used external pneumatic compression (EPC) as prophylaxis against deep vein thrombosis, there is an increasing amount of evidence that it works as well as or better than prophylactic heparin. In neurosurgical and urologic patients where any bleeding complication would be especially undesirable, EPC may find its greatest usefulness. The major deterrents to more widespread use of this technique would seem to be as follows: (1) patient comfort; (2) cost of the equipment; and (3) difficulties associated with the application and movement of the equipment.[16]

PREOPERATIVE WORKUP

Elderly patients must be more carefully evaluated before surgery than are their younger counterparts. The aged cannot be specifically evaluated by age group or by general appearance. One patient may appear older than his stated age and yet have excellent function of all organ systems, whereas another appears younger than expected and yet has severe coronary artery or renal disease. Every attempt should be made to eliminate unexpected pathologic conditions preoperatively. Although the yield may be relatively small, it has become increasingly our practice to consider an upper gastrointestinal series, lower gastrointestinal series, gallbladder evaluation, intravenous pyelogram, SMA-12, complete blood cell count, electrolyte determination, electrocardiogram, chest x-ray examination, and proctoscopy as a "routine workup" for the patient over 65 years of age who is to undergo elective major surgery. In this group the axiom that "it is easier to stay out of trouble, than it is to get out of trouble" is especially true.

At this time when greater and greater reliance is being placed on the laboratory evaluation of the patient, it is important to emphasize the role of the physical examination in the diagnosis of disease in the aged surgical patient. Probably the greatest return in terms of treatable previously unrecognized and often asymptomatic disease on physical examination is that of the peripheral vascular system. This is also that area of the anatomy that is best assessed by physical examination and yet most overlooked. The asymptomatic carotid stenosis and abdominal or popliteal aneurysm are forerunners of their complications, which are potentially lethal or nearly totally disabling. All are probably present for long periods before their complications occur. Elaborate descriptions of liver size, heart murmurs, or the optic fundus are frequently present in the physical examination with no mention of the auscultatory findings over the carotid or the size of the abdominal aorta. The former findings are interesting, contribute to a diagnosis, and are important, but they frequently lead to no important treatment, in contrast to the latter. The physical examination in the aged therefore should be complete, but with special emphasis on those areas in which degenerative and neoplastic disease are common.

Greater use of noninvasive or less invasive diagnostic procedures has recently expanded rapidly because of the availability of new mechanical devices and specialists experienced in their use. Almost every blood vessel in the body can now be examined by arteriography, either for evidence of intrinsic disease, displacement by extrinsic disease, or development of tumor vasculature. Fiber-optic endoscopy of the upper gastrointestinal tract with routine biopsy provides an increasingly reliable method of diagnosis. Use of an instrument to cannulate the common bile and pancreatic ducts is becoming routine in many hospitals. Fiber-optic colonoscopy in the hands of an expert has almost eliminated the need for transabdominal colonic polypectomy in our institution. The procedure requires elaborate cleansing and much patience, but these considerations are minor when weighed against those of general anesthesia, celiotomy, and colotomy in the aged. This technique will be elaborated further under operative treatment.

Percutaneous liver biopsy and liver biopsy through the peritoneoscope have permitted the establishment of metastatic disease in the liver without formal laparotomy with increasing frequency. A common diagnostic problem, namely obstructive as opposed to hepatogenous jaundice, has recently been elucidated further by the radiologist. The percutaneous transhepatic cholangiogram using a thin-walled (Chiba) needle has proven to be very safe and effective in our institution.[17]

POLYSURGERY AND A PREOPERATIVE PLAN

Since each operation performed has potential complications, no matter how small the statistical incidence, the mature surgeon weighs the question of multiple operations at one sitting carefully. A cholecystectomy that might be accompanied by an appendectomy on a patient at 35 years of age should not be performed on a patient 75 years of age. The 75-year-old patient has almost no statistical chance of developing appendicitis and will not tolerate a wound infection as well as his younger counterpart. An asymptomatic solitary large gallstone should be left undisturbed at the time of an emergency procedure for a perforated ulcer for similar reasons. A significant complication of either procedure may lead to others and start a chain of events that cannot be reversed.

As much as is possible preoperatively, all alternatives for intraoperative management should be evaluated in light of the patient's total picture. The surgeon dealing with this group should be completely familiar with all of the techniques available for staging standard approaches to a surgical problem. The Hartmann procedure, for example, is useful in the management of neoplastic and inflammatory lesions of the lower sigmoid colon when an anastomosis is considered undesirable or the distal sigmoid cannot be brought up to the skin.[18] In most instances it is wise to adhere to the preoperative estimate of what the patient will tolerate rather than to extend the procedure because the patient seems to be doing well. The ability to tolerate the procedure is an unreliable guide to the patient's postoperative course. The operation that combines the least morbidity consistent with the patient's life expectancy and other diseases, together with the greatest chance of success, is our goal.

At certain ages many operations commonly performed in the pregeriatric period are probably rarely indicated; that is, their potential benefit is exceeded by the risk, and in most cases alternative nonsurgical plans of management are available. Examples might be varicose veins in the absence of ulceration, hemorrhoids, and an asymptomatic 3 cm solitary gallstone. A long list could be compiled but would be heavily dependent on specific information about each patient.

Local anesthesia seems to be better tolerated by the older patient, and it is our routine practice to use it, for example, on all types of inguinal hernia in older men. Premedication with moderate amounts of meperidine hydrochloride and a tranquilizer are essential components of this plan. These patients can usually eat lunch and can walk to the bathroom shortly after their operation. Special benefits of this technique are the absence of postoperative delirium or episodes of urinary retention.

The use of prophylactic antibiotics has been avoided for many years, since it was shown that the practice frequently led to the overgrowth of more resistant strains of bacteria with an actual increase in the number of surgical infections. More recently it has been suggested that if antibiotics are administered preoperatively and intraoperatively as well as postoperatively to those patients who are considered to have a high risk of infection or in whom an infection might result in severe morbidity or mortality (vascular case), the incidence of infection may be decreased. It is our present practice, for example, to begin broad-spectrum antibiotic coverage preoperatively on the patient who is to undergo an abdominal perineal resection or vascular surgery where a prosthetic graft is to be used.

OPERATIVE CARE

Intraoperative monitoring

The same careful monitoring that is essential in the postoperative period is also critically important in the operative period. The usual monitoring of pulse, cuff blood pressure, and electrocardiogram should be carried out on all patients. If the operative procedure is lengthy or if the field is to involve the pelvis, a Foley closed urinary drainage system will also be needed. The urine collection bag, if true monitoring of urinary output is to be done, should be at the head of the operating table. Temperature monitoring should probably be used for all major cases, since significant hypothermia is a common sequela of a long operative procedure in which viscera are exposed. It is not uncommon at the end of a long vascular case where multiple units of blood and many liters of crystalloid have been used to find a rectal temperature of 94° F or lower. Immediate postoperative temperatures of 90° F have been noted on two recent cases of ruptured abdominal aortic aneurysm. This degree of hypothermia in itself can lead to death secondary to ventricular fibrillation (said to occur at 89° F). Thus any and all measures to maintain a reasonable body temperature are indicated and include (1) warming of *all* fluids (both blood and crystalloid); (2) maintaining a reasonable operating room temperature; (3) attempting to maintain the viscera within the abdominal cavity or covered with warm laparotomy pads; (4) use of warm saline lavage of the abdominal cavity where not contraindicated; and (5) the shortest operative time possible.

More sophisticated monitoring in the critical elderly patient should be available for ideal operative care. The use of continuous arterial and venous pressures including pulmonary artery pressures can be an invaluable adjunct to the usual monitoring devices; as their availability increases, they will become more routine for any critically ill elderly patient undergoing major surgery.

Choice of incision

The single most important factor in choosing the incision is the consideration of ease of proper exposure. Each surgeon will develop favorite incisions for specific surgical procedures; however, the habitus of the individual patient should be considered rather than relying on the same incision for all patients. A cholecystectomy in a patient with a very narrow costal margin can usually be carried out more easily through a vertical incision, which should be used rather than the subcostal incision. In the very obese patient with a pendulous apron, a supraumbilical transverse incision can often be substituted for a vertical incision and thus avoid the deep fat of the apron and the common wound seromas and infections. So, although exposure must be the foremost consideration in the choice of an incision, the individual patient's body build should be carefully evaluated as well.

Specific operative procedures

A brief review of all types of operative procedures would be impossible in a book covering all areas of geriatric care; furthermore, it would lead to a rather worthless outline without depth in any one area. Therefore certain important areas in geriatric surgery will be covered with some degree of detail.

Colonic polyps. Tremendous advances have been made in the treatment of colon polyps as a result of the development of the fiber-optic colonoscope. This is of great benefit to the elderly patient in whom a major abdominal operation for removal of a 2 to 5 cm polyp might carry significant morbidity and definite occasional mortality. A 150-cm colonoscope is used and usually allows complete evaluation of the colon up to the cecum. Occasionally a 180-cm colonoscope is necessary to reach the cecum in patients with elongated colons. The sigmoid sheath is rarely used today. Now polyps that would have been followed with lower gastrointestinal examinations every 6 months or polyps that would have required transabdominal polypectomy can be removed with a snare by an experienced colonoscopist. Polyps removed are then examined histologically, and in general, if a focus of carcinoma does not involve the stalk, the elderly poor-risk patient can probably be considered cured. In the younger patient, invasion beyond the basement membrane should be considered the point at which resection is then undertaken.

In the hands of an experienced colonoscopist the procedure of polypectomy can be carried out without significant morbidity and almost no mortality. Wolff and Shinya[19] have reported 499 polypectomies with no deaths and only two significant complications (bleeding in one and localized limited perforation in another). Certainly, in the treatment of polyps in the elderly, colonoscopy has made possible a tremendous reduction in morbidity and mortality.

Acute colonic obstruction. Carcinoma, diverticulitis, and volvulus are the three most common causes of acute large bowel obstruction. Although these are pathologic states that can affect all ages, they are of special importance in the elderly because of the higher mortality associated with them. Acute large bowel obstruction is usually accompanied by a combination of pain and constipation. Unfortunately, in elderly persons constipation is a rather ordinary situation and often does not cause appropriate concern. Vomiting is often a late finding, although in 31% of a combined series[20] that we contributed to, it occurred early presumably as a result of a reflex response to colon distention. It is interesting that diarrhea can be a part of the presenting symptom complex (19% of patients); this is probably related to a combination of hyperperistalsis with emptying of the colon distal to the obstruction and also passage of liquid stool around a partial obstruction. Two thirds of the patients in our combined series were over 60 years of age, with a large number in their seventies and eighties. Proper diagnosis is accomplished by a lower gastrointestinal series; it is essential that this be done before an upper gastrointestinal series. The latter, done as an initial study, can convert a partial obstruction to a complete obstruction by means of inspissated barium occluding a narrowed colonic lumen.

It is rare that a proctoscopic examination is necessary for diagnosis; however, it is of extreme importance in proper treatment of sigmoid volvulus. This entity is of particular interest because of its frequency in the elderly, chronically constipated patient. Its diagnosis is initially based on the characteristic plain film (Fig. 17-2), which has been described as a "bent inner tube sign." It is usually advisable to confirm this diagnosis with a lower gastrointestinal series (Fig. 17-3), since colonic ileus can occasionally give a similar plain film appearance.

Initially treatment should be proctoscopic tube decompression, unless there are findings that suggest strangulation (abdominal tenderness, rigidity, or leukocytosis). If there is difficulty decompressing by proctoscopic techniques, colonoscopy can be also used and may help avoid emergency surgery. This technique also allows a direct view of the sigmoid mucosa, confirming viability.[21] If a bloody, foul-smelling material is evacuated at the time of decompression or if it is impossible to straighten the twisted segment, surgical exploration is necessary. In our series 17 patients had successful tube decompression with only one death. It is important to plan on elective surgery when the patient is stable because recurrent volvulus is the rule rather than the exception. Drapanas and Stewart[22] found a rate of 2.9 episodes of volvulus per patient in their series of 40 patients. Elective surgical treatment has usually consisted of sigmoid resection; however, in the poor-risk pa-

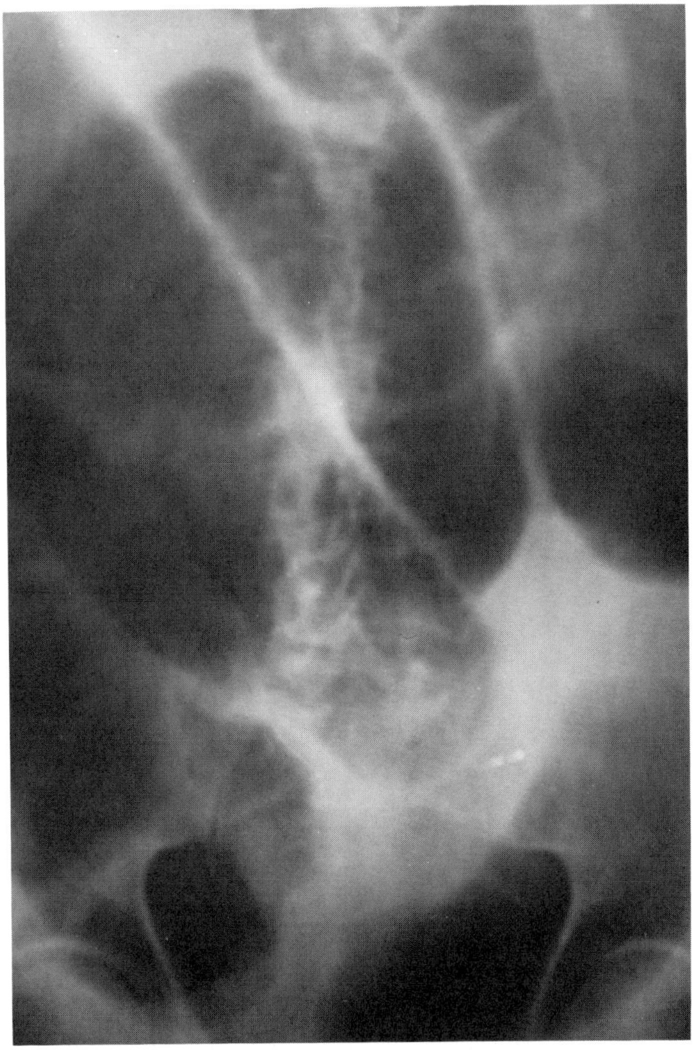

Fig. 17-2. Characteristic bent inner tube sign of sigmoid volvulus.

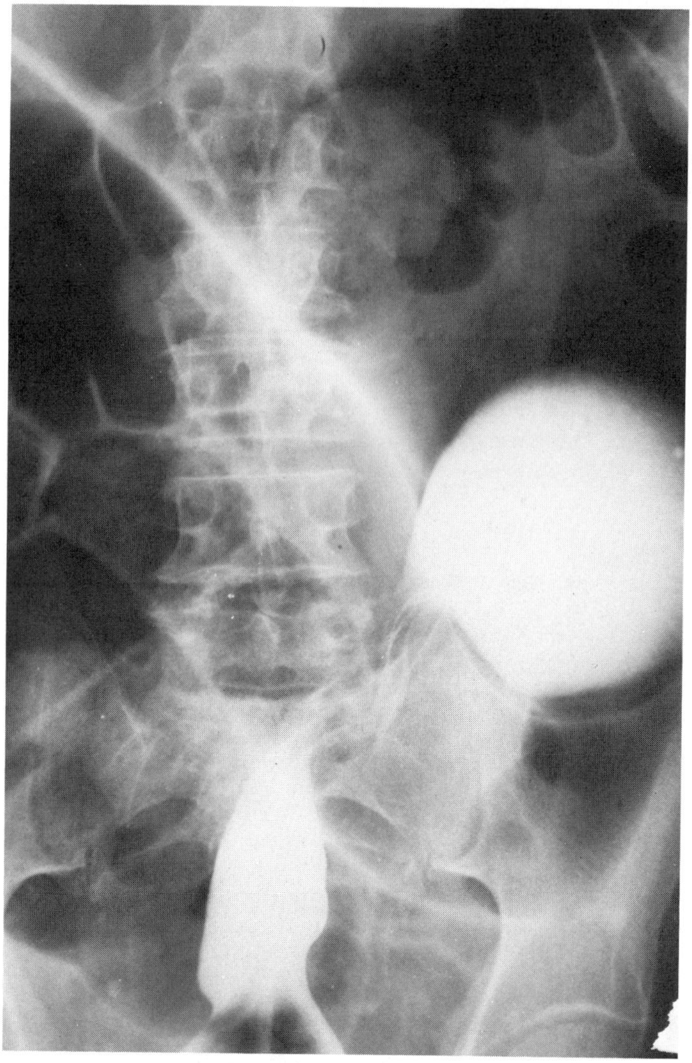

Fig. 17-3. Bird's beak sign of sigmoid volvulus.

tient the use of Foley catheter fixation to the abdominal wall has been reported as an alternative.

Acute colonic obstruction caused by diverticulitis and carcinoma present a similar clinical picture, and it is often difficult to differentiate these two diagnoses with a lower gastrointestinal examination (Fig. 17-4). It is not really necessary to have a definite diagnosis; it is only necessary to know that there is an organic obstruction in the sigmoid in urgent need of decompression. This is carried out quickly and simply by way of a small right upper quadrant transverse incision with a loop colostomy without exploration. In 8% of the patients, however, there will be an associated perforation. One half of these will be found in the cecal area, and in those cases a right transverse colostomy will be totally inadequate therapy. It will be necessary in this small group of patients to exteriorize the cecal perforation as the decompressive procedure. In the 40% of cases that perforate in the region of the sigmoid obstruction, right transverse colostomy with drainage will often be adequate therapy; however, there is a definite place for resection with a Hartmann procedure in these cases. Overall, the mortality for acute large bowel obstruction is extremely high (37% in our combined series), whether the patients are treated in a private, county, or Veterans Administration hospital.

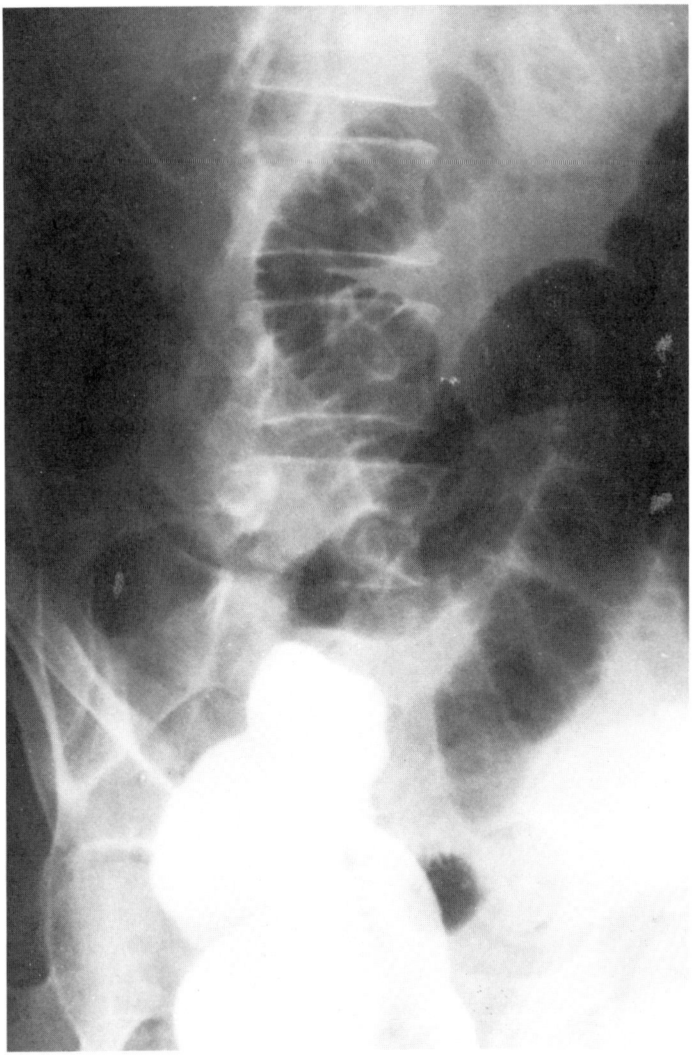

Fig. 17-4. Obstruction secondary to carcinoma, which can be difficult to differentiate from diverticulitis.

This is probably related more to the age of the patients and their associated medical diseases than to the type of management. The only hope for a significant reduction in mortality lies in an earlier diagnosis of the condition at a stage before true complete obstruction occurs, allowing for controlled one-stage resection.

Cecal volvulus. Although cecal volvulus is considered a type of colonic obstruction, its clinical presentation is truly unique. Approximately 40% of these patients are over 50 years of age[23] and are often quite elderly. The majority of patients will have cramping pain, and almost all will have abdominal distention. Interestingly, because of the acute presentation and the low level of the obstruction, vomiting is not a common symptom. Plain x-ray films are often diagnostic, showing the dilated cecum in the midline, but lower gastrointestinal examinations are necessary to confirm the diagnosis.

Although laporatomy is usually required for cecal volvulus, colonoscopy has been used successfully at our institution in poor-risk patients.[24] The usual surgical procedure is resection with primary anastomosis; however, cecostomy tube fixation can also be used in the poor-risk patient.

Acute diverticulitis. Acute inflammation is certainly the most common complication of diverticular disease. Acute diverticulitis can appear in middle age patients, but the majority of cases occur in the elderly. Patients usually have left lower quadrant pain, some change in bowel habits with either constipation or diarrhea, and fever. Physical examination reveals left lower quadrant tenderness and guarding. Many patients demonstrate a tender mass either on abdominal, rectal, or pelvic examination. Treatment is initially medical with bowel rest (nothing by mouth, nasogastric decompression if vomiting or distention occurs) combined with broad spectrum gram-negative antibiotic coverage. Lower gastrointestinal barium studies are contraindicated in this acute phase but can be done when the acute symptoms have resolved. Interestingly, lower gastrointestinal radiographic examinations often fail to reveal such conditions as sinus or mass. Thus the diagnosis is clinical. The outlined treatment program should be continued despite failure of radiographic confirmation.

Surgical intervention is essential in patients who do not respond to the medical program and who develop progressive sepsis or peritonitis. The Hartmann procedure (two-stage procedure with resection, closure of rectal stump, and sigmoid end colostomy as first stage and reanastomosis at second stage) is the ideal operation since it allows direct visualization and resection of the pathologic condition and is accomplished in only two stages.[25] There definitely are patients with a severe form of phlegmonous rectosigmoid inflammation in whom the standard three-stage therapy (transverse colostomy, stage 1; resection and anastomosis, stage 2; closure colostomy, stage 3) is still preferred. This type of diverticulitis has been described by Morgenstern as "malignant" diverticulitis[26] and is usually seen in the elderly and best treated with the conventional three-stage procedure.

Colon ileus. Colon ileus (pseudoobstruction of the colon) is an entity that is being recognized more frequently and will be seen in the geriatric patient. Its occurrence in Parkinson's disease has long been recognized. It has been thought to result from a combination of the basic degenerative disease and from the medical therapy. Colon ileus also occurs with pancreatitis, with blunt abdominal trauma associated with rib and spinal fractures, in postoperative pelvic surgery, and after acute appendicitis. Regardless of the underlying etiology, recognition of this entity is important because it can completely mimic an acute large bowel obstruction caused by carcinoma or diverticulitis of the sigmoid. Lower gastrointestinal examination in all patients with a dilated colon (Fig. 17-5) should be done to recognize this entity. The usual therapy is nonsurgical and includes nasogastric decompression, careful monitoring and replacement of fluids and electrolytes (especially potassium, which often plays a role if severe hypokalemia is present), and frequent rectal tube insertions. It is not only important to recognize this entity to differentiate it from a true colon obstruction, but it is also important to recognize the rare sequelae of this process, that is, cecal perforation. Sixteen cases of cecal perforation[27] have been reviewed occurring in association with colon ileus so that although it is uncommon, it is not rare. We have had two cases of cecal perforation[28] associated with adynamic ileus, and we believe that some important guidelines should be laid down. Once the diagnosis of colon ileus has been made, careful nasogastric decompression, intravenous fluid with potassium and magnesium therapy (if indicated), rectal tube decompression every 2 hours, positional change, and discontinuation of anticholinergic and antiparkinsonian medication should be instituted. The patient should then be observed with frequent physical examinations, white blood cell counts, and abdominal plain films.

When the cecum is greater than 10 cm in diameter, the patient must be considered at risk of cecal perforation. If the conservative measures of nasogastric decompression (to eliminate further swallowed air) and rectal tubes have not been successful in reducing cecal size, then the patient should undergo emergency colonoscopy with intubation of the cecum to allow decompression. This procedure can be carried out in the unprepared patient since the large size of the colon allows for easy passage of the colonoscope despite the presence of stool.[29] Occasionally repeat colonoscopy with further cecal decompression is necessary before the colon ileus resolves. This simple method of management should effectively prevent the dreaded complication of cecal blow-out without requiring the usual transverse colostomy or cecostomy.

Retained common duct stones. Any surgical innovation that lessens the need for major abdominal surgery is of great significance, particularly to an elderly poor-risk patient. The treat-

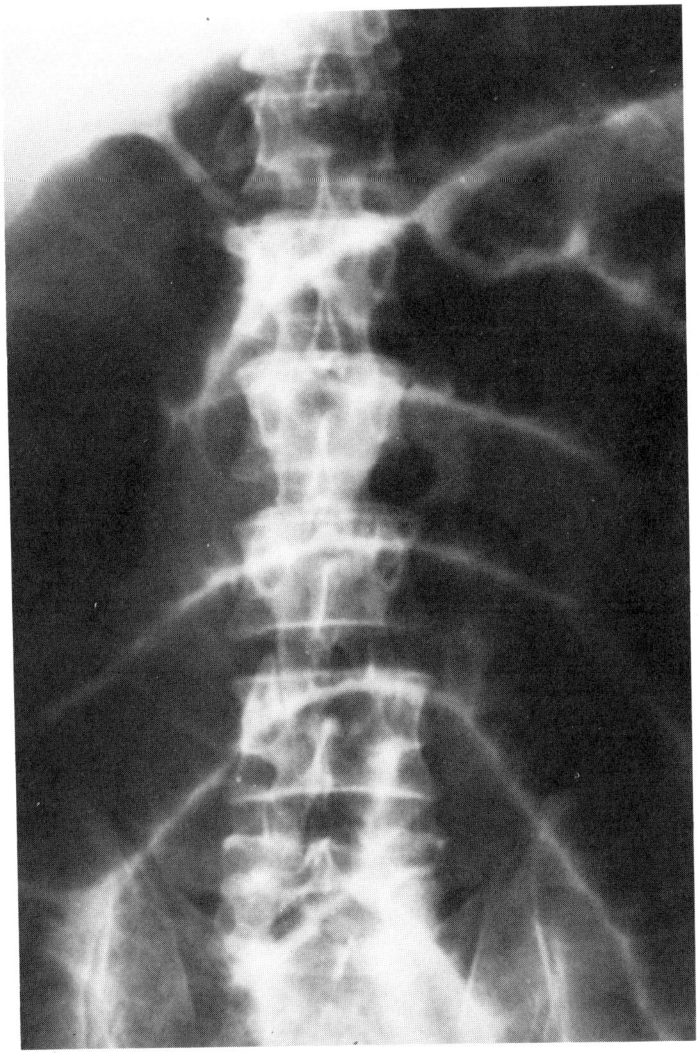

Fig. 17-5. Ileus with large and small bowel distention.

ment of retained common duct stones has undergone tremendous change in the last 5 years with the development of safe nonoperative techniques. The importance of these techniques is realized when one considers that there are approximately 5000 patients out of the 333,000 patients in whom cholecystectomies were done each year in the United States who will need secondary surgical procedures for removal of retained common duct stones.[30] Many of these, of course, are geriatric patients.

Various nonoperative techniques have been tried, beginning in 1891 with ether instillation, flushing with large volumes of solution G (used for dissolution of calcium-containing urinary calculi),[31] and more recently flushing with heparin[32] or cholate solution.[33] All of these techniques have had some success; however, the more recent mechanical approaches have the most promise.

Mazzariello[33] has reported the largest experience using a special forceps passed through the well-formed T tube tract with a success rate of 92% in 204 patients. Our technique and the one that is used more commonly in the United States[30] entails the use of a steerable No. 13 French catheter, which passes through a No. 14 T tube tract. Through this is passed a Dormia stone basket (identical to that used to remove ureteral stones), which engages the stone for removal.

Larger stones can be crushed and then withdrawn or pushed through into the duodenum. This technique carries a high success rate without significant morbidity (prophylactic antibiotics are generally used to reduce the chance of introducing infection) and can avoid reoperation in over 90% of patients with retained common duct stones. To make this technique feasible the surgeon should use at least a No. 14, preferably a No. 16 T tube, and should bring the T tube to the skin with a short tract at a right angle to the common duct. The use of this technique should greatly reduce the 5% mortality that reoperation for retained common duct stones carries and should prevent an elderly frail patient from undergoing additional major surgery.

In poor-risk elderly patients who have retained common duct stones and who do not have a T tube (months or years after biliary surgery), medical treatment has been carried out using chenodeoxycholic acid with some success. The other nonoperative method is endoscopic papillotomy. Although this is available, it has serious potential morbidity (hemorrhage and perforation) reported at 8% and mortality of 1.5% and should be used cautiously by endoscopists trained and experienced with this technique.[34]

Ascending cholangitis. Acute suppurative cholangitis is an entity that can affect any age group; however, the majority of patients are elderly. (Hampson's series of patients average 71 years of age[35]; Ostermiller's series average 74 years of age.[36]) The clinical diagnosis is based on recognition of Charcot's triad, which includes jaundice, upper abdomen pain, and chills with fever. Reynolds and Dargan[37] added shock and central nervous system depression, arriving at the presently recognized pentad of symptoms. The cause of the obstruction is usually choledocholithiasis, but it may be caused by benign or malignant strictures, or even pancreatitis.

It is important to recognize that there are patients with mild forms of cholangitis who do not develop the true urgent condition known as acute obstructive suppurative cholangitis.[38] These patients with lesser forms may only have a few symptoms of the pentad, with fever of undetermined origin or right upper quadrant pain and tenderness, and their condition will be mistaken for the usual cholecystitis. Thus if a patient has typical cholecystitis but moderate hyperbilirubinemia (Dow's series had bilirubin levels averaging 10 mg/100 ml)[39] and a temperature in the 101° to 104° F range with typical spiking (pus under pressure), cholangitis should be the diagnosis. At this point rapid therapeutic and diagnostic steps are indicated. Blood cultures should be drawn, since these will usually be positive (75% of our patients[40]) and can guide antibiotic therapy within 24 hours. A positive culture can also help to differentiate acute hepatitis in the obstructive phase and cholangitis.

Antibiotic therapy should begin immediately and should cover *Escherichia coli* and *Klebsiella*, which are the most commonly cultured pathogens (ampicillin, cephalothin, or cefamandole). Usual basic therapy with intravenous hydration, nasogastric decompression, and hourly monitoring of urine output is instituted. Vitamin K is often needed if there is complete long-standing ductal obstruction, and steroid administration may be indicated if the patient is hypotensive.

The decision to operate at this point is based on whether the patient's condition is improving significantly. As long as the patient's condition is improving, conservative therapy can be continued. Surgical intervention is carried out on an emergency basis if there is shock or delirium or if the patient's condition is not improving.

Surgical intervention, whether carried out on an urgent or elective basis, should be accomplished during the patient's present hospitalization. There is no place for discharge with elective exploration scheduled in 3 months as might be done for a patient with a resolving uncomplicated cholecystitis. The surgical treatment in the acutely ill patient should be rapid T tube decompression of the common bile duct. Cholecystotomy is *not* a method of adequate common duct decompression in this disease state. Whether one does a complete procedure (cholecystectomy, careful common duct exploration, and then placement of a T tube) depends on the status of the patient. In a stable patient undergoing elective surgery, the full procedure is, of course, carried out.

The mortality for the full-blown syndrome has been reported by Dow and Lindenauer as 61%.[39] This included a 100% mortality in non-surgically treated patients and 40% in surgically treated patients. The high mortality in these correctly treated patients probably represents uncontrolled sepsis with the fatal sequelae of multiple hepatic abscesses. To prevent this, early aggressive surgical therapy is essential and can lead to an acceptable mortality. Twenty-one surgical patients at our institution with documented cholangitis were managed with the foregoing protocol with only three deaths—certainly an acceptable mortality.

Acute mesenteric vascular occlusion. Acute mesenteric vascular occlusion affects primarily the elderly (Pierce and Brockenbrough's series[41] noted 75% of patients were over 70 years of age) and carries a mortality between 80% and 100%. It certainly could be considered the most fatal of the surgical diseases affecting the geriatric age group.

When one analyzes the etiologies involved in this syndrome, it is somewhat of a surprise to find that most cases are not caused by thromboses or emboli but are caused by an entity called *nonocclusive mesenteric infarction*. This entity probably accounts for 50% of cases of mesenteric infarction.[42] It often occurs in association with low flow states such as congestive heart failure, myocardial infarction with congestive failure, severe dehydration, and hemorrhage with hypotension. Digitalis has been incriminated as one possible cause and is thought to increase mesenteric vascular resistance. Diuretics, particularly thiazides, have also been thought to cause some mesenteric vascular spasm resulting in such decreased intestinal blood flow that necrosis develops.

The next most common cause of mesenteric infarction is thrombosis, occurring superimposed on an atherosclerotic superior mesenteric artery. Embolic occlusion accounts for less than 10% of the patients in most series, which is unfortunate because this group of patients can definitely be helped with rapid surgical therapy. Mesenteric venous thrombosis occurs with about the same frequency as arterial emboli and is now being seen less frequently. Wilson and Block[43] have suggested that control of intraperitoneal infection with antibiotics and other surgical resources might account for this decreasing incidence of venous thrombosis.

The high mortality in this disease spectrum is partly related to the difficulty in early diagnosis. These patients often have vague abdominal pain, vomiting, and diarrhea, and their condition can often look like diverticulitis or an incomplete small bowl obstruction. Upper gastrointestinal or rectal bleeding, diffuse abdominal rigidity, and severe hypovolemia and acidosis are all late findings that usually indicate full-blown infarction.

Management is by rapid stabilization and exploratory laparotomy. Angiography, in general, is not needed and can waste extremely valuable time. On exploration if there is a slightly bluish small bowel but no gross infarction, there is an excellent chance for salvage. If there are good pulsations to the level of the intestinal wall without any venous thrombi, one can consider the process to be nonocclusive and should close the abdomen. Management would then include the administration of low molecular weight dextran, maintenance of good cardiac output with isoproterenol (Isuprel) or dopamine, and provision of adequate intravascular volume. With this plan of management we have been able to prevent necrosis and obtain a low mortality.

On exploration, if there are scattered areas of gangrene throughout the small and large bowel with good pulsations and no venous thrombi, the diagnosis is again nonocclusive mesenteric infarction. This situation is almost always fatal, and if the entire small bowel is involved, closure without resection is indicated, since the mortality is 100% regardless of what is done.

Recognition of embolic as opposed to thrombotic occlusion is of extreme importance because vascular management of the two is different. If the area of dusky or infarcted small intestine begins several inches beyond the ligament of Treitz (usually 12 inches), embolism is generally the cause since occlusion usually occurs distal to the first two jejunal branches. This calls for rapid exposure of the superior mesenteric artery at its junction with the transverse mesocolon. Embolectomy of many of the distal branches should be done, including the right colic, ileocolic, and jejunal branches. Proximal superior mesenteric artery embolectomy is then done, and the arteriotomy is closed. At this point it is valuable to cover the bowel with moist warm laparotomy pads and to wait for 30 minutes to determine how much of the bowel is truly necrotic. Saving an additional several inches of ileum can make a tremendous difference in the degree of postoperative diarrhea and is well worth a period of 30 minutes of close observation with renewed blood flow. After this period all grossly necrotic bowel is resected, and anastomosis is carried out.

Thrombotic occlusion, on the other hand, occurs with duskiness or necrosis extending all the way to the ligament of Treitz, since the occlusion occurs at the origin of the superior mesenteric artery. Treatment should be saphenous vein bypass from the aorta to the superior mesenteric artery distal to the occlusion. Dacron grafts could be used, but the risk of contamination is significant, even when the bowel is only severely ischemic. Second–look procedures (12 to 24 hours after the initial operation) are often helpful in picking up small areas of additional necrosis, which can then be resected before significant peritoneal soilage occurs.

The preceding program of operative management will make possible the salvaging of more of these patients; however, mortality will continue to remain high because of the advanced state of necrosis of the small bowel in the majority of patients. Effective improvement of the now dismal treatment results in this disease will require better recognition of patients with intestinal angina. These patients have postprandial abdominal pain and weight loss (average 12.8 kg),[44] and their condition can only be discovered through the use of angiography. Revascularization in this elective situation can be accomplished with an acceptable mortality (4 deaths in 23 operated patients in a recent series)[44] and can prevent the 95% mortality of complete vascular occlusion.[45]

Rectal prolapse. Rectal prolapse, although not limited to the elderly, occurs primarily in patients in their seventies and eighties. The following is the simplest and most widely used classification[46]:

Type I (false prolapse). This is a protrusion of rectal mucosa for a distance of 1 to 3 cm. This type is most commonly associated with severe hemorrhoidal disease.

Type II. This is essentially an intussusception of all layers of the rectum and rectosigmoid through the anal canal but without a sliding hernia of the pouch of Douglas.

Type III (complete or true). This is a sliding hernia of the pouch of Douglas together with the intussusception described in type II.

The best explanation of the etiology of this disease is that it is an intussusception of the rectosigmoid brought on by prolonged marked straining. All the other changes that occur (cul-de-sac sliding hernia, loss of angle of rectum with anal canal, looseness of supporting structures of rectum, weakness of pelvic diaphragm, and incontinence) can be considered secondary. Altemeier et al.[47] consider the sliding hernia to be the primary pathologic condition; however, intussusception is probably more widely accepted as the basis for the disease.

One of the major problems associated with prolapses of types II and III is incontinence. This is an inevitable result of having the anal sphincter constantly dilated by the protruding intussusceptum. Although Altemeier et al. indicate that most of the patients in their series regain continence postoperatively, the general experience would indicate a high rate of continued incontinence in these elderly patients, particularly in those with neurologic deficits.

Surgical correction of prolapse is indicated, since although often it will not correct incontinence, it will correct the protruding mass of rectum and rectosigmoid, which is certainly bothersome both to patients and to those caring for them. There have been over 50 surgical procedures devised to treat prolapse,[48] which is an immediate indication that none of the procedures is completely ideal. For the type I (false) prolapse a radical hemorrhoidectomy (Whitehead procedure) is adequate and gives good results. It is generally accepted that for the extremely poor-risk patients with types II and III prolapse, an anal encircling procedure can be carried out safely under local anesthesia. The encircling can be done with silver wire (Thiersch's operation) or monofilament nylon.[49] Regardless of what material is used, breakage, impaction, protrusion, and infection are unfortunately the usual outcome with time.

The transabdominal approach with anterior resection and fixation probably has the lowest rate of recurrence; however, because of its magnitude, this procedure should be reserved for the excellent-risk patients.

Perineal one-stage repair as described by Altemeier[47] has an exceedingly high success rate (only three recurrences in 106 patients); however, it has the inherent morbidity of a pull-through anastomosis (four perineal abscesses). We have used a transsacral repair similar to that described by Davidian and Thomas[50] in which the levators are approximated in front of the rectum, recreating the acute angle of the rectoanal junction. This has the advantage of a simple transsacral approach and avoids the morbidity of resection and anastomosis. Long-term evaluation of this procedure will be necessary; however, it seems to provide an approach with low morbidity and low recurrence. (Davidian and Thomas report no recurrence in 30 patients.)

Lower extremity gangrene and amputation. Regardless of the advancement in vascular surgery, major lower limb amputations will continue to be necessary in those elderly patients with gangrenous foot changes without reconstructable vascular occlusions. These elderly patients are often diabetic (incidence ranges from 38% to 65% in various series), and the average age is about 65 years.

When the patient with a gangrenous foot is evaluated and an amputation is decided on, several decisions must be made before surgery is undertaken. First is the patient's condition suitable for a major surgical procedure at this time? Many times local refrigeration can be used to isolate the gangrenous foot while the patient's cardiac, renal, and other parameters are stabilized. Once the patient's condition will allow an amputation, the level at which amputation will be carried out must be determined. Maintenance of maximum length is of great importance; however, achieving a usable stump that will heal well is also equally important. Determining the level of amputation in these patients can often be extremely difficult, especially in those patients without distal pulses. Use of noninvasive methods, such as the Doppler pressure method, has not resolved the question, and no patient should be denied conservative amputation based on Doppler studies alone.[51]

It should be mentioned that one report[52] indicates success with use of Doppler studies in predicting level of amputation. However, the principle of a forefoot amputation as a trial despite low Doppler pressures is still preferred. For isolated gangrene of a toe, when the foot is warm, ray resection with the distal one third to one half of the metatarsal can often give excellent results. This is certainly the procedure of choice in the patient with foot pulses and isolated gangrene of one digit. Simple disarticulation of a toe, leaving the cartilaginous metatarsal head, is a poor amputation and will usually not heal because of the inadequate blood supply of the cartilage.

When several digits are gangrenous but the foot is otherwise viable with good pulses and no evidence of infection, a transmetatarsal amputation can often be successful. This is certainly worthy of a trial in this type of patient because it will maintain a potential for ambulation without prosthesis.

Unfortunately, the majority of the patients seen will have rather extensive gangrene of the foot without foot pulses and will not be suitable candidates for these limited amputations. In these patients the decision is usually between a below-the-knee as opposed to an above-the-knee amputation. The dilemma the surgeon faces is this: If the knee is sacrificed, good wound healing will surely result, but the patient may be unable to walk again; if the knee is saved, the functional result will be better, but the risk of wound problems is far greater (necrosis and infection). Formerly the decision for a below-the-knee amputation was only made in a patient with a palpable popliteal pulse; however, today a below-the-knee amputation should be considered in all patients. Use of a long, well-vascularized posterior flap is probably the most important technical point making this approach possible. Immediate postoperative prosthesis technique has been reported effectively to allow early ambulation, lowered wound pain, and better wound healing. This technique, however, is not widely available. Even in the bedridden patient, preservation of the knee joint can be of great aid in terms of providing leverage that can allow the patient far greater mobility for transfer from bed to wheelchair. Thus preservation of the knee joint should be considered in most patients undergoing amputation whether they are ambulatory or not. This philosophy is now well established, and Condon and Jordan[53] have shown that healing rates in diabetic patients without popliteal pulses are similar for below- or above-the-knee amputations.

Cholecystectomy. Cholecystectomy is probably the most frequently performed major operative procedure in the geriatric age group. Decisions regarding surgery in symptomatic patients are usually not difficult; however, recommendations in the elderly asymptomatic patient with cholelithiasis require extremely careful evaluation if mortality in this age group is to be kept at a minimum. In general, if a patient's overall medical status is good, cholecystectomy should be recommended both to avoid the inflammatory complications as well as the development of carcinoma of the gallbladder. (Glenn and Hays[54] noted gallbladder carcinoma in 10% of patients who were more than 65 years of age.) Asymptomatic patients over 80 years of age can probably be treated without surgery with reasonable safety, since the mortality from the operation begins to approach that of the disease without operation.

Another area of debate is early as opposed to late surgery for acute cholecystitis. Presently, our policy would strongly favor (based on the work of Glenn and Hays and recent studies) early cholecystectomy for most cases of acute well-documented cholecystitis.[55] This approach requires definitive prompt diagnostic evaluation within 48 to 72 hours, including ultrasonograms, intravenous cholangiograms, upper gastrointestinal series, intravenous pyelograms, and a lower gastrointestinal series when indicated. During the diagnostic period, a fluid and electrolyte imbalance can be corrected. Ideally early cholecystectomy should be carried out within 72 hours; however, surgery after the third day can certainly still be carried out safely. Cholecystostomy still has a place in the critically ill patient[56]; however, cholecystectomy can usually be carried out and is definitely preferred.

Surgical approach by way of a subcostal route is our preferred incision because of excellent exposure, low wound complications, and reduced incisional pain. Cholecystectomy is carried out using a combination of the classic, antegrade, and retrograde techniques thus reducing the chance of an inadvertent ligation of the right hepatic artery. A cystic duct cholangiogram is routinely done and can eliminate a large number of common duct explorations for previous "classic" indications.

Frequently exploration of the common bile duct for equivocal indications such as minimal jaundice, alkaline phosphatase elevation, pancreatitis, small stones, and dilated common bile duct can be avoided by the use of a cystic duct cholangiogram. In these cases if a high-quality cystic duct cholangiogram is normal, exploration should be unnecessary. Exploration with definite indications such as cholangitis, severe jaundice, positive intravenous cholangiogram, and palpable stone should, of course, be carried out but should be preceded by the cystic duct cholangiogram. This approach allows the surgeon to know where the stones are and also allows visualization of the ampulla before manipulation causes spasm. Use of this general approach will reduce the need for common duct explorations and increase their yield.

POSTOPERATIVE CARE

The aim of postoperative care is to assist the patient as quickly and safely as possible through the period of physiologic stress brought on by his disease and the operation. Although many geriatric patients tolerate extensive procedures with surprising ease, others will run a stormy course, taxing the skill and knowledge of the most experienced practitioner. In general, with advancing age there is a decreased ability of body systems, especially the cardiovascular, pulmonary, and renal systems, to cope with stress. This is reflected in the generally higher mortality in the geriatric age group for major surgical procedures (Tables 17-2 and 17-3). Mortality and morbidity rates will be kept to a minimum by taking maximum advantage of the information obtained in the preoperative workup.

Immediate postoperative monitoring

During the period of the actual operative procedure, careful minute-to-minute monitoring and control of physiologic functions by the anesthesiologist is taken for granted. This same type of monitoring and control should be continued in the immediate postoperative period until the patient has recovered from the anesthetic and is "stable." For this purpose a well-staffed and equipped recovery room is a must when major surgery is performed.

Pulse, blood pressure, temperature, and respiratory rate and depth should be monitored in every patient. Automated systems are available for monitoring these functions, but a concerned, experienced nurse can do them manually just as effectively and may also pick up the patient who "just doesn't look right" before one of these parameters changes greatly.

Electrocardiogram monitoring should be done on a geriatric patient after all major procedures and after those minor procedures where preexisting cardiac disease is known. Hourly urine output monitoring with an indwelling catheter should also be carried out after most major procedures.

Central venous pressure monitoring should be considered in those situations where large volumes of fluid may be required and when limited cardiac and pulmonary reserve is known to exist. Central venous pressure is of help in gauging the rate and volume of fluid replacement, but it is not totally reliable for always giving adequate advance notice of impending volume overload. We have seen patients pass from a state of hypovolemia with a low central venous pressure to a state of severe pulmonary edema before a significant elevation in central venous pressure was recorded. This is most likely to occur when large volumes of electrolyte solution are used. It is now possible to obtain an earlier and more reliable warning of this complication by means of a pulmonary wedge pressure measurement. This is done by passing a balloon-tipped catheter, as described by Swan et al.[57] from the arm through the right side of the heart and out into a peripheral pulmonary artery. By inflating a balloon, a pulmonary wedge pressure can be measured that approximates left atrial pressure. Thus an earlier warning of impending left ventricular failure will be obtained as the left atrial pressure "backs up" through the lung.

Appropriate laboratory studies should be included in recovery room monitoring where indicated. These generally include hemogram and electrolyte and blood gas studies.

Postoperative problems

Hypotension. Hypotension, when seen in the immediate postoperative period, is most often related to hypovolemia, either from continued postoperative bleeding or insufficient replacement during the operation. Rapid replacement of fluid and blood under careful observation will usually lead to a return to normal blood pressure. Vasopressor agents should not be used for postoperative hypotension unless there is evidence of adequate blood volume, such as a normal or elevated central venous or pulmonary wedge pressure.

When hypotension that responds to fluid replacement recurs, consideration should be given to occult postoperative bleeding, and reexploration may be necessary.

Hypothermia. Temperatures in the 90° to 94° F range will frequently be seen immediately after extensive surgical procedures. Further temperature lowering must be prevented, since bradycardia, cardiac irregularity, and cardiac arrest may occur in the 88° to 89° F range. Such hypothermia should be treated by warming all intravenous fluids and blood and by the use of warming blankets and mattresses.

Respiratory problems. Respiratory difficulty in the immediate postoperative period is often related to the incomplete reversal of muscle relaxants or to the continuing effect of anesthetic agents. Underlying pulmonary disease must also be considered. It is our policy not to remove endotracheal tubes after surgery until adequate ventilation is certain. If uncertainty exists, arterial blood gas measurement while the patient is breathing unassisted should be done to enable a safe decision to be made. If continued respiratory assistance is necessary, endotracheal tubes may be left in place for 3 to 5 days; they are surprisingly well tolerated. If a further period of respiratory assistance is needed, a tracheostomy should be done, since continued vocal cord pressure against the endotracheal tube may cause permanent damage. When either an endotracheal or tracheostomy tube is left in place for long periods of respiratory assistance, low-pressure cuffed tubes should be used to prevent tracheal erosion with either fatal hemorrhage or delayed tracheal stenosis. Scrupulous care of these tubes is essential to minimize contamination of the lungs. Sterile gloves must be worn when the trachea and bronchi are suctioned, and suction catheters are used once and discarded. Tracheal cultures should be taken periodically and appropriate antibiotics used. Adequate humidity must be delivered by the respirator to prevent inspissation of bronchial secretions. Mucolytic and bronchial dilating agents are used only when indicated.

When prolonged respiratory assistance is required, we prefer the use of a volume-limited respirator, since it will ensure adequate tidal volume despite changes in pulmonary compliance. Pressure-limited respirators may not deliver adequate volume with decreasing pulmonary compliance.

Oxygen concentration delivered by the respirator should be no higher than that necessary to maintain arterial Po_2 at an acceptable level. Inspired oxygen concentrations of 40% or less can be tolerated indefinitely, but higher concentrations run the risk of causing "oxygen toxicity" with alveolar collapse, interstitial edema, and hyaline membrane formation. When inspired oxygen concentrations greater than 50%

are required to maintain arterial oxygen concentration at an acceptable level, positive end expiratory pressure (PEEP) should be considered. This means that the respirator, at the end of expiration, does not allow intrapulmonary pressure to return to atmospheric pressure (generally 5 to 10 cm H_2O above the atmospheric pressure). PEEP does not "push" fluid out of the alveoli but does tend to open and keep open alveoli that have collapsed and thus permit ventilation of perfused alveoli. Caution should be exercised when instituting PEEP, especially in the face of hypovolemia, since alveolar pressure may exceed pulmonary capillary pressure, thus blocking blood return to the left side of the heart, leading to hypotension.

Respiratory alkalosis with a low P_{CO_2} will frequently be found in patients who are using a respirator. When the P_{CO_2} drops below 30 mm Hg, dead space added to the respirator line between the patient and the Y junction of the inspiratory and expiratory lines will correct this problem.

Once the patient has been extubated, every effort must be made to prevent pulmonary problems. Deep breathing and coughing at regular intervals should be encouraged. Early ambulation should be practiced because it stimulates breathing and the upright position itself increases lung capacity up to 15% to 20%, thus decreasing the chance of atelectasis. Intermittent positive-pressure breathing (IPPB) treatments, the use of "blow bottles," and the use of various inspiratory incentive devices will also aid in preventing and correcting atelectasis. Abdominal distention should be prevented by the use of a nasogastric tube, and tight abdominal dressings and binders should be avoided, since both tend to force the diaphragm up and promote atelectasis.

Pain medication should be used extremely sparingly because, in addition to suppressing the cough reflex, it causes decreased ventilatory effort in the "too comfortable" patient. Geriatric patients in general require much less narcotic than their younger counterparts to remain acceptably comfortable. They must, however, receive enough pain medication so that incision pain will not prevent deep breathing and coughing.

Nasotracheal suctioning can be used effectively to stimulate coughing and to remove tracheobronchial secretions. Bedside bronchoscopy may also be used to remove secretions from the more peripheral bronchial tree.

Despite these precautions, there will be a group of patients who will develop significant pulmonary complications, which are especially hazardous in the elderly patient with marginal pulmonary reserve. Major areas of atelectasis, pneumonia, and congestive heart failure are the most common causes of postoperative respiratory distress in this age group. There are patients, however, who develop respiratory distress that may be fatal, in whom the exact etiology is not precisely discernible. The terms *posttraumatic pulmonary insufficiency, shock lung, adult respiratory distress syndrome* (ARDS), and *wet lung* are among the names applied to this situation. Early recognition of this syndrome is difficult. Tachypnea and agitation are seen early and, in time, cyanosis with laborious, grunting respiratory effort. In the early stages (even before clinical symptoms or x-ray changes) arterial blood gas determinations will frequently demonstrate surprisingly low P_{O_2} values, often in the 30 to 40 mm Hg range. Additionally, a respiratory alkalosis with a low P_{CO_2} will be found. If the disease progresses, the arterial P_{O_2} level will fall, despite increasingly higher inspired oxygen concentrations, and eventually P_{CO_2} levels will begin to rise with the development of respiratory acidosis. In the early stages the chest x-ray film is normal, but with progression, perihilar and eventually diffuse infiltrates develop. The lungs of these patients are wet and heavy and it is believed that there is both a ventilation and a perfusion abnormality.

The mechanism of injury is poorly understood, but several possible causes are suggested including overinfusion of electrolyte solution, leading to pulmonary edema; reflex pulmonary vascular spasm, leading to pulmonary edema, caused by cerebral anoxia (similar to the acute pulmonary edema seen with head injury); microemboli from transfused blood; fat emboli; "oxygen toxicity"; disseminated intravascular coagulation; vasoactive "toxins" released from areas of sepsis remote from the lung; and direct lung injury such as with aspiration or burns.

In essence, the treatment of this condition is fluid restriction, diuresis, and mechanical ventilation. Fluids are usually restricted to between 1000 and 1500 ml per day, and diuresis using either furosemide or ethacrynic acid is undertaken. Relatively high tidal volumes should be used on the respirator (generally 12 to 15 cc/kg of body weight), and positive expiratory pressure will frequently be necessary. In some cases, high doses of steroids may be of value.

Appropriate antibiotics as determined by periodic tracheal cultures should be used. The use of salt-poor albumin to increase intravascular oncotic pressure is of questionable value. We have found the administration of heparin to be of no value in this situation.

Thrombophlebitis and thromboembolism. A common and potentially serious postoperative complication is the development of venous thrombosis. Statistics vary greatly, but autopsies reveal that up to 80% of all hospitalized patients may develop this complication.[58,59] It may occur in superficial veins, but generally only thrombosis of the deep venous system of the legs and pelvis is serious because of the potential for pulmonary embolization and of developing late venous stasis sequelae.

Many factors may predispose a patient to the development of venous thrombosis, including (1) reduction of venous flow rate because of inactivity at bed rest, congestive heart failure, local venous compression, hypovolemia, etc.; (2) direct injury to the vein wall from the surgical procedure, from indwelling venous catheters, or from adjacent inflammatory reactions; and (3) hypercoagulable states, such as seen with visceral malignancies, polycythemia, or after injury.

Although superficial phlebitis with obvious pain, tenderness, and erythema over the palpable thrombus is easily diagnosed, deep vein thrombosis, especially if located in the calf or distal thigh, is frequently difficult or impossible to diagnose clinically.

There may be no subjective symptoms at all, but a complaint of a vague ache or tightness in the leg should raise a suspicion. Fever, tachycardia, and leukocytosis can be caused by deep vein thrombosis, but all of these findings are frequently seen in the postoperative period and are hard to interpret.

Examination of the leg may reveal slight swelling and possibly pitting edema. Slight prominence of the superficial venous system may be seen, as may a slight cyanosis or rubor. The involved leg may be appreciably warmer than its fellow. Tenderness to gentle palpation and calf pain produced by dorsiflexion of the foot (Homans's sign) should be looked for. These latter two findings should be interpreted with caution because they depend on subjective patient interpretation and are thus subject to considerable error.

When ileofemoral thrombosis is present, the diagnosis is generally much more obvious, since both subjective symptoms and physical findings are much more significant.

Because of the difficulty in making a clinical diagnosis of deep vein thrombosis, several diagnostic aids are available as follows:

1. Doppler ultrasound equipment, for use at the bedside to detect abnormal venous flow patterns. It is most accurate in diagnosing thrombosis in large veins of the thigh.
2. Injection of radionuclide-tagged fibrinogen, urokinase, streptokinase, or white blood cells into high-risk patients and watching for the development of "hot spots" over the venous system, since these materials are incorportated into clot formation. This method is most effective in finding thromboses in the veins of the calf. (By using radionuclide-tagged fibrinogen it has been estimated that between 20% and 30% of postoperative patients develop deep vein thrombosis.)
3. Lower limb and pelvic venography looking for venous filling defects or total obstruction (Fig. 17-6). This method has proved to be reliable, is simple to perform, and is relatively free of risk. When a diagnosis of deep vein thrombosis is suspected but not clinically definite, we use venography to establish the diagnosis before undertaking therapy.

Prevention of deep venous thrombosis is important, and several steps should be taken to attain this goal. Early ambulation, elevation of the foot of the bed, and active and passive exercises of the legs in bed are effective in preventing thrombosis.[60] Made-to-measure graduated elastic support of the legs is also of value. (The application of ready-made elastic stockings or poorly applied elastic bandage is risky because they frequently are tighter proximally on the leg than distally, thus promoting rather than preventing stasis.)

Currently under investigation is the use of low-dose heparin, warfarin (Coumadin), and aspirin. Although early reports are encouraging,

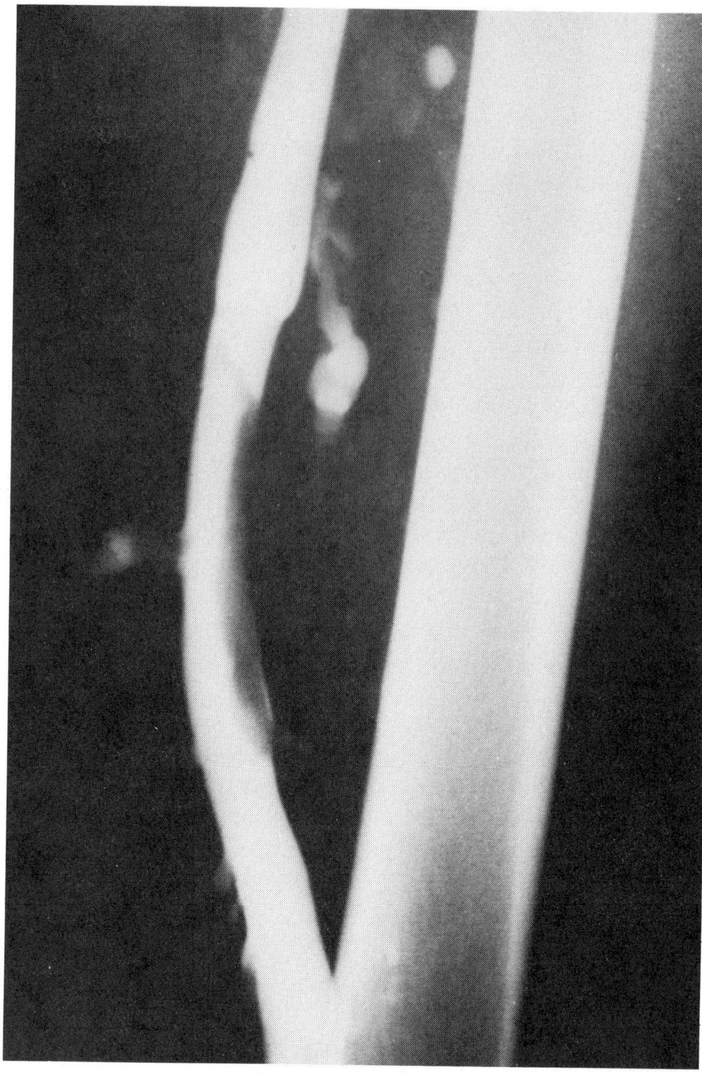

Fig. 17-6. Venogram showing large thrombus in femoral vein as well as thrombi in collateral veins.

their true value and risks have not been fully established. We have had several major bleeding complications associated with the use of low-dose heparin. For this reason, we recommend its use only in patients with a high risk of thrombophlebitis.

Treatment of superficial thrombophlebitis is usually simple, with rest, elevation of the feet, and local heat application being sufficient. Anticoagulation may be necessary when the process is widespread or progressive.

The treatment of deep venous thrombosis is designed to minimize the immediate risk of pulmonary emboli and the long-term risk of venous stasis problems. Adequate anticoagulation to prevent further propagation of soft nonadherent clots is the most important feature of the treatment. Intravenous heparin is given every 4 hours or by continuous infusion in dosages sufficient to maintain the partial thromboplastin time (PTT) at 2 to 2½ times the normal control (usually 5000 units every 4 hours). PTT determinations are done once daily when a stable heparin dosage has been achieved. Heparin administration is continued for 7 to 10 days (a minimum of 10 days if a pulmonary embolus has been diagnosed). Several days before discontinuing heparin administration a prothrombin-depressing drug such as Coumadin is given orally and continued for 3 to 4 months.

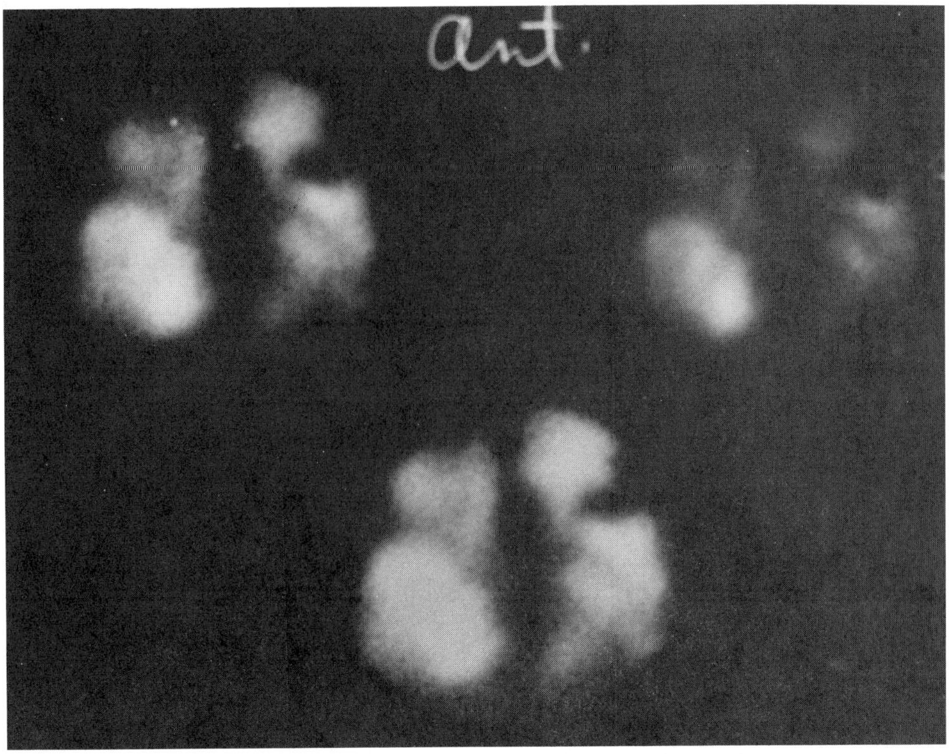

Fig. 17-7. Lung perfusion scan with defects characteristic of multiple pulmonary emboli.

When the symptoms and signs of the phlebitis are subsiding and the patient has been started on a regimen of orally given anticoagulants, ambulation is begun with made-to-measure graduated elastic stockings. Sitting with the legs down is not permitted. Elastic support is maintained as long as there is any tendency for edema formation when the patient is up and about.

Some controversy over the treatment of ileofemoral thrombosis exists. The thrombolytic agents urokinase and streptokinase have been used to hasten clot dissolution. Venous thrombectomy using balloon-tipped and suction catheters is also suggested by many. Neither of these methods, however, has been demonstrated to be superior to the use of heparin alone, either in preventing recurrent pulmonary emboli or in assuring long-term venous patency. We have, however, used venous thrombectomy in the face of phlegmasia cerulea dolans with impending gangrene of the leg in an effort to salvage the limb.

The most feared complication of deep thrombophlebitis is pulmonary embolism. Statistics again vary greatly, with autopsy analysis indicating between 1.8%[61] and 64%[62] incidence of pulmonary emboli. Fatal emboli are found in from 0.073% to 0.54% of all surgical patients.[63] Although the initial embolus may be rapidly fatal (about 5%),[64] most often it is small and produces relatively minor or no symptoms. The classically described symptoms of pulmonary embolism include the acute onset of pleuritic chest pain and dyspnea followed by hemoptysis. Physical examination may reveal a pleuritic friction rub, rales, tachycardia, split-second pulmonic sound, elevated central venous pressure, and a variable drop in blood pressure. The electrocardiogram may show right heart strain and ischemia, whereas the chest x-ray film may show a classic wedge-shaped opacity, an area of hyperlucency (Westermark's sign), or, more often, an ill-defined opacity. Blood studies may show an increase in lacticdehydrogenase and hypoxemia.

However, in the usual case symptoms, signs, and laboratory data are not absolutely diagnostic. Much has been written about the use of the lung perfusion scan in this situation to make an absolute diagnosis. Although the lung scan is of help (Fig. 17-7), considerable judgment must be used in interpretation in the geriatric patient in whom emphysematous blebs, old scarring, and recent areas of atelectasis or pneumonia may all present an identical picture. Pulmonary angiography, although much more specific, is rarely warranted in making the diagnosis of a small pulmonary embolus. In cases where clinical and laboratory suspicion of a pulmonary embolus exists along with evidence of a deep thrombophlebitis, treatment with heparin should be started immediately. The rates of recurrent pulmonary emboli while the patient is receiving heparin therapy vary from 0%[65] to 18%,[66] but most are in the 2% to 5% range.

Distress following a pulmonary embolus may require the use of vasopressor agents, atropine, papaverine, assisted ventilation, and closed cardiac massage. Pulmonary embolectomy may be necessary if shock persists despite these supportive measures. Embolectomy should never be undertaken without diagnostic confirmation by pulmonary angiography. Femoral-arterio-venous partial bypass done under local anesthesia may sustain such a patient until the diagnosis is confirmed and the operating room prepared. Pulmonary embolectomy is usually accomplished by opening the pulmonary artery while the patient is on cardiopulmonary bypass and removing the embolus under direct vision. A more simple method of removal of the offending embolus has been tried using a steerable catheter with a suction cup on its tip, which is passed into the pulmonary artery from the femoral vein. When the cup is placed in contact with the embolus, suction is applied and the instrument is withdrawn along with the embolus.[67]

Vena cava interruption just below the renal veins should be undertaken to prevent recurrent pulmonary emboli in the following cases: when an embolus occurs in the presence of adequate anticoagulation; when there is a contraindication to the use of anticoagulants (such as gastrointestinal bleeding or an allergy to the anticoagulant); in cases where there are septic pulmonary emboli; where pulmonary hypertension exists following multiple small emboli; and when pulmonary embolectomy has been necessary. Several methods of interruption are used, including ligation, suture plication, total and partially occluding clip application, and transvenous placement of a vena cava umbrella[68] or balloon.[69] Currently, we prefer the transvenous vena cava umbrella as the method of choice in most cases. This can be done under local anesthesia with little risk or discomfort to the patient.

Acute renal failure. Acute renal failure is a complication that must be carefully watched for in the geriatric patient in whom preexisting renal disease is not uncommon. Whereas oliguric renal failure (urine output less than 400 ml per day) is most commonly seen, nonoliguric (or high output) renal failure is not uncommon. Both will demonstrate azotemia with blood urea nitrogen levels over 30 mg/100 ml and serum creatinine levels over 3 mg/100 ml.

The most common cause of oliguria with some degree of azotemia seen in the postoperative period is fluid and electrolyte depletion. To differentiate this and "organic" renal failure a therapeutic test of blood volume expansion to the upper limits of the normal range, using extremely careful monitoring, should be tried. Whole blood, serum albumin, and crystalloid solutions may be used as volume expanders. In the usual situation it is our practice to give between 500 and 1000 ml of 5% dextrose in water over a 1-hour period along with an osmotic diuretic agent, such as 12.5 to 25 gm of mannitol given intravenously. Urine output should increase to greater than 40 ml per hour within 1 to 2 hours. If the response is not obtained, 40 to 200 mg of furosemide is then given intravenously in an effort to increase urine output. If this also fails, organic renal failure must be considered to exist.

If total anuria exists, one must be certain that postrenal obstruction of urine flow, that is, prostatic obstruction or bilateral ureteral obstruction, does not exist. Total renal vascular obstruction and renal cortical, medullary, and papillary necrosis can also produce total or nearly total anuria.

Primary renal failure is most often seen postoperatively in the geriatric patient when there has been a period of shock and especially if preexisting renal disease is present. It may also occur after the use of nephrotoxic aminoglycoside antibiotics, the use of the anesthetic agent methoxyflurane (Penthrane), and prolonged use of alpha-adrenergic vasopressor agents. Disseminated intravascular coagulation (such as is seen in the septic patient or after incompatible blood transfusion) and the release of myoglobin after extensive muscle injury may also lead to renal failure.

The pathophysiology of renal failure may be related to a combination of factors including shunting of blood away from the renal cortex caused by release of vasoactive substances (i.e., angiotensin), direct renal tubular cell injury, and physical obstruction of renal tubules by precipitated material and cellular debris.

Treatment of oliguric renal failure consists of the removal of continuing etiologic factors, fluid restriction, reduction of catabolism, and control of hyperkalemia and azotemia. In most cases 500 to 600 ml of fluid plus the volume of measured losses (i.e., gastrointestinal, urine, drain site, etc.) is given daily either orally or intravenously. If possible, 100 to 200 gm of glucose per day is given to reduce protein catabolism. Daily weights should be measured, and a drop of between ⅓ and ½ pound per day will be seen if good control is attained.

Temporary control of hyperkalemia may be obtained with intravenous administration of sodium bicarbonate, calcium chloride and hypertonic glucose with 1 unit of insulin per 3 gm of glucose. The ion exchange resin polystyrene sodium sulfonate (Kayexalate), given orally or by enema, will produce a more lasting reduction of serum potassium levels.

Early consideration should be given to the use of dialysis (either peritoneal dialysis or hemodialysis) when organic renal failure exists. It is our impression that the early use of dialysis maintains the patient in a better overall condition and may shorten the period of renal failure.

Postoperative delirium. Often geriatric patients will develop a degree of delirium in the postoperative period, especially while in the intensive care unit. This may range from mild confusion to total psychotic disorientation. Many factors, both environmental and physiologic, probably play a role, including preexisting senility, fluid and electrolyte imbalance, the effects of various medications, loss of normal sleep cycle caused by frequent, necessary nursing care interruptions, and loss of ability to keep track of time by normal change in light. These latter two conditions are especially common in intensive care units where there is 24-hour activity, the lights may be on day and night, and few if any windows are present.

Although the condition is distressing to relatives and friends, it is benign and will clear as physical recovery proceeds. Transfer out of the intensive care unit to the relatively normal environment of the regular ward seems to be the most effective therapeutic measure in hastening the recovery from this type of delirium.

Postoperative sepsis. The most common sites for postoperative infection are the urinary tract, the surgical wound, and the respiratory tract. In the last 6 months of 1979 at St. Francis Hospital, Evanston, Illinois, of all patients undergoing major surgery (including clean, clean contaminated, and contaminated cases) 5.3% developed a significant urinary tract infection, 4.9% developed a wound infection, and 4.0% developed a respiratory infection. Urinary tract infections were twice as common in the geriatric age group as in the younger age group and were directly proportional to the need for bladder catheterization. A single catheterization was followed by a 25% incidence of infection! For this reason catheterization should be used only when absolutely necessary. Sterile technique is a "must," and closed drainage systems should be used on indwelling catheters. Appropriate antibiotics as determined by urine culture should be used to control the infections.

Wound infections occurred with about equal frequency in the elderly and younger age group for equivalent procedures, in our recent evaluation, and varied from 12% in colon resections to 7.5% in cholecystectomies and 0.5% in inguinal hernia repairs. A reduction in wound infections will be brought about by careful preoperative cleansing of the skin, careful handling of tissues at the operating table, along with complete hemostasis and wound irrigation. If a large "dead space" is present in the wound, we prefer the use of a closed suction system to many catgut sutures. Wounds frankly contaminated at the time of surgery should be left open and closed several days later.

The preoperative and continued administration of antibiotics has been demonstrated to reduce the incidence of wound infection.[70] This should be used only in the case where a high incidence of wound infection is expected (i.e., colon resection) or where a wound infection might lead to a disaster (i.e., over a prosthetic vascular graft). The preoperative use of antibiotics effective against colonic anaerobic bacteria (i.e., erythromycin) may also reduce postoperative wound infections after colon resection.[71]

Adequate drainage is the primary treatment of a wound infection and should be done promptly because the elderly tolerate infection poorly.

Fluid, electrolyte, and nutritional maintenance. Fluid and electrolyte management in the elderly is rendered more difficult by the reduced adaptive capacity of bodily systems, leaving a relatively narrow margin between too little and too much treatment. The preoperative state of nutrition, the extent of the operative procedure, and postoperative problems will all influence the management program.

Normally, for several days after injury the body will retain water and sodium in response to outpouring of aldosterone and antidiuretic hormone. For this reason excessive fluid administration must be avoided in the elderly patient with reduced cardiovascular function. Only enough fluid should be given to provide for adequate urine output, insensible fluid losses, and other measured or estimated external losses. When external losses are not great, fluid requirements for 24 hours usually range from 1500 to 2500 ml. Considerably more fluid may be required if excessive "third space" fluid sequestration occurs, such as in a distended bowel or inflamed subcutaneous tissues. Particular care must be exercised in fluid administration as sequestered fluid is remobilized. Monitoring central venous pressure, pulmonary wedge pressure, urine output, and other procedures as previously outlined will guide fluid management.

Sodium and chloride requirements in the immediate postoperative period are theoretically minimal. It has been our experience, however, that if little or no sodium chloride is given at this time, a prolonged hyponatremia and hypochloremia will persist after the period of normal physiologic salt retention. Therefore, in the usual case we give approximately 75 mEq of sodium per day. If external losses are present (i.e., nasogastric suction, excessive diarrhea), additional salt will be given. If prolonged excessive external losses are present, it is wise to send a sample to the laboratory for accurate determination of salt concentration.

Potassium is not retained postoperatively, and usually 40 to 60 mEq will be given if adequate urine output exists. Excessive external losses must be replaced. Serum potassium levels must be maintained, especially if digitalis is being given because digitalis intoxication may occur in the face of hypokalemia.

Magnesium generally need not be given unless prolonged intravenous therapy is anticipated. In this situation 5 to 10 mEq of magnesium as sulfate per day will prevent depletion.

Caloric requirements after most operative procedures will usually be met by giving 100 to 150 gm of glucose. This will keep protein and fat catabolism to a minimum. However, a weight loss of up to ½ pound should be expected.

GENERAL POSTOPERATIVE CARE

Many factors are involved in the care of the postoperative patient. Only a few will be briefly mentioned here.

The geriatric patient, in general, requires more nursing care than the younger patient. Ambulation, which should be begun early, frequently will require the assistance of one or two people for several days but is essential. Aid may also be required at meal times. Skin care must be performed to prevent decubitus ulcers, which are most common over the sacrum, trochanter, and heels. This requires careful washing and lubrication of the skin, frequent change of position, and when necessary, the use of alternating air-pressure mattresses, sheepskins, and foam pads.

Nausea in the postoperative period and especially after abdominal surgery should be treated with nasogastric tube decompression and not by antiemetic medication. Nasogastric decompression will prevent vomiting with possible aspiration, the development of acute gastric dilatation, and the development of abdominal distention with resultant interference with respiration. Nasogastric tubes should not, however, be left in place unnecessarily, since they do cause local throat irritation and may eventually lead to esophageal ulceration. When prolonged intestinal decompression is anticipated, consideration should be given to the placement of a gastrostomy tube at the time of surgery.

Drains placed at surgery should be cared for with sterile techniques. They may be covered with sterile dressings or, when large volumes of fluid are lost, with sterile adherent collecting bags. (This also allows precise measurement of fluid loss.) Drains should be removed as soon as useful function no longer exists, which is usually on the second or third postoperative day.

Most often skin sutures may safely be removed about 1 week postoperatively. However, in the poorly nourished and septic patient and in the patient receiving steroids, we leave the skin sutures in for a longer period of time, since these patients have a high incidence of fascial disruption and may be spared a total evisceration if the skin remains intact. Evisceration, should it occur, is usually treated by immediate surgical repair. Occasionally in the extremely poor-risk patient evisceration may be handled nonoperatively by returning the viscera to the abdominal cavity and holding them in place with sterile saline-soaked dressings and adhesive strapping.

Today increasing emphasis is being placed on discharge planning.[72] This should begin several days before the patient is ready to leave the hospital and can be frequently done with the help of hospital social service departments. This preplanning will help to shorten the hospital stay and will assure the patient of a prepared environment whether it be in his own home or a nursing home.

REFERENCES

1. U.S. Department of Commerce, Bureau of Census: Current population reports, Series P-25, No. 870, Washington, D.C., Jan. 1980.
2. U.S. Department of Commerce, Bureau of Census: Current population reports: population estimates and projection, Series P-25, No. 704, Washington, D.C., July, 1977, p. 13.
3. Commission on Professional and Hospital Activities: Professional activity study, Ann Arbor, Mich., 1975.
4. Estes, W.L.: Reduction of mortality in surgery of the aged, Pa. Med. **52**:937, 1949.
5. Haug, C.A., and Dale, W.A.: Major surgery in old people, Arch. Surg. **64**:421, 1952.
6. Bosch, D.T., Islani, A., Tarr, C.T.C., and Beling, C.A.: The elderly surgical patient, Arch. Surg. **64**:269, 1952.
7. Cohn, R., Close, M.B., and Mathewson, C.: Operations upon the aged, Calif. Med. **86**:299, 1957.
8. Cole, W.H.: Medical differences between the young and the aged, J. Am. Geriatr. Soc. **18**:589, 1970.
9. Glenn, F.: Pre- and postoperative management of elderly surgical patients, J. Am. Geriatr. Soc. **21**:385, 1973.
10. Gordon, D.W.: Post-hospital discharge: patient care and utilization of services and facilities, Inquiry (Blue Cross Association) **10**:41, Dec., 1973.
11. Butler, R.N., and Lewis, M.I.: Aging and mental health, St. Louis, 1973, The C.V. Mosby Co.
12. Skinner, J.F., and Pearce, M.L.: Surgical risk in the cardiac patient, J. Chronic Dis. **17**:57, 1964.
13. Tarhan, S., Moffitt, E.A., Taylor, W.F., and Ginliani, E.R.: Myocardial infarction after general anesthesia, J.A.M.A. **220**:1451, 1972.
14. Dudrick, S.J., and Douglas, W.L.: Long-term parenteral feeding, Hosp. Practice, **3**:65, Oct., 1968.
15. Kakkar, V.V., et al.: Efficacy of low doses of heparin in prevention of deep vein thrombosis after major surgery, Lancet, **2**:101, July, 1972.
16. Coe, N.P., et al.: Prevention of deep vein thrombosis in urological patients: a controlled randomized trial of low dose heparin and external pneumatic compression boots, Surgery **83**:2, Feb., 1978.
17. Jain, S., et al.: Percutaneous transhepatic cholangiography using Chiba needle, Br. J. Radiol. **50**:175, 1977.
18. Hartmann, H.: Cong. Franc. Chir. **30**:411, 1921.
19. Wolff, W.I., and Shinya, H.: A new approach to colonic polyps, Ann. Surg. **178**:367, 1973.
20. Greenlee, H.B., et al.: Acute large bowel obstruction comparison of county, Veterans Administration and community populations, Arch. Surg. **108**:470, 1974.
21. Starling, J.R.: Initial treatment of sigmoid volvulus by colonoscopy, Ann. Surg. **190**:36, 1979.
22. Drapanas, T., and Stewart, J.D.: Acute sigmoid volvulus, concepts in surgical treatment, Am. J. Surg. **101**:70, 1961.
23. Howard, R.S., and Catto, J.: Cecal volvulus, Arch. Surg. **115**:273, 1980.
24. Ghazi, A., Shinya, H., and Wolff, W.I.: Treatment of volvulus of the colon by colonoscopy, Ann. Surg. **183**:205, 1976.
25. Nunes, G.C., Robnett, A.H., Kremer, R.M., and Ahlquist, R.E.: The Hartmann procedure for complications of diverticulitis, Arch. Surg. **114**:425, 1979.
26. Morgenstern, L., Weiner, R., and Michel, S.L.: 'Malignant' diverticulitis, Arch. Surg. **114**:1112, 1979.
27. Adams, J.T.: Adynamic ileus of the colon, Arch. Surg. **109**:503, 1974.
28. Eider, M.: Adynamic ileus of the colon with perforation: a report of two cases, St. Francis Hosp. Q. Bull. **5**:10, 1973.
29. Kukova, J.S., and Dent, T.L.: Colonoscopic decompression of massive nonobstructive cecal dilation, Arch. Surg. **112**:512, 1977.
30. Burhenne, H.J.: Nonoperative retained biliary tract stone extraction, Am. J. Roentgenol. Radium Ther. Nucl. Med. **117**:388, 1973.
31. Sasson, L.: Dissolution and flushing techniques for removal of retained common duct stones, Am. J. Gastroenterol. **51**:394, 1969.
32. Sohrabi, A., Max, M.H., and Hershey, C.D.: Cholate sodium infusion for retained common bile duct stones, Arch. Surg. **114**:1169, 1979.
33. Mazzariello, R.: Review of 220 cases of residual biliary tract calculi treated without reoperation: an eight year study, Surgery **73**:299, 1972.
34. Fischer, M.G., and McSherry, C.K.: Endoscopic papillotomy—a plea for rational restraint, Arch. Surg. **114**:991, 1979.
35. Hampson, L.G., Dickison, J.C., and Robertson, H.R.: Emergency surgery involving the biliary tract, Surg. Clin. North Am. **40**:1171, 1960.
36. Ostermiller, W., Jr., Thompson, R.J., Jr., Carter, R., and Hinshaw, D.B.: Acute obstructive cholangitis, Arch. Surg. **90**:392, 1965.
37. Reynolds, B.M., and Dargan, E.L.: Acute obstructive cholangitis, Ann. Surg. **150**:299, 1959.
38. Boey, J.H., and Way, L.W.: Acute cholangitis, Ann. Surg. **191**:264, 1980.
39. Dow, R.W., and Lindenauer, S.M.: Acute obstructive suppurative cholangitis, Ann. Surg. **169**:272, 1969.
40. Cacioppo, P.L., and Mason, J.H.: Ascending cholangitis, an urgent surgical problem, Geriatrics **28**(3):156, 1972.

41. Pierce, G.E., and Brockenbrough, E.C.: The spectrum of mesenteric infarction, Am. J. Surg. **119**:233, 1970.
42. Mattox, K.L., and Guinn, G.A.: Mesenteric infarction, Am. J. Surg. **126**:332, 1973.
43. Wilson, G.S.M., and Block, J.: Mesenteric vascular occlusion, Arch. Surg. **73**:330, 1965.
44. Zelenack, G.B., et al.: Splanchnic arteriosclerotic disease and intestinal angina, Arch. Surg. **115**:497, 1980.
45. Hildebrand, H.D., and Zierler, R.E.: Mesenteric vascular disease, Am. J. Surg. **139**:188, 1980.
46. Beahrs, O.H., Theuerhauf, F.J., Jr., and Hill, J.R.: Procidentia: surgical treatment, Dis. Colon Rectum **15**:337, 1972.
47. Altemeier, W.A., Culbertson, W.R., Schowengerdt, C., and Hunt, J.: Nineteen years' experience with the one-stage perineal repair of rectal prolapse, Ann. Surg. **173**:993, 1971.
48. Thomas, C.G.: Rectal prolapse (symposium), Cont. Surg. **17**:54, 1980.
49. Baker, W.N.W.: Results of using monofilament nylon in Thiersch's operation for rectal prolapse, Br. J. Surg. **57**:37, 1970.
50. Davidian, V.A., and Thomas, C.G.: Transsacral repair of rectal prolapse, Am. J. Surg. **123**:231, 1972.
51. Gibbons, G.W., et al.: Predicting success of forefoot amputations in diabetics by non-invasive testing, Arch. Surg. **114**:1034, 1979.
52. Pollock, S.B., and Ernst, C.B.: Use of Doppler pressure measurements in predicting success in amputation of the leg, Am. J. Surg. **139**:303, 1980.
53. Condon, R.E., and Jordan, P.H.: Below-knee amputations for arterial insufficiency, Surg. Gynecol. Obstet. **130**:641, 1970.
54. Glenn, F., and Hays, D.M.: The scope of radical surgery in the treatment of malignant tumors of the extrahepatic biliary tract, Surg. Gynecol. Obstet. **99**:529, 1954.
55. Jarvinen, H.J., and Hassbocka, J.: Early cholecystectomy for acute cholecystitis, Ann. Surg. **191**:501, 1980.
56. Hinchey, E.J., Elias, G.L., and Hampson, L.G.: Acute cholecystitis, Surg. Gynecol. Obstet. **120**:475, 1965.
57. Swan, H.I.C., et al.: Catheterization of the heart in man with use of a flow-directed balloon-tipped catheter, N. Engl. J. Med. **283**:447, 1970.
58. Secker-Walker, R., and Potchen, E.J.: Radiology of venous thrombosis: current status, Radiology **101**:449, 1971.
59. Sevitt, S., and Gallagher, N.: Venous thrombosis and pulmonary emboli: a clinicopathologic study in injured and burned patients, Br. J. Surg. **48**:475, 1961.
60. Tsapogos, M.J., et al.: Postoperative venous thrombosis and the effectiveness of prophylactic measures, Arch. Surg. **103**:561, 1971.
61. Pulvertaft, R.J.V.: Postoperative pulmonary embolism, Ann. R. Coll. Surg. Engl. **1**:181, 1947.
62. Freiman, D.G., Suyemoto, J., and Wessler, S.: Frequency of pulmonary thromboembolism in man, N. Engl. J. Med. **272**:1278, 1965.
63. Gjores, J.E.: The incidence of venous thrombosis and its sequelae in certain districts of Sweden, Acta Chir. Scand (Suppl. 206), 1956.
64. Thomas, D.P.: The management of pulmonary embolic disease, Am. J. Med. Sci. **259**:157, 1970.
65. Barrett, D.W., and Jordan, S.C.: Anticoagulant drugs in the treatment of pulmonary embolism: a controlled trial, Lancet **1**:1309, 1960.
66. The urokinase pulmonary embolism trial: a national cooperative study, Circulation **47** (Suppl. 2):1, 1973.
67. Greenfield, L.J., Reif, M.E., and Guenter, C.E.: Hemodynamic and respiratory responses to transvenous pulmonary embolectomy, J. Thorac. Cardiovasc. Surg. **62**:890, 1971.
68. H., Robinson, R., Michie, D., and Jude, J.R.: Transvenous caval interruption with umbrella filter, N. Engl. J. Med. **286**:55, 1972.
69. Hunter, J.A.: Surgery of venous and thromboembolic disease, Surg. Clin. North Am. **51**:99, 1971.
70. Chetlin, S.H., and Elliott, D.W.: Preoperative antibiotics in biliary surgery, Arch. Surg. **107**:319, 1973.
71. Nichols, R.L., et al.: Effect of preoperative neomycin-erythromycin intestinal preparation on incidence of infectious complications following colon surgery, Ann. Surg. **178**:453, 1973.
72. Podolsky, R., and Mason, J.H.: Geriatric discharge planning and follow-up, Ill. Med. J.**157**(5):291, May, 1980.

CHAPTER 18 · ANESTHESIA

Robert B. Dodd

PREOPERATIVE EVALUATION

Most anesthesiologists in the United States use the classification of the American Society of Anesthesiologists in their preoperative evaluation of patients. This classification, which was originally designed to standardize physical status categories for statistical studies and for hospital records, is used with marked consistency by anesthesiologists around the country.[1] There are five categories in the classification:

Class 1. A normally healthy patient
Class 2. A patient with mild systemic disease
Class 3. A patient with severe systemic disease that is not incapacitating.
Class 4. A patient with an incapacitating systemic disease that is a constant threat to life.
Class 5. A moribund patient who is not expected to survive for 24 hours with or without operation

(Emergencies are designated by adding the letter E following the numerical classification.)

Although age, per se, is not one of the criteria for classifying patients,[1] there is evidence that diseases exist in the older age group even though they may be asymptomatic. Beecher and Todd[2] reported that 45% of all deaths from anesthetics occurred among patients over 50 years of age, who comprised only 35% of the surgical population in the hospitals studied. Coronary atherosclerosis is the largest cause of death in the United States and is responsible for one third of all deaths and two thirds of fatalities from cardiovascular disease.[3] Since symptoms of coronary disease do not appear in over 75% of patients until multivessel obstruction develops, most patients over age 50 have varying degrees of impaired cardiac function, which may be silent clinically and could be considered class 2. Patients over the age of 70 usually have some disorder (or disorders) of the body systems, which limits their activity but is not incapacitating. Most of these patients will be classified as class 3. Being over 70 years old has, indeed, been identified as one of the major cardiac risk factors in patients undergoing noncardiac operations.[4] In a study of the outcome of surgery in patients over 80,[5] there seemed to be a difference in mortality between those classified as class 2 (1%) and those in class 3 (4%). Of 14 patients in class 4, 25% died as did the only class 5 patient. There appeared to be an increasing mortality with increasing age in this group, 13% for patients over 95 years of age. In this series and others,[6,7] sex was not a risk factor. Poor health before surgery and emergency procedures are major risk factors.[5,6]

Since anesthesia risk is greater for the older patient, the most important preoperative judgment is an estimation of the patient's physiologic age. There are "young" nonagenarians and "old" sexagenarians. The amount, if any, of preoperative sedation and the method and agent(s) used for anesthesia should be governed by this evaluation. How badly worn is the machinery? How will it respond to the reversible poisoning by the drugs used in anesthesia and to the trauma of operation?

In the following discussion, physical examination of the patient has been largely ignored. It is assumed that the patient will have been examined completely by the attending physician. The anesthetist should always examine the patient's airway, including jaw mobility and dentition, and the heart and lungs. Other parts of the body may be examined according to their pertinence to the anesthetic technique used or to protection of the patient (paralyzed limbs, ectropion, etc.). Preoperative evaluation also relies heavily on observation of the patient and his behavior, the medical history, and pertinent laboratory results.

Central nervous system status

The patient's general mood is a valuable clue to how he will withstand the surgical procedure. The cheerful patient who wants to live, and knows why he wants to live, is a relatively good risk. This type of person is interested in people, aware of current events, and sensitive to matters of his personal hygiene. He may not be as young as he feels, but he can be considerably "younger" than others having a decade or two less chronologic age. Those with parkinsonism may be difficult to judge in this regard. Their masklike facies do not reflect emotions well, and their appearance of debility can be misleading. If they have no other serious organ system disorder, they are not unusually poor risks. Control of the symptoms of parkinsonism by treatment with amantadine hydrochloride (Symmetrel), levodopa (Dopar, Larodopa) or a combination of levodopa and carbidopa (Sinemet) may produce a variety of adverse neurologic, gastrointestinal, psychiatric, and cardiovascular reactions. These, however, are masked or do not appear under general anesthesia. Because levodopa has a short duration of action, patients may continue receiving therapy before surgery as long as oral intake is allowed and resume therapy as soon as possible postoperatively to prevent a recurrence of symptoms.[8]

If the patient's responses during the preoperative interview are inappropriate, the cause should be found and, if possible, circumvented. The patient may be hard of hearing or may have a residual aphasia from a stroke and still be acute in other faculties, or he may have a general brain deterioration. Knowledge of these disorders is important in predicting his response to depressant drugs. The patient with chronic brain syndrome can be considered to have partially induced anesthesia and will require a lower dose or concentration of general anesthetic drugs to achieve clinical anesthesia. Careful consideration should also be given to the amount, if any, of sedation used. When a patient's grasp of reality is tenuous, it seems illogical to jeopardize that hold with a depressant or dissociative drug. The elderly patient should be given as much information about routines surrounding his operation as he can assimilate comfortably. The type of information and the amount must be tailored to the patient's ability to comprehend. He will want to cooperate if he knows what to expect and understands that the anesthetist is part of a team devoted to getting him well.

Some of the psychic and sensory residuals of stroke have been mentioned, but a history of stroke is important in other regards. It is an index of the degree of atherosclerosis present and the brain's tolerance to it. Whether the stroke was due to hemorrhage or thrombosis should be considered in anesthetic management. The patient's chief protection is careful monitoring of the blood pressure during anesthesia and trying to keep the readings in a range of about 20% variation from the average preoperative systolic pressure. The preferred method of maintaining this homeostasis is the use of intravenous fluids, such as preloading prior to the vasodilatation produced by spinal anesthesia, but small doses of vasopressors may be used instead. The technique of induced hypotension should be considered only if the risk of bleeding, either from volume loss or from blood obscuring the operative site, is felt to be greater than the risk of another stroke. The use of extreme hyperventilation by control of respiratory activity is not recommended, except when indicated in intracranial operations, since a lowered carbon dioxide tension in the blood decreases cerebral blood flow.

Another consideration concerning the patient with a history of stroke is the amount of residual motor impairment. If a long time has elapsed since the stroke and the degree of functional return is maximal, the primary consideration is protection of the palsied or paralyzed extremity during positioning for operation. If the patient is relearning the use of a limb, the safety of block anesthesia should be weighed against the possibility of slowing the patient's recovery by temporarily removing his conscious control of his limb. This is especially true in spinal block anesthesia, in which deafferentation is profound and moderately prolonged.

The presence of glaucoma should be noted. If there is increased intraocular pressure, special precautions must be taken to prevent any pressure on the eyeball that might be transmitted to the optic disk, causing visual impairment or blindness. Some of these patients who have become resistant to pilocarpine or physostigmine eyedrops are treated with eyedrops containing a long-acting cholinesterase, echothiophate (Phospholine) or demecarium (Humorsol). Echothiophate has caused prolonged apnea following administration of succinylcholine through its lowering of plasma cholinesterase levels.[8,9] Drugs acting in this manner should be discontinued 3 weeks to 1 month prior to elective surgery.[9] Carbonic anhydrase inhibitors, such as acetazolamide (Diamox), do not pose any special problems except those associated with hypokalemia, which can be managed if discovered before surgery. There seems to be no danger to glaucoma patients from dosages of atropine used in preanesthetic medication. Because of the loss of tone in the lids with aging, which tends to cause inversion or eversion of the lower lid, special precautions must be taken to protect the lids and the underlying conjunctiva and cornea. Tear production is stopped or markedly reduced during anesthesia. If the anesthetist is not able to frequently inspect the eyes and gently massage the upper lids, artificial tears or ointment should be instilled and the lids should be taped shut. The use of eye patches is not recommended as the lids might become open under the patch without being noticed, leading to severe abrasions of the conjunctiva and cornea.

Many older patients receive mood altering drugs. Lithium salts have a remarkable effect in calming manic excitement, and maintenance administration of the drug decreases the number of future manic and depressive episodes. Therapy with lithium is monitored by its concentration in the plasma. Although lithium is said to potentiate the actions of anesthetics and muscle relaxants in experimental animals, there are no clinical reports of adverse reactions under anesthesia when the plasma level of lithium was below the toxic level of 1.5 mEq/liter.[10] Since the possibility of drug interaction does exist, the last two doses of lithium might be withheld prior to an elective procedure to allow plasma levels to fall to a concentration where anesthetic interactions should not occur. Tricyclic compounds, such as imipramine (Tofranil) and amitriptyline (Elavil), are used to treat depressed patients. These drugs are said to cause cardiovascular instability and arrhythmias under anesthesia.[8] Except for the usual restrictions on oral intake prior to anesthesia, these drugs need not be discontinued. Electrocardiographic monitoring for arrhythmias should now be routine. Monamine oxidase (MAO) inhibitors are also used as mood elevators. The anesthetist should know if the patient is taking an MAO inhibitor. They enhance the effect of sympathomimetic amines, causing hypertensive crises, and interfere with the detoxification of other drugs, resulting in a prolonged recovery from anesthesia. Meperidine (Demerol) is specifically contraindicated in patients taking MAO inhibitors because its administration may result in excitation, sweating, rigidity, hypertension or hypotension, and even coma.[8] A patient who has taken MAO inhibitors within the past 2 weeks should not undergo elective surgery. If surgery is necessary, one should avoid narcotics, treat hypertension with direct-acting vasodilators, for example, nitroprusside (Nipride), and treat hypotension with intravenous fluids or careful administration of a direct-acting vasopressor, for example, phenylephrine (Neo-Synephrine) by intravenous drip. The MAO inhibitors marketed in this country are furazolidone (Furoxone), isocarboxazid (Marplan), pargyline (Eutonyl, Eutron), phenelzine (Nardil), procarbazine (Matulane), and tranylcypromine (Parnate).[11] The mood altering substance taken most frequently by geriatric patients is a nonprescription drug, alcohol. The clinical observation that acute alcoholic intoxication lowers the anesthetic dose requirements and that sober chronic alcoholics require higher anesthetic doses has been supported by laboratory studies in mice.[8]

Cardiovascular status

The patient with congestive heart failure is not a candidate for elective surgery. Patients whose congestive failure is still evident preoperatively are much more likely to develop postoperative failure and pulmonary edema than those who are no longer in failure or have no history of heart failure.[6]

Patients with jugular venous distentions and/or a third heart sound are at increased risk for postoperative cardiac death. Judicious use of digitalis preparations, diuretics such as furosemide (Lasix), and vasodilators such as nitroglycerin and the nitrate compounds can improve cardiac performance preoperatively and reduce the risk of surgery in these patients. Digitalis is recommended preoperatively when there is a history of previous congestive failure, cardiac dysfunction as evidenced by the signs of impaired ventricular response mentioned above, nocturnal angina (a symptom related to depressed ventricular function), atrial fibrillation or flutter with a rapid ventricular response, or frequent episodes of paroxysmal atrial or junctional tachycardia.[3] Digitalis therapy should be carefully monitored because of the numerous factors enhancing the potential for digitalis toxicity in the perioperative period.

Recent myocardial infarction, within 6 months preceding surgery, is a lethal risk factor in analyses of cardiac complications following noncardiac surgery.[6,7,12] Unfortunately, the advent of new anesthetic agents and techniques and more sophisticated monitoring has not lowered the reinfarction rate. Tarhan,[7] who studied reinfarction in patients undergoing noncardiac surgery in the same institution in 1967 and 1968 and again in 1974 and 1975, found the incidence of reinfarction to be 27% to 37% when the previous infarct was within 1 week of surgery and 11% to 16% in the period from 4 to 6 months. Mortality from reinfarction was 69%. After 6 months, the risk of myocardial infarction is stable at about 5% whether the patient has a history of infarction or not.[6,7] Although Tarhan's earlier study indicated a high risk of reinfarction with anesthesia and surgery during the 6-month post-infarction period, the proportion of patients with myocardial infarction zero to 3 months and 4 to 6 months preceding surgery was the same for the 1974 and 1975 study as it had been in 1967 and 1968. It is concluded that the only way to prevent reinfarction during anesthesia and surgery is to postpone elective surgery for at least 6 months after a myocardial infarction. The choice of anesthetic technique apparently is not a factor in postoperative cardiac death. Conduction anesthesia (spinal, epidural, upper extremity block) was associated with a lower incidence of heart failure,[6] but there was no difference in the occurrence of postoperative myocardial infarction and death.[6,7] If heart failure is present or thought to be hazard, spinal or epidural anesthesia for operations below the umbilicus and conduction anesthesia for operations on the arm might be indicated.

The exercise tolerance of the patient with cardiac disease should be learned by asking questions such as what the patient's usual daily activities are and how easily he tires. Physical testing of the patient is generally unnecessary.

An electrocardiogram should be made before the operation to aid in preoperative assessment and as a reference should cardiac complications develop later. Nonspecific T wave and S-T segment changes in a stable electrocardiogram are relatively unimportant for evaluation compared with a thorough history and physical examination. New ischemic patterns, however, should be checked with serial tracings before an elective procedure is performed. The electrocardiogram does give very helpful information about the heart's conduction mechanism. Atrial premature contractions are a benign finding unless they occur frequently, in which case they might indicate impending atrial fibrillation or supraventricular tachycardia.

Electrocardiographic abnormalities, particularly arrhythmias, have been designated as risk factors associated with postoperative cardiac death.[6,12] Electrocardiographic abnormalities that are significantly correlated with postoperative cardiac death are more than five premature ventricular contractions per minute documented at any time preoperatively and rhythm other than sinus on the preoperative electrocardiogram.[6] Occasional premature ventricular contractions as a solitary finding usually do not require treatment preoperatively, as they often become less frequent or disappear under general anesthesia.

As of this writing, there is no drug commonly used in treating heart disease that should be withdrawn prior to surgery. Beta-adrenergic blockade with drugs such as propranolol (Inderal) is used in the treatment of angina pectoris, hypertension, and cardiac arrhythmias. Since propranolol is an indiscriminate beta-adrenergic blocker with a relatively short biologic half-life, second generation beta blockers have been developed in an attempt to overcome the disadvantages of chronic propranolol therapy. Like propranolol, all the newer agents produce dose related decreases in $beta_1$ mediated heart rate and contractility. These beta blockers are atenolol (Tenormin), metoprolol (Lopressor), nadolol (Corgard), and timolol (Biocardrin). Only atenolol and metoprolol spare the $beta_2$-adrenoreceptors, located chiefly in the bronchial and vascular musculature, but this selectivity disappears as the dose of these drugs is increased.

Only nadolol has a long half-life (17 to 24 hours) compatible with a single daily dose schedule. There is ample evidence that patients treated with a beta-adrenergic blocker can be safely anesthetized and, in fact, there may be some danger to suddenly withdrawing the drug.[8] The presence of antiarrhythmics, such as lidocaine (Xylocaine), procainamide (Procan, Pronestyl), phenytoin (Dilantin), and quinidine, cause no concern to the anesthesiologist, except for the organic condition necessitating their use. Nifedipine (Procardia) and verapamil (Calan, Isoptin), classified as calcium channel blockers, are approved for the treatment of vasospastic and classical effort-associated angina. Verapamil, but not nifedipine, is effective intravenously in breaking supraventricular tachycardia and decreasing the ventricular response to atrial fibrillation. Disopyramide (Norpace) and verapamil are incompatible in the treatment of arrhythmias because of their combined effects in depressing myocardial function. Both verapamil and nifedipine can enhance the myocardial depression produced by beta blockers and can increase the risk of heart failure in patients on that therapy. Both agents increase serum digoxin levels in pateints receiving that drug.[13] If the patient is stabilized on calcium channel blocker therapy, it may be continued preoperatively, but the anesthesiologist should be informed since these agents alter the body's response to anesthetics and other vasoactive drugs. If calcium channel blocker therapy has just been introduced into the treatment of a patient receiving digitalis and/or a beta-adrenergic blocker, it should be discontinued before the operation. Digitalis preparations used in the treatment of supraventricular arrhythmias and heart failure, as has been noted, have a limited margin of safety in the perioperative period. The likelihood of digitalis toxicity increases with decreases in serum potassium; such decreases may result from respiratory alkalosis produced by hyperventilation or from metabolic alkalosis due to gastric drainage.

It now appears that antihypertensive drugs should not be withdrawn prior to surgery. In a prospective study, Goldman and Caldera[14] found that untreated or inadequately treated hypertensive patients have larger absolute decreases in blood pressure during anesthesia than do adequately treated hypertensive patients. The mortality in the study groups, which also included normotensive patients who were not receiving therapy and patients receiving diuretics who had no history of hypertension, was not related to hypertension or its control. It was concluded that this reflected the anesthesiologist's ability to prevent marked intraoperative blood pressure changes. Clonidine (Catapres) was not used in the aforementioned series. The withdrawal of clonidine has been reported to result in severe rebound hypertension, so patients should be maintained on this drug as long as oral medications are allowed.[8] The thiazide diuretics, which are used alone or in conjunction with other drugs in the treatment of hypertension, tend to deplete the body of potassium. Serum potassium levels should be checked preoperatively. If the potassium level is markedly decreased, elective surgery should be postponed until potassium can be repleted by an oral supplement. Hypokalemia in the perioperative period is associated with altered response to nondepolarizing muscle relaxants, cardiac arrhythmias, and digitalis toxicity.

The type and condition of permanent pacemakers should be evaluated to learn if the pacemaker is capturing consistently and going at the stated rate. Patients undergoing transurethral resection of the prostate where electrocautery is necessary often have a pacemaker. Since the indifferent electrode is placed under the buttocks and the electrocautery is also over a foot away from the pacemaker, difficulties have not been encountered. Other precautions suggested for the use of electrocautery when the patient has a pacemaker are changing the pacemaker to the fixed mode and limiting the frequency and duration of electrocautery to 1-second bursts longer than 10 seconds apart.

Since depression of the hypothalamo-pituitary-adrenocortical response to stress may be manifested by cardiovascular collapse, the question of management of patients who have been receiving steroid therapy will be discussed here. If the patient is receiving steroids, the drug should be continued. There is disagreement as to how to manage patients whose steroid therapy has been discontinued from 2 to 12 months preoperatively.[8] If the patient who is to undergo major surgery has received systemic doses of drugs affecting the pituitary-adrenocortical axis during the preceding year, prophylactic hydrocortisone should be administered preoperatively and during the perioperative period. This eliminates one of the variables should the patient become "shocky" during or after surgery. The question of how to handle minor operations of short duration remains moot. A single dose of hydrocortisone should not be harmful, but some would call it a needless expense.

Finally, Goldman et al.[4] equated a poor general medical condition preoperatively with intraperitoneal, intrathoracic, or aortic operations as cardiac risk factors in patients undergoing noncardiac surgical procedures. Factors of "poor general medical condition" were an arterial oxygen tension of less than 60 torr or a carbon dioxide tension greater than 50 torr, a potassium level of less than 3 mEq/liter or a bicarbonate level less than 20 mEq/liter, a urea nitrogen concentration of over 50 mg/100 ml or creatinine concentration greater than 3 mg/100 ml, abnormal glutamic oxaloacetic transaminase level, signs of chronic liver disease, or a patient bedridden from noncardiac causes.

Respiratory status

The other respiratory systems, in common with the other body systems, deteriorates with age. Niesenbaum[15] has reviewed the anatomic and physiologic changes to be found with aging and the effects of pulmonary disease in the aged compared with those in younger patients. He concludes that "senescence and [pulmonary] disease are not synonymous although at times they present similarities." As an example, when there is barrel chest deformity, this does not necessarily mean that clinical emphysema is present.

The appearance and breathing pattern of the patient should tell the anesthetist whether significant pulmonary disease exists. If the patient is in a relaxed position and can speak in complete sentences without stopping to take a breath, disabling pulmonary disease is not present or is well controlled. The patient suffering from chronic breathing difficulty will assume a military posture or will bend slightly forward and will have poor breath control during conversation. Pursing of the lips with each expiration is another sign of advanced lung disease. The patient should be able to walk the hospital corridor at a reasonable pace or climb a short flight of stairs without becoming dyspneic.

If the patient is being treated for emphysema, bronchitis, or asthma, the anesthetist should know the regimen of treatment. The anesthetist should also find out how long the patient has been receiving treatment; the types of drugs used, their dosages, and routes of administration; and whether the patient has ever been hospitalized for lung disease. This will provide important information as to the patient's respiratory status to guide preoperative preparation and operative and postoperative management. The asthmatic patient who developed the initial symptoms after the age of 50 has a poor prognosis. Preanesthetic medication and the plan of anesthetic management should be aimed at preventing an asthmatic attack. Response to therapy is not good in these patients, and complete relief from status asthmaticus is rare. A history of smoking, especially if associated with cough or shortness of breath, seems to be at least as important in one study as one of working in various dust-laden environments. All the workers studied smoked, and none of them had the disabling form of coal workers' pneumoconiosis—progressive massive fibrosis.[16] A history of respiratory failure or of episodes of failure is ominous and almost precludes the possibility of recovery from major intraabdominal or intrathoracic surgery.

Although they are not sophisticated enough to pick up beginning lung disease nor pathophysiologic mechanisms, the most informative pulmonary function tests in evaluating how a patient with lung disease will tolerate anesthesia and surgery are the forced vital capacity (FVC), the amount of air that the patient can exhale after a maximum inspiration, and the volume of this (FVC) air that can be expelled in one second (FEV_1). This test can be done at the bedside with simple equipment and interpreted by the anesthetist or attending physician. If the test reveals significant obstructive disease, treatment should be instituted preoperatively to bring the patient to maximal improvement if time allows. If a bronchodilator improves function during the test, it can be added to the treatment regimen. Blood gas analyses are not necessary to make the diagnosis but add information as to the seriousness of the disease. They should be done preoperatively as a baseline in patients with severe obstructive or restrictive pulmonary disease who are to undergo major intraabdominal or intrathoracic operations.

If the patient has obstructive respiratory secretions, it is best to clean out the tracheobronchial tree before major surgery. Therapy consists of deep breathing exercises, a bronchodilator if indicated, ultrasonic nebulization, postural drainage by elevating the foot of the bed, and chest physical therapy (percussion of the chest with the cupped hand), especially if the secretions are tenacious. One week of therapy might be required depending on improvement in the patient's symptomatology and pulmonary function tests. The patient is taught deep breathing exercises preoperatively and is told he will be expected to do as well postoperatively. Currently, the most popular aid in this exercise is the incentive spirometer, which indicates the goals to be reached in the postoperative period. The effectiveness of this exercise seems to be in direct proportion to the amount of encouragement and reinforcement that the patient receives from the respiratory therapist on each postoperative day.[17] During the postoperative period, other than ultrasonic nebulization and deep breathing exercises, more vigorous therapy is usually withheld unless there are signs of atelectasis. Intermittent positive pressure breathing (IPPB or IPPV) has lost its popularity in perioperative management of pulmonary patients, particularly in the postoperative period except for continuous ventilation via an endotracheal tube. Because of fright or pain, the deep breath given by the machine does not have the patient acceptance that voluntary deep breathing has. IPPB also carries an increased risk of aerophagia and gastric dilatation. Furthermore, it has been shown that IPPB causes a decrease in functional residual capacity and a decrease in arterial oxygen tension immediately following therapy in the postoperative period.[18]

Extracellular fluid volume status

The status of the extracellular fluid compartments can be assumed to be normal in the healthy-appearing candidate for elective operation if the results of routine laboratory tests are normal. The patient with a broken hip who has been transported from a nursing home or who has been living alone presents a different problem. If the patient is somnolent or confused, he may have an extracellular fluid volume deficit brought on by lack of fluid intake after the injury, superimposed on loss of fluid and blood into the injured area and on a habit pattern of borderline nutrition. This patient will also tend to become hypotensive or faint when he is moved or is propped up in bed. His response to intravenous infusion of a balanced salt solution, of ionic composition approximating that of plasma, is often dramatic. His preinjury mental status may be restored in an hour or less. If rehydration is to be accomplished that rapidly, the effects of the fluid load should be monitored by central venous pressure measurement.

The patient with acute intestinal obstruction often has a massive extracellular fluid volume deficit. Except in the few cases when preoperative diagnoses such as bowel infarction are made, surgery should be delayed until the extracellular fluid volume can be restored to a state at which the patient is alert and maintains a normal blood pressure. The intravenous administration of solutions for volume and electrolyte replacement should be monitored by central venous or pulmonary wedge pressure measurement and by measurement of constant urinary bladder drainage to an output of a minimum of 1 ml/kg per hour.

A hemoglobin level of 10 gm/100 ml is the usually accepted minimum in a patient who is to undergo general or spinal anesthesia for an elective operation causing little blood loss. If the blood loss is expected to be 500 ml or more, it is preferable to give such a patient preoperative transfusion rather than to correct the anemia during the operation. The preoperative transfusion(s) should be packed red blood cells rather than whole blood unless the anemia was caused by recent acute blood loss. A further reason for using red blood cells, except when whole blood is needed to replace rapid blood loss, is that plasma volume in "anemic" cachectic people is usually normal or slightly expanded.[19] Giving these patients whole blood when the deficit is red blood cell mass only may lead to circulatory overload.

ANESTHETIC MANAGEMENT

The following discussion will not dwell on the pharmacology and pharmacodynamics of drugs used in anesthesia but will stress certain facets of anesthetic management that are particularly applicable to the geriatric patient.

Drugs used before anesthesia

The drugs used in preanesthetic medication are a part of the induction of surgical anesthesia and should be ordered with that in mind. Narcotic and sedative drugs are used to calm the patient so that he will accept the strange surroundings of the operating room suite in a tranquil mood. The dosages of drugs used for this purpose should be reduced by one third to one half the amount that would be given to a younger person of the same size. If the patient is so obtunded that the operating room scene will not be frightening or if he has been receiving narcotics regularly for pain, no medication may be necessary.

I usually give a narcotic before anesthesia. This is often supplemented with hydroxyzine hydrochloride (Vistaril), in a dosage range of 25 to 50 mg intramuscularly, or diazepam (Valium), in a dosage range of 2.5 to 5 mg intramuscularly. Both are nonphenothiazine tranquilizers that enhance the effects of depressant drugs so that smaller doses are required to produce a given degree of sedation or analgesia. A narcotic is used for its analgesic and its hypnotic effect. There is discomfort associated with the induction of anesthesia, for example, from the hard operating or examining table and the placement of needles for infusion or block anesthesia. Another reason for giving a narcotic is that it may provide some residual analgesia during the early part of anesthesia so that lower concentrations of anesthetic may be needed to produce adequate anesthesia. If the patient appears too frail to tolerate a narcotic, a small dose of hydroxyzine or diazepam or no preanesthetic medication is used. Diphenhydramine hydrochloride (Benadryl) is occasionally used in 25 to 50 mg dosage intramuscularly for the patient with asthma or multiple allergies or both. It produces sedation in addition to having an antihistaminic action.

The advisability of administering belladonna alkaloids prior to anesthesia to geriatric patients is questionable. In elderly people the nasal mucosa and glands atrophy, and the secretions along the respiratory tree are more viscous.[15] The antisialagogic action of atropine sulfate or scopolamine hydrobromide will make the secretions even more tenacious and difficult to expel or remove. In the dosage used and when given preoperatively, atropine sulfate provides little protection against vagal reflexes during anesthesia. If such difficulties arise during anesthesia, it may be given intravenously with good therapeutic effect.

Choice of anesthetic agents and techniques

Block anesthesia should be used when feasible in the elderly patient who is a fair to poor risk (physical status 3, 4, or 5). The agent of choice is the one that the anesthetist prefers. When there is increased risk, it seems illogical to anesthetize the entire body when only a portion requires anesthetization. Upper extremity operations and extraperitoneal operations below the umbilicus are in this category. The exceptions may be extremely short procedures, including diagnostic procedures to be followed at a later date by definitive operation under spinal anesthesia, for example, cystoscopy followed by transurethral resection of the prostate.

Brachial block, utilizing the axillary approach, usually provides excellent conditions for arm operations, and the surgeon may use a tourniquet to provide a bloodless field. The tourniquet technique of intravenous block anesthesia usually has a higher success rate than specific nerve block techniques. It is particularly well suited to relatively short procedures on the arm that require a tourniquet. The advent of small gauge (20 to 22 G) plastic intravenous cannulae has nearly obviated the earlier problem of veins tearing under the pressure of the injected solution.

Spinal anesthesia is usually preferred to peridural anesthesia or individual nerve block anesthesia for extraperitoneal operations below the umbilicus. Spinal anesthesia is more dependable, more predictable, and takes less time to induce. It is most frequently used in inguinal hernia repairs, anorectal operations, prostatic resections, hip pinnings, and amputations of the leg. It is less frequently used for gynecologic perineal repairs, short anorectal procedures with the patient in lithotomy position, cystoscopy and fulguration of bladder tumors, and open reductions of leg fractures. The choice of anesthesia for insertion of a hip prosthesis is open to debate. When spinal anesthesia is used, these patients often require fairly heavy sedation to withstand the discomfort of the lateral position, the manipulation, and the noise of the procedure. A light general anesthesia alone would seem preferable.

General anesthesia, usually administered through an endotracheal tube, is preferred for intraabdominal operations. In the geriatric age group extensive exploration is generally indicated, and spinal anesthesia is rarely satisfactory. If the number of spinal segments anesthetized permits thorough abdominal exploration without discomfort to the patient, blood pressure and respiration will have to be supported artificially. If too few segments are anesthetized, the patient will need additional sedation, often to the point of general anesthesia.

A thiobarbiturate such as thiopental sodium (Pentothal sodium) or thiamylal (Surital) given intravenously is generally used for induction of anesthesia. Only a "sleep dose," generally 50 to 250 mg, should be used, and anesthesia should be maintained by agents that are eliminated mainly through the lungs. Patients with clinical heart disease or advanced respiratory disease should receive oxygen by mask prior to and during the barbiturate injection.

Nitrous oxide in concentrations of 50% to 60% with oxygen is used as a carrier gas during maintenance of anesthesia unless the patient requires more oxygen. With nitrous oxide present, lower concentrations of the more potent agents are required to maintain surgical anesthesia. Nitrous oxide is also used as a principal agent, with its analgesia supplemented by narcotics given intravenously in small doses. Although morphine or meperidine (Demerol) may be used, fentanyl (Sublimaze) is preferred by most anesthesiologists because its short duration of action allows close control of dosage.

The potent inhalation agents may be used with nitrous oxide or with oxygen alone. They are, in order of their introduction into clinical practice in the United States, halothane (Fluothane), enflurane (Ethrane), isoflurane (Forane), and methoxyflurane (Penthrane). All are nonexplosive halogenated hydrocarbons and are metabolized to some extent in the body. The biodegradation products resulting from anesthetic concentrations of methoxyflurane have been shown to be nephrotoxic, and there is no indication for its use in this age group. Conversely, the flurry over the danger of hepatotoxicity from halothane has now died down, and the agent is being used extensively.

Isoflurane was introduced into clinical practice in the United States in 1981, after an exhaustive period of investigation covering 16 years.[20] The earlier findings in laboratory animals, human volunteers, and selected patients were generally confirmed by a multi-center clinical evaluation performed before the introduction isoflurane into general use.[21] A brief comparison of isoflurane and the other two commonly used agents seems appropriate. Isoflurane's lower blood solubility facilitates control of anesthetic depth and speeds awakening from anesthesia, as compared to halothane and enflurane. Both isoflurane and enflurane are mildly pungent, while halothane is not. This pungency limits the rate of induction with isoflurane, even though its blood solubility is about half that of halothane. Myocardial depression is not a constant finding with isoflurane, whereas both halothane and enflurane cause depression. Although all three agents depress blood pressure, enflurane and isoflurane increase heart rate. With isoflurane, the degree of increase in pulse is less in the over 60 age group. Of the three, arrhythmias secondary to the presence of epinephrine are least likely to occur with isoflurane. Isoflurane and enflurane potentiate the effect of muscle relaxants more than halothane. Cerebral blood flow and intracranial pressure may be increased less by isoflurane than by the other two agents. This might allow better control of intracranial pressure during operation. The rapid emergence from isoflurane anesthesia might facilitate the neurological evaluation of a patient following intracranial surgery. Biodegradation of isoflurane is one tenth that of enflurane and one hundredth that of halothane, so that the possibility of nephrotoxicity or hepatotoxicity, which is small with all agents, is least with isoflurane.

Although it is superior in many ways, isoflurane has two disadvantages relative to enflurane and halothane. It is more expensive and it has received far less clinical use. Further experience may reveal some presently unknown noxious effects.[20]

All patients receiving nitrous oxide mixtures should breathe pure oxygen for several minutes at the termination of anesthesia. This is especially true when an endotracheal tube has been used, since tracheal suction and extubation may produce transient hypoxia.

A dissociative agent, ketamine (Ketaject, Ketalar), has proved to be most useful in pediatric and geriatric patients. It is a potent analgesic that may be administered by the intravenous or intramuscular route. Hallucinations on emergence from ketamine anesthesia, which have caused problems in the general patient population, have a low incidence in these age groups. In elderly patients, ketamine's use as an analgesic or as an induction agent has reduced this incidence to a rarity. The only procedures for which ketamine is sometimes used as the sole anesthetic agent in this age group are burn debridements and dressings. Its principal use is as an analgesic to allay the discomfort of the patient when his position is changed, for example, moving a patient with a broken hip from the bed to the operating table for insertion of a prosthesis or positioning the patient in bed to induce spinal anesthesia for hip pinning. Remarkably small doses are needed–25 to 75 mg intravenously (usually 30 to 50 mg). Ketamine is useful in these situations because the patient's blood pressure is generally well maintained during the movement. The manufacturers of ketamine recommend that it not be used in patients in whom a significant elevation of blood pressure would constitute a serious hazard. In the dosage range used we have not encountered this problem. The lack of hypotensive effect makes ketamine an excellent induction agent for patients in borderline shock who require an emergency operation. In rare situations in which the patient's lack of cooperation precludes securing an intravenous port, the intramuscular route may be used and generally requires about three times the expected intravenous dose. An intravenous infusion can be started after the drug takes effect. Ketamine is not used for patients with increased intracranial pressure.

Diazepam is a useful intravenous adjunct to provide light sedation to patients having operations under conduction anesthesia, such as transurethral resection of the prostate or hip pinnings under spinal anesthesia and permanent pacemaker insertion under local anesthesia. Systemic blood pressure and cardiac rhythm are rarely affected by small increments (2.5 mg) of the intravenous preparation.

As with the local anesthetic agents, the muscle relaxant of choice is the one that the anesthetist prefers. Succinylcholine chloride. *d*-tubocurarine chloride, and pancuronium bromide (Pavulon) are well tolerated when judiciously given. An overdose is easily attained if the anesthetist uses the same dosage in milligrams per kilogram of body weight per minute that would be used for a younger patient. One must assume that the skeletal muscle mass in the geriatric patient has decreased in size and vigor until clinical signs prove otherwise. A peripheral nerve stimulator (e.g., hand twitch in response to intermittent or sustained stimulation of the ulnar nerve) should be used in making this assessment, particularly in prolonged intraabdominal operations. The muscles of the abdominal wall, which must be relaxed for intraabdominal manipulations, are respiratory muscles. If they are relaxed, the patient cannot ventilate adequately without assistance from the anesthetist.

Monitoring

It is standard clinical practice to record the blood pressure, pulse rate, and respiratory rate at regular intervals throughout anesthesia and to take more frequent readings when anesthetic or operative conditions indicate. In addition the heart tones and breath sounds should be constantly monitored by precordial or esophageal stethoscope. This provides more information concerning the patient's cardiovascular and respiratory status than any other single monitor. Changes in the heart's rate, rhythm, and output may be detected as well as changes in breath sounds caused by secretions or increased airway resistance.

Oscilloscopic monitoring with the electrocardiograph should be routine. The electrocardiograph is very helpful in long operations and when atrioventricular conduction abnormalities or clinical heart disease are present. In addition to displaying arrhythmias, it may reveal electrolyte disturbances or myocardial ischemia.

Monitoring of the body temperature has now become routine during anesthesia lasting longer than a few minutes. The thermistor may be placed in the nose, esophagus, rectum, or axilla or on the tympanic membrane or the skin under the patient. Body cavity temperatures are more accurate, but any site used consistently is useful in indicating changes or trends. The possibility of malignant hyperpyrexia in the elderly is remote but cannot be ignored. The body temperature of a patient under general anesthesia usually falls slightly and may fall to dangerously low levels during long operations in cold operating rooms, particularly when large volumes of cold blood or fluid are given intravenously without prior warming. A blood warmer should also be used to warm fluid or blood given an extensively burned patient. Another method of preventing heat loss, during debridement of burns and the taking or application of skin grafts, is to turn off the air conditioning in the operating room. The patient who has a high fever may be cooled during anesthesia by intravenous administration of refrigerated fluids or by passing the fluids through a blood-warming coil placed in an ice bath.

Central venous pressure (CVP) should be measured in patients who will be receiving large volumes of fluid, blood, or both intravenously and in patients who have recently had heart failure. It is especially helpful when combined with continuous urinary output measurement. Patients with a low CVP, less than 5 cm of water or saline solution, should not be treated unless there are other signs of extracellular fluid deficit, such as hypotension, tachycardia, or oliguria. Treatment in this case is administration of fluid and blood. If the CVP rises sharply with the rapid infusion of fluids, it means that the right heart cannot handle the load and the infusion rate should be greatly decreased. If the heart is inefficient because of arrhythmia, the arrhythmia should be treated. If digitalis is needed, a small dose of a rapidly acting preparation should be given. The response to a fluid challenge is much more important than isolated CVP levels. The CVP will read 5 to 10 cm H_2O or more, higher than the true level if the patient is on a ventilator using high tidal volumes. Vasopressors also produce high CVP readings. Thus therapy need not be started because a CVP is low or discontinued because it is high. If the CVP is low and remains low following a fluid challenge that does not produce a rise in systolic blood pressure, one must consider the possibility that the right heart is functioning well and that the left heart is failing or in failure. Placement of a Swan-Ganz catheter into the pulmonary artery will provide information for the diagnosis and help monitor therapy.

Pulmonary wedge pressure (PWP) is the back pressure in the blood vessels of the lungs as measured through a catheter (Swan-Ganz) in a balloon occluded pulmonary artery. This pressure is measured by an electronic pressure monitor and reflects left ventricular function. The PWP is very helpful in patients with severe coronary heart disease who are to undergo major surgery. It is also helpful in the timing of a needed operation in a patient who has had a recent myocardial infarction. A reading of less than 10 torr suggests hypovolemia, whereas a reading of over 20 torr may indicate overload and/or left ventricular failure. As with the CVP, the response of the PWP to a fluid challenge is more revealing than isolated readings. In operations where the patient's condition indicates the use of a Swan-Ganz catheter, it is best to have it inserted preoperatively to provide baseline readings and to assist in determining whether the patient is in optimal shape for the operation.

Direct arterial blood pressure measurement through a small (20 G) plastic cannula, usually in the radial artery, is being used more frequently. The cannula provides a continuous monitor of the patient's blood pressure and a port from which to draw blood samples for gas or other analyses. It is indicated in resections of the abdominal aorta, intrathoracic vascular operations and in operations in which the blood pressure is deliberately lowered. The indwelling arterial cannula is very useful in obtaining arterial blood for the perioperative management of a patient with chronic pulmonary disease who is undergoing major surgery.

Fluid management

If there is no contraindication, the patient should be allowed clear liquids by mouth until 5 hours before the operation. If fluid intake has been restricted and repeated enemas have been given in preparation for diagnostic procedures followed closely by the operation, the administration of dextrose in a balanced salt solution should be started intravenously early on the day of the operation. Such a patient often becomes hypotensive when anesthetized if he has not received fluid replacement.

The geriatric patient requires fluid and electrolyte replacement in amounts similar to those used for younger patients. During an extensive operation there will be significant tissue fluid loss, which should be replaced. As stated earlier, the patient's response to this shifting fluid load should be monitored closely by CVP, PWP, and urinary output measurement.

Postanesthesia care

This brief discussion covers only that portion of time during which the patient is emerging from anesthesia in the postanesthesia recovery unit. Every patient who has had general anesthesia should receive oxygen until he is fully responsive. The preferred route is by nasal cannula ("prongs"), usually at a flow rate of 5 liters per minute. If the patient has severe chronic lung disease, a 2- to 3-liter flow might be indicated lest higher concentrations depress respiration.

The nasopharyngeal catheter is more efficient when optimally placed but is usually not tolerated for as long a period of time, and if inserted too far, it may cause gastric dilatation or rupture.

If there is any doubt about the effectiveness of the patient's respiratory effort, his ventilation should be assisted by intermittent positive-pressure breathing with a humidified oxygen mixture by way of an endotracheal tube until that doubt is removed. Patients who have had intrathoracic operations, particularly open heart procedures, may require respiratory assistance for days. In the postanesthesia recovery unit the decision concerning when to discontinue respiratory assistance and (or whether) the patient should have his endotracheal tube removed will usually be based on clincial judgment supported by spirometric and respiratory effort measurements, and arterial blood gas measurements.

Geriatric patients rarely request pain medication during their stay in the postanesthesia room unless they are truly suffering. The aftereffects of anesthesia and surgery usually keep them somnolent but arousable. If the pain seems disproportionate to the operation, other sources of discomfort should be sought. If the patient is just restless, a small dose of hydroxyzine or diazepam might suffice. If the patient does require pain relief, a small dose of morphine (3 to 5 mg) or meperidine (15 to 25 mg) will usually put the patient at ease.

CONCLUSION

In the clinical practice of anesthesia, the geriatric patient is an ideal example of the necessity for a careful preoperative evaluation on which to base a plan for maintenance of the patient's respiratory and circulatory homeostasis through the surgery and the immediate postoperative period.

REFERENCES

1. Owen, W.D., Felts, J.A., and Spitznagel, E.L., Jr.: ASA physical status classifications, Anesthesiology **49:**239, 1978.
2. Beecher, H.K., and Todd, D.P.: Study of deaths associated with anesthesia and surgery, Ann. Surg. **140:**2, 1954.
3. Rose, S.D., Corman, L.C., and Mason, D.T.: Cardiac risk factors in patients undergoing noncardiac surgery, Med. Clin. North Am. **63:**1271, 1979.
4. Goldman, L., et al.: Multifactorial index of cardiac risk in noncardiac surgical procedures, N. Engl. J. Med. **297:**845, 1977.
5. Djokovic, J.L., and Hedley-White, J.: Prediction of outcome of surgery and anesthesia in patients over 80, J.A.M.A. **242:**2301, 1979.
6. Goldman, L., et al.: Cardiac risk factors and complications in non-cardiac surgery, Medicine **57:**357, 1978.
7. Steen, P.A., Tinker, J.H., and Tarhan, S.: Myocardial reinfarction after anesthesia and surgery, J.A.M.A. **239:**2566, 1978.
8. Cullen, B.F., and Miller, M.G.: Drug interactions and anesthesia: a review, Anesth. Analg. **58:**413, 1979.
9. Duncalf, D., Goldman, K.S., McNeil, J.M., and McCammon, R.M.: Symposium on ocular care of the hospitalized patient, Anesthesiology Rev. **7:**51, 1980.
10. Havdala, H.S., Borison, R.L., and Diamond, B.I.: Potential hazards and applications of lithium in anesthesiology, Anesthesiology **50:**534, 1979.
11. Physician's Desk Reference, Oradell, N.J., 1982, Medical Economics Co., p. 1457.
12. Cooperman, M., Pflug, B., Martin, E.W., Jr., and Evans, W.E.: Cardiovascular risk factors in patients with peripheral vascular disease, Surgery **84:**505, 1978.
13. Food and Drug Administration: New angina drugs, FDA Drug Bull. **12:**1, 1982.
14. Goldman, L., and Caldera, D.L.: Risks of general anesthesia and elective operation in the hypertensive patient, Anesthesiology, **50:**285, 1979.
15. Niesenbaum, L.: Problems of pulmonary disease in the aged, Geriatrics **23**(7):127, 1968.
16. Morgan, W.K.C., Lapp, N.L., and Seaton, D.: Respiratory disability in coal miners, J.A.M.A. **243:**2401, 1980.
17. Lederer, D.H., Van de Water, J.M., and Indech, R.B.: Which deep breathing device should the postoperative patient use? Chest **77:**610, 1980.
18. Dutton, R.E., Browner, B.D., and Powers, S.R., Jr.: Lung volumes and blood oxygenation after intermittent positive pressure breathing, Arch. Surg. **114:**568, 1979.
19. Peden, J.C., Jr., Maxwell, M., Ohin, A., and Moyer, C.A.: A consideration of indications for preoperative transfusions based on analysis of blood volumes and circulating proteins in normal and malnourished patients with and without cancer, Ann. Surg. **151:**303, 1960.
20. Eger, E.I., II: Isoflurane: a review, Anesthesiology **55:**559, 1981.
21. Forrest, J.B., et al.: A multi-centre clinical evaluation of isoflurane, Can. Anaesth. Soc. J. **29:**S1, 1982.

CHAPTER 19 · ORTHOPEDICS

Michael Devas

The many years' experience of an extensive geriatric orthopedic practice at Hastings, England, and a liaison with the geriatric physician and the rehabilitation team have engendered a philosophy for the treatment and management of the elderly patient with an orthopedic lesion. In this chapter the emphasis will be on the proper approach to the problems of the elderly; only those orthopedic conditions that need special regard, or treatment differing from that in the younger patient will be discussed.

PRINCIPLES OF GERIATRIC ORTHOPEDIC CARE

In the elderly, a return to function is a return to independence. The longer an elderly person stays in a hospital, the more difficult it is to achieve a level of rehabilitation that will enable the patient to live independently. Elderly people are to be treated with the most intense effort possible, and nowhere is it more necessary to practice the art of medicine to its fullest extent.

Geriatric orthopedic problems can be divided into two main groups: acute, in which most of the patients suffer from fractures that require immediate treatment; and chronic, in which arthroses and other degenerative conditions often necessitate total joint replacement or other large surgical procedures. In both groups, but especially in the former, it must always be remembered that bed rest, even for only a short time, has a deleterious effect on the patient and that the patient may have one or more illnesses other than the orthopedic complaint.

In treating a geriatric patient it is important to realize that most elderly women suffer from some degree of osteoporosis. Osteoporosis is not a contraindication to surgery, and, furthermore, it adds urgency to rehabilitation, particularly after a fracture. This is because bed rest or immobilization in any form will increase osteoporosis, making it imperative to get the geriatric patient up and about as quickly as possible.

In the elderly the most important orthopedic physical sign is to see the patient walking. Without walking true independence cannot be achieved. The longer the patient is confined to bed the greater becomes the problem of achieving independence. In considering the treatment of many geriatric patients the surgeon must determine not whether the patient is fit for surgery but whether it will be safe to treat the patient in bed. Most serious fractures in the elderly can and should be treated by early surgery and internal fixation so that the patient may walk forthwith. In the fit adult, conservative treatment of fractures is considered the safest and best method because the time spent in bed has no ill effect and the morbidity of surgery is avoided. The reverse is true in the elderly. Morbidity from lying in bed for weeks or months far outweighs the morbidity of properly performed surgery. Furthermore, the elderly often have little time to live and do not wish to spend most of their remaining time lying in bed. All elderly people are jealous of their independence and accept the inevitability of death, but until it occurs they wish to have a satisfactory quality of life.

Old people need intensive rehabilitation because loss of muscle strength and tone is a concomitant of the aging process. Loss of strength and muscle tone enhances osteoporosis; this is

□ Michael Devas' chapter has its foundation in his extensive experience as head of a geriatric orthopedic unit at the Royal East Sussex Hospital in Hastings, England. Some of the approaches and methods described may be at variance with those commonly in use in the United States. However, the coordinated approach to the overall health care of the geriatric patient with an orthopedic disorder should be of profound interest to gerontologists everywhere. It may well serve as a model to those who plan geriatric services. THE EDITOR.

another most important reason to get geriatric patients up and walking without delay.

The skeletal system developed to enable humans to stand upright, and in so doing gravity had to be resisted by muscular activity. Without the necessity to be upright muscles lose their strength and tone. Therefore the best preventive measure and the best rehabilitation is to keep the patient up and walking. Practically all muscles are used in controlling posture while standing or walking. Bed rest for the elderly is little more than rehabilitation for the grave.

Isometric exercises are beneficial, but the elderly find it somewhat bewildering to try to gain proficiency in contracting muscles. The difficulty is overcome by simple physical therapy exercises that cause muscles of the body to contract. Such exercises should be routine for all patients, especially those who are for some reason confined to bed or a chair and cannot walk immediately. The simplest method of achieving these isometric contractions is to have the patient lie in a supine position and gently raise weights held in each hand. The weights are varied to the individual's capability. Thus a 1-pound weight held in each hand by the side and then raised against gravity to the upright position will contract practically all the muscles of the legs and trunk. Such exercises are no substitute for walking but are essential when the latter is not possible.

Osteoporosis, from the orthopedic viewpoint, may almost be considered a natural concomitant of old age, but this is not true of osteomalacia, which is often present as well, particularly in elderly people who have not had a proper diet. The osteoporotic and osteomalacic bone is weaker than bone with osteoporosis alone; not only may Looser's zones appear, with characteristic linear cracks in the bone, but also fractures will occur more readily.

The weakness that osteoporosis engenders can allow a bone to be stressed to the limits of its strength and, as soon as this happens, pain will occur. This is because small microfractures occur, for example, in the vertebrae, and the patient will experience pain that may radiate around the concerned dermatome. At this early stage there will be no radiologic changes of note, and because the pain is relieved by rest the paradox occurs that the relief of the pain will increase the osteoporosis. Later the vertebra will compress, giving rise to the classical osteoporotic compression fracture. Sometimes osteoporotic bone will collapse gradually with little or no pain, giving rise to the number of crush fractures demonstrated in radiographs, that have caused the patient no symptoms of note.

Thus the almost inevitable osteoporosis of the elderly makes them susceptible to fractures from the simple activities of living; prolonged rest will also increase osteoporosis with a consequent increase in the risk of a fracture when activity is at last resumed.

It will be shown later that in the elderly increased activity occasioned by a painful joint with a prosthetic replacement may also lead to fractures. This type of fracture is caused by increased use and therefore increased stress on a bone weakened by disuse. In the young patient a limb encased in a cast will show disuse osteoporosis. The same condition, but to a much greater extent, occurs in the elderly, often on top of idiopathic osteoporosis. Therefore prolonged immobilization of a limb must be avoided if any other quicker method of treatment is available. In a geriatric patient the immobilization of a limb in a plaster cast for too long a period may cause so much osteoporosis that the limb is painful when used, presenting a clinical picture almost indistinguishable from Sudek's atrophy. Activity causes pain, and as a result, the patient is even more inactive. This vicious circle of pain on activity, demanding more rest with a consequent increase in osteoporosis can only be broken by intense remedial treatment.

All these points emphasize that the challenge an elderly person presents to the orthopedic surgeon is both urgent and difficult and necessitates great skill and ingenuity in choosing the correct treatment. To deny the elderly patient an operation is often to deny hope as well. Yet with all the concomitant ailments of old age, surgery is sometimes risky; however, when considered in the context of the patient, the patient's quality of life, and the risks of prolonged bed rest it is always the correct choice.

FRACTURES NEAR THE HIP

The most common acute orthopedic condition in the elderly is a fracture near the hip. If there is a clear understanding of the proper principles to be used in the treatment of such a fracture, then the same principles can be applied to most other geriatric orthopedic conditions, acute or chronic. Therefore the treatment of this injury will be discussed in full, although the actual type of operation is of no importance provided it obviates the fracture and allows the patient to walk forthwith.

Hospital services vary from country to country. In many places geriatric orthopedic units are considered to be a most suitable adjunct to the rehabilitation of the most ill of the many elderly patients admitted with fractures. Such a unit is described later.

Etiology

There are two groups of elderly patients who sustain fractures near the hip. The first group consists of otherwise extremely fit individuals who have had a true accident, such as being knocked down in the street or tripping over some obstacle while engaged in an active life. In the second group of elderly patients the fracture is a symptom of impending dissolution; these patients present the most serious problem to the physician because the so-called accident was probably occasioned by a mild cerebral vascular accident, a drop attack, giddiness, or even a fall in the bedroom or kitchen for no apparent reason. It is in this group of patients that the prognosis is by far the worst. Between these two groups there are those patients who cannot be fitted into either group at the time of admission, but in whom progress soon indicates the true state of affairs. The history of the actual occurrence causing the fracture may be of no help in determining the general condition of the patients in this group. For example, a patient who lives alone, falls, and is not found for several hours and suffers from hypothermia as a result. However fit the patient was, and if it was a true accident, the hypothermia will give the patient an almost moribund appearance, making it difficult for the clinician to determine a prognosis at this stage. However, by the time the patient has been warmed (this must be confirmed by obtaining a rectal temperature) and an operation has been performed to deal with the fracture, the patient's appearance may be so changed that a good prognosis is obvious.

The art of diagnosis is most needed with the old person after an injury because a full clinical examination, laboratory investigations of the blood, or radiographic examination of the lung fields, and so on may show little or no abnormality. Usually taking the patient's medical history and the conversation necessary to obtain it, either before or after surgery, will demonstrate the patient's state and level of activity before the accident.

The clinical examination can be extremely deceptive, particularly if the patient is in pain. To examine a fractured hip by feeling for abnormal movements or crepitus is to be decried. Observation and gentle palpation should be sufficient to indicate the site of the fracture. In the control of pain it must be remembered that morphine must not be given too freely to the aged and that meperidine is usually sufficient to control muscle spasms and pain, after which the leg may be positioned comfortably with pillows or sandbags. Should pain continue thereafter, traction is necessary. This must be done by simple methods using neither skeletal traction nor adhesive plaster but by binding on some type of nonslip traction bandages and putting only a small amount of weight at first over the pulley. No attempt should be made to try and reduce the fracture by traction. This will be done if necessary under general anesthesia in the operating room.

Good quality radiographs are most important. The anesthetist will wish to see the condition of the chest, and the orthopedic surgeon will need a clear delineation of the whole pelvis for comparison of the two hips and detailed views of the fracture.

The laboratory investigations will include blood hemoglobin estimation, blood typing, and blood urea and serum electrolyte level determinations. Arrangements will then be made for the patient to be operated on at a suitable time within 24 hours of the injury. Experience has shown that this is satisfactory and allows sufficient time for proper assessment and preparation of the patient in a calm and unhurried manner. Longer delay should not be tolerated unless the patient has some condition that necessitates treatment before surgery such as heart failure or diabetes, neither of which should take more than 24 to 48 hours to control. It is also important to remember that if a patient is considered moribund and too ill to undergo surgery, the condition must be reviewed every few hours. The patient may be much better after a rest in a warm hospital bed with careful nursing attention, and surgery may then be decided on and a successful outcome obtained, despite a poor prognosis, a short life expectancy, and the risk of the operation. There is no worse treatment of elderly patients than to allow them to die with a painful fracture of the hip left untreated by the surgeon through mistaken kindness. The orthopedic surgeon who has a high mortality because he operates on as many old people with fractures as he can will be compensated by having many more grateful patients than the surgeon who does not do so. That the patient's last few days or weeks of life should be spent bedridden with great pain on movement is a sorry reflection on medical skill.

Generally it is convenient to start an intravenous infusion at the time of admission because most patients are usually dehydrated. Preparation should be made for a blood transfusion to be given before, during, and after the operation.

Operative approach

There are two fractures that occur near the hip. One is the fracture of the femoral neck, and the other is the trochanteric fracture. Further division into the level of the fracture in the femoral neck or determining whether the fracture is intertrochanteric or pertrochanteric is unnecessary. In the elderly person there is no place for the use of internal fixation for the fractured neck of the femur; it should always be treated by excision of the upper fragment and replaced by a prosthesis. This is because the failure rate for internal fixation is too high to be acceptable, and it is more difficult to rehabilitate a patient after a pinning procedure than after a prosthetic replacement. The ill geriatric patient should undergo a single operation without risk of a second, such as from a failed pin, so that medical rehabilitation can proceed uninterrupted by such complications as avascular necrosis of the femoral head. The trochanteric fracture should be treated by implantation of a form of pin and plate, skillfully introduced and adequately fixed under radiographic control.

These two methods will obviate the fracture; as a result the patient may walk the following day. No technique should be used for a fracture near the hip that does not allow immediate walking because that would leave the patient to recover from both the fracture and the operation.

Anesthesia

The anesthetic plays a very important part in the well-being of the patient, more so, perhaps, than was realized in the past. There is growing evidence that mental disturbance may be caused or increased by a general anesthetic, particularly if there has been any degree of oxygen deprivation. This means that epidural or spinal anesthesia has to be considered. There is a good case to be made for the use of these anesthetics, but they take a certain time to prepare, set up, and administer and can cause considerable discomfort when positioning the patient with a fracture. Therefore a general anesthetic is still preferred, provided the anesthetist concentrates more on techniques that obviate pain than on deep anesthesia and keeps the patient fully oxygenated throughout the operation and in the recovery room. The patient should be awake as the last stitch is tied and carefully watched thereafter, especially in the recovery room.

There is one other factor of great importance favoring a use of general anesthetic; that is the practice of sucking out the bronchi, sometimes during and always at the end of the operation. This clears phlegm and secretions, and if the patient has a bronchopneumonia at induction, it may be greatly improved at the end of operation.

FRACTURES OF THE FEMORAL NECK

Operative approach

The use of the correct approach to the hip is particularly important. An anterior-lateral incision allows excellent access to the hip, easy removal of the femoral head and upper fragment of the neck, and equally easy insertion of the prosthesis. This incision is much less likely to be contaminated by incontinence than is the posterior approach; it is easily and simply dressed after the operation. The scar heals well despite any of the patient's activities that may delay healing of the scar resulting from the anterior approach, particularly in the obese, because it is near the inguinal crease. What is more important, the prosthesis does not dislocate after its proper insertion through the anterior-lateral approach.

Choice of prosthesis

The prosthesis should be one that can be cemented in place. A prosthesis, rigidly fixed at surgery, increases the patient's confidence in the implant—perhaps by allowing more proprioception—than does a prosthesis that relies on bone formation to hold it firmly in place. The morbidity of cement is not sufficiently high to cause anxiety in this respect, provided a proper technique is used and the anesthetist avoids those anesthetic agents that might contribute to a drop in blood pressure. It is always necessary to warn the anesthetist that cement is to be inserted. Cement that is firmly pressed into the femoral shaft may cause some amount of fat embolism. This can be avoided by passing a soft catheter made of a material unaffected by the cement (e.g., polythene) down the neck of the femur and into the femoral shaft just below the point where the lower tip of the prosthesis will lie. Suction is applied to the catheter to remove the semiliquid fat that lies within the shaft. Suction is maintained while the cement is gently eased into the femoral neck and sucked down the shaft to the correct depth using the least amount of tamponade. The catheter is then withdrawn and the prosthesis inserted with steady pressure rather than fierce hammer blows on an impactor. Two or three gentle taps with the impactor at the end will ensure that the prosthesis is properly seated.

Part of the capsule may be excised if it impedes the speed and accuracy of the operation. No attempt need be made to repair the capsule because dislocation will not occur with the anterior-lateral approach, provided the correct size of prosthesis is used. To verify this it is important to fit the chosen size into the acetabulum as a final check, holding the stem while this is done. Some resistance in withdrawing the head of the prosthesis from the acetabulum indicates a snug fit. Secure hemostasis must be obtained, and the wound should have at least two suction drains.

The wound is dressed with a simple adhesive, occlusive dressing, and no bandages are applied. The following day the patient should stand and walk.

Acetabular erosion

The results of hemiarthroplasty in the treatment of fractures in the neck of the femur are very good, but the late results are marred by pain and disability in a number of patients who have developed acetabular erosion. Because of the patients' high survival rates, this has become an increasingly important problem, one that must be solved if the quality of life returned to the patient by early surgery and rehabilitation is to be preserved.

Experience has shown that the Thompson, Austin Moore, and similar prostheses, made in one piece out of solid metal with sizes graduated in eighths of an inch, are no longer satisfactory. This is because of acetabular erosion, which can occur at practically any age but certainly occurs far more frequently in the more active and usually younger patients.[2]

It has been shown that the late complications of hemiarthroplasty are dominated by acetabular erosion, occurring in 16% of replacements, of whom at least half had symptoms necessitating revision. Obviously if all patients remained active and could carry on indefinitely the number would be greater, but even so this percentage is unacceptable.

The cause of acetabular erosion is not yet fully understood. It is possible that there are several different reasons: (1) the prosthetic head may be too small or too large for the acetabulum by a sixteenth of an inch in 50% of the operations in which an ordinary Thompson or Austin Moore prosthesis is used; (2) the femoral neck and upper shaft are resilient and like all other bone will bend slightly with each footfall, whereas the cemented metal prosthesis takes the impact of the footfall from the uppermost third of the femur and transfers it directly to the acetabulum; (3) the acetabular floor may have been damaged by an accident. It is almost invariable that the elderly person, who has not had a stress fracture of the femoral neck, falls directly on the hip, and the impact of the fall causes the fracture of the femoral neck, which must be resisted by the acetabulum when the femoral head impinges on it. A total hip replacement is indicated when a damaged acetabulum is discovered during surgery. From experience the most important cause of acetabular erosion is thought to be a femoral prosthetic head that is slightly too small and causes point bearing in the acetabulum, that is, the small head articulates with the acetabulum in one small place instead of over the whole surface.

A total hip replacement instead of a hemiarthroplasty in each patient is usually not indicated because it involves considerable extra time during surgery and a second cementing after preparing the acetabulum to hold the cup in place. This part of the operation is considerably more traumatic to the patient than a simple femoral head replacement. There is further morbidity from loosening of the replacement, especially the acetabular component.

To combat acetabular erosion, the requisites for prosthetic replacement of a fractured neck of a femur need to be revised. A suitable prosthesis must have the following: (1) 1-mm gradations; (2) a method for accurately sizing the required prosthetic head; (3) double articulation with a cushion (of high-density polythene); (4) ease of total hip replacement; and (5) a constant distance from the top of the head to the shoulder. Such prostheses are at present under trial.*

Pertrochanteric fracture

In the pertrochanteric fracture the lateral incision is used. The patient is positioned on a suitable table so that the achieved reduction can be checked radiographically, using both anterior-posterior and lateral projections or an image intensifier. The guidewire should lie snugly up the center of the neck of the femur, and by accurate measurement a size of nail should be chosen so that the tip of the nail lies within 1 cm of the top of the femoral head.

The plate must be securely screwed to the bone by at least five screws. Each drilled screw hole should be of the correct size for the screws used and threaded by means of a tap. This enhances the grip of the screws in osteoporotic bone and also means that ordinary screws (as opposed to self-tapping screws) can be used. No plate should ever be left with one or more holes unfilled because a screw has failed to bite and grip the bone satisfactorily. When this occurs a small, high-density polythene plate can be put on the inner side of the femur shaft into which the screw can be made to pass, providing a highly satisfactory grip when tightened. A polythene plate should be used routinely on at least some of the screws in patients for whom any anxiety exists concerning the screws holding the plate firmly against the femoral shaft.

Should the fracture be somewhat lower than usual, a seven-holed plate or longer may be used. It is vital that a really secure grip be obtained because, as with the fractured neck of the femur that has been replaced, the patient is to walk the following day and the fracture fixation must be sound.

The wound is closed using suction drainage and dressed with an occlusive, adhesive dressing.

Fluid and blood replacement

Most elderly patients on admission after a fracture near the hip need an intravenous infusion to restore or maintain fluid balance and electrolyte levels. Some patients may have lain for several hours unattended and need to have the fluid that was lost during that time replaced. However, during the hours before surgery the geriatric patient is generally disinclined to drink much, and fluids by mouth are of course barred for the necessary period before a general anesthetic is administered.

The hemoglobin content will have been estimated on admission, although at this stage it may not be accurate because of systemic shock causing hemoconcentration. The incipient anemia that is so often present in this age group needs to be corrected to improve the prognosis for rehabilitation. According to the findings the necessary amount of blood is cross-matched before surgery, but the blood loss at operation is also considered. If the patient is very anemic, concentrated red cells may be given before surgery. It is better to use this method for correcting a very low hemoglobin content because it avoids excessive input of fluid, which can be deleterious, particularly to those patients with anemia accompanied by incipient heart failure. By increasing the hemoglobin content of the blood before anesthesia is administered, there is again improved oxygenation of the brain.

Blood lost during surgery is replaced slowly. Another hemoglobin estimation is done 48 hours later and more blood may then be given if necessary. There is no doubt that a geriatric patient who is not anemic has a greater chance of successful rehabilitation than one whose deficit has not been corrected. The intravenous infusion is always kept open with bland fluids, such as saline solution or glucose, until the patient is able to drink freely. If there is a possibility of any complication occurring, the infusion is continued. Tubes into or out of the patient, when properly secured, are no bar to early mobilization.

*The "Hastings hip" has been under trial for 5 years with no acetabular erosion reported. The hip is manufactured by Thackray's of Leeds, England.

Catheterization

Although the anterior-lateral or lateral incision recommended is less likely to be contaminated by urine if the patient is incontinent, it is still a possibility. Bed sores are encouraged by incontinence, and the discomfort of a wet bed can disturb and make more irritable the patient with some degree of brain failure. Therefore it is wise always to catheterize the patient before surgery. This particularly applies to women, but there is a growing tendency for this to be done in men also, even before elective procedures, especially if there is any evidence of prostatic enlargement.

Any patient in whom the urea content of the serum is raised should be catheterized to ensure there is no possibility of partial urine retention; such patients in general will need a high fluid intake, and careful management of output is essential and easily controlled in the catheterized patient.

Use of antibiotics

There is a difference of opinion over the use of antibiotics as a routine preventive measure in geriatric orthopedics, but it is strongly recommended here. Only one patient who has developed severe sepsis out of many hundreds of others who have not is sufficient to make most surgeons believe that antibiotic cover should be given. Whatever added cost or morbidity that the antibiotic may cause is completely outweighed by the benefit, not only in preventing wound sepsis but also in controlling bronchial or pneumonic infections and urinary problems. This means that a wide spectrum antibiotic, such as cephalosporin, is best used. It must be remembered that many elderly patients, particularly where a wound is accessible, find it an irritation; their wandering fingers can interfere, explore, and scratch the wound, despite close supervision. Walking the day after the operation will also put a slight strain on the wound, which might become superficially infected were it not for the antibiotic. Usually 4 to 7 days is sufficient antibiotic therapy. Primary wound healing is most important, and nothing should be left undone to stand in its way.

Postoperative progress

The crucial period occurs after surgery. The operation has obviated the fracture near the hip, and the patient may walk. All the staff concerned must have absolute confidence in this program because if there is doubt in the mind of any member of the team, the doubt will be sensed by the patient to the detriment of quick progress.

The patient is first put in a sitting position in a chair. The vacuum drains are tied to the patient's chair, as is the urine bag if the patient has a catheter. To help the patient walk the same routine must be used by every member of the team who treats the patient. First a walking frame of suitable height is chosen. The patient is then made to put the hands on the front ends of the arms of the chair and asked to bend forward as far as possible and at the same time to push up on the hands. Some help may be necessary and should be given by gentle lifting under each armpit. Once the patient is upright and beginning to balance, one hand is moved and then the other from the arm of the chair to the walking frame. The patient is then encouraged to stand up as straight as possible. This achieved, a few tentative steps are taken. The patient is then allowed either to walk backward to the chair or the chair is brought to the patient. Later the patient is taught to do a complete walking turn back to the chair, then to turn around and sit down by first bending forward and moving one and then the other hand from the frame to the arms of the chair.

It is usually at this stage that the patients who were in the first group, those who were in good health and who had a true accident, will show themselves to be capable of walking independently within a few days. They may then be allowed to go home and the stitches removed at a later date. The vacuum drains are usually removed 48 hours after surgery, or when there is less than 50 ml of serosanguineous fluid in the suction bottle after 12 hours.

Those patients who have other geriatric problems should be under the care of their geriatric physician or, if such a center exists, should be transferred to a geriatric orthopedic unit.

Care of the bladder

On admission the patient's bladder may be distended because of urine retention, or distention may occur later. A catheter is passed into the bladder, using full aseptic precautions; the bladder is emptied, and a urine specimen is sent to the laboratory for testing. After surgery the catheter is removed as soon as the patient can sit out of bed and normal micturition can be attempted. If this fails, the catheter is replaced and spigoted, and the bladder is emptied at definite periods to maintain bladder tone. After 2 days another attempt at normal micturition should be made. Sometimes in the decrepit patient it may take 1 or 2 weeks for a normal pattern of micturition to be established.

In elderly men the same principle should apply, but if micturition is not established fairly quickly, the advice of a urologist should be obtained.

A slight amount of cystitis will encourage both urine retention or frequency. Once the infection is controlled, bladder function should return to normal. However, many elderly women may continue to have difficulty with incontinence, in which case a strict bladder voiding routine by day and night will improve continence. This may also be helped by the administration of anticholinergic agents.

Care of the skin

At the time of admission and initial assessment, the skin must be carefully examined to determine if there has been damage to the skin, predisposing the patient to bedsores. Lying immobile on a hard floor for only a short while after the accident can cause an elderly person's skin to break later at the site where the pressure was applied. The patient must be nursed on a suitable type of bed to avoid continued pressure, and the pressure areas should be treated as regularly as possible, at least hourly. The use of air beds, water beds, and sheepskins is beneficial. The best skin care is having the patient mobile in and out of bed, thus avoiding further pressure areas.

FRACTURES IN GENERAL

The detailed description of the patient with a fracture near the hip serves as a good example of the principles underlying the orthopedic treatment of all elderly people and should be applied to all other fractures.

All fractures that can be obviated by surgery should be so treated, but the methods used in the healthy adult may not necessarily be the best for the aged person. Furthermore, the activities of the geriatric patient are much less than those of the young adult so that the methods that would not be acceptable for strong, young patients may be used with great success in the elderly.

Fractures of the femoral shaft

The very high fracture of the shaft of the femur is best treated by a pin and long plate rather than by intramedullary fixation because there is often an unseen crack extending up to the great trochanter, making adequate fixation of the intermedullary pin in the proximal fragment of the femur impossible.

Lower down, the fracture of the femoral shaft in the elderly is often spiral, but it does not contraindicate internal fixation with an intramedullary nail. However, the procedure can be done much more simply than in the younger adult. The patient is placed on the operating table with a tourniquet around the upper thigh and the knee flexed over the end of the operating table. An incision is made to the medial side of the patella and the patellar ligament. The patella is retracted laterally, and a hole is made between the femoral condyles; the guide wire for the intramedullary nail is passed up the femoral shaft. Simple traction by the surgeon is usually sufficient to reduce the fracture to allow the guide wire, under x-ray control, to pass into the proximal fragment. The intramedullary nail is then passed up the shaft from below. If the fracture seems secure, the hole between the femoral condyles is plugged with bone cement. It is wise to rebate the cancellous bone just above the cortical bone to ensure that the cement has an adequate grip. The knee is cleared of debris and sewn up. This is a quick, simple procedure that takes only a few minutes. Should it be impossible to reduce the fracture, particularly a transverse fracture, a small incision is made anteriorly in the thigh over the fracture. By inserting two fingers in the incision the fracture can be reduced. With an oblique fracture, the nail, although achieving lateral stability, will allow shortening by overriding the bone fragments, one on the other; to prevent this, cerclage by strong wires or springs through a small lateral incision is satisfactory. After this is accomplished, it is safe to allow walking forthwith. In the very osteoporotic femur even the largest Küntscher nail may be too loose; in this case two nails can be "stacked" to give better grip.

Supracondylar fractures of the femur

The supracondylar fracture may be a simple fracture of the lowermost third of the femur, or, as is often the case, the fracture line may extend down to the knee, separating the femoral condyles. Conservative treatment is long, tedious, and fraught with all the complications of bed rest in the elderly, and because of the proximity or involvement of the knee, movement after enforced immobilization is poor. Internal fixation is therefore doubly important. A nail plate is applied through a lateral approach, but because of the extension between the femoral condyles, a bolt with a washer is applied to the medial femoral condyle to hold the two condyles firmly together. This is done by having the nail threaded on its inside so that the bolt can be screwed into it along the guide wire passed from the lateral side. Excellent compression can be obtained. If the bone is osteoporotic or if some of the screws pass through some of the fracture line, high-density polythene washers applied on the medial side of the femur maintain a firm screw fixation of the plate.[3] The wound is closed as usual, and, because it is often easier to perform this operation using a pneumatic tourniquet, a firm pressure bandage is applied; further bandages or support from toes to knee prevent distal edema.

Early movement of the knee is allowed, stiffness is avoided, and the patient may walk forthwith.

Fractures of the patella

To avoid prolonged cast fixation the shattered patella should be excised and the quadriceps expansion carefully sutured if it is damaged. A pressure dressing of the Robert Jones type is put on, which supports the knee sufficiently to allow early walking with a frame.

The patella that has a transverse crack but no separation often needs no more than a firm supporting bandage, after which the patient can perform straight leg raising and may then walk, perhaps with a walking frame, and need not be admitted to the hospital. If the patella is separated by a transverse fracture, internal fixation with a bolt and washers and repair of the lateral extension into the quadriceps expansion should be done; again walking is achieved with a pressure dressing.

Fractures of the tibia

The fractured shaft of the tibia is easily treated by an intramedullary nail inserted in a manner similar to that described for the femur but through a small incision medial to the patellar ligament, exposing the upper tibial plateau outside the joint proper. With the knee bent over the end of the table, a suitable point at the front of the tibial plateau is broached; an intramedullary nail can be dropped down easily. The fracture generally reduces itself with the simple effect of gravity pulling on the foot and lower calf. This procedure is not difficult; it must be remembered that the upper part of the tibia is slightly angled backward so that a hole made at the front of the tibial plateau is over the center of the medulla of the tibial shaft.

Fractures of the tibial plateau

Fractures of the tibial plateau should be bolted so that the fracture is compressed. The technique is no different from that used for any other age group, but the program after surgery can be much more brisk with early movement and assisted walking.

Fractures near the ankle

An elderly person who is decrepit does not tolerate the below-the-knee walking plaster cast at all well. Consequently, even the simple Pott's fracture, which might necessitate such a cast, is best treated by screwing the fractured malleoli in such a way as to achieve firm fixation. Long screws may be used, one of which may pass up the shaft of the fibula. It is helpful to use a polythene washer between the head of the screw and the tip of the malleolus. The medial malleolus, again using a similar polythene washer, is screwed back onto the lower shaft of the tibia. The patient is then allowed to walk with no more than a firm pressure dressing and some suitable bootee, such as may be made in any physical therapy department. The more severe the Pott's fracture, the more important it is to try and achieve sound fixation. This also applies to the fracture just above the ankle in the lowermost part of the tibia, which is extremely difficult to treat. Sometimes it is possible to fix this fracture with a plate, even if it is often insufficiently secure to allow the patient to be free of plaster. A below-the-knee cast that is applied after a short interval will provide sufficient external support.

Fractures of the foot

Foot fractures in elderly persons are rarely that incapacitating as to necessitate their admission to the hospital; they can mostly be treated by supportive strapping and bandaging at home.

Fractures of the upper limb

In the elderly a severe fracture of the neck of the humerus may cause so much pain that the patient is incapable of leading an independent existence. It is an axiom in the treatment of these fractures that early movement is essential to prevent stiffness of the shoulder, but if the patient is so severely incapacitated that this is impossible, it is wise to operate. A simple procedure is to approach the head of the humerus through the most anterior fibers of the deltoid muscle and, after carefully drilling a hole in the most lateral part of the head of the humerus, to insert an intramedullary pin through the hole and down the shaft to hold the head in place. This usually gives substantial relief of pain, allows early movement, and enables the patient to go home soon.

Humeral shaft fractures

Humeral shaft fractures are extremely disabling, and the standard methods of conservative management are always to be abandoned in favor of internal fixation. The approach is similar to that for the fractured neck of the humerus, and again it is often possible to achieve a blind intramedullary fixation under radiologic control. If not, the usual methods of open reduction are used.

Fractures near the elbow

A shattered elbow should be treated with a firm pressure dressing and a collar and cuff sling, and the patient should be encouraged to do early movements. To try and internally fix such a "bag of bones" usually ends in a surgical disaster; for this condition prudence is as yet the best treatment. However, the fractured olecranon should always be fixed so securely that no plaster is needed and elbow movements can start forthwith.

Fractures of the radius and ulna

After the reduction of a fracture of the radius and ulna, a plaster cast has to extend from the hand to the axilla, which may be unacceptable in the very aged. Internal fixation of both bones, using plates and screws or intramedullary rods, is then indicated.

Colles' fracture

Colles' fracture is extremely common, and if patients are treated properly, good results will occur. A plaster cast should be applied after a careful reduction of the fracture by closed methods under radiologic control. All patients, as soon as they have recovered from the reduction of the fracture, preferably the same day, must start active movements of the fingers, elbow, and shoulder. They should attend therapy sessions throughout the period that the plaster cast is on; this rarely need be longer than 5 weeks. If such activity is maintained, when the plaster is removed the patient should have full movement of the fingers; the slight residual stiffness of the wrist is soon overcome by active use.

It is quite common for a Colles' fracture to displace somewhat after the initial reduction. A subsequent remanipulation may not improve matters very much and may be detrimental to function. A slight residual deformity may not interfere with function, whereas repeated striving after perfect position may leave a wrist lacking full movement.

SPINAL INJURIES

Cervical spine

Many old people suffer from spondylosis (or osteoarthritis) and disc degeneration of the cervical spine, with or without symptoms. Degenerate discs may bulge posteriorly to form bars anterior to the cord. These can become hard and fixed but not necessarily calcified, so that they are not visible on plain radiographs but are demonstrated by myelography. The posterior longitudinal ligament lies behind the bodies of the vertebrae and covers the posterior aspect of this bar. The bars may not give rise to overt symptoms but can cause sufficient pressure on the cervical cord to produce pyramidal signs and weakness of the lower limbs and upgoing plantar reflexes. This predisposes the patient to two different types of injury. First, the resulting unsteadiness is a frequent cause of falls; a very careful medical history is needed to discover this because patients are likely to say that they tripped over something or give a similar story. In fact the fall will have been caused not by an obstruction, such as a rug, but by the unsteadiness or inability to lift the feet properly. Another way in which falls occur in the otherwise healthy old person with this neck condition is in a public place when a minor unintentional jostle by a passerby may put the patient off balance. An aged individual cannot recover from a jostle that a fully normal person would hardly notice. It is in this type of patient that looking up can cause a fall, not only because the cord gets an increase in pressure but also because the eyes, on which greater reliance for balance is placed, are no longer of help. Here it is important to note that good eyesight is very important; vision must always be carefully checked and corrected as necessary.

If an accident, especially an acceleration injury in an automobile mishap, occurs, immediate tetraparesis may result or sometimes complete tetraplegia. The elderly patient who has survived such an accident and has been brought to the hospital with tetraparesis will almost certainly not have a very unstable injury to the neck, else a tetraplegia would be present. Nevertheless, the investigation, after the full careful clinical examination, must include radiography of the cervical spine. The usual investigations will also be done and the clinical examination repeated at frequent intervals to assess the continuing paresis, which not only may vary but may become dramatically worse if spinal cord edema occurs and spreads. However, in general an increasing paresis for several hours after the injury indicates that edema is the cause and, on reduction of the edema, recovery should occur. If plain radiography of the cervical spine shows no injury but severe neurologic changes that have remained constant are present, myelography should be considered. At this stage a neurosurgeon should be asked to advise because, in the rare case where surgical exploration is indicated, it should be done by a surgeon well-versed in cervical cord surgery, with the orthopedic surgeon available to stabilize the cervical spine thereafter.

In the absence of an unstable fracture, conservative treatment should be by simple means; head traction is difficult to manage in the elderly. It is better to accept a lesser degree of immobilization of the neck for the sake of better mobilization of the patient. Early rehabilitation is indicated from the earliest moment, and a full exercise regimen should be started. These are best achieved by the use of a cervical collar. The outlook, if recovery does not occur within a few days, is poor.

Thoracic spine

Elderly people commonly suffer from two forms of thoracic spinal fractures—those occasioned by the spontaneous collapse of an osteoporotic vertebra and those caused by a fall; very often there is a combination of these two. The pain is severe, and the patient is scared and anxious. After admission to the hospital the patient is laid flat in bed without boards under the mattress. Pillows are then added in numbers compatible with comfort, the patient having been given mild analgesics. By increasing the pillows, in 2 or 3 days the patient is sitting up in bed. Elderly people are frightened when told they have a fractured spine or a broken back; it is better to be euphemistic and to attribute the severe pain to heavy bruising of the bone or some such diagnosis. The patient should also be told that once sitting in bed has been achieved sitting in a chair is to be tried. Again, the patient is warned that there will be pain, which should be accepted in the interest of avoiding other complications. Reassured, the patient does not then mind sitting out of bed, and because the weight above the fracture is not altered by standing, the patient will soon walk. It is good practice to use analgesics of a strength that does not interfere with the patient's mental capabilities. Should stronger drugs be needed to control the pain, longer bed rest may have to be allowed.

A ready-made orthopedic corset should be given to the patient when sitting has been achieved and a custom-made model ordered for further use, which may be prolonged in the severely osteoporotic patient.

Fractures of the pelvis

Fractures of the pelvis are common and often occasioned by some trivial fall. Frequently the initial diagnosis may be that of a fractured hip. Because the latter is not observed on the radiograph, a crack fracture in the ischiopubic ramus may be missed. Sometimes one and sometimes all four rami are fractured, but normally such fractures are stable; the patient can be treated in exactly the same way as that described earlier for the compression fracture of the vertebra. The patient should walk with a walking frame as soon as possible; rarely is it necessary to delay the patient in bed for more than a few days.

Stress fractures

The elderly are susceptible to stress fractures, especially of the femoral neck, pelvis, tibia, and more rarely, tibia and fibula combined. Often these occur in patients with marked osteoporosis, but stress fractures will also occur with some unusual, if not abnormal, activity such as a holiday with the family when there is more than usual activity. The symptoms in the femoral neck may be slight, a dull ache getting slightly worse with exercise and improved with rest. If diagnosed, internal fixation at once (using one or two thin pins) relieves pain and anxiety. Only too often, however, catastrophe occurs; the stress fracture breaks, and the patient falls to the ground. If the patient's medical history is not taken carefully, the preexisting symptoms will be missed and the fracture considered the result and not the cause of the fall.

The stress fracture of the pelvis is diagnosed by a similar medical history and confirmed by clinical examination and radiography. No treatment other than a level of activity that does not produce pain is needed.

The tibia may cause problems. Although the stress fracture is usually in the uppermost one third, it may be anywhere in the shaft. If radiologically it looks unstable or liable to break completely, internal fixation should be done, usually as for an ordinary fracture.

A valuable adjunct to diagnosis is the radioisotope bone scan, which will reveal a stress fracture considerably earlier than a normal radiograph. The pattern can be at times so distinctive that it is a definite confirmation of the clinical diagnosis.

Stress fractures must be recognized because they may have medical-legal implications when, for example, a fracture of the femoral neck causes the patient to fall and neglect may be alleged if it occurs when the patient is under some form of care. Furthermore, with advanced osteoporosis tibias and femurs have been known to break when the patient is assisted out of bed.

SCINTIGRAPHY

Radioisotope bone scans are very useful in investigating problems in the elderly, particularly when the clinical problem does not give easy access to a firm diagnosis. This particularly applies to fractures, metastatic deposits, rheumatoid disease, and metastatic bone disease. Technetium is injected in a pyrophosphate base and deposited in areas in which osteoblastic activity is present. It has a low radiation effect on the body. Where osteoblastic activity is present, there is seen to be a "hot spot" with much increased absorption, thereby causing increased radiation and a dark area on the scintigraphic printout. It is interesting that bone scans will give a positive answer sometimes well before plain radiography will demonstrate a lesion, whether it be a stress fracture or a metastatic deposit. Because of the surgical interference, there is a "hot spot" for about a year after a total joint replacement, but thereafter positive findings may confirm loosening or low grade infection long before anything is apparent on plain radiographs.

PATHOLOGIC FRACTURES

Malignant disease involving the bones of an elderly person is usually, but not always, metastatic from a known or hidden primary lesion. The exceptions are myelomatosis and, more rarely, sarcoma secondary to Paget's disease.

Because a malignant deposit often erodes and weakens the bone in which it is growing, pain may be severe, not only where a pathologic fracture has occurred but before; the weakened bone giving pain in the same way that a stress fracture causes pain; thus the bone is in an overstressed condition. Some tumors growing within a bone may give pain in their own right, which is not only distressing but disabling to the patient. Often only a vigorous surgical attack will prevent the geriatric patient from living out his life bedridden and in great discomfort.

Fractures of the spine

Pathologic fractures of the spine occur with either an everincreasing backache or incipient or established paraplegia. The origin of the tumor may be either metastatic or sometimes a direct spread from carcinoma of the lung, pancreas, or other organ.

The body of the vertebra may be involved, with subsequent crushing and collapse, or the vertebral arch may be affected. This may not be readily demonstrated in ordinary radiographs, and a tomograph may be helpful. Also the tumor may itself invade the spinal canal and cause paraplegia because of direct compression of the spinal cord.

Radiotherapy should be used for the patient with increasing severe backache produced by a metastasis. However, if the pain has become extremely severe and especially if there is danger of collapse and paraplegia, it is proper to stabilize that part of the spine before radiotherapy is given; this is not only to ease the pain but because it takes at least 6 weeks from the end of the radiotherapy course for the bone to start hardening again so that its structural stability is assured. Stabilization can be done simply by putting in spinal plates, such as those of Meurig Williams, without using a bone grafting procedure. A further advantage is that the patient can be treated more easily and efficiently by the radiotherapist when plaster casts or plaster beds are not needed.

The patient who has incipient or complete paraplegia is to be considered an extreme emergency. A myelograph must be done at once and the usual laboratory tests performed to assess the patient's general condition and to prepare the patient for surgery. When the clinician has established the level of the pressure site and determined that the paraplegia is not caused by avascularity of the cord from the metastatic deposit blocking the blood supply, the patient is subjected to decompression of the spinal cord. Adequate provision for blood transfusion must be made. The shorter the time between the onset of paraplegia and decompression, the better the chance of recovery; thus if the patient has only the early signs of the condition, such as slight weakness or an upgoing plantar reflex, myelography and decompression should be done. If the bladder has been paralyzed for any length of time, it is unlikely to recover after decompression. Although it is accepted that decompression will rarely cause recovery from paraplegia if it has existed for more than a few days, it is still worth doing, especially if the patient is in pain; plates should be used to stabilize the spine. Not only does this relieve pain but also the general condition of the patient is materially improved, both physically, which includes ease of nursing and a lessening of the risk of pressure sores, and mentally. The patient finds it easier to accept the condition knowing that everything possible has been done.

Decompression is done by excising the laminae from the level of the block, determined by the myelograph, upward until free pulsation returns. Once the laminae in the upper thoracic spine have been freely removed, no further surgery to reconstitute the posterior parts of the vertebrae is needed because of the support of the rib cage; in the thoracolumbar and lumbar spine it is wise to bridge the gap left by the decompression with spinal plates of correct length to stabilize the spine if it appears to need it at the time of the operation. The metal implant in no way prevents proper radiotherapy, which usually follows any orthopedic treatment of metastatic tumors.

Portions of the tumor should be examined histologically because it is possible for the elderly person to have had one primary tumor treated previously, whereas the metastasis may come from a hitherto unsuspected tumor. If the tumor bleeds freely during surgery, myeloma is suggested. It is wrong to delay decompression while investigations are done to determine the nature of the primary and secondary tumors if it is not already known. The histology of the tumor is the only absolute method of diagnosis.

After surgery the patient is nursed in bed with no form of fixation but with great care taken to prevent bedsores and urinary stasis by frequent attention to the skin and by turning the patient. An automatic turning bed, which tilts from side to side, is a valuable adjunct to treatment.

No patient with paraplegia caused by a metastatic, malignant disease should be refused surgery. To live out the remaining few weeks of life paralyzed from the waist down and incontinent is a terrible insult to human dignity. In addition, a suspicion that an operation might have helped adds grievously to the burden.

Fractures of the limbs

Pathologic fractures of the limbs can be subdivided into those that are about to occur and those that have occurred. Both are in urgent need of treatment. The pathologic fracture of the neck of the femur should be treated by excision and replacement, as for an ordinary fracture; cement and metal do not detract from the normal efficacy of radiotherapy or cytotoxic drugs. The fractures that occur in long bones, including the humerus, femur, and tibia, should all be internally fixed by the usual methods. A skeletal survey should be done to diagnose other symptomless deposits that may be worth prophylactic treatment by various means, such as an intramedullary nail. The radiotherapist will always appreciate being able to treat a patient knowing that not only is there no danger of a pathologic fracture occurring, but also that the radiographic fields are not obscured by plaster casts.

There need be no fear of the tumor fungating through the wound, even if it is resistant to radiotherapy. It occurs so rarely, and then only in the final stages of the disease, that this slight risk is worth taking for the present comfort of the patient.

CHRONIC ORTHOPEDIC CONDITIONS

Fractures, especially those near the hip in the elderly, have been discussed in detail to show the principles behind the management of the geriatric orthopedic patient; such elderly patients will also suffer from all the orthopedic problems seen at earlier ages. The operative treatment is rarely different, with the exception of the management not only of the problem but also of the patient as a whole.

It is not proposed, therefore, to discuss in detail the operations or orthopedic lesions except insofar as the methods or care are altered to benefit the elderly patient.

Osteoarthritis

Age is no bar to surgery. Once a joint has become sufficiently painful or disabling to spoil the quality of life, there should be no hesitation in doing a total joint replacement. The risk of a major operation to restore function in the arthritic joint of an elderly person may be undertaken with confidence because nowhere is such a patient safer than in the hands of a competent anesthetist in the operating room. There is normally no place in the elderly for lesser procedures such as osteotomy of the femur or tibia, which used to be done before total hip or knee replacements were satisfactory.[4] Osteotomy usually requires considerable treatment and care after surgery and takes much longer for the end result than does a total replacement. Also the reliability of osteotomy is less than that of a properly done joint replacement. The hip prosthesis, which has now been followed up for many years, has been shown to be successful as has the knee prosthesis, which if properly chosen is almost equally successful and can be used in the elderly with great success.

One of the problems of arthroplasty is loosening of the components. The actual wearing out of the movable parts has not shown itself to be a problem of any note, but after an indefinable amount of use one or other component becomes loose, either in the cement or the cement in the bone, causing pain that may be sufficiently severe to indicate revision of the arthroplasty. However, this is not so common in the elderly because of the decline in activity that occurs. Falls and injuries can matter a great deal and can cause loosening. This matter must always be remembered as a problem; no elderly patient who is at all unsteady or suffering from lack of balance and has had a total joint replacement should be allowed to continue without all preventive measures being implemented, especially the use of a cane. If loosening does occur, it can often be confirmed by the use of scintigraphy, as described above.

The late complications of arthroplasty are greatly decreased if there is no likelihood of infection. If infection occurs in an elderly patient after a total joint replacement, it is a disaster of great magnitude and must be avoided by taking every precaution possible. Thus it is imperative that if total hip replacements are to be done, operating room conditions must be sound. Whereas it is not always necessary to have a clean air operating room, this should certainly be insisted on if the room is shared with other surgical disciplines and if surgery for sepsis is sometimes performed there.

Particularly in the elderly patient with rheumatoid arthritis strict instructions should be given that if the patient having had a total hip replacement is to undergo any further surgical procedure that might entail a bacteremia the patient should be given a course of antibiotics for 2 or 3 days to cover the bacterial invasion and to prevent an infection occuring at the junction of the bone and cement. Even dental extractions or simple genitourinary procedures like catheterization should be covered in this way. All rheumatoid patients at any age should, of course, follow this regimen, and certainly any patient on steroids for other reasons, such as asthma, who has also had a joint replacement, should have a similar antibiotic regimen during periods of possible bacteremia. The osteoarthritic patient is less likely to suffer from a metastatic infection, but if there is any anxiety, antibiotics should be used.

The smaller joints do not as yet lend themselves to trustworthy replacement as, for example, the shoulder, elbow, wrist, or ankle. In most patients there are other methods of treatment still in use. For example, the wrist and ankle do very well after arthrodesis. If the ankle is fused by means of compression clamps, the patient can walk soon after, which is a prerequisite of most elective geriatric orthopedic operations, and need not be immobilized for a long time after the operation. The wrist may also have internal fixation of one form or another so that little if any external immobilization is needed. The shoulder, if extremely painful, is often extremely stiff and of little value to the patient, who often does better with an excision of the joint rather than arthrodesis, which is cumbersome and protracted with practically every surgical method available. The elbow usually will respond to an excision of the head of the radius, and removal of loose bodies, providing a reasonable range of motion with not too severe pain. Most of the joints described here are of course in patients with rheumatoid arthritis with many joints involved. This makes it imperative to treat some, if not all, the joints to preserve function.

Osteoarthritis of the hip. The normal, conservative treatment methods for osteoarthritis of the hip by a cane, analgesics, and physical therapy often have little effect on the elderly person. Once the disease has advanced so as to prevent the enjoyment of life or has become a disability rather than an inconvenience, the patient may be subjected to total hip replacement. The only difference between this operation, apart from the technique itself, and that done for the fracture near the hip is that there is ample time beforehand for the patient to be assessed by the anesthetist and for the usual blood investigations to be carried out.

The surgical technique used should be one that will allow the patient to be out of bed as soon as possible. Many of the hip prostheses are modifications of the McKee or Charnley designs, and, provided the patient is allowed up immediately after the operation, there is probably little to choose between them. If there is a choice of techniques, one requiring a shorter bed rest than the other is preferred. There are the usual good indications to allow the patient to walk on the day after operation. It is most important in hip arthroplasty not to measure the range of movement achieved at 3 to 6 months after the operation, which is of little consequence to the geriatric patient, but to ensure that the hip allows the patient to do all the activities of daily living. Time and energy wasted treating patients to obtain a range of movement that they do not need is detrimental; the sooner the patient is at home living normally, the more successful is the operation.

The operation must be covered by the administration of an antibiotic, but the routine use of anticoagulants has not yet been shown to be necessary, provided the patient is kept active both before and after the operation.

Osteoarthritis of the knee. The knee has many more types of replacement prostheses than has the hip, but for the elderly person the choice of replacement should be one that takes all the weight off the joint surfaces but does not necessitate too much bone removal, as does the hinge type of prosthesis. Furthermore, the prosthesis must stabilize the knee in all planes other than the normal range of movement. The arthritic condition often so damages one or the other tibial condyle that there is much laxity in the lateral ligaments; also the cruciate ligaments may be degenerated.[5]

The patient who needs a knee replacement must be warned that it is less easy in a knee to restore movement that has been absent for a long time than it is in the hip, although a moderate flexion contracture can be overcome. A painful, stiff knee will generally become painless, with a useful but by no means full range of movement. This careful explanation beforehand avoids future disappointment and leaves patients contented with satisfactory function.

Rheumatoid arthritis. Rheumatoid arthritis can be either a burned-out condition or a moderately acute form with an onset in later life. The latter form is properly treated by the rheumatologist, but it may leave the patient with all the problems seen in the younger patient. For the elderly with joint destruction from rheumatoid arthritis there should be no hesitation in employing all surgical methods necessary, from synovectomy of the joints that remain with thickened synovia that do not respond to medical treatment to arthroplasty and arthrodesis of the various affected joints. It must be remembered that patients with long-standing rheumatoid arthritis have diseased joints with ligaments often much laxer than is found in patients with primary osteoarthritis.

The elderly patient with rheumatoid arthritis, if previously treated by cortisone derivatives, must be carefully watched during and after the operation, and hydrocortisone should be readily available for intravenous administration should the patient develop a hypotensive crisis or some other complication of adrenal failure.

One part of the body affected in the elderly by rheumatoid arthritis is the neck; careful investigation, particularly of the upper cervical spine, should always be made if there are any symptoms localized to that area. Progressive subluxation at the atlantoaxial joint can be dangerous to life. It is not uncommon but is a hazard not to be left untreated. Often rest for several months in a cervical collar is all that is necessary, provided there is adequate clinical and radiologic supervision. If conservative treatment fails, it will be necessary to perform an occipitocervical fusion. Usually it is sufficient to freshen the base of the occiput and the spinous processes and laminae of the second and third cervical spines, or lower if necessary, and to insert bone chips into the bed thus provided. After immobilization for 6 to 12 weeks in a well-fitting cervical collar, the neck will be stabilized sufficiently, even though bony union between the graft and the occiput is not always present then or later; the strong fibrous tissue between the skull and the graft is sufficient to prevent further subluxation.

Spinal stenosis. Stenosis, or narrowing of the spinal canal can be congenital, but most commonly it is caused in two ways by osteoarthritis. The most common way, perhaps, is by osteoarthritis of the facet joint, allowing a forward slip and a subsequent spondylolisthesis, usually at the L4-5 level. The other way it occurs is by direct narrowing of the spinal canal by osteoarthritic facets sinking inward and encroaching on the canal; this may cause pressure on cord, corda equina, or nerve roots. The spondylolisthetic type is easily confirmed by radiculography, but the other variety, although it can often be shown on radiculographs, is better demonstrated on a computed tomograph (CT scan). The narrow spinal canal will suffer stenosis more easily, and therefore earlier, than the larger canal. Sometimes a superimposed disc degeneration or protrusion produces the symptoms that would not have occurred in an otherwise normal canal. Spinal stenosis is being found more often now that there are an increasing number of elderly people blessed with both longevity and activity.

The symptoms are highly characteristic and may easily be mistaken for intermittent claudication. The patient may complain of severe backache that only occurs with or during activity, causing that activity to cease and the patient to rest, usually by sitting down. Indeed it is generally said that on sitting down the pain ceases. However, the most important part of the patient's medical history is the description of the weakness, numbness, or other vague statements about the feeling in the legs after walking a short distance. Although not paralyzed, one or both legs feel to the patient that they will not support the body any longer, and the patient must sit down. Soon this feeling passes and walking may be continued only for the same cycle of symptoms to be repeated. Examination of the patient reveals only too often no physical signs whatsoever. This must not deter the physician from making the diagnosis.

The stenosed lumbar spine is narrower when the patient is erect than when the patient is sitting with the lumbar spine slightly flexed. In this position there is less pressure on the intervertebral spaces; it has been suggested that this allows the posterior bulge of the disc to be reduced, thus alleviating the pressure in the canal and on the structures within it. This accounts for the peculiar symptoms that occur with activity and the necessity for sitting to ease the pain or other sensations quickly.

Treatment includes establishing the level of the stenosis by radiculography or a CT scan and then decompressing the spinal cord at that level. If necessary, a protruding disc is removed and the spine stabilized thereafter with a large, flat graft from the ilium with the cortex inward, leaving plenty of space for the spinal cord, which should be protected from the graft by layers of gelatin foam.

The method of grafting should incorporate fixation so that the patient may be allowed up within a few days after the operation without detriment to the grafting procedure.

CT SCANNING

CT scanning is a helpful method for investigating certain conditions of the elderly. It is perhaps the only investigation that will show lumbar stenosis properly, delineating the actual areas of pressure and the extent of the bone mass that is causing the problem.

The CT scan uses x-rays, penetrating the patient with heavy dosage. The beam traverses the patient segmentally, while a computer builds the images on a screen. This can then be altered by the computer into different orientations and preserved on videotape.

The investigation is expensive because of the initial outlay on apparatus, installation, revenue, and servicing costs; consequently it is only available at large medical centers and should only be used on those patients in definite need of its help.

In the elderly orthopedic patient CT scanning is best reserved for those patients with either undiagnosed lesions in which the scan will help establish the diagnosis or in those mechanical conditions caused by bony impingement on other structures, particularly in the spinal cord. The computer will allow the viewer, by reorientating the message received, to move up (or down) the spinal column as though within a tunnel. The dramatic pictures, showing even a single osteophyte pressing on a nerve, are extremely helpful in this particular condition. Nevertheless, many patients with lumbar stenosis can have the diagnosis confirmed by simple radiculography.

VASCULAR DISEASE

When a patient with vascular disease is referred to the orthopedic surgeon, it is because the condition has gone so far that amputation is necessary. This may be an emergency because of gangrene, which, because of its associated toxicity, renders the patient extremely ill, especially so if diabetes is also present. Even so, the limb should be ablated at the lowest level and, if possible, the knee preserved. Often by using a long posterior flap, a high below-the-knee amputation will be successful when other techniques, such as using equal flaps, would fail. Techniques suited to the younger patient are unnecessary, such as forming a synostosis between the cut ends of the tibia and fibula. What is important is to obtain primary wound healing. If it is apparent during surgery that amputation below the knee will fail, either a through-the-knee or a low thigh amputation should be chosen. Whatever the method and whatever the level of amputation used, geriatric patients should be provided with some form of early walking aid so that they may walk within a few days after the amputation. The immediate postoperative fitting technique, in which an exoprosthesis is applied to the stump by means of a plaster cast, can be highly satisfactory in specialized centers in which a full team of trained personnel exists; but where such facilities are unavailable, early walking is as good. It can be left safely to the physical therapist to teach the patient how to use the early walking aid.[6]

The principles of early walking are perhaps poorly understood. Most geriatric patients who require amputation suffer from vascular disease not only in the part affected but throughout the body. This means that they are frequently somewhat confused, although this may not show through the illness and toxicity before the amputation. Memory and orientation may be poor, and the ability to cope with such a traumatic experience will be limited. Therefore the early walking aid must be cosmetic and extremely light. It should be easily put on, safe, and there must be a knee hinge. Although the most important physical sign in the elderly may be to see the patient walk, there is no doubt that the normal habitat of that same patient is the chair. To sit with an unhinged pylon is both distressing and ugly.

It is particularly important that instead of a rocker there should be a foot on which a shoe may be put. The elderly person, particularly when confused, who attempts to walk and sees one foot properly encased in a shoe and an odd-looking apparatus on the other is not in the least encouraged. Two feet with two shoes give an appearance of a return to normal and provide great encouragement to the patient who can now believe that the absolute loss of independence that the amputation caused is now over and a return to function and independence lies ahead.

ASSESSMENT OF GERIATRIC PATIENTS

Before elective surgery

Before an elective operation of some magnitude an elderly person must be properly assessed. It is important to know the patient's background domestically, socially, physically, and mentally. Many old people live in straitened circumstances. With inflation, fixed incomes become less valuable; gradually the patient moves into less and less amenable accomodations. The patient may even end in an apartment high up in a house with no elevator. Nourishment may be poor with vitamin deficiencies and anemia.

Relatives may or may not be available to help in the home or to do the shopping. Eyesight and hearing may be poor, and the quality of existence, only acceptable while otherwise active, becomes intolerable when an osteoarthritic hip or knee confines the patient to a greater and greater extent.

To assess patients before surgery a special clinic is useful. The clinic is run by a team of therapists under the direction of a unit manager or orthopedic nurse who coordinates the work and collates her own findings with those of the therapists.

The manager and therapists at the clinic are able to make a complete mental, physical, and social assessment of the needs of each particular patient. The surgeon's notes and recommendations are reviewed and acted on; when necessary the patient is referred to the anesthetist or the social worker. Usually the assessment is done about 6 weeks before the patient is to be admitted to the hospital for the operation.

The procedures are explained and fears allayed. It is, for example, proper to explain that it is routine for tubes to be going in and out of various parts of the body after surgery; otherwise, on waking the patient may believe that something has gone wrong and that all is lost. These small details are an essential part of a good geriatric orthopedic service.

The patient first sees a therapist who will discover the activities the patient can do and also those that are necessary for an independent existence. For example, if patients live in single story housing, there is no point in teaching them how to use stairs. A program of exercises will be given to strengthen the muscles that will have to work the new joint. Because the patient knows that the operation is near these are done as assiduously as the mentality of the patient will allow. This is a beneficial aspect of an assessment clinic and is important particularly before a joint replacement is performed to reduce flexion or other deformities. It is at this stage that the patient will be told about getting out of bed the day after the operation and the reasons for doing so. Forewarned, especially about there being some discomfort or pain, the patient will cooperate fully.

Details of the assessment are kept in the case notes. Routine or special investigations are arranged at this stage so that on admission there need to be no delay before the operation, including having blood of the correct group available for transfusion. Finally the date of admission is arranged with the social and family circumstances in mind so that the projected date of discharge will be when help at home is readily available.

After surgery the assessment is continued daily and the patient's progress monitored. This is to ensure that the predictions, such as physical ability, date of discharge, and arrangements for domestic help, are adhered to, or any alteration noted and the program amended.

After emergency admission

Patients who have had an emergency admission obviously cannot be assessed beforehand; because they may be ill, in pain, and confused it may take several days to obtain a clear and accurate insight into their general condition, both clinically and socially. The program of aftercare can be radically altered in the light of the knowledge obtained by the team; what at first may have appeared to be a difficult social problem may be resolved by this early attention to detail. Relatives, friends, and neighbors who are available to give information or to help the patient upon discharge are seen. The therapist will assess the capabilities of the patient and may do a home visit to assess the various aids needed to improve the home, such as double bannisters, pull-rails in the bathroom, good lighting, removal or adjustment of worn or loose carpets, and so on, including an attempt to find the cause of the fall. Financial aspects are not neglected, and decisions have to be made as to whether or not the patient should continue to live alone. Alternative or sheltered accommodations may have to be found. If the patient is already in sheltered accommodations before an emergency admission, it is usually necessary to find different accommodations in which there will be increased care and attention, because, however good the surgery, the capabilities of the patient are decreased, and it is rare for such patients to achieve the same level of independence as before the fracture.

GERIATRIC ORTHOPEDIC UNITS

Admission units

It is becoming more necessary, with the increasing age of the population, and therefore of patients, to involve the geriatric physician at the earliest possible stage in the treatment of the geriatric orthopedic emergency. To this end admission units have been, and should be, developed wherein the patients are at once under the care of both disciplines. This makes for efficient medical treatment from the time when the patient is first seen for any of the many other conditions that beset most elderly people with a fracture and for total care from the moment of admission. In ideal circumstances the patient should remain in such a unit until it is obvious that there is either no need for further geriatric supervision or that, despite obviating the fracture, the patient will need longer geriatric rehabilitation than usual.

Rehabilitation units

The problems of the elderly vary not only from continent to continent and country to country but even in some measure from one district to another. No geriatric orthopedic unit should be planned on any particular format but must always be designed to overcome the problems of the local geriatric orthopedic patients.[7]

However, there are some basic principles that should be common to all such units. Without doubt the most important is the cooperation between the geriatric physician and the orthopedic surgeon. Provided this close liaison comes from the management level, the rest of the team will work smoothly with all their attention directed to the patients and not distracted by any feelings of split loyalties.

Perhaps the second most important feature of a geriatric orthopedic unit is the surgery done on the patient. This must be of such a quality that the fracture is obviated by the operation; it must never be considered that the unit is for failed patients or failed surgery. Therefore the patients, although having had surgery recently, are merely recovering from the operation and not from the fracture. In other words the patients must be in a position to be surgically rehabilitated by the team in a very active environment.

Another important principle to follow is that a geriatric orthopedic unit is for the most ill patients who need urgent efforts to ensure that they are rehabilitated quickly; otherwise this may not be possible and not only is independence not achieved but the quality of life is reduced.

It is necessary to have a properly organized team within the unit, whose duties each member must know exactly. To achieve this a weekly round is made in the unit, at which both physician and surgeon attend with all members of the team. During rounds all decisions are made for the future program, either for the coming week or for a period as necessary. The nurse in charge of the ward will report on the patient's progress, bearing in mind a special reference to nocturnal behavior. The therapists will report on the patient's ability to walk and to achieve the activities of daily living such as going to the bathroom, dressing, toilet, feeding, and later the ability to manage in the kitchen unit. The medical social worker will report on the home conditions, the financial problems, the necessity of having relatives or other help at home, whether temporarily or permanently, and the possibility for the patient to live on one floor, even if this means having a bed brought downstairs. All decisions and information are recorded by the unit secretary.

In the unit the patients come under the day-to-day care of the geriatric physician and medical staff who are adept at dealing with all the other illnesses that are always present in the feeble geriatric patient who is an orthopedic emergency. They will have assessed the general state of the patient in regard not only to physical health but also to mental capabilities. A simple test of the mentality is recorded on admission and regularly thereafter. An increasing score in the test is a good prognostic sign, whereas a deteriorating score often indicates that the patient has brain failure that may ultimately preclude an independent existence.

There are many common conditions that may weigh against quick rehabilitation. The most common, anemia of a simple iron deficiency type, should have been rectified temporarily by transfusion, but further treatment must be given to prevent a recurrence. Pernicious anemia is a common finding, as are ischemic heart disease, cerebral vascular disorders, bronchitis, genitourinary conditions, and dementia. Postural hypotension may detract from the ability to walk, but once diagnosed suitable supports of the legs and abdomen will completely change the apparently poor prognosis.

In the geriatric orthopedic unit all the patients have a bedside locker and wardrobe in which they keep their clothes. Initially it is usual for the patient to need help dressing, but every patient must be fully dressed and sitting out of bed for as long as possible during the day. After the midday meal patients may rest on their beds but again fully clothed. This is most important because elderly persons in bedclothes and dressing gown feel that their proper place is in bed, whereas when dressed their proper place is up. In addition, wearing shoes rather than slippers indicates to the patient that they are ready and able to walk. The simple recurrent exercise of dressing restores the patient's morale to a far greater extent than does any verbal assurance of a rapid return home.

Many elderly patients are deaf; the strange surrounding and turmoil of the acute care ward, the operation, the drainage tubes, the intravenous infusions, and so on engender confusion, particularly so if patients cannot hear what is said. Great attention must be paid to making sure that the patients understand what is to be done and what is going to happen to allay their natural apprehension.

Remembering that it is only the ill patients who are transferred to the geriatric orthopedic unit, it is usually found that the average stay is about a month. Some patients achieve independence sooner than this or at least a level of independence that will enable them to go to a sheltered accommodation for a further period of time. Before the patient is discharged, a full discussion takes place with the team to ensure that the patient is fit and capable of living alone. When indicated, it is better to err on the side of the patient's opinion rather than on that of the team, particularly when the patient is desperately anxious to get home and there is only marginal doubt as to the patient's capabilities. Sometimes a trial discharge is arranged in which the patient may go home, but the bed is kept in the unit for a few days. If the patient finds or relatives find that the patient cannot manage, the patient can return to the unit for further rehabilitation. Although the patients are up all day, the unit is not a convalescent ward and is staffed as an acute geriatric unit.

Unfortunately there are some who do not make sufficient progress to be able to achieve an independent existence. When the team members agree that the orthopedic condition is not holding the patient in the hospital, the geriatric physician will accept responsibility for the patient.

Although it is an important orthopedic principle in general to achieve full movement in a joint that has been operated on, in the elderly this is not necessarily so. After a fracture the function of the hip should be assessed as part of the function of the whole patient; this means that there is no necessity to achieve a full range of movement in the hip provided the patient is able to perform the activities of daily living. It is a waste of elderly persons' time to try to achieve a full range of movement in any joint as long as what movement they have is sufficient for their ordinary activities.

Finally there are those patients for whom the skills of resuscitation and rehabilitation are of no avail. Death is a natural part of existence and to many old people comes as a friend. Once death is imminent no steps should be taken to prolong life unnecessarily. The patient should be allowed to die in comfort, with dignity and without pain. All drugs are stopped except those for comfort, and the patient is treated with tender loving care. No team of physicians and surgeons is infallible. It is a salutory experience to stop administration of all drugs to a patient and to find, a week later, that the patient is a great deal better, with hope again of an active life.

CONCLUSION

The elderly person has only a short while to live and does not wish to spend that time burdened by ailments so debilitating that life cannot be enjoyed. The elderly person knows that death is inevitable; frank discussions on the risks of an operation are received with gratitude and the operation accepted with alacrity. Only too often is the surgeon more frightened of the patient's death than is the patient to whom it might occur.

REFERENCES

1. Devas, M.B. editor: Geriatric orthopedics, London, 1977, Academic Press, Inc.
2. Devas, M.B., and D'Arcy, J.C.:Treatment of fractures of the femoral neck by replacement with the Thompson prosthesis, J. Bone Joint Surg. (Br.) **58B**:279, 1976.
3. Gallannaugh, C.: Supracondylar fractures of the femur

in the elderly: treatment by internal fixation, Injury **5**:259,1974.

4. Devas, M.B.: High tibial osteotomy for arthritis of the knee. A method specially suitable for the elderly, J. Bone Joint Surg. (Br.) **51**:95, 1969.
5. Attenborough, C.G.: Total knee replacement using the stabilized gliding prosthesis, Ann. R. Coll. Surg. Engl. **58**:4, 1976.
6. Devas, M.B.: Early walking of geriatric amputees, Br. Med. J. **1**:394, 1971.
7. Devas, M.B., and Irvine, R.E.: The geriatric orthopedic unit, Br. J. Geriatr. Pract. **6**:19, 1969.

CHAPTER 20 · UROLOGY

Richard M. Pearson

Significant strides have been made in the diagnosis and management of urologic problems in the older patient. This success has come from research into the basic pathophysiology of urinary disease in the aging population, from improvements in diagnostic techniques and diagnostic equipment, and from development of improved techniques and instrumentation for treatment. The scope of these advances is so broad as to preclude any complete coverage of the topic in a limited space. What can be presented, however, is a broad description of the diagnostic and therapeutic modalities available, with specific information to guide the thoughtful clinician to optimal patient management.

Emphasis will be on appropriate consideration of signs and symptoms, choice and efficacy of diagnostic procedures, and therapeutic alternatives. This problem-oriented approach to the management of urologic diseases is especially useful in the older population because major problems fall into a limited number of areas. Thus the majority of major urologic problems in older persons may be categorized into neoplasms, abnormalities of urine emptying or storage, and sexual dysfunction in the male. By proceeding systematically, the geriatrician will be able to characterize the general problem, consider a limited number of likely diagnoses, and proceed with appropriate diagnostic studies.

DIAGNOSTIC CONSIDERATIONS

Multiple sophisticated imaging techniques can be brought to bear on urologic problems. The techniques include contrast radiography, computed tomography (CT), radionuclide studies, and ultrasonography. The excretory urogram (intravenous pyelogram) continues to be the mainstay of radiographic diagnosis of diseases of the upper urinary tract. High doses of contrast media and tomography provide superior imaging of small renal lesions or lesions that might otherwise be obscured by poor delineation from adjacent structures. High dose infusion urography is generally well tolerated by the elderly patient. However, special attention must be given to the dehydrated patient, the diabetic patient, or the patient with previous acutely compromised renal function. In these patients, further preparatory dehydration or the contrast media itself may acutely diminish renal function.

Whereas excretory urography provides excellent anatomic detail, radionuclide studies provide excellent functional information. Radionuclide studies have additional advantages of requiring no special preparation and of much lower radiation exposure confined to the urinary tract. Radionuclide studies provide information regarding renal blood flow, relative renal function, and degree of upper tract obstruction. Bone imaging is invaluable for detection of bony metastases and for assessment of response to treatment of metastatic disease. Multiple radiopharmaceuticals are available, many specifically designed for enhancing some particular aspect of renal diagnosis.

CT has been of particular value in urologic diagnosis because of its special ability to detect retroperitoneal pathologic conditions both within and outside the urinary collecting system. The presence and extent of retroperitoneal masses and metastases can be carefully determined. It is a valuable adjunct in characterization of renal masses and may be the preferred method for visualization of the adrenal gland. The capability of projecting a three-dimensional relationship between the primary lesion and surrounding tissue makes CT scanning particularly useful to the urologic surgeon in the planning and execution of radical operative procedures. The presence of perirenal or pararenal processes such as hemorrhage, abscesss, or urine can be determined.

Ultrasound scanning of the abdomen is a useful adjunct to other diagnostic approaches. As a single study, ultrasonography has significant limitations. However, combined with radiographic imaging and endoscopy, ultrasonography may obviate the need for additional, more invasive, more costly procedures. Ultrasonography is particularly useful in the evaluation of renal masses, obstructive uropathy of the upper urinary tract, renal size, and disease within the perinephric space.

Endoscopy is irreplaceable for accurate evaluation of the lower urinary tract and for allowing access to retrograde studies of the upper urinary tract. The quality of both diagnostic and therapeutic endoscopic instruments continues to improve. Current instruments are far lighter, smaller, and equipped with greatly improved optical systems. These features enhance patient comfort and the urologist's ability to accurately diagnose. Although other diagnostic studies can determine the *presence* of a lower urinary tract obstruction, it remains for endoscopy to determine the *nature* of the obstruction. Cystoscopy is by far the most accurate method for detection and evaluation of tumors of the bladder. Additional diagnostic studies may be necessary for evaluation of the extent of the tumor. Endoscopy combined with direct vision, cold knife urethrotomy is assuming an increasing role in the management of urethral stricture disease and is replacing the time-honored modality of urethral stricture dilatation. Endoscopy coupled with laser technology is being used on a limited basis for removal of small bladder neoplasms. Intraoperative renal endoscopy (nephroscopy) is increasingly important in the optimal diagnosis and management of lesions of the renal pelvis and calices, including calculi, suspected renal neoplasms, and essential hematuria.

In the female, endoscopy of the lower urinary tract can usually be accomplished without difficulty in an office setting. After intraurethral application of a suitable topical anesthetic, a small diameter endoscopic instrument can be easily introduced into the short, straight female urethra for rapid examination of the lower urinary tract. The particularly anxious individual may require cautious intravenous administration of sedatives. Concomitant use of a sedative requires more careful attention to the patient's overall status. Endoscopic examination of the male, even with topical anesthesia, is frequently uncomfortable. The patient should be apprised of this fact, and the cooperative patient may certainly be studied in the office. Less cooperative patients and those fearful of even minor discomfort will require hospitalization for regional or general anesthesia. When such anesthesia is necessary, the appropriate endoscopic therapy is usually combined with diagnostic cystoscopy, as in the case of transurethral resection of the prostate gland. Following office endoscopy the patient should be alerted to expect minor voiding discomfort with urgency, burning, and possibly minimal hematuria. Many urologists routinely prescribe anticholinergic agents, topical bladder anesthetics such as the azo dyes, or minor antimicrobials after office endoscopy to maximize patient comfort and to minimize iatrogenic urinary tract infection.

For many years the diagnosis of disturbances in urinary storage and emptying was hampered by inability to monitor the functioning of the lower urinary tract. Endoscopy and radiology made possible the delineation of the form of the lower urinary tract; but function does not always follow form, and often therapy was inappropriate. The functioning of the lower urinary tract can now be measured by the application of principles of *urodynamics*. Urodynamics seeks to describe micturition and storage of urine in terms of the physical principles that govern the flow of all liquids. Urinary retention and urinary incontinence are such major problems of the elderly that urodynamic studies are particularly appropriate in the evaluation of these patients. Urine flow rate, intrinsic bladder detrusor muscle function, bladder proprioception and compliance, urethral resistance, and function of the striated urinary sphincters can be measured, and the results of these measurements applied clinically to improve the status of the patient.

NEOPLASMS

Neoplastic lesions of the genitourinary tract produce symptoms of obstruction, capsular distention, or invasion of adjacent structures. Such symptoms are likely to occur late in the disease process and are not reliable early indicators of neoplasia. Similarly, the mass effect produced by urinary tract neoplasms is of little aid in early detection. Renal neoplasms do not produce a palpable mass until late in the disease. A bladder tumor rarely ever presents as a palpable abdominal mass; by the time a hard prostatic mass is discovered, metastases are frequently present. A bladder mass is almost never palpable in the presence of bladder tumor, and discovery of a hard prostatic mass is frequently associated with metastatic carcinoma.

Hematuria is a more reliable indicator of early neoplasm of the urinary tract than are pain and mass effect. For this reason, the physician must search carefully for hematuria and must aggressively diagnose its cause once it is discovered. Hematuria may be either gross or microscopic, and either initial, terminal, or total. Microscopic hematuria may often be associated with benign prostatic hyperplasia or inflammatory disease of the bladder, but under these circumstances it is also associated with voiding symptoms. Gross, total, painless hematuria is particularly significant in that it is a harbinger of potential carcinoma of the bladder or kidney.

Neoplasms of the kidney

Renal cell carcinoma. Renal cell carcinoma (adenocarcinoma) is a common malignancy with a high mortality. Renal cell carcinoma represents the majority of primary renal tumors and occurs most commonly in the sixth and seventh decades of life. The disease is twice as common in males as in females.[1] In most cases excretory urography will reveal a renal mass effect, distorting either the intrarenal collecting system or the renal outline. Diagnostic procedures must include nephrotomography, ultrasonography, CT scanning, and possibly renal angiography.

The major diagnostic dilemma is in distinguishing renal cell carcinoma, simple renal cyst, and hemorrhagic renal cyst. Renal cell carcinoma will be a solid mass, with or without a hemorrhagic center, and will demonstrate internal echos on ultrasound examination. Renal cysts are hollow and do not demonstrate internal echos. Hemorrhagic renal cysts have features of both carcinoma and simple cysts. Following excretory urography and ultrasound examination, the addition of cyst puncture and aspiration, CT scanning, and/or renal angiography raises the diagnostic accuracy to 98.5%.[2] Except in rare circumstances, simple renal cysts do not require treatment. The 1.5% of undiagnosed lesions require exploration.

The accepted treatment for nonmetastatic adenocarcinoma of the kidney is radical extirpation of the kidney, perirenal fat, and surrounding Gerota's fascia. Every effort should be made preoperatively to exclude the possibility of metastatic disease through use of radionuclide bone scanning, whole lung tomography or CT scanning of the lungs, and liver scanning if hepatic enzymatic studies are abnormal. Accurate staging of the lesion is important for appropriate management as well as prognostication. When distant metastases are present at the time of surgery, the 5-year survival rate is less than 10%.[3] Metastatic disease occurring after radical nephrectomy is in some instances isolated and amenable to excision. The 5-year survival rate in this group increases to 33%.[4] When tumor is confined to the kidney at the time of the nephrectomy, the 5-year survival rate approaches 80%.[3]

The therapeutic effect of regional lymphadenectomy at the time of radical nephrectomy is controversial. Regional lymphadenectomy with the removal of lymphatics on the aorta (for left nephrectomy) or vena cava (for right nephrectomy) appears to benefit some patients.

In the presence of known metastatic disease palliative nephrectomy is indicated for relief of hemorrhage, pain, or local problems caused by the tumor mass. The 1-year survival rate after palliative nephrectomy is poor. Approximately 40% of patients with metastatic disease at the time of initial diagnosis die within 2 years regardless of treatment.[5] Palliative nephrectomy should be reserved for that patient in whom the operative procedure will definitely improve the quality of life.

Presently there is no consistently effective chemotherapy, hormonal therapy, radiotherapy, or immunotherapy for metastatic renal cell carcinoma. Limited subjective remissions have been reported in small numbers of patients following use of progestational agents. Radiation therapy does not appear to be useful in the primary management of renal cell carcinoma although it may be of value in palliation of symptomatic metastases. Currently efforts are being made to invoke antitumor immune response by embolization and infarction of the carcinoma before nephrectomy.

Transitional cell carcinoma. The other common primary renal neoplasm is transitional cell carcinoma of the renal pelvis or calices. With rare exception, transitional cell carcinoma of the ureter is managed in a fashion identical to that outlined for the kidney parenchyma. As with renal cell carcinoma, transitional cell carcinoma of the kidney is more common in males and may reflect the preponderance of cigarette smoking in males. Diagnosis is usually made on the basis of an excretory urogram that demonstrates a filling defect within the renal collecting system associated with gross or microscopic hematuria. Appropriate diagnostic studies such as retrograde pyelography may be necessary to distinguish a neoplasm from a necrotic renal papilla, clot, or uric acid calculus. Brush biopsy of the renal pelvis or cytologic examination of the urinary sediment by the Papanicolaou technique may be diagnostic.

Accepted therapy of transitional cell carcinoma of the kidney and/or ureter is total nephroureterectomy with removal of a cuff of bladder tissue. If a cuff of bladder at the ureteral orifice is not excised, the incidence of tumor recurrence in the bladder following nephroureterectomy is high. After nephroureterectomy patients must be followed for extended periods with urinary cytologic examinations and endoscopic examinations of the bladder. Survival is dependent on the extent of muscle invasion by the primary tumor at time of diagnosis, with 5-year survival ranging from 91% for no muscle invasion to zero for distant metastasis.[6]

Neoplasms of the bladder

Transitional cell carcinoma of the bladder is much more common than the infrequent adenocarcinoma or squamous cell carcinoma. Transitional cell carcinoma of the bladder is primarily a disease of the elderly and is statistically associated with tobacco use and with occupational exposure to aniline dyes, rubber, leather, paints, and organic chemicals. Animal experimentation suggests a relationship between bladder carcinoma and artificial sweeteners, including saccharin. Prospective studies of the risks associated with artificial sweeteners in humans have not been done.

Management is predicated on the stage and grade of the neoplasm. Low grade neoplasms tend to be papillary in character and noninvasive, whereas high grade tumors tend to be sessile and invasive. Transitional cell carcinoma of the bladder is frequently multicentric, occurring and recurring at multiple sites, suggesting that a field effect is involved in the pathophysiology of tumor development. The tumor may be completely asymptomatic unless the lesion occurs in the trigonal area, in which case the patient may experience urgency and frequency. Hematuria, either gross or microscopic, is an indication for endoscopy to rule out bladder carcinoma. Irritative bladder symptoms are also an indication for endoscopy in the older patient, especially if no other reasonable cause is apparent.

Small, papillary, low grade lesions that are noninvasive may be managed by endoscopic resection of the tumor in combination with frequent cystoscopic examination as often as every 3 months. Intravesical chemotherapy with thiotepa is useful as adjuvant therapy for grossly visible or microscopic tumor following resection. The typical therapeutic dose is 60 mg instilled in the bladder for approximately 1 hour at the time of surgery and then repeated at 1-month intervals for up to 1 year.[7] Other agents that have been used locally include bleomycin, doxorubicin, and epodyl. Large, sessile, invasive, high grade tumors of the bladder require radical cystectomy and ileal conduit urinary diversion frequently combined with preoperative radiation therapy and postoperative systemic chemotherapy. Preoperative irradiation with 2000 to 4000 rads may downstage the bladder tumor. Such radiation probably destroys microscopic metastases in the immediate region of surgical resection and reduces the ability of residual cells to implant if they are liberated into the patient during surgical manipulation. Results of treatment of invasive bladder carcinoma with radiation therapy alone are poor, with only a 36% 5-year survival rate and with recurrent tumor developing in 56% of the patients.[8] Pelvic lymphadenectomy with total cystectomy does not significantly increase operative morbidity or mortality and allows for cure of a small number of patients who have only local lymphatic metastatic disease. The 5-year survival following cystectomy for invasive bladder carcinoma is approximately 50%.[9] Partial cystectomy, rather than total cystectomy, should be approached cautiously and should be reserved for patients who have isolated low grade disease in an easily accessible portion of the bladder.

Painful local metastasis from transitional cell

carcinoma may be managed with local radiation therapy or systemic chemotherapy. The most promising single chemotherapeutic agent for metastatic bladder carcinoma is cisplatin. If there is tumor spill at the time of cystectomy or significant local metastatic disease, the urologic surgeon may elect to begin systemic chemotherapy as an adjunct to the surgical procedure before the documentation of any distant metastasis.

Neoplasms of the prostate gland

Carcinoma of the prostate gland is the second most common neoplasm of American men and is a major cause of cancer death in older men. It is rapidly losing its reputation as an "innocuous" malignancy. The tumor metastasizes to the obturator and hypogastric and iliac lymph nodes and by hematogenous spreading passes to the bony pelvis, spine, femurs, and ribs. Early diagnosis of prostatic carcinoma is dependent on careful rectal examination. Prostatic carcinoma is characteristically firm and dense to palpation. All suspicious prostate lesions should be biopsied. Transrectal and transperineal needle biopsy of the prostate gland is easily performed. Serum acid phosphatase is a valuable biochemmarker for adenocarcinoma of the prostate gland. Elevated levels of the marker signify local or distant extension of the tumor beyond the confines of the prostate capsule. Radionuclide bone scanning is a more sensitive indicator of metastatic disease than are radiographic bone surveys. However, because the bone scan detects all active bone lesions, radiographic confirmation may be necessary to distinguish metastatic disease and traumatic or inflammatory bone disease.

Staging of prostatic carcinoma has undergone major changes. Clinically unsuspected disease found at the time of prostatectomy is classified as A-1 if the lesion is well differentiated and less than 5% of the tissue is occupied by a neoplasm.[10] Unsuspected, poorly differentiated tumors occupying larger portions of the prostatic gland are classified as A-2. Stage B-1 describes prostatic carcinoma limited to one lobe of the prostate gland, and stage B-2 designates a tumor involving both prostatic lobes that is confined to the prostate gland. Stage C disease represents local extension beyond the prostate gland, and Stage D identifies distant lymph node or bony metastasis.

There is no single treatment for adenocarcinoma of the prostate gland. Patients with stage A-1 disease probably require no additional treatment. Radical prostatectomy remains the treatment of choice for patients with stage B-1 disease. Radical prostatectomy for stages A-2, B-2, and C disease has been unsuccessful. Virtually all patients experience erectile impotence following radical prostatectomy, 10% have total urinary incontinence, and approximately 40% have stress urinary incontinence.

External beam radiation or interstitial irradiation with ^{125}I seeds has been introduced as a treatment for adenocarcinoma of the prostate gland because of the morbidity associated with radical prostatectomy. Candidates for ^{125}I implantation are patients with B lesions or with well-defined C lesions. Implantation is usually combined with a staging pelvic lymphadenectomy. Proper seed placement allows a tumor radiation dose of 16,000 to 18,000 rads over a 1-year period in an effort to achieve good local control. External beam radiation delivers a tumor dose of 5000 to 7000 rads to the prostate gland and periprostatic tissue. The long-term therapeutic effects of radiation for prostatic carcinoma are uncertain. Five-year tumor-free survival after ^{125}I implantation is 58% compared with 53% five-year tumor-free survival for external beam radiation.[11] Complications from irradiation include irritative bowel and bladder symptoms, urethral stricture, rectal ulceration, and prostatocutaneous and prostatorectal fistulae. However, erectile potency is preserved in the majority of the patients who were potent preoperatively, in contrast to the universal impotence associated with radical prostatectomy.

Prostatic carcinoma is a hormonal dependent tumor, and 70% to 80% of patients with symptomatic metastatic disease initially respond to bilateral orchiectomy or estrogen administration. There is not, however, any evidence that hormonal manipulation prolongs survival. Because high doses (5 mg per day) of diethylstilbestrol are associated with increased cardiovascular related deaths, orchiectomy is the therapy of choice for patients with severe cardiovascular disease. Patients without severe cardiovascular disease may be managed successfully with either orchiectomy or smaller doses (1 to 2 mg per day) of diethylstilbestrol. Gynecomastia caused by estrogen administration can be avoided by pretreatment irradiation of the breasts. Controversy surrounds the timing of initial estrogen therapy. Early therapy affords a longer symptom-free period but later offers little relief when the neoplasm becomes refractory to estrogens. Delayed estrogen therapy, beginning at the onset of bone pain, affords a shorter symptom-free interval but provides more effective long-term palliation.[12] Nonhormonal chemotherapy for carcinoma of the prostate gland is currently being evaluated. Two cytotoxic agents, 5-fluorouracil and cyclophosphamide, have demonstrated remission effects in some patients who have become refractory to estrogen therapy.

Prostatic carcinoma may produce obstruction of either the ureters or the urethra. Urethral obstruction is managed with routine transurethral resection of the prostate gland. Orchiectomy is the treatment of choice for ureteral obstruction from prostatic carcinoma with a reported response rate of 88%.[13]

Neoplasms of the testicle

The most common testicular neoplasm in the older population is seminoma, which usually occurs after age 50. Approximately 10% of seminomas are classified as anaplastic and often are more advanced at first appearance than plain seminomas.[14] These neoplasms usually appear as a nonpainful testicular mass. Immediate exploration is advisable through an inguinal incision with high ligation of the spermatic cord. Therapy depends on the stage and cell type of the neoplasm. Radiation therapy is the treatment of choice for seminoma, with a 5-year survival rate of 90% to 95%. Irradiated areas should include the inguinal, periaortic, mediastinal, and supraclavicular lymph nodes. CT scanning is particularly useful in the identification of lymph node extension. Whether anaplastic seminoma should be managed in a different fashion is not known and is currently under investigation.

Neoplasms of the penis

Squamous cell carcinoma of the penis is an uncommon lesion in the United States. This neoplasm is found in uncircumcised men and is often associated with poor hygiene. Almost all chronic lesions of the penis require biopsy and histologic examination. Physical examination of the older male should always include complete retraction of the foreskin and careful examination of the foreskin and glands for any suspicious lesion.

Squamous cell carcinoma is the most common penile cancer, occurring most often on the glans and less commonly on the prepuce or shaft. The patient may complain of a palpable penile mass, pain, purulent or serosanguineous discharge or lymphadenopathy.[15] Invasive lesions of the distal penis should be treated with partial phallectomy with an adequate tumor margin. Partial penectomy allows for later directional control of the urinary stream. Post-operative sexual intercourse is usually impossible, and the psychologic impact may be dramatic. Less disfiguring, more conservative treatment methods such as local excision, fulguration, and radiation therapy are risky and should probably be reserved for younger men. Patients with large tumors that extensively involve the glans or with tumors that have extended into the shaft should be treated with total penectomy. Inguinal lymphadenopathy may be associated with penile cancer either because of metastatic disease or because of the inflammation associated with the primary lesion. Lymphadenopathy remaining 6 to 12 weeks following surgical treatment of the primary lesion must be considered to be metastatic disease and is an indication for ilioinguinal node dissection.

Ilioinguinal node dissection is a major operative procedure with significant complications including deep venous thrombosis, chronic lymphedema of the lower extremities, and skin slough at the operative site. Despite the magnitude of the operative procedure it should not be delayed out of fear of operative or postoperative complications, since 50% of patients with nodes containing tumor can be cured by lymphadenectomy, whereas all untreated patients will die of metastatic disease within 3 years.[16]

URINE STORAGE AND URINE EMPTYING PROBLEMS

Elderly patients frequently have symptoms of both urinary obstruction and urinary incontinence. Rather than designating such patients as either incontinent or obstructed, it is more clinically useful to characterize the problems as either failure of urine storage or failure of urine emptying. The routine urologic history that elicits such symptoms as frequency, urgency, and incontinence is not particularly useful unless the physician listens with the concept of normal urodynamics in mind and is able to enlarge on the patient's history by asking specific, relevant questions that further characterize the patient's problem. A brief discussion of the types of urodynamic measurements available will also allow for introduction of specific terminology.

Urine flow rate is the volume of urine voided per unit of time, usually expressed in milliliter per second. It is not equivalent to either velocity or energy of the urinary stream. By means of suitable electronic urine flow meters now available, the urine flow rate may be instantly and graphically displayed as urine voided (in milliliters per second) versus time (in seconds). This study is completely noninvasive and requires only that the patient stand or sit on a suitable commode chair and void in his or her normal fashion. The graphic display of this information allows the determination of intermittency of voiding, of hesitancy in initiating the urinary stream, of postvoid dribbling, and allows the calculation of average urine flow rate and peak urine flow rate. Peak urine flow rate is a better indicator of bladder outlet obstruction than is average urine flow rate. The geriatrician is able to see graphically the way in which the patient voids and can compare that information with the patient's history.

The static function of the bladder detrusor smooth muscle is measured by means of a *cystometrogram*. Bladder pressure and the presence or absence of a normal bladder detrusor reflex contraction are recorded as the bladder is filled through a urethral catheter. Depending on the information needed, the bladder may be filled during cystometry with either carbon dioxide or water, and the fill rate may be slow or rapid. If one wishes to determine bladder capacity, bladder proprioception, and bladder compliance, then slow filling with water is most useful. If one is interested primarily in determining the presence or absence of an adequate bladder detrusor contraction, then rapid bladder filling with carbon dioxide combined with provocative measures such as bethanechol administration, standing, coughing, or heel jouncing may be used during cystometry.

The patient with completely normal bladder detrusor function is able to inhibit the onset of the bladder contraction during bladder filling to the point of significant pain. Failure to inhibit is defined as detrusor hyperreflexia (in the presence of obvious neurogenic disease), detrusor hyperactivity, or detrusor instability (in the absence of obvious neurogenic disease). Patients with normal detrusor function are described as normoreflexic, and patients with diminished or absent detrusor function are described as being hyporeflexic or areflexic, respectively.

Normal micturition requires that the striated portion of the external urinary sphincter relax simultaneously with bladder detrusor contraction to allow for complete bladder emptying. Striated sphincter relaxation can be measured by *electromyography* (EMG) of the striated muscle, accomplished by superficial insertion of a small wire or needle electrode in the periurethral area. Lack of coordinated function between the bladder detrusor muscle and the striated sphincter is referred to as detrusor sphincter dyssynergia. Dyssynergia may also occur between the bladder detrusor and the smooth muscle sphincter at the bladder neck, but this smooth muscle activity cannot be monitored by EMG and can only be demonstrated by voiding cystourethrography with fluoroscopy.

An approximation of intrinsic urethral function can be obtained by means of the *urethral pressure profile*. The profile of pressures along the urethra, urethral length, and urethral closing pressure can be measured by a number of techniques, each of which can be accomplished easily with existing urodynamic instruments and each of which has its own limitations. In general, urethral closing pressure is at a minimum at the external urethral meatus and is at a maximum in the mid urethra "continent zone." Urethral pressure profilometry is most useful in assessing an individual patient before, during, or after some specific surgical or pharmaceutical therapy to determine whether objective improvement in urine storage or emptying has occurred. It is less useful in comparing an individual patient with a set of normal values for maximum urethral length or maximum urethral closing pressure, since the range of normal values is large.

By placement of a small pressure monitoring catheter into the bladder via the urethra, with intraabdominal pressure recorded by means of an intrarectal balloon catheter, and with EMG activity of the striated sphincter monitored, a dynamic (rather than static) voiding study (*micturition study*) may be obtained in which urine flow rate, bladder pressure, intraabdominal pressure, and striated urethral sphincter function are simultaneously measured and displayed on a multichannel strip chart recorder. The micturition study is especially useful in the assessment of complicated problems with incontinence or obstruction.

Urodynamic testing

Urodynamic testing makes possible the determination of whether obstruction or incontinence exists and of lower urinary tract events that contribute to the disorder. However, urodynamic studies alone cannot determine the location or the cause of the incontinence or obstruction and, therefore, must be used in conjunction with other established urologic diagnostic techniques such as endoscopy and radiography. The urine flow study is useful as a screening procedure in almost every elderly patient with any complaint of voiding difficulty or incontinence. If the flow study is normal, then further evaluation for obstruction may be minimized; if the study is abnormal, then appropriate diagnostic studies can be selected and unsatisfactory empirical treatments may be avoided.

Long-standing bladder outlet obstruction in men or women may lead to detrusor instability (hyperreflexia). Clinically, relief of the obstruction frequently rsults in the eventual resolution of the detrusor instability. However, it must be emphasized that detrusor instability can occur independent of obstruction, and the presence of detrusor instability does not imply obstruction, nor does the presence of obstruction with urgency and urge incontinence imply detrusor instability. Because detrusor stability or instability is an intrinsic function of the bladder detrusor muscle and because bladder outlet obstruction and incontinence additionally involve urethral sphincter mechanisms, detrusor function and outlet obstruction must be evaluated separately.

Largely because of the information now available through urodynamic studies, certain longstanding misconceptions can be accurately dispelled. Misconceptions about the significance of certain urinary symptoms and findings existed because of our initial inability to characterize the mechanisms of normal micturition. Urinary frequency may be either motor or sensory in origin. If detrusor hyperreflexia exists, then motor frequency is present and the patient will usually have nighttime frequency (nocturia) as well as daytime symptoms. Sensory frequency is associated with urinary tract infection, trigonitis, and urethral hypersensitivity syndrome in women; and detrusor hyperactivity is not present. *Nocturia* is simply nighttime frequency and must be distinguished from frequency secondary to insomnia or excessive fluid intake during the night. Urgency is a sufficiently strong desire to urinate that no significant delay can be tolerated by the patient. It differs from frequency. Most patients with true urgency will, on proper questioning, admit to occasional episodes of urge incontinence. Hesitancy and a decreased urinary stream are indications of bladder outlet obstruction. Such symptoms may or may not coexist with urinary frequency and urgency and have a different pathophysiology. The unobstructed patient with frequency will have a small urinary stream simply because small volumes are being voided.

Bladder outlet obstruction in the male

Bladder outlet obstruction in the male is most commonly caused by benign prostatic hyperplasia or dysfunctional bladder neck obstruction (bladder neck contracture). The patient will have symptoms of hesitancy; decreased urinary stream, often associated with frequency; nocturia; and urgency. Uroflowmetry should be performed to demonstrate decreased peak urine flow rate and average urine flow rate with prolonged voiding. Such patients notoriously overestimate the force of their own urinary streams. There is no direct correlation between the size of the prostate gland and the presence or degree of obstruction. The size of the prostate gland should be considered by the clinician when determining the type of operative approach to use if obstruction exists, but obstruction may be present with a small prostate gland and may be absent with a large prostate gland.

The presence of residual urine indicates that the bladder has failed to empty and may be a symptom of severe bladder outlet obstruction; it may also indicate the presence of an inadequate detrusor contraction without obstruction. The absence of residual urine does not mean that the patient is unobstructed, and this misconception should be laid to rest. Severe outlet obstruction may coexist with the absence of residual urine. Symptoms of frequency and nocturia indicate that detrusor instability has developed. However, prostatic obstruction can exist without detrusor instability, and if the urine flow rate shows an obstructed pattern, the patient should be advised to have appropriate treatment. The patient with frequency and urgency, both signs of detrusor instability, who is unobstructed should have cystometry to document the presence of detrusor instability and to guide appropriate therapy.

Prostatectomy should be advised when obstruction is objectively documented regardless of prostate gland size. Absolute indications for operative therapy are evidence of deterioration of the upper urinary tracts and recurrent urinary tract infection. The size of the prostatic adenoma will usually dictate the choice of operative procedure. Usually small prostate glands are easily managed by transurethral resection, and because of improvements in instrumentation, including the continuous flow resectoscope, certain larger glands may be removed transurethrally. For very large adenomas, open prostatectomy by either the retropubic, suprapubic, or perineal approach is indicated. Postoperative measurement of the urine flow rate will allow documentation of the patient's improvement and will screen for such postoperative complications as severe urethral stricture or bladder neck contracture.

Bladder neck dysfunction in the male is diagnosed by a decreased urine flow rate. Closure of the bladder neck concomitant with bladder detrusor contraction, as demonstrated by a voiding cystourethrogram, indicates that the bladder is functionally obstructed. Patients with this difficulty frequently have a lifelong history of a noncompetitive stream.[17] Indicated treatment is incision of the obstructing bladder neck. The patient who has been followed for a long period and has a diagnosis of abacterial prostatitis should be suspected of having dyssynergic bladder neck obstruction.

Bladder outlet obstruction in the female

The symptoms of bladder outlet obstruction in the female are not so well defined as in the male. Symptoms vary widely, pointing up again the necessity of an adequate urodynamic evaluation of such patients. Urethral calibration is a static measurement of a dynamic structure. The size and shape of the urethra during voiding bears little or no relationship to the static configuration. The presence of residual urine is evidence of voiding dysfunction but does not necessarily indicate the presence of an outlet obstruction. As in the male, the absence of residual urine does not exclude a significant bladder outlet obstruction. Endoscopic examination in the female cannot determine or exclude the presence of a bladder outlet obstruction because observation of the urethra is being done in a static fashion. Finally bladder trabeculation in the female is most commonly associated with detrusor instability rather than outlet obstruction.

As in the male, the optimal screening test for bladder outlet obstruction in the female is the urine flow rate. An acceptable maximum urine flow rate and flow pattern essentially exclude bladder outlet obstruction, and an abnormal flow rate or pattern indicates the necessity for further urodynamic studies. Cystometry may indicate the presence of inadequate detrusor contraction or detrusor areflexia. If detrusor function is normal, voiding cystourethrography is then useful for determining whether a proven obstruction is located at the bladder neck or in the distal urethra.

Distal urethral obstruction in the female is a dynamic process and does not correlate well with the urethral diameter as measured by calibration. Office dilation of distal urethral obstruction does not produce any measurable urodynamic improvement.[18] Richard Turner-Warwick advocates treatment of distal obstruction by overdilatation of the urethra to approximately 40 to 45 French in a stepwise fashion, under anesthesia.[19] Proximal obstruction at the level of the bladder neck is managed by incision of the bladder neck. Great caution should be exercised because incision results in permanent incompetence of the internal urinary sphincter, and the risk of incontinence is significant since only the distal urinary sphincter remains.

Male incontinence

If neurogenic bladder disease is excluded, the majority of males with urinary incontinence are postprostatectomy patients. The majority of these patients have persistent detrusor instability and may have residual prostatic obstruction.[20] Detrusor instability associated with obstruction will revert to normal in 60% of cases within a year of the time that the obstruction is relieved. Patients with persistent detrusor instability and no outlet obstruction are candidates for treatment with anticholinergic drugs to suppress detrusor hyperreflexia.

In the absence of detrusor instability, men with postprostatectomy incontinence demonstrate pure sphincter incompetence secondary to operative injury. Patients with pure sphincter incontinence must be managed with implantation of an antiincontinence prosthesis. The Kaufman prosthesis is a gel-filled, silicon device that produces compression of the urethra after implantation through the perineum. Its advantages include simplicity of placement and operation. However, the degree of compression is difficult to control and late failures may occur for an overall success rate of approximately 50%. The Brantley Scott artificial urinary sphincter is a more sophisticated device consisting of several components. An inflatable occlusive sphincter is placed completely around the bulbous urethra and is fluid coupled to the control mechanism. A pressure regulating balloon reservoir and the control mechanism are placed in the retropubic space and inguinal region, respectively. A constant pressure of 50 to 70 cm of water is applied by the pressure regulating balloon and control assembly to the urethral cuff to occlude the urethra and to maintain continence. Voiding is accomplished by operation of a small intrascrotal pump that temporarily deflates the urethral cuff to allow urethral opening and normal voiding. In properly selected patients the success rate with the artificial urinary sphincter is 90%.

Female incontinence

In women the smooth muscle bladder neck sphincter is stronger and more capable of maintaining continence than is the urethral sphincter mechanism. Women with stress incontinence have incompetence of both the bladder neck and distal urethral mechanism associated with coughing, lifting, and similar provocations. Urethral competence is the sum of several factors. First the urethral closing pressure as measured by urethral pressure profilometry results from intrinsic urethral smooth muscle contraction, from urethral striated muscle contraction, and from the pressure of the vascular bed of the urethra. Second the urethra must be anatomically situated within the abdomen so that the proximal urethra receives any sudden increase in intraabdominal pressure, such as that associated with coughing, and closes as a result. Third the urethral closing pressure increases with increasing functional urethral length.

In uncomplicated stress incontinence the peak urine flow rate will frequently be elevated since urethral resistance is decreased. The presence of significant residual urine indicates the coexistence of factors other than those of simple stress incontinence and warrants further investigation. Detrusor instability is frequently associated wth stress urinary incontinence. Provocation cystometry with rapid filling, bethanechol administration, cystometry in the standing position, and cystometry with coughing and heel jouncing should be carried out to elicit the presence of detrusor instability. Patients with urge incontinence and patients who have had a previous failed procedure for correction of their incontinence should have a complete urodynamic evaluation. Endoscopy must be performed to evaluate urethral length, urethral tone, and urethral blood supply and to rule out sources of sensory urgency such as cystitis, urethritis, and trigonitis.

Stress urinary incontinence is managed by surgical repositioning of the urethra. Multiple surgical approaches, both abdominal and transvaginal, are well recognized. The essential element in any operative procedure for correction of stress incontinence is repositioning of the urethra into the pelvis so that the proximal urethra is capable of receiving sudden increases in intraabdominal pressure. Detrusor instability associated with stress incontinence rarely improves after correction of the stress incontinence. It is therefore important to identify this condition preoperatively so that the patient can be adequately counseled regarding the expected results of operative therapy.

Minimal pure stress urinary incontinence may be successfully managed for a number of years by administration of sympathomimetic agents that increase the maximum urethral closing pressure by increasing the resting tone of the urethral smooth muscle. Phenylpropanolamine and ephedrine, administered in a dosage of 25 mg, three to four times a day, is effective. The use of such drugs in patients with hypertension, cardiovascular disease, and glaucoma requires special attention.

Neurogenic incontinence

Neurogenic incontinence may be iatrogenic, produced by administration of drugs that either block the bladder neck and urethral mechanisms and produce sphincter incompetency or that interfere with normal detrusor function and lead to urinary retention and overflow incontinence. Drugs that promote urinary retention and overflow incontinence include opiates, anticholinergics, antihistamines, and sympathomimetic drugs. Phenothiazines and many peripheral and ganglionic blockers such as alpha-methyldopa, which is useful in the management of hypertension, may lead to urinary incontinence. Initial management of incontinence in such patients should be the discontinuance of the possible offending drugs.

Cerebral lesions including cerebral vascular accidents, extensive cerebral vascular disease, parkinsonism, and cerebral neoplasms produce detrusor hyperreflexia. Incontinent patients with such lesions should have cystometry to detect detrusor hyperreflexia and then appropriate anticholinergic drug therapy to reduce the hyperreflexia. Patients with multiple sclerosis may have either detrusor hyperreflexia or detrusor areflexia; cystometry is essential to classify the nature of their disorder and to determine appropriate treatment.

Patients with lower spinal cord lesions, including central herniated nucleus pulposus, will demonstrate detrusor areflexia. Detrusor areflexia is also frequently seen in elderly women without an identifiable cause. The majority of such cases may represent the long-term sequelae of chronic overdistension of the bladder and infrequent voiding with disruption of the innervation of the bladder and fibrosis within the bladder wall. This "myogenic" bladder responds poorly to therapy. If the patient has noninfected residual urine, no incontinence or discomfort, and no deterioration of renal function, then treatment need be only careful observation. For the patient with retention, incontinence, or recurring infection therapy with bethanechol chloride in a dosage of 100 to 200 mg per 24 hours in four divided doses is indicated. Phenoxybenzamine, an alpha-adrenergic blocker, may be administered with bethanechol chloride to decrease bladder neck resistance and to maximize bladder emptying. Phenoxybenzamine produces orthostatic hypotension and must be used selectively in higher doses. Repeated urethral dilatations in patients with areflexia or myogenic bladders are probably of no benefit and may worsen the situation by introducing trauma and infection.

SEXUAL DYSFUNCTION

Evaluation

Erectile impotence is the inability to obtain or maintain an erection suitable for vaginal penetration and intercourse and is common in the older male population. Ejaculatory impotence is the inability to ejaculate and is an uncommon problem, usually associated with significant spinal cord disease or direct injury to the sympathetic trunk. The physician should be acutely aware that inability to maintain an erection is functionally as significant as the inability to obtain an erection. Many patients who complain of erectile impotence will describe partial incomplete erections of short duration and of insufficient rigidity to allow vaginal penetration. In obtaining a history from a male with impotence the interviewer must ask appropriate questions to elicit detailed information about the quality of the erection and the difficulty associated with intercourse. Even the best history is not always reliable. Patients frequently have a poor understanding of their own sexual abilities and function. They are not aware of what constitutes normal erectile function and may be unable to ascertain whether they are normal or abnormal. The successful diagnosis and management of impotence in the married male inevitably must include physician interaction with the spouse. The initial interview and examination may not be the ideal time for a conversation with the wife, but it is an appropriate time to indicate to the patient that his wife must be involved in the ultimate resolution of the problem.

Patients with long-standing, insulin-dependent diabetes mellitus and patients who have had radical pelvic surgery have obvious causes for their impotence, but the majority of patients have no clear-cut cause for impotence. Physicians who initially direct their efforts toward establishing causal factors will frequently be frustrated as will the patients. In those patients who have no obvious cause for impotence, the first priority should be to establish whether indeed organic erectile impotence exists. Efforts to detect occult vascular disease, diabetes, or hypogonadism in the patients with psychogenic impotence are wasted. A much heralded statistic is that 90% of all impotence is psychogenic. Objective evaluation of impotent males for the past decade has failed to bear out this statistic, and probably 50% or more cases of impotence have an organic cause.

It is the belief of this author that the initial diagnostic evaluation of the impotent male should be nocturnal penile tumescence (NPT) monitoring. In all males with normal erectile function, normal erections occur during REM (rapid eye movement) sleep. Two small strain gauges placed at the base and tip of the penis record the erections. NPT monitoring provides a graphic display of nocturnal erection patterns, including measurements of maximum circumferential increase of the penile tip and base, the number of nocturnal erections, and the duration of each erection. Normal data for these factors have been established. NPT is best accomplished in a hospital-based laboratory, usually in conjunction with a sleep disorders laboratory. In this setting, the additional useful information about the relationship between NPT and REM sleep can be obtained and valuable information regarding depression or anxiety obtained. The usefulness of NPT data from home monitoring or routine hospital room monitoring is compromised by lack of control over equipment calibration, erroneous gauge placement, malingering by the patient, inability to assess rigidity, and, especially in the hospital room, disturbed sleep.

The patient in whom NPT studies demonstrate abnormal erectile function can then be subjected to appropriate studies to determine the cause of impotence. Such studies include measurement of penile blood flow and penile blood pressure using the Doppler technique; EMG and nerve conduction studies to detect neuropathies; possible cystometry to detect neurogenic disease in the cauda equina region; serum testosterone level determination; glucose tolerance test; and psychiatric evaluation. Patients who have normal NPT studies can be immediately referred for sexual or psychiatric counseling and can be spared the expense of metabolic and vascular evaluations.

Treatment

Sexual counseling is appropriate for those patients who appear to have no serious underlying psychiatric problem but suffer from "performance anxiety." Patients with depression and similar problems or with serious marital problems should be referred for psychiatric evaluation and therapy.

An occasional patient will be found to have a significantly decreased serum testosterone level. Testosterone therapy should not be instituted empirically but should be based on measurements of serum testosterone. Oral androgen preparations are frequently unreliable for androgen replacement because of poor and erratic gastrointestinal absorption and because of poor patient compliance. Replacement therapy should be with parenteral testosterone in the form of testosterone cypionate or testosterone enanthate, 300 to 400 mg administered intramuscularly monthly. Males receiving parenteral testosterone therapy should have frequent rectal examinations since carcinoma of the prostate gland is known to be androgen-dependent. Evidence of vascular disease or of a significant neuropathy will be present in most patients with organic impotence. Since neither of these problems is medically reversible, treatment of the associated impotence is usually surgical. The patient with vascular impotence and other indicators of peripheral vascular disease may require pelvic angiography. Revascularization of the distal penile blood supply for impotence has not proven successful. However, the patient with significant aortoiliac occlusive vascular disease should have corrective vascular surgery initially; if there is no improvement in erectile impotence, later operative therapy directed at the penis can be instituted.

Operative insertion of a penile prosthesis is the definitive therapy for the majority of patients with organic erectile impotence. Many excellent penile prostheses are available, both inflatable and noninflatable. The noninflatable prostheses are either rigid or semirigid, allowing for flexion of the penis at its base to improve patient comfort, acceptance, and concealment. These prostheses produce an excellent functional and cosmetic result and are usually well accepted by the sexual partner. All may be inserted through a small incision in the perineum or dorsum of the penis. Patients with symptoms of bladder outlet obstruction should have the obstruction evaluated before insertion of a penile prosthesis. Insertion of a noninflatable prosthesis makes subsequent urethral instrumentation or transurethral resection difficult and mandates the use of a perineal urethrostomy to accomplish these procedures. Patients in whom repeated urethral instrumentation is necessary, as with severe urethral stricture disease or recurrent bladder tumors, are poor candidates for a noninflatable prosthesis.

The inflatable penile prosthesis developed by Brantley Scott, M.D., affords an excellent cosmetic result together with the advantage of producing an erection only when it is desired. As with the noninflatable prosthesis, the inflatable prosthesis can be inserted through a modest infrapubic or scrotal incision. The prosthesis has three components: paired inflatable cylinders, which are inserted in the corpora cavernosa; a fluid reservoir, which is placed in the prevesical space; and a small inflation/deflation pump, which is concealed in the scrotum and which when operated transfers fluid from the reservoir to the cylinders to produce an erection. Functional and cosmetic results reported in a large series are excellent.[21] The inflatable penile prosthesis, because it is a mechanical device, has a small mechanical failure rate of approximately 2%. Design and implantation of the prosthesis is such that minor revision after a mechanical failure is simplified.

Chronic malcontents, patients with serious psychologic disorders, and patients receiving high dose steroids or chemotherapy are poor candidates for prostheses.

CONCLUSIONS

The major urologic problems facing the aging population are neoplasia, failure of bladder emptying and bladder storage, and sexual dysfunction. Accurate, specific radiographic, endoscopic, and urodynamic diagnostic techniques can be brought to focus on these problems. A problem-oriented approach to the elderly patient with urologic disease will allow for the effective and expeditious use of these diagnostic modalities.

The problem-oriented approach begins with effective history taking. The geriatric physician must be armed with sufficient knowledge of the spectrum of urologic disease to ask those penetrating questions and to seek out relevant signs that will quickly lead to the appropriate diagnosis.

Therapeutic advances have clearly paralleled diagnostic advances both in instrumentation and techniques. The clinician who is aware of the therapeutic choices can evaluate a patient in the light of those choices and choose the optimal care for each patient. The adage that physicians must treat patients rather than disease is nowhere truer than in geriatrics.

REFERENCES

1. American society: cancer statistics, CA **30:**23, 1980.
2. Lang, E.K.: Roentgenologic approach to the diagnosis and management of cystic lesions of the kidney: is cyst exploration mandatory? Urol. Clin. North Am. **7:**677, 1980.
3. Skinner, D.G., et al.: Diagnosis and management of renal cell carcinoma. A clinical and pathological study of 309 cases, Cancer **28:**1165, 1971.
4. Skinner, D.G., and deKernion, J.B.: Clinical manifestations and treatment of renal parenchymal tumors. In Skinner, D.G., and deKernion, J.B., editors: Genitourinary cancer, Philadelphia, 1978, W.B. Saunders Co., p. 127.
5. Mostofi, F.K.: Pathology and spread of renal cell carcinoma. In King, J.S., Jr., editor: Renal neoplasia, Boston, 1967, Little, Brown & Co., p. 41.
6. Batata, M., and Grabstald, H.: Upper urinary tract urothelial tumors, Urol. Clin. North Am. **3**(1):79, 1976.
7. Soloway, M.S.: Rationale for intensive intravesical chemotherapy for superficial bladder cancer, J. Urol. **123:**461, 1980.
8. Cummings, K.B., et al.: Observations on definitive cobalt 60 radiation for cure in bladder carcinoma: 15 year follow up, J. Urol. **115:**152, 1976.
9. Grossman, H.B.: Current therapy of bladder carcinoma, J. Urol. **121:**1, 1979.
10. Walsh, P.C.: Radical prostatectomy for the treatment of localized prostatic carcinoma, Urol. Clin. North Am. **7:**583, 1980.
11. Herr, H.W.: Iodine 125 implantation in the management of localized prostatic carcinoma, Urol. Clin. North Am. **7:**605, 1980.
12. Blackard, C.E.: The Veterans Administration Cooperative Urologic Research Group. Studies of carcinoma of the prostate: a review, Cancer Chemother. Rep. **59:**225, 1975.
13. Michigan, S., and Catalona, W.J.: Ureteral obstruction from prostatic carcinoma: response to endocrine and radiation therapy, J. Urol. **118:**733, 1977.
14. Johnson, D.E., Gomez, J.J., and Ayala, A.G.: Anaplastic seminoma, J. Urol. **114:**80, 1975.
15. Hanash, K.A., Furlow, W.L., Utz, D.C., and Harrison, E.G., Jr.: Carcinoma of the penis: a clinicopathologic study, J. Urol. **104:**291, 1970.
16. Skinner, D.G., Leadbetter, W.F., and Kelley, S.B.: The surgical management of squamous cell carcinoma of the penis, J. Urol. **107:**273, 1972.
17. Turner-Warwick, R.: A urodynamic review of bladder outlet obstruction in the male and its clinical implications, Urol. Clin. North Am. **6:**171, 1979.
18. Turner-Warwick, R., et al.: A urodynamic view of the clinical problems associated with bladder neck dysfunction and its treatment by endoscopic incision and transtrigonal prostectomy, Br. J. Urol. **45:**44, 1973.
19. Farrar, D., and Turner-Warwick, R.: Outflow obstruction in the female, Urol. Clin. North Am. **6:**217, 1979.
20. Worth, P.: Urinary incontinence in the male, Urol. Clin. North Am. **6:**199, 1979.
21. Furlow, W.L.: Inflatable penile prosthesis: Mayo Clinic experience with 175 patients, Urology **13:**166, 1979.

CHAPTER 21 · PERIPHERAL VASCULAR DISEASE

Jess R. Young

ARTERIAL DISEASE

This discussion of arterial disease is divided into two sections: the general approach to the elderly patient with suspected arterial disease and the treatment of specific organ systems affected by arterial disease.

General approach

Evaluation of elderly patients with arterial disease should be tempered with caution. They are less tolerant of stress and of excesses of treatment than are younger patients. Stress should be minimized even at the expense of selecting treatment that is less than curative. Phrased differently, one should attempt to do the least that is necessary rather than the most that is possible.

Evaluation of the elderly patient should answer the following questions:

- Are the complaints due to arterial disease?
- If they are, need the condition be specifically treated?
- If so, should primary treatment be medical or surgical?
- If surgery is indicated, can the patient tolerate the surgical procedure?
- If he can, what is the minimal surgical procedure that will suffice?
- Once an operation is decided on, what elements of care are especially important to the elderly patient?

Are the complaints due to arterial disease? To many the pathophysiology of arterial disease seems to be clouded by mysticism such that when no other diagnosis readily fits the patient's complaints, the condition must be due to "poor circulation." We frequently see patients with thrombophlebitis, varicose veins, lymphedema, fibrositis, night cramps, restless legs, and peripheral neuropathies who are referred as having arterial insufficiency of the legs. Primary eye disease, migraine, brain tumor, postural hypotension, hyperventilation, cervical myalgia, and Bell's palsy are seen with a presumptive diagnosis of extracranial cerebral ischemia. Diverticulitis, gallbladder disease, renal colic, peptic ulcer, and irritable bowel are referred as symptomatic aortic aneurysms.

The patient with arterial disease must be separated from this larger group, using the tools of history, physical examination, a knowledge of differential diagnosis, and when appropriate, angiography.

Need the condition be specifically treated? Granting that an arterial abnormality has been found, there are many situations when specific treatment need not be given immediately, and in some cases ever. The elderly patient will die eventually, frequently of some condition other than the presenting one. It may be better to allow the patient to live with a minor disability or even a minor threat to his life than to precipitate his death in an attempt to cure him.

A tortuous aorta masquerading as an aortic aneurysm or an elongated innominate or carotid artery bulging the right side of the neck needs no treatment other than explanation.[1] A calcified aorta is merely a calcified aorta and does not require arteriography or surgery. In the absence of significant claudication of the involved arm, the inappropriately named subclavian steal is no more than an interesting and dramatic collateral pathway. Small aortic aneurysms, particularly if fusiform, in an elderly patient do not require immediate surgery. One-block claudication that might put a 40-year-old person out of work rarely causes significant inconvenience to a retired person whose avocation is quiet activity.

Should primary treatment be medical or surgical? A surgical approach may be technically impossible, physiologically useless, inferior to corresponding medical treatment, or obligatory.

From a technical viewpoint, acquiring a source of blood is always possible by going sufficiently proximal in the arterial tree. However, if the extent of arterial involvement is such that this new blood supply cannot be directed into an outflow tract adequate to supply the ischemic part, a revascularization procedure becomes impossible. This decision can usually be made from the arteriograms.

A surgical procedure is physiologically useless when reconstitution of an interrupted blood supply will not change the existing pathophysiology. For example, carotid endarterectomy will not improve a completed stroke, renal artery repair will not improve an inherently nephrosclerotic kidney, and arterial reconstruction in the leg will not reverse frank gangrene.

In some instances medical treatment is superior to surgical treatment. Cessation of smoking in patients with thromboangiitis obliterans (Buerger's disease) is more effective than sympathectomy.[2] Type III dissecting aneurysms frequently may be readily controlled by a hypotensive regimen not requiring surgery.[3] Patients with claudication, particularly of recent origin, will at times improve sufficiently on a progressive walking program so that surgical repair is not required. In a patient with transient ischemic attacks caused by emboli from an ulcerated arteriosclerotic plaque in the internal carotid artery, the total risk may be less by treating the patient with aspirin than by surgery if he also has class IV angina.

However, surgery is the treatment of choice in many instances. Large or enlarging aneurysms, most instances of extracranial cerebral artery disease, and progressive claudication or severe ischemia in most patients require surgical correction if it is technically possible.

In summary, when there is a choice of procedure, elderly patients are entitled to a serious consideration of a medical regimen before some surgical procedure is decided on.

Can the patient tolerate the surgical procedure? It is not possible to be dogmatic about the contraindications to surgery in patients with arterial disease. A decision for or against an operation must be based on such factors as the physiologic age of the patient and a calculation of his current ability to withstand a major stress. Imminently fatal diseases such as metastatic cancer, severe renal failure, severe emphysema, or incapacitating heart disease are obvious contraindications to elective surgery. As an example, in patients with aneurysm the danger of surgery must be weighed against the danger of rupture of the aneurysm. Patients with mild angina or emphysema might not be considered operable if the aneurysm were small, but patients with severe angina or moderate renal failure might be operated on if the aneurysm were large.

More specifically, a history of myocardial infarction without residual angina is not considered a contraindication to vascular surgery nor is the mild angina of effort. In the instance of a recent myocardial infarction, a 3- to 6-month recovery period is desirable before undertaking arterial surgery. The patient with a history of several myocardial infarctions and significant angina pectoris must be considered a poor risk for surgery, and elective procedures should be avoided. In recent years, a more definitive evaluation of many of these patients is being done through coronary angiography followed by surgical improvement of the blood supply to the heart when indicated. Such patients may then become candidates for elective arterial surgery elsewhere.[4]

Diabetes mellitus is not a contraindication to surgery. However, because of the high incidence of arteriosclerosis in the small vessels of the calf in patients with diabetes, the chance of a successful vascular procedure is less in a diabetic patient than in a nondiabetic individual.

Renal insufficiency (usually a result of nephrosclerosis) demands serious evaluation if an intraabdominal procedure is planned. Although cross-clamping of the aorta does not adversely affect total renal flow, there are changes in the relative flows to the cortex and the medulla. This, combined with the overall stress of an aortic procedure, may cause acute failure of a kidney with borderline function.

One of the most serious problems encountered in the consideration of a patient for vascular surgery is decreased pulmonary function due to obstructive emphysema. In these patients with severely diminished pulmonary function, postoperative atelectasis and pneumonia with secondary severe respiratory failure are so common that this disorder is not only a serious deterrent but occasionally is an absolute contraindication to vascular repairs.

What is the minimal surgical procedure that will suffice? In the younger patient, particularly during the working years, the goal is to restore him to as close to normalcy as possible. In the older patient, the physician should be content with achieving preservation of organs and attaining reasonable mobility. For example, if a leg is ischemic because of both iliac and superficial femoral artery disease, repair of the iliac component alone will probably result in preservation of the limb and perhaps the ability to walk one or two blocks before claudication occurs.[5] This is often an entirely adequate result. There is little to gain in also repairing the femoral artery occlusion so that the patient may attain the ability to walk twenty-blocks that he would never attempt.

In considering the procedure to be employed, the practical aspects of duration of the procedure (partly of the surgeon involved) and anticipated blood loss must be considered. Elderly patients do not tolerate prolonged anesthesia well and are less tolerant of multiple transfusions than younger patients.

What elements of care are especially important to the elderly patient? If the final decision is that a surgical approach is the treatment of choice, some elements of care should receive special attention in the elderly patient.

1. Smoking should be discontinued, preferably at least 1 month prior to the procedure. If significant emphysema and/or pulmonary fibrosis is present, chest physical therapy should be employed for several days prior to anesthesia.
2. Fluid intake should be normal or slightly restricted but certainly never excessive. To be oversolicitous to the elderly patient may result in overtreatment with excess loading of their less elastic homeostatic mechanisms.
3. Hypoxia and hypotension are poorly tolerated by the older person's cardiopulmonary system.
4. Careful monitoring of electrolyte balance is imperative. Sodium and chloride imbalances occur easily, frequently with corresponding changes in potassium levels and cardiac arrhythmias. Metabolic acidosis is easy to achieve but may be difficult to correct.
5. The response of the elderly to drugs is sometimes slow and at times unpredictable. Multiple drug therapy should be avoided.
6. Because the elderly patient is frail, experienced care becomes more important. Anesthesia departments, recovery rooms, and intensive care units staffed by personnel who have day-to-day experience with vascular surgery can provide better care for the geriatric patient than those who, however knowledgeable, do not have extensive experience.
7. Suitable equipment (monitors, respirators, blood gas laboratories, adequate blood banks) are obligatory and supporting services (internists, cardiologists, chest physical therapists) must be available.
8. The most effective team consists of the internist, anesthesiologist, and surgeon who have frequently worked together and have come to an agreement on the care of the various aspects of the surgical care of the "arterial patient."

Treatment of specific organ systems

Although in a vascular practice a great variety of conditions are seen, such as arteriovenous fistulae, renovascular hypertension, vascular insufficiency of the bowel, and aneurysms in the smaller vessels of the extremities, only the three areas that make up the bulk of arterial disease in the elderly patient will be discussed in this chapter—ischemia of the lower extremities, aortic aneurysm, and extracranial cerebral ischemia.

Ischemia of the lower extremity. Since *ischemia* is a relative term, a prime consideration in the evaluation of these patients is a determination of the degree of the ischemia. Severity may range from intermittent claudication of varying degrees through pain at rest and ulceration to frank gangrene. In addition, acute ischemia may occur.

Intermittent claudication. When the patient

complains only of claudication, the decrease in blood flow to the leg is not sufficient to threaten gangrene. Claudication is annoying but disabling only in patients whose occupations require prolonged walking. However, it is important to stress that claudication indicates the presence of significant arteriosclerosis in the leg, and the patient is therefore a candidate for more severe ischemia in the future.

Palpating peripheral pulses is the most important single maneuver in establishing the diagnosis of occlusive arterial disease. Unfortunately, the art of pulse palpation is not one that is usually well taught in medical school or in postgraduate training. Nutritional changes, including loss of hair on the dorsum of the foot and toes and trophic changes of the nails and skin represent end-stages of ischemia. Postural color changes are a good indication of the adequacy of arterial circulation. When ischemia is moderate or severe, the feet will blanch when they are elevated (elevation pallor) and become excessively red or cyanotic when they are dependent (dependent rubor). A delay of more than 15 seconds in the time required for the veins on the dorsum of the foot to fill after the legs have been changed from the elevated to the dependent position usually indicates ischemia.

The diagnosis of occlusive arterial disease can be established in 95% of the cases without the aid of special laboratory procedures. If further information is needed, a variety of noninvasive instrumentation is now available, ranging from simple devices to be used in the physician's office to more complicated and expensive instruments suitable only for the vascular laboratory. One of the best and simplest methods is to measure the systolic pressure at the level of the ankles with a Doppler ultrasound instrument, then compare the pressure with the brachial systolic pressure.

Arteriography is the only method available at this time to precisely locate anatomic disease and therefore is an essential guide to the vascular surgeon. Arteriography is not done unless the patient is being considered for surgical revascularization.

A patient whose only complaint is claudication may be considered a candidate for revascularization if (1) the claudication is economically disabling, (2) the claudication progressively worsens, or (3) certain avocations are so important to the patient that the inability to walk distances becomes psychologically destructive.

Pain at rest and ischemic ulceration. Progressive arteriosclerosis may further decrease the blood supply to the limb of a patient with intermittent claudication to the point that the circulation cannot meet the metabolic demands of the leg even at rest. Ischemic fissures and ulcerations occur on the heels, toes, and other pressure points of the foot. The patient will have pain or numbness in the leg even when not walking, and especially if the leg is elevated when lying in bed at night. At this stage gangrene is imminent. If amputation is to be avoided, some form of revascularization is imperative, and arterial reconstruction should be done if at all possible.

Gangrene. Once a part has become gangrenous, recovery of that part will not occur. Simple amputation of the dead toe or forefoot is usually impossible, since the adjacent tissues have a borderline blood supply and the increased vascular demand required to heal the amputation wound cannot be met by the involved tissues. Hence the amputation wound becomes gangrenous, and the process repeats itself. It is commonly known that amputation well above the involved area, where the blood supply is adequate, will result in primary healing of the wound. Many surgeons, to ensure primary healing, select a very high site for amputation, with the result that more than 50% of the amputations of the leg done today for ischemia are above the knee—many unnecessarily.[6]

Since the advent of vascular surgery, some of these legs can be revascularized so that, at worst, a below-knee amputation may be done, and sometimes a transmetatarsal amputation will heal. In a suitable patient it is obviously desirable to convert what would be a crippling above-knee amputation to a below-knee amputation that most elderly people can manage or, even better, to a transmetatarsal amputation where the disability is trivial.

Acute ischemia. Acute ischemia may be the result of an embolus from a proximal source or the result of an acute thrombosis-in-situ superimposed on moderately severe arteriosclerosis. In either event the occlusion causes a sudden loss of blood supply to the leg for which the patient is unprepared. Unlike progressive arteriosclerosis, where collateral arteries have had time to develop, there are few secondary pathways available for immediate use in the case of an acute occlusion. Some patients are able to compensate to some degree within a few hours, however, if given the opportunity.

It has been our practice to treat acute arterial occlusions for 3 or 4 hours with intravenously administered heparin, low molecular weight dextran, and elevation of the head of the bed.[7] If the leg improves during that time, we will watch it for a longer time, offering more opportunity to correct the cause of the embolus and to prepare the patient better for arterial embolectomy. Occasionally, no operation is required.

If the limb does not improve within 3 or 4 hours, however, emergency surgical treatment is obligatory.

Selection of procedure. The elderly patient who is considered a poor surgical risk because of age or serious associated disease may be successfully treated with the use of the less traumatic extraanatomic bypasses (axillofemoral and femorofemoral), since surgical dissection is minimal and the procedure can be done under local anesthesia if necessary. The results approach those observed with the standard aortofemoral bypass.

There has been a trend to establish techniques that permit anastomosis to smaller and smaller vessels. Aortoiliac reconstructions were extended to aortofemoral and aortopopliteal levels; common femoral to superficial femoral repairs were carried to femoropopliteal levels. Recently there has been an effort to establish popliteal-tibial grafts, even as far distally as the ankle.[8-12]

Continued patency of a reconstruction depends on a high volume flow, which in turn is related to the size of the outflow bed and the peripheral resistance. The more distal the anastomosis the smaller will be the outflow bed and the greater the chance of early or late occlusion of the repair. In aged individuals the terminal vessels are commonly sclerotic with many patchy areas of occlusion, and therefore small vessel repairs are usually less successful in this age group.

It may be necessary to employ a distal repair in an attempt to save a limb. However, many legs in a critical condition will show, in addition to their superficial femoral artery disease, varying degrees of involvement of the profunda femoral artery. If this is the case, revascularization of the profunda artery alone will frequently preserve the life of the limb and should be done before attempting the more difficult distal repair.

Whatever surgical procedure is selected, it must be such that there are no areas of occlusion or significant stenosis proximal to the repair, since any interference with the inflow volume seriously threatens the continued patency of a more distal repair. Therefore, angiography of both the aortoiliac tree and the femoropopliteal-tibial vessels is essential in evaluating anatomic feasibility of any vascular reconstruction.

Sympathectomy. The value of sympathectomy is questionable. There is little if any sympathetic effect on vessels in the leg other than those in the skin, and, in addition, the sympathetic chain in the elderly patient is frequently so atrophic that it is difficult to identify. Improvement in the foot of an elderly patient after sympathectomy is not easy to recognize, but the operation is frequently done for pain at rest, minor ulceration, or minor gangrene if no other procedure is available.

Aortic aneurysm

Abdominal aortic aneurysm. The abdominal aortic aneurysm is the most common aneurysm and, with the possible exception of a cerebral aneurysm, also the most deadly, since most abdominal aortic aneurysms ultimately rupture. The key factor in considering an elderly patient for aneurysmectomy is to weigh the risk of rupture of the aneurysm to the life of the patient against the risk of the operative procedure to the life of the patient.

Although somewhat contradictory papers have been written on the natural history of abdominal aneurysm, there is reasonable evidence that aneurysms less than 5 cm in transverse diameter are less likely to rupture than larger aneurysms.[13] Therefore, in a poor-risk patient, surgery should be deferred if the aneurysm measures less than 5 cm and particularly if the aneurysm is calcified and can be seen on an x-ray film. Such a patient should be observed by physical examination and lateral radiographs of the abdomen at 3-, 6-, or 12-month intervals, depending on how long the aneurysm has been known to be stable. If the aneurysm is not calcified, ultrasound is useful to determine the size of the aneurysm and to follow the patient with serial examinations. Once the aneurysm starts to enlarge or becomes symptomatic, immediate repair should be done.

The possibility of rupture of aneurysms larger than 5 cm is high. An untreated ruptured aneurysm is essentially 100% fatal. For patients with a ruptured aneurysm who are able to live long enough to reach the operating room, the in-hospital mortality rate is still 50%. In elective aneurysmectomy the mortality rate should never exceed 10% and probably should not be more than 5% when surgery is in experienced hands.[14] Age itself is not a contraindication to surgery,[15] and any aneurysm larger than 5 cm should be repaired in a healthy patient regardless of age. One cannot be dogmatic concerning the importance of associated diseases. Patients with mild angina or emphysema should be considered candidates for elective surgery if the aneurysm is 5 to 8 cm, and patients with severe angina, emphysema, or renal disease should be operated on if the aneurysm is larger than 8 cm, if it is enlarging under observation, or if it has become symptomatic.

Because the incidence of severe coronary artery disease has been found to be about 80% in patients with abdominal aortic aneurysms,[4] routine coronary angiography followed by surgical improvement of the blood supply to the heart when indicated should be seriously considered in this group of patients.

Thoracic aortic aneurysm. Although it was originally thought that the incidence of rupture of thoracic aneurysms was about the same as that of abdominal aneurysms, this has not proved to be true. Thoracic aortic aneurysms tend to enlarge more slowly, and thus rupture is less frequent. In addition, surgery carries a greater risk than that for abdominal aneurysms. We are inclined to observe an elderly patient who has a thoracic aneurysm unless the aneurysm enlarges, as shown on periodic radiographs, or becomes symptomatic.

Cerebral ischemia. Many thrombotic cerebral vascular accidents are caused by occlusive arteriosclerosis of the extracranial arteries. Also many patients experience premonitory transient ischemic attacks prior to a completed stroke. These attacks are caused by small emboli that break off from a rough or ulcerated arteriosclerotic plaque usually located in the bulb of the common carotid artery or within the proximal 1 or 2 cm of the internal carotid artery itself. These small emboli transiently occlude a terminal vessel in the ipsilateral cerebral cortex or eye. When this happens, the patient may experience transient episodes of motor or sensory weakness in an arm or leg, partial or complete transient blindness, or temporary aphasia.

Although there may be many such episodes before a completed stroke, it cannot be emphasized too strongly that only one such episode may occur before acute thrombosis and a completed stroke supervenes.[16] Therefore arteriography should be done as soon as possible in patients with transient ischemia, and significant stenosis or ulceration should be corrected by endarterectomy. It is important to operate on these patients prophylactically before a completed stroke has resulted, since rarely it is possible for surgery to bring about improvement of a patient after the stroke. In fact, blood flow restoration in a patient with a recently completed stroke can result in significant worsening of the patient by hemorrhage into an area already softened by infarction.[17]

Carotid endarterectomy is a minimally stressful surgical procedure that can be readily done in patients whose associated disease might contraindicate more extensive procedures. Both short-term and long-term results are excellent, and the 5-year recurrent stenosis rate is minimal.[18] Confidence in this procedure has steadily increased. In the early years of carotid endarterectomy the procedure was done only for severe stenosis. Now endarterectomy is also done for minimal but ulcerated lesions in patients with transient attacks. Asymptomatic patients with severely stenotic lesions are candidates for endarterectomy if they are to undergo some other major surgical procedure that might result in hypotension and subsequent thrombosis of a carotid artery.

The indications for surgical treatment of vertebral artery stenosis are not as clearly defined as those of carotid artery stenosis. The symptoms are less distinct than those of carotid insufficiency and may be confused with vestibular vertigo, postural hypotension, hyperventilation syndrome, and other conditions. There are few patients with vertebrobasilar insufficiency whose disease is confined to the vertebral arteries alone. Usually an associated carotid artery stenosis is present, and in the presence of both vertebral and carotid artery stenosis, symptoms attributable to basilar artery insufficiency are generally relieved by correction of the carotid lesion alone.[19]

The subclavian (vertebral) steal is a condition in which, in the presence of an innominate or subclavian artery occlusion, the collateral supply to the deprived arm occurs by way of the contralateral vertebral artery, through the basilar artery, down the ipsilateral vertebral artery, and into the occluded subclavian artery distal to the occlusion. Although the collateral pathway is not infrequently seen, the condition rarely if ever affects circulation to the brain, and cerebral symptoms from an occluded innominate or subclavian artery are rare. Surgical correction should be done only if symptoms of arm claudication warrant it.

Conclusion

There should be no hesitation in operating on the geriatric patient who really needs arterial repair. However, the demands of the elderly person for normal function are less, and it is frequently acceptable to do less and to be more cautious than one might be with a younger individual.

VENOUS DISEASE

Varicose veins

More than eight million Americans suffer from varicose veins. Heredity is the most important factor in the development of varices, but they can develop in elderly people because the veins tend to lose their elasticity with aging and the muscles supporting them weaken.

Elastic stockings will counteract the stasis and swelling of varicose veins. For patients with mild to moderate varices, a light support hose or panty hose bought in a department store may be sufficient. For more severe varices, it may be necessary to purchase a heavier stocking.

The injection of solutions to thrombose the vein (sclerotherapy) is not as widely used as it once was. However, it is still a valuable procedure for smaller varicose veins and for "spider-burst" skin veins.

As a rule, ligation and stripping of varicose veins is not necessary if the patient is willing to wear the appropriate elastic support stockings.

Thrombophlebitis. The incidence of thrombophlebitis is higher in elderly individuals. The patient with superficial thrombophlebitis usually has a red, warm, painful, tender area under the skin along the course of a vein. It may occur in a varicose vein. Edema is not present. Since emboli do not result from superficial thrombophlebitis, anticoagulants are not required. Treatment consists of heat, rest, and elevation of the extremity until most of the pain and tenderness are gone.

Deep thrombophlebitis may result in minimal physical findings or edema, distended superficial veins, a reddish cyanotic color, and pain and tenderness. The key to early diagnosis is a high index of suspicion. The diagnosis can be confirmed by venography. Now available in many hospitals are new, accurate methods of diagnosis that produce less discomfort to the patient, including radioactive fibrinogen studies and noninvasive studies such as impedance phlebography and the use of the Doppler technique.

Since deep thrombophlebitis can result in pulmonary emboli, anticoagulants are required. Heparin and warfarin (Coumadin) are given for the first 7 to 10 days; then warfarin alone is given for the next 3 to 6 months.

Chronic venous insufficiency. Chronic venous insufficiency is the end-result of incompetency of the valves of damaged veins. The damaged valves usually result from a deep thrombophlebitis, but occasionally severe varicose veins can result in chronic venous insufficiency.

The clinical picture is characterized by edema and induration in the lower third or more of the leg. Chronic edema that is not controlled by elastic support can lead to fibrosis, induration, and inflammation (chronic stasis cellulitis). Often a characteristic brownish pigmentation will develop in the distal third of the leg because of capillary rupture and hemosiderin deposits. Dermatitis and stasis ulcers frequently occur if proper care is not given the leg.

Chronic venous insufficiency can be prevented if patients wear adequate elastic support on the involved leg below the knee when edema is present with severe varicose veins or following deep thrombophlebitis. The elastic support, whether it is a stocking or a wraparound bandage, should be strong enough to prevent edema. The elderly patient may need assistance in putting on these supports. They should be removed at night and can be omitted periodically to see if edema recurs. They can be discontinued whenever the leg remains free of edema.

REFERENCES

1. Buxton, J.T., Jr., and Stallworth, J.M.: Tortuous innominate arteries simulating aneurysms, J.A.M.A. **184:**1048, 1963.
2. Schatz, I.J., Fine, G., and Ehler, W.R.: Thromboangiitis obliterans, Br. Heart J. **28:**84, 1966.
3. Wheat, M.W., Jr.: Treatment of dissecting aneurysms of the aorta: current status, Prog. Cardiovasc. Dis. **16:**87, 1973.
4. Hertzer, N.R., et al.: Routine coronary angiography prior to elective aortic reconstruction, Arch. Surg. **114:**1336, 1979.
5. Humphries, A.W., and Young, J.R.: Experiences with aortoiliac and femoropopliteal endarterectomy, Surgery **67:**34, 1969.
6. Davies, E.J., Friz, B.R., and Clippinger, F.W.: Amputees and their prostheses, Artif. Limbs **14:**19, 1970.
7. Young, J.R.: Sudden arterial occlusion: medical aspects, Cardiovasc. Clin. **3:**159, 1971.
8. Imparato, A.M., Kim, G.E., Madayag, M., and Haveson, S.: Angiographic criteria for successful tibial arterial reconstructions, Surgery **74:**830, 1973.
9. Kahn, S.P., et al.: Femorotibial vein bypass, Arch. Surg. **107:**309, 1973.
10. Kaminski, D.L., et al.: Femoral-tibial bypass grafting, Arch. Surg. **104:**527, 1972.
11. Dillihunt, R.C., and Ray, F.S.: Femoral to anterior tibial artery bypass utilizing the tibial tunnel technic, Am. J. Surg. **127:**492, 1974.
12. Reichle, F.A., and Tyson, R.R.: Bypasses to tibial or popliteal arteries in severely ischemic lower extremities, Ann. Surg. **176:**315, 1972.
13. Sommerville, R.I., Allen, E.V., and Edwards, J.E.: Bland and infected abdominal aortic aneurysms: a clinicopathologic study, Medicine **38:**207, 1959.
14. Yasharr, J.J., Indeglia, R.A., and Yashar, J.: Surgery for abdominal aortic aneurysms: factors affecting survival and long-term results, Am. J. Surg. **128:**398, 1972.
15. Esselstyn, C.B., Jr., et al.: Aneurysmectomy in the aged? Surgery **67:**34, 1970.
16. Whisnant, J.P.: Epidemiology of stroke: emphasis on transient cerebral ischemic attacks and hypertension, Stroke **5:**68, 1974.
17. Wylie, E.J., Hein, M.F., and Adams, J.E.: Intracranial hemorrhage following surgical revascularization for treatment of acute strokes, J. Neurosurg. **21:**212, 1964.
18. Thompson, J.E., Austin, D.J., and Patman, R.D.: Carotid endarterectomy for cerebrovascular insufficiency: long-term results in 592 patients followed up to thirteen years, Ann. Surg. **172:**663, 1970.
19. Humphries, A.W., et al.: The relief of vertebrobasilar symptoms by carotid endarterectomy, Surgery **57:**48, 1965.

CHAPTER 22 · GYNECOLOGIC DISORDERS

Samuel D. Soule

Aging begins with fertilization of the freshly extruded ovum. When the female infant is born, she may be considered to be 9 months old. Growth, maturation, and concomitant aging proceed progressively to senility and death. As actuarial statistics reveal that more and more of the population reach older and older ages, the geriatric female of today must be viewed from the point of view of her relationship to the environment rather than merely as a chronologic entity. The woman of advanced years not only is to live longer, but she should be comfortable, useful, and happy as long as life continues.

The aging woman goes through perimenopausal trials in her forties, followed by a postmenopausal phase of the climacteric in her late forties or fifties. Ultimately, in her sixth decade she may be considered to be geriatric. Unlike some of the medical modalities that more frequently relate to specific disease entities, gynecologic disorders often refer to the central nervous system or the endocrine chain. Dysfunction in the complex hormonal gonad end-organ system may tax diagnostic acumen as keenly as does specific organic pathologic states.

The female reproductive system is dependent on hormonal function initiated in the hypothalamus, mediated through the anterior pituitary gland to the ovaries and on to the reproductive end-organs. This is manifested by the cyclic character of genital change noted throughout the reproductive phase of a woman's life. The hypothalamic-pituitary axis appears to remain functionally intact well into old age. Although no histologic changes have been described in studies of aging persons, there is a growing literature that describes hormonal and chemical changes in the geriatric population.

It is axiomatic that regressive changes associated with the aging process occur in all organs and tissues of the body. The progressive decrease of gonadal endocrine stimulation to the female generative tract results in the observed changes in end-organ tissues. Atrophic changes in stroma, changes in fat distribution, vascular and pigment variations, and aberrant calcium metabolism are noted.

Age alone is no longer a contraindication to definitive therapeutic modalities. Preoperative preparation, both constitutional and local; surgical skills; and infinite improvements in anesthesia allow an active approach to many disorders previously not treated surgically. Recognition of dysfunctional conditions may result in need for medicinal and psychiatric therapy.

GENERAL PHYSICAL CHANGES

During and after the menopause there is progressive atrophy of tissues. Specific gynecologic examples include the following: Vulvar hair becomes sparse and gray; the vulva becomes pallid and the labia shrunken; the vaginal wall becomes thin and atrophic and pale in color; progressive subcutaneous atrophy may cause shortening and narrowing of the vaginal canal; and the vault may become obliterated. Normal moisture lessens, and the fully stimulated cytogram of a younger person is gradually replaced by a completely atrophic basal cell cytogram. The cervix becomes atrophic and occasionally completely stenosed. The corpus decreases in size, the myometrium becomes replaced by fibrous tissue, blood vessels sclerose, and the endometrium is thin and atrophic. With progressive decrease in ovarian function the ovaries decrease in size and the stroma becomes compact.

Relaxation of the pelvic floor, including urethrocele, cystocele, rectocele, enterocele, or varying degrees of uterine prolapse *may* have an origin in congenital weakness. However, most of such conditions relate to childbearing injuries, with subsequent aggravation by the loss of tissue tone incidental to aging.

Neoplasms and endocrine, metabolic, and excretory system disorders have significance in the gynecologic care of aging women. Organic disease and dysfunctional disorders of old age are insidious in onset and usually slow in progression. This is in striking contrast to the more acute processes of earlier years. On rare occasions acute specific infection of the vulva and vagina may occur. The thin atrophic vaginal membrane of the aging female is not an appropriate medium for growth of bacteria or for monilial or trichomonal infections.

Estrogen therapy has been recommended to stay the development of some of the degenerative changes in the geriatric female. Osteoporosis and some of the genitourinary and vaginal symptoms related to hormone deficiency usually respond well to such therapy. Although an extensive literature has been developed on the relationship between estrogens and endometrial cancer, there is no uniform acceptance of such an association. An acceptable regimen is predicted on the premise that estrogen therapy will be advised when the situation demands such therapy. Physical examination to rule out absolute contraindications is necessary. Liver disease, cardiovascular disease or previous myocardial infarction, venous thrombosis, possibly diabetes mellitus, marked fibrocystic disease, or previous breast or other malignancy may contraindicate estrogen therapy. Dosage should be kept as low as possible, and administration should be cyclic rather than continuous for indefinite periods of time. The addition of progestin for the last 5 to 7 days of each cycle of estrogen is advocated by many authors. Any bleeding during or after hormone administration demands a definitive diagnostic procedure. Periodic follow-up with cytology, endometrial biopsy, or colposcopy is mandatory for any woman receiving hormone therapy. It may be properly inferred that I do not ascribe to either the "estrogen never" or the "estrogen forever" philosophy.

The geriatric female should not be denied estrogen therapy when its use is indicated. The benefits of replacement therapy far outweigh any risk.

POSTMENOPAUSAL BLEEDING

The climacteric is a normal physiologic state of a woman's life welcomed by most emotionally stable women. Secondary endocrine readjustments are associated with progressive ovarian quiescence. The age at which the menopause occurs varies with different women. Although it is impractical to set a specific time limit, any bleeding that occurs more than 1 year after cessation of menstruation must be considered to be abnormal. Periodic examination for early detection of coexistent organic problems accompanies education of patients regarding the physiology of the menopause.

Benign conditions associated with postmenopausal bleeding include senile vaginitis, urethral caruncle, cervical erosion or ulceration associated with descensus uteri, cervical or endometrial polyps, senile endometritis, endometrial hyperplasia, and systemic disease. Endometrial hyperplasia is not uncommon in elderly patients. It may occur along with atrophic or senile ovaries but always raises the suspicion that there may be a granulosa cell or thecal cell tumor of the ovary. Prolonged estrogen therapy as an anabolic agent in geriatric care is sometimes associated with bleeding. In a large proportion of cases the endometrial histology is retrogressive in character relating to the menopausal period, but in others the endometrium undergoes an active glandular proliferation that may predispose to carcinoma. The malignancies that most frequently cause postmenopausal bleeding are vulvar, cervical, and endometrial carcinoma and granulosa or thecal cell tumor of the ovary. More rare tumors have been described also.

After careful inspection and palpation, complete diagnostic procedures are carried out. Vaginal, cervical, and endometrial cytology may be diagnostically informative. Biopsy and curettage are employed as indicated. Colposcopy and hysteroscopy are more current additions to the gynecologist's armamentarium; these diagnostic procedures have added immeasurably to our diagnostic skills and make for improved therapeutic procedures. Urinary and rectal areas are studied for etiologic evidence.

Treatment depends on diagnosis. Local benign conditions respond to appropriate treatment, which may be local or systemic. Adequate treatment of prolapse or surgical intervention should be instituted as indicated.

VULVA

The progressive atrophic changes in the entire vulvar and perineal area described before are under hormonal control. As estrogenic influence diminishes with advancing age, atrophic changes become increasingly manifest. *Pruritus vulvae* is a common symptom that warrants a careful search for an underlying cause. The gynecologist often is the primary physician consulted for this condition. Constitutional diseases such as diabetes, pernicious anemia, hepatitis or other liver conditions, leukemia, or drug reactions, must be ruled out. Leakage of urine due to urethral or bladder disease is a frequent cause of local vulvar irritation.

Senile atrophy, including so-called *atrophic vaginitis,* is a common finding in the group of degenerative diseases that includes leukoplakia, kraurosis, and lichen sclerosus et atrophicus. Pruritus, burning sensation, and marked dryness are presenting complaints. Leukoplakia is first seen as hyperkeratosis, which progresses to atrophy. If there is a real difference between leukoplakia and kraurosis it lies in the advanced atrophy of kraurosis. There is a definite relationship between these atrophic lesions and epidermoid carcinoma in that 50% of carcinomas develop in an atrophic background. Lichen sclerosus et atrophicus is a similar atrophic lesion, characterized by patchy isolated papules, which eventually coalesce to form nodules. This lesion is more edematous and less fibrotic and is considered to be without the malignant potential of leukoplakia or kraurosis.

In general, treatment should be gentle and consist mainly of cleanliness, nutritional supplementation, sedation, and soothing local applications. Many conditions respond to careful local hygiene with either starch baths or a cool, dry, bland starch powder. Others subside with topical application of a nongreasy soothing cream containing estrogenic substances. Estrogen administered orally must be monitored carefully because of potential constitutional contraindication.

Basal cell carcinoma is a rather indolent malignancy that is found occasionally in the vulva of elderly women. Less frequently melanoma, intraepithelial carcinoma, Paget's disease, and carcinoma of Bartholin's glands are observed.

True invasive carcinoma of the vulva is predominantly a disease of elderly women. The tumor usually arises in the anterior half of the vulva, from the labia majora or minora, the clitoris, or the vestibule of the vagina. It forms a flat, infiltrative or ulcerative type of growth, although it may be predominantly exophytic. The symptoms are usually pruritus with vulvar irritation, a mass or ulceration, bloody discharge, and pain as a late complaint. Extension to regional lymph nodes frequently occurs at an early stage of the disease. Prognosis depends to a large extent on the presence or absence of metastases.

Radical vulvectomy and bilateral dissection of superficial and deep nodes should be performed in every case if the patient's condition permits. The extent of the dissection and whether gland dissection is performed depends on the extent of the parent lesion, the character of the tumor, and the condition of the patient. Despite the advanced age of patients with vulvar carcinoma and the not-infrequent presence of constitutional hazards such as diabetes, obesity, and vascular disturbances, which render them poor surgical risks, they tolerate radical surgery well, and age is not a contraindication to operation. Radiation therapy is extremely disappointing and should be employed only when surgery is absolutely contraindicated.

RELAXATION OF THE PELVIC FLOOR

Relaxation of the pelvic floor may occur in nulligravid or even virginal women. However, the more frequently observed relaxations are seen in postmenopausal women who have had considerable attenuation of supporting structures or childbirth lacerations in earlier years. The atrophic changes incidental to the aging process lend themselves to aggravation of previously minimal weakness in the levator musculature and enveloping fascial layers.

The elderly woman may note bearing-down discomfort—a sense of weight in the pelvis—or protrusion of a mass as an acute symptom complex. In such cases the physician may be dealing with an acute herniation subsequent to lifting or straining in an individual in whom the criteria for such a breakthrough were present but in whom an acute trauma induced the integumental herniation. More often there is a gradual progressive increase in discomfort, an increasing degree of prolapse, and eventual disability requiring definitive attention.

Cystocele

A cystocele is a relaxation of the anterior vaginal wall: it is usually the result of childbirth trauma and is a defect in the pubovesical and pubocervical fascia. There is usually a coexistent urethrocele. The symptoms are a mass protruding from the vagina, an annoying sense of weight in the pelvis, dysuria, and often repeated urinary tract infections.

Rectocele

A rectocele is a prolapse of the posterior vaginal wall. Its cause lies in attenuation or laceration of the rectovaginal fascia, separation of the levator muscles, and perineal laceration. Bulging of the anal pouch and rectum through these attenuated structures produces symptoms of bearing-down pressure, protrusion of a mass through the vaginal opening, and faults with defecation. Such a bulging mass must be distinguished from a frequently associated cystocele and enterocele.

Enterocele

An enterocele, which is a true hernia, is a protrusion through the pelvic outlet by way of the vagina. The peritoneal sac may contain omentum or gut. In rare instances the hernia occurs in front of the uterus; more often it is bounded anteriorly by the posterior surface of the uterus, laterally by the sacrouterine ligaments, and posteriorly by the rectum. Uterine prolapse of varying degree usually accompanies an enterocele, and a rectocele is almost always an associated finding. Obstetric trauma is the most frequent etiologic factor.

Symptoms of an enterocele are essentially the same as those of a rectocele. In addition, the symptoms and danger of entrapped gut with strangulation and incarceration are a possibility.

Careful rectal examination of posterior wall relaxation enables the examiner to differentiate between a rectocele and an enterocele.

Cystocele, rectocele, and enterocele require no surgical treatment if of minor degree and asymptomatic. Surgical repair is indicated when the relaxation is of greater extent, when it is becoming progressively larger, or when it is causing discomfort or disability. When other conditions that require surgery are present, the associated findings should be corrected.

Stress incontinence

In general genitourinary symptoms are related in part to old parturition trauma, previous surgery, or postradiation tissue changes and in part to the progressive atrophy due to diminishing hormone stimulation to this anatomic area. Stress incontinence, also described as *partial incontinence,* is that condition in which urine is lost involuntarily with a sudden increase in intraabdominal pressure or with straining, coughing, or sneezing. The incontinence is due to weakness in the supportive structures of the vesical neck.

The diagnosis is made from the history and the physical examination. During pelvic examination a bearing-down effort or coughing may cause a leaking or even projectile expulsion of urine. Often this does not occur until the patient stands and makes an expulsive effort. Splinting the paraurethral tissues with two examining fingers or a partially opened dressing forceps, or other paired long-bladed instrument, may give the support necessary to alleviate the incontinence. Differential diagnosis between stress incontinence and other genitourinary conditions that may cause loss of urine should be made prior to definitive treatment. Examination of urinary sediment for infection, endoscopic and cystoscopic examination, or cystographic and cystometric studies may be indicated in any one given case.

There is no one completely satisfactory treatment for this condition. When the degree of disability warrants, surgical correction is preferred. Careful study of the anatomic defect should allow the surgeon to decide whether local repair via vaginal approach is preferable to a suprapubic procedure. Most often vaginal surgery is employed first. Recurrence of stress incontinence warrants suprapubic vesicourethral suspension. All these operative procedures employ the same basic technique of freeing the vesical neck and urethra and reestablishing the vesicourethral angle from above. The differences in procedure relate to suture material, number of sutures, and location of the anchoring stitches. It is recommended that these geriatric women be given estrogen for several weeks prior to surgery to increase the tone and viability of the tissues to be manipulated. Diethylstilbestrol, estradiol, or conjugated estrogen may be prescribed with attention to tolerance of such medication by patients in this age group.

Prolapse of the uterus

Prolapse of the uterus is that condition in which the uterus occupies a position below its normal level in the pelvis. *Prolapse* is synonymous with *descensus*. The cause of prolapse most frequently is the attenuation or laceration of the supporting structures of the uterus during childbirth. The occurrence of these conditions in nulligravid women and the absence of them in many women who have had extremely traumatic deliveries emphasizes the fact that an inherent fault in the tissue tone exists in some patients. It is most unusual for prolapse to occur as a primary condition in geriatric females. The loss of tone and the general tissue atrophy that occur in the postmenopausal woman favor a progressive increase in the degree of prolapse so that eventually a symptomatic and disabling condition exists. In first-degree prolapse the cervix does not yet descend outside the introitus, and symptoms of minimal to moderate pelvic pressure are noted. Increasing bearing-down discomfort and protrusion of the cervix through the vaginal orifice characterize a second-degree prolapse. A complete extrusion of the cervix and corpus is a third-degree prolapse, also known as *procidentia*. A cystocele and a rectocele usually accompany second- and third-degree prolapse.

Aside from the physical discomfort of pressure symptoms and presence of a protruding mass, there are dangers to allied organs because of prolapse of the uterus. Prolapse of the bladder gives rise to incomplete emptying and residual urine with accompanying pyelonephritis as an ultimate complication. Associated rectocele causes difficulty with fecal evacuation. Protrusion of the cervix makes it prone to dryness, subsequent excoriation, and infection. The prolapsed vaginal membrane often becomes thickened and leathery.

Treatment of prolapse of the uterus in the geriatric female depends on the degree of prolapse, the severity of symptoms, and the condition of the patient. In the geriatric age group, first-degree prolapse is best treated by periodic examination for aggravation of the relaxation and by reassuring the patient that the symptom complex is not serious. Similarly, a second-degree prolapse does not usually warrant definitive treatment unless the symptoms are increasingly disabling. Operation is recommended for complete prolapse unless the general condition of the patient contraindicates such care. With current progress in anesthesia, early ambulation, and careful preparation of the patient for surgery, vaginal hysterectomy is usually well tolerated. Less frequently, colpocleisis or, in ideal situations, Watkins' interposition operation may be the preferred procedure.

Palliative measures, reserved for the patient who is an extremely poor surgical risk or for the very aged, may keep a patient comfortable by relieving the irritation that causes ulceration of protruding structures and by diminishing the tension on uterine supports. The soft rubber doughnut pessary or a modified Gellhorn pessary may raise the uterus and maintain the fundus in an elevated position. Such devices must be removed at frequent intervals and the vaginal wall inspected for pressure ulceration. The use of cleansing douches or vaginal instillation of antibacterial suppositories or creams may be necessary.

VAGINA

The vaginal membrane is a modified epithelium. It is subject to the same changes observed in the vulva. The depletion of estrogenic stimulation to the vaginal membrane causes an atrophic thinning of tissue, an altered bacterial flora, and a change toward more alkaline pH. Punctate hemorrhagic areas are frequently noted, especially at the vault. An epithelial discharge is not infrequent. Vaginal dermis is almost entirely of the basal cell type. Therapy is indicated if there is an associated pruritus or concomitant genitourinary symptoms.

Vaginal pruritus is often associated with a watery or even bloody discharge. Culture for specific organisms and Papanicolaou smears to rule out malignancy should precede local application of estrogen cream or suppository. Estrogens administered by mouth must be prescribed cautiously to all senescent individuals.

Vaginal infection with *Monilia (Candida)*, a more frequent condition observed in younger age groups, is unusual in the geriatric patient except in those with diabetes or receiving antibiotic therapy. Similarly, trichomoniasis and *Haemophilus* infection are seldom seen.

Carcinoma of the vagina is an extremely rare

tumor in this age group. When it occurs, it is most likely to be a metastatic lesion or a direct extension from a lesion of the cervix. Diagnosis is made by biopsy, and appropriate treatment would depend on the parent lesion.

CERVIX

The atrophic changes described before in the external organs of reproduction also take place in the cervix. With progressive atrophy the stroma of the cervix is replaced by connective tissue. The endocervical glands tend to seal over, and the cervical canal may become totally stenosed. Such a senescent change may be a serious complicating factor when secretions are trapped in the endometrial cavity. Such may occur in endometrial carcinoma, hematometra associated with estrogen administration, or pyometra occurring with infection.

Benign endocervical polyps are seen in elderly women. Evulsion or excision should be done in every case. A thorough investigation of the endocervix and endometrium must complement such an examination to rule out multiplicity of growths or associated malignancy.

Although 60% of cases of cancer of the cervix occur prior to 60 years of age, 5% to 10% are found in those over 70 years of age. The structure and behavior of cervical carcinoma are not significantly influenced by age, although the course appears to be more indolent in senescence. As part of the general education of all segments of society, more elderly women report more regularly for periodic examination. Furthermore, education to be wary of any abnormal bleeding, watery discharge, or pain, when combined with Papanicolaou smears at all ages, will result in fewer advanced clinical stages coming under observation.

Treatment currently consists of local treatment with radioactive agents and deep therapy with transabdominal radiation. Radical surgery may be employed occasionally in certain specifically selected cases.

CORPUS UTERI

As a woman becomes progressively more menopausal, the uterus involutes until it becomes a fibrotic structure scarcely larger than the cervix. Concomitantly, the endometrium becomes markedly atrophic. The senile endometrium is normally composed of atrophic glands, which are not infrequently cystic. Senile endometritis, occasionally with pyometra, occurs in this age group.

Hyperplasia of the endometrium in elderly patients, even many years after the menopause, is evidence that the endometrium never loses its capacity to respond to hormonal stimulation. An inactive cystic endometrial pattern is noted frequently in the well-established postmenopausal phase. This response is probably induced by the persistent minimal estrogenic production from ovaries that arc not entirely quiescent.

Glandular hyperplasia of the endometrium in the postmenopausal woman suggests a persistent endogenous source of estrogen such as granulosa or thecal cell tumor of the ovary or an adrenal source of gonadal hormone. Also, exogenous administration of estrogenic hormones may result in bleeding from glandular hyperplasia. There is suggestive evidence that adenomatous endometrial hyperplasia is a precursor of adenocarcinoma of the endometrium.

Carcinoma of the endometrium

Carcinoma of the endometrium exceeds cervical cancer in frequency in the older age groups. Since the incidence of uterine cancer reaches its peak in the age group of the middle sixties, it may be presumed that the increasing longevity of the population is an important factor in the rising incidence of this cancer.

Carcinoma of the body of the uterus may be associated with either an inactive or a hyperplastic endometrium. Although there is no direct proof that estrogens cause cancer of the uterus, it is difficult to negate the conclusion that they are intimately associated with some cases, particularly in the case of estrogen-producing tumors of the ovaries associated with endometrial carcinoma.

The usual presenting symptom is postmenopausal bleeding. An enlarging corpus noted during periodic examination may be suspicious, although often there is no gross change in the uterus. Diagnosis is made by cytology, endometrial biopsy, or curettage.

Treatment of carcinoma of the endometrium is tempered to some degree by the physical status of the patient. Ideally, preliminary intracavitary radiation is followed by external radiation. In selected cases preliminary radiation may not be feasible, and primary hysterectomy becomes the treatment of choice. Postoperative transabdominal radiation is then considered.

Sarcoma of the uterus comprises less than 5% of uterine malignancies and has its greatest incidence in the fifth and sixth decades of a person's life. It is exceedingly rare for malignant change to occur in a leiomyoma after the menopause. When it occurs, leiomyosarcoma usually takes origin directly from the myometrium.

Mixed mesodermal tumors are a specialized form of sarcoma. When they occur in the postmenopausal period, they are usually a corporeal growth.

OVARY

The senile ovary is a markedly atrophic organ and becomes convoluted and sclerotic. Germinal inclusion cysts are the only form of ovarian cyst that increase in frequency with advancing age. The dysfunctional types of ovarian tumor and endometrial cysts of the ovaries are characteristic of the reproductive period of life. Ovarian enlargement discovered in the postmenopausal period must be treated as a malignancy until proved otherwise because of the high degree of malignancy noted in this age group. Surgery is advisable after thorough study has been done to determine the possibility of metastatic disease.

At least 50% of granulosa cell tumors occur after the menopause and have been reported in women 70 to 80 years of age. Patients who have not menstruated for years and who are not receiving estrogens may complain of bleeding. Granulosa cell tumors are estrogen producing. This hormone influence is evidenced by vaginal cytologic or endometrial histologic study. These tumors are often tiny and often not detected by manual examination. For the geriatric age group, laparotomy with removal of the uterus and both adnexa is advisable. With removal of the tumor, patients often experience a sound menopause with characteristic vasomotor phenomena. Malignancy is reported in 5% to 25% of these tumors.

Thecoma of the ovary is even more characteristically a tumor of the senescent female. It is generally a solid tumor, is fibrous, and has a tendency toward lipid deposit. Thecoma is a biologically active tumor and is associated more frequently with endometrial carcinoma than is granulosa cell tumor. Symptoms and treatment are the same as for granulosa cell tumor.

Finally, the Brenner tumor has a predilection for the postmenopausal period. Cystic endometrial hyperplasia has been observed with this tumor, even in the advanced age group.

CONCLUSION

The needs of the aging female increase as the span of life is prolonged. The perspective of the practitioner must be broadened to encompass these needs, being equally mindful of the advances in the skills of the medical and surgical armamentarium.

Progressive atrophy of the genital tract leads to a physiologic change in visible and palpable organs. However, any discharge, bleeding, ulceration, or mass must be investigated to a definitive diagnosis prior to any therapeutic trial.

Abdominal laparotomy and vaginal surgery are not contraindicated by age, provided preoperative evaluation indicates a suitable risk.

Steroid therapy, primarily with estrogenic substances, must be guided by the constitutional indications and contraindications to such medication.

REFERENCES

1. Birnbaum, S.J.: Geriatric gynecology. In Chinn, A.B., editor: Working with older people, Public Health Service Pub. No. 1459, vol. 4, Washington, D.C., 1971, Government Printing Office.
2. Brewer, J.I., and DeCosta, E.J.: Textbook of gynecology, Baltimore, 1967, The Williams & Wilkins Co.
3. Greenblatt, R.B., and Stoddard, L.D.: The estrogen-cancer controversy, J. Am. Geriatr. Soc. **26**:1, 1978.
4. Longcape, C.: Hormones: beneficial or dangerous to the aged? J. Am. Geriatr. Soc. **26**:145, 1978.
5. McKeown, F.: Pathology of the aged, London, 1965, Butterworth & Co. Publishers, Ltd.
6. Notelowitz, M.: Gynecologic problems of menopausal women. 1. Changes in the genital tissue, Geriatrics **33**(8):24, 1978.
7. Notelowitz, M.: Gynecologic problems of menopausal women. 2. Treating estrogen deficiency, Geriatrics **33**(9):35, 1978.
8. Notelowitz, M.: Gynecologic problems of menopausal women. 3. Changes in extragenital tissues and sexuality, Geriatrics **33**(10):51, 1978.
9. Parsons, L., and Sommers, S.C.: Gynecology, ed. 2, Philadelphia, 1978, W.B. Saunders Co.

CHAPTER 23 · ORAL CARE OF THE GERIATRIC PATIENT

Saul Kamen

A recent experience epitomizes the interface between the physician and dentist in the clinical management of the geriatric patient.

A 68-year-old man is scheduled for a triple coronary bypass following several episodes of acute angina pectoris. A few days before his hospital admission a cusp of a maxillary second molar fractures, leaving a sharp, knifelike edge of enamel and resulting in thermal sensitivity. He pays an emergency visit to the dentist, who examines the tooth and performs a vitality test, both of which indicate that the pulp is undergoing devitalization and that an abscess may be forming. The dentist calls the patient's cardiologist, who advises that definitive treatment, such as root canal treatment or extraction, could be inordinately stress producing and might trigger another anginal episode, thus delaying the impending cardiac surgery. The patient, already anguished at the prospect of serious surgery, is now increasingly anxious because of the complication of dental infection. And the dentist, complying with the recommendation of the cardiologist, is forced to temporize, albeit aware that the oral infection, if uncontrolled, might jeopardize not only the patient care plan but the postoperative course of events and the successful outcome of the cardiac surgery.

This case history is introduced at this point not for the purpose of problem solving but to establish the basic principle that the mouth can play a particularly significant role in the total health status of the elderly patient and that poor oral health may become one of the "contingencies of living" that Alex Comfort alludes to in his sociogenic view of aging.

Although the salutary effects of water fluoridation and preventive dentistry campaigns are beginning to show some positive results, it is still a sad fact that of the approximately 50% of Americans over 60 years of age who have retained some or all of their natural teeth, 90% will have some degree of periodontal disease—the loss of the supporting structure of the teeth—and a significant incidence of dental decay. Apparently in the past four centuries we have not progressed far from Shakespeare's description of the seventh age of man as "sans teeth, sans taste, sans eyes, sans everything" *(As You Like It)*. In this context it is certainly appropriate to examine the reasons for the poor oral health of the elderly and how the interdisciplinary cooperation of physicians and dentists can aid in its amelioration.

Poor oral health diminishes the quality of life of the affected individual throughout life. Consider the many functions of the mouth. In the infant it is the organ of both expression and sustenance. With it the young baby expresses hunger, fear, pleasure, anger, and, often wreathed with smiles, love and joy. Masticatory efficiency is manifested early in life and persists throughout growth and development as the primary factor in the proper functioning of the digestive process. As the child grows into young adulthood the appearance of the mouth plays a most important role in the entire physiognomy and sometimes makes all the difference between social acceptability and rejection. The attractive smile, so frequently exploited by the media, becomes a keystone in the development of personality and temperament. Thus from childhood through old age, self-esteem and a good self-image are dependent on the arrangement of the teeth and jaws. Masticatory efficiency, speech, and appearance are the basic triad of functions that determine the status of oral health.

Although we should never underestimate the functions of the mouth, it may nevertheless be said that the presence of teeth is not absolutely essential for the preparation of food for digestion. Indeed we all know of individuals who function quite well in the edentulous state and who will not accept prosthetic replacements. It is quite true that the diet for the completely edentulous patient without dentures can be modified for purposes of ingestion of food, but there are two important reservations that should be considered. First, while the nutritional benefit may be the same, the *enjoyment* of the performance of eating is undoubtedly diminished, and second, many edentulous individuals who for one reason or another cannot wear dentures are embarrassed or reluctant to engage in the social contact of mealtime with friends and as a result become isolated.

How then can the physician lend his skills to improving the oral health of his patient? The achievement of this objective requires an understanding of the biologic, physiologic, psychologic, and pathologic effects of aging on the oral apparatus; the ability to perform an adequate evaluation of the mouth and its adnexae; and an appreciation of the medical-dental interactions in the clinical management of the compromised individual.

NORMATIVE AGING CHANGES OF THE ORAL APPARATUS

The most obvious changes that affect the mouth and its adnexae occur in the surrounding integumentary tissues. As with all of the aging processes, individuals are not affected uniformly or at the same rate. Nevertheless, the loss of intracellular water and subcutaneous fat is an inexorable physiologic fact of aging and results in the infolding of the epithelium with subsequent wrinkling of the facial skin. This usually begins with crow's-feet of the forehead and gradually progresses to encompass the entire facial features. The dentist is particularly concerned with the deep wrinkles forming around the mouth, extending from the alae nasi to the corner of the lips and thence to the chin. Adding insult to injury, in the edentulous patient there is usually a collapse of the vertical dimension, the distance between the tip of the nose and a point on the middle of the chin. Some gnathologists attribute this to changes in the temporomandibular joint (TMJ) concomitant with osteoporosis. The ultimate effect of the contracture may be the purse string, or feathered, mouth, in which it appears as if a drawstring has been pulled tightly through the lips (Fig. 23-1). The dentist tries to mitigate these adverse changes

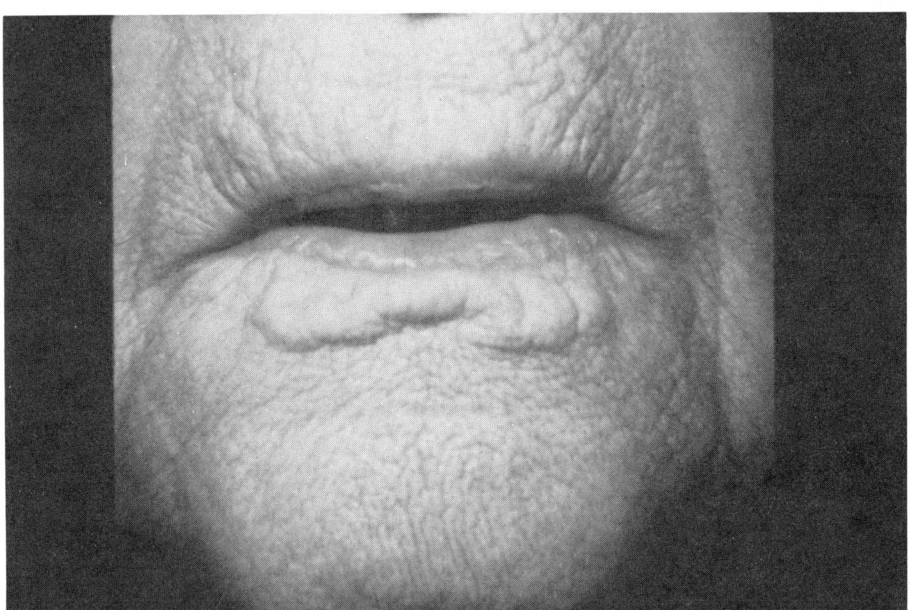

Fig. 23-1. Purse string mouth—the effects of aging on the surrounding integument and orbicularis oris musculature.

as he constructs his prostheses; cosmetic rehabilitation is one of the great challenges in the art of the prosthodontist.

The change in water balance also affects salivary gland function, with a varying degree of diminution of saliva and mucus. This is exacerbated by the xerostomic drug effects that elderly patients are subject to.

Normal changes manifested in the lips, primarily as a result of diminished peripheral vascular function, include a thinning of the vermillion border and an atrophic, pale appearance.

Turning our attention to dentition, the biologic effect of aging on the teeth can be readily observed. The enamel loses its translucency, and the teeth darken. Attrition (Fig. 23-2,*A*) is the wearing away of the occlusal and incisal surfaces of the teeth as the result of many years of mastication. Abrasion (Fig. 23-2,*B*) is the indentation of enamel at the junction of the crown and root and is chiefly caused by mechanical factors such as adverse toothbrushing habits. Erosion (Fig. 23-2,*C*) is similar in appearance to abrasion but is caused by the chemical constitutents of the diet and saliva. Unlike these regressive changes, which may be considered normal, cervical caries, which are distinct pathologic entities are seen in the same illustration (Fig. 23-2,*D*).

The foregoing processes, along with extrinsic staining, occur by and large in most elderly individuals, but it would be a mistake to believe that they inevitably lead to tooth loss. It can be stated almost categorically that with our current knowledge people should be able to retain most of their natural teeth throughout life. Refinements in our concepts of diet, saliva, and plaque (the sticky film consisting of bacterial substrate and mucin that is essential for the process of decay) make it possible to institute measures of prevention that can literally save teeth from dental disease for a lifetime.

The soft tissues of the mouth undergo subtle changes during aging that may also be considered within normal limits. Thus the Fordyce granules of the buccal mucosa lining the lips and cheeks may become more numerous and prominent, but these small sebaceous glands are entirely benign. The oral mucosa becomes thin and pale in appearance, reflecting diminished peripheral circulation. The tongue becomes fissured, and there is a progressive defoliation of the papillae, giving it a smoother appearance on its dorsal surface, while varicosities appear more frequently on the ventral surface. The gradual loss of taste buds may result in alterations in taste, ranging from a mild *dysgeusia* (distortion

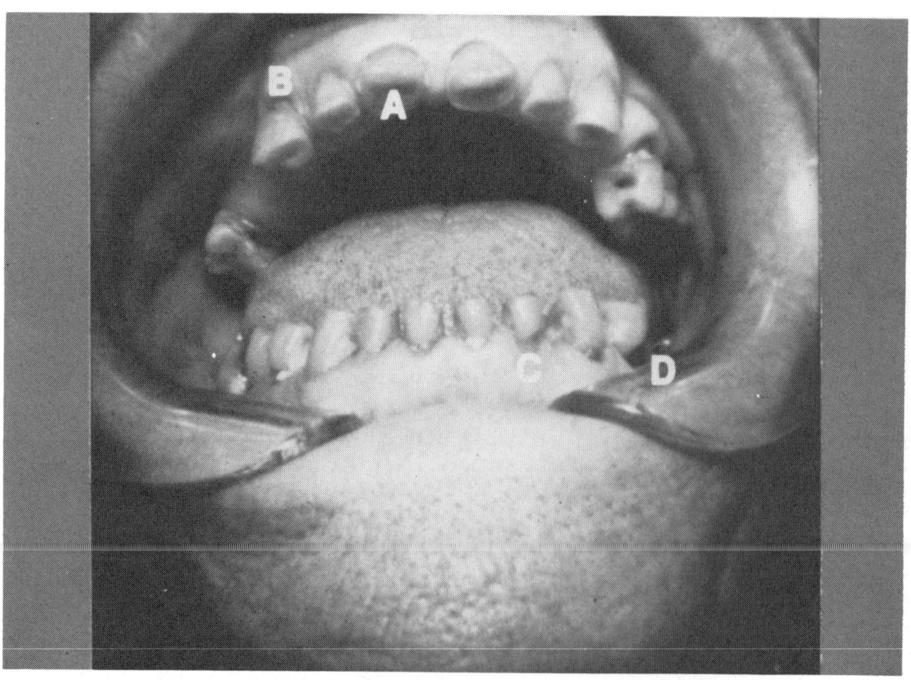

Fig. 23-2. The aging dentition: **A,** attrition; **B,** abrasion; **C,** erosion; **D,** cervical caries.

of taste) to a marked *ageusia* (loss of taste), particularly in systemic disorders such as hypothyroidism.

Exostoses of the palate (torus palatinus) and sometimes of the mandible may be considered normal, for they occur with considerable frequency from adulthood on and are benign. They may interfere with the construction of prostheses and will then require surgical ablation.

Because of the prevalence of edentulousness in the over-65 age group, we should also consider the effect of loss of teeth on the maxilla and mandible. We have already noted that peri-

A

B

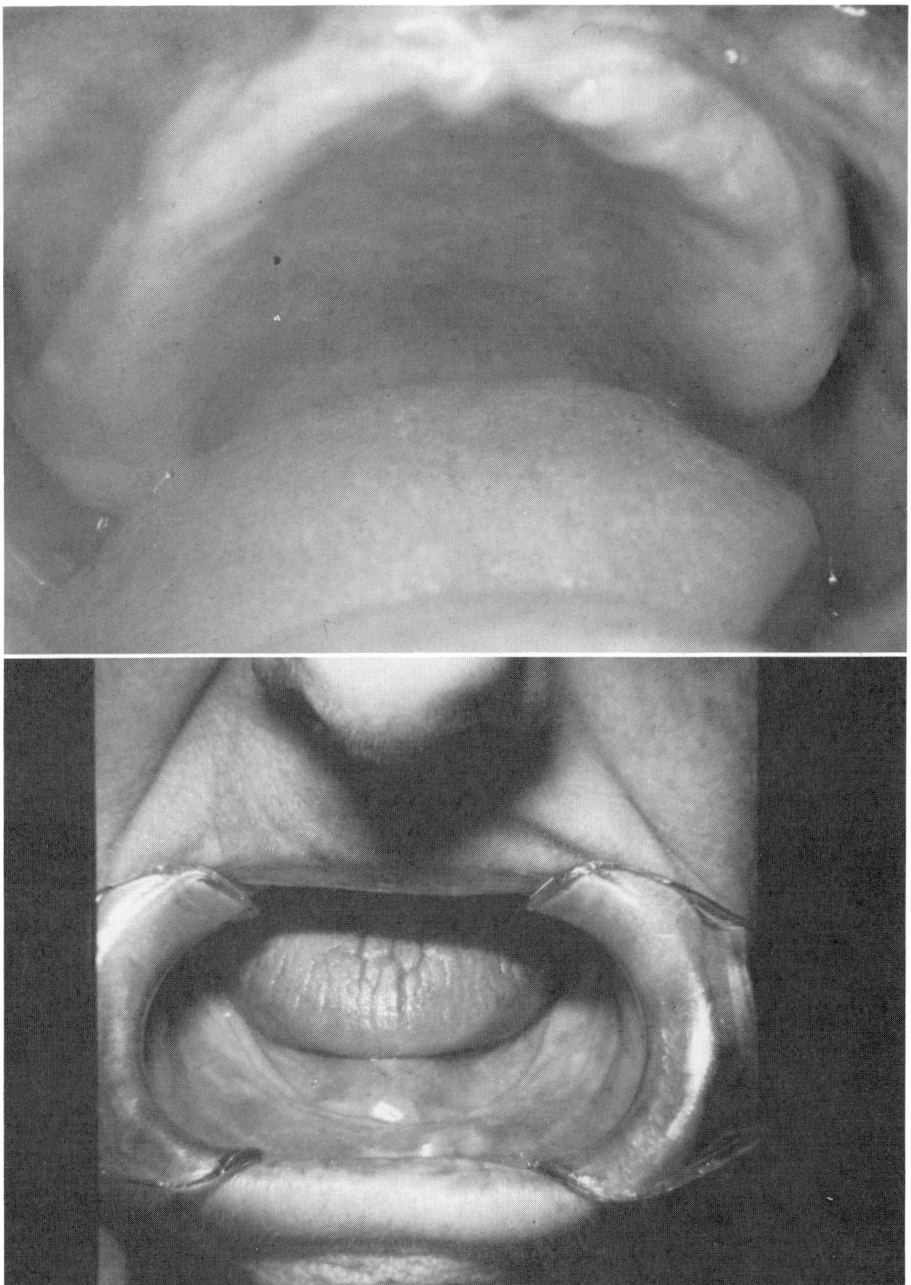

Fig. 23-3. Effects of aging in the edentulous patient. Note atrophy of the alveolar ridges in **A,** maxilla, and **B,** mandible, in a 73-year-old female with diabetes and osteoporosis.

odontal disease (pyorrhea alveolaris), the primary cause of tooth loss, affects the supporting structure of the teeth and thereby reduces the height of the alveolar ridges. Concomitant with this process, osteoporotic changes accelerate osseus remodeling, and atrophy of both alveolar ridges occurs with the mandibular bone being resorbed at four times the rate of the maxilla (Fig. 23-3). In extensive mandibular atrophy the mental foramen assumes a more superior position on the crest of the ridge, resulting in a dehiscence that can be quite painful in the presence of an overlying denture.[1] Such problems, of course, are within the province of the prosthodontist.

The effect of dentures on mastication, as might be expected, results in compromised oral function. A 10-year longitudinal study at the Veteran's Administration outpatient clinic in Boston showed that whereas masticatory function remained constant for all persons with complete or partially compromised natural dentition, tooth loss and replacement by removable prostheses resulted in lowered efficiency of deglutition, as measured by a Swallowing Threshold Test Index, and mastication, as measured by a Standardized Masticatory Performance Test.[2] This study further demonstrated that impaired dentition required increased effort to adequately pulverize food. Indeed, this author is aware of an incident in which a diner in a restaurant suddenly collapsed and died. The death certificate stated cardiac arrest as the cause of death. The body was subsequently exhumed, and the autopsy revealed a bolus of food lodged in the pharynx. With the development of the Heimlich maneuver such accidents can be aborted if there is a suspicion of asphyxiation, for which the denture wearer should certainly be considered at higher risk.

In summary, normal anatomic and physiologic changes in the oral cavity include the following:

1. A reduction in the thickness of epithelial and connective tissues causing a thinning of the oral mucosa
2. A decrease in salivary flow as well as qualitative changes in the nature of the saliva
3. Diminished potential for healing
4. Reduction and/or alterations in taste perception
5. Fissuring of the tongue
6. White, hairy tongue resulting from accumulation of keratin on the filiform papillae of the dorsal surface
7. Varicosities of the ventral surface of the tongue and of the lips
8. Tori of the palate and mandible
9. Regressive alterations in the enamel of the teeth, that is attrition, erosion, and abrasion
10. Calcification and obliteration of the pulp chambers and root canals
11. Recession of the gingivae and diminution of the periodontal support of the teeth

REGIONAL EXAMINATION OF THE MOUTH

The physician's evaluation and diagnostic workup will be inadequate if it fails to include a regional examination of the mouth and surrounding tissues. Tunnel vision, that is, bypassing the mouth and looking only at the throat, is poor preventive medicine, for the mouth of the compromised elderly patient is a common site of pathologic conditions. It will take but a few extra minutes to perform a systematic regional assessment in the following sequence:

1. The face should first be examined, both anteriorly and from the side, observing for asymmetry, pigmentations, masses, ulcers, and inflammatory lesions or lacerations, describing the location, size, and depth of deviations. Be particularly alert for lesions, such as basal cell carcinomas, which frequently occur in areas adjoining the mouth (Fig. 23-4).
2. Palpate the cervical chain of lymph nodes, starting with the posterior cervical region through the submandibular, sublingual, and anterior cervical areas.
3. Palpate the submandibular duct with the index fingers of both hands.
4. Compress the lips gently to palpate for masses and observe for normal and abnormal changes.
5. Proceed to the teeth, noting the presence of decay or loose teeth.
6. Examine the buccal mucosa, observing for color, masses, or inflammatory lesions. Note particularly the patency of ducts by gently milking the parotid gland (Stensen's duct) and the submandibular gland (Wharton's duct).
7. Examine the tongue, both the ventral and

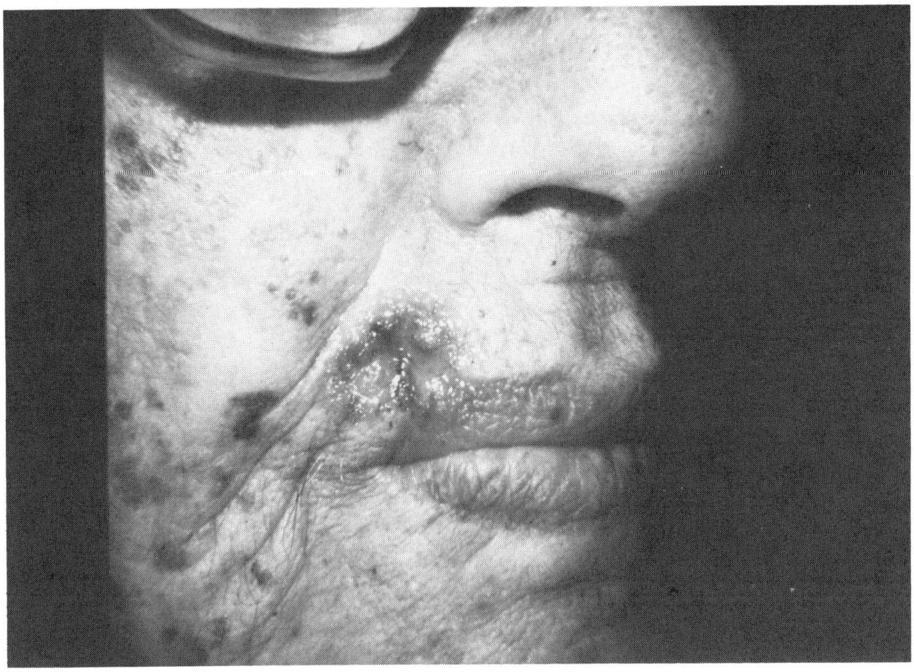

Fig. 23-4. Basal cell carcinoma.

dorsal aspects. The normal diminution of foliate papillae results in a smooth appearing, depapillated dorsal surface. The circumvallate papillae, a V-shaped chain in the rear of the tongue, may appear hypertrophied and are sometimes the cause of cancerphobia, which should be allayed. This is also a good occasion to question the patient as to any alterations in taste, an area of evaluation that is often ignored. Varices are a normal finding on the ventral surface.

8. Grasp the tongue with a 2-inch × 2-inch gauze pad and carefully examine the lateral borders, the base, and the floor of the mouth.
9. In the edentulous patient, examine the alveolar ridges, palpating for any unusual lumps and bumps.
10. Examine the palate. The torus palatinus is seen in a small percentage of elderly patients, both with natural dentition or edentulous, and should be considered within normal limits.

If the patient is wearing dentures, the regional examination should be concluded with an examination of artificial replacements. The physician should inquire as to the patient's comfort and should emphasize at this point the importance of frequent examination by the dentist.

DENTURES

A denture is a removable prosthetic appliance replacing missing teeth. Used in the completely edentulous maxilla or mandible, it is called a full or complete removable denture. Where there are some remaining teeth a partial denture usually consists of a metal framework with clasps and an acrylic base in which the teeth are secured.

Although approximately 50% of those over 65 years of age in the United States are completely edentulous, not all those who are so affected wear dentures; indeed, many of the elderly who have prostheses are unable to wear them. As with any prosthetic replacement the ability of the patient to adapt to these devices is as important as the technical construction, perhaps more so. The physician may be the recipient of complaints from patients who are new denture wearers and should encourage these patients to practice patience and forbearance and above all cooperation with the dentist. This reinforcement can be of invaluable assistance to both patient and dentist in the critical "breaking in" period.

There is a common misconception among elderly denture wearers that once they are edentulous and have had dentures inserted they no longer need periodic dental exminations. Statistically, 8% of such patients will visit the dentist only once in 5 years, whereas 70% will visit a physician at least once a year. Perhaps one reason for this is that medicare reimburses the medical patient but has few or no dental benefits. Nevertheless, because of changes in the oral mucosa with aging these tissues become more vulnerable to deteriorating processes, with resultant pathologic effects. The most common denture induced lesions are denture sores (decubitus ulcers), denture stomatitis, papillary hyperplasia of the palate, and epulis fissuratum, which will be described subsequently.

ORAL PROBLEMS OF THE OLDER PATIENT

Pathologic conditions of the hard and soft tissues of the mouth occur with greater frequency but not exclusively in aging individuals. There is scarcely a pathologic condition, with the possible exception of iatrogenic lesions resulting from dentures, that may not be observed in the young as well as the old. It is somewhat ironic that patients who develop oral lessions will often consult the physician, who is generally ill-trained in this area, rather than the dentist. The internist and family doctor, therefore, should learn to recognize common oral problems of the geriatric patient, such as the following (not necessarily described in order of incidence or prevalence).

Pathologic conditions of the hard structures

The chief disorder affecting the teeth has earned the ignominious eponym of senile caries. This may be defined as decalcification, or decay, affecting the tooth at the cervical area, that is, at the junction of the crown of the tooth and the gingival epithelium. This type of decay differs from that found in children and adults in several respects. In the younger age group decay occurs primarily in the occlusal and interproximal aspects of the tooth surface. Recent studies indicate that the bacterial spectrum implicated in coronal caries consists of gram-positive cocci, whereas the predominant flora in cervical caries is *Actinomyces* viscosus, an anaerobic filamentous organism.[3] The chief etiologic factors in cervical caries in the aged are probably the qualitative and quantitative changes in the composition of saliva that predispose the tooth to a thick mucinous plaque with a high cariogenic potential. Complicating this process is the soft, easy-to-chew diet which older people resort to because of compromised dentition and which is generally high in refined carbohydrates. Add to these factors gingival recession, which is both physiologic and pathologic, and the lack of dexterity required for good oral hygiene and the end result is a vicious cycle depicted in the following schema of cervical caries and periodontal disease.

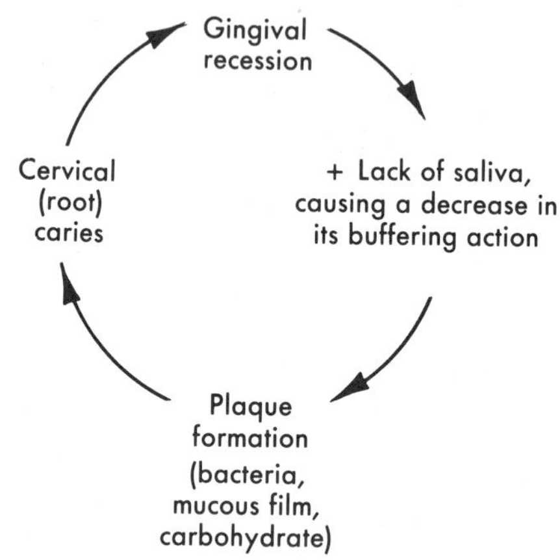

When the physician performs a regional examination and observes caries he should refer the patient to the dentist for the treatment of such lesions. Neglected decay may otherwise progress at a rapid rate, invade the pulp, and lead to abscess formation. In the patient who suffers from cardiac disease or who is otherwise debilitated, this may be a significant focus of infection and can have serious consequences. Unfortunately, by the time the infection becomes acute and the patient is referred to the dentist much damage may have already been done. Good preventive medicine requires an assessment of the dentitional status as part of the diagnostic work-up.[4]

Caries. The loss of teeth through decay, once considered inevitable in the course of aging, can now be prevented with modern dental care. "A clean tooth never decays" may be a slight exaggeration but is nevertheless fundamentally true. The physician can be an influential reinforcer of the dentist's instructions to brush and floss, the two mechanical methods that remain the mainstay of preventive dentistry. If the patient suffers limitation of functions because of stroke, arthritic disorders, or other physically disabling conditions, the dentist may recommend a battery operated toothbrush or various adjuncts in manipulating the conventionl toothbrush.

Since it has been established that senile caries have an unequivocal cause-effect relationship with salivary function, an artificial saliva that ameliorates the xerostomic effects of physiologic aging and of the drugs commonly used by the elderly has recently been developed.[5] This is now commercially available over the counter as Xerolube; it is claimed to palliate the discomfort of dry mucosa and to remineralize decalicified enamel. It should be noted that this solution contains a significant amount of sodium, and patients on a sodium-free regimen should be cautioned to expectorate after rinsing.

Another method of prevention is the use of a toothbrush dipped in 3% hydrogen peroxide and covered with a stabilized water-free 0.4% stannous fluoride gel[6] with instructions to use as a dentifrice and to swish it over the teeth.

There are many other oral hygiene devices on the market, and the physician is advised to refer inquiries as to their efficacy to the dentist.

Although it has not yet been clearly established that decay or periodontal disease is a consequence of the decline in immune function accompanying aging, one may hypothesize that a decrease in immunocompetency favors the proliferation of bacterial agents in the plaque, which is a prerequisite of these diseases. It remains to be shown whether or not the increased incidence of these disorders is caused by a decline in immune function.

Periodontal disease. The basic cause of periodontal disease (pyorrhea) is the presence of plaque and calculus. These result in gingival inflammation, recession of the gums, pocket formation, and the loss of the bony support of the teeth. Estimates of the incidence of periodontal disease in the over-65 age group range as high as 90%, and there is no doubt that it is the most important cause of the loss of teeth. This disease is often an insidious process beginning in middle age and is accelerated by systemic disorders, such as diabetes, osteoporosis, and metabolic deficiencies. The same etiologic factors for decay such as limited manual dexterity, poor oral hygiene, and malnutrition are also involved in periodontal disease. The most important health measure to reduce the level of periodontitis is the preventive removal of food plaque and calculus. For the patient with stroke, arthritic disorders, and other conditions resulting in limited range of motions, the dentist can suggest modifications in toothbrushes and other oral hygiene adjuncts.

Pathologic conditions of the soft tissues

Without engaging in an exhaustive taxonomy of lesions of the oral mucosa, we shall limit this section to the most common problems seen in the elderly.

Denture ulcer. This is probably the most common lesion seen in the mouth of the edentulous, denture wearing patient. It appears as a circumscribed inflammatory lesion of varing size with a central ulceration surrounded by raised borders and upon careful examination is found to be contiguous with the border of the denture (Fig. 23-5). If this is overextended, it will create a pressure atrophy of the soft tissues akin to the decubitus ulcers found in other areas of the body. It can be quite painful but will usually disappear within a short time after the denture is adjusted. If it persists it should be differentiated from aphthous ulcers, neoplasms, and other lesions, which sometimes require histologic evaluation. The neglected denture ulcer may hypertrophy and form a redundant mass of epithelial tissue called the epulis *fissuratum*.

Denture stomatitis and papillary hyperplasia. Denture stomatitis, or denture sore mouth, is a generalized, inflammatory area of tisue (Fig. 23-6) usually overlying the hard palate. The gross appearance is granular, differentiating it from the warty, sometimes pebbly surface in papillary hyperplasia. In either case these must be viewed as reactive inflammatory lesions that are almost always associated with poor cleaning of the dentures or ill-fitting dentures. Both denture stomatitis and papillary palatal hyperplasia may be considered benign, but as the patient becomes more prone to debilitating disease, concomitant with diminished immunocompetence, bacterial and fungal invasion are encouraged and may result in candidiasis.

Angular cheilosis. The terms *cheilosis*, *cheilitis*, and *perleche* have been used interchange-

A

B

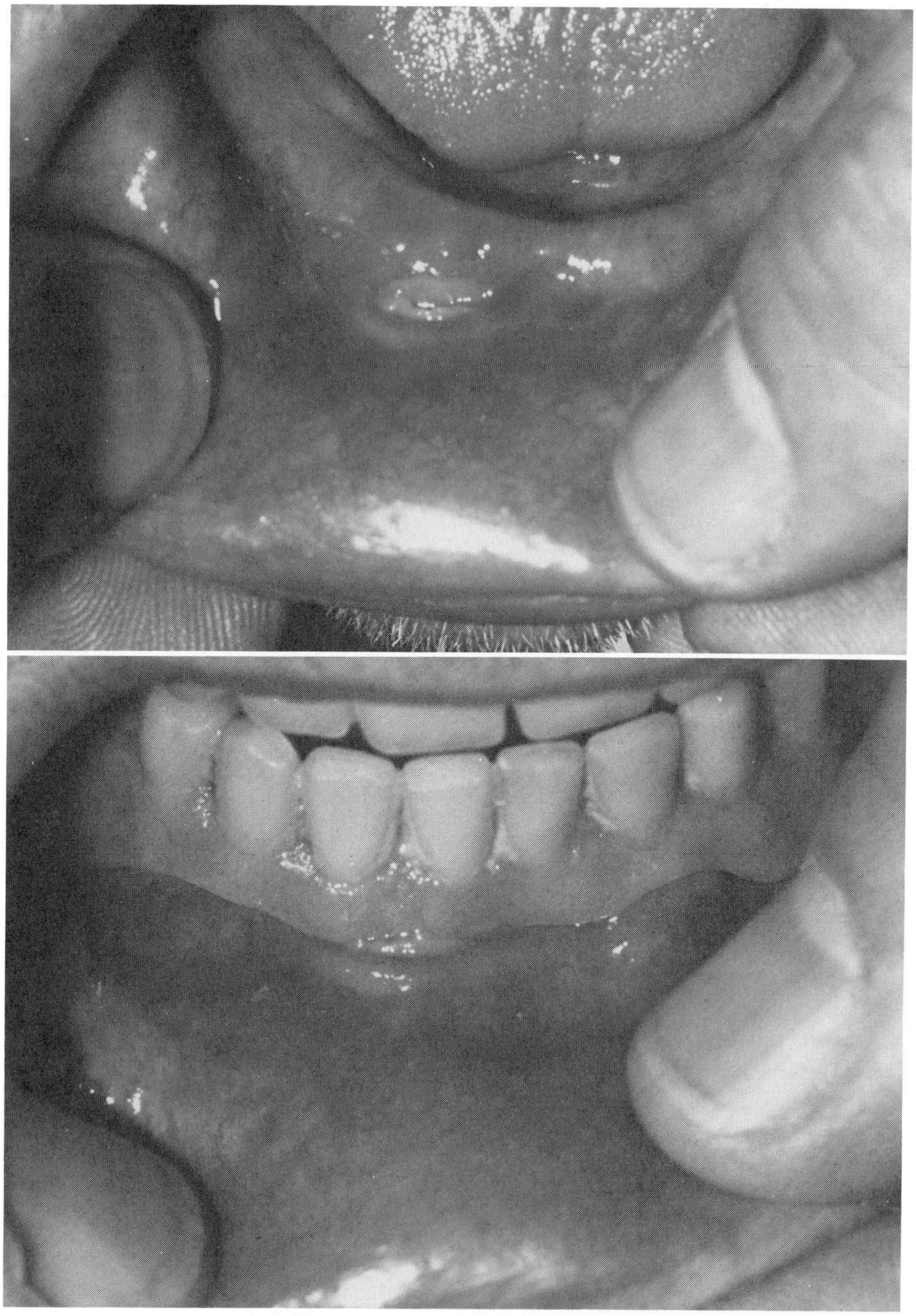

Fig. 23-5. A, Denture ulcer on alveolar ridge. **B,** Note contiguous border of the denture in the same patient.

ably to describe an inflammatory fissuring and maceration at the commissure of the lips. It may be unilateral or bilateral and has been attributed to the following three factors: (1) The overclosure of the jaws as previously described; (2) riboflavin deficiency; and (3) xerostomia. This combination of events favors the growth of *candida albicans*, a natural inhabitant of the oral ecology that combines with other organisms to generate a secondary infection. Treatment consists of prosthetic rehabilitation, dietary management with vitamin B complex, and the use

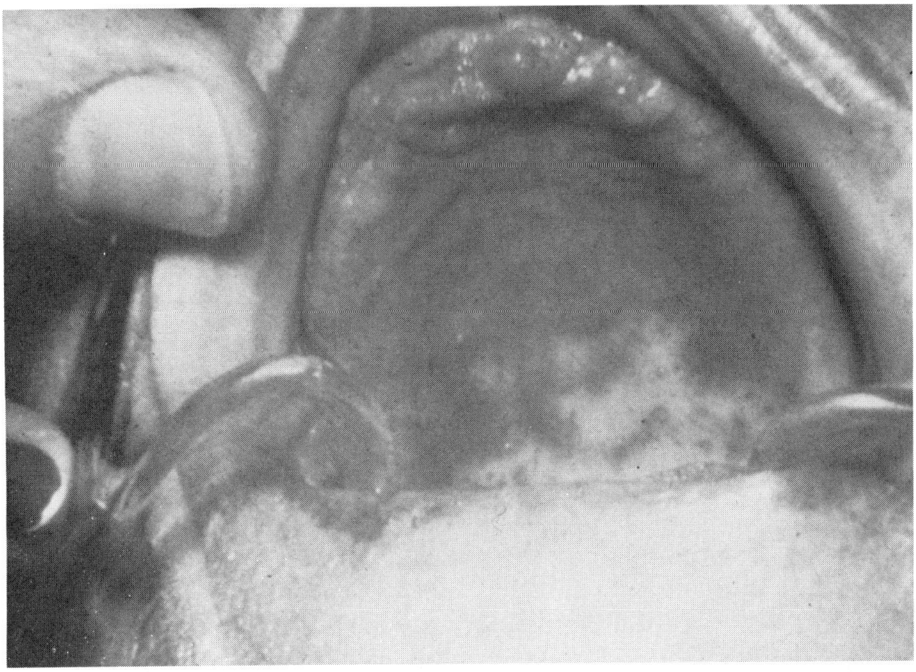

Fig. 23-6. Denture stomatitis. This 71-year-old female patient has been wearing a denture for 23 years and refuses to take it out at night.

of an antibacterial antifungal ointment such as nystatin-neomycin-triamcinalone acetonide (Mycolog).

Geographic tongue. The older patient is often subject to cancerphobias and may suddenly become aware of a long-standing condition-known as geographic tongue. The typical appearance of this benign anomaly is that of multiple areas of atrophied filiform papillae surrounded by raised yellowish-white borders. Geographic tongue should be differentiated from benign migratory glossitis (erythema migrans), which also demonstrates depapillated areas but without the definitive borders and which is more often symptomatic. Geographic tongue may arise from childhood on; it wanes and recurs and changes its shape from time to time. It is considered entirely benign and does not require therapeutic intervention.

Candidiasis (moniliasis). As has been stated previously, *Candida albicans* is a normal component of the oral flora but rarely manifests itself in pathologic form in the healthy older patient. In the presence of cachexia, malnutrition, and lowered resistance to infection, however, the monilial organisms predominate. Other factors favoring growth of the fungus are long-term antibiotic therapy, diabetes, corticosteroid therapy, and cancer chemotherapy.

Candida rapidly colonizes and forms a white, cheesy coating over erythematous, epithelial areas, sometimes covering broad surfaces of the oral mucosa, including the palate, tongue, and buccal surfaces. The presumptive diagnosis is made when the superficial white, curdlike deposit is removed with a cotton swab or gauze, revealing the inflamed underlying tissues. Microscopic examination demonstrating the elongated hyphae of the fungal organism confirms the diagnosis but is not always necessary. It is preferable to begin an antifungal regimen, such as nystatin (Mycostatin) oral suspension (100,000 units/ml) with instructions to swish 2 ml of the medication over the tissues every 4 hours for 2 minutes and then swallow. Treatment should be continued for at least 2 weeks and may sometimes require 4 to 6 weeks or longer for tenacious infections.[7]

Candida albicans is the dominant organism in two inflammatory conditions resulting from ill-fitting dentures or poor cleaning of dentures, denture stomatitis, and papillary hyperplasia, which have been previously described.

Lichen planus. Recent studies implicate this dermatologic lesion of the oral mucosa as a frequent concomitant of diabetes mellitus in older patients. The chief forms of this fungal disorder in the mouth are a classic type consisting of lace-like white lines (Wickham's striae) in an annular pattern on the buccal mucosa and an erosive form that is more inflammatory in appearance and can occur on the tongue, lips, palate, gingiva, buccal surfaces, and floor of the mouth. We also recognize other lesions that may be lichenoid, but must be differentiated from lichen planus per se. When the oral manifestations are a component of a severe dermatologic attack affecting other areas of the body, the institution of steroid therapy combined with antibiotics may be indicated.

Burning mouth syndrome. This is a phenomenon that occurs primarily but not exclusively in postmenopausal women, the cause of which includes a combination of organic and psychogenic factors. The chief complaint is pain, ranging from mild discomfort to a truly burning sensation. Estrogen imbalance, xerostomia, iron deficiency, and malnutrition may all be involved, and the locus may be generalized throughout the mouth or more usually confined to the tongue. In the latter case, glossitis (inflammation of the tongue), glossodynia (painful tongue), or glossopyrosis (burning tongue) may be involved. It is not uncommon for this condition to arise concomitantly with depression, and the clinician should tactfully inquire into emotional factors that may be contributory. Vitamin deficiency, particularly of the vitamin B complex may be suspected, either as a causal factor or as a consequence of malnutrition resulting from the inability to take adequate sustenance. Iron deficiency anemia, pernicious anemia, Sjögren's syndrome, Mikulicz's disease, and Plummer-Vinson syndrome should be ruled out in the differential diagnosis. Dryness of the oral mucous membranes (xerostomia) may be associated with the burning mouth syndrome and may be verified by the observation of absent or scant salivation.

Treatment of burning mouth syndrome remains one of the baffling challenges to the dentist and oral pathologist. A history of xerostomic drugs, such as antihistamines, tranquilizers, and atropine-like compounds, dictates that such medications be discontinued if at all possible and substitute therapy sought. Treatment with estrogens and vasodilators such as nicotinic acid may be instituted, although these drugs have their own serious side effects. Saliva stimulants, such as citric fruit drops, lemon swabs, and even sialagogues, are rarely successful. Palliative relief may be temporarily obtained by the use of demulcent agents such as 10% glycerin in distilled water with instructions to swish and expectorate. More positive results have been reported with the use of an artificial saliva (Xerolube), which was developed by Dr. Ira Shannon, a dental researcher with the Veterans Administration. This is an over-the-counter item that is dispensed in a flip top bottle, with directions to squeeze a few drops into the mouth, swish, and swallow or expectorate. Since there is a significant sodium content in the solution, it is advisable to have the patient who is on a sodium-free diet expectorate after application.

Despite all of these efforts this painful condition may persist, and in some cases psychiatric counseling may be indicated. I know of one such case in which electroconvulsive therapy was employed as a final resort but only provided transient relief.

Oral cancer. The physician should be aware that approximately 26,000 cases of oral cancer occur each year with 8000 reported fatalities. More than 90% occur in persons over age 45, with the average age being 60. Unfortunately, most oral cancer is painless in the early stages when it is highly curable, but by the time it metastasizes to the cervical lymph nodes of the neck the prognosis is, at best, dubious. Because oral cancers are usually visible and accessible, the alert physician, as well as the dentist, is in a position to make an early diagnosis by cytologic investigation or biopsy.[8]

Most oral cancers are of the squamous cell type, with the following sites of occurrence:

Tongue, 52%
Floor of the mouth, 16%
Alveolar mucosa, 12%
Palate, 11%
Buccal mucosa, 9%

As has been stated, the first sign of oral cancer may be the appearance of a lump in the neck. If the lesion is located in the posterior aspect of the tongue or in the pharyngeal region, the patient may complain of earache. This may be followed by dysphagia, dysphasia, and difficulty in chewing as the lesion progresses. A history of excessive smoking and drinking is frequently elicited. Early changes in the mucous membranes may appear as white lesions—leukoplakia—but the propensity of these for malignancy remains somewhat controversial. On the other hand, erythroplakia—red plaques or patches of ulceration—are more indicative of malignancy. The presence of ulcers, masses, and pigmented areas calls for palpation to detect induration and infiltration of adjacent tissues. Squamous cell carcinomas may appear as an exophytic mass or may rapidly become invasive as endophytic neoplasms involving nerves, periosteum, bone, and blood vessels. The endophytic ulcerating lesion metastasizes to the regional lymph nodes of the neck, worsening the prognosis, and usually requires hemimandibulectomy and radical neck dissection followed by radiation therapy. Although the patient may survive for several years, the quality of life is adversely affected.

Adenocarcinomas are cancers of the minor salivary glands and include several histologic types, such as adenoid cystic carcinomas, mucoepidermoid carcinomas, and malignant mixed tumors. The junction of the hard and soft palate is a frequent site of this neoplasm. On palpation the tumor may feel firm or fluctuant and be covered by intact mucous membrane. It is painless and slow growing but gradually invades adjacent hard and soft tissues, sometimes extending into the maxillary sinus. Treatment of adenocarcinomas of the salivary gland type consists of surgical excision followed by adjuvant radiation therapy to prevent recurrence.

Kaposi's sarcoma (multiple idiopathic hemorrhagic sarcoma) is a slow growing but widespread neoplasm most common after the fifth decade of life. Its characteristic appearance is that of bluish nodules of the skin with hemorrhages somewhat resembling hemangiomas. Organs that may be simultaneously affected include the colon, the breasts, the prostate gland, the tongue, tonsils, the palate, and the pancreas. Radiation therapy is the method of choice.

Benign oral tumors and tumorlike conditions should be differentiated from malignancies. Of these benign lesions the most common are the mucocele, a bluish retention cyst located most often on the lower lip or the floor of the mouth; papillomas, which are benign epithelial projections; fibromas—lesions sometimes seen as a result of biting on the buccal mucosa; hemangiomas; and lymphangiomas.

The management of oral cancer is truly interdisciplinary and should ideally be guided by a team of head and neck specialists. The physician is advised to refer patients with suspected neoplasms to a competent oral pathologist for evaluation and histologic examination. Regional head and neck tumor centers are now more readily available, and the oral pathologist will usually refer the patient to the team conference. The ideal head and neck team of specialists consists of one or more oral pathologists, oral surgeons, prosthodontists, plastic surgeons, general surgeons, head and neck surgeons, psychiatrists, internists, radiologists, nurses, and social workers. The decisions such a team will make require ethical, moral, and psychosocial considerations as well as the technologic aspects of surgery and rehabilitation.

MEDICAL-DENTAL INTERACTIONS

There is scarcely an adverse effect of aging that is not reflected in some manner in the mouth and its adnexae. Here we shall elaborate on the most frequent situations in the experience of the dental service of a rehabilitation-oriented skilled nursing facility that consistently required consultations with the medical staff.

Patients with cardiac deficits

The greatest danger in the dental treatment of patients with a wide range of congenital or acquired heart disease is the possibility of bacterial endocarditis as a consequence of dental manipulations. This includes seemingly innocuous procedures, such as filling or cleaning teeth, as well as surgical operations. It may be true that only a small incidence of subacute bacterial endocarditis (SBE) in such patients has been reported following dental treatment, but for those affected the morbidity can be quite significant. Sufficient experience has been amassed to heed the advice and guidelines of the American Heart Association, as delineated in the July, 1977, issue of the Journal of the American Dental Association,[9] as follows*:

Regimen A. For most congenital heart disease (ventricular septal defect [VSD], tetralogy of Fallot,

*Bacterial endocarditis. A committee report of the American Heart Association, J. Am. Dent. Assoc. **95**:600, 1977.

aortic stenosis, pulmonic stenosis, complex cyanotic heart disease, patent ductus arteriosus, or systemic to pulmonary shunts), rheumatic or other acquired valvular heart disease, idiopathic hypertrophic subaortic stenosis, mitral valve prolapse syndrome with mitral insufficiency, the following may be used:

Penicillin

1. Parenteral-oral combined: Adults—aqueous crystalline penicillin G (1,000,000 units intramuscularly) mixed with procaine penicillin G (600,000 units intramuscularly). Administer 30 minutes to 1 hour before the procedure and then administer penicillin V, 500 mg orally every 6 hours for eight doses.
2. Oral: Adults—penicillin V (2 gm orally) 30 minutes to 1 hour before the procedure and then 500 mg orally every 6 hours for 8 doses.

FOR PATIENTS ALLERGIC TO PENICILLIN:

Use either vancomycin (see regimen B) or use: Adults—erythromycin (1 gm orally) 1½ to 2 hours before the procedure and then 500 mg orally every 6 hours for 8 doses.

Regimen B. For high risk patients such as those with prosthetic heart valves who require extensive dental procedures, especially extractions or periodontal surgery:

Penicillin plus streptomycin

Adults—Aqueous crystalline penicillin G (1,000,000 units intramuscularly) mixed with procaine penicillin G (600,000 units intramuscularly), plus streptomycin (1 gm intramuscularly). Administer 30 minutes to 1 hour before the procedure, then penicillin V 500 mg orally every 6 hours for eight doses.

FOR PATIENTS ALLERGIC TO PENICILLIN:

Adults—vancomycin (1 gm intravenously over 30 minutes to 1 hour). Start initial vancomycin infusion 30 minutes to 1 hour before the procedure followed by erythromycin 500 mg orally every 6 hours for eight doses.

In occasional patients receiving continuous oral penicillin for secondary prevention of rheumatic fever, alpha hemolytic streptococci, which are relatively resistant to penicillin, may be found in the oral cavity. In such patients, it is advisable to switch to the oral erythromycin protocol as outlined for the penicillin-allergic patient. In addition, the clinician should be aware that erythromycin-resistant streptococci have been reported.

I would be remiss if I did not emphasize the fact that too often the physician only becomes aware of dental disease when it threatens the patient after cardiac revascularization. The cardiologist should insist that the patient have good dental attention—it makes no sense to have the patient give up smoking and then let the patient walk around like a time bomb with dental infections that can be lethal catalytic agents.

Another question that frequently arises between dentist and physician is the use of local anesthetic agents with epinephrine. In most cases of heart disease or hypertension the use of epinephrine is not contraindicated, but the dentist should consult the patient's physician on this point.

Patients with cerebral vascular accident (CVA)

A severe cerebral vascular accident resulting in hemiparesis will in many cases demonstrate profound effects on the mouth of the patient. The most obvious manifestations are deficits in deglutition and speech, in both of which dentition plays an important role. In the denture wearing patient, the neuromuscular imbalance may seriously impair the function of the prostheses and diminish their usefulness. Nutritional intake, so important in the rehabilitation process, will require modification because of inadequate masticatory performance. Loss of the swallowing reflex may result in the pooling of saliva and drooling, with subsequent angular cheilosis at the commissure of the lips.

Even as the patient makes a gradual recovery, it will be noted that stroke frequently has adverse effects on oral hygiene, particularly on the affected side of the body. This results primarily from reduced efficiency of the natural detergent mechanism, in which the orobuccal musculature and the tongue both play important roles. The observant clinician will discover that there is usually an increase in plaque, debris, and tartar on the affected side, sometimes exacerbated by the inability of the patient to perform manual procedures of oral hygiene.

When the dentist calls on the physician for advice on the management of the patient with stroke the following factors should be considered:

1. The dentist should be informed if the patient is receiving anticoagulant therapy. If oral surgery is planned, it will be necessary to monitor hemostasis before such treatment is begun.
2. The dentist should be advised to minimize stress, for example, short appointments, use of tranquilizers, etc.

3. The dentist should be cautioned against the use of drugs, such as meperidine (Demerol), which may be contraindicated in conditions apt to be accompanied by increased cerebral spinal fluid pressure.
4. The dentist should be advised to employ maximum evacuation of fluids and solids to avoid aspiration in the presence of dysphagia.

There is a tendency among many dentists, on eliciting a history of anticoagulant therapy, to request the patient's physician to interrupt therapy before dental surgery. Without entering into the complexities of the coagulation process, we now know that it is not necessary to place all patients at high risk for thrombus formation; indeed it is poor practice to do so. The wise dentist will ask the physician to monitor hemostasis by checking prothrombin (PT) time 2 or 3 days before dental surgery. If the PT time equals or is less than 1½ times the normal, routine oral surgery may be performed, followed by suturing, and, if necessary, the application of a clotting agent such as absorbable gelatin sponge (Gelfoam) or the use of a thrombin saturated pad.

Patients undergoing radiation therapy

Radiation therapy can result in xerostomia and rampant cervical caries. The physician should always consult with the dentist before initiating radiation therapy to the head and neck. The dentist will recommend a daily regimen of topical fluorides and the removal of all mobile and infected teeth before therapy; otherwise, osteomyelitis and subsequent sloughing of alveolar bone may occur.

In patients scheduled for oral surgery who have already received head and neck irradiation, the following protocol should be used:

1. Administer preoperative penicillin (regimen A) the morning of surgery, followed by 4 days of postoperative antibiotic therapy.
2. Advise the dentist to limit the number of extractions to two or three teeth at a time.
3. Attempt primary closure if possible; employ chromic sutures if necessary.

Patients with diabetes

The most common question arising in dental treatment for the diabetic patient is whether to employ antimicrobial prophylaxis. It will be noted that the diet controlled adult diabetic can be treated without the use of antibiotics. Nevertheless, if an extensive surgical procedure is planned, antibiotic prophylaxis should be prescribed both preoperatively and postoperatively. The insulin dependent diabetic should be advised to eat a normal breakfast and take the customary dose of insulin before the dental visit. If the patient is advised not to have breakfast, for example, if a general anesthetic is planned, the patient should take one fourth to one half the normal dose of insulin. For the brittle diabetic, antibiotic prophylaxis is essential.

All diabetic patients should be referred to the dentist for continued, consistent observation. Dental infections such as gingivitis, periodontitis, and acute alveolar abscesses may cause a detectable elevation in blood sugar. Reciprocally, the diabetic state may also cause an exacerbation of periodontal disease leading to loss of teeth.

Patients with Parkinson's disorder

Oral manifestations in Parkinson's disorder include bruxism, dysphagia, dysphasia, drooling, and impaired masticatory efficiency. The masked facies so often accompanying the neuromuscular deficits should be noted in the regional evaluation.

The dental implications in Parkinson's disorder are profound, and the subsequent impaired functions of the dentition seriously aggravate the quality of life.[10] The physician may be called on to advise the dentist in the following areas:

1. Inform the dentist of extrapyramidal side effects of Parkinson's disorder—dyskinesia, xerostomia, etc.
2. If indicated advise against the use of epinephrine in local anesthetics, which may result in a stress reaction. Suggest the use of appropriate sedative/tranquilizing agents to minimize stress.
3. Advise the dentist to employ adequate suctioning to avoid aspiration of water and/or solids in the course of treatment.

Patients with Paget's disease (osteitis deformans)

This is an osseous disorder of unknown causes characterized by generalized skeletal deformities. The process by which this condition progresses involves recurrent episodes of osteoclastic activity resulting in sclerotic reossification.[11] These stages are readily observed in the skull plate as areas of osteolysis and condensation resulting in the typical "cotton wool" appearance.

The incidence of Paget's disease increases with age, ranging from 3% of persons over 40 years of age to as much as 10% in nonagenarians.[12]

Since most cases of Paget's disease are asymptomatic, suspicion may first be aroused by oral manifestations occurring early in the disorder in the jaws and skull.[13] These include a sudden flaring of the teeth, particularly in the maxilla, because of the flattening and widening of the palatal bones, sometimes accompanied by enlargement of one or both maxillary ridges. The edentulous patient's dentures will rapidly become ill-fitting as the disease progresses, requiring frequent reconstruction. The prosthodontist will observe the development of a prognathic occlusal relationship in most cases as the patient assumes an acromegalic appearance.

Periapical radiographs reveal pulpal calcifications, generalized hypercementosis, loss of lamina dura, blunting of root apices, and a stepladder effect of the body trabeculae.

Additional symptoms that may appear as the bony sclerosis impinges on associated nerves include atypical facial neuralgias, deafness, blindness, facial paralysis, dizziness, and emotional instability. These findings warrant the ordering of blood tests, in which normal calcium and phosphorus levels and elevated serum alkaline phosphatase may be expected.

The dentist should advise the patient that dentures may require modification or reconstruction. Because the bones become excessively vascular, precautions to minimize bleeding and infection should be taken in the event of oral surgery.

The current treatment for Paget's disease involves some medications that may interact with dental procedures. Patients receiving long-range aspirin therapy may develop platelet deficiencies resulting in a tendency to hemorrhage after prophylaxis or oral surgery. If the patient is receiving corticosteroids to suppress inflammation, one may expect immunoincompetence and the necessity for precautionary measures after invasive dental procedures. Delayed healing may well be a consequence in such patients.

Patients with iatrogenic oral manifestations

The pharmacodynamics of drugs for the elderly has been described elsewhere in this text (see Chapter 15). Because of increased vulnerability with aging, the mouth may be the site of adverse drug effects reflected both in the dentition and oral mucosa. These reactions are not necessarily confined to the oral cavity and usually involve many different organs and tissues. In addition to adverse effects there are other predictable side effects that accompany certain therapeutic agents, for example, xerostomia. The physician is advised to include a copy of *Accepted Dental Therapeutics* in his library.[14]

DEGENERATIVE JOINT DISEASE (DJD)—OSTEOARTHRITIS, OSTEOARTHROSIS

The pathogenic mechanism of DJD is not primarily inflammatory in nature and consists of a fragmentation and splitting of articular cartilage in the involved joints. Among predisposing factors for DJD are age, trauma, and wear, tear and possibly genetic factors.[15]

When DJD involves the TMJ, the effects are usually unilateral and include joint pain, stiffness after rest, limitation of motion, and deviation to the affected side on opening the mouth. The patient may complain of earache and/or painful muscle spasm. Crepitation may be demonstrated on auscultation.[16]

Radiographs may disclose osteophytic spurs, subarticular cysts, or pseudocysts resulting from cortical erosion of the condyle and sometimes osteosclerosis of the condyle. Since a definitive diagnosis is dependent on radiographic findings, it may be necessary to substantiate the disorder with tomograms.

Treatment of DJD entails judicious use of analgesic and anti-inflammatory agents. Aspirin remains the drug of choice unless and until gastrointestinal side effects are noted,[17] in which case one of the proprionic acid derivatives, for example, ibuprofen or naproxen, may be employed. Indomethacin is an effective drug, but one must be aware of its side effects—nausea, gastrointestinal bleeding, or headache. In the same family of drugs is a relatively new compound, tolmetin, also more potent than the propionic acid derivatives and with fewer side effects than indomethacin. Another effective an-

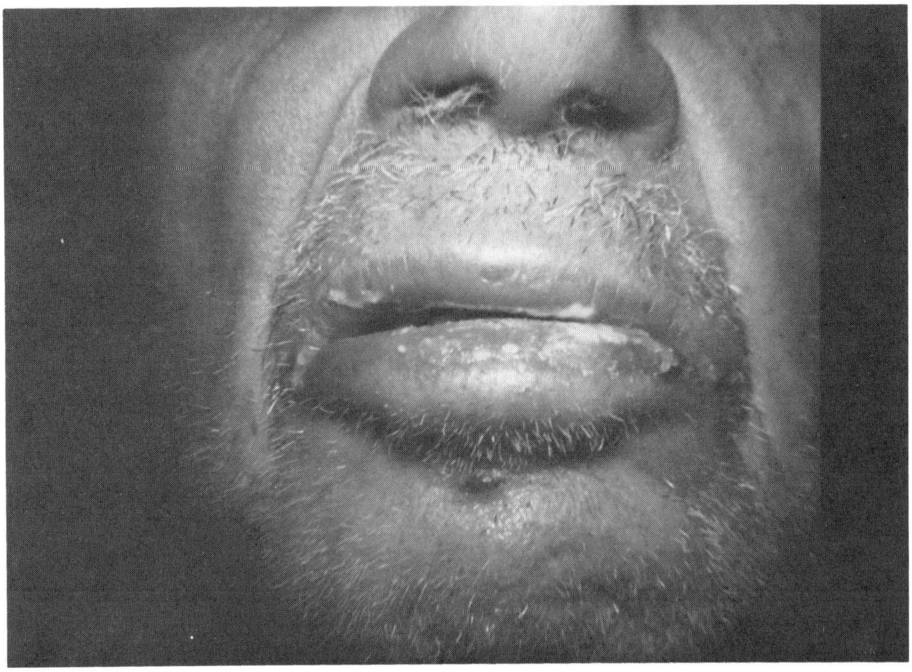

Fig. 23-7. Urticarial reaction on lips of a patient receiving antigout medication.

tiarthritic drug is phenylbutazone, but it has to be carefully monitored, for, in addition to gastrointestinal complications, cases of bone marrow failure and cardiac complications have been reported. If the above regimen proves ineffective, intraarticular injections of steroids may be used but should be limited to three or four per year.[18] Physical therapy, including range of motion exercises, may be prescribed. In cases of severe synovitis the use of a bite-opening removable appliance such as a Hawley-type retainer or Omnivac mouthguard may be of some value. Finally, although condylectomy has been resorted to in the younger patient, it is certainly too heroic and controversial for geriatric patients and is contraindicated.

Psoriatic arthritis

TMJ involvement in psoriatic arthritis has been described by Franks.[19] The dermatologic lesions are scaly and erythematous and may be observed as psoriasiform areas on the tongue. When these lesions are located in the periauricular area or on the scalp, TMJ function may be affected in varying degrees with unilateral, episodic pain, and limitation of motion. Spontaneous exacerbations and remissions coincide with the course of the skin manifestations.

TMJ symptoms are relatively mild and can usually be managed with physical therapy and nonsteroidal antiinflammatory medications.

Gout

TMJ involvement in gout is rare but has been reported in at least one article.[20] This author has seen one indirect oral manifestation, this being a severe urticarial reaction to allopurinol involving the mouth, adjacent tissues, and extremities (Fig. 23-7).

The diagnosis of myofacial pain disorder (MPD) syndrome involves an assessment of multiple subjective and objective factors. History, radiography, tomograms, and careful regional examinations are essential. When the patient's history and evaluation demonstrate rheumatic disease, its potential effect on the TMJ must be weighed, interdisciplinary consultation sought, and appropriate treatment rendered.

DIET AND DENTITION

In January 1977, a report of the Senate Select Committee on Nutrition and Human Needs noted that 6 out of the 10 leading causes of death in the United States are linked to diet (cardiac disorders, stroke, arteriosclerosis, cancer, cirrhosis of the liver, and diabetes), that is, 50% of all deaths. Perhaps one reason that the elderly are prone to malnutrition is that it is easier to consume and masticate nonnutritious foods excessively high in salt, sugar, fat, and cholesterol. The elderly, and especially the poor elderly, may subsist on pulverized meat high in fat content, refined carbohydrates, processed fruits and vegetables, and even commercial baby foods when they suffer the loss of masticatory efficiency. Nutritional counseling that ignores the level of masticatory performance may therefore fall on deaf ears and empty mouths. In 1976 bananas were the favorite form of fresh fruit (36% of the fresh fruit market) and probably constitute the favorite snack of the edentulous elderly. Soft drinks, calorie-filled and nutrient-empty, are cheaper and more available than milk, so that between 1960 and 1976 Americans as a whole cut back on their combined whole and skim milk consumption by about 5 gallons per person, while intake of soft drinks increased by 19 gallons apiece.[21] Thus the current per capita consumption of calcium, so essential for bones and teeth, no longer meets the recommended daily dietary allowance from childhood through old age.[22]

The three main reasons for the prevalence of malnutrition in the elderly stated in the Older Americans Act of 1965 were poverty, lack of skills and knowledge in the selection and preparation of well-balanced meals, and isolation, which diminishes the incentive for cooking an attractive and nourishing meal. Perhaps we should add a fourth factor—the loss of the enjoyment of eating because of impaired denti tion.

> From the nutrition-oriented health care perspective, 100 percent of the malnutrition seen in the elderly today is secondary to disease or disability—physical, emotional, or attitudinal. Examples of this include altered metabolism accompanying disease and the inability to obtain food, prepare meals, or even feed oneself because of a physical handicap. *Other impairments to food consumption by the elderly are the absence of teeth or poorly fitting dentures*, the lack of desire to feed oneself, the "avoidance of protective foods," and the ingestion of harmful foods through habit. (italics ours)*

*From Watkins, D.A.: Nutritional needs of the elderly. In Toga, C.J., Nandy, K., and Chauncey, H.H., editors: Geriatric dentistry, Lexington, Mass., 1979, Lexington Books, p. 224.

ORAL HEALTH CARE FOR THE INSTITUTIONALIZED ELDERLY

There are now more nursing home beds than general hospital beds in the United States, about 1.5 million versus 1 million. Although only 5% of the over-65 population reside in such facilities, it is nevertheless a sobering fact that 20% to 25% of this age cohort will spend some time in long-term care units before their ultimate demise. Since the medical director is responsible for the overall supervision of health care in these institutions, he should be aware of the existing requirements for medicare certification as promulgated by regulations enacted in 1974. Under these guidelines the nursing home must conform to the following minimal standards for the oral health of its residents.

1. The operator must retain a dental advisor or consultant.
2. There must be an annual dental examination of all residents.
3. The facility must have written oral hygiene policies.
4. The operator must provide transportation for residents requiring dental care, and emergency care must be available on a 24-hour basis.

In addition to these regulations, medicaid provides dental benefits to nursing home residents in 11 states. It must be remembered that medicare has little or no dental benefits, and it is only in those states that have medicaid funding that some progress has been made in elevating the standards of oral health care in nursing homes. On the whole, however, these guidelines are observed more in the breach than in performance. Neglect of oral health, which was cited by the Senate Special Committee Hearings on Aging in 1975 as one of a litany of nursing home abuses, continues to this day and it will require major efforts on the part of government and accrediting agencies to reverse this deficiency. The conscientious medical director should consult local dental societies or the American Society for Geriatric Dentistry* for advice on establishing oral health care programs to implement existing regulations.

*The American Society for Geriatric Dentistry, 1121 W. Michigan Avenue, Indianapolis, Ind.

CONCLUSION

With the explosiveness of a Mount St. Helens the demographic pendulum is swinging toward an exponential increase in the over-65 population of the world. Belatedly, medical practice and the medical school curriculum are beginning to take note of inadequacies in the training of physicians to cope with the manifold problems of this age group. To the science of medicine the art of gerodontics—dentistry for the elderly—now adds a significant dimension for the optimal health care of the elderly. It is hoped that this chapter will make a modest contribution toward this mutually desired goal.

REFERENCES

1. Rowe, N.H.: Dental surgery. In Cowdry, E.V., and Steinberg, F.U., editors: The care of the geriatric patient, ed. 4, St. Louis, 1971, The C.V. Mosby Co., p. 302.
2. Feldman, R.S., Kapur, K.K., Alman, J.E., and Chauncey, H.H.: Aging and mastication: changes in performance and in the swallowing threshold with natural dentition, J. Am. Geriatr. Soc. **28:**97, 1980.
3. Keyes, P.H., and Jordan, H.V.: Periodontal lesions in the Syrian hamster, Arch. Oral Biol. **9:**377, 1964.
4. Buch, J., Basavaraju, N.G., Charatan, F.B., and Kamen, S.: Preventive medicine in a long term care institution, Geriatrics, **31**(2):99, 1976.
5. Shannon, I.L.: A saliva substitute for dry mouth relief, Harvard University, Veterans Administration geriatric symposium, Boston, 1977.
6. Keyes, P.: National Institute of Dental Health, Bethesda, Md. Personal communication, November 2, 1979.
7. Holroyd, S.V.: Clinical pharmacology in dental practice, ed. 2, St. Louis, 1978, The C.V. Mosby Co.
8. Baker, H.W., et al.: Oral cancer, Professional education publication, 1973, American Cancer Society, Inc. 1972.
9. Bacterial endocarditis. A committee report of the American Heart Association, J. Am. Dent. Assoc. **95:**600, 1977.
10. Kamen, S.: Tardive dyskinesia—a significant syndrome for geriatric dentistry, Oral Surg. **39**(1):52, 1975.
11. Handy, R.: The signs and treatment of Paget's disease, Geriatrics **32**(6):89, 1977.
12. Akin, R.K., et al.: Paget's disease of bone: report of case, Oral Surg. **39**(5):707, 1975.
13. Marks, J.M., and Dunkelberger, F.B.: Paget's disease, J. Am. Dent. Assoc. **101:**49, 1980.
14. Council on Dental Therapeutics: Accepted dental therapeutics, ed. 37, 1977, American Dental Association.
15. Scott, J.T., et al.: Copeman's textbook of the rheumatic diseases, ed. 5, New York, 1978, Churchill-Livingstone.
16. Marbach, J.J.: Arthritis of the temporomandibular joints, Bull. Rheum. Dis. **27**(8):918, 1977.
17. Huskisson, E.D.: Anti-inflammatory drugs, Semin. Arthritis Rheum. **7**(1):1, 1977.
18. Harrison's principles of internal medicine, ed. 9, New York, 1980, McGraw-Hill, Inc.
19. Franks, A.S.T.: The temporomandibular joint arthrosis associated with psoriasis, Oral Surg. **19:**301, 1965.
20. Kleinman, H.Z., and Ewbank, R.I.: Gout of the temporomandibular joint, Oral Surg. **27:**281, 1969.
21. Brewster, L., and Jacobson, M.F.: The changing American diet. Monograph of the Center for Science in the Public Interest, Washington, D.C., 1978.
22. Slesinger, D.P., McDivitt, M., and O'Donnell, F.M.: Food patterns in an urban population: age and sociodemographic correlates, J. Gerontol. **35**(3):432, 1980.
23. Watkins, D.A.: Nutritional needs of the elderly. In Toga, C.J., Nandy, K., and Chauncey, H.H.: Geriatric dentistry, Lexington, Mass., 1979, Lexington Books, p. 224.

CHAPTER 24 · CARE OF THE FOOT

Arthur E. Helfand

Foot problems in the elderly and the ability to remain ambulatory are major concerns in any geriatric comprehensive care program. Although the foot itself is seldom the cause of mortality, it is often the site of morbidity, disability, impairment, and limitation of activity. Many initial signs of systemic disease, the complications of systemic disease, and the residual processes of such change are often manifested in the foot. Examples of this include diabetes mellitus, peripheral arterial occlusion, and the various changes associated with musculoskeletal and metabolic diseases, such as gout, rheumatoid arthritis, and degenerative joint disease. Disuse and age are also significant factors in producing foot pain in the elderly. Repeated trauma and microtrauma, static and dynamic stresses imposed by weight bearing and foot wear, and the rigidity and atrophy associated with age additionally contribute to the development of keratotic lesions and fixed joints, which limit the ambulatory status of the patient.

The ability of an individual to remain ambulatory may be the only dividing line between institutionalization and remaining an active and viable member of a community and society. Thus not only is the foot frequently a mirror of health, but it can enhance and provide a partial means to protect some of the social needs of patients in future years.

In managing geriatric patients and their foot problems the years of neglect, abuse, and the almost total lack of foot health education and preventive measures in younger years must be considered. In addition, consideration must also be given to the functional needs of elderly patients and the adaptive measures that should be undertaken to help them maintain one of their primary goals, that of remaining ambulatory and being able to care for themselves.

Prevention should be the primary approach to providing foot care for the elderly. As part of that concern, attention must be given to some other key aspects of geriatric care. These include the fact that the average geriatric patient is usually being treated for one or more systemic diseases at any given time. He is usually taking one or more drugs and may have a higher sensitivity to medications in general. The elderly patient is generally more susceptible to foot infection from minor trauma, which is related to decreased arterial supply and sensation. The elderly person usually has a lower threshold to emotional and physical stress, is more likely to injure his lower extremities, is generally at greater risk than the nongeriatric patient, and has tissues in the foot that do not repair readily. All these factors demonstrate the need for early management and preventive foot care if complications are to be avoided.

Elderly patients complaining of foot discomfort and pain should receive a careful evaluation and examination. The case review should include the social status of the patient in relation to his functional needs. A review of the present complaint, past podiatric and general history, and a systems review to provide evidence of other than local pathology should be included. Particular attention should be given to conditions such as gout, diabetes mellitus, neuropathy, peripheral arterial disease, and arthritis. Occupational relationships should be identified that focus on weight-bearing periods, excessive stress, and environmental factors.

Appropriate consideration should be given to the identification of toenail changes and deformities, the relationship of hyperkeratotic lesions to overt foot deformity, pedal pulses, and changes in sensation to the whole foot or to part of it. Biomechanical evaluation of the patient's pedal structures should be completed when the symptoms and findings are related to musculoskeletal problems. Observations should be made in the non–weight-bearing attitude, in stance using the normal angle of gait for the particular individual, and during the dynamic phases of walking. Other elements of such an examination should include locomotor coordination, general posture, limb size, and symmetry, gait studies, ranges of motion of all pedal joints, the relationship of limitation and deformity to the normal anatomic planes, and observation of overt joint deformity.

Palpation of the foot should identify areas of sensitivity, the quality of pain-free motion, osseous abnormalities, and the presence of extraneous masses and swellings. Manual muscle testing should be included, and grading of muscle groups should be recorded. Muscle tone, strength, mass, and mechanical direction should be related to work tolerance and correlated with neurologic testing.

Inspection of footwear should be included to identify wear patterns, shoe last compatibility, shoe structure in relation to patient needs, and the presence or absence of shoe corrections and modifications that may have been prescribed many years ago. Radiographic examination may be required of both pedal extremities to provide comparison and this may include weight-bearing and non–weight-bearing studies.

When care programs are developed for the elderly, it is essential that the life patterns of the patient be considered, that is, the living environment. Patients who are caring for themselves at home and patients who reside in institutions, such as homes for the aged, nursing homes, or boarding homes, must have therapy directed to their functional needs and within the confines of their economic status so that their dignity can be preserved. The balance of this chapter will attempt to present those common foot conditions that are not described elsewhere in the text and will focus primarily on local deformities.

ABNORMALITIES OF TOENAILS

Toenails have a tendency to become thickened and deformed. The gradual thickening, or onychauxis, is related to repeated microtrauma of the matrix, vascular insufficiency, and nutritional changes in the growth process. A comparison of toenails and fingernails will usually identify considerable differences in the same patient. With thickening, deformity becomes more evident. In cases where mycosis is present, the deformity may be increased. The nails usually become brittle and lose their translucent character. Loosening of the nail from the bed, starting at the free edge, or onycholysis, is common. Subungual debris is considerable and can itself be the source of pressure, pain, and a focus for both mycotic and bacterial infections. The patient's inability to see properly or to bend usually delays treatment. In situations in which the condition is permitted to persist without appropriate care, the deformity increases, and the toenails become long and tend to curl in an anterior-posterior manner. This condition is aggravated by pressure from footwear and is referred to as *ram's horn nail*, or *onychogryphosis*. Management consists of periodic and appropriate debridement and the use of an emollient to hydrate and lubricate the adjacent periungual structures. When the nail plate is excessively thickened or larger than the nail bed and soft tissues, hyperkeratosis or callus forms in the medial and lateral nail grooves and produces pain. Debridement of the tissue and nail plate is required to provide patient comfort.

Sudden trauma to the nail plate generally produces a subungual hematoma. Pain is severe, and evidence of hemorrhage is usually noted under the nail plate. X-ray examination should be undertaken to rule out a fracture of the distal phalanx. Management during the first 24 hours usually consists of drilling a small hole in the nail plate to permit the fluid to escape. If a longer period of time has elapsed, it may be best to protect the part and provide the patient with an analgesic. The hemorrhagic area will frequently grow forward with the nail plate. In cases in which the trauma has been significant, the nail may shed, with new nail generating posteriorally. Some thickening of the nail usually results when trauma to the matrix cells is significant. With trauma, inflammation of the posterior nail fold, or onychia, may also be present. Mild saline soaks or povidone-iodine (Betadine) compresses and other infection-preventing measures should be instituted.

The true ingrown toenail occurs when a segment of nail penetrates the adjacent soft tissues. In the elderly, it is usually induced by improper self-care attempts. When the nail penetrates the soft tissue, an abscess usually results.

Left untreated, an associated paronychia may develop. Unless the segment of nail is removed, treatment of the infective process is protracted and generally unsuccessful. Should the segment of nail not be removed, periungual and ulcerative granulation tissue will develop even after a short period of time. Initial treatment should consist of drainage of the abscess or excision of the nail segment. Mild saline or povidone-iodine (Betadine) compresses and antibiotics usually resolve the acute manifestations. When the involution of the toenail, that is, a downward and inward pinching of the nail plate on the soft tissue, is partly responsible, surgical excision and destruction of the matrix is generally the treatment of choice.

If granulation tissue is present, surgical excision should be considered. Topical caustics such as silver nitrate may also be used. The prime complication is associated with peripheral arterial occlusion and the possible development of necrosis. When surgical excision of even a small segment of nail needs to be completed, excision of a portion or of the total matrix may be appropriate to prevent future exacerbations of the problem. It should be noted that hypertrophy of the medial and lateral nail lips may also precipitate the condition. If surgical repair cannot be considered, the debridement or thinning of the nail plate or the excision of small segments of nail periodically may be required to maintain a pain-free state and prevent infection and ulceration. Nail packing of cotton, wool, or plastic may be used to protect the soft tissue.

Sometimes patients may have pain under the nail plate. The prime differential diagnosis includes subungual melanoma, hematoma, and heloma. Heloma is the most common condition and usually is related to a subungual exostosis, spur, enlarged tuft of the distal phalanx, and external shoe pressure. If a neoplasm can be identified, surgical excision should be considered. If the heloma is pressure related, partial avulsion or debridement of the nail plate is indicated, followed by debridement of the hyperkeratotic lesion. Appropriate shoe modifications or other orthotic devices are indicated. When conservative treatment is chosen, the use of tube foam and removal of the distal portion of the upper part of the shoe may also be required. It should be noted that a glomus tumor, although rare, should also be considered if the pain is acute and not relieved when pressure is removed.

Onychomycosis is a fungus infection of the nail plate and bed and is far more common in toenails than fingernails. There is no question that the environmental factor of footwear and continued microtrauma is related to its etiology. In the elderly the lack of vascular supply to the nail bed usually increases the deformity and limits the prognosis for total remission. The infection generally originates at the free edge of the nail, with onycholysis resulting. Subungual debris accumulates, and the infection progresses toward the posterior nail wall and the matrix. When the matrix cells are involved, excessive deformity results. The nail destruction is characterized by an opaque, yellowish discoloration and a characteristic musty odor. The mycotic nail remains a focus of infection as long as the condition is active. Once hypertrophy of the nail plate takes place with matrix involvement, the deformed nail usually remains as a residual, even if the organisms are destroyed. At times the nails may have a granular appearance. Onchomycosis is particularly prevalent in the elderly and chronic in nature. The clinical picture needs to be differentiated from psoriatic involvement. Management should be instituted when the condition is diagnosed. Culture and smear may not always identify a singular organism.

Management should include surgical debridement of the infected and deformed nail and the use of appropriate antifungal agents. The success of systemic antifungal agents is directly related to the vascular supply to the nail bed. This treatment has had a limited response in the elderly and in toenail infections. Topical applications of Haloprogin solution appear to be the most appropriate form of management when combined with periodic debridement. Total remission should not be expected when the matrix cells are infected. However, because of the communicable nature of the disease, treatment should be instituted. In cases in which the deformity is excessive and the vascular supply to the part adequate, total surgical removal of the nail and destruction of the matrix may prove to be the more logical approach to long-term remission, when postoperative care also includes systemic antifungal agents.

Two additional clinical manifestations should also be identified: Beau's lines, which are transverse interruptions in nail growth associated with acute changes in the vascular supply to the matrix and onychorrhexis, which represents exaggeration in the longitudinal attachments of the inferior nail plate to the superior nail bed. Both entities should be noted for future reference.

CUTANEOUS LESIONS

Hyperkeratosis and keratotic lesions represent a significant clinical entity in the elderly as well as a source of pain and limitation of activity. Keratotic lesions may present as space replacements for atrophied tissue or a lack of soft tissue mobilization. Lesions may also be present as a hyperplastic response of tissue to pressure and friction; particularly over weight-bearing areas and joint deformities. Increased hyperkeratosis is also related to a lack of hydration and of lubrication in the aging skin.

The types of primary lesions that occur are tyloma (callus) and various varieties of heloma (corn), such as heloma durum, vasculare, molle miliare, neurofibromas, and intractable lesions, which are generally neurovascular in character. The sites of prevalence generally include the plantar metatarsal heads, dorsal interphalangeal articulations with associated contractures, the medial aspect of the first metatarsal head, marginal heel, and other points of marked internal or external pressure. Fissures are also associated with hyperkeratosis, particularly at the calcaneal area. Secondary bacterial infection and ulceration are usual complications in these cases.

Clinical evaluation usually involves differential relationships between dermatologic causes, biomechanical factors and deformities, and space replacement activity. In most cases, however, various forces on the foot, such as compressive, tensile, and shearing, and their relationship to friction, tissue elasticity, and fluid movement must be considered in the management of these conditions. Deformity, when complicated by the use of an ill-fitting shoe, can magnify pain, aggravate the lesions, and lead to decreased ambulation.

It should be noted that these lesions are symptoms, and when left untreated, they can result in counterpressure and ultimate ulceration.

Therapeutic approaches involve attempts to hydrate and lubricate the skin with appropriate emollients. Keratotic lesions should be debrided to minimize pressure points, and shoe last modifications should be utilized when practical. If gross deformity exists, surgical consideration should include not only the deformity itself but the patient's functional needs, activity requirements, living situation, systemic condition, and ability to adapt to structural change. In situations in which a definitive approach is not feasible, periodic debridement may be the only way to manage the patient to maintain comfort and ambulation and to prevent complications.

It is important at this point to impart concern for foot health education as a means of prevention. The United States Public Health Service publication, *Feet First*, represents a realistic approach for the elderly, the diabetic, and the patient with peripheral arterial disease. Methods of unsupervised self-care as an approach to definitive care and the use of commercial corn cures or other products should be avoided. When such products are employed, secondary chemical burns, infections, and extensive tissue destruction usually result. The expense of aftercare far exceeds projected management costs for the initial problem.

Local hyperhidrosis and/or bromhidrosis need to be managed with appropriate foot powders, astringents, and deodorant agents. Anhidrosis, xerosis, and dryness need to be managed with hydration and lubrication.

Tinea pedis, if identified in the elderly, can usually be managed with topical medication. Any one of the clinical manifestations may be present such as hyperkeratotic, intertriginous, acute vesicular, or subacute vesicular. Onychomycosis can be the precipitating factor or develop from an untreated dermatologic infection. One of the prime complications is associated scratching and the possible break in the skin, with resultant secondary bacterial infection. The prime differential diagnosis should also include contact dermatitis and eczematous reactions.

DEFORMITIES

Digitus flexus, or hammertoe, may be present on any one or all of the lesser toes. The deformity results from a variety of factors that may include atrophy or contracture of the interossei, rotational deformities, enlarged interphalangeal joints, hyperostosis, and condylar prominence and as the end-result of arthritic changes. Pain is usually the result of inflammatory changes and may be associated with bursitis, capsulitis, or tendonitis. Heloma formation is common dorsally or distally. Ulceration with possible sinus formation may result with continued pressure. Management consists of care in footwear, the use of protective shields, orthodigital and silicone molds, and consideration of surgical procedures to manage or modify the deformity.

Hallux valgus, or bunion, is a symptom complex. It usually involves some inward deviation of the first metatarsal (varus), outward deviation of the great toe (valgus), rotational deformity of the great toe, lateral displacement of the plantar sesamoids, tendon contractures, and adventitious bursa formation. The pain that develops is inflammatory and a result of repeated microtrauma to the soft tissues. Degenerative joint changes may be present with acute inflammation from time to time. Even if symptoms are not paramount, the patient may be concerned with the cosmetic appearance of the foot. Therapy in the geriatric patient should be directed toward symptomatic relief rather than toward modifying the cosmetic concerns of the patient. Because of the general long-standing character of this condition in the elderly and its possible hereditary and degenerative etiology, conservative therapy should be considered initially. A bunion last shoe can be prescribed to accommodate the deformity. Orthoses and shields can be constructed to modify the pressure to the joint. Local steroids and physical measures, such as ultrasound or whirlpool, can be employed to manage the acute and subacute inflammatory processes. Proper concern should also be directed to compensate biomechanically for the associated foot changes, which are etiologic factors.

Many surgical procedures are available for the surgical revision of this joint. Justification for surgical intervention should be based on the symptoms present, the patient's functional needs, and the general medical condition of the patient. Concern should also be directed toward the patient's ability to adjust to the gait changes that will occur after the surgical revision of a major propulsive joint, the postoperative care, and the postoperative management of related foot problems.

Hallux limitus appears clinically and radiographically as a monoarticular arthritis of the first metatarsal-phalangeal joint. When no motion is demonstrable, the condition is known as *hallux rigidus*. Clinically, there is significant limitation of extension of the great toe because of dorsal lipping and spur formation of the great toe joint. Movement creates a chronically inflamed joint, resulting in pain with motion. Treatment after appropriate x-ray examination consists of analgesics and antiinflammatory drugs administered for pain, physical modalities such as whirlpool and ultrasound treatment for pain, local steroid injections, and orthoses or shoe modifications to limit movement at the great toe joint. Surgical revision should be considered when conservative measures fail, in keeping with the functional needs of the patient.

At times, repeated microtrauma to the plantar surface of the first metatarsal head can result in clinical inflammation of the sesamoids in the flexor hallucis brevis tendon. Sesamoiditis can generally be managed with local steroid injections and physical modalities, together with padding and an orthosis to suspend pressure and weight bearing from the area of involvement.

Digiti quinti varus, or tailor's bunion, is a condition similar to hallux valgus and bunion involving the lateral aspect of the foot. In this case the fifth metatarsal demonstrates a varus deformity. The principles of management are similar to those of hallux valgus. However, the pain is not usually as acute because of the different requirements in gait and function. Many patients will also complain of pain in the ball of the foot. This condition has been termed *metatarsalgia* by many, which merely means pain in the metatarsals.

An attempt should be made to identify the cause of the symptoms, some of which include shortening of the first metatarsal segment, or ray, hypermobility of the first segment, loss of the plantar foot pad, traumatic anterior metatarsal bursitis, tendonitis, tenosynovitis, or fasciitis, and the various forefoot and rearfoot compensatory factors.

Treatment should be directed toward the cause, and in this particular case, comparative weight and non–weight-bearing x-ray studies are of great value. Physical modalities including ultrasound and whirlpool are indicated during the acute stages. Local steroid injections and orthotic compensation for the biomechanical changes will help to prevent exacerbative phases. If there are changes in the metatarsal length pattern that produce a maldistribution of weight transmission during function, orthoses that are functional in nature and that either diffuse or redistribute dispersed weight may be the primary vehicles of choice.

MISCELLANEOUS FOOT PROBLEMS

Interdigital neuroma or neuritis generally produces a burning pain that is aggravated by compression from footwear. The patient complains of pain, radiating from the metatarsal head to the distal portion of the toe. The entrapment neuritis may respond to conservative therapy such as local anesthetics, local steroid injections, and physical therapy. Orthotic devices can also be employed to change the intermetatarsal head relationship in conjunction with changes in the shoe last. If the neuritis does not respond to conservative treatment, surgical removal may be required.

Heel pain may be the result of many factors. Included may be pressure on the posterior-superior surface of the calcaneus, known as *Haglund's disease*. This tends to produce a bursitis either between the Achilles tendon and the skin or between the tendon and the posterior surface of the calcaneus. Calcaneal spurs may be demonstrated on x-ray film, generally involving the medial, plantar tuberosity. This may produce pain associated with a subcalcaneal bursitis. Often there is an etiologic association with plantar fasciitis, resulting from microtrauma and continual pull on the posterior attachment of the plantar fascia.

Management of the posterior calcaneal lesions involve heel elevations, physical therapy such as ultrasound, steroid injections, and surgical intervention if the bony prominence cannot be managed with a conservative approach. Plantar heel pain may be treated with physical modalities, such as ultrasound and whirlpool, to reduce the inflammation; steroids during the acute phases; analgesics and muscle relaxants to control pain; and heel cups, heel pads, shoe modifications, and orthoses to control the pull on the plantar fascia by changing the degree of weight borne on the medial tuberosity. In most cases nonsurgical management is successful. If it is not, excision of the bony enlargement should be considered.

Trauma can produce fractures of the bones of the foot. Treatment consists of immobilization followed by appropriate postfracture care. In many cases, immobilization can be achieved by materials other than plaster casts, such as surgical shoes, adhesive strapping, padding, shoe modifications, splinting of toes, and the use of rigid or semirigid protective materials, such as Silastic and silicone.

There is a large variety of foot conditions in the elderly that are residuals from youth and occupational activities. Some of these conditions have been classed under various clinical entities such as pes planus, pes valgus planus, imbalance, subtalar or calcaneal varus, forefoot varus, equinus, and plantar flexed ray syndromes. In any case the residual pain is chronic in nature and modified by the functional needs of the patient. If deformity exists, compensation is probably the best approach. If pain is persistent, arthritic and soft tissue inflammation should be considered. In most cases physical therapy and exercise are of great value.

Shoe selection should meet the functional needs of the elderly patient. Orthoses should be functional and provide accommodation and compensation for the problem. Shoe modifications often can be the simplest and most economic approach. The value of adequate footwear that gives support and protection is increased by the use of molds, inlays, and shields, which diffuse, disperse, and redistribute weight transmission. When recommending a shoe for an aged patient, the clinician must use a different approach, depending on whether the person lives at home and has a normal life-style or is confined to an institution with activity limited. The prime concerns should involve personal comfort, protection, support, and last compatibility and a shoe that will be functional, permit modifications for existing deformities, and permit the use of orthoses if needed. It should be noted that the "orthopedic shoe" is not corrective but rather compensatory in nature, particularly in the elderly patient. Care must also be exercised in their use so that they do not become the "catch-all," replacing other forms of appropriate therapy. If the deformity is extensive, such as the residual or advanced arthritic changes, if surgical revision is not possible or needed to maintain the patient in a functional norm, and if a commercial last is not available, the "molded shoe" provides a viable alternative and should be considered.

The shoe always should be considered as an article of clothing and should meet functional needs. Slip-on lasts are more acceptable to most elderly patients who are unable to bend to tie laces. In all cases, however, full foot covering, particularly for the heel and long plantar areas of the foot is advisable during ambulation to provide stability and to minimize the falls that can occur when footwear is improper.

Some of the external shoe modifications that can be used for the elderly include the following: medial and lateral heel wedges to improve structural stability; medial sole wedges where there is evidence of significant subtalar restricted motion; lateral sole wedges to help compensate for a residual in-toe gait or to modify a poststroke gait; metatarsal bars to transfer weight from the metatarsal heads to the metatarsal shafts; bars to modify supination; the Thomas heel to compensate for and assist medial structural deformity and rotation; the reversed Thomas heel to assist lateral stability; long counters to add medial stability to fixed and rotational foot deformities; medial and lateral heel flares or wedgies to make the entire plantar surface weight bearing; hallux limitus stiffeners to help limit dorsiflexion and extension of the first metatarsal-phalangeal joint; rocker bars to prevent flexion and extension of the shoe; custom-molded shoes; cork buildups for short limbs; and special soles to help in weight diffusion. Some of the internal shoe modifications include the following: longitudinal or scaphoid pads to provide soft tissue replacement and weight diffusion, possibly with cutouts for painful plantar lesions; calcaneal bars and heel pads for calcaneal pain and bursitis; heel lifts for minimal limb shortening; and tongue pads to compensate for some shoe last-to-toe incompatibilities.

The materials used for foot orthoses vary from rigid, such as metal and plastic, to soft, such as felt, latex, foam, and cork, to semirigid, such as leather, Silastic, Plastazote, and dynamic molding compounds. In any case, the choice of shoes is related to the selection and type of foot orthoses, and attention must be paid to shoe last compatibility, shoe volume, and the materials and additions to the shoe itself.

CONCLUSION

Foot problems in the elderly are the end result of a lifetime of disease, untreated deformity, trauma and abuse, a lack of health education, and lack of preventive measures in earlier years. Treatment approaches are modified by aging and disease. An attempt has been made in this chapter to present some of the more common foot problems that are primarily local in nature. The information is not intended to be all inclusive but rather to add to the information in other chapters, such as dermatology and the management of diabetes mellitus. It is intended to raise the index of suspicion for a pathologic condition in the presence of patient complaints, deformity, and pain.

It should be noted that the podogeriatric management of these conditions has as its prime concern the total patient and the appropriate use of all health care and related personnel, the patient, and his family in an evolution of a team approach to patient care so that comprehensive services can be brought to and planned for the elderly.

REFERENCES

1. Brachman, P.R.: Mechanical foot therapy, Chicago, 1966, Podiatry Books Co.
2. Brachman, P.R.: Foot orthopedics, Chicago, 1966, Podiatry Books Co.
3. Cailliet, R.: Foot and ankle pain, Philadelphia, 1968, F.A. Davis Co.
4. Giannestras, N.J.: Foot disorders, medical and surgical management, ed. 2, Philadelphia, 1973, Lea & Febiger.
5. Gibbard, L.C.: Charlesworth's chiropodical orthopedics, London, 1968, Baillière, Tindall & Cassell, Ltd.
6. Helfand, A.E.: Podiatrist looks at public health in diabetes and arthritis control, Public Health News, State of New Jersey Department of Health, June, 1965.
7. Helfand, A.E.: Practice guide for podiatric programs in extended care facilities: J. Am. Podiatry Assoc. **56**:220, 1966.
8. Helfand, A.E.: Podiatry in a total geriatric health program, common foot problems in the aged, J. Am. Geriatric Soc. **16**:593, 1967.
9. Helfand, A.E.: Rules for foot health in aging, J. Practical Nurs. **18**:25, May, 1968.
10. Helfand, H.E.: Clinical podogeriatrics, Baltimore, 1981, The Williams & Wilkins Co.
11. Inman, V.T.: DuVries' surgery of the foot, ed. 3, St. Louis, 1973, The C.V. Mosby Co.
12. Kelikian, H.: Hallux valgus, allied deformities of the forefoot and metatarsalgia, Philadelphia, 1965, W.B. Saunders Co.
13. Levin, M.E., and O'Neal, L.W.: The diabetic foot, ed. 3, St. Louis, 1982, The C.V. Mosby Co.
14. Lewin, P.: The foot and ankle, ed. 4, Philadelphia, 1959, Lea & Febiger.

15. Mennell, J.M.: Foot pain, Boston, 1969, Little, Brown & Co.
16. Samitz, M.H., and Dana, A.S., Jr.: Cutaneous lesions of the lower extremities, Philadelphia, 1971, J.B. Lippincott Co.
17. Samman, P.D.: The nails in disease, London, 1965, William Heinemann Medical Books Ltd.
18. U.S. Department of Health, Education and Welfare: Long-term care facility administration, Case study manual, Pub. No. 384-034/922, Washington, D.C., 1970, U.S. Government Printing Office.
19. U.S. Department of Health, Education and Welfare: Feet first, Pub. No. 388-126, Washington, D.C., U.S. Government Printing Office.
20. Weinstein, F.: Principles and practice of podiatry, Philadelphia, 1968, Lea & Febiger.
21. Yale, I.: Podiatric medicine, Baltimore, 1974, The Williams & Wilkins Co.

PART III DISORDERS OF THE NERVOUS AND SENSORY SYSTEMS

CHAPTER 25 · PSYCHOLOGIC ASPECTS

Martha Storandt

It has only been since the 1940s that psychology has turned to systematic study of the human organism in the last half of the life span. Many questions still remain; many areas of research are plumbed only partially; little exists in the way of comprehensive theoretic frameworks on which to hang the bits and pieces of knowledge that have been obtained. Thus, if the reader finds that questions concerning the psychologic aspects of the treatment of the geriatric patient are unanswered in this chapter, it may be that the answers are unavailable. However, space limitations may necessitate some omission of information. The reader searching for more detailed information on a particular issue in gerontologic psychology is referred to two recent, comprehensive reviews: *Aging and Behavior*[1] and *Handbook of the Psychology of Aging*.[2]

The following discussion refers to the "elderly person" or the "geriatric patient" and might be taken to imply that all older adults are alike. Nothing could be further from the truth. Many old people may have certain abilities, needs, and problems in common, but each geriatric patient is an individual. In fact, individual differences *increase* in old age. Thus each patient must be treated in terms of the specific circumstances of his or her own particular abilities, medical condition, environment, and life history.

SENSATION

Psychology studies the behavior of the human organism in relation to its environment. Basic to this relationship is the ability of the individual to sense and perceive the surrounding world. Changes in sensory and perceptual abilities that occur as a function of increased age influence a wide range of the behaviors and attitudes of the geriatric patient. For example, a hearing loss in an elderly person may be followed by a withdrawal from interpersonal relationships because of the difficulty experienced in communicating with others. Such withdrawal may lead to isolation, loneliness, depression, and severe loss of morale. Even a relatively mild hearing loss may serve to handicap the older adult performing the variety of cognitive processes that have substantial verbal components.[3] Thus a knowledge of the sensory capabilities of the elderly person may expose a chain of events that points the way to simple and effective therapeutic intervention.

Vision

Vision is the most thoroughly studied sense with respect to age related patterns of differences and will be described here in more detail than the other senses.

Illumination. As the individual grows older, decreased pupil size, loss of lens transparency, increased thickness of the lens, and thickening of the capsule allow less light to reach the retina. Thus the absolute threshold for vision is raised. This reduced retinal illumination can be corrected partially by increasing the level of illumination at which the elderly individual performs visual tasks. For example, the 65-year-old person needs about twice as much illumination as the 20-year-old adult just to compensate for decreased pupil size.[4]

Accommodation. The ability of the eye to discriminate detail of near objects is related to the ability of the lens to change its refractive power. With increasing age the elasticity of the lens decreases, and elderly people experience increasing farsightedness, or presbyopia. Accommodative power of the lens is at a peak of approximately 20 diopters at about 5 years of age and decreases linearly until about 60 years of age, when it reaches a value of approximately 0.5 diopter. Little change is seen beyond 60 years of age. This loss of accommodative power is recognized most frequently in the forties as an inability to see well enough to read. The arms are too short to hold the newspaper far enough away! This condition can be corrected by glasses.

Visual acuity. Visual acuity, the ability to distinguish detail at a distance, increases throughout childhood until it reaches a peak in young adulthood. There is a slight decline from young adulthood to the fifties, which is followed by a more rapid decline in the sixties and seventies. Hirsch[5] reported a decline from a median Snellen decimal of 1.20 in the forties to less than 0.50 at 80 years of age. Most elderly people require correction by glasses for this loss of visual acuity.

Color vision. The ability to discriminate color reaches its peak in the twenties and after that follows a course of steady decline. This is especially true of the colors at the blue end of the spectrum. With increasing age the lens of the eye tend to yellow. Blues and violets are filtered out and thus are more difficult to differentiate than are colors at the red end of the visible spectrum. This has practical implications for the aged patient who may be taking a variety of medications. If the patient codes the pills or capsules by color and takes two of the purple ones instead of two of the blue ones, the course of treatment could be altered drastically.

Hearing

Auditory acuity declines with increased age, just as does visual acuity. This condition is called *presbycusis*. However, loss of auditory acuity is not constant across all frequencies but is more severe for high tones. Presbycusis is seen to a greater degree in men than in women.

Speech intelligibility, as well as auditory threshold and pitch discrimination, is affected with increased age. Some consonants, especially s, z, t, f, and g, are high frequency in nature and have little acoustic power. Since high frequency sounds are more difficult for the elderly person to hear, difficulty in word discrimination may occur and understanding of normal conversation may be affected.

Elderly people are susceptible to the problem of masking. All of us have had the experience at large parties of being unable to hear a conversation going on very close to us when the background noise level is high. The noise masks the weaker consonants, which carry much information. Since older adults have decreased auditory acuity, the problem is more severe for them. It can be alleviated simply by reduction of background noise levels.

Hearing aids can be of benefit in some kinds of hearing losses. However, the elderly individual must be carefully and patiently trained in the use of the aid. Hearing aids do not operate efficiently on dead batteries or with ear pieces plugged with ear wax. Lipreading is a solution favored by some older adults with hearing losses. Those in the environment of such an individual must be careful to speak directly to the older person.

Taste

The number of taste buds declines with increased age, beginning in the middle years and becoming more obvious after age 60.[6] Although elderly people can identify the basic qualities of sweet, salty, bitter, and sour, their threshold of recognition is increased, that is, they require more concentrated solutions to determine the particular taste. This may explain the comment of one nursing home dietician who, beset with resident complaints about the food, observed that they all liked the chili! Food complaints by older persons may be related to nonsensory factors such as diseases of the mouth, poorly fitted dentures, diets that are contrary to food preferences but are required for a particular health condition such as cardiovascular disease or diabetes, lack of economic resources to purchase preferred food, or lack of social stimulation at mealtimes—a problem for elderly individuals who live alone.

Olfaction

Although the evidence is somewhat contradictory, it appears that smell sensitivity may decrease with age,[7] probably as a result of changes in the olfactory bulb and tract.[8] It is not clear to what extent generalized health problems play a role in the decline in smell sensitivity, which has been observed, and individual differences among the old are extensive.[9] Increased olfactory thresholds would reduce the ability of older adults to discriminate food odors and, in combination with decreases in taste sensitivity, would contribute to changes in food preferences and eating patterns. The older adult's ability to discriminate fruit odors, in comparison to odors of other foods, may explain the preference for fruits found in one study.[10]

Somesthetic senses

Older adults appear to decline somewhat in terms of sensitivity to pain. More importantly, they may be less willing to report pain. Decreases in tactile sensitivity occur in some older adults and may be seen primarily in areas of hairless skin such as the palms of the hands and the soles of the feet. The ability to sense vibration declines somewhat with age, primarily in the lower extremities. No changes in sensitivity to temperature have been substantiated.[11]

Disturbances related to loss of sensory abilities

It is known that sensory deprivation can produce hallucinations as well as intellectual and perceptual deterioration in normal individuals.[12] Some of the commonly observed eccentricities or emotional disturbances of elderly patients may be related directly to decreased sensory stimulation. For example, families or those charged with the care of aged patients sometimes complain of nocturnal restlessness in the elderly individual. The geriatric patient receives a reduced amount of stimulation under normal conditions of illumination and noise background. The patient is deprived even further when lights are low and all is quiet. This frightening experience and its behavioral consequences may be eliminated by the presence of a night-light.

Another example relates to loss of auditory acuity. Suspiciousness may be increased to paranoid dimensions by loss of hearing. If the elderly person cannot hear the conversations of others accurately, it is possible that the older adult will impute hostile motives where none exist in reality, especially if the older adult is of a suspicious nature to begin with.

More severe loss of the ability to interact with the environment has been the focus of a treatment technique designed for regressed senile patients. Sensory retraining, as described later in this chapter, provides a structured experience in the exercise of the senses to improve perception of the environment, both physical and human.[13]

SLOWING OF RESPONSE TIME

One of the best-documented changes that occurs with increased age is the slowing of response time. Although a small portion of this loss in speed may be attributable to reduced peripheral nerve transmissions, it appears that slowness in old age is related primarily to more central physiologic mechanisms.

The effects of loss of speed can be minimized by habits of exercise, opportunities for practice, and motivational patterns.[1] For example, the older adult may reduce the speed of performance to achieve greater accuracy. By being coaxed to worry less about correctness, greater speed can be obtained—*if* speed, not accuracy, is desired.

Furthermore, individual differences in psychomotor speed are great. Many older adults can perform more rapidly than some young adults. However, loss of speed is common and may account for a portion of the measured deficits in other functions such as learning and problem solving. Such slowing with increased age must be taken into account in almost all facets of the treatment of the geriatric patient.

LEARNING AND MEMORY

The adage, "You can't teach an old dog new tricks," is not true. Older persons can and do learn. However, they frequently take longer than do young persons. Older adults need more time both to study the material to be remembered and, perhaps more importantly, more time to give their response when asked to demonstrate their learning.[14]

Conditioning

There are two types of conditioning: classical and instrumental. In Pavlovian classical conditioning an unconditioned stimulus such as a puff of air to the eye produces an involuntary response, an eyeblink. If the puff of air is paired over a number of trials with a conditioned stimulus, a buzzer for example, eventually the buzzer by itself will elicit the response of the eyeblink. Such involuntary conditioned responses are acquired more slowly by older adults and are extinguished or lost more rapidly than by younger adults.[15]

The principles of instrumental conditioning indicate that if a response which occurs voluntarily from the individual's repertoire of behaviors is *rewarded*, it will occur more frequently. It is as if the individual says, "I was rewarded for doing this before; therefore, if I do it again, I'll be rewarded again." As in classical conditioning, the acquisition of instrumentally conditioned responses occurs more slowly in the aged person. However, even the severely memory-disoriented elderly patient, such as those found in psychiatric wards, can be instrumentally conditioned to make at least simple responses, given appropriate reinforcers.[16] Once acquired by the elderly individual, such an instrumentally conditioned response, unlike a classically conditioned response, is more difficult to extinguish than it is in the young person.

Memory

Difficulty with memory is popularly thought to be one of the major psychologic problems associated with normal old age. It should be pointed out, however, that memory and learning are extremely difficult to differentiate. There can be no memory if learning has not occurred first. On the other hand, learning is assessed by determining how well information is remembered.

The major difficulty in memory that elderly individuals experience may be at the point of registration. Older adults do relatively well in remembering things like phone numbers for the time that it takes them to dial the number. Their strategy here is probably like that of younger adults: rehearsal. By saying the number over and over again to one's self it can be recalled long enough to be used, but as soon as the number is dialed it is forgotten. But when information is to be remembered for longer periods of time, it must be processed more "deeply" at the time that it is learned. Elaboration and association with related information already in the person's memory help the long-term retention of new material. It would appear that older adults do not process new information as thoroughly or effectively as do younger adults; therefore, the information is less likely to be available later.[17]

Motivation

Motivation influences learning. If the individual is highly interested in the material to be learned, it is thought that learning will be enhanced. Frequently older persons do perform better on tasks that are personally relevant to them in comparison to their relatively poor performance on meaningless tasks. For example, if an elderly woman is asked to memorize a list of nonsense syllables, frequently used in laboratory studies of learning and memory, she may do very poorly. If instead she is asked to memorize the ingredients of a recipe she has been trying to get from her neighbor for many years, her performance may be outstanding. The difficulty of the task also limits the learning performance of older adults. Frequently they will refuse to attempt difficult tasks at all.[18]

There is an optimum level of motivation. Beyond such a point, motivation may become anxiety provoking and act as a detriment to performance. Eisdorfer[19] has suggested that some learning situations produce a state of psychophysiologic arousal in elderly individuals, which is extreme and which detracts from their ability to perform when learning is required. The response of the elderly adult is inhibited. There is no response. The task is discontinued.

Learning aids

There are many aids to learning that the older adult can be taught to use to improve learning performance in daily life. These include simple strategies of organization, such as categorization and indexing, which assist the older person in organizing the material to be remembered.[20,21]

Mediational techniques or mnemonic devices may improve memory performance. If the task is to remember two things that go together, a visual picture of the two related together or a verbal phrase relating the two objects improves performance. Elderly people do not use such mediational techniques spontaneously and must be provided with them or given practice in forming them.[22,23]

Note writing is an obvious aid to memory. However, the few studies of note writing as an aid to memory in older adults indicate that they do not employ this technique spontaneously. Even when attempts were made to train the older adults in note writing, they frequently did not use their notes. They could see no reason for using the notes (perhaps denial of memory difficulties) or found their own handwriting unreadable.[24]

Older individuals learn better in a supportive context[25] and appear to do better when the presentation of the material is not only visual but also auditory, that is, when the individual not only sees the item to be remembered but also says it or hears it said or described aloud.[26] The elderly person should avoid the interference of extraneous material when attempting to learn something new. The principle is to learn one thing at a time and learn it well before going on to something else.[1]

These aids, in addition to slow pacing of the learning and appropriate levels of motivation and task difficulty, can improve greatly the learning and memory performance of the older adult.

INTELLIGENCE

It would appear that little if any loss occurs in the normal elderly individual when intelligence is measured in terms of stored information.[27] Most verbal abilities are maintained and may even increase in the later years of life. This is especially true for individuals of initially high or average ability.[15] For example, older people perform best on the Information, Vocabulary, and Comprehension subtests of the Wechsler Adult Intelligence Scale (WAIS). These tests all involve verbal abilities and are influenced to a substantial extent by experience and education.

Perceptual-integrative intelligence, on the other hand, appears to decrease with age. Poor performance by older adults is seen on the WAIS subtests of Digit Symbol, Picture Arrangement, and Block Design—measures that depend on the processing of novel information. This decline in perceptual-integrative performance in older adults is based in part on their slower speed of performance. Although older people do not need more time than allotted to perform these tasks used to measure perceptual-integrative intelligence, they do not solve the problems as rapidly as do young people and therefore do not obtain as many "bonus points," which are awarded, usually to the very bright, for rapid performance.[28]

Horn and Cattell[29] have suggested two components to intelligence: fluid and crystallized. Fluid intelligence is probably biologically based, whereas crystallized intelligence depends on the interaction of the organism with its environment and represents the acculturation factor in intellectual functioning. It would appear that crystallized intelligence is maintained in old age, whereas fluid intelligence may decline, perhaps reflecting decreased efficiency of the central nervous system.

PERSONALITY

Personality theorists have devoted their greatest efforts in the past to the study of the development of personality in childhood. Few have examined the normal course of personality change, if there indeed is any, in the adult years.

To complete his eight stages of man, describing the developmental tasks of the individual, Erikson[30] described two stages of personality development that span the period of life from the twenties to death. In the stage of *generativity* the task of the individual is to contribute to the continuation of the species by means of nurturance of the new generation. This stage applies most obviously to young adulthood and the middle years of life. In the final stage of personality development, the stage of *ego-integrity*, the individual's task is to develop a sense of worth of his or her own life—a sense of uniqueness and wisdom but of oneness with other cultures and historic periods. If a sense of ego-integrity is not obtained, the individual is left with a sense of despair and a fear of death. This developmental task of later life remains theoretic in nature, since little research has been generated to substantiate its generality or mechanisms.

Studies using objective measures of personality have reported little in the way of age differences. Even large-scale longitudinal studies show little change in personality.[31] Therefore it would appear that stability in basic personality is the rule throughout the adult years. Major differences are between individuals, not within individuals over time.

Successful aging

Great emphasis has been placed by social gerontologists on the study of successful aging. Much of the impetus for this research was from Cumming's and Henry's disengagement theory,[32] based on an empirical study of a large sample of elderly people in Kansas City. Their work suggested that disengagement was a process of *mutual* withdrawal of the individual from society and of society from the individual. The quantity and quality of relationships that the older individual has with others in the social world change as the individual grows older. Processes of psychologic and social disengagement are the means whereby the individual *and* society prepare for the final disengagement of death of the person and, as such, provide for an orderly end to the individual's life span.

The universality of disengagement as an optimum process of aging has been questioned by subsequent research. Whether an individual will follow a path of engagement or disengagement in the later years probably is related to lifelong personality styles and characteristics.[33] The nature of the activities from which the individual disengages appears to be related to the maintenance of high morale. A high level of noninterpersonal activity was seen by Maddox[34] as associated with good morale, whereas decline in interpersonal involvement seemed less negative in its implications. Lowenthal and Haven[35] have suggested that the elderly person may be relatively isolated in a social sense and still maintain good morale as long as a confidant, a person with whom the older adult can share personal concerns on an intimate basis, is present. It may be that the quality, as opposed to the quantity, of social interaction contributes to life satisfaction.[36]

Good health is a major contributor to a sense of well-being in later life. By maintaining good health the older adult can continue in those social and nonsocial activities that are important to him or her.[37] Other factors that influence life satisfaction in old age include socioeconomic variables such as education and previous occupation (persons with lower socioeconomic status experience less life satisfaction), marital status (the married are somewhat more satisfied), and the availability of transportation and good housing.[38]

Rigidity and cautiousness

It is an oversimplification to say that older people are rigid, dogmatic, and resistant to change. Although stereotypic dogmatism may be greater in older adults, intolerant attitudes and dogmatism based on anxiety and insecurity appear to be less.[39] Rigidity can take many forms. The older person may be rigid about some things but quite flexible about others.

Older adults are described frequently as more cautious than young people, and, indeed, they do appear to be so in many settings. Older persons appear to value accuracy and frequently avoid mistakes by refusing to respond at all—an error of omission as opposed to an error of commission. They also demonstrate a greater need for certainty before venturing a response and, in fact, may avoid decision making altogether to eliminate the risk of negative consequences. However, one study found older adults to be no more cautious than young adults when the risk was appropriate in terms of the payoff.[40]

Sometimes an increased need for certainty is not expressed overtly by the elderly individual. Indeed the older person may even minimize or deny a lack of self-confidence. The sensitive geriatrician is aware of the elderly patient's increased need for certainty. The caregiver should provide appropriate structure and direction, rather than assuming that the older patient will determine it on his own. This is *not* to say that older persons are incapable of self-determination and decision making or should be treated in an authoritative manner. Rather explanations and instructions should be explicit and clear as opposed to ambiguous, sketchy, or generalized.

This admonition applies particularly to staff in acute care facilities where the emphasis is on the efficient application of treatment procedures. Many negative emotional reactions by elderly patients in such settings are unnecessary and could be avoided if sufficient explanations are given beforehand. Thus, in the long run, the time devoted to careful psychologic preparation of the patient is well spent, since it eliminates the necessity of dealing with problems after they develop.

Depression

Many older individuals, especially white males, do appear to experience increased depression in the later years of life as evidenced by increased suicide rates (Fig. 25-1), clinical reports, and psychometric testing. Evidence from the Minnesota Multiphasic Personality Inventory (MMPI) indicates that older adults more frequently have peak scores on the depression scale than on any of the remainder of the clinical scales. However, it has been suggested that this peak, at least in aged psychiatric patients, is related to a decrease in other kinds of symptomatology.[41] Thus other psychopathologies are less prominent, leaving depression as the most obvious emotional disturbance.

The higher suicide rates of older men compared with those of older women may be related

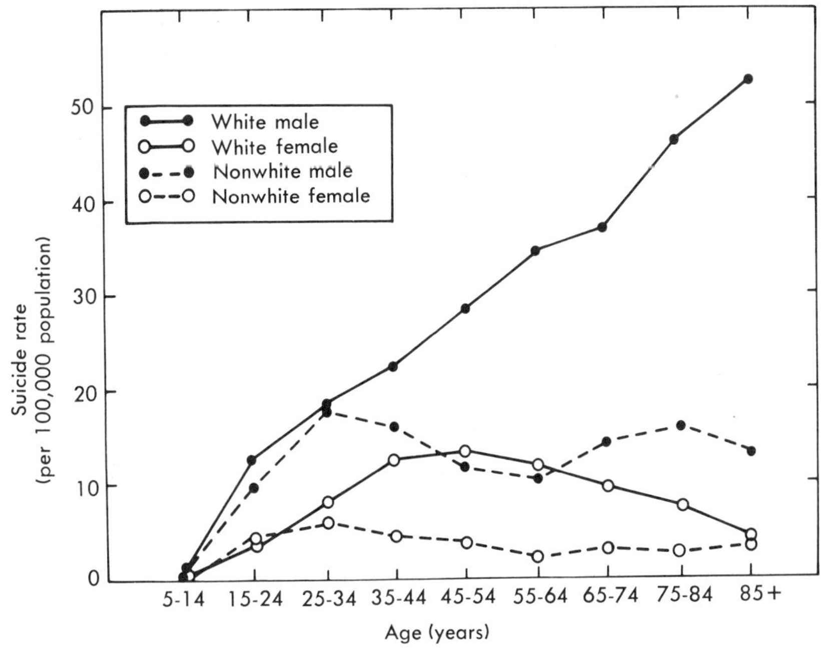

Fig. 25-1. Suicide rates by age, sex, and color in the United States, 1969. (Data from United States Department of Health, Education, and Welfare: Vital statistics of the United States, 1969, vol. II. A. Mortality, Rockville, Md., 1974, National Center for Health Statistics.)

partially to sex differences in methods of self-destruction. Men more frequently employ violent, irreversible means of committing suicide, whereas women take a more passive approach, for example, an overdose of barbiturates. Thus more women are rescued from suicide attempts.[42]

Depression seen in old age is frequently exogenous, or reactive, in nature as opposed to endogenous. Exogenous depressions arise in response to events that occur outside the individual. Endogenous depressions, on the other hand, have no observable external causes; they are thought to be related to intrapsychic or internal characteristics of the individual. Older persons experience many losses, ranging from loss of personal significance or loss of the work role at retirement to the death of a spouse or serious ill health. Such depressions can be alleviated frequently by drug therapy or psychotherapy, usually supportive in nature (see Chapter 26).

Facing death

Only recently have researchers begun to investigate, from a scientific point of view, the meaning of death to the individual. However, an understanding of the process of dying and of attitudes concerning death is of great importance both for older adults themselves and for those in the health care professions who most frequently deal with the dying. Medicine emphasizes the maintenance of life and, in its fight to prevent death, has ignored the fact that it can only be postponed, never eliminated.

Older adults are better prepared for their own death and have less fear of it than those in younger age groups.[44] They have reconciled themselves to mortality. However, the aged *are* concerned about being in control of the conditions under which they die. One highly intelligent and remarkably active octogenarian complained bitterly of his physician's lack of understanding of the needs and problems of the older patient. He wanted a geriatrician who "knew something about older people." Furthermore, he contemplated suicide while he was still able to make such a decision and take the appropriate action. The implication was that he did not wish to be left in the hands of those who would allow him to linger for a long period of time as a vegetating, ineffectual, psychologically dead organism.

With respect to the psychologic needs of terminal patients, the pioneering work of Kubler-Ross[45] has demonstrated that the terminal patient goes through five stages in coming to grips with the inevitability of death. These include, in order of appearance, denial, anger and rage, bargaining, depression, and, finally, acceptance. She has demonstrated that individuals facing death generally want, and freely join in, an opportunity to discuss the approaching end of their lives with others. It is not a taboo subject for them. The terminally ill desire an opportunity to set their lives in order, to discuss their concerns with those who are important to them, and to come to grips with remaining, unsolved problems they may have so that they can meet death with dignity and acceptance. Frequently, however, they are denied this opportunity, since those around them are often less adept in facing the issues surrounding the dying process.

To foster sharing of attitudes and concerns, discussions of death should be made a part of the curriculum in schools for health care professionals and should be the subject of periodic inservice training programs. If death can be faced openly by those who deal with it on a daily basis, perhaps methods of meeting it in a psychologically prepared state will become more obvious and widespread.

Sexuality

The bumper sticker reads, "I'm not a dirty old man, I'm a sexy senior citizen." Until very recently, it was considered inappropriate and distasteful to suggest that older adults have sexual needs and interests or that they engage in sexual intercourse. However, research has shown that sexual activity may be maintained, in some individuals at least, well into the eighties.[46-49]

The age related patterns of sexuality are different for men and women. Men reach a peak of sexual activity in the teens and follow a path of slow but steady decline thereafter. Masters and Johnson[48] have suggested a number of explanations for this age related pattern of decreased sexual activity in the male. The causes include poor health, concern with career and economic activities, fatigue, overindulgence in food or alcohol, fear of failure, and boredom with his partner. However, they also emphasize that older couples may continue to enjoy sexual relations well into old age, given a positive attitude toward the aging process, good health, and a life history of regular and satisfying sexual activity.

Age related patterns of sexual activity in the female follow a somewhat different course. Although the woman is less sexually active, she does not appear to experience the same decline with age as does the man. When sexual activity does cease for the woman, frequently it is due to impotence on the part of her partner or to widowhood.[49] Although menopause brings with it a cessation of the ability to bear children, it does not herald the cessation of sexual activity in the female. Some women report a heightened awareness and enjoyment of sexual activity in the postmenopausal period.

Many institutions caring for geriatric patients have not yet been able to reconcile in any practical way the remnants of sexual taboos with more recent scientific knowledge of sexuality in old age. Staff and family members are taken aback at the suggestion that unmarried or even married couples who are nursing home residents be allowed privacy and freedom of sexual expression. Masturbation is seen as an undesirable behavior, an activity to be suppressed and eliminated. Such restrictive policies deny the sexuality of the geriatric patient and produce still another loss to add to an already lengthy list.

Some geriatric health professionals are becoming more aware of the sexual needs of their patients. Physicians, for example, may temper their instructions to older patients with cardiovascular disorders to "take it easy" with an explanation that, in most instances, moderate, relaxed, tension-free sexual intercourse is possible after a period of recovery from acute phases of cardiac illness. Care should be taken to prepare, in a psychologic sense, the elderly patient scheduled for prostatectomy, mastectomy, hysterectomy, or the like to prevent subsequent emotional disturbances associated with sexual identity.

PSYCHOLOGIC THERAPIES FOR THE AGED

Until recently little emphasis has been placed on active psychologic treatment of older people. Many mental health professionals have been pessimistic about the possibility of such treatment, seeing it as difficult to provide and even as a waste of scarce resources, since the elderly individual has few remaining years, in comparison with younger clients, in which to reap the benefits of a successful therapeutic program. Instead a course of custodial care has been followed. Such a pessimistic attitude on the part of mental health practitioners has its roots in reality. Many chronic psychiatric conditions are difficult to alleviate, given present treatment techniques. But nonaggressive treatment of aged patients may stem from the pervasive negative attitudes that American culture has about old age. Such pessimism is undeserved. Positive outcomes for actively treated geriatric patients have been demonstrated.[50] Furthermore, those in the helping professions have an ethical obligation to provide the best in care to all.

In addition to traditional individual and group psychotherapy, several innovative treatment programs for geriatric patients, particularly those demonstrating intellectual deterioration, have been described in recent years. One review listed 10 such treatment methods, which are described here.[51]

Reality orientation. In a daily classroom setting small groups of severely to moderately deteriorated patients are taught, primarily by repetition, basic information such as name, place, and time. This learning is augmented by 24-hour-a-day follow-up on the part of the entire staff, in which each contact with the patient is used to orient the person to the surrounding environment.

Attitude therapy. Attitude therapy is a technique of behavior modification frequently used in conjunction with reality orientation. One of five major attitudes (kind firmness, active friendliness, passive friendliness, no demand, or matter-of-fact) is prescribed, based on an evaluation of the major behavior pattern of the individual patient. For example, if the patient is withdrawn and apathetic, an attitude of active friendliness may be prescribed. *All* staff who come into contact with this patient would make special efforts to spend time with the patient, offer praise, and make sure the patient never fails. The basic purpose of attitude therapy is to reinforce or increase desirable behavior and extinguish or eliminate undesirable behavior.

Remotivation. When a patient successfully completes a program of reality orientation, the next step is a remotivation group. The purpose of remotivation groups is to promote patient discussion of topics relating to the real world and to improve interpersonal relationships and communications. These small groups of five to twelve persons generally meet once a week for an hour at a time and are led by nonprofessional workers, such as aides and attendants, who are closely attuned to ward climate and topical issues.

Resocialization. Another group technique used with institutionalized geriatric patients is resocialization, a discussion group program that has as its purpose the expansion and broadening of available choices. It focuses strongly on interpersonal relations and feelings within the group and the reliving of happy experiences from the past, as well as the problems of living in a community. The leader takes a more interpretative approach in this group than in remotivation groups.

Reinforcement therapy. Programs of both individual and group behavior modification, such as token economies, are useful with geriatric patients. Since the principles of learning dictate that a rewarded behavior will increase in its frequency and a behavior that is not rewarded will decrease, a wide variety of behaviors are amenable to behavior modification through reinforcement therapy. These include simple self-care tasks, such as dressing and brushing the teeth, as well as more complex social behaviors such as interpersonal communication, acceptance of responsibility, or helping another patient. Behavioral techniques have been shown to be useful in the management of chronic pain and physical problems.[52]

Several cautions must be observed in applying the principles of behavior modification. The behavior to be modified must be specified carefully. An appropriate reinforcement or reward must be determined. Effective rewards are often highly specific to the individual. The staff must have a commitment to the program of modification so that each time the behavior to be reinforced does occur it is rewarded as quickly as possible. Long delays between the behavior and the reward make it more difficult to establish the behavior. Similarly, with a program of extinction of an undesirable behavior care must be taken to eliminate all rewards for the behavior. The behavior modification program will not be effective if some staff ignore the targeted behavior while others reward it.

Milieu therapy. In milieu therapy, or the

therapeutic community, it is assumed that all aspects of the patient's social milieu can be therapeutic and contribute in a positive way to treatment. Emphasis is placed on providing a climate in which the patient can gain awareness of self and can try out new behaviors or develop new skills. Patients themselves are allowed and expected to participate in the decisions of the ward or "community" and to take responsibility for themselves. There is a blurring of the usual authoritative, hierarchical structure typical of institutional settings.

PREVLAB. The Prevention of Loneliness, Anxiety, and Boredom program introduces into the environment high-interest items that are humorous or gimmicky, can be handled by the patient, stimulate or appeal to the senses, or have cultural or historic interest. Such items may be made part of the decor of the building itself or can form a part of a portable kit, which can be passed from one patient to another. The purpose of these items is to stimulate and improve conversation among patients and those with whom they come in contact, both staff and visitors.

Sensory retraining. Sensory retraining can be conducted either in small groups or with single individuals. The purpose of this technique, used with regressed geriatric patients, is to provide the opportunity to improve interaction with the environment through the senses. The patient is provided with activities and objects that stimulate or exercise the senses. Objects to be used are varied but might include mirrors and colorful objects that would stimulate the eyes, bits of fabric and solid material to provide tactile stimulation, or records and musical instruments to exercise the auditory sense.

Self-image therapy. By means of a group reading of a book, selected by the group, a cohesiveness is developed to provide the geriatric patient with a sense of belonging and security. Then the therapist can help the patient to explore the reality of the patient's self-image, especially if it is distorted, and to develop a sense of self-respect with emphasis on the patient's assets as opposed to liabilities.

Reality therapy. This five step individual therapeutic program concentrates on reinstituting satisfying interpersonal relationships and on satisfying needs in the real world through a rationally formulated plan to alter or change behavior as opposed to a denial of the real world.[53] After a period in which the patient and therapist develop a sense of involvement, the patient is taught to look critically at his or her behavior, judging its worth and benefits to the self and others. In the third step, the patient makes a rational decision to change some behavior. Then the patient and therapist develop a realistic plan to change the target behavior and, finally, implement the plan. This technique is thought to be especially appropriate for the apathetic, dejected, institutionalized aged patient.

• • •

In addition to the techniques just listed, other treatment procedures applied to younger persons may be appropriate for elderly individuals as well. Family or marital therapy may be successful in dealing with intergenerational struggles or in easing the transition of the elderly couple into the postretirement period.[54] Individual counseling conducted by telephone may be the only therapy available to the elderly person with a transportation problem. Sensitivity training or human awareness groups can provide a useful experience to adults of all ages, young and old, who are in search of more meaningful interpersonal relationships. Behavior modification procedures such as desensitization and modeling can be used to reduce anxiety in old age and to institute adaptive behaviors.

In summary, many treatment techniques are appropriate to and successful with the geriatric patient. Psychologic disturbances in later life are not necessarily incurable.

REFERENCES

1. Botwinick, J.: Aging and behavior, ed. 2, New York, 1978, Springer Publishing Co., Inc.
2. Birren, J.E., and Schaie, K.W., editors: Handbook of the psychology of aging, New York, 1977, Van Nostrand Reinhold Co.
3. Granick, S., Kleban, M.H., and Weiss, A.D.: Relationships between hearing loss and cognition in normally hearing aged persons, J. Gerontol. **30**:434, 1976.
4. Crouch, C.L.: The relation between illumination and vision, Illuminating Engineering, **40**:747, 1945.
5. Hirsch, M.J., cited by Weumouth, F.W.: Effect of age on visual acuity. In Hirsch, M.J., and Wick, R.E., editors: Vision of the aging patient, Philadelphia, 1960, Chilton Book Co.
6. Arey, L.B., Tremaine, M.J., and Monzingo, F.L.: The numerical and topographical relations of taste buds to human circumvallate papillae throughout the life span, Anat. Rec. **64**:9, 1936.
7. Hinchcliff, R.: The pattern of the threshold of percep-

tion for hearing and other specific senses as a function of age, Gerontologia **2**:311, 1958.

8. Liss, L., and Gomex, F.: The nature of senile changes of the human olfactory bulb and tract, AMA Arch. Otolaryngol. **67**:167, 1958.
9. Engen, T.: Taste and smell. In Birren, J.E., and Schaie, K.W., editors: Handbook of the psychology of aging, New York, 1977, Van Nostrand Reinhold Co.
10. Schiffman, S., and Pasternak, M.: Decreased discrimination of food odors in the elderly, J. Gerontol. **34**:73, 1979.
11. Kenshalo, D.R.: Age changes in touch, vibration, temperature, kinesthesis, and pain sensitivity. In Birren, J.E., and Schaie, K.W., editors: Handbook of the psychology of aging, New York, 1977, Van Nostrand Reinhold Co.
12. Suedfeld, P.: Introduction and historical background. In Zubek, J.P., editor: Sensory deprivation: fifteen years of research, New York, 1969, Appleton-Century-Crofts.
13. Richman, L.: Sensory training for geriatric patients, Am. J. Occup. Ther. **22**:254, 1969.
14. Arenberg, D., and Robertson-Tchabo, E.A.: Learning and aging. In Birren, J.E., and Schaie, K.W., editors: Handbook of the psychology of aging, New York, 1977, Van Nostrand Reinhold Co.
15. Botwinick, J.: Cognitive processes in maturity and old age, New York, 1967, Springer Publishing Co., Inc.
16. Ankus, M., and Quarrington, B.: Operant behavior in the memory-disordered, J. Gerontol. **27**:500, 1972.
17. Craik, F.I.M.: Age differences in human memory. In Birren, J.E., and Schaie, K.W., editors: Handbook of the psychology of aging, New York, 1977, Van Nostrand Reinhold Co.
18. Hulicka, I.M.: Age differences in retention as a function of interference, J. Gerontol. **22**:180, 1967.
19. Eisdorfer, G.: Arousal and performance: experiments in verbal learning and a tentative theory. In Talland, G.A., editor: Human aging and behavior, New York, 1968, Academic Press, Inc.
20. Hultsch, D.: Adult age differences in the organization of free recall, Dev. Psychol. **1**:673, 1969.
21. Hultsch, D.: Adult age differences in free classification and free recall, Dev. Psychol. **4**:338, 1971.
22. Hulicka, I.M., and Grossman, J.L.: Age-group comparisons for the use of mediators in paired-associate learning, J. Gerontol. **22**:46, 1967.
23. Canestrari, R.E., Jr.: Age changes in acquisition. In Talland, G.A., editor: Human aging and behavior, New York, 1968, Academic Press, Inc.
24. Jerome, F.A.: Decay of heuristic processes in the aged. In Tibbits, C., and Donahue, W., editors: Social and psychological aspects of aging, New York, 1962, Columbia University Press.
25. Ross, E.: Effects of challenging and supportive instructions in verbal learning in older persons, J. Educ. Psychol. **59**:261, 1968.
26. Arenberg, D.: The effects of auditory augmentation on visual retention for young and old adults, J. Gerontol. **32**:192, 1977.
27. Botwinick, J.: Intellectual abilities. In Birren, J.E., and Schaie, K.W., editors: Handbook of the psychology of aging, New York, 1977, Van Nostrand Reinhold Co.
28. Storandt, M.: Age, ability level, and method of administering and scoring the WAIS, J. Gerontol. **32**:175, 1977.
29. Horn, J.L., and Cattell, R.B.: Age differences in fluid and crystallized intelligence, Acta Psychol. **26**:107, 1967.
30. Erikson, E.H.: Childhood and society, ed. 2, New York, 1963, W.W. Norton & Co., Inc.
31. Costa, P.T., and McCrae, R.R.: Objective personality assessment. In Storandt, M., Siegler, I.C., and Elias, M.F., editors: The clinical psychology of aging, New York, 1978, Plenum Press.
32. Cumming, E., and Henry, W.: Growing old: the process of disengagement, New York, 1961, Basic Books, Inc., Publishers.
33. Neugarten, B.L., Havighurst, R.J., and Tobin, S.S.: Personality and patterns of aging. In Neugarten, B.L., editor: Middle age and aging, Chicago, 1968, University of Chicago Press.
34. Maddox, G.L.: Fact and artifact: evidence bearing on disengagement theory from the Duke Geriatrics projects, Hum. Dev. **8**:117, 1965.
35. Lowenthal, M.F., and Haven, C.: Interaction and adaptation intimacy as a critical variable, Am. Sociol. Rev. **33**:1, 1968.
36. Conner, K.A., Powers, E.A., and Bultena, G.L.: Social interaction and life satisfaction: an empirical assessment of late-life patterns, J. Gerontol. **34**:116, 1979.
37. Markides, K.S., and Martin, H.W.: A causal model of life satisfaction among the elderly, J. Gerontol. **34**:86, 1979.
38. Larson, R.: Thirty years of research on the subjective well-being of older Americans, J. Gerontol. **33**:109, 1978.
39. Riegel, K.F., and Riegel, R.M.: A study of changes of attitudes and interests during later years of life, Vita Humana **3**:177, 1960.
40. Okun, M.A., and Elias, C.S.: Cautiousness in adulthood as a function of age and payoff structure, J. Gerontol. **32**:451, 1977.
41. Gynther, M.D., and Shimkunas, A.M.: Age and MMPI performance, J. Consult. Psychol. **2**:118, 1966.
42. Birren, J.E.: The psychology of aging, Englewood Cliffs, N.J., 1964, Prentice-Hall, Inc.
43. Butler, R.N., and Lewis, M.I.: Aging and mental health, ed. 2, St. Louis, 1977, The C.V. Mosby Co.
44. Bengtson, V.L., Cuellar, J.B., and Ragan, P.K.: Stratum contrasts and similarities in attitudes toward death, J. Gerontol. **32**:76, 1977.
45. Kubler-Ross, E.: On death and dying, New York, 1969, Macmillan, Inc.
46. Kinsey, A.C., Pomery, W.B., and Martin, C.E.: Sexual behavior in the human male, Philadelphia, 1948, W.B. Saunders Co.
47. Kinsey, A.C., Pomeroy, W.B., Martin, C.E., and Gebhard, P.M.: Sexual behavior in the human female, Philadelphia, 1953, W.B. Saunders Co.
48. Masters, W.H., and Johnson, V.E.: Human sexual response, Boston, 1966, Little, Brown & Co.
49. Pfeiffer, E., Verwoerdt, A., and Wang, H.: Sexual behavior in aged men and women, Arch. Gen. Psychiatry **19**:753, 1968.
50. Storandt, M., Siegler, I.C., and Elias, M.F., editors: The clinical psychology of aging, New York, 1978, Plenum Press.

51. Barns, E.K., Sack, A., and Shore, H.: Guidelines to treatment approaches: modalities and methods for use with the aged, Gerontologist **13:**513, 1973.
52. Richards, W.S., and Thorpe, G.L.: Behavioral approaches to the problems of later life. In Storandt, M., Siegler, I.C., and Elias, M.F., editors: The clinical psychology of aging, New York, 1978, Plenum Press.
53. Glasser, W.: Reality therapy, New York, 1965, Harper & Row, Publishers.
54. Herr, J., and Weakland, J.: Counseling elders and their families: practical techniques in applied gerontology, New York, 1979, Springer Publishing Co.

CHAPTER 26 · PSYCHIATRIC ASPECTS

Monica D. Blumenthal

The specialty of geriatric psychiatry is not very old, having had its start in 1955 with the seminal work of Martin Roth[1] who differentiated between organic and affective disorders in a psychogeriatric hospital population. The fact that up until that time it had not been clearly understood that these two groups of patients could be distinguished tells us something about the nature of the field. For a long time the development and the practice of geriatric psychiatry have been hindered by many prejudices about the character of mental life in old age. It has been thought, and incorrectly so, that the marked mental decline, which is called *senility* by lay persons, was an inevitable accompaniment of increasing years. Now we know this is not the case, but the legend that it is true has permeated the thinking of many and has often led physicians and their co-workers to assume that nothing can be done for the elderly person who is showing symptoms of mental decline.

There are many differences between geriatric psychiatry and the psychiatry of young people and adults, although there are also many similarities. Many of the illnesses are the same, although some occur more frequently in older people and others are more commonly found among the young. Senile dementia, for example, is found almost exclusively among the former, whereas schizophrenia almost always begins before old age. In this chapter, the most common psychiatric illnesses of the old and the important differences between young and old in patient management will be stressed. Differences between the two groups are due to their history, their social roles, the effect of aging on normal physiology, problems generated by managing multiple illnesses and conditions in one person, and differences in diagnosis and treatment.

Changes in social roles are particularly important in managing older patients and will be considered first in this chapter followed by a discussion of the depressive illnesses, paranoid states, and the irreversible and reversible organic brain syndromes.

CHANGES IN SOCIAL ROLES

Retirement. In the United States, the old have been distinguished by a lack of respect, a lack of money, and a lack of roles. Until very recently, we have had a mandatory retirement policy in this country, which meant that a very high percentage of workers were forced out of their jobs at 65 years of age. In the last few years, laws concerning mandatory retirement have been changed so that retirement has been deferred until age 70 in private industry and indefinitely in government. The effect of previous policies has been that at the present time, only one out of five older men works, and it is expected that the figure will drop to one out of six shortly. This is in contrast to conditions at the turn of the century when two out of every three men who were 65 years old or older were still working. The physician must recognize that the reason most older men do not work is a matter of social policy rather than of personal incapacity. This policy has important effects on the psychologic and social well-being of many who have been affected by it. Not all people are influenced by social policy; private entrepreneurs and some professionals such as physicians have escaped the influence of mandatory retirement, but most workers have been greatly influenced by these regulations.

There are many advantages to having a job, but the greatest of these is the money that can be obtained through work. Elderly couples who still include a wage earner are better off financially than almost all of their fellows. For those who are retired, the sad fact is that income usually drops to one half of preretirement income, an amount which often does not cover the basic necessities of life—food, housing, and medical care. One of the difficulties is that the majority of Americans are dependent on Social Security payments for their major retirement income. For the average person, these payments are small, although they do increase with inflation. Unfortunately, most private retirement plans provide fixed incomes, and those individuals who are fortunate enough to have private pension plans available to them often derive relatively little benefit from them because of the extremely rapid erosion of such incomes by inflation. Poverty among the elderly is pervasive; indeed, one quarter of the over-65 population has an income at or below the official near-poverty level, \$4040 a year for a couple in 1975.[2] The poverty of many older Americans is an important consideration when one is dealing with elderly people. Lack of money may make it impossible for them to pursue favored hobbies, engage in recreational activities, buy medication, or even to pay for adequate diets. There is little doubt that the resulting deprivation can influence a patient's state of mind and even lead to illness due to lack of medication or adequate diet. Not that most older Americans see themselves burdened or put upon by a lack of money; the most common feeling of the old seems to be that they are better off than most of their fellows, a sentiment which is more a tribute to the toughmindedness of the old than to any social or fiscal reality.

Lack of employment has other effects than those engendered by relative poverty. A job in the everyday world is an important source of self-identity for most men and many women. Many people think of themselves in terms of their roles; men often think of themselves in terms of their work roles, and Americans as a whole are apt to favor producers over those who are no longer considered productive. The older individual who has come to the end of his working life may think less of himself because he no longer occupies a productive role. Some exworkers miss the organization and structure given to their time by their occupations; others miss the social aspects of the work place. The loss of structure that a job gives to a person's time may become an important issue in the minor depressions which sometimes follow retirement. The task of the physician in dealing with such a depression may include helping the patient to put a schedule back in his life, to find new social relationships, and to enter new activities. Assisting the patient to think out and follow a regular series of activities, which provide structure for his time, often helps the patient regain a comfortable and satisfying existence. It makes sense for the physician to prescribe activities including exercise and participation in church or hobby groups and senior citizen centers with a view to regularizing the patient's existence and helping him develop a self-imposed structure for his time. The activities should, of course, be congenial and interesting for the patient.

The fact that some patients develop depressive episodes in making the transition to retirement does not imply that most older people are unhappy with retirement. Most people make this change successfully in spite of the fact that some run into genuine psychologic difficulty with this change, just as some young people are troubled by the transitions of adolescence and others fail to negotiate successfully the changes brought about by marriage and parenthood.

Social losses. Other roles are lost by the old besides those associated with working. Many older people suffer attrition of their social circle due to the ravages of illness and bereavement. The loss of social support and social interaction is often crucial for the aging individual. Someone to talk to, someone with whom to share a social hour, a confidant to participate in life's pleasures and problems are important ingredients in successful living. Many older people lose such relationships, and this becomes a critical problem for those who are the last survivors of a diminishing social circle. Relatives are also a major support system for the elderly. However, it is estimated that 20% of older people have no surviving children. It is also known that social support from relatives is a major factor in the wellbeing of older people who suffer from some disability. Very little is known about how older people who have no living children manage, although it is known that older people without living relatives have much higher rates of institutionalization than those who do. The problem of how elderly people without children manage will increase in importance as the cohort of those who were young adults during the great depression pass through old age. Many who struggled through those times had no children or few; many are left now without any.

It is important, if possible, to encourage older people to interact with others and to seek new friends in senior citizen centers, through volunteer organizations, churches, and in the entire array of social activities open to the older individuals. This is simpler, however, for those who are among the young-old, 65 to 75 years of age, than for those who are the old-old, those 75 years and older. Among the latter, at least 42% have difficulties with ordinary activities of everyday living such as bending, walking, or climbing stairs.[3] In addition, among the old-old, there are many who are not able to drive a car and still more who can no longer afford to maintain one. Among these, problems in mobility may substantially interfere with social life and other activities of daily living. Of course many among the old-old are still quite able and some among the young-old have already developed the mobility problems that are more characteristic of the older group; but in general greater age is associated with greater mobility problems. It is helpful for the physician and his co-workers to remember that such problems with mobility may interfere substantially with efforts to resocialize the individual. Making new friends often involves being able to get to new places or to continue activities at old ones and the difficulties with transportation characteristic of most cities and even more suburban communities, coupled with personal mobility problems and the lack of money to take taxis, may create almost insurmountable barriers to the older individual's expanding his dwindling social resources.

Bereavement. For the older person bereavement may be a major problem that can generate or unmask substantial psychiatric difficulties. Whereas the process of mourning is entirely normal as discussed later in this chapter, the physician should be aware that bereavement may produce pathologic grief reactions and that a death in the family may uncover psychologic deficits which were not apparent as long as the marriage endured. Marriage, in addition to its emotional and social meanings, usually carries with it a division of labor, which facilitates the execution of the many activities necessary to sustain life and make it comfortable. We are used to thinking of a division of labor among the married, a sharing of the so-called instrumental roles. Among the middle-aged and older, it is common to find that the wife cooks, does the housework, sews on the buttons, and is responsible for the food shopping while the husband manages the car, the finances, and repairs around the house. As people become older their needs for personal care often increase; an elderly person may not be able to get into the tub without assistance, may be too deaf to answer the phone, or may not be able to read the label of a medication bottle. If the person has been undergoing some deteriorating disease of the brain, he may require considerable assistance from the spouse with decision making and instrumental tasks such as dressing, bathing, and shopping. If death overtakes the more capable spouse, the bereavement may suddenly seem to precipitate the surviving partner into a state of substantial helplessness of rather sudden onset. Such situations pose a difficult problem for the physician, since there is no question that bereavement itself will produce behavioral decompensation in some older people. The question then becomes how much of the behavioral disturbance is a temporary situation caused by stress and grief and how much is an uncovering of behavior already present before the death of the spouse, which had been hidden because the well partner managed the ailing spouse's deficits successfully. The physician must evaluate how much of the deficit can be expected to continue as permanent disability. Usually the best approach to such problems is to take as complete a history as can be obtained from the patient and from some competent outside observer (preferably a close relative) to supply appropriate supports to manage the immediate situation and to wait for the evolution of the case over the next few months. With time the diagnostic issues often become substantially clearer. Such issues will be discussed further in the section on management of the patient with organic brain syndromes.

PSYCHIATRIC DISORDERS

Several major psychiatric disorders are common in old age. These are the affective disorders, the organic mental disorders including both the chronic and acute forms, anxiety disorders, hypochondriasis, paranoid states, medication abuse, and character disorders. Also included are mental illnesses acquired at a much earlier age with which some persons have grown old. Elderly patients with schizophrenia usually fall in this category.

Affective disorders

The affective disorders constitute the most common mental illness of the elderly. The common affective disorders among the old as among the young consist of the major affective disorders, bipolar affective disorder (manic depressive disease), major depressive disorder (either a single episode or recurrent disease), minor affective disorder, chronic depressive disorder, and atypical depressive disorders. For the physician, the most important distinction to be made is the one between a major depressive episode and chronic, probably characterologic, depressive conditions. Recognized and properly treated, a depressive illness need not be more than a passing incident in the life of the older person; misdiagnosed, it leads to invalidism and death.[4,5] Depressive illness is extremely common among the old. Although those over age 65 form fewer than 11% of our population, they account for 25% of our suicides, many probably due to depressive illness.

Symptoms. Many old people with depressive illness have symptoms similar to those found in young persons with depressive illness. Vegetative symptoms found at all ages include loss of appetite, weight loss, sleep disturbance with multiple awakenings during the night and final waking too early in the morning, loss of libido, fatigue, and weakness, not to mention the inevitable constipation. Among the elderly, weight loss may be severe and dramatic. Feelings of sadness, apathy, or irritability; loss of interest in friends and in everyday pursuits; a sense that ordinary activities require great effort; and feelings of self-reproach, helplessness, and worthlessness are among the psychic symptoms of depression common to young and old. When an older patient has such typical symptoms, the diagnosis should be easy. Sometimes, however, older patients with depression have symptoms that differ from those seen among the young.

Older patients who suffer from depressive illness may appear in the doctor's office complaining mainly of physical illness. The illness may affect almost any system, but cardiac, gastrointestinal, or musculoskeletal complaints are most common. The patient may indeed suffer from physical illness referable to the symptoms-generating system, but the patient's complaints are intractable, do not diminish in response to reassurance or appropriate treatment, and seem out of proportion to the degree of illness. Some of these patients will turn out to have a true hypochondriasis, which must be managed by special techniques,[6] but some will respond very well to antidepressive pharmacotherapy and emotional support provided by the physician. Most hypochondriacal elderly patients deserve a trial of antidepressant pharmacotherapy.

In addition to the hypochondriacal presentation of some elderly patients, some patients in this age group develop depressive illnesses that appear to mimic dementias. Memory loss, impaired concentration, and loss of function including personal untidiness are associated with depressive illness in all age groups. Among the elderly such symptoms may become so severe that the patient appears for all the world to be a disoriented dement.[7] Some patients even develop soft neurologic signs such as the inability to perform constructional tasks or mild aphasias.

It is important to remember that untidiness, impaired concentration, and apparent memory loss in a previously well functioning young person always lead to surprise and the suspicion that something is radically wrong, a suspicion that leads to every effort to establish a diagnosis. When symptoms of untidiness, impaired concentration, and memory loss are seen in an old person, however, it is easy to succumb to the notion that the patient is falling prey to a dementing illness or, worse yet, attribute these symptoms to old age, a thought unlikely to lead to strenuous diagnostic effort. So preconceived notions may interfere with our best diagnostic efforts. In any case, patients with so-called depressive pseudodementias are sometimes difficult to distinguish from patients who are suffering from a mild to moderate organic brain syndrome with depressive symptomatology. A trial of treatment with antidepressants is often the best way to clarify the issue.

Elderly patients in contrast to those who are younger seem to be more likely to suffer from serious depressive illness in which the patient becomes almost mute, refuses to eat or drink, and takes to bed. These depressions are life threatening. Most old people tolerate dehydration and malnutrition badly, and serious depressions must be treated promptly in an inpatient setting. Such patients often have delusions, particularly somatic delusions, that is, erroneous beliefs that they have cancer or are suffering from an intractable illness of one kind or another. Sometimes delusions are of guilt, for example, one old man with a psychotic depression believed that he was responsible for the downfall of all the prostitutes in the world. Paranoid delusions are not uncommon in severely depressed elderly patients. Often such delusions include the belief that food and medications are poisoned. Vigorous measures to maintain nutrition and hydration may be required in addition to antidepressants or electroconvulsive shock therapy (ECT).

Drug-induced depression. There are several important considerations in diagnosing depressive illness in elderly patients. The first is the possibility that the depression may be drug induced. Elderly patients often suffer from multiple medical illnesses that are treated with a variety of drugs, many of which may produce depressions. These drugs are outlined below*:

Depression-inducing drugs

1. Analgesics: phenacetin
2. Antianxiety agents and CNS depressants: benzodiazepines
   a. Chlordiazepoxide
   b. Diazepam
   c. Phenobarbital and other barbiturates**
3. Antiarthritic agents
   a. Phenylbutazone
   b. Indomethacin**
4. Antibiotics
   a. Aminoglycosides
   b. Sulfonamides
5. Anticonvulsants
   a. Succinimide derivatives
   b. Carbamazepine (Tegretol)
6. Antihypertensives
   a. Alpha-methyldopa**
   b. Clonidine**
   c. Hydralazine
   d. Propranolol**
   e. Reserpine**
7. Antiparkinsonism drugs
   a. Amantadine
   b. Levodopa
8. Antipsychotics
   a. Phenothiazines, especially fluphenazine
   b. Haloperidol**
   c. Thioxanthenes
9. Appetite suppressants
   a. Amphetamines**
   b. Fenfluramine
   c. Phenmetrazine**
10. Cardiovascular drugs
    a. Digitalis
    b. Procainamide (Pronestyl)
11. Miscellaneous drugs
    a. Alcohol
    b. Choline
    c. Corticosteroids
    d. Disulfiram
    e. Oral contraceptives
    f. Physostigmine
    g. Methyl mercury
    h. Organopesticides

In our experience reserpine has been the most common offender. With the many antihypertensives available, it is hardly ever needed. Indeed, many older people suffer from overtreated hypertension, which can be well controlled with diuretics alone. If a patient with a depressive illness is taking a drug known to cause depression, a good first step is to take the patient off the possibly offending drug. Often the patient will manage nicely without it. In many cases removing the patient from a drug known to cause depression will solve the problem. Signs of diminishing depression will appear in 1 to 2 weeks, often with quite remarkable improvement within a month. Some patients whose depression appears to have been caused by a depression-generating drug will require treatment with a tricyclic antidepressant. In our experience this is particularly true when the offending agent has been reserpine, propranolol, or digoxin.

Depression and physical illness. A second consideration in assessing the older patient with

*From Blumenthal, M.D.: Geriatrics **35**:34, 1980.[12]
Based on data from Hendrie, H.: Psychiatr. Clin. North Am. **1**:3, 1978[8]; Drug induced depression (Editorial), Lancet **2**:1333, 1978[9]; Salzman, C., and Shader, R.I.: J. Am. Geriatr. Soc. **26**:303, 1978[10]; Whitlock, F., and Evans, L.E.J.: Drugs **15**:53, 1978.[11]

**Drugs more frequently implicated as a cause of depression.

depressive illness is whether the depression is associated with a physical illness. There are a number of physical illnesses that appear to generate depressive illness. The approach is to identify the physical illness in question and treat it. Cancer, particularly cancers of the head of the pancreas, endocrinopathies, especially hypothyroidism, hyperthyroidism (which often presents in an apathetic form in this age group), and adrenal dysfunction (both Addison's and Cushing's diseases), all are known to be associated with depressive illness. Hypoglycemia can also lead to a disorder mimicking depressive illness, as can hyperparathyroidism. Clearly the treatment of depression associated with these diseases should consist of a search for the primary disorder and the appropriate treatment for that disease. Often remission of the depression will occur with these measures. The depressive illness may have to be treated in the usual manner if it does not respond to treatment of the primary illness.

Depression often accompanies other illnesses such as rheumatoid arthritis, Parkinson's disease, and diseases of the brain including senile dementia and cerebral arteriosclerosis. In the case of these diseases, the depression must almost always be treated as a separate entity. The illnesses known to be associated with depressive disease are listed below:

Illnesses associated with depressive disease*

- Endocrinopathies and metabolic disorders
  - Hyperthyroidism
  - Hypothyroidism
  - Addison's disease
  - Cushing's disease
  - Diabetes mellitus
  - Hypoglycemia
- Viral infections
  - Influenza
  - Hepatitis
  - Viral pneumonias
- Rheumatoid arthritis: systemic lupus erythematosus
- Cancer: carcinoma of the head of the pancreas
- Central nervous system disorders
  - Parkinson's disease
  - Cerebral arteriosclerosis
  - Senile dementia
  - Normal pressure hydrocephalus
  - Focal lesions of the nondominant lobe
  - Subarachnoid hemorrhage
- Disabling disease of all kinds
- Metal intoxications
  - Thallium
  - Mercury

*From Blumenthal, M.D.: Geriatrics **35**:34, 1980.[12]
Based on data from Hendrie, H.: Psychiatr. Clin. North Am. **1**:3, 1978[8]; Drug induced depression (Editorial), Lancet **2**:1333, 1978.[9]

Depression secondary to disease is often more refractory to treatment than primary depressive illness, although good results can frequently be obtained. In treating a secondary depression, proper attention to the primary illness is essential. In managing depression associated with disability, adequate rehabilitation is crucial. In addition, the patient's social support system must be understood and bolstered as much as possible if the patient with depression and medical illness or disability is to have the best chance at recovery.

Among elderly persons who have symptoms of depressive illness, many will have suffered from obvious precipitating factors. Bereavement; loss of status, prestige, and income; illness; and loss of mobility are but a few of the many events that may precipitate depression. Many older people suffer from a series of losses that culminate in a reactive depression. The presence of precipitating factors should not lead the physician to the conclusion that biologic treatment is unwarranted. Many reactive depressions respond nicely to antidepressant therapy. Nevertheless, some elderly patients will have feelings of existential sadness, which may be entirely appropriate to their situation. Sadness per se is not an illness and should not be confused with the more complex picture presented by affective disorder. Both patients with affective disorders and existential sadness can be helped by the opportunity to ventilate their problems and by practical help with environmental conditions.

There is one other important point: a depressive illness must have an onset. Occasionally, an older patient has many of the symptoms of a depressive disorder, but careful inquiry will uncover the fact that nothing about the patient has really changed. He or she is exactly the way they always were only now, because of some factor such as increasing dependency, someone in the environment wishes to have the patient improved. Such patients are most frequently brought by their families and usually see little wrong with their own behavior. Generally such people are suffering from a defect in their character structure, which is quite acceptable to them even if it is entirely unacceptable to others. When the patient lacks a genuine desire to change, there is usually relatively little that can be done to remedy the situation. Some frank honest discussions with the patient and the family may be helpful, but these are usually more helpful to the family than to the patient. It is important for the physician to recognize patients with character disorders because they will not respond to conventional antidepressant therapy, and there is no point in exposing them to the risks of the drugs. The most that can be hoped for is that with supportive care from the physician these patients will be able to diminish the stridor with which they place their demands on the family so that a slightly more amiable adjustment can be made.

Treatment of affective disorders. The basic management of depressive disorders in the elderly patient is very much like the management of depression in younger patients with some important differences, including modification of dosage schedules and assessment of side effects. The first step is to take an accurate history and allow the patient to ventilate his troubles and difficulties. Many people will improve with such simple measures. Others will not. When the physician has ascertained that neither drug intoxication nor underlying disease is responsible for the depressive episode, pharmacologic treatment of the illness should be considered. As a rule, the tricyclic antidepressants are the drugs of choice. Monoamine oxidase inhibitors can be useful, but compliance problems in elderly persons are substantial and the risk of drug interactions or drug-food interactions is higher than with tricyclic drugs. Electroconvulsive therapy is often the safest, most effective treatment of serious depression in this age group, but it is rarely the first treatment used mainly because there is so much prejudice against it.

The appropriate therapeutic dose for the older person shows much greater variability than is true for younger persons, and the maximum dose must be approached much more cautiously. While young and middle-aged people can readily be started on 75 mg per day of a tricyclic such as imipramine or amitriptyline, it is well to start the elderly person on as little as 10 mg twice daily. This dose can be increased to 10 mg three times a day in 2 or 3 days, followed by 10 mg four times a day after which the patient can be increased to 50, 75, 100, and 150 mg daily. Tricyclic drugs are best administered in divided doses to the older person, since side effects, particularly orthostatic hypotension, may be associated with blood level peaks of the drug, which are considerably higher if a single daily dose is adopted. Some older patients will require higher doses of tricyclic antidepressants than these, but the vast majority of patients will develop limiting side effects long before high doses are reached, and many will recover from their depressive illnesses on daily doses of as little as 40 mg of tricyclic daily. Determining the appropriate dose depends mainly on the appearance of intolerable side effects.

Side effects of tricyclic antidepressants. In choosing a tricyclic antidepressant several things should be kept in mind. Clinicians often choose amitriptyline for its sedating side effect in patients who show depression and agitation and imipramine for patients who show psychomotor retardation. These drug choices are appropriate for the old as well as the young, but the anticholinergic side effects of the drug may be a more important consideration in some patients than the sedating side effects. The anticholinergic activities of tricyclics are responsible for some of the more serious side effects produced by these drugs and these can be particularly dangerous in the elderly—urinary hesitancy leading to urinary obstruction, exacerbation of glaucoma, constipation and occasional ileus, and more distressing than these, the development of anticholinergic psychoses, which may mimic worsening depressive illness. Following is a list of the commonly used antidepressants in order of their anticholinergic effects*:

- Most anticholinergic
  - Amitriptyline (Elavil)
  - Nortriptyline (Aventyl)
  - Doxepin (Sinaquan)
  - Imipramine (Tofranil)
- Least anticholinergic: desipramine (Norpramin, Pertofrane)

Desipramine, which is the least anticholin-

*From Blumenthal, M.D.: Geriatrics **35**:34, 1980.[12] Based on data from Synder, S., and Yamamura, H.I.: Arch. Gen. Psychiatry **34**:236, 1977.

ergic of the available tricyclics, is not currently available in a 10 mg tablet and so is not practical for some geriatric patients who cannot tolerate 50 mg a day but require more than 25. The physician should be aware of other anticholinergic drugs that the patient is taking so that a combined regimen, which includes several anticholinergic drugs, does not tip the patient into a toxic confusional state.

A second major side effect of the tricyclic antidepressant drugs is orthostatic hypotension in a substantial number of patients. Many elderly patients suffer from idiopathic orthostatic hypotension, and still more have orthostatic hypotension caused by disease or drugs used to control various medical problems. Asymptomatic orthostatic hypotension is not necessarily directly dangerous to the patient, but it does increase the risk of stroke, myocardial infarction, and other diseases resulting from low perfusion pressures. Symptomatic orthostatic hypotension, in which the patient complains of dizziness on standing or getting out of bed or when being raised from a lying to a standing posture, can be destructive to the patient. Falls, which frequently result in fracture, are a major health hazard to the elderly. In addition, the patient who suffers from dizziness on rising is likely to suffer a loss of confidence, to become less mobile, and to develop an unnecessary level of invalidism. Every elderly patient receiving tricyclic medication should have regular assessments of orthostatic hypotension; that is, the patient's blood pressure should be obtained in the lying position after 5 minutes rest and then in the standing position within the first 60 seconds after rising. A drop of greater than 25 mm mercury systolic, or 10 mm diastolic, or a complaint of dizziness elicited from the patient immediately after standing all require a reduction in dose. Often if the patient is followed closely, he will develop tolerance to the side effects of the drug and drug doses can be increased later. Doxepin is said to produce the least orthostatic hypotension and amitriptyline the most.[14]

The tricyclic antidepressants are well known to have cardiac effects; in particular, they may exacerbate some arrhythmias (although in some cases they may have an antiarrhythmic effect). The drugs decrease the inotropic action of the heart and so may aggravate congestive heart failure. They are likely to increase conduction time.[15,16] Congestive heart failure, left bundle branch block, and premature ventricular beats are generally thought to be contraindications to the use of these drugs. The contraindications should not be regarded as absolute if tricyclics are needed to alleviate a serious depression, which does not respond to ECT, or if the patient suffers from relapse a short time after ECT. Under the circumstances tricyclics may be used in patients whose cardiac condition would generally preclude the use of these drugs. In these cases, however, the drugs should be instituted in the hospital under careful supervision and monitoring with serial electrocardiograms. In some cases the insertion of a pacemaker may be necessary to make drug therapy possible.

The maximum dose for an older individual must often be determined through an assessment of side effects. In our clinic we usually stop increasing the dose if an orthostatic hypotension of 30 mm Hg systolic supervenes or if the systolic drop is 20 mm and the patient complains of dizziness on standing. Urinary hesitancy can usually be treated with bethanechol chloride, and urinary obstruction is rarely a reason to cease treatment although occasionally it creates a problem. More commonly tricyclics must be stopped because of cardiac complications, particularly the development of first-degree heart block. In such patients a pacemaker may be justified to allow continuation of the treatment. Increased intraocular pressure is rarely a problem.

Lithium is an appropriate drug for the treatment of manic depressive disease in the old as well as in the young. The treatment is more dangerous in the elderly and must be modified if it is to be successful. Starting doses in elderly persons should be no more than 300 mg a day. Loading doses should not be used. The usual therapeutic blood levels of 1.0 to 1.5 mEq/liter of lithium are likely to produce toxic symptoms in the old, and it is best to maintain blood levels between 0.5 and 0.7 mEq. Some octogenerians will show a therapeutic response at drug levels as low as 0.3 mEq. Blood levels should be followed every second or third day while therapeutic levels are being developed and once a month thereafter. Lithium excretion is directly proportional to creatinine clearance, which is often reduced in the older patient, and daily maintenance doses of 150 to 600 mg are usual in this age group.

Symptoms of lithium toxicity include nausea, vomiting, diarrhea, tremors, light-headedness, and confusion. In older patients confusional states occur more frequently than in younger people and may occur even with the individual's blood levels in the therapeutic range. This side effect often requires the cessation of treatment.

Electroconvulsive shock therapy (ECT). When tricyclic medication cannot be taken or produces no effect, ECT should be undertaken. The risks of the procedure are very little over and above the risks of the anesthesia and the muscle relaxation necessary to carry out the shock treatments. It is well tolerated by most elderly patients, the risk being mainly the risk of anesthesia. It is probably safer for many patients than the tricyclic antidepressants; however, the treatment has had such a "bad press" that many patients are fearful of it and refuse it as an initial treatment.

Memory loss and disorientation are common side effects of ECT during treatment; however, these tend to remit quickly, particularly when the newer techniques of ECT involving only unilateral, nondominant treatments are used. Contemporary methods of applying shock under anesthesia with muscle relaxation have eliminated much of the fear and all of the danger of fracture and injury that attended methods used several decades ago. Nevertheless, many persons still feel very apprehensive about the idea of ECT and require much reassurance before they will consent to it. In spite of this, the treatment may be lifesaving in patients who are suicidal or who are suffering from dehydration and malnutrition concomitant to severe psychomotor retardation or paranoid delusions involving food and water. Many patients will relapse rather quickly after ECT and require maintenance tricyclic therapy to maintain their remission.

Paranoid states

It is not unusual for an older person to display paranoia, which may vary from mild suspiciousness to a flamboyant delusional system. Paranoia in itself is not diagnostic of anything, and the syndrome has been recently reviewed by Eisdorfer.[17] Paranoid states and psychoses may occur in isolation, or they may be accompaniments of depressive illness, late onset schizophrenia, or organic brain syndromes. The treatment must vary with the underlying illness.

In all cases of paranoia, and particularly in those where there is neither depressive illness nor an underlying organic brain syndrome, it is important for the physician to establish rapport with the patient. For this reason, it is best not to confront the patient with his delusional system directly, since the patient is likely to find this highly threatening and will tend to sever his relationship with the physician when confrontation is used as a mode of approach early in the treatment. Nevertheless, the physician should not commit the contrary error of reinforcing the patient's delusions by agreeing with the patient and pretending that the delusions are correct. The best approach is to reassure such patients that you understand their ideas are very real to them and may be very frightening, but that you yourself do not share the notion that they are correct. It is important to convey to the paranoid patient that you are genuinely interested in his welfare and are going to try to help him. Having established rapport with the patient, the physician must then assess the individual carefully to see if the source of the delusions can be identified. If the patient is worried that someone is stealing his money, and it is obvious that there has been some confusion in the patient's financial affairs, it may be helpful to provide the patient with realistic assistance.

It is also helpful to assess the extent of the paranoia. Some patients will have mild symptoms, which consist mainly of the patient suspecting thievery while searching for articles that have been misplaced or lost. Such patients often respond to explanations and reassurance. Some patients exhibit only suspiciousness that may be based in reality. Complaints that children are trying to obtain the patient's money, that potential employers are prejudiced against people of their age, and that agencies have no interest in their case must always be taken seriously. Children do sometimes steal their parent's money, employers are often prejudiced, and agencies do show disinterest in their clients. Environmental manipulations in such situations may be quite helpful.

Other patients show highly organized delusional systems. These patients may or may not have additional evidence of thought disorder, disturbed affect, or hallucinations. Some of these patients will have a history suggestive of depression. Others will show a pattern of thinking similar to that of schizophrenia, while a third group will manifest cognitive changes characteristic of organic brain syndromes. In each case, treatment of the paranoia requires dealing with the underlying disease as well as with the paranoid symptoms. In many cases, especially those patients treated as outpatients, the use of neuroleptic drugs will be necessary although reassurance should always be tried first. If the patient suffers from an underlying organic brain syndrome, the dosage of neuroleptic required will probably be very small: 0.5 to 4 mg of haloperidol daily, 2 to 5 mg of thiothixene, or 50 to 100 mg of thioridazine may be ample.

When the patient is not suffering from an organic brain disorder or a depression but the paranoid state appears de novo, the situation with regard to drug treatment may be quite different with drug doses approaching those used in younger people. The relationship of paranoid psychosis in old age to the schizophrenias that occur in younger people is problematic, since the etiology of the former is not well understood. There does appear to be an association between paranoid psychosis and deafness. The constellation of a fairly serious psychosis occurring in older people has been noted by the British who have labeled the syndrome *paraphrenia;* these older people have had a lifelong history of being somewhat peculiar and suspicious and in a large majority of the cases are deaf.[18] The literature indicates that treatment may be difficult and the outcome poor, but so far the condition has not been sufficiently studied to allow one to draw any definite conclusions.

Many paranoid patients respond well to supportive care, environmental manipulation, and neuroleptics. Institutionalization is rarely required, but often the patient will require extended contact with the physician. Elderly paranoid patients are rarely dangerous but are often frightened and anxious. Like younger paranoid patients they usually welcome relief from their symptoms, and it is often difficult to establish a relation of trust between patient and physician. A devoted family member who encourages the patient to pursue treatment and accompanies the patient to the clinic can be of extraordinary assistance to the physician in the management of such cases.

Anxiety states

Anxiety states are common in the elderly, althought at least one author has suggested that they are less common than one might expect.[19] Little is known about the epidemiology of disorders or whether the old are more subject to anxiety than the young, but anxious elderly people are common in clinical practice. Symptoms in this age group may be quite variable. Some patients will present with circumscribed phobias—fears of going out alone, of riding in elevators, and of staying by oneself (especially at night) are common. Some anxious patients will present with nonspecific symptoms only: general complaints of "nerves" and feelings of going to pieces, falling apart, apprehension, and anxiety. Attempts to make the patient specify the source of the feelings may be fruitless. Other patients present largely with somatic complaints; concerns related to cardiac function, bowel function, and genitourinary symptoms are particularly common. Still other patients present with mainly motor symptomatology, such as sweating, tremor, dry mouth, and blurring of vision. In all cases the patient is uncomfortable and, nowadays at least, generally expresses a strong desire to have the physician do something about it.

Like the paranoid syndromes, anxiety per se is not the diagnosis of any particular condition and is a frequent concomitant of other psychiatric disorders. Anxiety can be a prominent part of depressive illness, particularly of the agitated depressions. Consideration of whether or not the patient has a depressive disorder should always be an important part of the evaluation of the anxious older patient. Anxiety is also common in patients with organic brain disease. This may be particularly confusing early in the illness when cognitive symptomatology is not marked. Since patients with organic brain disease tend to tolerate the minor tranquilizers and sedatives poorly, a careful search for cognitive impairment should always be conducted in the elderly patient.

Anxiety can also be a major symptom of physical illness in the elderly, so a careful search for physical disease is as important for the elderly patient with anxiety as it is for the elderly individual with an apparent organic brain syndrome. This is particularly true in the patients with somatic manifestations such as palpitations, which may be due to intermittent arrhythmias and which can be caused by neurologic disease, genitourinary symptoms, and preoccupation with the bowels, which may be secondary to changes produced by diverticulitis or neoplasm among others.

In approaching the elderly anxious patient,

the physician should develop interviewing habits that are conducive to obtaining good rapport with the patient. An interview with an older patient should be a two-sided affair with a genuine interaction between patient and physician. It is important to set the patient at ease and to convey a genuine sense of warmth and concern. The physician who is too harassed to be able to listen in a relaxed manner or who personally feels pessimistic about the outcome is unlikely to be able to provide the necessary atmosphere of loving concern and relaxation. Any information available to the physician from the social worker or ancillary medical personnel should be shared with the patient and used as tool for further discussion. Older patients are less likely than their younger fellows to be able to present themselves accurately. They are also more likely to leave out important symptoms and to assume that the physician has information that he may not have. They are more likely to attribute pathologic symptoms to age and less likely to have an accurate conception of good health. Any assistance that the physician can give to help the patient develop his story will be greatly appreciated. Older patients tend not to be very psychologically oriented and it is often necessary for the physician to suggest to the patient that feelings are important health issues which need to be discussed.

The older patient, and not only the anxious one, will generally respond favorably to a more informal social atmosphere than is usual in a medical practice. Physical contact in the form of a handshake or a pat on the back or the knee is more welcome by the old than by the young. More than one elderly patient has given me a hug or a kiss, and I have found myself welcoming these demonstrations of affection in spite of the fact that I am generally a somewhat reserved and private person. Somehow these gestures have an entirely different meaning when one is dealing with a 70-year-old than when one is managing someone several decades younger. I often offer the patient a cup of coffee or Sanka during a consultation and turn my time with the patient into a more social occasion than would be appropriate for a younger person. These amenities are particularly important in dealing with the anxious patient for whom a non–drug-oriented approach will frequently be more advisable than reliance on medication.

In assessing the older anxious patient it is important to remember the many losses to which an individual is vulnerable at this time in life. Anxiety may be a response to loss of a friend or a spouse, to reduced income, to impaired health, to diminished reserves, and to a decline in coping capacity.

The old may become anxious because they are afraid they will be burdensome to their family, or they may become anxious because they are afraid there will be no one there to assist them when they need it. However, the older patient may be reluctant to mention these concerns spontaneously and may require substantial encouragement. Nevertheless, anxiety in response to such losses can usually be managed by psychotherapeutic means alone. The opportunity to discuss the situation, the possibility of exploring alternative solutions, and even the chance to describe a difficult situation that must be endured often are sufficient for the elderly patient to be able to gain better control of his anxiety. Usually, however, the amelioration of symptoms does not occur immediately in response to a psychotherapeutic approach but develops over several sessions as the patient develops confidence in the physician and in their relationship.

When the patient is subject to environmental stress, environmental modification may be a useful approach in helping the patient deal with his symptoms. Many patients are concerned that their symptoms imply serious physical illness. An explanation of how the mind can influence the body with emphasis on the extremely common nature of these symptoms is always helpful. Reassurance as to the lack of physical illness or the limitations of its extensiveness is also helpful. The patient is better able to cope with definite information than with vague information or no information at all. Nevertheless, it is always important for the physician to emphasize that the symptoms are real and have a physiologic basis, even though the basis may be a response by the nervous system to stress. Most patients do not accept being told that something is "all in your mind." They can feel their symptoms and know they are real; in spite of this, they can usually accept explanations that teach them how their brain is able to influence physiologic actions.

Many anxious old patients are treated with psychotropic medication, and if the underlying disorder is a depression or an organic brain syndrome, this may well be necessary. Usually psychotropic medication is not necessary if the patient is suffering from an uncomplicated anxiety disorder. It is helpful to remember that the effectiveness of the antianxiety agents is relatively brief and that they should not be extended over indefinite periods of time. Many of the problems of elderly people are long-term and may be expected to continue. In such cases it is much wiser to try a psychotherapeutic approach than to begin the patient on a drug regimen that will have to be terminated when the problem is essentially unchanged. If there is a time-limited stress or if it is thought that the patient will make some psychotherapeutic progress over a period of several weeks or a few months, then it may be helpful to institute a brief trial of minor tranquilizers or sedatives. The antianxiety agents comprise a broad range of drugs including the benzodiazepines (chlordiazepoxide, diazepam, and oxazepam) and the propanediols (meprobamate and tybamate). Several of these are not useful in the elderly. Barbiturates are poorly tolerated and often cause paradoxical reactions. They probably should not be used in the elderly. Meprobamate has a weaker sedative effect than the benzodiazepines, but its addicting potential is close to the therapeutic dose and it is probably not advisable to use this drug on elderly persons. Of the available drugs the benzodiazepines are probably the most useful in the patient who is not suffering from an organic brain syndrome, although the pharmacokinetics of these drugs are probably different in older than in younger people and there is a tendency for these drugs to cause depressive and confusional states. If they are used at all, the patient should be started on very small doses, for example, 2 mg two or three times a day of diazepam or 5 mg three times a day of chlordiazepoxide. Oxazepam has the shortest half-life in the group and may be useful as a hypnotic, although flurazepam (Dalmane) has been more commonly used in this age group.

When anxiety is an accompaniment of organic brain syndrome, it is usually best to treat it with small doses of neuroleptics. Thioridazine is particularly helpful, since it has a sedative action as well as an antianxiety effect. The rationale for using neuroleptics rather than the more conventional antianxiety drugs is that most of the latter tend to exacerbate the confusion and cognitive impairment of this group. More detail about the use of neuroleptics in the patient with organic brain disease is given later in this chapter.

ORGANIC BRAIN SYNDROME

Little that is written about organic brain syndrome is truly useful to the practicing physician. In the past a great deal has been made out of the difference between acute organic brain syndrome and chronic organic brain syndrome. The former was defined as having a sudden onset and as being reversible; the latter as having a slow onset and being irreversible. Unfortunately, the correlation between onset and reversibility is not absolute, and acute brain syndromes can have slow, gradual onset, as when they are associated with anemia. Chronic brain syndromes may have a sudden onset, for example, those that occur after surgery or after shock following cardiac arrhythmias. The terminology has been abandoned by the American Psychiatric Association, but the language and its attendant implications remain to do a considerable amount of damage in practice. The most important distinction that the physician must make is between organic brain syndromes that are reversible and those that are not. This is not always an easy distinction, and it is toward making this distinction that most of our effort will be devoted.

The British have bypassed the confusion implicit in the terms *chronic* and *acute* organic brain syndrome by talking about *brain failure* instead, and it is useful to think in these terms. Brain failure neither implies that the condition is permanent or passing nor that the condition is due to a structural change in the brain. This is excellent for our purposes, since many old people who seem to be suffering from symptoms that might have been called *brain syndrome* are not suffering from any structural change in the brain but have brain failure due to reversible causes.

Characteristics of brain failure. What are the symptoms of brain failure? The outstanding characteristic is one of confusion. The older individual does not know where he is, is not oriented in time, suffers from a memory deficit, is not able to employ his cognitive capacity, seems to be suffering from poor judgment, may show some change in mood, and has an impaired ability to abstract, learn, and be attentive. A set of 10 questions (listed below) has been developed;

these are useful for establishing whether or not the individual is confused.

Where are we now? (place orientation)
Where is this place located? (place orientation)
What month is it? (time orientation)
What day of the month is it? (time orientation)
What year is it? (time orientation)
How old are you? (memory)
When is your birthday? (memory)
Who is president of the United States? (general information and memory)
Who was president before him? (general information and memory)

These ten questions have been used repeatedly, but it should be clear to the physician that the responses to these questions do not necessarily establish whether or not the individual does indeed suffer from an organic brain syndrome. More detailed mental status examinations such as described by Strub and Black[20] are more helpful in assessing the details of cognitive change than are the briefer versions.

Persons with organic brain syndromes are classically described as suffering from disorientation; problems with attention; memory impairment, especially recent memory; judgment impairment; and affective change (often and incorrectly described as having lability of affect, that is, going readily from tears to laughter and back again). They are also described as suffering from a decrease in information, having impaired ability to abstract and losing specific cognitive capacities such as the ability to do mental arithmetic. The individual with a genuine organic brain syndrome, one that is based in structural change in the brain such as that due to senile dementia or multiinfarct dementia, may or may not have any specific symptom. Memory loss is exceedingly common among these patients, and indeed memory loss may be the only symptom, in which case the disorder is referred to as an *amnestic syndrome*. The latter will not necessarily develop into a true dementia, but not all patients who are suffering from a deteriorating disease of the brain have prominent memory loss early in the course of the disease. Symptomatology probably depends on what part of the central nervous system is affected. Some patients have symptoms that can be attributed mainly to deficits in frontal lobe function. Such patients may be profoundly disinterested in activities that used to engage them avidly. They may be untidy and may appear to lose their social graces, and a previously thoughtful individual may appear to become totally insensitive to the people around him. One rabbi's daughter developed a frontal lobe syndrome and took great delight in using mildly obscene words much to the horror of her refined and pious sisters. The patient had not the foggiest notion that her language was in any way upsetting.

Occasionally patients with frontal lobe syndromes become quick tempered and abusive, but often their memories are surprisingly intact in spite of the fact that they may become totally unable to care for themselves because of their profound apathy and inability to plan. One of the major defects in patients with frontal lobe problems is their loss of ability to respond to words normally. Most of us manage our lives by responding to a set of inner verbal instructions; we make lists, develop plans, and use words as guides to organize our behaviors. The patient with frontal lobe damage may lose the ability to respond to such plans, both his own and other peoples. When one makes a request of such a patient, the patient will often say, "Yes, of course" and repeat the request but fail to comply. Such patients may be severely handicapped in spite of the retention of many cognitive abilities.

Other patients suffer from parietal lobe symptomatology. Such patients may have left-right confusion, be unable to calculate, may have serious difficulty with the rules of grammar, forget the names of their fingers, and be unable to understand grammatically complex statements. These deficits may be quite out of proportion to the amount of memory loss from which the patient suffers. The difficulties that characterize such patients are quite different from those afflicting patients with mainly frontal lobe symptoms. Patients with parietal lobe deficits may be highly motivated and work hard at the problems they have been asked to solve. Such patients may manage in their own living situations considerably better than the patient who suffers from the apathy of a frontal lobe syndrome in spite of the fact that the cognitive capacities of the latter appear considerably greater than those of the former.

It had been thought in the past that it was inevitable that all persons would suffer from mental deterioration if they only lived long enough. We know now that such is not the case. The best evidence available seems to indicate that normal old people maintain their intelligence very well except for the last year of life when a decline in intelligence often occurs. It is true that old people seem to undergo a decline in their capacity to solve complex and abstract problems, a characteristic often referred to as fluid intelligence; however, crystallized intelligence or the ability to perform on such tests as vocabulary, general information, social situations, esoteric analogies, arithmetic problems, and controlled associations seem to remain intact with only minimal decline throughout life.[22]

Irreversible brain failure

Unfortunately, a substantial number of older people suffer from progressive intellectual deterioration, about 5% among all those 65 years old and older and about 25% among those 80 and over. There does not appear to be an increase in the number who suffer from such decline after age 80; however, it is now known that such intellectual decline represents illness. The most common cause of decline is senile dementia of the Alzheimer's type or primary neuronal degeneration. It is now generally thought that senile dementia represents the same illness that appears as Alzheimer's disease in those who are somewhat younger. Senile dementia has a definite neuropathologic picture consisting of senile plaques, neurofibrillary tangles, and granulovacular degeneration in the cells. A rough correlation exists between the extent of the pathology and the extent of mental deterioration measured on specific tests of mental function.[23]

The cause of Alzheimer's disease or senile dementia is not known. Several hypotheses concerning its etiology are under investigation. These include aluminum metabolism,[24] immune and autoimmune processes,[25,26] and latent viruses.[27] There may also be a genetic component in some cases.[28] The exact relationship between senile dementia and Alzheimer's disease is not clear. Many clinical and pathologic studies have been unable to distinguish the two, so at the present time clinicians often treat the two conditions as though they were the same illness.

The second major cause of mental decline in late life is multiinfarct dementia. Here the pathologic change is due to multiple infarcts of brain, either because of arteriosclerotic processes or, probably more commonly, due to multiple emboli, most usually from the common carotids or from the heart. Clinically, multiinfarct dementia is not easy to distinguish from senile dementia, but in a typical case the individual with multiinfarct disease is more likely to have a history of stepwise decline in functioning, a history of transient ischemic attacks or small strokes, and associated atherosclerotic disease in the carotids or a cardiac condition such as auricular fibrillation, which lends itself to the development of showers of emboli. Such patients are said to be more likely to have focal neurologic signs and histories of diabetes, hypertension, or hyperlipemia. Patients with multiinfarct disease are said to have a more fluctuating course, that is, to show more variability in their condition from day to day, to be more likely to preserve insight into their condition, and to be more apt to show lability of affect. Few studies correlating clinical conditions with autopsy materials have been carried out so definitive descriptions of the syndrome are yet to be written. In any case, autopsy studies show that among patients who suffer from mental deterioration, about half suffer from senile dementia of the Alzheimer's type, about a fifth suffer from multiinfarct disease, roughly the same number have pathologic findings showing that both diseases contributed to the condition, and the remainder fall into a variety of categories.[29] These studies make it clear that most deteriorating disease in the old is not due to arteriosclerosis as had been thought previously.

It is often considered a truism that senile dementia of the Alzheimer's type begins with a personality change. While this is true for some patients, other patients may have remarkably intact personalities in the face of profound cognitive impairment. Such persons may be deceiving to the casual examiner because their remaining social graces and manners give the appearance of mental intactness. It is important to remember that patients who suffer from true brain disease may present a variable picture, particularly early in the illness. After the illness has run its course, such patients tend to look quite similar with marked disorientation, profound memory loss, severe impairment of the activities of daily living, marked incapacity to abstract or to learn new materials, and often incontinence of both bowel and bladder. Early in their illness, however, such patients may have quite heterogeneous symptoms, and it is important to remember that not all patients progress at the same pace or follow the same course; therefore it is not inevitable that someone who presents initially with mild impairment of memory will reach a terminal state of dementia.[30] It is important to plan for patients as they are rather than as one expects them to be 5 to 10 years in the future. Many patients with moderately severe organic brain syndromes manage quite well in community settings, particularly if there are adequate social supports and the patient is not given to wandering or to dangerous behavior such as fire setting, hostility and abusiveness, or incontinence. It is not necessary for every person with an organic brain syndrome to be institutionalized, and much agony can be prevented if the physician will refrain from making such a suggestion before it is truly necessary.

Reversible brain failure

More important than the differentiation of multiinfarct dementia and senile dementia is the problem of distinguishing between the true degenerative illnesses and the so-called pseudodementias or reversible brain failures. It is important for the physician to understand that in old age confusion or deterioration of mental function often becomes one of the primary symptoms of many systemic diseases. At the same time, the more classic symptoms of illness are apt to disappear or become less dramatic. For example, it is estimated that 25% of persons with digitalis toxicity show confusion, and it may be the major symptom.[31] Similarly, 25% of those with myocardial infarction may have symptoms of confusion and be without chest pain. This tendency for physical illness to present as mental aberration is one that must be constantly in the physician's mind when he deals with older persons, particularly those who are 75 years old or older. Unfortunately decisions about institutionalizing patients have been made when the patient's main problem was not a mental one, but one secondary to physical disease. Some of the major causes of physiologic and pathologic conditions that lead to an appearance of dementia in some patients are listed below:

Causes of reversible pseudodementias

1. Medication
   a. Errors in self-administration
   b. Iatrogenic drug intoxication
2. Metabolic imbalance
   a. Hypercalcemia
   b. Hypocalcemia
   c. Hyperglycemia
   d. Hypoglycemia
   e. Hyperthyroidism
   f. Hypothyroidism
   g. Hypernatremia
   h. Hyponatremia
   i. Azotemia
3. Depressive illness
4. Undernutrition
5. Tumors
6. Hepatic conditions
7. Cardiac conditions
8. Vascular conditions
9. Febrile conditions
10. Pulmonary conditions
11. Postsurgical dementia
12. Posttraumatic dementia
13. Psychosis
14. Sensory deprivation

One of the difficulties in diagnosing reversible brain disease is that there are no symptoms that necessarily distinguish between reversible and irreversible brain failure. If a patient is suffering from a delirium, a condition which generally implies remedial illness, there are helpful signs. For example, the delirious patient generally has a fluctuating level of consciousness. Typically such a person is also hallucinating and delusional, but many persons with a reversible brain syndrome are not delirious, but are fully conscious. Such syndromes are generally referred to as *pseudodementias*. The behavior of people with pseudodementias cannot be systematically distinguished from those with organic brain disease. For this reason, a careful search for causes of reversible brain failure should be undertaken in everyone who presents with cognitive symptomatology.

Drug intoxication. The first and probably most common condition that must be considered when evaluating the patient with brain failure is drug toxicity. Older patients commonly have multiple illnesses and older patients commonly are placed on multiple medications by their physicians. In addition, because of diminishing renal function, liver function, and frequently, a smaller body mass not to mention changes in drug binding and distribution, the older individual is far less able to manage drugs than a younger person who has greater physiologic reserve in his excretory and metabolic capacity.[32] Consequently, older people frequently become drug intoxicated on drug regimens that would be entirely suitable for younger persons. When the drugs become multiple, the likelihood of drug toxicity is multiplied. In our experience, the most common offenders in causing brain failure in older people have been the minor tranquilizers such as chlordiazepoxide (Librium) and diazepam (Valium), sedatives and hypnotics, antihypertensives, digoxin, and the anticholinergics. The major tranquilizers or neuroleptics, such as the phenothiazines and butyrophenones, also present a problem. Usually the patient with drug intoxication is receiving multiple medications. (See chapter 15.)

The physician must also remember that when medication schedules become complex, there is a good chance that the older person will get confused about what pill is to be taken when, and that confusion about the medication schedule may lead to serious errors in self-administration. In addition, the elderly patient in consultation with his friendly local pharmacist may add over-the-counter medications to his regimen, confusing medication issues even further. The first step in the evaluation of the patient with confusion is to take a complete drug history. It is best if the patient brings all the medication he is currently taking with him. When the list of drugs has been completed, the physician must ruthlessly eliminate all that are not essential to the patient's survival. It is amazing how many drugs people can do without. British studies have indicated that of all patients receiving digitalis preparations, 70% no longer required them. It is almost always possible to remove drugs from patients judiciously and cautiously and then to determine, by means of careful monitoring, whether or not they are really needed.

Metabolic disturbances. Next to drugs, the physician must be aware of the possibility that the patient is suffering from a metabolic disturbance. Dehydration with elevated potassium, sodium, and blood urea nitrogen (BUN) is a common problem among older people. Hypokalemia, often secondary to diuretics, is also common. Disturbances in calcium metabolism, both hypocalcemia and hypercalcemia, are less frequent, but sufficiently common that they should be considered. Both hypoglycemia and hyperglycemia may cause a reversible dementia, the latter most often being secondary to diabetes and the former most commonly secondary to overtreatment of diabetic conditions. The older patient is often an individual who eats irregularly and inadequately, making him a poor candidate for insulin and the longer acting oral hypoglycemics. Often older patients continue to take hypoglycemia-inducing medication, irrespective of whether or not they are eating, and the consequences can be seen in confusional states that clear up when the patient's proper regimen is resumed. However, the older person who has become confused due to some reversible cause usually takes a good deal more time to fully regain his mental functioning than it takes for him to lose it. Patience is a good watchword in dealing with this population.

In addition to the metabolic consequences of diabetes, difficulties with thyroid function are quite common in older persons presenting with behavioral problems. Both hyperthyroidism and hypothyroidism can lead to brain failure, and hypothyroidism at least, can lead to permanent dementia if not treated properly and promptly. Hypoparathyroidism and hyperparathyroidism can also lead to a pseudodementia, although they are far less common than thyroid conditions. It should also be remembered that nutritional deficiencies are not unusual in the older patient. Thiamine, folic acid, and vitamin B_{12} may all be deficient, and both calories and protein may be insufficient in the diet. An occasional older person will be found to be scorbutic.

Azotemia also creates a situation in which the patient may present with brain failure. Older people commonly suffer from elevated BUN either due to dehydration, urinary tract infections, or obstructive uropathy either structural or neuropathic. The older patient, like the younger, may develop mental changes secondary to hepatic failure.

Infections. If the patient does not have a metabolic condition that is causing the brain failure, serious consideration must be given to whether or not the person has an infection. Pneumonias, urinary tract infections, and viral infections all can precipitate a confusional state in the older individual. Indeed, since older people often do not develop elevated temperatures or pain with their infections, the infection may be missed unless the clinician makes a careful search for it.

Relatively minor infections can cause a substantial decrease in mental functioning in the vulnerable person.

Decreased cerebral perfusion. Since the brain is an organ that requires 20% of the total circulation to maintain its function, one might suspect that it would be extremely sensitive to physiologic conditions which interfere with its circulation, and indeed it is. Brain failure can be generated by congestive heart failure, myocardial infarctions, pulmonary disease that interferes with adequate oxygenation by the lung, and anemias that reduce the oxygen-carrying capacity of the blood.

The clinician must, of course, be aware of potentially reversible neurologic disease such as syphilis, brain tumors, and meningitis (which may present quite indolently), as well as the relatively rare low pressure hydrocephalus syndrome. More commonly, the astute clinician may discover a subdural hemorrhage secondary to one of the many falls to which this patient population is so susceptible.

Depressive pseudodementia. Having considered all this, the clinician must remember that one of the most common causes of a dementia-like syndrome in patients who do not have an apparent mental illness is depression. It has previously been mentioned in this chapter that depressive illness in some elderly persons is likely to mimic the dementias. When confronted with an individual who appears to be suffering from brain failure, in the absence of overt physical illness and a prolonged downhill course, it is reasonable to consider that the condition may be due to a depressive illness, particularly if the individual shows signs of apathy, irritability, dysphoria, paranoia, or somatic symptomatology. It is also helpful to remember that patients with cerebral vulnerability are likely to be sensitive to drug toxicity and that caution in instituting tricyclic drug therapy is indicated in these patients.

Sensory deprivation. The final situation which should be considered in relation to the organic brain syndromes is that of sensory deprivation. Older people are more likely to suffer from serious visual problems and/or deafness than are those who are younger. It has been demonstrated that there are many persons with visual and hearing deficits among those with severe organic brain syndrome.[33] In addition, it is extremely difficult to evaluate the mental status of someone who can neither see nor hear. Obviously, if the central nervous system does not receive inputs, it cannot respond to them. There is no systematic evidence that persons who have visual and auditory deficits and brain failure will improve if prosthetic devices are supplied, but it seems reasonable that some will do so. It is true that older people who are placed in situations where there are inappropriate or insufficient sensory stimuli will deteriorate rapidly. Recovery room and intensive care units where continuous light and noise are coupled with sedating drugs make it difficult for patients to differentiate between stimuli and background noise, often precipitating confusional states. Elderly people frequently develop deliria in these settings, which resolve when more appropriate stimulation is supplied and sedation is reduced, although sometimes the deliria produced in the recovery room will take several weeks to clear completely.

Assessing reversible brain disease. It is relatively simple to evaluate the patient for pseudodementia provided one uses a systematic approach. It is necessary to measure electrolytes, BUN, serum creatinine, glucose, SGOT, alkaline phosphatase, and serum albumin levels and to do complete blood counts, serum folate and vitamin B_{12}, serology, thyroid function studies, ECG and chest film, in addition to urinalysis and urine culture. A routine medical history and physical examination should be completed as well as a psychiatric evaluation. This relatively simple assessment uncovers most of the causes of reversible brain failure. A few causes of reversible brain failure such as subdural hematomas, brain tumors, and low pressure hydrocephalus will require a more elaborate examination. Patients with a gait disturbance generally deserve the attention of a neurologist unless the physician specializes in geriatric care, as will those patients who show abnormalities on the brief neurologic assessment, which should accompany the medical examination. Such a schema should lead to the discovery of most of the conditions that can produce a pseudodementia. CT scans and EEGs are useful supplements to the routine investigation and should be performed in all patients who have focal neurologic symptoms, localizing cortical signs, a relatively brief duration of illness (less than 4 years), a history of falls, or a history compatible with multiinfarct disease. Whether CT scans should be performed in all patients is a matter for debate, since their considerable expense has led the medical economists to decry their widespread use. Certainly the procedure itself, unlike the invasive tests that it replaces, is never harmful to the patient although a few individuals may be too restless to tolerate it well.

Diagnosis of irreversible brain disease

A diagnosis of a permanent dementing illness should never be made until the presence of reversible brain syndrome has been eliminated. If it is clear that the patient's symptoms cannot be attributed to any intercurrent illness or intoxication, the diagnosis of irreversible brain disease may be made. It is probably a mistake to assign a definite etiology to the brain disease while the patient is still alive. The most common cause of irreversible brain disease will be senile dementia of the Alzheimer's type. This illness usually begins slowly and insidiously, often with a personality change or with memory loss. It often progresses to a stage where more focal symptoms predominate, and it is not unusual for the patient to develop language disorder, apraxias, and other localizing cortical signs before severe and global dementia begins. The decline is generally gradual and without sudden changes, although the course may be quite variable in length. Unfortunately, the natural history of senile dementia of the Alzheimer's type has not been well described, and relatively little is understood about early or mild cases.

If the patient has a picture consistent with multiinfarct dementia, that diagnosis must be considered, although again, the diagnosis cannot be made with certainty until autopsy unless infarcts are present on CT scans, which is not always the case. If the patient has a history of heavy alcohol intake, the diagnosis of organic brain syndrome secondary to alcoholism must be considered. If the patient also has parkinsonism, dementia secondary to Parkinson's disease must be considered as a diagnostic possibility, although it may be that eventually research will determine that the dementia accompanying Parkinson's disease is only an associated Alzheimer's dementia.[34] Pick's disease is another degenerative disease of the brain, which may begin in later life although it is most likely to have its origin between the ages of 50 and 60 years. Pathologically, it is characterized by marked atrophy of the frontal and temporal lobes. Clinically, the illness is likely to start with frontal lobe symptomatology, although in practice it is difficult to distinguish from senile dementia of the Alzheimer's type. Huntington's chorea, another cause of degenerative brain disease, is extremely rare although possible in old age. This illness is usually accompanied by a movement disorder and a strong family history. Equally rare is Creutzfeldt-Jakob disease, which usually runs a rapid course with approximately half the patients being dead within 9 months and the great majority within 2 years. The physician should also consider the possibility of Wernicke-Korsakoff's psychosis, which may be a consequence of alcoholism.

Management of the demented patient

Management of the patient with a true organic brain disease or irreversible brain failure presents a challenge worthy of the physician's best efforts.[35] The first step in management is to develop a detailed picture of the patient's illness. This involves not only information concerning physical illness discussed earlier under the reversible brain syndromes, but also information about the patient's living situation, social supports, and capacity to manage activities of daily living in the home environment. The deteriorating patient who lives with a healthy and willing spouse or child presents a very different management problem from an individual with the same capacities who lives alone or with an individual who is also in deteriorating health. These considerations are important because often persons with deteriorating brain disease are in their eighties or even older; their children, as well as their spouses, may be suffering from a variety of physical, mental, and financial problems common in older persons. Sometimes the social, physical, and mental problems of the caretakers are sufficiently severe that they are unable to provide caretaking services. The social and economic resources of the caretaking system all must be taken into account before a suitable plan can be made. The assistance of a social worker skilled in managing the problems of the elderly is an invaluable asset in this process.

Having evaluated the capabilities of the patient's social supports, it is important to assess how the patient's disabilities fit with the capacities of the support system. Obviously, if the patient requires assistance with bathing and if the caretaker has arthritis which prevents him or her from bending over, help must be supplied if this patient is to be comfortably maintained at home. If the patient has lost the capacity to drive and the patient's wife has never learned, it may be necessary to make some arrangements by which the wife can be brought to a store so that she can manage her shopping. If ample social resources are available to provide support for a caretaker whose charge requires incessant watching, the situation is quite different from the one in which the caretaker is housebound by the mentally ailing charge. In the latter case, arrangements should be made if it is at all possible to provide relief so that the caretaker can maintain his own well-being by periodic escapes from the caretaking situation.

In managing the patients themselves, careful attention should be paid to their physical well-being. Just as physical illness can produce pseudodementia in a patient who is not suffering from degenerative brain disease, the presence of a physical illness or of a drug intoxication can exacerbate the behavioral deficits of the individual with true disease of the central nervous system. Maintaining these people in optimal physical health often makes the difference between their being able to manage in the community or not. Overmedication is particularly harmful to these patients whose central nervous systems seem to be extremely sensitive to drug toxicity. Having considered the patient's physical health, the physician should determine whether or not the brain failure is being aggravated by the presence of a concurrent depression. If the patient shows depressive symptomatology, a cautious trial of tricyclic antidepressants is in order. Often a patient will respond remarkably to such a regimen.

Psychosis superimposed on the organic brain syndrome is another factor likely to make the patient decompensate. The presence of hallucinations, delusions, and paranoia is almost always an indication for psychopharmacologic treatment. Often patients will show a considerable improvement in their cognitive capacity when their psychoses are brought under control. Again, modest drug doses are in order. Haloperidol, 0.5 to 4 mg twice a day, and 25 to 150 mg thioridazine per day given in divided doses are indicative of the dose range that is generally useful. The physician should choose a neuroleptic on the basis of the side effect. Drugs such as trifluoperazine are likely to produce parkinsonism in elderly patients and are best avoided. In many patients, the parkinsonism produced is reminiscent of idiopathic Parkinson's disease with its associated retropulsion and falling. This side effect may become extremely difficult to manage and will not necessarily disappear when drugs are discontinued. Thioridazine is likely to cause orthostatic hypotension, a problem that can be managed if drug doses are increased slowly and orthostatic hypotension is carefully monitored. It has the advantage of being somewhat sedating, a characteristic which may be desirable in the management of an agitated, hyperactive patient. Haloperidol is usually less sedating. For reasons which are not entirely clear, haloperidol and thioridazine have been the most used drugs in the elderly in the United States, but both drugs are effective and useful. Haloperidol, however, may be more likely to produce tardive dyskinesia because of its high affinity for dopaminergic receptors and should be used with caution.

A third difficulty, which can sometimes be managed by the judicious use of neuroleptics, is the problem of day/night confusion, which often occurs together with a fourth serious problem, wandering. Many patients who are severely deteriorated develop disturbances in their day/night patterns of wakefulness. Such patients may wander around the house intermittently all through the night, causing the family considerable distress due to loss of sleep. Small doses of thioridazine at night may be quite effective in providing the patient and family a good night's sleep. Usually 25 to 100 mg is sufficient. Other sedating neuroleptics are equally useful.

Wandering is a symptom that develops quite frequently in patients with severe organic brain syndromes. These patients develop the urge to walk. They are apt to set out on their journeys any time of day or night, and they are likely to get lost once they have left familiar surroundings. Frequently, they are returned by the police. This situation often causes the family a great deal of distress, since such patients must be watched constantly. Wandering is a condition which can often be controlled by late afternoon, early evening neuroleptics such as thioridazine.

It should be remembered that the barbiturates, nonbarbiturate hypnotics, and the diazepam sedatives are all best avoided in this group of patients. The barbiturates are likely to cause paradoxical responses, and sedatives and hypnotics are likely to impair cognitive functioning still further.

More important than anything else in managing these patients is the support, education, and encouragement that the physician can provide the family. It is difficult to care for a mentally deteriorating person, and this care may be physically wearing and psychologically devastating. After all, the disoriented person who no longer knows his spouse may have been once the mainstay of the caretaker's existence. In the United States, it is often difficult and sometimes impossible to find a placement or assistance with home care for the severely impaired individual, particularly if he is doubly incontinent. The physical and emotional resources of the family may be stretched beyond belief. Even if the physician is not able to provide material assistance, his understanding ear may make the difficult and strenuous task of caretaking easier for the distraught family. The physician can usually help the patient's familiy to understand the nature of the patient's condition. Many families are profoundly puzzled by neuropsychologic deficits such as apathy, perseveration, and personality change. Explanations of the relation between brain and behavior and discussions of what may be expected of the patient may be extremely helpful to the family.

SUMMARY

Elderly people are particularly vulnerable to mental illness. Much mental illness in this age group is complicated by physical illness and its treatment, and much of mental illness is amenable to treatment and amelioration. The basic elements of the evaluation of mental change in the older person must include a thorough medical evaluation, a good drug history, and a careful psychiatric assessment. A careful social evaluation is an integral part of the assessment. The conscientious physician will find that it is possible to do a good deal for many patients, and their families will greatly appreciate his efforts.

REFERENCES

1. Roth, M.: The natural history of mental disorder in old age, J. Ment. Sci. **101**:281, 1955.
2. National Council on the Aging, Inc.: Fact book on aging: a profile of America's older population, Washington, D.C., Feb., 1978, The National Council on the Aging, Inc.
3. Nagi, S.Z.: An epidemiology of disability among adults in the United States. Milbank Mem. Fund Q., Fall, 1976, pp. 439-467.
4. Post, F.: The functional psychoses. In Isaacs, A., and Post, F., editors: Studies in geriatric psychiatry, New York, 1978, John Wiley & Sons, Inc., pp. 77-94.
5. Hall, P.: Differential diagnosis and treatment of depression in the elderly, Gerontologia Clinica **16**:126, 1974.
6. Busse, E., and Pfeiffer, E.: Mental illness in later life, Washington, D.C., 1973, American Psychiatric Association.
7. Post, F.: Dementia, depression and pseudodementia. In Benson, D., and Blumer, D., editors: Psychiatric aspects of neurologic disease, New York, 1975, Grune & Stratton, Inc., pp. 99-120.
8. Hendrie, H.: Organic brain disorders: classification, the "symptomatic" psychoses, misdiagnosis, Psychiatr. Clin. North Am. **1**:3, 1978.
9. Drug induced depression (Editorial), Lancet **2**:1333, 1977.
10. Salzman, C., and Shader, R.I.: Depression in the elderly. II. Possible drug etiologies: differential diagnostic criteria, J. Am. Geriatr. Soc. **26**:303, 1978.
11. Whitlock, F., and Evans, L.E.J.: Drugs and depression, Drugs **15**:53, 1978.
12. Blumenthal, M.D.: Depressive illness in old age: getting behind the mask, Geriatrics **35**(4):26, 1980.
13. Snyder, S.H., and Yamamura, H.I.: Antidepressants and the muscarinic acetylcholine receptor, Arch. Gen. Psychiatry **34**:236, 1977.
14. Goldberg, H.L., and Finnerty, R.J.: Cardiovascular effects of tricyclics. Presented as a Scientific Exhibit at the American College of Physicians 60th Annual Session, San Francisco, Calif., March 26-29, 1979.
15. Carney, M.W.P.: Comments: tricyclics and the heart, Br. J. Psychiatry **134**:637, 1979.
16. Jefferson, J.W.: A review of the cardiovascular effects and toxicity of tricyclic antidepressants, Psychosom. Med. **37**:160, 1975.
17. Eisdorfer, C.: Paranoia and schizophrenic disorders in later life. In Busse, E.W., and Blazer, D.G., editors: Handbook of geriatric psychiatry, New York, 1980, Van Nostrand Reinhold Co., pp. 329-337.
18. Bridge, T.P., and Wyatt, R.J.: Paraphrenia: paranoid states of late life. I. European research, J. Am. Geriatr. Soc. **28**:193, 1980.
19. Jarvik, L.F.: Anxiety and stress in the aged. In Diagnosis and treatment of anxiety in the aged. I. Anxiety in the aged. A symposium sponsored by the Department of Psychiatry, University of Arizona College of Medicine, and the Professional Services Department of Roche Laboratories, Division of Hoffman-LaRoche, Inc., Tucson, Ariz., Nov. 16-17, 1977.
20. Strub, R.L., and Black, F.W.: The mental status examination in neurology, Philadelphia, 1977, F.A. Davis Co.

21. Luria, A.R.: The working brain: an introduction to neuropsychology, New York, 1973, Basic Books, Inc.
22. Botwinick, J.: Intellectual abilities. In Birren, J.E., and Schaie, K.W., editors: Handbook of the psychology of aging, New York, 1977, Van Nostrand Reinhold Co., pp. 580-605.
23. Blessed, G., Tomlinson, B.E., and Roth, M.: The association between quantitative measures of dementia and of senile change in the cerebral grey matter of elderly subjects, Br. J. Psychiatry **114**:797, 1968.
24. Crapper, D.R., and DeBoni, U.: Aluminum and the genetic apparatus in Alzheimer disease. In Nandy, K., and Sherwin, I., editors: The aging brain and senile dementia, New York, 1977, Plenum Press, pp. 229-246.
25. Cohen, D., and Eisdorfer, C.: Serum immunoglobulins and cognitive status in the elderly. I. A population study, Br. J. Psychiatry **136**:33, 1980.
26. Nandy, K.: Immune reactions in aging brain and senile dementia. In Nandy, K., and Sherwin, I., editors: The aging brain and senile dementia, New York, 1977, Plenum Press, pp. 181-196.
27. Gajdusek, D.C.: Unconventional viruses and the origin and disappearance of kuru, Science **197**:943, 1977.
28. Larsson, T., Sjogren, T., and Jacobson, G.: Senile dementia. A clinical, sociomedical and genetic study, Acta Psychiatr. Scand. (Suppl. 167) **39**:1, 1963.
29. Tomlinson, B.E.: Morphological changes and dementia in old age. In Smith, W.L., and Kinsbourne, M., editors: Aging and dementia, Jamaica, New York, 1977, Spectrum Publications, pp. 25-56.
30. Nott, P.N., and Fleminger, J.J.: Presenile dementia: the difficulties of early diagnosis, Acta Psychiatr. Scand. **51**:210, 1975.
31. Brocklehurst, J.C.: Textbook of geriatric medicine and gerontology, ed. 2, New York, 1978, Churchill Livingstone, Inc.
32. Vestal, R.E.: Drug use in the elderly: a review of problems and special considerations, Drugs **16**:358, 1978.
33. Kay, D.W.K., Beamish, P., and Roth, M.: Old age mental disorders in Newcastle upon Tyne. II. A study of possible social and medical causes, Br. J. Psychiatry **110**:668, 1964.
34. Boller, F., Mizutani, T., Roessmann, U., and Gambetti, P.: Parkinson disease, dementia and Alzheimer disease: clinicopathological correlations, Ann. Neurol. **7**:329, 1980.
35. Miller, E.: The management of dementia: a review of some possibilities, Br. J. Soc. Clin. Psychol. **16**:77, 1977.

CHAPTER 27 · OPHTHALMIC ASPECTS

David W. Meltzer

The importance of vision for the maintenance of a normal way of life is obvious, and a change in vision is usually evident to that affected individual. He may seek medical assistance earlier than he would for slowly developing disease elsewhere in the body.

The conditions causing the deterioration of vision in the aged are of several different varieties. There may be functional changes such as modification of the patient's refractive status. Increasing need for glasses with advancing years has become one of the most universally accepted manifestations of aging. Senile tissue degenerations, which are easily recognized and constitute some of the most characteristic signs of aging, are obvious around the eyes, occurring in the tissues of the lid, the orbit, and the conjunctiva. Distinct pathologic lesions in the eye are often the cause of visual disturbances, and some of these, particularly vascular lesions, are manifestations in the eye of systemic disease. Others, such as glaucoma and cataract, are characteristic of the eye.

EXTERNAL CHANGES

Although it does not profoundly affect vision as do most eye conditions, senile atrophy of the various tissues surrounding the eyeball is characteristic of the aging process and may cause a distinct change in facial appearance. The tissues of the lids and orbit may become atrophic, resulting in drooping of the lids, exaggerated wrinkles, entropion, or inturning of the lower lid (Fig. 27-1), or ectropion, or eversion (Fig. 27-2).

The lids are subject to the usual tumors of the skin, some of which are encountered more frequently in the elderly patient. Benign tumors include seborrheic keratoses, cutaneous horns, and keratin cysts. Xanthelasma is a cutaneous deposition of lipid material occurring most commonly at the inner portion of the lids (Fig. 27-3). Basal cell carcinoma is the most common neoplasm of the lids, and its frequency increases with age (Fig. 27-4).

Atrophic changes of the conjunctiva may cause conjunctivitis with secondary infection. A most annoying result of this is profuse shedding of tears, which is so frequently observed in very elderly persons.

Two benign lesions of the conjunctiva that occur more frequently in aged persons than in younger individuals are pinguecula and pterygium. Pinguecula is a benign, degenerative, slightly elevated, yellow mass at the limbus (corneoscleral junction), usually on the nasal side. Pterygium is a benign triangular fold of conjunctiva, which may progress onto the cornea and reduce vision (Fig. 27-5).

Conjunctival tumors, which occur more frequently in the elderly than in younger individuals, include benign papillomas, carcinoma in situ (often referred to as "Bowen's disease"), and squamous cell carcinoma. The benign papillomas and the carcinoma in situ lesions are relatively common in a busy ophthalmologic practice, whereas squamous cell carcinoma is, fortunately, quite rare.

Continued transparency of the cornea is necessary for good vision. Most corneal disease cannot be considered to be primarily the result of aging. The deposition of lipid material around the periphery of the cornea gives rise to the characteristic arcus senilis, which does not interfere with vision (Fig. 27-6).

Idiopathic dystrophic changes of the corneal endothelium characteristically occur in the fifth

□ I wish to express my gratitude to Dr. T.E. Sanders and Dr. M.E. Smith who authored earlier editions of this chapter. The majority of the earlier text remains.

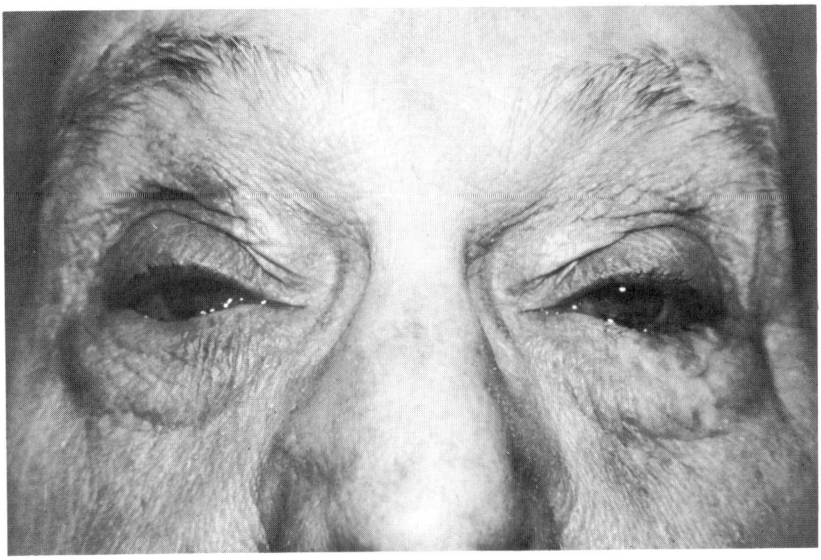

Fig. 27-1. Senile entropion of both lower lids.

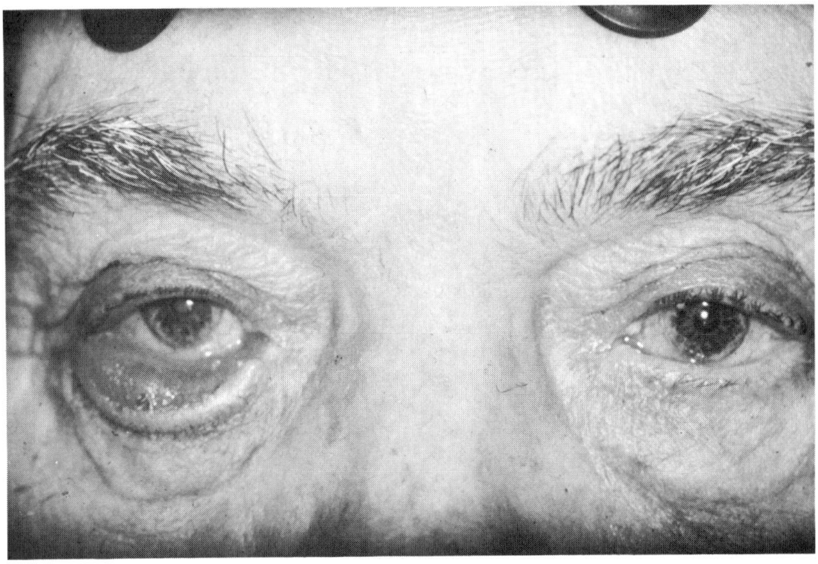

Fig. 27-2. Ectropion of the right lower lid.

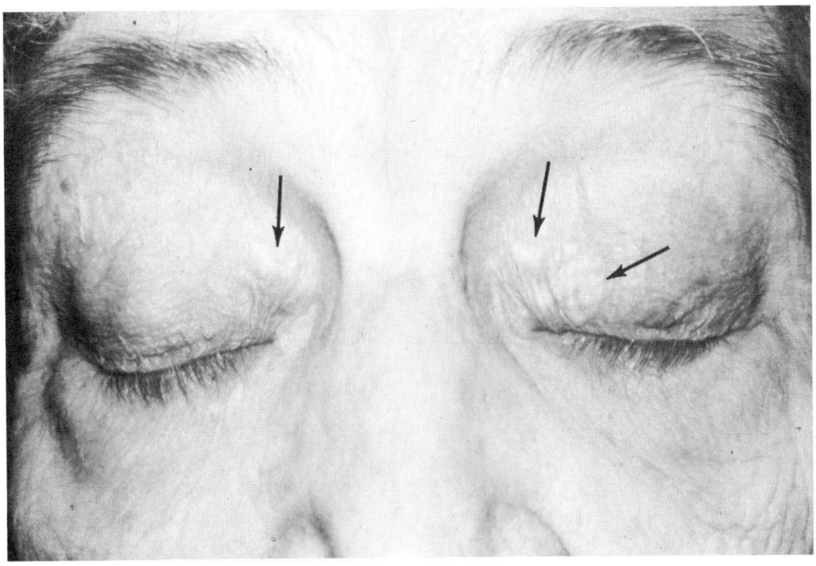

Fig. 27-3. Xanthelasmas of both upper lids.

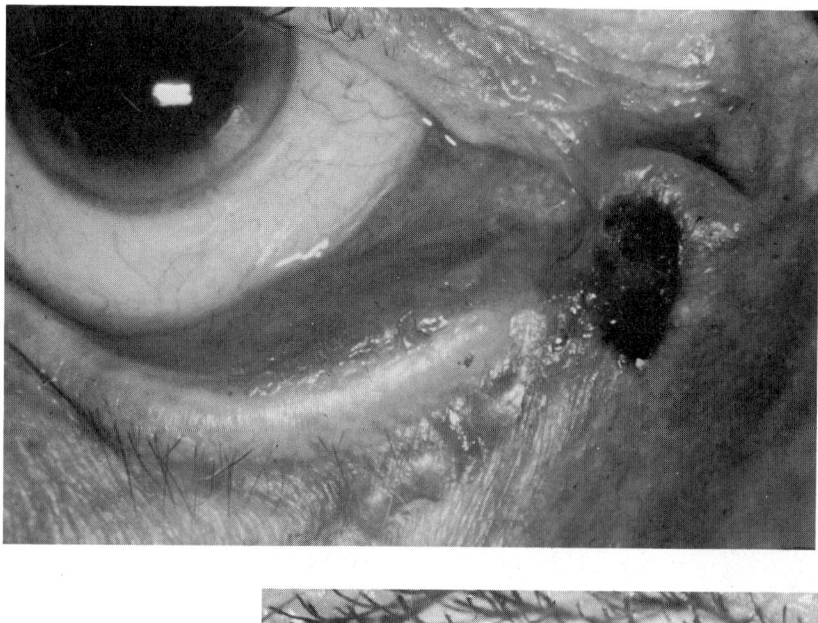

Fig. 27-4. Basal cell carcinoma at the inner canthus.

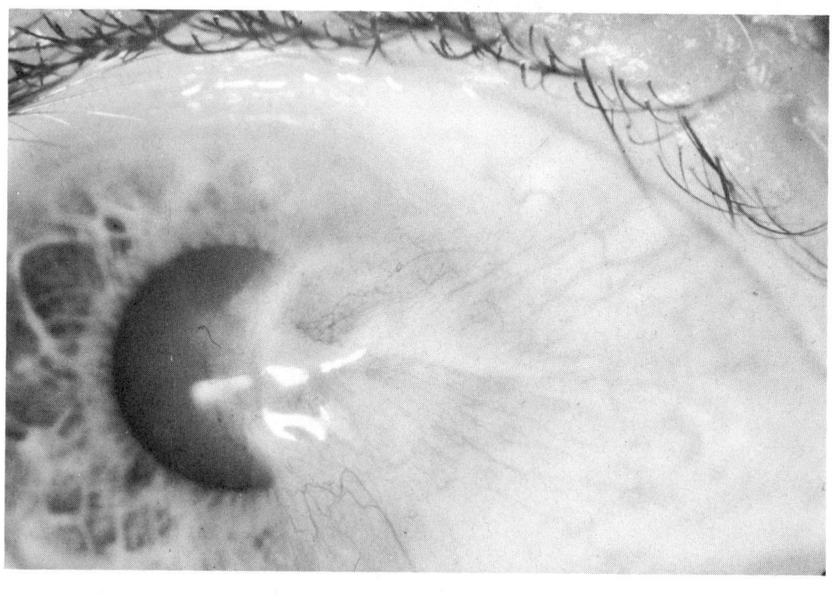

Fig. 27-5. This pterygium has grown over the cornea and encroached on the visual axis.

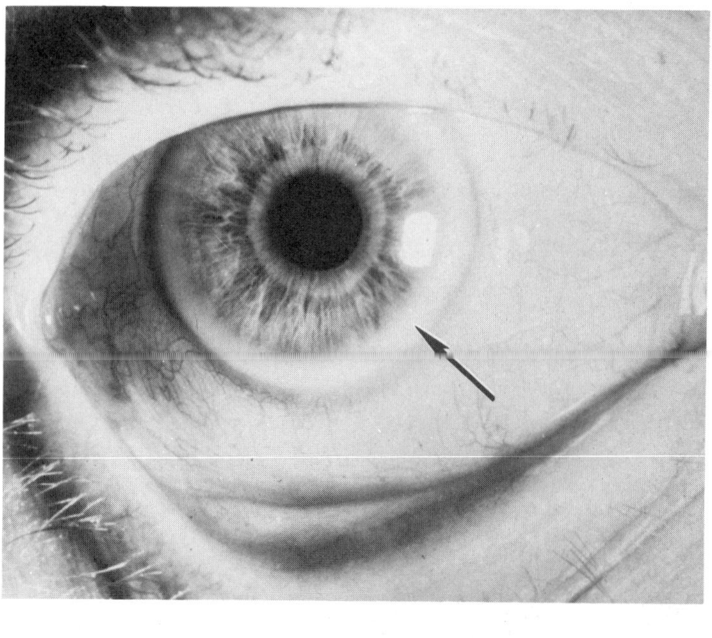

Fig. 27-6. Arcus senilis around the periphery of the cornea (arrow).

to seventh decades and at times progress to chronic corneal edema, decreased vision, and discomfort. Corneal transplantation is often necessary in these cases.

CONDITIONS INVOLVING THE LENS

In several respects the lens of the eye is a unique structure. Embryologically it originates as a hollow vesicle formed by a pouching-in of surface ectoderm. Proliferation of lens fibers occurs in the equatorial region. The newer fibers are laid down around the older fibers, which migrate toward the center. This embryologic growth of the lens continues throughout life, with the central fibers gradually forming a denser central nucleus. The lens is surrounded by a cuticular capsule and is completely avascular. All of its metabolic interchange must occur by diffusion through the membrane of this capsule. The fibers are so arranged that the lens is completely transparent, and any loss of this transparency will result in loss of vision.

Presbyopia

The near point of accommodation is that distance from the eye at which near objects such as print can be easily seen. In childhood this is extremely short, but with each year the near point slips farther away. By the time a person reaches his middle forties, the print usually must be held too far away for the eye to read it easily and comfortably. This is presbyopia, or "old vision." Although this condition may not affect distance vision, it necessitates a convex lens for reading comfort. The near point continues to recede, necessitating a stronger reading glass every few years for the next two decades. In the case of many individuals, this need of a glass for reading is the first intimation of old age, particularly if bifocals are needed.

Presbyopia is probably caused by two factors. As was already noted, the older fibers migrate toward the center of the lens, where they become denser and more rigid, thereby making curvature of the lens more resistant to change by action of the ciliary muscle. A second factor is probably an increasing loss of effectiveness of the ciliary muscle itself.

Cataract

Cataract is defined as an opacity in the lens of the eye. Cataracts may be congenital or may develop from many causes such as trauma, inflammation, various sytemic diseases such as diabetes mellitus, and drug treatment such as administration of topical or systemic corticosteroids. By far the most common cause of cataract is aging.

Cataract is treated by surgical removal of the opaque lens. Such procedures were described over 200 years ago. At present approximately 400,000 cataract operations are performed yearly in the United States, making it one of the most common major surgical procedures. It is also one of the most successful; approximately 97% of patients enjoy improved vision postoperatively.

Cataract surgery may be performed in several ways. The first procedures described involved not removal, but dislocation of an opaque lens so that a clear zone of vision was provided around the lens. The first true extractions were performed in an extracapsular fashion; that is, the capsule of the lens was opened and cortical material aspirated. This often resulted in prolonged inflammation caused by retained lens material. Often an opaque membrane developed in the pupillary space of the remaining capsule, which had to be secondarily incised.

Since about 1940 most surgeons have turned to intracapsular extraction in which the lens is removed entirely. Today the most popular instrument for such lens removal is the cryoprobe, which adheres to the lens by freezing.

About the same time that the intracapsular method became popular, exact suturing of the corneal incision (about 180 degrees of the limbus) was perfected. Previously the wound was not supported by sutures. This necessitated a long period of bed rest with bilateral bandages until the wound became well healed. At the present time there are many types of wound suturing with various suture materials. All of these result in a tight secure wound, which enables the patient to become ambulatory within 24 to 48 hours. Obviously this is of greatest importance to the postoperative care of the elderly patient. With the elimination of bilateral bandages, the disorientation and mental confusion so often seen previously have disappeared. Adequate wound closure also reduces the postoperative complications to a great degree. The enzyme alpha-chymotrypsin has been found to have a specific dissolving effect on the suspending ligaments of the lens. In many cases its use results in a much easier removal of the lens. The use of the operating microscope has also made the surgical procedure far more exact.

In the last decade a new technique, phacoemulsification, has rekindled interest in extracapsular procedures. In this method an ultrasonic probe breaks the lens into tiny fragments that are then aspirated with the same probe. The advantage, indeed the raison d'être, for the procedure is that the incision is tiny, thus reducing the convalescent period. There are, however, disadvantages. Lack of surgical exposure makes the technique difficult in some cases, and the ultrasonic energy needed to break up the hard nuclear sclerotic lenses found in elderly patients may damage the cornea. With the great progress in suture materials and technique there is less relative advantage to a 3 mm incision versus a 12 mm one. Thus the initial great enthusiasm for phacoemulsification has been tempered. It remains a very useful technique, however, in selected cases.

Cataract surgery involves, as we have said, removal of the opaque lens from the eye. The lens provides optical power, and so its removal necessitates replacement of that optical power if the patient is to achieve new visual potential. The simplest optical correction that can be provided is spectacle correction with the thick "cataract glasses" familiar to all who deal with elderly patients. Such glasses do provide the necessary optical power, but they place that power far anterior to its original location within the eye. This results in vision that, although clear, is magnified (1.3 times) and distorted (e.g., doorways appear to bow inward). In addition, because of the magnification peripheral vision is markedly reduced. Visual disorientation often results and may never be overcome, particularly by the elderly patient.

Aphakic magnification and optical distortion are minimized by placing the substitute optical element in a position as close as possible to that of the original lens. Contact lenses provide such correction. Both hard and soft contact lens materials are available and provide a wide range of parameters allowing successful fit of many pa-

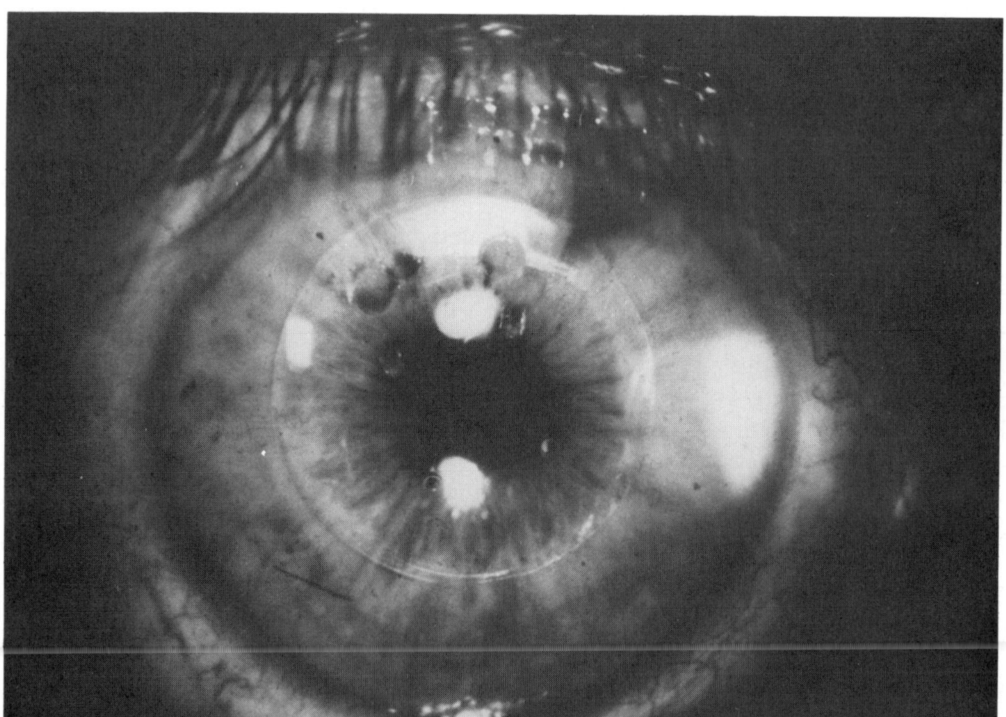

Fig. 27-7. Intraocular lens sutured in place in the iris plane. Intracapsular cataract extraction preceded lens insertion.

tients. Nevertheless, it will be appreciated that many elderly patients are unable to manage the daily insertion and removal required by traditional contact lenses. A recent development is the extended wear contact lens that can be left in place for several weeks. Unfortunately, the convenience of this modality is counterbalanced to some extent by the need for frequent office examinations.

In 1949 Ridley, in England, pioneered another approach to aphakic correction by placing a plastic prosthetic intraocular lens in the eye of a patient. Since that time the lenses and surgical techniques have been refined, so that today intraocular lens implantation is a common, successful procedure (Fig. 27-7). Approximately 30% of all cataract operations in the United States now include placement of an intraocular lens. There are many styles of lenses available, and depending on the style, the cataract extraction itself may be performed by either intracapsular or extracapsular technique. It is even possible to use phacoemulsification, although the small wound created by the phacoemulsifier usually has to be enlarged to permit insertion of the intraocular lens.

There is another group of techniques for optical correction after cataract surgery that have recently become available. These are the various refractive keratoplasties in which the cornea itself is reshaped. There are several different techniques, but in essence, the anterior portion of the cornea is cut away, frozen, reshaped on a lathe, and sutured back into position. This is clearly a drastic procedure, but it offers an alternative form of correction in selected cases.

DISORDERS OF THE VITREOUS

The posterior segment of the eye is filled with a viscid gel-like mass, the vitreous body, consisting of an inert fiberlike network filled with fluid. As a person grows older, there is a tendency for the vitreous body to shrink and become more liquid. During this process, vitreous opacities may form, which cause the common, so-called floaters noted by many aging individuals. Shrinking of the vitreous body may pull on the retina at points of adhesion. Retinal traction may cause the perception of light flashes by the patient which are often described as "lightning flashes." At times these adhesions are dense enough to cause breaks in the retina, which may lead to retinal detachment. Although detachment of the retina is not necessarily a disease of the aged, some of the underlying causes resulting from vitreous degenerative changes are surely related to aging. Other factors are localized degenerative changes in the retina itself.

Some recent advances have been made in the treatment of retinal degenerations and detachments. The peripheral retinal degenerations often can be prevented from developing into frank detachments by the creation of a delimiting chorioretinal scar by several means such as xenon arc photocoagulation, laser beam treatment, or cryotherapy.

Vitreous hemorrhage may result from a retinal tear across a vessel, bleeding from neovascular tissue such as in proliferative diabetic retinopathy, or as a manifestation of hypertension. Recurrent hemorrhage leads to opacified vitreous with subsequent visual loss. Until recently there was little to offer such patients.

Over the last decade, however, great progress has been made in the technique and instrumentation for vitreous surgery. Thus it is now possible to excise opacified vitreous. It is even possible in selected cases to peel membranes off the retina itself.

VASCULAR DISEASE

The retina

"Arteriosclerosis" refers to a variety of processes in which there is hardening and thickening of the arterial wall. These changes in the arterial wall may be caused by atherosclerosis or may be the result of diffuse arteriolar sclerosis.

In atherosclerosis there is deposition of lipids associated with degenerative changes occurring in large- and medium-sized arteries, such as the central retinal artery and its branches immediately adjacent to the optic disc. These changes may give rise to occlusion of the central retinal vein or artery, with subsequent sudden, almost complete loss of vision. Arteriolar sclerosis results from prolonged vascular hypertension and is characterized by irregular fusiform attenuation of the retinal arteries, producing the so-called copper-wire appearance. Hemorrhages and exudates may occur, with consequent retinal damage and visual loss. It should be emphasized that vascular changes of the retina may be of both hypertensive and atherosclerotic types and that both of these may occur simultaneously.

Another type of retinal vascular disease of increasing importance is diabetic retinopathy, which may result in slowly progressive but at times complete blindness. The fundus usually has a characteristic appearance. Small, round hemorrhages and hard exudates are found, generally in the macular region (Fig. 27-8). The basic lesion has proved to be a capillary microaneurysm, which gives rise to localized edema and hemorrhage. The hemorrhages may become massive, leading to scarring and retinal detachment.

For years the condition, which is characterized by short periods of complete loss of vision in one eye, has been known as *amaurosis fugax*. However, by the methods of ophthalmodynamometry, it has become possible to measure the retinal arterial blood pressure. In the eye with amaurosis fugax this pressure is generally distinctly lower than that in the unaffected eye. This has been shown usually to be the result of carotid artery occlusive disease on the side of the affected eye. This finding is extremely valuable diagnostically, as amaurosis fugax may herald a true stroke with permanent neurologic cardiovascular deficit. Carotid endarterectomy or antiembolic medical therapy is often indicated in such patients.

Obviously all these vascular conditions are local manifestations of underlying systemic disease. The appearance of the ocular fundus as seen with the ophthalmoscope may be of diagnostic and prognostic importance. Management of retinal vascular disease must be based on medical therapy of the systemic disease; however, retinal damage often is permanent and not amenable to treatment.

The choroid

Vascular alterations in the choroid are much less obvious with an ophthalmoscope than are those in the overlying retina. Choroidal vascular changes are usually not clinically significant except in the area of the macula. The area of central vision is the fovea centralis, which includes a small amount of surrounding retina known as the macula. This area is completely devoid of

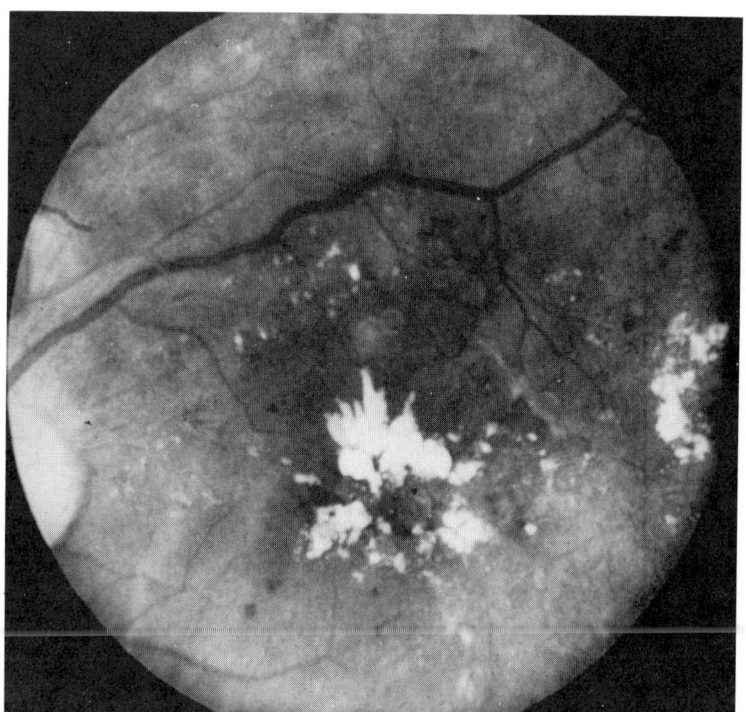

Fig. 27-8. Diabetic retinopathy. The white areas are exudates; dark spots are intraretinal hemorrhages.

retinal circulation, and therefore all of its nutrition is derived from the underlying capillary layer of the choroid.

Changes in the capillary layer of the choroid and/or the pigment epithelial layer of the retina are probably the source of one of the most common causes of visual deterioration in the aged—senile macular degeneration. Patients with this condition complain of a slowly progressive impairment of central vision, which usually leads in its later stages to loss of reading vision. Peripheral vision is retained so that complete blindness does not result. The earliest ophthalmoscopic changes consist of a subtle migration of pigment around the fovea centralis, which progresses to clumping of the pigment with some white scarring (Fig. 27-9).

A second type of senile macular degeneration has a more sudden onset and is caused by a hemorrhage from the choroidal capillaries under the retina at the macula (Fig. 27-10). The hemorrhage organizes to form an elevated mass with degeneration of the overlying retina. This type of macular degeneration is known as *disciform macular degeneration*.

An advance in the evaluation of retinal and choroidal vascular disease is fluorescein angiography. Fluorescein is injected into the patient's antecubital vein, and within a few seconds the intravascular fluorescein can be visualized in the retinal and choroidal vessels with the use of blue filters. Many diseases can be categorized according to their distinctive fluorescein angiographic appearance.

Patients with diminished central vision (e.g., macular degeneration) can often be helped with a variety of visual aids including magnifiers, strong reading glasses, telescopes, and even television magnification of reading materials. Until recently, however, there was no real treatment for senile macular degeneration. The advent of laser photocoagulation in conjunction with fluorescein angiography now allows successful treatment of a small fraction of these cases.

The optic nerve

Although it is often difficult to evaluate, mild reduction of visual acuity may be caused by arteriosclerotic optic atrophy. This condition is caused by changes in the small nutrient arteries entering the optic nerve from the surrounding

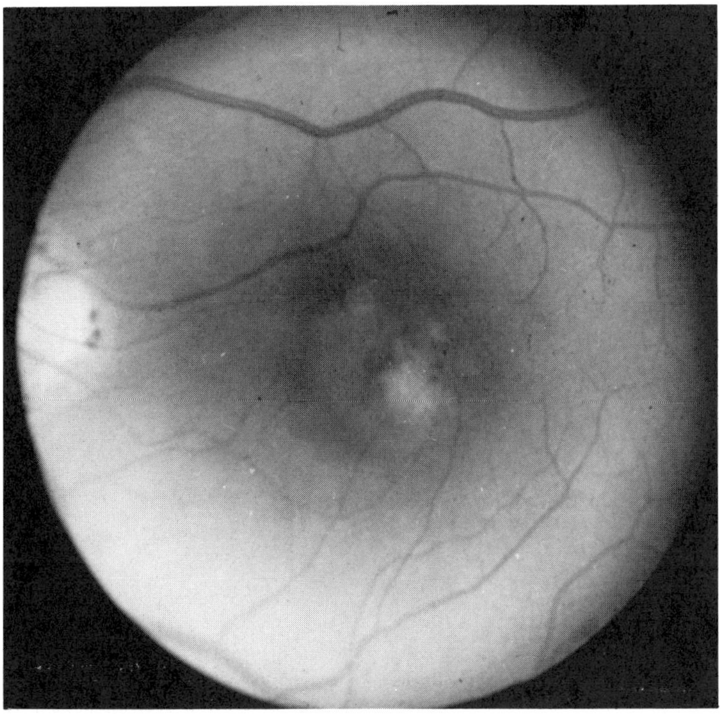

Fig. 27-9. The macula shows the "mottled" appearance of depigmentation and hyperpigmentation of senile macular degeneration.

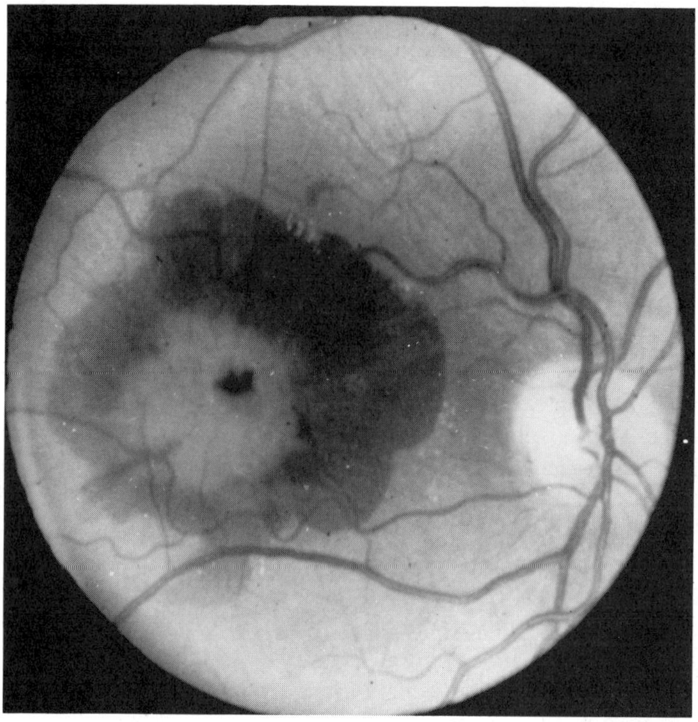

Fig. 27-10. Acute intraretinal and subretinal hemorrhage in the macular region.

optic nerve sheaths. Sudden profound loss of vision may be seen in the elderly patient from optic nerve involvement in temporal arteritis (giant cell arteritis). Under ophthalmoscopic examination the nerve head appears to be slightly edematous and slightly pale and may have one or two surrounding hemorrhages. Loss of vision is often complete and irreversible. Therapy with large doses of systemic steroids may have a beneficial effect if started very early in the course of the disease.

GLAUCOMA

Increased intraocular pressure is the common characteristic of a group of diseases called glaucoma. The cause of various glaucomas may be different, but all types are probably caused by some impairment in the outflow of aqueous humor from the eye.

Although increased intraocular pressure from impairment in the outflow of aqueous humor is common to all glaucomas, it is possible by other diagnostic measures to separate glaucoma into several varieties. Congenital glaucoma is the result of an embryologic developmental defect in the angle of the anterior chamber. Glaucoma may also occur secondary to trauma or to a number of intraocular diseases including tumor, vascular disease, and inflammation. In most cases of secondary glaucoma the causative lesion is obvious, with the treatment directed not only to lowering the intraocular pressure but also to elimination of the primary etiologic factors.

There are two types of so-called primary glaucoma. Although these may occur in any age group, the incidence of both types—chronic simple glaucoma and angle-closure glaucoma—definitely increases with each decade of life. These two types are distinct in their mechanisms, manifestations, and management.

Chronic simple glaucoma

Chronic simple glaucoma is the most common of all glaucomas. It is characterized by a slow, insidious increase in intraocular pressure. Usually subjective symptoms are not noticed by the patient until visual field loss has occurred. Early detection in this type of glaucoma is most important and can be best accomplished by routine measurement of intraocular pressure (tonometry) for all patients old enough to cooperate. Generally if a borderline or slightly elevated

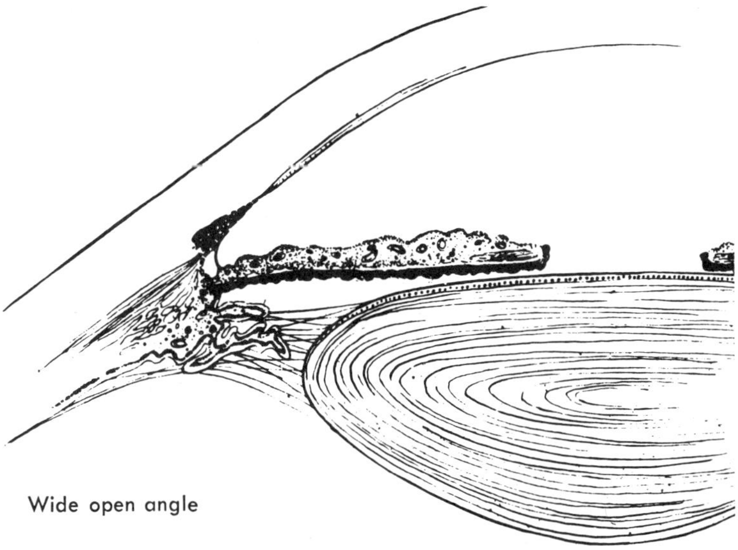

Fig. 27-11. Wide open angle of an eye that is normal or that is affected by chronic simple glaucoma.

pressure is found, the patient must be observed for some time before the diagnosis of chronic simple glaucoma is definitely established. However, if the characteristic field loss and optic nerve changes are present, the diagnosis is definite and treatment is usually started.

Chronic simple glaucoma is essentially a medical disease. In most cases elevated tension can be normalized over long periods by the use of several topical agents. The first drug used topically to control glaucoma was pilocarpine hydrochloride. It is still the most commonly employed of all antiglaucoma agents. If pilocarpine hydrochloride is ineffective, stronger miotic agents such as physostigmine (eserine), demecarium bromide (Humorsol), or echothiophate iodide (Phospholine iodide) may be used. In many cases a 1% or 2% solution of epinephrine may be used successfully and be more acceptable to the patient because of the absence of miotic effects. More recently a beta-adrenergic blocking agent, timolol (Timoptic), has also proved useful in topical therapy.

If topical medication is ineffective in lowering the intraocular pressure, it may be necessary to add such systemic medication as acetazolamide (Diamox) to the regimen. Such drugs inhibit the enzyme carbonic anhydrase and thereby suppress the formation of aqueous humor. It is important to remember that certain side effects such as drowsiness, tingling in the extremities, and the formation of kidney stones may occur in patients receiving acetazolamide.

In advanced cases of glaucoma, surgery may be indicated to prevent further visual loss. There are a number of operations designed to increase aqueous drainage from the eye. The most commonly employed operations result in a fistula that drains the aqueous humor externally under the conjunctiva.

The fundamental pathologic change in chronic simple glaucoma is probably a degenerative change in the outflow channels of the eye. These changes inhibit the rate of flow of the aqueous humor through the outflow channels, resulting in the rise of the intraocular pressure, with subsequent damage to the optic nerve (Fig. 27-11).

There is now good evidence that chronic simple glaucoma is genetically determined. This genetic aspect is related to the discovery that in patients with chronic simple glaucoma, increased intraocular pressure develops after 3 weeks of ocular instillation with corticosteroid drops. Offspring of parents with chronic simple glaucoma also show this steroid responsiveness. It is postulated that the chronic simple glaucoma patient is a homozygote for the abnormal gene. Any individual with a family history of this condition should be considered a candidate for chronic simple glaucoma and should receive a complete evaluation at periodic intervals. Furthermore, recent studies have shown that there is an increase in the frequency of glaucoma among diabetic patients.

Angle-closure glaucoma

Angle-closure glaucoma is much less common than chronic simple glaucoma and is the result of an anatomic defect in the angle of the anterior chamber. The base of the iris is attached to the ciliary body to form a narrow cleft between the iris and the trabecular structures. This narrowing of the periphery of the anterior chamber is often indicated grossly by a shallow anterior chamber. However, the area can be directly studied with the gonioscope and the narrow angle evaluated (Fig. 27-12).

When first examined, most of the people with narrow angles do not have glaucoma. However, an increase in intraocular pressure may be induced by a variety of provocative tests. In many other cases the condition may progress spontaneously to occlude the aqueous humor outflow. If this happens suddenly, an attack of acute congestive glaucoma results with severe ocular pain, pronounced loss of vision, and occasionally nausea. Examination shows the cornea to be cloudy, the pupil in middilatation, and the intraocular pressure very high. With the gonioscope the angle can be seen to be completely occluded. With many patients the attack may be subacute, characterized by mild ocular pain, headache, and halos seen around lights as a result of the corneal edema. Chronic angle closure may occur as repeated attacks and may simulate chronic simple glaucoma, but the differentiation can usually be made by gonioscopy.

In chronic simple glaucoma the pathologic process in the outflow channels is permanent and irreversible. In angle-closure glaucoma the glaucomatous state can be completely reversed if the angle is opened by intensive miotic therapy and administration of acetazolamide or osmotic agents, such as glycerin orally or mannitol intravenously. The only adequate and permanent treatment of angle-closure glaucoma is surgery. An iridectomy, usually done peripherally, will open the angle and prevent further angle closure. Not only is this operation useful in the treatment of angle closure but also it will prevent future attacks. Thus it is often used in the second eye after an acute attack in the first eye, as a prophylactic measure, since the disease is bilateral.

• • •

The aging process in most individuals causes a slow but steady decrease in visual efficiency. The backgrounds of these visual disturbances are many and varied. Although many of these processes are distinct physiologic and pathologic processes, others are merely local manifestations of tissue degeneration seen elsewhere in the body. Because of its structure and its accessibility to examination, the eye is a favorable organ for accurate observation and diagnosis. The cause of most visual disturbances can be ascertained by adequate examination. Although a careful examination by an ophthalmologist is usually necessary for an exact diagnosis, the nature of these conditions should be understood by all physicians who care for the aging patient.

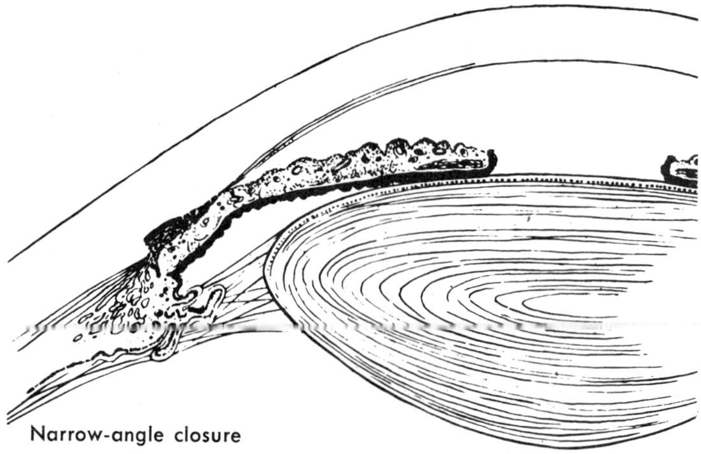

Fig. 27-12. Iris root against the outflow channels in angle-closure glaucoma.

Although many of the conditions causing visual loss in the aged are characteristic of this age group, some of these conditions start in younger persons and progress into old age. It is most important therefore that these processes be recognized early so that their destructive effect on vision may be minimized. Although many visual disturbances are primarily the result of aging, the effects of heredity and environment may modify their clinical course in individual patients. Psychologic changes occurring in the elderly patient may often modify his reactions to his visual problems (see Chapter 25).

REFERENCES

1. Becker, B.: Diabetes mellitus and primary open-angle glaucoma, Edward Jackson Memorial Lecture, Tr. Am. Acad. Ophthalmol. Otolaryngol. **75:**239, 1971.
2. Becker, B., and Ballin, N.: Glaucoma and corticosteroid provocative testing, Arch. Ophthalmol. **74:**621, 1965.
3. Becker, B., and Hahn, K.A.: Topical corticosteroids and heredity in primary open-angle glaucoma, Am. J. Ophthalmol. **57:**543, 1964.
4. Cinotti, A.A., and Patti, J.D.: Lens abnormalities in an aging population of nonglaucomatous patients, Am. J. Ophthalmol. **65:**25, 1968.
5. Gass, J., and Arnold, M.: A fluorescein angiographic study of macular dysfunction secondary to retinal vascular disease, Arch. Ophthalmol. **80:**535, 1968.
6. Hogan, M.J., and Zimmerman, L.E.: Ophthalmic pathology, an atlas and textbook, ed. 2, Philadelphia, 1962, W.B. Saunders Co.
7. Kolker, A.E., and Hetherington, J.: Becker-Shaffer's diagnosis and therapy of the glaucomas, ed. 5, St. Louis, 1982, The C.V. Mosby Co.
8. Kornzweig, A.: Diagnosis and treatment of common eye diseases in the aged: guidelines for the practicing physician, J. Am. Geriatr. Soc. **21:**512, 1973.
9. Kornzweig, A.L., Eliasoph, I., and Feldstein, M.: Retinal vasculature in macular degeneration, Arch. Ophthalmol. **75:**326, 1966.
10. Kornzweig, A.L., Feldstein, M., and Schneider, J.: The eye in old age. IV. Ocular survey of over one thousand aged persons with special reference to normal and disturbed visual function, Am. J. Ophthalmol. **44:**29, 1957.
11. McDonald, J.E., and Johnson, M.O.: Glaucoma screening in office of general practitioners and internists: a study of 10,090 patients, Am. J. Ophthalmol. **59:**875, 1965.
12. Newell, F.W.: Ophthalmology—principles and concepts, ed. 5, St. Louis, 1982, The C.V. Mosby Co.
13. Teeters, V.W., and Bird, A.C.: A clinical study of the vascularity of senile macular degeneration, Am. J. Ophthalmol. **75:**53, 1973.
14. Wise, G.N., Dollery, C.T., and Henkind, P.: The retinal circulation, New York, 1971, Harper & Row, Publishers.

CHAPTER 28 · NEUROLOGIC ASPECTS

William B. Hardin, Jr.

No neurologic disorder can be attributed exclusively to senium. So-called senile dementia occurs as well in persons under sixty years old; and strokes, unfortunately, occur at any age. There are, of course, neurologic conditions whose incidence increases with age. Some of these conditions will be discussed in this chapter.

The neurologic history of the geriatric patient requires a different perspective by the examining physician. For example, more time and attention should be devoted to medical histories of elderly patients than is generally given to histories of younger patients because the former often have longer and more complex medical records. Accidents, diseases, operations, and the varieties of drugs taken now and over the years contribute to the solution of what might otherwise be a confusing array of neurologic findings.

Unlike the child or young adult, the elderly person has acquired skills and accomplishments that provide an historic background against which his current performance can be more accurately judged. The patient should not be viewed as a mere isolate in his environment, since many puzzling neurologic conditions have an heredofamilial base and are solvable in some instances by paying sufficient attention to family and environmental ties. Even when it is not possible to examine the patient's parents or siblings, the physician may clarify a perplexing neurologic problem merely by examining children and grandchildren, thereby obviating the need for extensive and costly laboratory procedures. Longer experience with life often brings about greater insight into illness. Thus if we were to take time to listen, we, as physicians, may hear patients correctly telling us their own diagnoses before we ever get them on the examination table.

The technique of the neurologic examination of an elderly person is essentially like that of anyone over the age of 6, except more attention is usually paid to analyses of higher order functions such as language, memory, abstract conceptualization, and temporal orientation. The physician, however, must allow more latitude in the interpretation of the physical findings because as the nervous system ages certain neurologic signs appear within a context of "normality" that might otherwise be unacceptable in younger persons. MacDonald Critchley, in his article on neurologic changes in the aged,[1] selected the following signs and symptoms as appearing most consistently in 80-year olds: presbyopia, presbycusis, reduced acuity of smell, reduced speeds and amounts of motor activities, delayed reaction times, slowness and narrowed compass of perception, small pupils with restricted amplitudes of pupillary reactivity, limited range of upward gaze, tendency to have a flexed posture of trunk and limbs, diminished perception of vibratory sense in the feet, reduction of fine finger coordination and agility, weakening of muscular power, reduction of muscle bulk (especially in the legs), and reduced or absent triceps surae tendon reflex. It is up to examining physicians to judge from their own experiences the degrees to which they will accept these signs while examining an elderly individual for the first time.[2]

With the exception of the optic nerve head, the central nervous system is largely encased in bone and is virtually inaccessible to direct study. Thus the usual methods of direct bedside examination are replaced by indirect ones in which gait and station, coordination, muscle strength, and general and special sensibility are evaluated. Such indirect methods require active participation by the patient. In addition to the general physical examination, the physician often listens over the cranium or blood vessels to detect bruits, palpates muscles to estimate their volume and tone, and inspects the body surface for enlarged nerves or local departures from the usual bilateral muscular symmetry.

Weakness of a limb may be attributable to local involvement of the motor nerve outflow, such as that which supplies an arm or a leg, or to interruption of the motor paths that descend from one side of the brain to connect with the motor outflow over cranial and spinal nerves. Because of the involvement of long tracts of the central nervous system, an entire side of the body may abruptly become paralyzed as in stroke. It is a physiologic fact that one side of the body is controlled by the opposite half of the brain. This necessitates a crossing of motor outflow paths from the cerebral hemisphere to the opposite spinal outflow mechanism. Similarly, the afferent inflow over sensory nerves eventually connects with sensory long tracts that decussate within the spinal cord to the opposite thalamus and cerebral cortex. Cerebellar controls are exercised homolaterally, whereas the primary mechanisms for speech are located in the left hemisphere of the brain in 95% of right-handed people and 55% of left-handed people. Language functions in women are less strongly lateralized to one cerebral hemisphere than they are in men.

Besides the necessity of locating the side of a lesion within the central nervous system, one must keep in mind the signs that isolate peripheral from central nervous system lesions. In general, peripheral sensory impairment occurs within the distribution of a specific nerve, nerve plexus, or consecutive spinal roots. For each pattern of nerve or root involvement, there is a characteristic area of sensory impairment. Flaccid paralysis with muscle atrophy in a nerve or root distribution is indicative of local motor nerve or spinal segment impairment. Absence of a related tendon jerk, such as the knee jerk, may indicate an interruption of the motor side, sensory side, or both sides of a local reflex arc. A unilateral lesion of a spinal segment frequently causes bilateral clinical signs, thereby allowing a differentiation to be made between it and lesions of the nerve or root, which are unilateral. Finally, the presence of an extensor plantar response (Babinski's reflex) is always indicative of a disturbance of pyramidal tract function somewhere along its course from the cerebral cortex through the spinal cord. Many excellent texts describing the technique and meaning of the neurologic examination are available.[3,4]

Diseases mentioned in the following sections were chosen either because they are most likely to be encountered in senium or because they present a characteristic problem of differential diagnosis or management. An effort is made preceding the discussion of each condition to present some statistical perspective that justifies inclusion of the condition as a problem of people over 65 years of age. Specific forms of treatment are discussed only in passing, since there are ample sources available to the reader.[5-7]

DEMENTIA

Perhaps the most subtle neurologic disease of the elderly is *dementia*. Popularly attributed to the infirmities of old age, dementia is probably the single necessary consequence of the aging brain. No organ works efficiently forever. Philosophically speaking, dementia represents the final running down of the individual's biologic clock, the intervals of which are measured in years rather than hours. Even though it occurs more precipitously in some cases than in others, the unwinding of this clock generally cannot be categorized as a disease but as the result of an incremental deterioration of a nervous system long active in the storage and analysis of diverse human experiences. Vascular and metabolic deficiencies advance the rate of deterioration, but progressive sensory insufficiency and increasing social and cultural isolation also contribute. In any event dementia may be considered as the end phase of a sociobiologic process as well as a rather indistinct pathophysiologic entity that justly falls within the meaning of the word *disease*.

Fortunately the severity of dementia and chronologic age are not necessarily predictably correlative, since the effects of aging on mental abilities are extremely variable. Many people remain creative, imaginative, resilient, and intelligent well into their eighth decade, while others show signs of mental incapacity before they are sixty. Generally speaking, apperceptive ability starts to decline early in adult life (thirties to forties) and continues on into senium. According to Adams and Victor,[8] the Wechsler Adult Intelligence Scale (WAIS) shows that vocabulary, fund of information, comprehension, object assembly, and picture completion hold up better as we get older, than does digit symbol, block design, similarities, digit reversal, picture arrangement, and arithmetic. Many old people become mentally rigid, conservative, opinionated, and suspicious of change. Mental energy and motivation may decline; whereupon agitated depression often appears to accompany the additional loss of functions precipitated by the onset of a neurologic disease.

Along with aging there are involutional changes in the nervous system. For example the weight of the brain diminishes in a linear curve by about 10% to 15% from age 25 to 90. Smaller brains decrease proportionately less than larger brains. Similarly there is gradual loss of the number of Purkinje cells of the cerebellum, motor neurons of the anterior horn of the spinal cord, sensory ganglion cells, and myelinated fibers in the pyramidal tract.[9,10]

On the physiologic side of the aging process, the peripheral nerve conduction velocities decrease by 10% to 15%. The electroencephalogram (EEG) of the elderly tends to show minimal slowing of the occipital alpha frequency and a slight reduction in wave amplitudes. Theta (4 to 7 Hertz) and delta (less than 4 Hertz) waves from the temporal lobes become more prominent. These reported EEG changes, however, have no predictive value as far as mental functioning or longevity are concerned. Visually evoked cortical responses (VER) undergo changes from age 1 month to 81 years according to Dustman and Beck (1969).[11] The VER in the geriatric population shows diminished amplitude, prolonged latency, and the addition of a number of small wave components. The VER is a relatively new technique for studying the brain, and the significance of these wave forms in senium is not yet understood.

We might anticipate a significant correlation between cerebral blood flow and aging, but, surprisingly enough, the answers are not as yet readily apparent. Using the nitrous oxide method of measuring total cerebral blood flow, Fazekas et al.[12] found blood flow and metabolic rate of the brains of persons between ages 90 and 102 to be significantly lower than that of persons 50 and younger but not significantly lower than a group of elderly people with a mean age of 68 years. Thus the cerebral blood flow must reach a plateau in senium at which point it ceases to correlate with continuing cerebral atrophy and neuronal loss. In a summary of these and other studies of regional cerebral blood flow and cerebral blood flow and intelligence, Torack[9] concludes, "The results of all types of assay appear to be in agreement that there is no abnormality of cerebral blood flow which can be used as a criterion of aging or as an indication of intellectual decline and premature death."

The prototype of dementia, either in senium or presenium, is Alzheimer's disease. It is exemplified clinically by a gradual loss of memory, judgment, and general intelligence as measured by tests of comprehension, general knowledge, and calculative and learning abilities. This decline is associated with loss of sociability, lability, shallowness of affect, and depression. As the condition advances, disorientation, delusions, and hallucinations replace the earlier signs of simple confusion. Aphasia, apraxia, or agnosia can also appear at this time, making speech and actions caricatural and inappropriate. Some persons more dramatically affected develop epilepsy, hemiparesis, or spontaneous choreiform movements, after which they sink into a state of complete helplessness, akinetic mutism, or coma.

The incidence of dementia in the elderly population varies according to the methods of investigation. Katzman[13] says that about 15% of people over 64 years old display signs of dementia, two thirds of these are mild to moderate and one third are severe. Other studies reveal the difficulties of making estimates of prevalence rates among urban versus rural and institutional versus noninstitutional populations. One thing is certain, and that is the likelihood of an increasing incidence of dementia as the mean age of the population of the country shifts toward senium.

An uncritical acceptance of the notion that an elderly patient with dementia has Alzheimer's disease or "hardening of the brain's arteries" and therefore has a hopeless prognosis may cause the physician to overlook the existence of an infectious, nutritive, metabolic, or surgically correctable condition. It is important to recognize that surgically amenable conditions such as anterior cranial fossa meningiomas, incisural block, or chronic subdural hematomas may be responsible for a deteriorating mental state.

One potentially correctable condition, known as normal pressure communicating hydrocephalus (NPH) is occasionally discovered in the elderly patient with hypertension. The syndrome is characterized by a 3- to 6-months progressive deterioration of mental status, of walking ability, and of urinary continence. During the symptomatic period, the ventricles dilate in the absence of a comparable degree of cerebral cortical atrophy, and spinal fluid does not flow properly out of the ventricles and up over the cerebral convexity. Curiously enough computed tomography (CT) scanning has revealed a related group of elderly individuals with chronic (usually insulin dependent) diabetes mellitus who have CT scans similar in appearance to the NPH group but not the typical clinical syndrome. They may, and usually are, neurologically asymptomatic. One logical but unproved hypothesis implicates the basement membrane of the capillaries of the arachnoid villae. Thickening of this membrane, with consequent reduction of cerebral spinal fluid absorption, may occur secondary to diabetes.

Other patients with dementia may have myxedema; diabetes mellitus; uremia; pulmonary insufficiency; hypertensive, renal, or hepatic encephalopathy; congestive heart failure; or central nervous system syphilis. In all such cases careful examination of the patient's mental status and medical history is necessary to rule out involutional depression, schizophrenia, long-standing mental retardation, Wernicke-Korsakoff disease, or specific disturbances of some higher order mental function caused by localized cerebral vascular disease. Thus the mere recognition of the presence of dementia demands a complete assay of the patient's medical status.

After potentially treatable conditions are excluded and historic evidence for truly progressive dissolution of mental integrity over an extended period is obtained, there remains the probable diagnosis of one of the several forms of degenerative dementias (Alzheimer's disease, arteriosclerotic disease, Pick's disease [lobar atrophy], subacute spongiform encephalopathy, parkinsonism-dementia complex, and a few rarities).

The diagnosis of degenerative dementia need not be one of exclusion, and it may be necessary to know the prognosis more exactly for family counselling or for legal reasons. Certain ancillary tests have distinct diagnostic value. The EEG may be unremarkable at the onset, but when followed serially it becomes diffusely slow and greatly disorganized, the rapidity of change generally paralleling the progress of the dementia.[14-16]

The pneumoencephalogram may reveal symmetrically enlarged ventricles or an excess of supracortical air shadows, either of which can indicate cerebral atrophy. CT scanning may clearly demonstrate ventricular dilatation and cortical atrophy without the patient having to suffer any significant risk or even pain. Compare the CT scan of a normal individual, Fig. 28-1, with that of a person with cerebral atrophy, Fig. 28-2.

Serial psychometric tests may help form a measurable basis on which to judge the rate of deterioration. In the course of degenerative dementias, language function often is impaired long before it becomes clearly evident to the examining physician. A number of sophisticated audiologic tests may be used to measure the patient's capacity for handling verbal language.[17]

When an early diagnosis is necessary, a surgical biopsy of the cerebral cortex may confirm the presence of a pathologic condition. In this connection, it is important to remember that generally applicable morphologic criteria that can be used to differentiate the pathologic atrophy of the senile brain from the results of normal aging do not exist.[18] Biopsies have their chief use in positively establishing diagnoses of Alzheimer's disease, Pick's disease, or the varieties of spongiform encephalopathy. The differentiation of senile dementia and the arteriosclerotic variety is less clear-cut, however. In a clinicopathologic study of a large series of patients with degenerative dementia whose mean age at death was 68 years, Corsellis[19] found 45% with primarily cerebral vascular changes, 34% with primarily Alzheimer's changes, and 21% with an equal combination of the two.

Management of all senile dementias is difficult. The physician's role is that of making an early and accurate diagnosis followed by family guidance and home care for as long as is feasible. By judicious use of phenothiazines for overac-

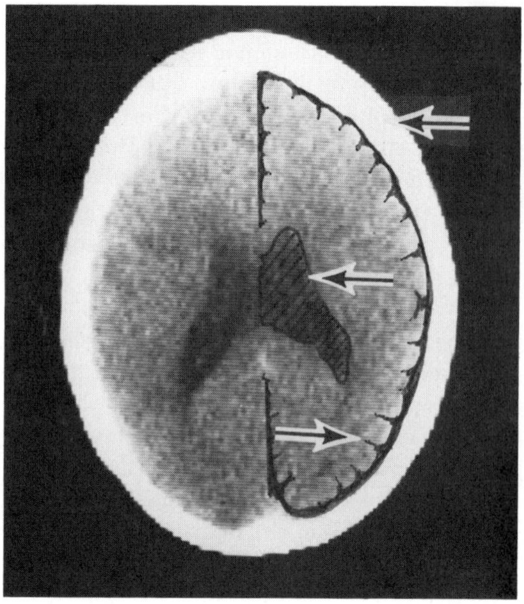

Fig. 28-1. Normal brain. Noncontrasted CT scan at 35 degree high ventricular level, retouched on the right to demonstrate skull (top arrow), lateral ventricle (middle arrow), and relatively small cortical sulci (lower arrow) enclosing gray area (right cerebral hemisphere).

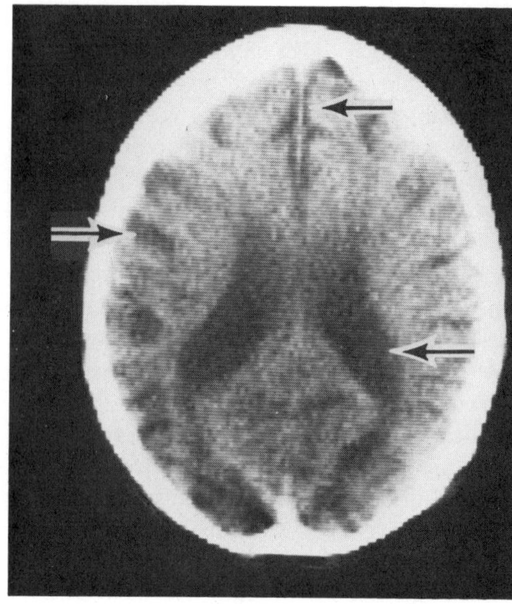

Fig. 28-2. Cerebral atrophy. Noncontrasted CT scan taken at 35 degree high ventricular level demonstrating enlarged cortical sulci (left arrow), widened frontal interhemispheric fissure (top arrow), and dilated ventricles (lower arrow). Could be case of Alzheimer's disease.

tivity; haloperidol for hallucinations and excited states; amphetamines and monoamine oxidase inhibitors for depression; and paraldehyde, chloral hydrate, and other sedatives for sleep and twilight restlessness the period of home care may be significantly prolonged. Many families will continue to provide care at home if the concerned physician offers advice and encouragement at intervals.

STROKE

About 250,000 people die from "stroke" annually. This number represents 11% of the total yearly deaths from all causes, exceeded only by heart disease and cancer.[20] Three fourths of all deaths from cerebral vascular disease are reported to be among persons 70 years of age or older. Stroke is the third leading cause of death among persons 55 to 74 years of age and the second leading cause of death among people 75 years of age and older. In addition to those who die from stroke, there are an estimated two million persons currently suffering the residuals of cerebral vascular disease, one third of whom have been made unemployable by their condition.[21] These statistics are undoubtedly tied to the increasing incidences of atherosclerosis, heart disease, and hypertension in an aging population, since the overwhelming majority of strokes are the end result of these diseases.

Stroke may be defined as an abruptly developing neurologic abnormality that is secondary to an occlusive or hemorrhagic vascular accident involving one or more of the vessels (arteries or venous structures) of the brain. On the basis of postmortem studies strokes have been traditionally classified as thrombosis, embolism, or hemorrhage; yet the clinical diagnosis of these categories of stroke, based only on the neurologic history and examination, can be inaccurate. For example, of 1000 cases of stroke studied, both antemortem and postmortem, Dalsgaard-Nielsen[22] found that the clinical diagnosis of hemorrhage was correct only 65% of the time and of infarction (thromboembolism) only 58% of the time.

Recognizing the limitations of stroke diagnosis, physicians prefer to classify strokes according to their temporal profiles. Thereby strokes are grouped as follows: (1) transient ischemic attack, (2) reversible ischemic neurologic deficit, (3) stroke-in-evolution, and (4) completed stroke.[23] In the transient ischemic attack (TIA) the neurologic deficit occurs abruptly, lasts a few minutes to 24 hours, and disappears completely. Reversible ischemic neurologic deficit (RIND) resembles TIA except that the neurologic deficit lasts from several more hours to 2 days before remitting beyond clinical detection. The stroke-in-evolution begins as a relatively small neurologic deficit, which subsequently increases stepwise over a period of several hours or days. The completed stroke (CS) is one in which the abrupt neurologic deficit remains stable over a long period (days to years) and does not completely regress over time. An understanding of the implications of these temporal categories is important for guiding the physician toward the appropriate diagnostic workup and treatment.

The physician, having concluded that the patient has had a cerebral vascular attack of some type, determines whether it is in the anterior (carotid) or posterior (vertebral-basilar) arterial circulations. Characteristic syndromes indicative of the anterior circulation include the following: (1) contralateral paralysis, weakness, or numbness; (2) dysphasia, apraxia, and confusion with dominant hemisphere involvement; (3) transient monocular blindness; and (4) homonymous visual field defects. Syndromes of vertebral-basilar artery disease tend to be bilateral or generalized. They include the following: (1) dysarthria and dysphagia; (2) vertigo, tinnitus, and deafness; (3) unilateral or bilateral sensory and motor deficits often associated with cranial nerve dysfunction; (4) generalized imbalance with unilateral limb ataxia; and (5) visual field defects. Figs. 28-3 to 28-7 are examples of vascular lesions in territories of the three cerebral arteries as shown by a CT scan of the cerebrum.

In addition to the medical history and physical examination of the patient with a stroke, the physician should obtain the following laboratory studies: complete blood count, urinalysis, SMA-12, serum electrolyte count, serologic test for syphilis, erythrocyte count, sedimentation rate determination, antinuclear antibody titers, platelet count, presence of fibrin split products, skull and chest x-ray examinations, electrocardiograms (and cardiac isoenzymes if abnormal), EEGs and CT scan of the brain with contrast. The radionuclide brain scan and spinal tap are often of supplemental help, especially if the other studies are equivocal or the patient is febrile. Oculoplethysmography and other methods using ultrasonography and visual imaging assist in determining the locations of stenoses within the multiple cranial probes, now used as a research tool for analyzing regional cerebral blood flow, will someday be put to more common use in the diagnosis of cerebral vascular diseases.

The reasons for most of these tests are self-evident. *Cerebral embolism* may be suspected with bruits in the neck vessels or atrial fibrillation. Isotope brain scans, as a rule, become abnormal between the second and fourteenth days after cerebral infarction. An abnormal scan result in 24 to 48 hours may indicate a brain tumor or arteriovenous malformation. Large embolic infarctions, however, have been known to show abnormal scan results within 24 to 48 hours. Welch et al.,[24] in a reappraisal of isotope brain scanning in cerebral vascular diseases, found only 33% of 162 patients with strokes to have initially positive brain scans. Within this group, however, the percentages of abnormal scans increased in proportion to the time intervals after the onset of stroke from 27% within the first 2 days of symptoms to 52% after the tenth day.

CT scans of the brain now supplement and may soon replace isotope brain scanning in the diagnosis of intracerebral hemorrhages and infarctions. CT scanning is the more sensitive technique, capable of delineating brain lesions as small as 1.5 cm and demonstrating cerebral, cerebellar, and brain stem infarctions within the first 24 hours.

Cerebral spinal fluid (CSF) is generally normal during the first 24 to 72 hours after a cerebral thrombosis; thereafter the total protein level may rise a bit above the normal of 20 to 45 mg/100 ml. Blood in the CSF after a nontraumatic lumbar puncture indicates intracerebral hemorrhage, subarachnoid hemorrhage, or a "red infarction" (occasionally seen with cerebral embolism). One should keep in mind that 20% of intracerebral hemorrhages remain encapsulated within the brain substance and that blood from a ruptured berry aneurysm may not reach the lumbar subarachnoid space for as long as 6 to 8 hours after the initial event.

Angiography is useful and may be essential in

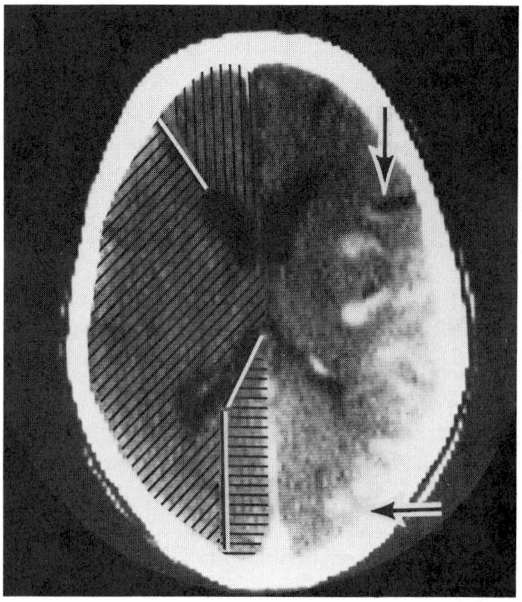

Fig. 28-3. Right middle cerebral artery territory infarction. Contrasted CT scan at horizontal pineal-trigone level demonstrating anterior (top arrow) and posterior (bottom arrow) extent of infarction. Photograph is retouched with hatched lines to demonstrate territories of anterior cerebral (vertical hatch), middle cerebral (slanted hatch), and posterior cerebral (horizontal hatch) arteries.

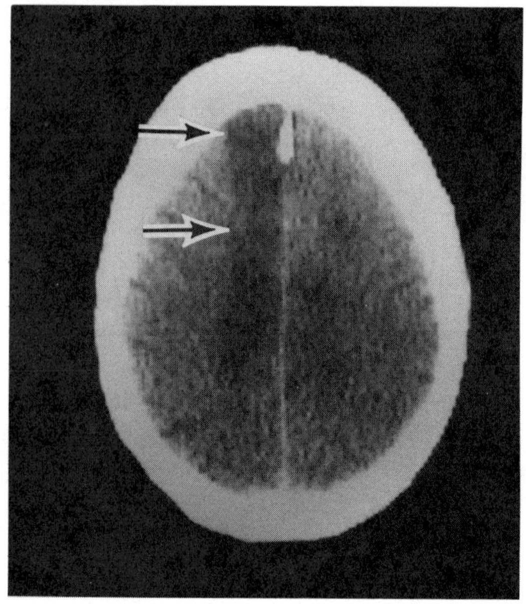

Fig. 28-4. Left anterior cerebral artery territory infarction. Noncontrasted CT scan at 25 degree supraventricular centrum semiovale level demonstrating anterior (top arrow) and posterior (lower arrow) extent of ischemic infarction as distinguished from the ventricular shadow and its opposite companion below.

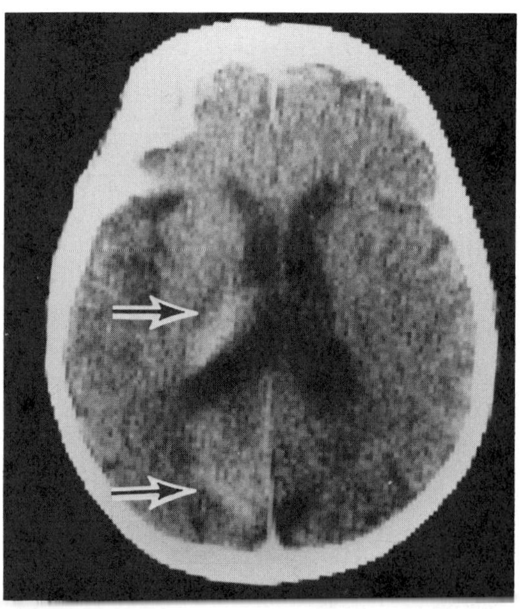

Fig. 28-5. Left posterior cerebral artery territory infarction. Contrasted CT scan at 25 degree midventricular level demonstrating infarcted area anterior to (top arrow) and posterior to (bottom arrow) confluence of ventricles.

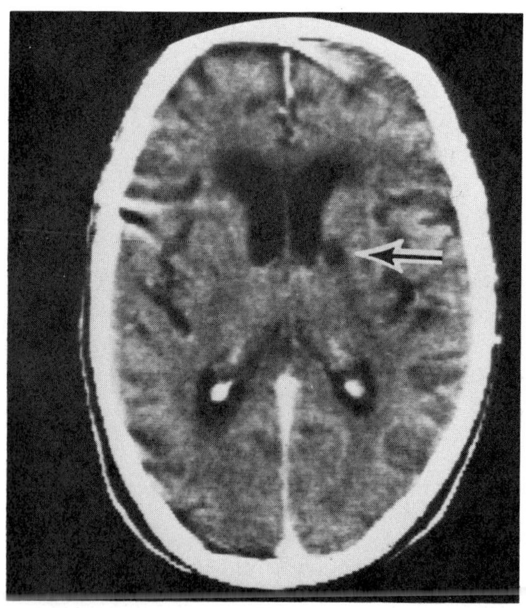

Fig. 28-6. Lacunar infarction precisely within the genu of the right internal capsule. Noncontrasted CT scan at 25 degree suprathird ventricle section with arrow pointing to lacuna (hole). The mechanisms of lacunar infarctions are not known exactly.

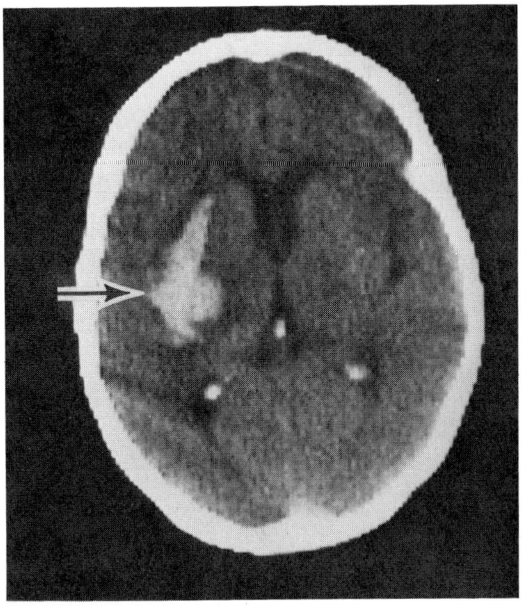

Fig. 28-7. Left intracerebral hemorrhage without rupture into ventricles. Noncontrasted CT scan at 25 degree pineal level shaped like hammerhead (arrow) and confined to substance of the insula, external capsule putamen, and posterior limb of internal capsule. Note some distortion of left ventricular system by mass effect. White dots are calcifications within the pineal (center) and choroid plexus (two lateral dots).

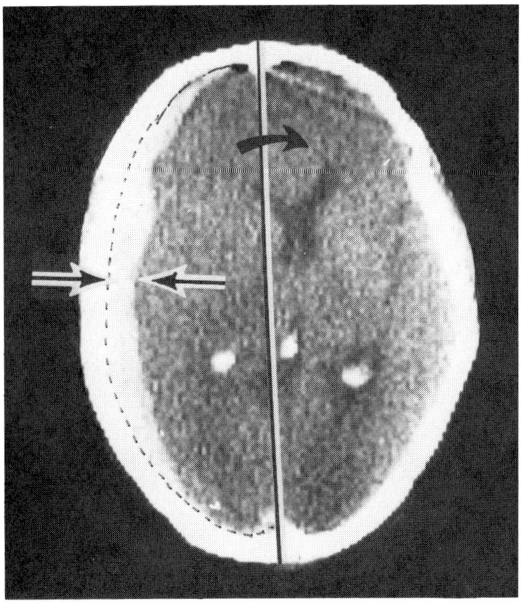

Fig. 28-8. Left subdural hematoma. Noncontrasted CT scan at 25 degree pineal level demonstrating brain shifted from left to right (top arrow) across the midline (retouched for emphasis) by an accumulation of venous blood in the subdural space (dotted line, opposing arrows).

the proper diagnoses of some cerebral vascular accidents. Nevertheless, angiography is indicated only if reconstructive vascular surgery is contemplated or if an intracranial mass lesion (tumor, subdural or epidural hematoma, or a surgically accessible intracerebral clot) is suspected. Angiographic signs of cerebral vascular disease include the following: (1) positive contrast images of berry aneurysms and arteriovenous malformations; (2) avascular areas indicative of blockage of blood flow through specific arterial channels or displacements of vessels; and (3) delayed rerouting of blood flow around or into infarcted regions indicating abnormal collateral circulation. In about 40% of cases of thromboembolic disease (including TIA), the lesion sufficient to explain the signs and symptoms lies in a surgically accessible neck vessel. This high incidence of neck vessel disease explains the shift in the trend of arteriography of cerebral vascular disorders away from direct percutaneous puncture of the neck vessels to visualization by means of catheterization through the axillary, brachial, or femoral arteries.[25]

The vast majority of stroke syndromes are managed medically and conservatively. Indications for surgical management of thromboembolic states are still not completely agreed on, but certain general principles seem to apply. For instance, surgery is best used to increase blood flow to noninfarcted areas by endarterectomies performed on stenotic arteries and to relieve further stenosis or fragmentation of ulcerated plaques of large neck vessels, thus reducing chance of thrombosis or embolism in the future. Surgery of extracranial vascular disease itself has an overall mortality of about 3% to 4%.[23] Thus surgery is generally performed on the selected patient with TIA who is at low risk. Surgery is also indicated for some nonthromboembolic vascular conditions such as the following: subdural (Fig. 28-8) and epidural hematomas; subarachnoid hemorrhages when an aneurysm can be demonstrated and the patient is not comatose; acute, intracerebellar hemorrhages; and selected cases of intracerebral hemorrhages (Fig. 28-7) when consciousness is preserved but the patient is gradually worsening.[25]

Medical management is determined by the presence or absence of associated pathologic conditions that may contribute to the total disability of the stroke patient. The incidence of hypertensive disease, cardiac disorders, and diabetes is especially high, and treatment is required. Anticoagulants may be administered either on a short-term (in-hospital) basis to stop or retard the stroke-in-evolution or on a long-term basis to the properly selected (nonsurgical) patient with TIA. Recent evidence from the Mayo Clinic suggests administering warfarin and similar anticoagulants for 3 to 6 months after a TIA.[26] Any longer use of anticoagulants results in no further statistically noticeable improvement of the morbidity or mortality of this group of stroke-prone patients. Most authorities do not carry out anticoagulation therapy in patients with completed strokes.[27] A possible exception to this is in the early management of cerebral embolism, with short-term anticoagulation therapy (heparin and warfarin for several weeks or months) until the source of embolization is believed to be resolved or eliminated. Anticoagulants are never administered when the presence of blood has been demonstrated in the cerebral spinal fluid.

In the last few years acetylsalicylic acid and other compounds such as sulfinpyrazone and dipyridamole have been used in patients with completed strokes and in TIA (without a demonstrated surgical lesion or in patients for whom warfarin-type anticoagulants are contraindicated). Although the results of group studies are still pending, there seems to be some justification for the use of these drugs in preventing subsequent strokes.

There is a 20% mortality in persons hospitalized with acute completed stroke. Not all of these by any means are caused by the stroke itself but by concurrent disorders such as myocardial infarction, pneumonia, and pulmonary embolism. Seizures complicate strokes in about 10% to 15% of cases (initially or during the first poststroke year). By far the majority of elderly persons with completed strokes who leave the hospital to resume their lives die, not from another stroke, but of heart disease. Debilitation secondary to depression undoubtedly takes it toll.

At the present time, the best "treatment" for strokes is prevention. Analysis of scores of patients with cerebral thromboembolic disease has revealed a list of so-called risk factors or associated conditions that occur in this population to an extent significantly greater than in the age-matched nonstroke population at large. These factors include the following: hypertensive disease with consistent blood pressure readings greater than 159/89; enlarged cardiac silhouette on chest x-ray film; electrocardiographic evidence of left ventricular hypertrophy, myocardial infarction, or intraventricular block; congestive heart failure; diabetes mellitus; angiographic evidence of a cerebral vascular anomaly or vascular stenosis; family history of strokes; history of angina pectoris or peripheral vascular disease; and TIA.[28] Of course the greatest risk factor for stroke, for which prevention has untenable consequences, is age itself. One is reminded here of the grimly humorous auto bumper sticker that reads, "Cancer cures smoking."

BRAIN TUMORS

Only 5 in 100,000 persons from all age groups in the United States die yearly of primary intracranial neoplasms, with the greatest number of such deaths occurring in the fourth and fifth decades of life rather than in senium.[29] Zimmerman[30] surveyed 5199 central nervous system masses of all kinds and found that 47% were primary intracranial neoplasms, whereas 20% arose metastatically from extracranial sites. The remainder were nonneoplastic space-occupying masses, such as abscesses, cysts, hematomas, and gummas. These data support the contention that primary gliomas are not a significant medical problem of the geriatric population as a whole. Nevertheless, the physician must constantly be on guard against the unexpected occurrences of secondary neoplasms and other space-occupying lesions such as chronic subdural hematomas and brain abscesses. The latter may closely simulate a cerebral tumor in the development of signs and symptoms yet give a gratifying response to surgery.

Most primary brain tumors found in the geriatric population are glioblastomas and astrocytomas, which almost always occur above the tentorium cerebelli within the substance of the cerebral hemispheres. By contrast, tumors metastatic to the central nervous system are found below the tentorium within the brain stem and cerebellum about one third of the time and within the cerebrum the remainder of the time. Metastases to the spinal cord are extremely rare. Malignancies of the lung in men or of the breast in women are those most likely to metastasize to the central nervous system in the general population. However, central nervous system secondary tumors from malignancies of the gastrointestinal and urinary systems are found more often in individuals over 65 years of age.[31,32]

The symptoms and signs of brain tumor are much the same whether the lesion is primary or secondary but differ according to the site of the mass and its rate of growth. A recent history of extracranial malignancy provides strong grounds for believing the recent onset of a central nervous system sign to be the result of a metastasis. As a tumor grows, it consumes space; and although headache, papilledema, vomiting, and stupor are important general signs, coincident and progressive neurologic deficit is the most significant portent of tumor. Progressive sensory loss, paralysis, visual impairment, aphasia, ataxia, imbalance, neural deafness, and convulsions may indicate a brain tumor. Thus an expanding intracranial mass lesion is to be suspected when one of these signs appears and increases in severity over time (even in a short time).

Central nervous system tumors declare their clinical appearance in three ways depending on whether they are supratentorial, infratentorial, or meningeal. Signs can develop insidiously over weeks or months but are occasionally abrupt and dramatic in onset. The latter kind of presentation is more indicative of a metastatic lesion. Supratentorial tumors tend to cause focal neurologic signs (paresis, apraxia, sensory disturbances, seizures) or general signs (diffuse weakness or proneness to fatigue, personality and cognitive changes). Headache, vomiting, and mental dullness may develop later. With infratentorial tumors, local signs of limb ataxia and cranial nerve dysfunction tend to occur along with the generalized signs of imbalance and increased intracranial pressure. Focal or lateralized paresis or sensory signs develop late if at all. With sarcoma or carcinoma of the meninges, diffuse, severe, unremitting headache is the rule, developing earlier than any other neurologic sign besides nuchal rigidity.

A suspicion of brain tumor can often be confirmed by ancillary diagnostic procedures. The following data are often obtained when there is a tumor: elevated spinal fluid protein level over 45 mg/100 ml; lymphocytic pleocytosis (over 5 lymphocytes/mm^3); normal glucose level (except in the case of carcinomatosis of the meninges, in which case it is low); negative test for lues; and normal bacteriologic studies. In addition, skull x-ray films may show a significant shift of the calcified pineal from its normal midline position and pressure demineralization of the dorsum sella. Slow-growing tumors, such as meningiomas and oligodendrogliomas, may contain patches of calcification that are x-ray opaque. The EEG may indicate an area of focal slowing overlying the tumor site. Changes in the EEG with serial examinations tend to correlate with the rapidity of tumor growth and surrounding brain edema. Radioisotope scans of the cranium using technetium pertechnetate (^{99}TC) or mercury chlormerodrin (^{203}Hg) also aid in the locating of tumors. CT scans yield positive results more often than ordinary radioisotope brain scans in the search for intracranial masses of all types, including tumors of the orbits or globes of the eyes. Fig. 28-9 demonstrates the appear-

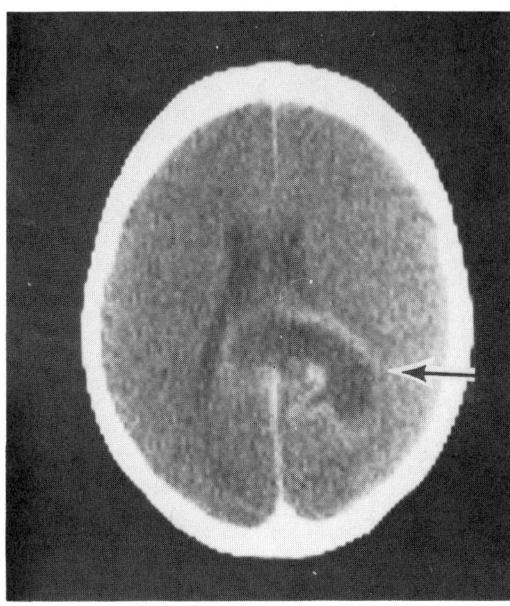

Fig. 28-9. Brain tumor (glioblastoma). Contrasted CT scan at 35 degree high ventricular level demonstrating "chick embryo-shaped" mass with halo (arrow) crossing the midline, via the corpus callosum, and displacing ventricular system.

ance of a brain tumor on a CT scan. When considering surgery or irradiation, the physician should delineate the extent and vascular supply of the tumor by cerebral angiography. The patterns of small blood vessels visualized during the capillary and venous phases of the arteriogram help delineate the extent of the tumor likely to be encountered at surgery.

A relatively new tumor biopsy technique of using the CT scanner and a coring needle has been developed, which allows the surgeon to take a piece of any tumor in any part of the brain through a small burr hole in the skull. The technique is faster, simpler, and safer than craniotomy. Furthermore the procedure can be done in the x-ray department.[33]

Once the presence of an expanding intracranial mass lesion has been ascertained, the question of management arises. Here the patient's age and physical status and the size and location of the mass are important surgical considerations. Meningiomas are generally amenable to surgery. They comprise about 15% of all primary intracranial neoplasms.[30] Subdural hematomas or hygromas (Fig. 28-10) have a good prognosis

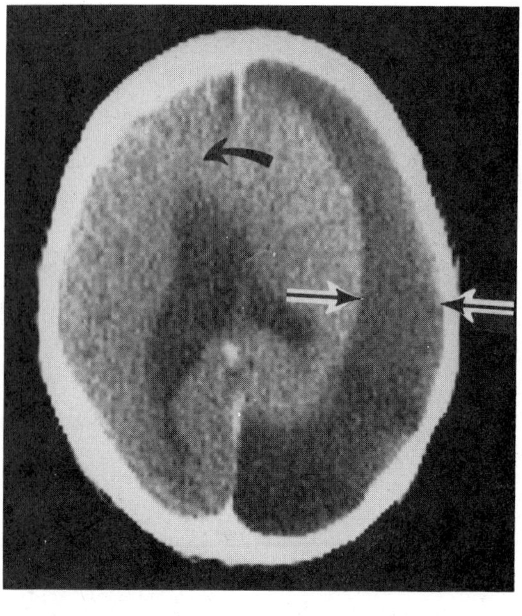

Fig. 28-10. Subdural hygroma. Noncontrasted CT scan at 35 degree high ventricular level demonstrating marked accumulation of cerebral spinal fluid between brain surface (inner straight arrow) and dura lying against inner table of skull (opposing straight arrow). Ventricles have been distorted (see Fig. 28-1) and shifted toward the left (curved black arrow).

at any age if discovered and treated before unconsciousness becomes prolonged. Primary gliomas, however, can rarely be removed surgically in their entirety, and metastatic lesions of the central nervous system are in more than one location 65% of the time. Surgery plus irradiation of gliomas yield a slightly longer survival time than surgery alone.[29] Chemotherapeutic agents continue to have disappointing results in the treatment of brain tumors in humans.[34]

It is important to recognize that extracranial neoplasms, including lymphomas, may cause diffuse and even focal neurologic signs in the absence of secondary metastases or direct extension to the brain.[35] Progressive multifocal leukoencephalopathy (PML) can occur along with carcinoma of the lung, sometimes preceding clinical symptoms of lung diseae by as much as 15 months.[36] These conditions are rarely encountered even in large medical centers. Not nearly so rare, however, is the incidence of invasion of the central nervous system by herpes simplex, cryptococcus organisms, or other infectious organisms during the course of treatment of a systemic malignancy. The cerebral spinal fluid generally shows moderate pleocytosis together with positive reactions to india ink staining, indicating the presence of a yeast infection. Spinal fluid is normal in cases of "remote" malignant encephalopathies such as PML and cerebellar cortical degeneration, sometimes referred to as paraneoplastic disease of the central nervous system.[37]

NEUROPATHY

Weakness is a common complaint of elderly people. However, what is meant by weakness is not always readily apparent. It may describe the fatigue that is caused by lessened cardiovascular reserve, diminished oxygen-carrying capacity of the blood secondary to anemia or pulmonary disease, diabetes mellitus or other systemic conditions, or it may be the primary symptom of a neurotic or depressive illness. More specifically, weakness may result from increased stiffness of the joints associated with arthritis or from muscle atrophy secondary to motoneuron disease or primary muscle fiber disease. Dysfunction of the basal ganglia of the forebrain and cerebellum, as well as of the suprasegmental motor neurons, cause disturbances of movement that are frequently interpreted by the patient as weakness.

A common cause of weakness, especially of a body part rather than of the body as a whole, is neuropathy. Neuropathy is an inclusive medical term for any dysfunction of a peripheral nerve secondary to disease or injury (including pressure). A long list of illnesses can be compiled in which neuropathy (peripheral neuritis) is frequently a complication.[38] It is important to bear in mind that peripheral neuritis is frequently the earliest and only indication that systemic disease is developing. For this reason every instance of peripheral neuritis must be explored carefully, lest a condition far more ominous than the demonstrated symptom be overlooked. Neuropathies can affect a single nerve (mononeuropathy), occur temporally and spatially scattered among many nerves (polyneuropathy or mononeuritis multiplex), or be confined to the distal portion of nerves so as to involve the limbs symmetrically (symmetrical distal polyneuropathy). Peripheral neuritis may be further described as sensory, motor, or mixed. Empirical groupings such as these relate fairly well to etiologic classifications such as alcoholic neuropathy and arsenical neuropathy, inasmuch as many diseases tend to involve the peripheral nervous system in a predictable manner.[39] Within the continental United States, diabetes mellitus is the most common cause of neuropathy in the elderly, followed by nutritional disorders associated with chronic illnesses and alcoholism.

The diagnosis of neuropathy requires two or more of the following clinical signs: pain, paresthesias, sensory impairment, local discomfort or projected sensations elicited by gentle percussion over the affected nerve, loss or reduction of myotatic reflexes, muscle weakness in accord with its nerve supply, or atrophic changes in skin and nails resulting from coincident involvement of postganglionic sympathetic axons.

The most common mononeuropathies of elderly persons are trigeminal and postherpetic neuralgia and facial nerve neuritis (Bell's palsy). *Trigeminal neuralgia* is characterized by paroxysms of severe lancinating pain experienced on one side of the face, either occurring spontaneously or related to touching the face, talking, or chewing. Sensory deficit is the exception rather than the rule in untreated patients. Causes of trigeminal neuralgia (tic douloureux) are unknown. A popular current theory claims that a "knuckle" of a redundant blood vessel presses itself into the trigeminal nerve root close to its emergence from the brain stem, thereby "irritating" the nerve from time to time. Plaques of demyelination have been found in the descending tract of the trigeminal nerve at postmortem in some instances of multiple sclerosis with tic douloureux. Most of the time no cause is determined, either surgically or at postmortem.

Preferred treatment for the most part is medical. The drugs presently used with good success are carbamazepine (600 to 1000 mg daily), phenytoin (400 to 600 mg daily), or chlorphenesin (800 to 1600 mg daily). If drug therapy fails to help over a period of time then one among various neurosurgical procedures must be done to relieve the patient of severe unsettling pain. Such procedures include the following (1) crushing or partial section of the trigeminal root (retrogasserian neurectomy); (2) application of a radio frequency current to the gasserian ganglion (or appropriate postganglionic branch of the trigeminal nerve complex); or (3) separating the trigeminal root from its presumably offending arterial compression (Jannetta procedure). Surgical treatment is more effective and more risky. Surgical mortality and postsurgical recurrence rates vary among different procedures (and surgeons). Trigeminal neuralgia often remits spontaneously, only to recur months or even years later. Part of management is to delay surgery while maintaining hope for a spontaneous remission.

"Shingles" is a somewhat more common neural affliction among the elderly than among others. A varicella zoster virus infection almost always clinically appears in the elderly as localized mononeuritis. Deep, aching, severe pain localized to some relatively small portion of the body or of a limb is the usual. For a week or more this may be the only symptom, and diagnosis remains obscure. Then a few (or perhaps many) small vesicular eruptions appear on the skin roughly corresponding to the area of pain, verifying the presence of varicella zoster virus. The patient should be told to anticipate several months or more of pain. It is important to realize that localized weakness may also be a prominent symptom in this condition and that the weak muscles need not be those beneath the painful skin area. Herpetic neuritis is often associated with cerebral spinal fluid pleocytosis, and meningitic symptoms may also be present. Rarely does clinically significant encephalitis appear. When it does it is usually benign and without residual central nervous system damage.

After the vesicles heal (with or without depigmentation or scarification), the individual may be left with a persistent, aggravating discomfort in the nerve distribution known as *postherpetic neuralgia*. There is no adequate therapy for this condition. Occasionally corticosteroids, administered during the infectious phase of the illness, may prevent or ameliorate postherpetic neuralgia. Chronic pain may be treated with analgesics and amitriptyline in combination with fluphenazine or hydroxyzine pamoate. As with trigeminal neuralgia, phenytoin and carbamazepine administration has been successful in some instances.

Acute idiopathic facial paralysis (Bell's palsy) occurs in all age groups, with peak incidence between ages 20 and 40. May et al.[40] found about 16% in his series to be over 60 years old. Usually the patient or a friend discovers the patient's face to be sagging on one side, and the patient is certain a stroke has occurred. Taverner (1955)[41] insisted that certain criteria be met before the term *Bell's palsy* is used as the diagnosis in a particular case of facial palsy. For example, its onset should be relatively abrupt, preferably within 24 to 48 hours; the paralysis should be limited to only one side of the face for any one episode; and there should be no signs or symptoms of cerebral or brain stem disease and no evidence of extraaxial posterior fossa lesions or of ear disease. May,[42] in a comprehensive review of the etiologic factors of facial paralysis, mentioned more than 60 causes, many of which initially appear as cases of typical Bell's palsy. May admitted that almost 10% of the 90 patients in his carefully studied series of patients with abrupt unilateral facial palsy were misdiagnosed as idiopathic.

A careful office examination of the patient with facial paralysis can be the most important method of determining the site of the offending lesion and, by implication, its cause. In *supranuclear* lesions of the facial nerve's central connections, there is usually good facial muscular tone; intact upper facial movements; and an asymmetrical voluntary smile. Often other neurologic abnormalities such as hemiparesis, monoparesis, aphasia, or cortical combined hemisensory defects are present. The cause in this instance is likely to be a cerebral vascular accident or tumor.

Within the brain stem there can be direct *nuclear* involvement of the seventh cranial nerve nucleus in the pons. Often the sixth and seventh cranial nerves as well as the corticospinal tract are involved so that signs of other neurologic deficits are present. Etiologic factors in this instance may be vascular, neoplastic, infectious, or demyelinating. Poliomyelitis, now rare, is sometimes a consideration.

Extrinsic to the brain stem but within the posterior fossa, mass lesions of the pontine angle produce involvement of vestibular and cochlear portions of the eighth cranial nerve, possibly the fifth, ninth, tenth, and eleventh nerves; taste; lacrimation; salivation; and facial motor portions of the seventh nerve all on the same side. Etiologic factors include neuromas, meningiomas, cholesteatomas, and of course trauma with fracture of the temporal bone.

A lesion at the level of the geniculate ganglion will cause hyperacusis, alter taste, diminish salivation and lacrimation, and cause hemifacial palsy. Herpes zoster oticus, temporal bone fracture, and idiopathic (Bell's) palsy are primarily responsible.

Lesions in the tympanomastoid region also cause hyperacusis, facial paralysis, and decreased salivation but leave lacrimation intact. Bell's palsy, cholesteatoma of the middle ear, fractures, or infections are usually responsible.

Extracranial lesions of the facial nerve may cause complete or partial (because of the involvement of individual branches) facial paralysis. All other facial nerve functions remain intact. Facial soft tissue trauma, tumors, parotid carcinoma, and pharyngeal carcinoma are the most common etiologic factors.

If we exclude stroke from the list of causes of facial palsy, then close to 90% of the remaining causes will be affections of the facial nerve within the temporal bone. Until recently (1971) more than 75% of these could further be grouped as idiopathic facial palsy. Adour et al.,[43] in a communication published in the *Journal of the American Medical Association*, proposed a viral cause of Bell's palsy. Adour explains that facial nerve function is compromised by means of a "mechanism" that reactivates the latent herpes simplex virus. Conditions favorable to this mechanism include pregnancy, menstruation, fever, dental extractions, exposure to cold or strong sunlight, and emotional shock. He speculates that the offending neurotropic virus probably resides within the gasserian or geniculate ganglion where it is protected from circulating antibodies, only to become activated under the appropriate set of circumstances. In this regard, pain, facial dysesthesia, and reduced sensitivity to pinpricks and corneal stimulation have been observed by many others who have studied large numbers of patients diagnosed as having Bell's palsy.

About 65% of patients will recover completely without any treatment, the remaining 35% have anywhere from "undetectable" or "minimal" residual denervation to complete and permanent denervation. Corticosteroids reduce pain and may hasten recovery, but whether they significantly alter the ultimate outcome is still, in my opinion, controversial.

Neuropathies that are generalized or else symmetrically distributed about the body's midline are likely to have metabolic, nutritional, autoimmune, or toxic etiologic factors. They are difficult if not impossible to distinguish merely on the basis of their signs or symptoms, since most patients will complain of numbness, tingling, pain and weakness and since signs will be those of impaired primary sensibilities (touch, temperature, or pain), weakness, hypotonia, and reduction of the myotatic reflexes. Sympathetic dysfunction; loss of vibratory, motion, and position senses; and perversions of touch, temperature, and pain stimuli are also reported. Once the diagnosis of distal symmetrical peripheral neuropathy is made, then a lengthy search for its cause may lie ahead of the investigator. It is safe to say (with few reservations) that virtually all the diseases a physician can think of have, at one time or another, been associated with peripheral neuropathy.[38,39]

To start the investigation, the physician looks for the simplest, most common causes (diabetes, alcoholism, drugs, heavy metal poisoning, polyarteritis, remote effects of carcinoma); and moves on to the more obscure and complex causes (amyloidosis, porphyria, dysthyroidism, paraproteinemias, heredo-degenerations). Diagnosing neuropathy is made easier by the technique of electroneurography, in which the conduction velocities of anatomically available mixed peripheral nerves are measured and compared against standard norms.[44] Excessive slowing of the nerve impulse along the entire length or even in the distal portions of a peripheral nerve is a nonspecific indicator of disease. Blockage or delay of the nerve impulse locally along a segment of the peripheral nerve indicates local pressure, infarction, or severance of the nerve.

There are several conditions resembling peripheral neuropathy that bear mentioning. Motoneuron disease, myasthenia gravis, and the myopathies may be superficially confused with peripheral neuropathies. These conditions are dealt with elsewhere in this book. Localized or projected pain without any objective neurologic sign of impairment may be impossible to diagnose.

Keep in mind that peripheral nerves are also the telephone lines to and from the central nervous system and the body's sensors, so that what "hurts" or "tingles" or "feels numb" may really be a pathologic condition in the skin, joint, muscle, or viscera or even within the central nervous system itself. A healthy peripheral nerve in these instances is merely doing its job of transmitting the message that something elsewhere is amiss. Demyelinating disease often appears as a sensory symptom of the hand or foot, but the causative lesion is almost always within the brain or spinal cord. Tabes is accompanied by numbness, sharp stabbing pains in the limbs, and trouble in walking. Reflexes will be absent at the knees and ankles, and pain, especially aching, slow, burning pain, cannot be felt when appropriate noxious stimulation is applied to the lower extremities. The causative lesions are not to be found in the peripheral nerves but in the spinal cord. Subacute combined degeneration (of the spinal cord in pernicious anemia) is almost always mistaken for peripheral neuritis at its onset. This is to be expected because the early symptoms are weakness, tingling paresthesia of the fingers and toes, and numbness. Reflexes may be severely reduced and, in the elderly, may even be absent at the knees and ankles. Vibratory sensation and touch localization are severely impaired in a distal to proximal distribution not unlike that of neuropathy. As the disease progresses, however, ataxia becomes more prominent, Babinski's signs appear, and visual and mental impairment occur, thereby clearly removing it from the category of neuropathy.

The syndrome of Guillain-Barré deserves special mention under the general topic of peripheral neuropathy. Guillain-Barré disease is an acute inflammatory polyradiculoneuropathy affecting children and adults of all ages. Its prominent pathologic features are segmental demyelination and perivenular lymphoid infiltration throughout the peripheral nervous system, with the most severe reactions being proximally located in the spinal nerve roots and cauda equina. The sympathetic chain and ganglia are involved, and lymphocytic infiltrates are found in the liver, spleen, heart, kidneys, and other organs, attesting to the systemic nature of the condition. The annual incidence rate among persons older than 40 is 3.3 per 100,000.[45]

The illness is ushered in by fairly rapid development (hours to weeks) of limb weakness, acroparesthesia, pain, dysphagia, loss of myotatic reflexes, and respiratory difficulty. Signs and symptoms reach their maximum in 1 to 30 days, with a median of 8 days, from which point improvement begins anywhere from 1 to 45 days (10-day median). Total recovery varies widely from weeks to years. The diagnosis is made by the dramatic clinical picture aided by the cerebral spinal fluid examination. Spinal fluid protein tends to be elevated (80% of the time), while the cell count is normal (85% of the time) if sampled about 2 weeks after the onset of symptoms. Spinal fluid gamma globulin is often disproportionately elevated. Curiously enough, the results of the spinal fluid tests bear no correlation to the severity or prognosis of the individual case. The recurrence rate is extremely low.

Treatment of the distal symmetric peripheral neuropathies is solely dependent on determining the etiologic factors. In some instances the disease found to be the presumed cause for the patient's neuropathy is poorly responsive to treatment or simply not treatable. The neuropathy may then progress along with the disease. Physical therapy measures and pain control are usually indicated along with liberal doses of multiple vitamins. In spite of the most conscientious efforts at diagnosis, a small contingent of inexplicable neuropathies will haunt the physician's practice and remain more or less resistant to therapeutic efforts. It is wise to follow the courses of these patients to await the belated arrival of clues that may in time secure the diagnosis.

MOVEMENT DISORDERS

Some neurologic diseases of senium are characterized by abnormal and involuntary movements of the body, many of which are presumed to be related to the loss of basal ganglia control.[46] The coarse rhythmic tremor of parkinsonism is both well known and distinctive.[47] *Athetosis* (slow writhing sinuous movements) and *chorea* (brief, dancing, jerky movements) of the trunk and extremities are only rarely the results of cerebral vascular disease in the elderly. Generally their cause is never discovered. *Habit tics* (stereotyped activity patterns that often mimic natural movements) are of equally obscure causes and are refractory to treatment. Another type of abnormal movement disorder of adults is *action dystonia*. In this condition brief episodes of uncontrolled movement often precede the initiation of a voluntary act.[48,49] *Meige's syndrome* ordinarily develops after a person reaches 60 years of age. It consists of involuntary asynchronous and arrhythmic forced blinking, wrinkling of the nose, pursing of the lips, and licking movements of the tongue. Like many involuntary movement disorders, Meige's syndrome does not respond to any form of therapy and must be tolerated as a continuing annoyance.

Parkinson's disease is by far the most common movement disorder encountered in the geriatric population, excluding people confined to hospitals for the chronically ill. It is estimated to occur in varying severity in 1 to 1.5 million people in the United States, principally elderly people.[49] In Peter Bent Brigham Hospital, Boston, the charts of 7941 persons over 61 years of age were reviewed, and 121 cases of parkinsonism (an incidence of 1.5%) were discovered.

The cause of the idiopathic variety of the disease is not precisely known but is related to the imperfect storage or use of biogenic amines by nuclei of the basal ganglia. Idiopathic parkinsonism is characterized by a slowly progressing rigidity of limb and trunk musculature with increasing poverty of voluntary movements. Cogwheel roughness may be detectable on passive movement of limbs about their joints. Flexion postures of trunk and limbs greatly shorten the patient's apparent height, and neck flexion may be severe enough to restrict forward gaze to a few yards. The face becomes expressionless. In other words, facies are frozen or masked; speech is in whispers and is muffled and monotonous;

and ocular mobility may become markedly circumscribed. Rhythmic tremors (four to six per second) of fingers, feet, head, and lips may occur but abate briefly during voluntary movement. A great many patients complain of excessive salivation, seborrhea, constipation, and urinary difficulties. In elderly individuals cognition and recall generally remain unaffected, but chronic brain syndromes and nonpsychotic depressions are commonly associated with Parkinson's disease, especially the rigid, nontremulous form of the disease.

A variety of parkinsonism known as *postencephalitic parkinsonism* was once prevalent but has become rare today. Because of the pandemic of influenza from 1916 to 1927, its onset was temporally asssociated with a history of influenza. Although it occurs infrequently at present, postencephalitic parkinsonism is still encountered. This variety differs from idiopathic parkinsonism in that torsion dystonic posturing, respiratory dysrhythmias, oculogyric crises, and sleep and personality disorders are seen in addition to the signs and symptoms of the idiopathic disease mentioned earlier. It has been postulated that some virus other than that of influenza may remain in the nervous system for long periods of time before causing its characteristic neurologic damage.

Levodopa, in doses of 3 to 8 gm administered daily (or 1 to 2 gm when used in combination with carbidopa), is helpful in relieving rigidity, bradykinesia, and tremor, as well as in moderating some of the other symptoms. Belladonna alkaloids and some antihistaminic compounds continue to be of value as supplementary drugs. Surgical treatment of selected cases of parkinsonism and of incapacitating essential tremor still has a place in therapy; however, young patients with other varieties of involuntary movement disorders respond to surgery better than do elderly persons with Parkinson's disease.[50]

The most troublesome, newly appreciated, movement disorder of the elderly is an iatrogenic condition known as *tardive dyskinesia*. Jeste and Wyatt[51] define tardive dyskinesia as "a syndrome consisting of abnormal stereotyped involuntary movements of the mouth, face, limbs and tongue which occurs rather late in the course of drug treatment [usually neuroleptic drugs], and in the etiology of which the [history of] drug treatment is a necessary factor." There are no specific clinical or laboratory tests that will definitely secure the diagnosis. The physician observes protruding, rolling, "fly catching" tongue movements; restless lip smacking and pouting; chewing, jutting, and retraction of the jaw; grimacing; puffing of the cheeks; choreoathetoid movements of the extremities; rocking and "caterpillar" movements of the trunk. The movements always disappear in sleep and are suppressed briefly by voluntary efforts to control them. Psychologic stress and voluntary movements of distant body parts temporarily aggravate them. Generally the patient has no other medical or hereditary condition that could explain the abnormal movements.

The prolonged use of phenothiazines, tricyclic antidepressants, levodopa, amphetamines, phenytoin, chloroquine, antihistamines, and even estrogens has been implicated in the causation of tardive dyskinesia. The elderly patient, more than young patients, is likely to develop permanent and irreversible dyskinesia with administration of these drugs. As more and more of these drugs enter the market and the periods of drug use increase, we are likely to see more patients in senium with this peculiar syndrome. Treatment is directed toward stopping or reducing the dose of the offending drug. Some patients respond to antidopamine drugs, while others respond to cholinergic agents. L-Tryptophan, an amino acid, has been given to dyskinesia patients recently with some reported successes.

Action tremor of the upper extremities, with or without an accompanying head tremor, is occasionally seen as an isolated phenomenon in the elderly. Usually it is seen as part of the syndrome of *benign essential tremor* appearing uncharacteristically late in life. It is important to distinguish benign essential tremor and Parkinson's disease, drug-induced tremors, dysthyroidism, hepatocerebral syndromes, alcoholic tremulousness, and the like. Benign essential tremor is usually distinguishable from parkinsonism by the absence of muscular rigidity and bradykinesia. In the early phases of these tremorous conditions, however, they may not be distinguishable. Essential tremor does not respond to levodopa, but the placebo effect of prescribing anything must be taken into account here, since the tremor of both parkinsonism and essential tumor are aggravated by anxiety and stress and mollified by serenity and relaxation.

The cause of essential tremor is unknown; in the majority of instances it is familial. Essential tremor is benign and rarely becomes incapacitating. Several ounces of ethanol in any form will stop the essential tremor for several hours, but propranolol, a beta-adrenergic blocking agent, is safer and ultimately more useful in controlling this variety of tremor.

SPONDYLOSIS

The process by which the interspaces between the individual vertebral bodies narrow (the result of degeneration of the intervertebral discs) and develop lipping (osteophyte formation) adjacent to the disc spaces is called *spondylosis*. The term vertebral osteoarthritis should be reserved for the inflammatory process affecting the synovial membranes of the diarthrodial facet joints. Facet joint arthritis, therefore, may occur as a primary condition (arthritis) secondary to denervation of pain fibers (Charcot joints) or to spondylosis or acute trauma.

Disc "spaces" make up 25% of the total height of the spine in the newborn and young adult. The water content of the disc of newborns is 88%, but by age 75 it is only 69%. Significant disc degeneration has already begun by the fourth decade of life. Desiccation of the disc is the essential etiologic factor of spondylosis. Water is bound to mucopolysaccharides (myxoid tissue), which provides the disc its elasticity. With dehydration the mucopolysaccharide content diminishes, collagen content increases, the nucleus pulposus disappears, and the disc becomes brittle, fibrous, and inelastic. Weight and shearing and bending forces cause bulging and hypertrophy of the anterior spinous ligament or extrusion of disc material to the side (so-called laterally herniated disc). Spondylosis has a predilection for the lower cervical, midthoracic, and lower lumbar interspaces.[52]

The neurologic picture of disc disease (spondylosis) varies in accordance with two factors: (1) the level of the offending spinal lesion (lumbar, thoracic, or cervical) and (2) the position of the compressing mass (midline or lateral). Keep in mind that segmental spinal roots exit above their respective vertebral bodies in the cervical region (i.e., C3 root exits via the foramen formed by the C2 and C3 cervical vertebrae). In the lumbar region the spinal roots exit below their respective vertebral bodies (i.e., L4 root exits via the foramen formed by L4 and L5 vertebrae).

The symptoms of a *laterally herniated disc* in the lumbar region are lateralized back pain, paraspinous muscle spasm, projected pain down into the ipsilateral lower extremity, variable weakness of the leg, and variable degrees of interruption of the myotatic reflex. Forward bending causes the ipsilateral knee to flex, while Kernig's sign (or other leg raising signs) is positive ipsilaterally. Leg pain is usually aggravated by sudden increases in intraabdominal pressure (coughing, straining, sneezing, etc.). Pain in the leg often worsens after falling asleep in the supine position as paraspinous muscles relax and allow the spine to lengthen.

The symptoms of a *centrally protruding disc* in the lumbar region are slower to develop as gradual stenosis of the vertebral canal occurs. Eventually, compression of the cauda equina roots, which exit below the level of the protruding disc, occurs. Intermittent claudication of the lower extremities resembling that of vascular insufficiency is not uncommon. Dysuria, leg dysesthesia, "restless legs," loss or impairment of myotatic reflexes bilaterally with low back pain and trouble walking occur. Sudden falls (without syncope) find the patient suddenly on the floor. Nocturnal pain is common with central disc protrusions in the lumbar region caused by a tug on the nerve roots by a relaxing and lengthening spinal column.

By far the vast majority of disc protrusions are in the lumbar region. Thoracic disc herniations sufficient to cause compression of the spinal cord are distinctly rare, estimated to occur once per million patients per year. The protruded thoracic disc in the thoracic region is usually central and impinges on the spinal cord, compressing it, causing cord edema, and interfering with its blood supply. There may be localized symptoms of root pain or segmental irritability, giving rise to a disturbing girdlelike sensation (pain, warmth, skin hypersensitivity) at or near the level of the offending disc. But more often, long tract signs and symptoms develop without a clear level. Thus sensory dysesthesia, pain, weakness, spasticity (of the legs) with hyperactive reflexes and Babinski's signs are present. Urinary urgency is a common complaint, and midback pain with coughing, sneezing, or reaching upwards may occur.

Disc protrusion at the cervical level is most likely to be at either the C4-5 or C5-6 level. At C4-5 a lateralized disc will impinge on the C5 nerve root, while a central disc protrusion will compress the cord at the C4 segmental level. Spur formation and hypertrophy of the anterior spinous ligament secondary to spondylosis are much more common than direct herniation of nucleus pulposus' fragments. In the cervical region basic syndromes caused by lateral "spurs" and central "bars" occur. Osteophytic spurs protrude laterally into a neural foramen, causing radicular pain, weakness, and impairment of the myotatic reflex arc within the cervical nerve root distribution. Segmental muscular atrophy, together with fibrillations, fasciculations, and reduction of the interference pattern may be detectable with electromyography.[44] With lateralized discs or spurs there is virtually no cord compression and no lower extremity symptoms.

The signs and symptoms of a central cervical disc or bar with cord compression develop slowly and insidiously, making initial complaints difficult to diagnose. Trouble walking or a tendency to stumble are often the earliest neurologic complaints, even though the patient may have had episodes of neck soreness and stiffness for 15 to 20 years. Reflexes in the lower extremities become hyperactive, and the ability to control the legs becomes more difficult as spasticity develops and Babinski's signs appear. Cremasteric and abdominal reflexes disappear as upper motor neurogenic bladder develops (urgency and frequency). Sensory symptoms can be present anywhere below the level of the cervical cord lesion. Because of the anatomy of the cervical cord, with its strong teetering dentate ligaments, compression of the dorsal columns (as well as of the lateral columns) tends to occur first with a ventrally compressing lesion. Therefore, dysesthesia of the feet with impaired vibratory perception may be the only sensory complaint. If the cervical lesion compresses the cord segment at the C5 level, then the biceps reflexes will be reduced and the triceps reflexes will become hyperactive. Lesions at higher cervical levels result in hyperactive reflexes in all the limbs with a normal jaw jerk, thus localizing the lesion below the pons and above the C5 segmental level. Cervical radicular pain in the arms, neck, or the occiput help to further localize the origin of leg and urinary complaints to the cervical level.

As expected, the neurologic signs of central or lateralized disc protrusions resemble those of any extradural mass, including tumors. It is therefore necessary to examine the patient with a variety of selected radiologic techniques such as plain spine x-ray examination, ordinary anterior-posterior and lateral tomograms, conventional myelography, epidural venography, or computer assisted transverse tomography, with or without contrast material in the spinal fluid.

As a rule, surgical intervention with decompression of the cord, cauda equina, or nerve root is the only definitive therapy. Where pain exists in the absence of objective neurologic, electromyographic or radiologic evidence of disease, it is usually best to recommend conservative (nonsurgical) therapeutic measures until such time as the offending disc or other lesion declares itself unequivocally.

SOME GENERAL CONSIDERATIONS

Many neurologic diseases of the elderly are not mentioned here, either because they are not prevalent enough to require specific comment or because they are unlikely to eventuate in a serious outcome. Some of these conditions are succinctly discussed by Carter.[53] For most of the neurologic conditions reviewed here, an early and correct diagnosis is imperative if the disease is to be managed properly. In this regard, Allison[54] has provided a comprehensive review of case taking, as well as criteria for neurologic and psychologic evaluation of the aged patient. Unlike the child or young adult, the elderly person is less likely to recover without specific intervention by a physician, and whatever the condition may be, it promises to add significantly to the cumulative disabilities of old age unless ameliorated.

It is important to note that the elderly person with an already compromised cerebral circulation or perhaps an incipient organic brain syndrome of other causes, may exhibit an alarming exacerbation of neurologic signs during bouts of pulmonary insufficiency, anemia, systemic viral disease, uremia or other metabolic derangements, or exposure to toxins or drugs. If the acutely developing systemic condition is remedied promptly, these exacerbations of latent neurologic disease are likely to be temporary.

Therefore the appearance of some neurologic signs in the presence of intercurrent disease should not necessarily be taken as an immediate signal to institute heroic diagnostic measures to uncover a stroke or brain tumor.

Numerous drugs and rehabilitative techniques that promise relief from particular conditions of the aged are available. Nevertheless, it is especially important in any illness to recognize and treat a concomitant depression that is commonly found in the elderly. Separated from his job and isolated from the social contacts that once played an important role in integrating his life pattern over many years, the aged, depressed patient has less will to overcome the obstacles of his increasing disability. Thus attention to mood and mental state is a sine qua non of good therapeutics in all neurologic conditions of the aged.

REFERENCES

1. Critchley, M.: Neurologic changes in the aged, J. Chronic Dis. **3**:459, 1956.
2. O'Leary, J.L.: Aging in the nervous system. In Lansing, A.I., editor: Cowdry's problems of ageing, biological and medical aspects, Baltimore, 1952, The Williams & Wilkins Co.
3. DeJong, R.N.: The neurologic examination, ed. 4, New York, 1979, Harper & Row, Publishers, Inc.
4. Crosby, E.C., Humphrey, I., and Laur, E.W.: Correlative anatomy of the nervous system, New York, 1962, Macmillan, Inc.
5. Conn, H.P., editor: Current therapy, 1980, Philadelphia, 1980, W.B. Saunders Co.
6. Freitag, J.J., and Miller, L.W.: Manual of medical therapeutics, ed. 23, Boston, 1980, Little, Brown & Co.
7. Samuels, M.A., editor: Manual of neurologic therapeutics, Boston, 1978, Little, Brown & Co.
8. Adams, R.D., and Victor, M.: Principles of neurology, New York, 1977, McGraw-Hill Book Co.
9. Torack, R.M.: The pathologic physiology of dementia, New York, 1978, Springer-Verlag, New York, Inc.
10. Wells, C.E., editor: Dementia, ed. 2, Contemporary neurology series, Philadelphia, 1978, F.A. Davis Co.
11. Dustman, R.E., and Beck, E.C.: The effects of maturation and aging on the wave form of visually evoked potentials, Electroencephalogr. Clin. Neurophysiol. **26**:2, 1969.
12. Fazekas, J.F., Kleh, J., and Witking, L.: Cerebral hemodynamics and metabolism in subjects over 90 years of age, J. Am. Geriatr. Soc. **1**:836, 1953.
13. Katzman, R., Terry, R.D., and Bick, K.L., editors: Alzheimer's disease: senile dementia and related disorders, New York, 1978, Raven Press.
14. Cotzias, G.C., Papavasiliou, P.S., and Gellene, R.: Modification of parkinsonism—chronic treatment with L-dopa, N. Engl. J. Med. **280**:337, 1969.
15. Friedlander, W.J.: EEG alpha rate in adults as a function of age, Geriatrics **13**:29, 1958.
16. Liddell, D.W.: Investigation of EEG findings in presenile dementia, J. Neurol. Neurosurg. Psychiatry **21**:173, 1958.
17. Rocca, E., and Calcaro, C.: Central hearing processes. In Jerger, J., editor: Modern developments in audiology, New York, 1963, Academic Press, Inc.
18. Tomlinson, B.E.: Observations on the brains of nondemented old people, J. Neurol. Sci. **7**:331, 1968.
19. Corsellis, J.A.N.: Mental illness and the ageing brain, London, 1962, Oxford University Press.
20. United States Department of Health, Education and Welfare: Vital statistics of the United States 1977, vol. 2, part B, Washington, D.C., 1980, U.S. Government Printing Office.
21. Kurtzke, J.F.: Epidemiology of cerebrovascular disease, New York, 1969, Springer-Verlag, New York, Inc.
22. Dalsgaard-Nielsen, T.: Some clinical experience in the treatment of cerebral apoplexy, Acta Psychiatr. Neurol. Scand. (Suppl. 108):101, 1956.
23. Toole, J.F.: Diagnosis and management of stroke. In Toole, J.F., and Patel, A.N.: Cerebrovascular disorders, New York, 1967, McGraw-Hill Book Co.
24. Welch, D.M., Coleman, R.E., Hardin, W.B., and Siegel, B.A.: Brain scanning in cerebral vascular disease: a reappraisal, Stroke **6**:136, 1975.
25. Carney, A.L., and Anderson, E.M., editors: Diagnosis and treatment of brain ischemia: CT, brain blood flow, brain hemodynamics, and carotid and vertebral artery surgery, Advances in neurology, vol. 30, New York, 1981, Raven Press.
26. Whisnant, J.P., Matsumato, N., and Elveback, L.R.: The effect of anticoagulant therapy on the programs of patients with transient ischemic attacks in a community, Rochester, Minnesota, 1950 through 1969, Mayo Clin. Proc. **48**:844, 1973.
27. McDevitt, E., and McDowell, F.H.: Anticoagulant therapy of the completed stroke, Geriatrics **23**:135, 1968.
28. Millikan, C.H.: The stroke-prone profile, Curr. Concepts Cerebrovascular Dis., **4**:17, 1969.
29. Bouchard, J.: Radiation therapy of tumors and diseases of the nervous system, Philadelphia, 1966, Lea & Febiger.
30. Zimmerman, H.M.: Brain tumors, their incidence and classification in man and their experimental production, Ann. N.Y. Acad. Sci. **159**:337, 1969.
31. Aita, J.A.: Neurological manifestations of general diseases, Springfield, Ill., 1964, Charles C Thomas, Publisher.
32. Adams, R.D., Hochberg, F., and Webster, H.: Tumors of the brain. In Harrison, T.R., et al., eds.: Principles of internal medicine, ed. 9, New York, 1979, McGraw-Hill Book Co.
33. Moran, C.J., Naidlich, T.P., Gado, M.H., and Marchosky, J.A.: Central nervous system lesions biopsied or treated by CT-guided needle placement, Radiology **131**:681, 1979.
34. Shapiro, W.R., and Ausman, J.E.: The chemotherapy of brain tumors: clinical and experimental review. In Plum, R., editor: Recent advances in neurology, Philadelphia, 1969, F.A. Davis Co.
35. Brain, L., and Norris, F., Jr.: The remote effects of cancer on the nervous system, New York, 1965, Grune & Stratton, Inc.

36. Richardson, E.P., Jr.: Progressive multifocal leukoencephalopathy, N. Engl. J. Med. **265:**815, 1961.
37. Verhaart, W.J.C.: Encephalopathy in general body malignant diseases. In Minckler, J., editor: Pathology of the nervous system, New York, 1968, McGraw-Hill Book Co.
38. Dyck, P.J., Thomas, P.K., and Lambert, E.H., eds.: Peripheral neuropathy, vols. I and II, Philadelphia, 1975, W.B. Saunders Co.
39. Wartenburg, R.: Neuritis, sensory neuritis, neuralgia, New York, 1958, Oxford University Press.
40. May, M., Hardin, W.B., Jr., and Sullivan, J.: Natural history of Bell's palsy, Laryngoscope **86:**704, 1976.
41. Taverner, D.: Treatment of facial palsy, Arch. Otolaryngol. **81:**489, 1965.
42. May, M., and Hardin, W.B., Jr.: Facial palsy: interpretation of neurologic findings, Trans. Am. Acad. Ophthalmol. Otolaryngol. **84:**710, 1977.
43. Adour, K.K., Bell, D.N., and Hilsinger, R.L., Jr.: Herpes simplex virus in idiopathic facial paralysis (Bell palsy), J.A.M.A. **233:**527, 1975.
44. Johnson, E.W., editor: Practical electromyography, Baltimore, 1980, The Williams & Wilkins Co.
45. Arnason, B.: Inflammatory polyneuropathies. In Dyck, P.J., Thomas, P.K., and Lambert, E.H., editors: Peripheral neuropathy, vol. 2, Philadelphia, 1975, W.B. Saunders Co.
46. Liversedge, L.A.: Involuntary movements. In Vinken, P.J., and Bruyn, G.W., editors: Disturbances of nervous functions, vol. 1, New York, 1969, John Wiley & Sons, Inc.
47. Werssowetz, O.F.: Parkinsonism, Springfield, Ill., 1964, Charles C Thomas, Publisher.
48. Martin, J.P.: The basal ganglia and posture, London, 1967, Pitman Books, Ltd.
49. Monroe, R.T.: Diseases of old age, Cambridge, Mass., 1951, Harvard University Press.
50. Cooper, I.S.: Involuntary movement disorders, New York, 1969, Harper & Row, Publishers, Inc.
51. Jeste, D.V., and Wyatt, R.J.: Tardive dyskinesia: the syndrome, Psychiatr. Ann. **10:**16, 1980.
52. Weinstein, P.R., Ehni, G., and Wilson, C.: Lumbar spondylosis, diagnosis, management and surgical treatment, Chicago, 1977, Year Book Medical Publishers, Inc.
53. Carter, A.B.: Neurological disease in the elderly, Practitioner **200:**765, 1968.
54. Allison, R.S.: The senile brain: a clinical study, London, 1962, Edward Arnold (Publishers), Ltd.

CHAPTER 29 · OTORHINO-LARYNGOLOGIC ASPECTS OF GERIATRIC CARE

Ben H. Senturia
Robert Goldstein
Webb S. Hersperger

Common otolaryngologic disorders, from impacted cerumen to malignancies, are often neglected by older people. Sometimes symptoms are dismissed by the older person because it is assumed that discomfort, loss of function, and changes in structure are the irremediable consequences of aging. Sometimes problems may be totally ignored for reasons associated with the stigma surrounding old age: fears of complaining too much, of "beginning to fail," or of "senility." In such cases the physician will need to elicit from a reluctant patient exactly what symptoms are present.

The sequelae of ear, nose, and throat diseases are especially serious because they disrupt the most characteristic human function—verbal communication. The inability to hear others or to speak to others may be the most devastating handicap of old age because it isolates the person who otherwise may have the physical and mental capacity to lead a happy and useful life. Withdrawal from the environment and from social stimulation can leave the communicatively handicapped person increasingly debilitated, depressed, and without much motivation for living.

DISEASES OF THE EAR

Disorders affecting the external ear

Impacted cerumen. Cerumen consists of secretions of the sebaceous and apocrine glands of the ear canals combined with exfoliated keratin from the surface of the skin that accumulates in the outer or cartilaginous canal. It is never present in the inner half or osseous part of the canal unless it is pushed there or accumulates as a result of pressure from the use of headphones or telephones.[1]

The wax is intimately adherent to the skin of the canal in older individuals and frequently must be separated under direct vision before it can be removed with a curette or by irrigation. Careful, slow, time-consuming efforts are necessary to separate the cerumen from the intact skin without causing discomfort and bleeding. Special wax-softening drops are not very effective and are of limited value because the chemical constituents of the keratin covering of the impacted cerumen are not very soluble. When drops are used, they should be continued for 3 to 7 days.

When the wax is loosened, mechanically or by drops, a small, dull curette should be inserted along the posterior canal wall to a point posterior or medial to the mass and rotated to engage the cerumen, which can then be withdrawn along the floor of the canal. If the wax has been pushed into the osseous canal, a metal syringe or an irrigating bottle containing 3% saline solution or warm water should be used to remove the wax from the canal. The water should be warm or tepid, otherwise dizziness may occur during irrigation. Lavage should not be performed if the patient has a history of perforation of the tympanic membrane, which could produce an infection of the middle ear if used. After irrigation, the ear canal should be carefully dried with a cotton-tipped applicator and the water removed from the inferior recess.

The older patient should be urged to have regular examinations by an otologist at intervals of 6 to 12 months (depending on the rate of accumulation of cerumen) to prevent buildup of cerumen and the accompanying pressure in the ear. The hearing loss associated with impacted cerumen is insidious and can result in serious difficulty with communication.

Indolent ulcer. Symptom-free indolent ulcers occur in the elderly and are usually confined to one ear. Occasionally there may be mild pain, a slightly moist or bloody discharge, and an unpleasant odor. Examination reveals a superficial to deep, punched-out area containing granulation tissue, usually located in the cartilaginous canal or at the junction of the cartilaginous and osseous canals. Diabetics are said to be particularly susceptible. These ulcers must be differentiated from neoplastic changes, osteomyelitis, and deep infection.

Healing usually occurs if the granulation tissue is gently curetted and the ear canal is packed with a combination of topical antibiotics and corticosteroids. If gram-negative bacilli are present, the condition must be observed very carefully and treated more actively with preparations containing polymyxin and neomycin.

External Otitis[1]

Furuncle and carbuncle. Painful, circumscribed, pustular lesions occur in hair follicles in the outer half of the ear canal. A single hair follicle is infected in a *furuncle*, while multiple hair follicles are involved in *carbuncles*. The etiologic organism is usually a *Staphylococcus*, and there is associated adenopathy depending on which canal wall is involved. When the lesion is on the anterior canal wall, a tender and enlarged preauricular node may be felt; if the posterior canal is affected, a postauricular gland is palpable on the mastoid process posterior to the canal. When the latter situation exists, the condition must be distinguished from mastoiditis.

In the mild furuncle, prompt response is usually obtained by snugly inserting into the outer third of the canal a wick of cotton impregnated with bacitracin and polymyxin B (Polysporin). Oral analgesics, sedatives, and a heating pad used for 30 minutes every 2 to 4 hours should be prescribed to control pain. Spontaneous resolution or drainage of the small core of the furuncle usually occurs after 24 to 48 hours. If spontaneous drainage does not occur but fluctuation is present, then consideration should be given to incising the small abscess.

Carbuncles require more active and prolonged local and systemic therapy. The presence of diabetes must be excluded in the older subject. If the patient does not respond, cultures should be obtained; consideration must be given to the possibility of a *Staphylococcus aureus* infection and a penicillinase-resistant antibiotic prescribed.

Cellulitis. Cellulitis is an infectious disease that can occur spontaneously or as a result of trauma; generally cellulitis is a result of a *Streptococcus* or a *Staphylococcus* infection. Frequently symptoms include fever, malaise, and marked erythema of the auricle and periauricular tissues. The condition may be triggered by scratching.

Treatment consists of the local application of warm, saline compresses (one teaspoon of salt to a glass of warm water) on a soft white handkerchief or cotton balls applied to the ear for 30 minutes every 4 hours. Oral penicillin is the antibiotic of choice, but erythromycin, clindamycin, cephalosporin, or trimethoprim-sulfamethoxazole may be used. If prompt improvement does not occur, then cultures should be obtained and consideration given to the possibility of a penicillin-resistant *Staphylococcus*. If the latter is present, then a penicillinase-resistant antibiotic should be given.

Erysipelas. This disease may involve the nose, face, or ears and is caused by a group A beta-hemolytic *Streptococcus*. It is commonly seen in the older patient, particularly in those who suffer from malnutrition. The skin lesion is very red, tender, and indurated and has a well-demarcated advancing border. Frequently there are associated systemic symptoms including high fever, headache, and malaise. It may be difficult to differentiate severe cellulitis and erysipelas of the ear. Penicillin-G is the drug of choice for treatment.

Necrotizing external otitis. Necrotizing external otitis[2] usually begins as a mild, diffuse external otitis during hot, humid weather, most often in a patient with diabetes or other systemic disease that causes a lowered state of cellular nutrition. *Pseudomonas* organisms appear primarily or secondarily as the infecting organism and are resistant to many of the antibiotics prescribed. Treatment of the ear canal is often inadequate, or the patient fails to follow instructions because of the small number of symptoms in the early stages. Then when granulation tissue and ulceration are found involving the ear canal, mastoid surgery is performed, complications ensue, and the patient's condition deteriorates. At this point, otitis media, mastoiditis, progressive cranial neuropathy, jugular vein and sigmoid sinus thromboses, and meningitis may occur if adequate vigorous treatment is not instituted. This condition occurs most frequently in elderly diabetics.

When the elderly patient with an ear infection is seen by the general physician and a localized ulcer or granulation tissue is found in the region of the isthmus of the ear canal, the patient should be referred to an otologist who is in a position to make an early differentiation between infection and malignancy. Culture and sensitivity of the organisms should be determined, and a biopsy of the tissue should be obtained. Then there should be aggressive and intensive treatment with appropriate topical and systemic antibiotics.

The ear canal should be packed at 24-hour intervals with selvedged gauze impregnated with an antibiotic containing polymyxin B or E and neomycin. The patient should be referred to an internist for immediate consultation regarding metabolic and hematologic status, and a complete glucose tolerance test should be obtained. If improvement does not occur promptly, then the patient should be hospitalized; the laboratory should be alerted and an infectious disease consultation requested. If there has not been adequate intake of fluids, infusion of saline solution or dextrose should be started and antibiotics administered. If no drug allergies or kidney diseases are present, it is preferred that carbenicillin, administered intravenously, and gentamicin administered intramuscularly, be prescribed and proper antibiotics applied to the lesion in the ear canal. If there is much edema of the skin of the ear canal, a combination of antibiotics and corticosteroids in a cream base should be applied. The patient should be alerted to the possible nephrotoxic and ototoxic action of the drugs being used.

The sensitivity of the organisms obtained from the ear should be monitored regularly to determine if bacterial resistance to the administered antibiotics is developing. Surgical intervention in the area of the ear canal and mastoid should be avoided for as long as possible if progress is being made in control of the infection. The use of alternative antibiotics such as tobramycin and ticarcillin should be discussed with an infectious disease consultant.

Infectious eczematoid dermatitis. In patients who have chronic otitis media or mastoiditis with suppurative drainage, the discharge will sensitize or infect the periauricular skin and produce an inflamed vesicular and crusted dermatitis. This weeping and vesiculation may be implanted on other parts of the face and body. The most frequently cultured organism is *Staphylococcus aureus*.

Examination reveals eczematous lesions in the periauricular area and wet, edematous, reddened skin in the ear canal. The lumen of the ear canal is usually filled with purulent secretions, and often there is evidence of granulation tissue in the middle ear region or in an old mastoidectomy cavity. Differentiation must be made between impetigo contagiosum, secondarily infected seborrheic dermatitis, and neurodermatitis.

Treatment must be directed towards the primary infection in the mastoid and middle ear and simultaneously to the skin of the external auditory canal and the periauricular area. Warm aluminum acetate or saline solution packs should be applied to the periauricular areas followed by a steroid-antibiotic cream.

Primary pruritus. Primary pruritus may occur without any obvious reason. It may be a manifestation of dry skin, contact and atopic factors, or a sign of diabetes, renal disease, or blood dyscrasia. Primary pruritus may be a symptom of various dermatoses, such as lichen chronic simplex, psoriasis, and pityriasis rosea.

Examination may not reveal any findings except mild erythema. On the other hand, there may be mild thickening and weeping of the skin suggestive of early neurodermatitis. Often the patient can be recognized as being under stress, showing anxiety and depression.

Treatment should consist of controlling erythema or vesiculation by the application of antipruritic agents such as aluminum acetate solution and steroids in a cream base. Mild sedatives and tranquilizers should be prescribed for tension.

Neurodermatitis. The primary finding in this disease is pruritus with secondary scratching, which traumatizes the skin; there follows thickening of the skin and the formation of small papules that form plaques and result in lichenification. The most common areas of involvement are the helix, concha, and the meatus of the auricle; there is a history of scratching with hairpins, matches, and paper clips. It is necessary to differentiate primary neurodermatitis, and psoriasis, seborrheic dermatitis, contact dermatitis, and lupus erythematosus.

When edema and weeping are present, warm or cold compresses may be of help. Nonfluorinated corticosteroid creams are helpful when applied to the skin. Aluminum acetate packs provide excellent temporary relief of the weeping and the excoriation. It is important to explain to the patient the psychogenic basis for most forms of neurodermatitis and to obtain consultation with a psychiatrist if improvement does not occur.

Actinic keratoses. Actinic keratoses appear in patients in the upper age group after excessive sun exposure; the auricle is a particularly vulnerable target. The lesions are flat, circumscribed, red, atrophic, scale-encrusted, and vary in size from 0.5 to 3 cm. The surrounding skin is generally freckled and furrowed. Differential diagnosis includes the red scaly plaques of chronic lupus erythematosus and seborrheic keratosis. In some of these ears, squamous cell carcinoma may develop.

Liquid nitrogen is the best therapy. Topical 5-fluorouracil in a cream base applied twice daily for 2 to 4 weeks is effective. It is essential that topical sunscreening preparations and protective clothing be used to minimize solar damage.

Cutaneous horns. These usually appear on actinic keratoses or other cutaneous lesions forming a growth of keratinous material on the skin surface. They should be excised and the tissue examined histologically.

Seborrheic keratoses. These are the most commonly found tumors in the elderly population. They are benign circumscribed lesions that occur on the auricle and periauricular areas and vary in size from 3 mm to 3 cm. Seborrheic keratoses are macular plaques that are greasy and have a "stuck on" appearance. The color may vary from light tan to dark brown and black.

Treatment consists of lightly freezing the lesions with ethyl chloride, nitrous oxide, or liquid nitrogen and then having the lesions scraped off with a sharp curette. Liquid nitrogen may be applied directly with a cotton-tipped applicator for 15 to 45 seconds, depending on the size and thickness of the lesion. Smaller lesions may be treated with light electric desiccation.

Nodular chondrodermatitis of the helix and auricle.[3] This lesion is usually a smooth, tender, raised, flat nodule, sometimes superimposed by a crust, which when removed, reveals a small ulcer. It usually occurs in older men around the age of 60. It is most frequently observed on the superior helix but may also be found on the anthelix and tragus. It has been attributed to the wearing of hats in men, but can be caused by tight earphones, headgear, etc. Patients usually complain of intense pain or tenderness out of proportion to the innocuous appearance of the lesion.

Initial treatment should be an injection of a corticosteroid. If the lesion and symptoms persist, then consideration should be given to surgical excision of the lesion. Use of anything that causes pressure on the auricle should be avoided.

Malignancy

Basal cell carcinoma. This is a nonmetastasizing epithelial tumor invading local structures. It generally grows slowly and is painless, unless it becomes secondarily infected. The lesions may be flat with a smooth surface or have a pearly, nodular appearance without pigmentation; they may be ulcerated. They can become extensive and involve the cartilage and the surrounding bone.

Wide local excision is advised; where available, use of the Mohs approach is desirable. X-ray treatment can be used in selected cases. Topical 5-fluorouracil can be used with some success in the treatment of these problems but must be carefully monitored.

Squamous cell carcinoma. This is a slow-growing tumor that occurs primarily in men, most frequently in areas of actinic damage such as the helix of the auricle. Examination shows an ulcerated tumor with surrounding induration, edema, and erythema and most often palpable periauricular lymph nodes. It is essential to obtain a biopsy.

Wide excision and removal of involved lymph

glands, parotid glands, and a radical neck dissection should be planned. X-ray therapy can be considered in selected cases. The Mohs technique of excision is particularly applicable in this area. When the disease involves the external auditory canal, radiologic visualization of the mastoid must be obtained and plans made for extensive excision of mastoid, parotid, middle ear, and contiguous soft tissues. If the neck is involved, a radical neck dissection should be planned and postoperative radiation considered. After the tumor has been removed, consideration should be given to the use of reconstructive procedures.

Disorders affecting the tympanic membrane and middle ear

Perforations of the tympanic membrane. Perforations of various sizes may occur as a result of many causes: direct injury from cotton-tipped applicators, pencils, etc., which are used to scratch the ear canal; a blow to the ear from a blunt instrument, a fall, or a slap to the side of the head with the hand; or from pressure changes in the middle or external ear as a result of barotraumatic change. These changes may be but are not always followed by bleeding, dizziness, or secondary infection. Depending on the size of the perforation, hearing may be mildly or moderately depressed. An otologic examination and an audiologic workup are desirable to help determine the extent of the damage. The situation or circumstances under which the perforation occurred may have been forgotten by the elderly patient; therefore when the patient is examined, careful observation of the status of the tympanic membrane must be determined. Obstructing wax in the ear canal should be removed cautiously without the use of irrigation and under good light.

It is important to determine whether there is significant conductive or sensorineural hearing loss because a large conductive hearing loss will indicate whether surgical correction or rehabilitation may be feasible.

When there is a small perforation of the tympanic membrane without middle ear complications, simple patching with tissue paper, fascia, or sclera (banked) (performed in the physician's office or hospital outpatient department) is effective for closing the perforation. A larger tympanic perforation will require myringoplasty under local anesthesia. If a small amount of granulation tissue is present around the periphery of the perforation, 10% silver nitrate may be applied to the granulation tissue and then neutralized with 70% ethyl alcohol.

In older patients with large perforations, cotton should be worn in the ear canal during exposure to low temperatures or cold wind to avoid vertigo. When it is necessary to remove retained water or secretion from the ear canal, the physician should remember that suctioning may cause severe vertigo, nausea, and vomiting.

Otitis media

Acute otitis media. An acute infection of the middle ear will ordinarily follow the usual course in the aging patient, beginning with pain, fever, and the occurrence of serous fluid, which may progress to seropurulent and then purulent secretion. Occasionally there is an insidious onset of effusion without pain or fever, and the patient is not aware of the effusion until hearing is decreased. At that time there is milky thickening and bulging of the eardrum and a conductive hearing loss of 30 to 40 decibels. Examination of the nose frequently reveals thick mucopurulent secretion in each nasal fossa.

It is important to obtain a culture of the nasal or nasopharyngeal secretion and wherever possible to prescribe specific antibiotics when the nature of the organism is determined. While waiting for the culture report, a broad coverage antibiotic such as ampicillin or tetracycline (250 mg, four times a day) should be prescribed and a vasoconstrictor sprayed into the nose four times a day. If prompt improvement of the ear infection does not occur in 24 to 48 hours, then myringotomy should be performed. Lidocaine hydrochloride injected into the skin of the ear canal usually provides good anesthesia so that an incision can be made into the posterior-inferior quadrant of the tympanic membrane. Iontophoresis may be of assistance in reducing the pain of myringotomy. A culture of the middle ear secretion should be made. The patient should be instructed to remove any secretion which accumulates in the ear canal three times a day with sterile cotton-tipped applicators. Sufficient oral analgesics should be prescribed to reduce associated pain. When the middle ear culture report is available, the progress of the otitis media should be reviewed to determine whether the antibiotic has been effective or should be changed.

Under proper care of the nose and the ear,

progressive improvement may be anticipated in 5 to 7 days. Depending on the response, medication should be continued for a total of 7 to 10 days.[4]

Otitis media with effusion. Failure of the patient and the doctor to insist on adequate care of acute otitis media is the most common cause of persistent otitis media with effusion. This occurs because the patient who is relieved of his pain feels that further medication and visits to the physician are unnecessary. A high percentage of such ears with fluid show positive cultures of *Haemophilus influenzae*, *Streptococcus pneumoniae*, etc., resulting in presistent smoldering fluid in the middle ear. The physician should not hope that the condition will spontaneously abate without active treatment but should persevere in the topical and systemic treatment of the ear, nose, and sinuses.

When persistent unilateral otitis media with effusion is present, consideration should be given to the possible presence of a neoplastic lesion involving the nasopharynx and eustachian tube. In their early stage these lesions cause no pain, produce minimal bleeding, and are not readily evident radiologically; they must be discovered with a postnasal mirror or a nasopharyngoscope.

Middle ear effusions that result from barotrauma during flying and do not improve promptly should be treated by an otologist. The middle ear should be inflated, and the patient should be taught to use Valsalva's technique if no acute nasal infection is present. Rarely is it necessary to perform a myringotomy and to insert a tube into the middle ear for aero-otitis media because the fluid is usually of low viscosity and will spontaneously drain down the eustachian tube if proper treatment is prescribed.

Allergic disorders involving the nose and middle ear do occasionally cause effusions and should be kept in mind. However, allergy has been demonstrated to play a minor role in the etiology of middle ear effusions.

Chronic otitis media and mastoiditis. The geriatric patient with chronic otitis media and mastoiditis gives a history of recurrent otologic infection and often of at least one surgical intervention. Hearing is usually reduced in the involved ear. Frequently there is evidence of chronic granulation tissue and some purulent secretion in the middle ear and mastoid. Cultures of the secretion in a high percentage of patients show *Pseudomonas* or *Proteus* organisms. From time to time, otomycosis is superimposed on the chronic drainage. Frequently the mastoidectomy cavity has been neglected so there is an accumulation of secretion, keratin, and cerumen with secondary ulceration of the epithelium lining the cavity. Occasionally there is keratoma (cholesteatoma) present in the ear canal, middle ear, and mastoid cavity.

It is important to approach the neglected external and middle ear and mastoid cavity with great care because any effort to remove the accumulated debris may disrupt the ossicular chain; energetic cleaning of the ear may produce dizziness as a result of stimulation of a fistula in the semicircular canal. Active bleeding from granulation tissue may occur following suction or attempted removal of granulation or polyps. To visualize the middle ear and mastoid cavity, it is often necessary to devote several sessions in the office in an effort to cautiously mobilize the keratin mass.

If a large polyp is present in the ear canal, the middle ear, or the mastoid, it should be carefully isolated and then, with good visualization and proper control, removed. The tissue should always be sent to the laboratory to rule out neoplastic changes. At the same time cultures of the secretion should be taken to determine the nature and sensitivity of the organisms involved.

After the middle ear and mastoid cavity have been thoroughly examined and hearing tests have been obtained, a decision must be made as to whether the patient has a good possibility of responding to conservative medical therapy or clearly requires surgical intervention. If the former approach is chosen, a broad coverage antibiotic that is effective against the organisms cultured should be prescribed. Some otologists prefer to pack the ear canal with one to three 12- to 18-inch-long selvedged gauze packs impregnated with an antibiotic-corticosteroid cream to control the granulation tissue and infection. The patient is seen again in 24 to 48 hours. More debris and cells containing granulations and infection can usually be located on the second visit, and slowly the entire disease process may be isolated. The cavity is repacked. After the second or third visit, ear drops containing antibiotics and corticosteroids may be substituted for the packs (5 to 10 drops four times a day for 5 minutes). If prompt improvement does not occur, then x-ray films of the mastoid should be obtained and discussions initiated with the patient, spouse, and family regarding surgical intervention.

In patients who have obvious inaccessible cholesteatoma or infected granulation tissue, audiologic and radiologic workups should be obtained promptly. Rarely must secondary intracranial disease be considered and neurologic consultation obtained.

In a patient with middle ear disease that has not been treated or has not responded satisfactorily to treatment, chronic middle ear changes may occur, often without the presence of a tympanic perforation. Fibrosing lesions involving the ossicular chain and tympanic cavity may cause atrophic changes of the tympanic membrane; osteitis may involve the ossicular chain, frequently causing disruption of the continuity of the ossicles; hyalin-collagen alterations may result in tympanosclerotic changes of the tympanic membrane and ossicular structures and may encroach on the middle ear space.[5] The studies of Etholm and Belal,[6] which include patients up to 96 years of age, showed arthritic changes in the ossicular chain that increased with advancing age, but these changes did not appear to impair sound transmission. Secondary calcifications, fibroses, etc., develop and cause reduced hearing, usually of a conductive type. Unfortunately, at the present time most of these lesions are not responsive to surgical intervention.

Otosclerosis. This is a bony disease that is more common in women, and involves the otic capsule and stapes. It is usually bilateral, but in one patient out of ten it may occur in only one ear. Although its most obvious manifestation is conductive hearing loss, as a result of fixation of the footplate of the stapes, there may also be involvement of other parts of the labyrinth that may yield audiologic findings indicative of sensorineural hearing loss.

A diagnosis of otosclerosis is usually easily made on the basis of the patient's medical history, ear examination, and audiologic evaluation. The primary conditions to be ruled out are middle ear fluid (particularly of the mucoid type in which fluid levels cannot be identified) and fixation or discontinuity of the malleus or incus. Slowly progressive Paget's disease in older patients may typically produce ossicular fixation and conductive hearing loss. Differentiation is usually made on the basis of examination and x-ray films of the skull.

Patients with a loss of air conduction of more than 35 decibels, good bone conduction in speech frequencies, and speech discrimination scores of 60% or better are candidates for surgery to restore useful hearing. Selected patients with greater losses may be candidates for surgery to improve the potential use of a hearing aid.

With few exceptions, the anesthesia of choice is a local one with proper preoperative sedation. There is no age limitation as long as the general condition of the patient is good. Goodhill[4] reports excellent results averaging 34.6 decibels for patients over 70 years old with profound mixed-type hearing losses.

Diseases affecting the inner ear

Hearing disorders

Basic hearing function and its disorders. The total auditory mechanism must perform two basic functions. It must gather in and register sound from the environment, and it must give meaning to the sounds that are received. In the normal functioning auditory system, sounds enter through the external auditory meatus and strike the tympanic membrane. The sounds vibrate the tympanic membrane, and the vibrations are transmitted to the fluid-filled cochlea or inner ear by means of a series of three ossicles—the malleus, incus, and stapes. The sensory hair cells of the organ of Corti in the cochlea play a key role in helping to convert mechanical sound energy into neural impulses. The neural impulses are then transmitted to the brain along the auditory nerve (eighth cranial nerve).

Ordinarily, most sound energy striking fluid will be reflected back into the air from which it arises. The principal function of the tympanic membrane and the associated middle ear ossicles is the efficient transmission of sound from the air to the fluid-filled cochlea with a minimum of loss of sound energy through reflection. Diseases or injury that interfere with normal tympanic and ossicular function, or blockage of the external auditory meatus that prevents sound from striking the tympanic membrane leads to a reduction in auditory sensitivity, which is properly designated as *hypacusis*. It is often spoken of as a conductive hypacusis or hearing loss because of the impairment in the sound conduction apparatus. The extent of hypacusis imposed by a faulty conductive mechanism can range from a negligible amount of hearing loss to one in which only intense sounds such as loud speech near the ear can barely be heard.

Diseases or injury can also interfere with the normal function of the sensory cells of the cochlea, with the normal function of the auditory nerve, or with both. The resultant damage can lead to an impairment in auditory sensitivity usually designated as a sensorineural hypacusis. Sensorineural hypacusis can range from negligible loss to total deafness, or *anacusis.*

Sensorineural impairments carry with them another kind of problem called *dysacusis*. Dysacusis can take many forms, the most important of which is less than normal understanding or discrimination of speech or other sounds when they are loud enough to be heard easily. The form of dysacusis known as loudness recruitment is common in persons whose sensorineural hypacusis is the result of impairment of the sensory cells of the organ of Corti. Although sounds must be made more intense to be heard, they are heard with disturbing loudness when the sounds are presented above the person's threshold of hearing. No hypacusis or loss of auditory sensitivity occurs with impairment of the central nervous system, but dysacusis in terms of impaired speech discrimination can occur.

Various combinations of conductive, sensorineural, and central nervous system problems can occur in the same person, and the resultant hearing disorders will of course reflect the contributions of each.

Nature of hearing disorders. The many, many things that can cause hearing disorders in young persons can, of course, cause hearing disorders in the elderly. The longer a person lives the greater the chance of having the hearing impaired by such things as otitis media, systemic viral infections, intense noise exposure, head trauma, and ototoxic drugs. Older persons could also have been born deaf and carry their deafness into their later years.

Nevertheless, age itself seems to be a factor in bringing about hearing losses in persons who have otherwise escaped auditory impairment from external causes. It has been claimed that the hearing tends to begin to deteriorate after the age of 50 years and continues to deteriorate gradually with increasing age. Nevertheless, many individuals 50 years old and older show little or no sensitivity impairment. Impairment great enough to interfere with communication does not occur in some persons until their eighties. It is probable that some of the deterioration of hearing with age is genetically determined; in some families the loss of hearing seems to begin in young adult life and middle age and to progress relatively rapidly to a severe hearing loss.

The gradual loss of auditory sensitivity with age without any apparent cause is usually of a sensorineural nature; that is, auditory tests show that the impairment is in the cochlea, the auditory nerve, or both. Sensitivity for high-frequency sounds diminishes first and most severely. Sensitivity later diminishes for the lower frequency sounds. The pattern of the hypacusis is approximately the same in both ears.

Although various manifestations of dysacusis accompany the sensorineural hypacusis, the most prominent complaint of the elderly person is an inability or difficulty in understanding speech. Words are distorted and tend to be a jumble of sounds. Younger persons with sensorineural disorders frequently have similar complaints, but in the older person poor speech discrimination is often out of proportion to the degree of hypacusis. It is probable that in these instances the dysacusis attributable to an impaired peripheral auditory system is compounded with a dysacusis stemming from a generalized impairment of the central nervous system.

This total picture of the gradually increasing sensorineural hearing loss, or hypacusis, and the inordinately poor speech discrimination has been called *presbycusis*. Another auditory problem that often adds to the difficulty of presbycusis is the problem of tinnitus.

ETIOLOGIC FACTORS. No one has clearly established the cause of presbycusis, and indeed, it may differ among individuals. A commonly accepted opinion is that the impairment of the sensory and neural structures of the ear, and perhaps of the brain, occurs because of alterations in normal metabolic processes, which, of course, may also affect other bodily structures and functions simultaneously. Either related to the metabolic alterations or independent of them are changes in the circulation that may have a particularly deleterious effect on the tiny blood vessels that nourish the cochlea and auditory nerve.

PREVALENCE. The prevalence of presbycusis has not been established to a satisfactory degree. At least three factors tend to compound the interpretations of hearing loss surveys that have been conducted. First, distinctions often are not made between a measurable hypacusis and a hypacusis that is severe enough to pose a significant handicap in verbal communication. Second, populations studied usually have been either of residents of homes for the aged, who, because of other infirmities, might also be expected to have hearing impairments, or of older persons attending state fairs or other large gatherings, who, because of their ability to get around well by themselves, might be expected to have healthy hearing. Third, it is difficult to separate presbycusis from other kinds of hearing disorders. The longer a person lives, the greater the possibility that hearing is impaired by some external cause.

The third factor is irrelevant in a sense, because whether the hearing disorder is strictly a function of aging or whether it was brought about by some external cause such as prolonged exposure to intense noise, hearing disorders are, in fact, far more prevalent among the aged than among persons less than 65 years of age.

Treatment of hearing disorders. It was mentioned earlier that medical and surgical treatment of hearing disorders in elderly patients is seldom effective. Some kinds of conductive hypacuses might be successfully cured or alleviated. Others are not amenable to treatment or else the person afflicted is unable to tolerate the treatment procedures.

Presbycusis and other forms of sensorineural disorders cannot be alleviated, and most elderly persons must resort to forms of therapy that help them compensate for hearing loss. The most common forms of therapy are (1) amplification of sound by a small wearable hearing aid; (2) auditory training, that is, training in the use of imperfect hearing, with or without a hearing aid, to improve the understanding of speech that is distorted by the ears and brain; and (3) training in the visual recognition of speech through speechreading, or lipreading, lessons. Ideally all three forms of therapy should be given in a unified program because they tend to complement or reinforce each other. For descriptive purposes, however, they will be treated separately.

HEARING AIDS. Persons who are acquainted with hearing aids through advertisements or through appealing feature articles in newspapers and magazines generally expect a hearing aid to solve all the communication problems of a hearing-handicapped person. Most professional workers outside the field of audiology and speech pathology share this view. A hard-of-hearing person, particularly an elderly person, who has worn a hearing aid realizes the näiveté of this view. Hearing aids are essential for most people with a handicapping hypacusis, and most of them can derive some benefit from a hearing aid if they are given proper guidance in its use, but *the hearing aid and the hearing aid user both have limitations* that do not allow the aid to give all the help that one would wish to derive from it. Among elderly persons the human limitations are much greater than the electroacoustic ones, and in this discussion as much stress will be placed on what cannot or should not be expected as on what can be done with hearing aids.

For practical purposes a hearing aid is a simple amplifier. Sounds entering its microphone are greatly amplified at the small loudspeaker or earphone that is inserted into the ear. Modern hearing aids are efficient amplifiers despite their small size. They can be designed to deliver enough sound energy so that the person with profound hypacusis but with some residual hearing can hear speech spoken into the aid. The person with absolutely no residual hearing can feel the vibrations of some of the low-frequency components of the speech that have been amplified thousands or millions of times. Persons with profound hypacusis or with anacusis will not understand any of the amplified sounds, but they can be aware that someone is speaking, can follow the rhythm of the speech, and can use the few cues that they receive from the sound or the vibration along with the visual cues they pick up from speechreading to derive some understanding of what is being said to them. The point made here is that a hearing aid should not be denied a person solely on the basis of the profundity of the hearing loss.

The small size of modern hearing aids is a mixed blessing. On the positive side, small size and correspondingly light weight make the hearing aid convenient and comfortable for a person to wear in the clothing or tucked behind the pinna, in the glasses, or even worn entirely within the pinna and ear canal. Because hearing aids are so small and can be disguised so easily, they are relatively inconspicuous. Even though hearing persons generally regard the visible aid with sympathy and understanding, many hard-of-hearing persons still consider hearing aids stigmatic. Hearing aids have indeed gained greater acceptance as they have become smaller and more easily disguised.

The small size of hearing aids and particularly of the microphones that pick up the sounds limits the quality of sound reproduction. The low- and high-frequency components of speech are not picked up or amplified nearly to the degree that the middle-frequency range is reproduced. Distortion of various sorts is introduced by the hearing aid, particularly at high levels of amplification. In general, speech coming out of a hearing aid is not as clear as the speech that is directed to it. In presbycusis, speech is further distorted by the faulty ear and possibly by the faulty brain of the listener. Thus the compounding of the physical and human distortion in the elderly person counteracts much of the benefit gained from amplification.

Tiny hearing aids necessarily have tiny switches that are needed for regulating the volume and, in some aids, the tonal quality of the reproduction. Batteries are correspondingly tiny, have a relatively short life, and must be replaced frequently. An elderly person whose coordination and dexterity may be less effective because of conditions such as arthritis or tremors may find it difficult to manipulate the small controls. Earmolds pose several problems. If they do not fit properly, they may allow some of the amplified sounds to escape from the ear canal. The sound returns to the nearby microphone of the hearing aid and is reamplified. This sets up a feedback loop that results in an annoying squeal. If the earmold does not fit properly, it should be modified or remade.

The small hole in the earmold, which conducts the amplified sound into the ear canal, can become clogged with wax or other debris. Unless the molds are cleaned regularly and thoroughly dried, they may seriously impede the sound. Older persons frequently find it difficult to maintain the cleanliness of their earmolds or may forget to do so. When the hearing aid loses much of its effectiveness because the mold is clogged, they suspect that the aid itself is malfunctioning, will go through needless trouble to have it repaired, or will put the aid aside and not use it.

Earmolds can also be irritating to the skin of the ear canal or can aggravate an existing skin irritation. This common annoyance in the elderly can restrict the usefulness of a hearing aid. Cleanliness of the earmold can do much toward preventing these irritations. Medical attention should be given to an ear with a persisting irritation.

These difficulties are given only as cautions and must not be interpreted as meaning that elderly persons should not have hearing aids. Elderly individuals themselves present strong impediments to the successful use of a hearing aid. If they have not used a hearing aid before, they feel incompetent to adjust to it and to the sounds, which are different from those to which they have been accustomed. If they have had poor experience in the past with the larger, more cumbersome aids and were never given any help in adjusting to an aid, their previous experiences make them hesitate to try the newer, smaller, more comfortable and more efficient hearing aids. They may balk at the cost of a hearing aid, and if their reluctance is based on more than cost, they will avoid being helped financially in the purchase of an aid.

Probably the biggest deterrent to an aged person's accepting a hearing aid is their unawareness of the extent of their communication handicap or their unwillingness to admit this disability. Some of the lack of awareness is understandable. Their hypacusis has probably progressed slowly over a long period of time. Over this period they have made certain compensatory adjustments of which they may not be cognizant. They watch the speaker more closely for visual clues, they sit close to the front in church, or dominate conversations so that they can be more knowledgeable of the topic of conversation and can get by on minimal auditory clues. They are unaware of the adjustments made by their family and friends who have learned to speak more clearly, loudly, and slowly to them. They engage the hearing-impaired individual in direct face-to-face conversation so that they have that person's complete attention. They turn down the radio or television so that he is not distracted by competing sounds.

If the elderly person's hypacusis is not profound, the low-frequency components of speech may be heard without too much difficulty—mostly the vowel sounds, which contain much of the energy of speech—but the consonant sounds that are more important for the intelligibility of speech may be missing, because they are usually less powerful than the vowels and contain more high-frequency sounds. It is in the high-frequency range that hypacusis is generally more severe. Thus the person may hear speech without really understanding it. If concentrating on the conversation, speech may be understood from speechreading as well as from auditory clues. If, on the other hand, the elderly person is absorbed in reading the evening newspaper, he probably will not understand what is being said to him and may even be oblivious to the fact that someone is talking to him. Thus when the elderly person in his reluctance to wear a hearing aid says, "I can hear everything I want to hear," the statement has a modicum of justification.

A point is reached, however, when the hypacusis is sufficiently troublesome so that all compensations on the part of the aged person and his family fail, and hearing amplification is needed, largely for the benefit of the other members of the family who are now reluctant to converse with that person. What procedures should be followed in providing help? Although many different professional and nonprofessional persons will be helping elderly patients with their hearing problems, three of them have key roles, which should follow in a certain sequence. (The sequence is not related to the importance of the roles because all of them are vital and indispensable.)

The first person in the sequence is the *otorhinolaryngologist*, who not only carries out the examination but also integrates the findings with those of other medical specialists who have been involved with the patient. The otorhinolaryngologists's first concern is with the control or eradication of any disease that is affecting the health of ears, nose, and throat and the patient's hearing. If treatment is indicated and if it is successful, sufficient hearing may be restored to obviate the need for a hearing aid.

If the patient's hearing disorder is of a sensorineural nature or is attributable to a conductive problem that cannot be remedied, the otorhinolaryngologist will refer the patient to an audiologist for a hearing aid evaluation and for guidance in the selection of an aid. First, however, the otorhinolaryngologist will determine if there is any reason why an earmold should not be used. If an earmold is out of the question for medical reasons, the audiologist will have to recommend a hearing aid in which sounds are delivered by means of a bone-conduction vibrator instead of an earmold placed in the ear canal.

The tasks of the *audiologist* are manifold. They include a thorough evaluation of the elderly patient's auditory function, an assessment of the patient's ability to benefit from amplification, and counseling of the patient and his family.

Many of the auditory tests used in a hearing aid evaluation are the same as those used for diagnostic purposes. Greatest attention is paid to the patient's ability to hear and to understand speech with a hearing aid. The principles of hearing aid evaluation and the exact procedures used vary with the individual audiologic service. Procedures range from selecting a specific brand of a hearing aid and specific tonal adjustments to simply making a decision about whether or not a hearing aid should be used and recommending a type of aid rather than a specific brand.

The most important decision by the audiologist is whether or not to recommend a hearing aid to the elderly patient. The decision is based partially on audiometric findings. Is the hypacusis sufficiently handicapping to warrant amplification of speech for the patient? Will the distorted sounds from the hearing aid reduce speech discrimination to the point that the beneficial effects of having louder speech delivered to the ear are offset? Will loudness recruitment counterbalance the benefits of amplification? Of course, if the hypacusis is severe enough so that the patient hears nothing without amplification, the negative aspects of using a hearing aid cannot be weighed as heavily.

The nonauditory factors may be even more crucial to a decision than the auditory ones. An important consideration is patients' actual need for amplification in daily living. If they are still very active socially or in an occupation, they may be extremely dependent on a hearing aid. If they are generally inactive and relatively isolated for reasons other than their hearing problem, they will have much less need and probably little desire for a hearing aid. If the patients are in generally poor health, they will probably have little or no motivation to use a hearing aid. If, however, care is dependent largely on how well others can communicate with them, a hearing aid may have to be recommended over their protests. The other problems mentioned previously, such as fingers gnarled by arthritis or a constant tinnitus, also have to be taken into consideration. If a hearing aid is recommended, the audiologist must also decide in which ear the hearing aid should be worn, or if hearing aids for both ears are desirable. The style of the hearing aid also should be determined.

Probably the most important job of the audiologist is the counseling of the patient. The audiologist must explain in simple terms the nature of the communication problem imposed by the hearing disorder, the kinds of help the patient can and cannot expect to derive from a hearing aid, how to go about purchasing an aid, and the kinds of audiologic help the patient should have in getting adjusted to the use of the instrument.

Counseling should be done not only with the patient but also with some interested family members. They should be present because most likely they will have to assist the elderly person in following the audiologist's recommendations. One should always keep in mind that the patient is being seen because a hearing problem is impeding the understanding of speech. How, therefore, can the elderly patient be expected to understand the oral counseling that is being given? A follow-up summary letter is helpful but does not obviate the need for the presence of a family member during counseling.

Advice given directly to the family may be of as much help to the patient as any hearing aid purchased. Families too often expect the hearing aid by itself to put them back in touch with the elderly member. They, too, must know the limitations of amplification and how best to structure situations so that spoken communication can be enhanced.

Families who have tried vainly for years to coerce an elderly patient to obtain a hearing aid unjustifiably expect the audiologist to accomplish the task after a brief encounter with the patient. The audiologist cannot always accomplish this, despite the belief that the patient could benefit appreciably from a hearing aid. The audiologist's wisest decision at times may be to accede to the patient's reluctance rather than to waste time, money, and emotional strength on a hearing aid that will never be used.

The audiologist's responsibility does not stop with recommendations and counseling. If the patient is advised to purchase an aid, that patient should be urged to return with the purchased hearing aid so that the audiologist can both determine whether or not it is giving the patient the kind of help that was anticipated and can help the patient in adjusting to the aid so that maximum benefit will be derived from it.

The roles of otorhinolaryngologists, audiologists, and hearing aid dealers are distinct but necessarily overlap considerably. Interaction between all three frequently is essential in the management of any one patient. Other professional persons such as social workers and psychologists may also be involved with elderly patients and their hearing aid needs, particularly when nonmedical and nonaudiologic aspects exert a strong influence on the successful use of a hearing aid.

AUDITORY TRAINING. Patients will derive more benefit from hearing aids if they are given some practice or training in listening to amplified sounds than if they attempt to wear it without any help. Many audiologists prefer to begin auditory training before a patient purchases a hearing aid. Training may begin with special high-fidelity amplifying units and the more conventional earphones. It can then be extended to units whose electroacoustic characteristics resemble those of hearing aids, or it can be done with recent-model hearing aids available to the audiologist. Training should continue with the hearing aid that the patient has purchased until the audiologist is confident that the patient is on the way to as successful a use of the hearing aid as can be expected.

There is no set procedure for auditory training. Frequently, however, it involves helping patients make distinctions between grossly differing sounds through their hearing alone and then helping them to develop their own clues for making finer distinctions, particularly between similar speech sounds. Auditory training does not improve the ears or basic auditory function. It can, however, improve the patients' listening in the sense that it makes them more alert to minimal distinguishing clues that they may have been hearing all along. Carefully graded and controlled training sessions can also help elderly patients become more accustomed to and tolerant of the imperfect amplifying system heard by their imperfect ears. Concentrated attention on incoming sounds, however imperfect they are, is the key to improved listening. The auditory training sessions, if properly handled, can give patients the confidence and motivation to perform a task that is difficult for them—attentive concentration. It is desirable to have elderly patient's family members present during the training sessions so that they may learn ways in which they may help and what can realistically be expected from the hearing aid.

SPEECHREADING. The process of speechreading, or lipreading, might better be termed *visual speech reception* because it involves a person deriving clues to what another person is saying from movements of eyes, tongue, cheeks, and throat, as well as from the lips. Clues are also given by expressions of the eyes, by tensions of the neck muscles, and by the actual movements of the muscles involved directly with speech. Nevertheless, in the process of visual speech reception, concentration on the lips is greatest, and it is from the lips that the principal clues are derived.

Just as auditory training cannot improve actual hearing, lessons in speechreading seldom improve the actual visual perceptual ability of hearing-impaired persons. Besides, many hearing-impaired persons unconsciously develop their own speechreading skills through necessity as their auditory sensitivity progressively diminishes. In a fashion similar to that in auditory training, lessons in speechreading can, however, make these persons more aware of the speech motions that they are already observing. The concentrated attention to both visual clues and auditory clues can do much to aid a patient in understanding the speech of others, even though the comprehension of speech through either channel alone may be limited.

The audiologist must be realistic in the recommendations and program for speechreading for elderly patients. These patients have no more motivation to engage in speechreading lessons than they have to use a hearing aid and to undergo auditory training. Many of them have poor vision, which makes extended attempts at training in speechreading impractical. Again, it is wise to involve the families of elderly patients in speechreading lessons. They can obtain a better understanding of the limitations of the speechreading skills of the elderly person. In addition, they can be given advice about making it easier for the elderly person to follow the speech movements of the family members by, for example, ensuring appropriate lighting of the face of the speaker or being careful in articulation of their own speech without using exaggerated expressions.

COMBINED HEARING THERAPY. Although hearing aids, auditory training, and speechreading lessons are treated separately in this chapter, they can be of great help to a patient if they are unified in a single program of hearing therapy. Benefits from each facet of therapy help the effectiveness of the other, probably more than in a simple additive manner. Sometimes the three facets must be supplemented by speech and voice training if the hearing impairment has led to deteriorating speech because the patients have been unable to monitor their own voices. Sometimes one facet may be eliminated. If vision is faulty, speechreading is impractical. If the sensorineural hearing impairment is such that it interferes with speech discrimination but hypacusis is not severe enough to justify a hearing aid, auditory training can be carried on without amplification.

A final caution is offered to professionals who work with older hearing-impaired persons. Do not abandon efforts to improve their communication through hearing before careful and serious attempts to help them have been exhausted. Many older persons *do* have the ability to adapt to new situations and to the new world of hearing through a hearing aid.

Vestibular disorders. True vertigo results from labyrinthine, retrolabyrinthine, or central nervous system vestibular disorders and is to be differentiated from various forms of spatial disorientation or ataxia caused by systemic vascular disorders or nonvestibular central nervous system diseases. In the geriatric patient, there are many causes of disequilibrium but surprisingly few cases of true vertigo as are seen so commonly in the younger adult subject. Thus true Meniere's disease is seen infrequently in the 50- to 70-year-old patient but frequently in 20- to 40-

year-olds. On the other hand, disequilibrium as a result of blood pressure changes and vascular lesions such as posterior-inferior cerebellar artery syndromes need to be watched carefully in the older patient. In the aging population, the intimate relationship between the eyes and the vestibular system must be kept constantly in mind. Poorly fitting glasses or eye disease may generate stimuli that affect the vestibular system.

Any patient who complains of dizziness should have a complete ear, nose, and throat examination, an audiologic evaluation, and a thorough otoneurologic survey including electronystagmography.

Tinnitus. Tinnitus is a common disease in older patients and deserves careful attention and evaluation. It may be a primary disease of the cochlea or may be secondary to local or systemic diseases. Tinnitus may be a consequence of impacted cerumen in the ear canal, lesions of the tympanic membrane, fluid in the middle ear, a laying down of cartilage and bone in the middle ear, or a result of organic changes in the cochlear or retrocochlear areas.

It is essential that a thorough otologic examination as well as a complete medical examination be performed on any patient with tinnitus.

If the medical consultant indicates that there is no hypertension or central nervous system disease and the audiologic and otoneurologic examinations show no significant disease, then the patient should be reassured. Mild sedatives should be prescribed for nighttime use; after careful consideration, low dosages of tranquilizers should be prescribed for short-term use.

The patient should be examined at regular intervals and an attempt made to understand all the factors contributing to the tinnitus. In recent years some effort has been made to evaluate the effectiveness of biofeedback for the relief of tinnitus and excellent results in some patients have been reported.[7] In the event of persistent or increasing tinnitus, a thorough neurologic evaluation and x-ray examination of the skull may be required. In rare cases, angiography of the carotid-vertebral vessels may be indicated.*

Acoustic neurinoma. Silverstein and Norrell[8] have recently explored the question of the diagnosis and treatment of neuromas in the elderly patient. Because these patients frequently have debilitating headache, facial pain, and ataxia, Silverstein and Norrell suggest that consideration be given to providing help in relieving these symptoms. On the basis of their experience Silverstein and Norrell recommend that a neurootologic surgeon and a neurosurgeon collaborate in performing subtotal intracapsular removal of the tumor. They operated on eight patients ranging in age from 66 to 83 years of age. These patients had a benign postoperative course similar to that of a patient undergoing mastoid surgery and left the hospital in 3 to 4 days after surgery. If rapid regrowth occurs, it is suggested that an intracapsular operation be reperformed through the previous operative defect.

*Some help may be obtained in understanding this pernicious problem through the American Tinnitus Association, P.O. Box 5, Portland, Ore. 97207.

DISEASES OF THE NOSE AND FACE

Epistaxis

In the elderly, a nosebleed can be severe enough to threaten life and can be challenging to treat. While in younger persons bleeding is usually from the anterior portion of the nose, posterior bleeding is seen more frequently in the elderly.

Trauma can be a significant cause of epistaxis because it may result in septal hematoma and an extravasation of blood between the mucoperichondrial flaps that cover the anterior portion of the nasal septum. Untreated, this problem leads to infection and necrosis of the cartilage, which may leave the victim with a permanent cosmetic deformity or saddle nose. In nasal trauma, it is as important to determine the condition of the internal nose as to evaluate the appearance of the external nose.

Septal perforation is another cause of epistaxis. Regardless of the cause of the perforation, attention will be directed to its presence by epistaxis, infection, crusting, a sensation of being unable to breathe through the nose, and sometimes whistling respiration.

Hypertension is a major cause of epistaxis among the elderly. Typically the nosebleed is posterior and frequently occurs in the middle of the night, causing the patient to wake gagging on a mouthful of blood.

Blood dyscrasias such as thrombocytopenia or leukemia are a source of epistaxis and can be difficult to treat. The use of medications containing aspirin or of anticoagulants such as sodium warfarin (Coumadin) or heparin may be an important factor; any patient with a difficult to control nosebleed should have a hematologic evaluation.

Tumors, both benign and malignant, within the nose and occasionally within the paranasal sinuses, can cause epistaxis. Radiography, polytomography, and occasionally computed tomography may be indicated to evaluate the sinuses.

In treating epistaxis, one must work efficiently and calmly and must seek the patient's confidence and comfort; it may be desirable to use a mild sedative. In taking the patient's medical history, it is important to find out where the bleeding first appeared; this frequently will indicate the proper side of the nose to be evaluated first. The patient should be in a sitting position, both for comfort and for the ease of evaluation by the physician. It is useful to have coaxial illumination for examination of the bleeding site; a headlight or head mirror will facilitate visualization for effective control of the bleeding. The patient should be instructed to blow the nose to remove blood clots before the bleeding site is sought. A vasoconstrictor such as .25% to .50% phenylephrine hydrochloride (Neo-Synephrine) solution and/or a topical anesthetic such as a 4% cocaine solution should then be applied.

If readily visible, the bleeding site may be controlled with chemical cautery, such as the application of silver nitrate, or electrocautery. Absorbable hemostat (Surgicel) or absorbable gelatin (Gelfoam) may be used as part of the packing within the nose. Strip packing, if used, may be ½-inch selvedged gauze applied in a switch-back fashion with bayonet forceps to allow adequate pressure and to decrease the possibility of the packing falling down the oropharynx. A useful technique for gauze packing is to impregnate the gauze with an antibiotic ointment to decrease the possibility of infection and to increase the ease with which the packing may be removed. Applying antibiotics to the pack eliminates the unpleasant odor that is sometimes associated with packing retained in the nose.

For posterior epistaxis, it may be desirable to do infracture of the inferior turbinate to visualize and to control the bleeding site or to use a postnasal pack of the classical type or one of the newer balloon control units that can be placed within the nose. One must be concerned about the possibility of necrosis where excessive and prolonged pressure has been applied.

Another way to control epistaxis is with salt pork, which can be kept frozen in the clinic or office, sliced in wedges and inserted into the nose. The hemostatic property of salt pork has been known for many years, although no one understands the mechanism. Some believe that epistaxis in patients with blood dyscrasias is more readily controlled by salt pork than by antibiotic-soaked gauze packing or cauterization.

Intractable bleeding may be controlled by ligating the appropriate blood vessel, which could be the internal maxillary, the anterior ethmoid, or even the external carotid artery. Other measures to control epistaxis include cryotherapy, embolization through the use of small pellets of absorbable gelatin or silicone, and occasionally septal dermaplasty; but these latter techniques are reserved for more difficult problems.

In the everyday prevention of nosebleed it is important to maintain adequate humidification during the winter months either through the use of humidifiers in the home or by spraying the nose several times daily with normal saline solution. The use of petrolatum (Vaseline) or boric acid and lanolin ointment (Borofax) will help maintain a moist nasal membrane. The patient should be urged to refrain from traumatizing the nose with the finger or applicator and to avoid the overuse of aspirin.

Atrophic rhinitis

Atrophic rhinitis[9] is a progressive, chronic disease in which the nasal fossae are greatly enlarged as a result of atrophic changes in the mucosa and underlying bone. Thick adherent crusts with a foul odor are formed in the nasal passages. Another name for atrophic rhinitis is *ozena*, derived from Greek, meaning stench. The etiologic factors are not entirely clear, although there are many theories. *Klebsiella ozenae and Corynebacterium diphtheriae,* in nontoxigenic form, have been cultured from the nose and are believed to be typical of this problem.

Histopathologic features vary and may include small islands of squamous metaplasia on the surface epithelium and in the lamina propria and an abundance of inflammatory and mast cells. There are many similarities between atrophic rhinitis and chronic rhinitis.

Normal airflow through the nose is markedly altered in atrophic rhinitis. The seromucinous glands function badly, circulation is poor, and inadequate moisture is produced. There is marked destruction of the nasal cilia, and crusts form on the nasal mucous membrane. The resulting sensation is a feeling of nasal obstruction despite the excessive airway. Nasopharyngitis or oropharyngitis and laryngitis sicca often accompany atrophic rhinitis.

Treatment usually consists of prolonged medical care, with surgery reserved for patients who are refractory to medical treatment. Among the most important considerations are discontinuance of vasoconstrictor nose drops and sprays and the use of cleansing nasal irrigations, such as normal saline solution, to control crust formation. Irrigation of the nose is greatly facilitated by a dental irrigator with a special tip. In this procedure, warm normal saline solution is flushed through the nose with the irrigator at its lowest setting.

Rarely there may be a purulent rhinitis or sinuitis along with the atrophic rhinitis. If such is the case, there should be a culture taken, sensitivity studies, and antibiotic treatment of rhinosinusitis.

Surgical management of atrophic rhinitis follows one of two general approaches. One procedure is endonasal microplasty, the objective of this procedure is to decrease the size of the nasal airway by inserting small pieces of bone in the floor of the nose or in the septum, possibly associated with reduction rhinoplasty. A second approach is that of temporarily closing the nostrils; the anterior nares are closed one at a time in the nasal vestibule area. When the nostril is reopened, the mucous membrane appears swollen and gradually returns to a normal appearance without nasal crusting and foul odor. After an interval of approximately 3 months, the opposite nostril is closed for a similar period of time.

Perforations of the nasal septum

Perforations of the nasal septum may result from trauma, such as nasal fracture, surgery, picking of the nose, septal hematomas or abscesses, application of chromic acid, syphilis, or cocaine usage. The patient frequently has a sensation of abnormal blockage of the nose and may sustain significant infection and bleeding from the edges of the perforation. Drying and crusting are significant, and whistling respiration is not unusual in these patients.

Medical treatment should include requesting the patient to refrain from picking the nose, to sniff salt water, to lubricate the nose with petrolatum or other emollient ointments, and to use antibiotic ointments, perferably with steroids, for short periods to decrease inflammation. Many techniques have been devised to repair perforations of the septum. The whistling sound associated with breathing can be altered by changing the size of the perforation in the septum; a significant degree of success has been obtained by enlarging the perforation. A more recent aid in closing perforations is the polymeric silicone (Silastic) collar button which allows more comfortable breathing; decreases the crusting, infection and bleeding; and returns many patients to a relatively satisfactory state of nasal health.

Abnormalities of the senses of taste and smell

Taste and smell are related chemical senses and, although it is possible to have malfunction in one or both of them, complaints are more frequently centered around a loss of olfaction. An acute loss of sense of smell can be related to an acute coryza; chronic losses often follow influenza-like viral infections, surgery, and radiation and may be related to high doses of aspirin or other drugs or to blockage of air currents through the nose from nasal polyps and space-occupying lesions. Head trauma and diseases such as cancer, liver disease, hyperthyroidism, hepatitis, or ileitis can alter taste and smell.

Mucormycosis (phycomycosis)

Mucormycosis, a serious and frequently life-threatening granulomatous fungal infection, initially appears as acute sinusitis. Frequently it is associated with facial cellulitis in diabetics who are poorly controlled and acidotic or in patients who have poor immunity. People who have received immunosuppressive therapy or who have lymphomas, leukemias, and connective tissue disorders are susceptible to the infection. Intranasal examination reveals a "black turbinate" resulting from necrosis of the tissue. The disease process, which can progress rapidly, may extend to the orbit or to the intracranial areas and cause death.

The organisms are widely distributed, being found in manure, soil, and in starchy foods; they are believed to enter the body through the nasal mucosa, invading and thrombosing blood vessels and infarcting the surrounding tissue. Diagnosis is established by identifying the organisms in tissue removed at biopsy.

Treatment includes use of amphotericin B as the drug of choice and wide and expeditious excision of all involved tissue; hyperglycemia must be corrected.

Facial trauma and surgery

Facial trauma. In the elderly, changes in vision and alterations in equilibrium contribute to falls and other accidents with consequent injury to the face. The use of anticoagulant medications and aspirin and the loss of tissue tone increase the tendency for bleeding and swelling in the traumatized tissues. Wiring of displaced facial bones in edentulous patients or in patients with full dentures requires a slight technique variation for satisfactory immobilization of the bone fragments. It is especially important to maintain ambulation in older patients, but in general they tolerate surgery and heal quite well.

Plastic and reconstructive facial surgery. Plastic and reconstructive facial surgery is of growing importance in the aging population. The physician's careful attention to the patient's desires, needs, and physical capabilities is essential. An aging individual with sagging jowls or "crow's feet" may seek a rhytidectomy on emotional, social, or professional grounds to maintain an appearance of vigor and vitality. The postsurgical defect following removal of a malignancy may require cosmetic or functional surgery such as closure of a hypopharyngeal fistula or construction of a neoglottis.

Recent developments such as microsurgery, free flaps, and myocutaneous flaps have significantly added to the surgeon's armamentarium and have improved reconstructive surgery significantly.

DISEASES OF THE THROAT, LARYNX, AND MANDIBLE

The aging larynx

Vocal strain occurs relatively frequently in the geriatric patient. The aging process affects voice pitch, quality, and volume and the rate of speech in varying degrees in different individuals. The voice, which can be described as tired, falters and occasionally fails. Wavering tone and decreased volume and carrying power all result in lessened intelligibility. Articulation may be significantly distorted by missing teeth or dentures or stroke. Chronic vocal strain and fatigue result from voice misuse. Cooper[10] has described a positive approach to voice therapy for organic lesions such as nodes, polyps, contact ulcers, bowed vocal cords, and for the tired voice.

Spastic dysphonia refers to a "strained, creaking and choking vocal attack, a tight and squeezed voice sound which is accompanied by extreme tension of the entire phonatory system."[11] This condition was long felt to be largely psychogenic but recently has come under further evaluation. It is now considered to have an organic cause, and recurrent nerve section is suggested in carefully controlled situations.[12]

Laryngeal dysfunction secondary to unilateral or bilateral cord paralysis entails special problems. Unilateral cord paralysis can have varying etiologic factors, of which approximately 30% are never identified precisely. After allowing a period of about 6 months for spontaneous resolution of the paralysis, it may be desirable to attempt to improve the voice and the effectiveness of the cough reflex by injecting polytetrafluoroethylene (Teflon) paste lateral to the paralyzed vocal cord. A test dose of gelatin may be used initially, followed by a permanent injection.

Bilateral abductor cord paralysis, while not affecting voice quality, may significantly affect the inspiratory function of the larynx and require corrective action. It may be desirable to perform a lateralizing procedure of the cord or perhaps a tracheostomy with the rehabilitative use of a valved tracheostomy tube such as a Kistner tube. A rehabilitated patient using this technique can function quite normally and frequently without others knowing that the tracheostomy exists.

Malignancies of the larynx are being treated with myriad approaches, but it is far beyond this chapter to enter into a discussion of specific techniques. There has been a significant improvement in rehabilitation of the voice following surgical removal of a malignancy. In addition to an electrolarynx and esophageal speech, there are multiple approaches to the surgical reconstruction of the speaking mechanism.

When a tracheostomy, a short- or long-term,

is necessary, the approach of the patient, the family, and the medical team will greatly affect the degree of success or failure of this procedure. Proper preoperative counseling of the patient is vital. It is necessary to explain the purpose of the procedure and that the patient will probably be without his voice until he can learn to occlude the airway and speak through his larynx or use esophageal speech. Having those close to the patient around when needed is an important factor in rehabilitation.

An important element in the basics of tracheostomy care is the type of the tracheostomy tube selected. In a patient undergoing irradiation therapy, a metal tube is not acceptable as it may alter the radiotherapeutic dose. After irradiation therapy has been completed, it is possible to use a metal tube. The diameter and length of the tracheostomy tube are important. The thickness of the tissue in the anterior neck, the diameter of the trachea, and the distance to the carina must be considered. A tube that is too long may touch the carina and cause coughing. It may dig into the anterior wall of the trachea, thereby becoming partially blocked, or it may dig into the posterior wall of the trachea, causing irritation, possible ulceration, or fistula formation in the esophagus. The largest diameter tube should be used to fully open the airway for efficient respiratory function.

Humidification of the patient's immediate environment is also important. It may be accomplished by nebulizing water with compressed air or oxygen through a cage over the tracheostomy. Dropping water or saline solution into the tracheal opening to maintain proper humidity also thins secretions and prevents crusting.

A fresh tracheostomy frequently requires more care than one that has had a chance to heal adequately and to which the patient has become acclimated. Secretions in a fresh tracheostomy are frequently more marked; however, suctioning should be reduced to a minimum as soon as possible so as not to remove any more cilia from the trachea than is absolutely necessary.

Many laryngectomy patients are able to function quite well without a tracheostomy tube in place unless their laryngectomy stoma starts to stenose.

Various techniques of neoglottic reconstruction have attracted widespread attention. It is now possible to develop voices that are superior to esophageal speech in a significant proportion of patients who have lost their voices as a result of cancer surgery or other causes.

Candidiasis

Candidiasis (moniliasis or thrush) is a common mucocutaneous infection caused by *Candida albicans* and other species of *Candida*. The fungus is present in the normal intestinal tract, and after prolonged or intensive treatment with antibiotics, especially in debilitated individuals, there may be a pathologic overgrowth of this organism. This appears to happen more frequently when tetracyclines are prescribed than with some of the other antibiotics. There may be widespread dissemination, including septicemia, and death may occur.

The typical clinical picture consists of white patches on the throat and hypopharynx with mild inflammatory reaction in the underlying tissues. After removal of the patches, a reddened surface remains. If the disease becomes systemic, there is a possibility of fatal outcome unless active therapy is initiated. The fungus is identified on Sabouraud's agar as a budding yeast. Diabetes favors the development of candidiasis.

Treatment is usually effective using a nystatin suspension, gentian violet, and for systemic infections, amphotericin B.

Temporomandibular joint syndrome

Temporomandibular joint (TMJ) syndrome or Costen's syndrome is defined as a dysfunction with severe pain in or about the TMJ, the ear, or contiguous structures. The TMJ is unique in that it has a fibrous disc or articular meniscus instead of the usual hyaline cartilage.

The movement of the joint is remarkable in that the upper portion glides anteriorly and the inferior compartment serves as a hinge with the two portions functioning simultaneously. Among the causes of TMJ dysfunction are contraction of the muscles in the area and dental malocclusion. Other causes are acute trauma such as a blow to the jaw, chronic trauma from clenching of the teeth, arthritis, or tumors in the area.

Symptoms referable to TMJ syndrome include tinnitus (usually a ringing type), a clicking or popping sensation when the jaws open or close, and vertigo. The latter may be related to the condylar head advancing over the damaged disc and returning to the mandibular fossa.

There may be increased sensitivity to sound or a sensation of impaired hearing, though the latter is very difficult to determine with the audiometer and may be more functional than organic. Pain and fullness in and about the ear are frequently present. In addition to the complete physical examination, it may be desirable to obtain x-ray films of the TMJ using the transcranial lateral oblique view.

Nonsurgical management includes symptomatic treatment such as heat, soft diet, physical therapy, analgesics or tranquilizers, dental splint, bite block, and biofeedback or psychotherapy. In the event that these are unsatisfactory, it is worthwhile to consider one of the many different surgical approaches that have been offered to alleviate this most uncomfortable problem.

REFERENCES

1. Senturia, B.H., Marcus, M.D., and Lucente, F.R.: Diseases of the external ear, ed. 2, New York, 1980, Grune & Stratton, Inc.
2. Chandler, J.R.: Malignant external otitis: further considerations, Ann. Otol. Rhinol. Laryngol. **86**:417, 1977.
3. Santa Cruz, D.J.: Chondrodermatitis nodularis helicis: a transepidermal perforating disorder, J. Cutan. Pathol. **7**:70, 1980.
4. Goodhill, V.: Ear diseases, deafness and dizziness, New York, 1979, Harper & Row, Publishers, Inc.
5. Paparella, M.M., and Shumrick, D.A., editors: Otolaryngology, Philadelphia, 1980, W.B. Saundners Co.
6. Etholm, B., and Belal, A., Jr.: Senile changes in the middle ear joints, Ann. Otol. Rhinol. Laryngol. **83**:49, 1974.
7. House, J.W., Miller, L., and House, P.R.: Severe tinnitus: treatment with biofeedback training (results in 41 cases), Trans. Am. Acad. Ophthalmol. Otolaryngol. **84**:697, 1977.
8. Silverstein, H., and Norrell, H.: Subtotal resection of acoustic neuromas in the aged patient. In Silverstein, H., and Norrell, H., editors: Neurological surgery of the ear, vol. 2, New York, 1979, Aesculapius Publishers, Inc., p. 262.
9. Goodman, W.S., and DeSouza, F.M.: Atrophic rhinitis. In English, G.M., editor: Otolaryngology, vol. 2, New York, 1979, Harper & Row, Publishers, Inc.
10. Cooper, M.: Voice problems of geriatric patients, Geriatrics **25**(6):107, 1970.
11. Arnold, G.E.: Spastic dysphonia. I. Changing interpretations of persistent affliction, Logos **2**:3, 1959.
12. Dedo, H.H.: Recurrent laryngeal nerve section for spastic dysphonia, Ann. Otol. Rhinol. Laryngol. **85**:451, 1976.

CHAPTER 30 · SEXUALITY AND THE AGED

Rose E. Boyarsky

Although an increased number of papers on the topic of sexuality in the aging population has been published in the last 5 years, Berezin[1] has noted that there seems to be little advance in our knowledge or scientific understanding over that which appeared in the previous 10 years. Thus, a pressing need for increased research and scientific understanding of sexuality and sexual behavior in the aged still remains. The many problems the physician is called on to treat in the elderly patient are frequently intertwined with the psychologic, physiologic, cultural, and sociological sequelae of sexual dysfunction. The physician treating the elderly individual is called on to treat all aspects of the ailing patient.

Scientific literature has obviously made the popular writer more aware of the outdated myths, social taboos, and cultural prejudice surrounding sexuality and the older person. Popular literature, however, has taken a tone of exhortation and demand that the elderly have a right to their sexuality, even that they must be functioning sexually. Scientific literature, on the other hand, remains too narrowly concerned with the physical and statistical observations of the organic-endocrine approach to sexual dysfunctions. More emphasis is needed on the study of the interrelationships of the organic-endocrine with the psychologic, sociologic, cultural, economic, and environmental causes of sexual dysfunctions. More emphasis must be put into the understanding that sexual behavior in the elderly is usually in the service of a love relationship and a continuing human need for closeness, tenderness, and affection. More emphasis must be put into understanding that continued sexual function is an important factor in the maintenance of self-esteem.

Evidence from many sources[2-6] indicates that, given a reasonably good state of health and a partner who is healthy, willing, and interested, there is no age limit to sexual functioning. This is a necessary but not a sufficient basis for the maintenance of sexual function in the elderly. The cultural, psychologic, social, and economic parameters of sexual functions must also be taken into consideration. For instance, sufficient health and desire may be present; privacy in a nursing home may be absent.

This chapter will discuss the normal physiologic changes in sexual function that occur as a result of aging, briefly discuss the sexual dysfunctions caused by organic-endocrine problems, and then go on to the psychologic, cultural, social, and economic influences on sexual function.

MALE PHYSIOLOGIC CHANGES

Most of the information concerning normal changes in the physiology of sexual function in the older male comes from the classic work of Masters and Johnson.[3] Their study of 39 sexually functioning men ranging in age from 50 to 89 years old, established the changes during the five phases of the male sexual response cycle. These changes, in the older male as compared to the younger, may be classed as quantitative rather than qualitative. In general the older male reacts more slowly and less intensively than he may have when younger. It must be emphasized that wide individual differences play a large part in any individual's response to sexual stimulation. There are some elderly men who react more rapidly, more frequently, and more intensively than some younger men. Each man is unique in his sex response cycle. He may exhibit some, all, or none of the following age-related changes at any specific sexual opportunity.

In general, for the man over 50 years of age,

it takes longer, given effective sexual stimulation, for erection to develop. Once developed, the erection may not be as full or firm as it had been in his younger days. In fact, full penile erection may not occur until just prior to the ejaculatory experience. The ejaculatory experience itself may be of lesser intensity and of shorter duration with fewer expulsive contractions propelling the seminal fluid.

The volume of the seminal fluid may be less, and indeed the demand to ejaculate may be lessened enough so that ejaculation may not occur at each sexual opportunity. Once ejaculation has occurred, particularly for the man over 60 years of age, detumescence is rapid. The refractory phase of the male sexual response, during which time the male is physiologically unable to ejaculate, tends to last for a longer period, extending at times up to several days.

These changes must be understood as the normal altering of the bodily functions and not as necessarily diminishing the subjective pleasure of sexual behavior.

MALE SEXUAL DYSFUNCTIONS

The sexual dysfunctions the physician is commonly called on to treat in the elderly male are

1. Diminished libido
2. Premature ejaculation
3. Retrograde ejaculation
4. Dyspareunia
5. Secondary impotence

Dimninished libido

Complaints of diminished or even total lack of sexual interest increase in the elderly population. This is often a cumulative result of overwork, alcoholism, marital or family conflict, economic or emotional stress, or a general debilitation following illness, poor nutrition, or fatigue. The physician would do well to explore some of the social and psychologic as well as the medical parameters of the older man's life to identify the source of the diminished libido.

A thorough drug history should be elicited from the older man complaining of decreased libido. There is a tendency for some of these men to drift into hypochondriasis and take many medications including an astounding mix of tranquilizers, tonics, stimulants, and antihistamines. Resorting to drugs to stimulate diminished libido merely increases the general sexual dullness.

There is debate about the existence of a hormonal male climacteric syndrome. Roughly from about the age of 40 years, the production of testosterone is gradually lessened. Since this is a gradual rather than abrupt change, the sequelae of decreasing energy and slowing sexual response cycle are undramatic and should be considered within normal limits. Hormonal insufficiency appears to have little if any effect on sexual potency in advancing age.[7] There are instances, however, of reported lowered libido corresponding to below normal levels of testosterone.

Premature ejaculation

For the man who in his younger years had a tendency to ejaculate prematurely, the advance of age might sufficiently slow the ejaculatory reflex so that rapid ejaculation no longer remains a problem. To his surprise he might even find that the ejaculation is occasionally absent. This can be explained to the older man as well as his partner as normal and therefore no cause for alarm.

There are a number of older males, who after a period of illness and prolonged sexual abstinence seem to develop too rapid ejaculation. To some extent this is related to the decreased frequency of sexual outlet. In some cases it is related to the anxiety and concerns about the rapid ejaculation. In other cases it is inexplicably related to the illness. In all cases treatment using either the squeeze technique developed by Masters and Johnson[8] or the start and stop technique developed by Semans[9] is indicated.

Retrograde ejaculation

This is a common complaint in the older diabetic and in men who have undergone surgical alteration of the bladder neck. Hotchkiss[10] reports occasional cases of retrograde ejaculation in males taking guanethidine for hypertension.

The elderly man facing major prostatic surgery should be warned that retrograde ejaculation will probably occur. A small amount of time spent explaining the cause of the expected retrograde ejaculation can relieve a good deal of concern, disappointment, and anxiety. It should be explained that this need not interfere with the sensation of orgasm, although there will be no emission sensation on ejaculation. This need not otherwise interfere with sexual interest or activity.

Dyspareunia

Painful erection, painful intromission, painful ejaculation, or pain along the urethra, penis, in the vas, testicles, or epididymis can lead the elderly man to avoid or greatly diminish his sexual activity. Dyspareunia can often be a symptom of infection, trauma, or inflammatory conditions.

Prostatic pain may result from spastic rather than rhythmic contractions of the prostate during ejaculation. It can often be relieved by testosterone replacement therapy. Prostatic pain can also be secondary to infection, benign prostatic hypertrophy, or carcinoma.[11]

Painful curvature of the shaft of the penis, Peyronie's disease, is a self-limiting disease of unknown etiology. Although the older man may be somewhat embarrassed by the resulting curvature, the pain usually disappears in 12 to 24 months. Afterwards he is usually not prevented from functioning sexually.

Secondary impotence

By far the greatest sexual complaint of the older male is secondary impotence. There is increasing debate among professionals as to the psychogenic versus organic etiology.[12] Depending on the characteristics of the population studied and on the setting in which they are studied, the incidence of organic impotence varies from 4% to 48%.[8,13-15] It seems obvious that the physician would suspect a higher percentage of organic causes of impotence especially in the age group over 40 years old.

Since abstinence, fear of failure, and focus on performance play such an important role in sexual dysfunction of the aging man, it may be difficult for the physician to separate physical from psychologic causes of potency problems. If a man has become impotent from physical causes and remains dysfunctional after the physical concerns for this dysfunction have been removed, it is necessary to consider the possible psychologic factors maintaining the disturbance. As a rule, if a man has an erection at any time, for instance, morning erections, he is physiologically capable of erections which are adequate for sexual functioning. Nocturnal penile tumescence measurements are now generally available and provide an effective and objective method to distinguish an organic from a psychogenic cause.[14,16] Referral to an appropriate mental health professional for treatment of psychogenic impotence is recommended.

An increasing number of men suffering problems of impotence elect surgery. Penile implants are available, which include the inflatable, the semirigid, and the flexible types.[17,18] In the hands of an experienced surgeon the success rate for penile implantation is over 90%.[19]

FEMALE PHYSIOLOGIC CHANGES

Finkle,[7] writing about sexual function during advancing age, as late as 1971, devoted most of his chapter to the function of the aging male because of the general lack of information concerning sexual function in the aging female.

Sexual problems for the female are complicated by the relatively rapid change in hormonal status occurring during the forties and early fifties. There are data indicating the desirability of hormone replacement therapy in maintaining the physical and psychologic well-being of the postmenopausal woman.[20,21]

Information concerning physiologic changes in the aging female during the sexual response cycle must be drawn from Masters and Johnson's studies.[3,8] Their findings are based on physiologic observation of 34 sexually functioning women between the ages of 51 and 73 years. As in the aging man, the changes due to aging in the woman should be considered quantitative rather than qualitative.

Normal aging changes in the female sexual response cycle resemble those in the aging male. With adequate steroid replacement therapy these changes are, to a large degree, delayed and attenuated. With aging there is a general lessening of the rapidity and degree of response to effective sexual stimulation. This should in no way be interpreted to mean that there must be a corresponding decrease in subjective sensual pleasure.

As the woman ages, there is a general lessening of muscle tension and vasocongestive response. It may take a longer period of time, after the start of effective sexual stimulation, for the production of vaginal lubrication. Once lubrication occurs, it tends to be somewhat less copious. The vagina of the aging woman tends to have less expansile capacity, with a measurable loss of length and width as well as elasticity. After 60 years of age there may be a modest loss in clitoral size. This corresponds to a general change in the distribution of fatty tissue in the older woman. Despite these changes, the clitoris remains the receptor of sensual stimuli exactly as it was in the younger woman. The orgasm for the older woman is usually of shorter duration and of lessened intensity, although it must be emphasized, not necessarily of lessened subjective pleasure. The return of the stimulated organs and tissue to prestimulative state is relatively rapid.

Physiologic changes with aging are both accelerated and more severe for the menopausal and postmenopausal woman who does not have the advantage of adequate estrogen replacement therapy. This is especially so for the woman with few sexual opportunities and no established habit of automanipulation. Lubrication can virtually cease, and atrophic vaginal changes can cause the occasional coital opportunity to be irritating and painful. Loss of the fatty tissue of the labia and clitoris may make genital play irritating. The uterus, instead of contracting intermittently may, with orgasm, go into a painful spastic contraction. Symptoms of bladder irritation may be present. Most of these symptoms can be alleviated with the administration of adequate amounts of topical or systematic estrogen under medical supervision.[3,20] There are a number of women who continue to function effectively without the need for steroid replacement and in spite of atrophic vaginal changes. This seems to be related to continued, frequent, and regular opportunity for sexual function.

FEMALE SEXUAL DYSFUNCTIONS

For the postmenopausal woman, sexual function can be seriously affected by decreased hormone levels and resulting dryness, thinning, and bleeding of vulval and vaginal mucosa. The three most common female sexual dysfunctions are:

1. Sexual avoidance
2. Dyspareunia
3. Lack of orgasm

Sexual avoidance

Sexual avoidance can be of cultural or emotional etiology. Avoidance may be related to dyspareunia and chronic lack of sexual satisfaction. Often the three dysfunctions—avoidance, dyspareunia, and lack of orgasm—must be treated at the same time on the level of physical relief from pain and psychologic relief from depression, guilt, and blame.

The most common causes of sexual avoidance in the older woman are psychologic. This may be a long-term negative or hostile relationship with a spouse or depression as a result of general and sexual involution.

Verwoerdt[22] points out that the real or fancied loss of any capacity, including sexual capacities, may give rise to a grief reaction, anxious concerns about disruptions to intimate relationships, and fears of loss of love. There then ensues a retreat into self-absorption and even hypochondriasis. This is where the physician is often consulted. It would be wise to inquire in detail into the sexual and marital relationships to understand the physical complaints and their relation to the older woman's psychologic state.

Dyspareunia

Painful sexual experiences for the elderly woman are most often a result of decreased sexual opportunity, decreased hormone production, and resulting atrophy of the genitourinary structures. Increased urinary tract infections such as cystitis, urethritis, and cystourethritis are reported by Kent[23] in women who remain sexually active. The urinary tract infections may result from a tendency for the older woman to engage in extended periods of intercourse because of delayed ejaculation.

The treatment of choice in these cases is systemic or topical hormone replacement combined with increased fluid intake and better hygiene along with specific medication to control the urologic infections.

Occasional cramping of the uterus at orgasm can also be attenuated by hormone replacement therapy.

Lack of orgasm

The older woman contending with depression, dyspareunia, infection, hostile relationships, or decreased physical well-being can hardly be expected to relax sufficiently during sexual activity to be orgasmic. This woman most often retreats from sexual opportunity or resigns herself to the situation rather than appearing at the physician's office to complain about the lack of orgasm. Often it will be her husband who complains of her lack of sexual interest or lack of sexual response.

Since decreased hormonal status of itself is not sufficient cause for lack of orgasm,[24] some time should be spent on a careful social and marital as well as physical anamnesis of the anorgasmic woman. Because treatment is time-consuming, it may often be best accomplished by referral to a marital or sexual therapist.

PHYSICAL INFLUENCES

Drugs

A number of drugs in common use can influence both sexual desire and potency. The elderly often have idiosyncratic responses to drugs. A list of drugs that adversely affect sexual function is available from many sources.[3,25]

Investigators have long pointed out the connection between alcohol and sexual impotence.[3,26] Lemere and Smith,[27] in their study of 17,000 chronic alcoholics, point out that in at least 8% of these men impotence is irreversible by virtue of permanent damage to the neurologic reflex subserving erection.

Estrogens prescribed for carcinoma of the prostate gland decrease both sexual desire and potency. Sedatives, large doses of alcohol, sympatholytic drugs such as guanethidine, and antihypertensive medications can be a cause for secondary impotence. Tranquilizers from barbiturates to meprobamate and antihistamines, which act to sedate, tend to decrease sexual interest and desire.

Little is known about the effect of drugs on the female sexual response.

The physician treating the elderly for sexual dysfunctions must take a careful history of drug use. The elderly patient should be made aware of the possible effects of a particular drug on sexual function when drug therapy is prescribed.

Cardiac disease

For the cardiac patient and his partner the resumption of sexual activity often provokes a good deal of concern and question. In general, exercise in moderation is beneficial. There are few activities done in moderation that physicians would prohibit to those recovering from heart disease.[28] Sexual activity for the cardiac patient can be considered another form of exercise to be pursued in moderation. The so-called "coital coronary" does occur but nowhere as often as myth would have us believe. Death can be precipitated also by masturbation. Death is more likely precipitated by extramarital liaisons in strange surroundings.[29] The vast majority of patients with coronary insufficiency can safely fulfill the demands of their usual sexual activity. The only large-scale study of death in cardiac patients during or after sexual activity was done in Japan.[30] Of 5559 cases of sudden death, 18 occurred as a result of heart disease during sexual activity. Over two thirds of these 18 deaths occurred during or after extramarital intercourse and the ingestion of rich foods and alcohol. In general, it would seem that previous levels of sexual activity may safely be resumed after convalescence from cardiac disease, gradually and carefully and avoiding stressful surroundings and sexual activity after overeating or alcoholic consumption. Nitroglycerin may be prescribed prophylactically or to treat pain if it occurs.[31]

Urologic conditions

The effect of kidney, bladder, prostate, or testicular diseases and surgery on potency and frequency of coitus in the elderly man has been studied.[2] Simple or radical perineal prostatectomy has a destructive effect on the potency of most but not all men. There is little effect on the libido. The younger and more sexually active man shows the greatest recovery of function. Most investigators find the incidence of urologic as well as nonurologic symptoms and diseases to be the same for potent as for impotent men.[2,32,33] These investigators found that impotence in the elderly man is usually independent of physical condition and that a willing sexual partner seems to be the most important factor in maintaining potency after urologic disease.

Retrograde ejaculation following surgery of the urinary tract has already been discussed.

CULTURAL INFLUENCES

American men have usually been given society's permission to be sexually active in a variety of ways. From the earliest years, a young boy is encouraged to touch his genitals in a socially acceptable fashion such as when urinating. Males learn to masturbate relatively early and continue to do so throughout much of their lives.[34] At all ages they are given permission to take the social and sexual initiative. As the male matures, his position, status, and wealth add to his sexual attractiveness, and he has little difficulty finding sexual partners.

To a great extent society regulates the modes of expression of the biologic sex drive. There is little tolerance shown for those whose sexual behavior violates cultural norms. These people are subject to contempt, ridicule, and even legal punishment; 30 years ago Kinsey described the discrepancy between legal and cultural norms and actual sexual behavior. In spite of the sexual freedom allowed the American male and the current cultural flux, taboos still exist in many subtle and explicit forms. Although throughout much of the rest of the world, the concept of sex as play is pervasive, contemporary (and historic) American society sees the purpose of sexual activity as procreation rather than recreation. The attitude is that sexual relations are permissible only between individuals in situations that could lead to socially approved pregnancies and that sexual contact between individuals over 50 years of age does not serve reproductive functions. Elderly people tend to share these prejudices.[36] The ethos is designed to place the physically disabled, the ill, and the elderly individual in the same asexual category.

As a result of the general climate of deprecation of sexual expression for people over 50 years of age and the demographic variables discussed next, the sexual freedom and activity of the elderly woman is most seriously affected.

For every 100 women over 65 years of age in the United States, there are presently only 72.7 men.[37] Two thirds of these women over 65 years old are widows. These women form the most sexually oppressed group in America. They suffer from loneliness and lack of companionship as well as sexual deprivation. They offer a challenge to society and medicine, who have lengthened but not necessarily enriched their lives. There is little opportunity for these women to express themselves sexually. In postmarital women the incidence of coitus decreases from 37% at 50 years of age to 0% at 65 years of age.[38] Society scoffs at their dating, especially if the man is appreciably younger. There are few available elderly men. These women are unable to take the social or sexual initiative. Extramarital liaisons are frowned on. Since sexual attractiveness for the woman is equated with youth, these women, just by virtue of being older, are no longer considered sexually attractive.

For the elderly woman who is married, sexual opportunity may be severely limited by a dysfunctional husband. In a study of married women who were no longer sexually active, it was found that the male factors were largely responsible for the cessation of sexual activity because the husbands had become ill, lost interest, or lost their sexual potency.[39,40] Those women who remained married with sexually functioning husbands showed little if any decline in sexual activity over a 10-year period.[40] This can be taken as an indication that the extent of an aging woman's sexual activity depends largely on the availability of a functioning sexual partner rather than on any decline in her own interest and capacity.

Summarizing the effect of aging and marital status on sexual activity, Pfeiffer et al.[40] found that, for the male, marital status had little effect on activity or interest. For the female, however, marital status had a considerable effect on activity. Generally speaking, the sexual activity of the man is greater than that of the woman, regardless of age or marital status in spite of the greater physiologic potential of the woman.[3,8] The role of the socially sanctioned sexually functional partner is probably the most powerful determinant of sexual behavior in the elderly woman.[4]

For both men and women a history of a high level of interest and activity in younger years is directly related to the maintenance of sexual interest and activity in older years. The practitioner should be aware that sex continues to play an important role in the lives of many elderly people within the wide range of individual differences which exist between people in any age group.

PSYCHOLOGIC INFLUENCES

Adverse psychologic influences on sexual interest and activity differ for men and women, yet probably lead to a single common pathway: depression. In spite of individual variation, it seems that depression often precedes sexual withdrawal for women, whereas sexual dysfunction often precedes depression for men.

Considered existentially, the involutional depression may have quite a realistic etiology.[41] In contemporary, youth-oriented American society, both elderly men and women are considered to have lost their usefulness, especially after retirement. The elderly individual is no longer valued for his opinion or learning, there is a loss of income, a loss of physical strength, and a loss of youthful attractiveness. Children no longer look to parents for support and guidance. Much of what had been a source of self-esteem and well-being is denied elderly people. It should be expected that they would mourn their losses while they are making adjustments to their changed life position.

Menopause and the "empty nest" syndrome

have frequently been blamed for depression,[42] yet it has been shown that for most people neither the menopause nor the end of active parenting has been experienced as a crisis. Some women feel a new sense of freedom and self-identity with the freedom from fears of pregnancy and the burdens of parenting. For both men and women the middle years can bring an enriched sense of self combined with an enhanced capacity to cope.[43]

Verwoerdt[22] points out that there are a number of psychologic reasons for increased sexual activity in the older adult. These are:

1. A lessening of earlier sexual inhibitions
2. Attempts to compensate for, or deny, age-related losses
3. A search for relief from boredom and monotony after retirement
4. Success in life's work resulting in increased self-esteem
5. Economic success
6. Family changes giving more privacy and leisure
7. Loss of concern about unwanted pregnancy
8. Decreased stress

Depression in later life frequently follows serious illness and is often associated with a cessation of sexual activity. Since depressive cycles tend to be self-perpetuating and since continued sexual relations can be an important source of self-esteem for the elderly individual, it is important that the physician recognize the syndrome and intervene. This cycle of depression is approximately the same for men and women; they merely enter the cycle at different points. Once caught, however, professional guidance is most often needed to relieve the problem.

Leviton[44] has some evidence that dysfunction or decrease in sexuality among the aged is at least partially implicated in the increased suicide rates in the elderly. He notes the palliative aspects of psychologic, medical, and surgical sexual therapy.

Depression can be manifested in feelings of hopelessness, sadness, anxiety, loss of self-esteem, and in psychosomatic and many other symptoms. Once started, the depressive cycle of lack of sexual activity can lead, for the man, to lowered libido and concerns about ability to perform sexually followed by active avoidance of sexual opportunity. The woman, wondering why her husband is avoiding sexual contact or is impotent during occasional sexual opportunity or reacts more slowly to opportunity, assumes her loss of youthful attractiveness as the cause. Her depressive cycle is thus accelerated, resulting on her part in a reactive loss of interest in sexual opportunity.

The resumption of sexual activity after a prolonged period of inactivity can be anxiety provoking, especially for men, possibly leading to potency problems, avoidance behaviors, and depression, further reducing the possibility of a return to effective sexual function. As soon as the man has doubts concerning his sexual potential and performance, he is well along the road to secondary impotence.

Erections are both reflexive and psychogenic.[45] The psychogenic factor can overrule the reflexive factor in the healthy man. When a man has doubts and concerns in regard to his ability to function sexually, he becomes a spectator watching himself to see if he will react to sensual stimulation rather than experiencing and enjoying the stimulation. These men will often say that they feel nothing. The psychologic stance of "spectatoring" acts to cut off awareness of feelings that seem to be a prerequisite for erection. It is particularly difficult for a man who has fears of performance and is spectatoring his sexual performance to understand that this is exactly what is interfering with his functioning. Professional guidance is required to help change the habits.

These factors can operate to interfere with erection at any age. It is particularly operative in the aging man, who for some reason has abstained from sexual activity for a period of time and who accepts on some level the cultural stereotype of getting close to the end of his active sexual life.

The woman, too, is subject to fears of performance and "spectatoring." She is more fortunate than the male in that she need not obtain an erection to function. On the other hand, spectatoring and fears for the woman result in lack of lubrication and possibly painful intercourse, in turn decreasing her desire for sexual opportunity. Exactly the same dynamics are at work, since lubrication in the woman is the physiologic analog of erection in the man.

Psychologically, fears and "spectatoring" by either sexual partner decrease sexual interest and opportunity, leading to increased fears and anxiety at any subsequent opportunity. Since continued sexual activity can provide a feeling of well-being, enjoyment, acceptance, and self-worth, it supplies some of the factors that can enter into the reversal of a depressive cycle. Careful but direct questioning into the current sexual status and the patient's satisfaction with this status can help the physician to diagnose the psychologic rather than physical roots of sexual dysfunction in the elderly person.

OTHER FACTORS

DeNicola and Peruzza[46] suggest the physician take a holistic care approach to the sexual problems of the elderly. The general condition of the older person, not simply disease or aging, may be the cause of sexual dysfunction. In addition to the endocrine-organic and psychologic factors, the physician must explore environmental, economic, technical, and occupational factors influencing sexual functioning.

An example of an occupational factor influencing sexual functioning includes exposure to CS_2 poisoning or industrial exposure to high frequency electromagnetic fields.

Environmental factors such as fatigue from conditions of commuting to and from work, lack of privacy in nursing homes, or even excessively or erroneously protective domestic surroundings can discourage or inhibit sexual expression.[47]

Economic factors resulting in lack of adequate housing or nutrition or an inability to live in a secure neighborhood may have an inhibiting effect on sexual desire as well as sexual opportunity. Widowhood and resulting economic privation is a common situation for many older women.

Technical factors such as disability because of spinal cord injury, arthritis, and so forth make special instruction and education for alternative sexual positions, techniques, and substitutions useful.

Interestingly enough it is the nonmedical community that is leading the way in correcting the environmental, technical, and economic influences on sexuality in the elderly.

Elderly Americans are exploring a variety of ways to meet their needs of intimacy and sexual expression inside a marriage, in nursing homes, in homosexual relationships, in long or short liaisons without consideration of marriage and in masturbation, coital and noncoital experience.[48,49]

CONCLUSION

Chronologic age per se is not a cause for an abrupt end to sexual activity. Most chronic physical illness does not completely remove sexual desire and interest. There is little evidence that inquiry regarding sexual activity and interests, appropriately introduced as a review of systems and conducted in an objective manner by a professional comfortable with the questions, evokes anxiety or evasion. On the contrary, patients seem relieved when the physician takes the initiative and asks pertinent questions. A few basic questions concerning present sexual activity and satisfaction with it often suffice. The questions must be posed in such a way as to make it easy for the patient to admit he or she has a problem. Once the presence of sexual dysfunction is established, the physician can give the information to help the couple understand normal aging changes. The physician is also in a position to assess the social, cultural, economic, technical, and environmental influences on the sexual dysfunctions. This may lead to an appropriate referral.

For both men and women the most important factor in the maintenance of sexual capacity and effective sexual function is the regularity of sexual outlet, whether coital, masturbatory, or fantasied. The most effective way to secure efficient functioning of an organ for the largest part of the life span is to use it.

REFERENCES

1. Berezin, M.A.: Normal psychology of the aging process, revisited—Sex and old age: a further review of the literature, J. Geriatr. Psychiatry **9:**189, 1976.
2. Finkle, A.L., and Prian, D.V.: Sexual potency in elderly men before and after prostatectomy, J.A.M.A. **196:**139, 1966.
3. Masters, W.H., and Johnson, V.E.: Human sexual response, Boston, 1966, Little, Brown & Co.
4. Newman, G., and Nichols, C.R.: Sexual activities and attitudes in older persons, J.A.M.A. **173:**33, 1960.
5. Pfeiffer, E., Verwoerdt, A., and Davis, G.C.: Sexual behavior in middle life, Am. J. Psychiatry **82:**1262, 1972.
6. Rubin, I.: Sexual life after 60, New York, 1965, Basic Books, Inc.
7. Finkle, A.L.: Sexual function during advancing age. In Rossman, I., editor: Clinical geriatrics, Philadelphia, 1971, J.B. Lippincott Co.
8. Masters, W.H., and Johnson, V.E.: Human sexual inadequacy, Boston, 1970, Little, Brown & Co.
9. Semans, J.H.: Premature ejaculation: a new approach, South. Med. J. **49:**353, 1956.
10. Hotchkiss, R.S.: Infertility in the male. In Campbell,

M.F., and Harrison, J.H., editors: Urology, ed. 3, Philadelphia, 1970, W.B. Saunders Co.

11. Boyarsky, S., and Boyarsky, R.: Office treatment of male sexual dysfunction, Urol. Clin. North Am. **7**:107, 1980.
12. Spark, R.F., White, R.A., and Connolly, P.B.: Impotence is not always psychogenic, J.A.M.A. **243**:750, 1980.
13. Jevtich, M.J., and Jarman, D.W.: Impotence: a challenge to the urologist, Program abstracts, 74th Annual Meeting, American Urology Association, New York, 1979, p. 121.
14. Blaivas, J.G., et al.: Comprehensive laboratory evaluation of impotent males, Program abstracts, 74th Annual Meeting, American Urology Association, New York, 1979, p. 121.
15. Shrom, S.H., Lief, H.I., and Wein, A.J.: Clinical profile of experience with 130 consecutive cases of impotent men, Urology **13**:511, 1979.
16. Beutler, L.E., Scott, F.B., and Karacan, I.: Psychological screening of impotent men, J. Urol. **116**:193, 1976.
17. Jonas, U., and Jacobi, G.H.: Silicone-silver penile prosthesis: description, operative approach and results, J. Urol. **123**:865, 1980.
18. Finney, R.: New hinged silicone penile implant, J. Urol. **118**:585, 1977.
19. Furlow, W.L.: Surgical management of impotence using the inflatable penile prosthesis: experience with 103 patients. Br. J. Urol. **50**:114, 1978.
20. Jern, H.Z.: Hormone therapy of the menopause and aging, Springfield, Ill., 1974, Charles C Thomas, Publisher.
21. Zussman, L.: The climacteric, Proc. R. Soc. Med. **66**:183, 1973.
22. Verwoerdt, A.: Normal psychology of the aging process revisited. Discussion, J. Geriatr. Psychiatry **9**:211, 1976.
23. Kent, S.: Urinary tract infections in women are linked to sexual activity, Geriatrics **30**(7):145, 1975.
24. Longcope, C.: Hormones: beneficial or dangerous to the aged? J. Am. Geriatr. Soc. **26**:145, 1978.
25. Glover, B.H.: Sex counseling of the elderly, Hosp. Pract. **12**:101, 1977.
26. Viamontes, J.A.: Alcohol abuse and sexual dysfunction, Human Sexuality **8**:185, 1974.
27. Lemere, F., and Smith, J.W.: Alcohol-induced sexual impotence, Am. J. Psychiatry **2**:130, 1973.
28. Likoff, W.V., Segal, B., and Galton, L.: Your heart, Philadelphia, 1972, J.B. Lippincott Co.
29. Massie, E., Rose, E., Rupp, J., and Whelton, R.: Sudden death during coitus—fact or fiction? Med. Aspects Human Sexuality **22**:22, 1969.
30. Ueno, M.: The so-called coition death, Jap. J. Leg. Med. **17**:333, 1963.
31. Friedberg, C.K.: Diseases of the heart, Philadelphia, 1966, W.B. Saunders Co.
32. Bowers, L.M., Cross, R.R., and Lloyd, F.A.: Sexual function and urologic disease in the elderly male, J. Am. Geriatr. Soc. **11**:647, 1963
33. Finkle, A.L., Moyers, T.G., Tobenkin, M.I., and Karg, S.J.: Sexual potency in aging males. I. Frequency of coitus among clinic patients, J.A.M.A. **170**:1391, 1959.
34. Kinsey, A.C., Pomeroy, W.B., and Martin, C.E.: Sexual behavior in the human male, Philadelphia, 1948, W.B. Saunders Co.
35. Kinsey, A.C., Pomeroy, W.B., Martin, C.E., and Gebhard, P.H.: Sexual behavior in the human female, Philadelphia, 1953, W.B. Saunders Co.
36. Post, F.: Sex and its problems. IX. Disorders of sex in the elderly, Practitioner **199**:377, 1967.
37. U.S. Bureau of Census: Statistical abstracts 1971, Washington, D.C., 1971, U.S. Government Printing Office.
38. Christenson, C.V., and Ganon, J.H.: Sexual behavior in a group of older women, J. Gerontol. **20**:351, 1965.
39. Pfeiffer, E., Verwoerdt, A., and Wang, H.S.: Sexual behavior in aged men and women. I. Observation on 254 community volunteers, Arch. Gen. Psychiatry **19**:753, 1968.
40. Pfeiffer, E., Verwoerdt, A., and Wang, H.S.: The natural history of sexual behavior in a biologically advantaged group of aged individuals, J. Gerontol. **24**:193, 1969.
41. Feigenbaum, E.M.: Geriatric psychopathology—internal or external? J. Am. Geriatr. Soc. **22**:49, 1974.
42. Lowenthal, M.F., and Chiriboga, D.: Transition to the empty nest-crisis, challenge or relief? Arch. Gen. Psychiatry **26**:8, 1972.
43. Neugarten, B.L.: Awareness of middle age. In Neugarten, B.L., editor: Middle age and aging, Chicago, 1968, University of Chicago Press.
44. Leviton, D.: The significance of sexuality as a deterrent to suicide among the aged, Omega **4**:163, 1973.
45. Bors, E., and Comarr, A.E.: Neurological disturbances of sexual function with special reference to 529 patients with spinal cord injury, Urol. Surv. **10**:191, 1960.
46. deNicola, P., and Peruzza, M.: Sex in the aged, J. Am. Geriatr. Soc. **22**:380, 1974.
47. Griggs, W.: Sex and the elderly, Am. J. Nurs. **78**:1352, 1978.
48. Wasow, M., and Loeb, M.: Sexuality in nursing homes, J. Am. Geriatr. Soc. **27**:73, 1979.
49. Cavan, R.S.: Speculations on innovations to conventional marriage in old age, Gerontologist **13**:409, 1973.

CHAPTER 31 · MUSCLE DISEASES OF THE AGED

Octavio de Marchena
Michael H. Brooke

While many diseases appear regardless of the patient's age, other diseases apparently tend to afflict age groups because of the relative vulnerability of that group to the disease. Muscle diseases are no exception; some are characteristic enough of the aged population to be considered in a chapter of this type.

Muscle itself undergoes changes with aging, and it is sometimes difficult to separate the effects of disease from those of senescence. In addition, muscle tissue contains many other components such as vascular and connective tissue, each of which suffers from its own set of diseases and dysfunctions. The muscle cell is wedded to the nervous system, and deficits in central nervous system function may produce muscle weakness without primary change in the muscle. Finally, muscles are dependent on systemic factors and may be secondarily affected by disturbances in the cardiovascular, endocrine, or other body systems.

Motor performance involves multiple integrated levels of the central nervous system. Even the simplest motor act requires immediate sensory data, experience, motivation, and complex coordination of multiple muscle groups. The elderly display a progressive decrease in the speed of movement and reaction time, disturbances in the smooth flow of motor performance, a decrease in the motivation for movement, and a reduction in the frequency of spontaneous movement.[1] Dysfunction in the motor unit is unlikely to be the major component of this deterioration, but it plays a role. The relative contribution of all the above factors has not been closely examined; however, such studies are essential in providing the foundation on which examination of muscle disease in the aged must be based.

Muscle strength decreases with age. The decrease is rather consistent, beginning in the mid twenties and continuing into late life. Various studies have put the decrease in strength to be in the range of 30% to 50% from ages 20 to 80 in otherwise healthy persons.[2,3] While decreases in fat-free mass and apparent muscle mass have been documented in old age, the correlation between these changes and increasing weakness is not very good.[4,5] Muscle strength does appear to be proportional to the active cross-sectional area of the muscle (total number of muscle fibers × average fiber area × percentage of activated fibers). Computerized tomography (CT) methods that provide a true cross-sectional area measurement of specific muscles may demonstrate a better correlation.[6]

Volitional factors limiting full muscle activation have been suggested as contributing to decreasing muscle strength in the elderly. All subjects have a proportion of muscle fibers that can be activated only with supramaximal stimulation of the nerve and that does not appear to be under volitional control. This results in a difference between the force generated by voluntary maximal contraction and that following electrical stimulation. The percentage of nonactivated fibers is higher in the untrained subject and probably higher in the aged.[9-11] However, even the maximal twitch tension produced following electrical stimulation decreases with age in some muscles. Campbell[12] noted a 32% decrease in twitch tension of the extensor digitorum brevis in a group of 60- to 96-year olds compared to a group 59 years old and younger. Most of the reduction in this study was felt to be caused by motor unit loss from denervation, a process that may not be true of all muscles.

Microscopic examination of muscle in the aged reveals a number of changes. A striking change is the reduction in the percentage of type II fibers and a decrease in type II fiber diameter. Larrson and Karlsson[8] measured fiber type percentages and area in the vastus lateralis of healthy sedentary males. The percentage of type I fibers in the vastus lateralis of the 20- to 29-year-old group of men was 39% ± 5%. In a group of 60- to 69-year-olds the percentage of type I fibers was 65%. The percentage area of type II fibers changed from 64% in the 20- to 29-year-old group to 44% in the 60- to 65-year-old group. This age related change is not limited to humans; it is also seen in rats and mice.[13] Type II fibers are involved in quick phasic voluntary movements and are distinguished biochemically by high glycolytic activity. In contrast, type I fibers are involved in slower more tonic movements and have a higher concentration of oxidative enzymes.[14] Type II fibers are sensitive to various factors. Disuse tends to reduce both type II fiber number and size; exercise tends to increase both. Several diseases and glucocorticoid excess have also been reported to decrease type II fiber number and size.[15] The reasons for the decrease in aging are not clear. Possibilities include the following:

1. A preferential loss of large myelinated units that preferentially innervate type II fibers. Large myelinated axons are lost in the aging process, accounting for the decrease in nerve conduction velocities with age; whether this is sufficient to decrease type II fibers selectively is not known.
2. "Functional" denervation as a result of disuse. Type II fibers are innervated by high threshold alpha-motor neurons.[17] The sedentary life-style of the elderly may lead to little activation of these fibers. That this may be a significant factor is emphasized by the reported reversal in type II fiber atrophy in older men involved in a rigorous exercise program.[18]

Can the decrease in the total type II fiber area account for the decrease in strength? Larrson[10] compared the decrease in strength in his elderly group with type II fiber area and found a strong correlation; that, however, did not completely explain decreased strength. He concluded that other factors, either motor unit loss or differences in activation, were also playing a role. Other researchers have suggested, however, that the change in the fiber type ratio may account for the increased endurance seen in elderly muscle as a greater percentage of the fibers would now be type I.[8,19]

Other changes described in aging muscle include evidence of denervation with angular fibers and fiber type grouping. The latter is usually felt to indicate denervation and reinnervation. Type grouping appears to be more common in distal than proximal muscles, perhaps because the longer peripheral nerves are more vulnerable to a lifetime of wear and tear than the shorter proximal ones.[20,21] Denervation may play an important part in the loss of strength in the distal musculature.[12] Other frankly degenerative changes include lipofucsin accumulation, ring fibers, vacuolation, sarcoplasmic masses, and an increase in connective and fatty tissue that may replace muscle.[22,23]

Biochemical changes are difficult to interpret; the levels greatly depend on the manner of measurement. Ermini and Verzar[24] found little change in the enzymatic behavior of myofibrillar proteins in the muscles of aged mammals but a decrease in energy metabolism manifested as a decrease and delay in the rephosphorylation of creatine after strenuous exercise. In contrast, Orlander et al.[25] found no major changes in energy metabolism in aged human muscle, although ultrastructurally, mitochondrial volume appeared to be reduced.

It would be of interest to know if the deterioration in muscle function and the associated histologic changes could be reversed. Vigorous activity has been suggested as a simple way to improve both muscle and cardiovascular function.[26] The elderly are able to improve maximal oxygen uptake with training,[27] although the improvement is smaller in old age, suggesting that the age decline cannot be completely removed by training. Trained older men do not appear to show the decrease in type II fiber number and size seen in sedentary older men. Orlander and Anniansson[18] also found higher oxidative enzyme activity in muscle biopsies of trained older men as compared to sedentary older men and an improvement in these activities with a rigorous training program.[28,29]

While helpful, none of these changes completely corrected the decrease in strength seen with aging, and further improvements may require better knowledge of the neuromuscular relationship during aging.

MYOPATHIES

Distal myopathy

Distal myopathy is characterized by the development in middle to late life of weakness of the distal musculature. Most cases reported have come from Sweden where the disease appears to be common. The cases reported by Welander[30] were characterized by onset from ages 20 to 77, with a mean age of onset of 47 years. Initial symptoms consisted of clumsiness in the hands that progressed to weakness and atrophy of the intrinsic musculature and extensors of the wrist. In a smaller group of patients weakness could begin in the feet, with dorsiflexors initially involved, or simultaneously in the hands and feet. Deep tendon reflexes were preserved, and there were no major sensory abnormalities. The progression was slow, and proximal weakness tended to be rare. Inheritance appeared to be autosomal dominant. The cases reported since then have been more heterogenous. Some patients have reported onset in childhood.[31] Markesberry et al.[32,33] have reported onset in a family with a similar clinical picture but for the early onset of weakness in the feet and progression to hand involvement. Age of onset in the patients was 46 to 51 years. The progression was also slow, but proximal weakness was more common. Cardiomyopathy was reported in one of his patients. Welander[34] has suggested that cases with an earlier, more severe, and generalized onset may represent the homozygous form.

Electromyograms (EMGs) have been reported to show low amplitude, brief duration motor unit potentials with polyphasic forms. Muscle biopsy showed variability in fiber size with necrosis, fibrosis, and internal nuclei. Vacuolar changes that appeared to be autophagic vacuoles have been reported in the Swedish cases and were common in the patients of Markesberry et al. Edstrom[35] noted early type I fiber atrophy.

The differential diagnosis includes differentiation from myotonic dystrophy, Charcot-Marie-Tooth disease, and the distal form of spinal muscular atrophy. Myotonic dystrophy may be distinguished by the presence of focal, neck, or sternocleidomastoid weakness or ptosis. Charcot-Marie-Tooth disease may be difficult to distinguish strictly on clinical grounds. In distal myopathy there is no evidence of sensory involvement or significant denervation in muscle biopsy, and nerve conduction velocities are normal. However, the neuronal form of Charcot-Marie-Tooth disease may also have normal nerve conductions, although the muscle biopsy reveals signs of denervation. Spinal muscular atrophy and motor neuron disease may appear with distal weakness. Again, muscle biopsy should allow differentiation.[33,35,36] Local nerve and cord disease may also be a possibility if sensory findings are not prominent.

Distal myopathy has a slow progression, particularly in familial cases, and is not generally disabling. No specific treatment is available. Bracing may occasionally be required.

Oculopharyngeal dystrophy

Oculopharyngeal dystrophy is a relatively rare myopathy accompanied by progressive ophthalmoplegia, ptosis, and dysphagia in middle to late life. The disease has an autosomal dominant inheritance and seems to cluster in some geographic areas. The largest documented group is found in families of French-Canadian background. Barbeau[37] traced these cases to a common French ancestor who arrived in Canada in the 1630s. A similar clustering has been described in Spanish-American families in the western United States.[14]

The onset of weakness may be as early as the third or fourth decades, but onset in the sixties is not unusual. Ptosis is usually the first symptom and may be asymmetric at first but eventually produces severe bilateral ptosis with limitation of extraocular movements in all directions; pupillary reflexes are spared. Dysphagia usually follows, although in some patients it may occur simultaneously or even precede ocular weakness. Facial weakness is usually present. In advanced cases proximal and generalized weakness may be noted. Dysphagia is the most disabling symptom and in severe cases may lead to considerable difficulties with eating, resulting in aspiration and emaciation. Progression is slow, and the disease is compatible with a normal life span. Most treatment is based on surgical procedures to control ptosis and lessen diplopia. In cases of oculopharyngeal dystrophy with severe dysphagia, cricopharyngeal myotomy has been reported to be helpful.[38] Some patients may require feeding by nasogastric tube or a surgical procedure such as a gastrostomy.

EMGs show small amplitude polyphasic potentials of short duration without any findings of denervation. Creatinine phosphokinase (CPK) levels can be elevated, but usually only mildly so, or may be normal. Muscle biopsy shows no pathognomonic findings but is notable for accelerated senescent changes. Rebeiz et al.[39] reported fibrosis, loss of myofibrils, sarcoplasmic masses, lipofucsin accumulation, and ring fibers. All these changes are present in aged muscle but at an earlier age than expected in these patients. Both clinically involved muscles and apparently uninvolved muscles were abnormal on biopsy. Studies of pharyngeal muscle have shown similar involvement of the striated muscle in the pharynx.[40] While esophageal manometry has suggested dysfunction of the lower esophagus, implicating a smooth muscle disturbance, no pathologic abnormality of smooth muscle has been found.

Dubowitz and Brooke[14] noted variability in fiber size with many small angulated fibers but no type grouping. A notable change in their biopsies was the presence of autophagic vacuoles in many fibers, appearing as punched out areas surrounded by filaments when stained red on the trichrome stain. Usually these vacuoles were seen within type I fibers. They also noted ringed, "moth-eaten," and whorled fibers. At least one report of transient marked inflammatory changes on muscle biopsy has been made.[41]

Differential diagnosis is not difficult with a good family history and typical presentation. Otherwise differentiation is needed from diseases producing ophthalmoplegia and dysphagia.

Myasthenia gravis (MG) may be limited to involvement of the ocular and pharyngeal musculature. However, lack of fluctuation of symptoms, failure to respond to cholinergic drugs, and the absence of a decremental response to repetitive stimulation should point away from myasthenia.

Ocular myopathy may be a variant of oculopharyngeal dystrophy. The onset is reportedly earlier in the second or third decade. Inheritance is not as clear; approximately 50% of the cases are sporadic, and the rest are reported to have both recessive and dominant inheritance patterns.[42] Face and limb muscles are also involved, although the disease is slowly progressive.

Oculocraniosomatic muscular disease can be accompanied by ophthalmoplegia and pharyngeal weakness, but onset is much earlier, often by age 20, and the associated changes, including pigmentary changes in the retina, cardioconduction defects, endocrine disturbances, and increased cerebral spinal fluid (CSF) protein, should allow differentiation. The biopsy is also distinctive, with many ragged, red muscle fibers containing abnormal lipid droplets and mitochondria and paracrystalline inclusions.

Myotonic dystrophy may have associated ptosis and mild dysphagia. The onset of symptoms in myotonic dystrophy should be earlier, and myotonia, demonstrated either clinically or on an EMG, is frequently present. Muscle biopsy can also be of assistance in these cases if doubt remains.

Endocrine myopathies

Endocrine myopathies are frequently included in the differential diagnosis of weakness and myalgias in the older patient. Endocrine dysfunctions that are associated with myopathy include thyroid, parathyroid, and both glucocorticoid and mineralocorticoid production.

Hypothyroidism is not an unusual condition in older patients and may be missed, particularly mild to moderate cases.[43,44] Muscular manifestations include development of myalgias and weakness. Proximal muscles of the pelvic and shoulder girdles are predominantly affected, although the weakness is rarely severe. In more advanced cases painful muscle cramps and stiffness may appear, precipitated by prolonged rest or exercise and made somewhat worse by cold weather.[45] Percussion of the muscle may elicit myoedema, producing a painless palpable mound that may persist for as long as a minute. Pseudohypertrophy may be present and can be localized or affect several muscle groups. Disturbances of the tendon jerk may be seen and consist of a prolongation of the total reflex time. Both contraction and relaxation are delayed, although the phenomenon is usually described as a prolongation of relaxation. Approximately 30% to 40% of hypothyroid patients have weakness, about three fourths have cramps, pain, and stiffness, and approximately one fourth have myotonia-like features.[46-49] EMG findings include decreased action potentials and polyphasia. Irregular high voltage potentials on electrode insertion occur in many patients, and tapping the muscle or tendon may produce repetitive trains of potentials in up to one third of patients.[46] The CPK level is elevated in almost all patients. The elevation can be substantial—up to 10 times normal.[50]

Muscle biopsy is neither consistent nor diagnostic. There may be variability of fiber size and increased central nuclei. Both type I and type II atrophy have been described.[14,51,52] The differential diagnosis involves ruling out other illnesses with muscle pains, cramps, and proximal weakness. In the elderly these include polymyositis, polymyalgia rheumatica, motor neuron disease, and other endocrine myopathies.[53] Thyroid function tests, including assays of thyroid-stimulating hormone (TSH), are preferred diagnostic tests. Treatment of thyroid deficiency reverses the signs and symptoms of hypothyroidism, including muscle manifestations.

Hyperthyroidism frequently produces weakness. As in hypothyroidism, proximal muscles are predominantly involved, particularly the shoulder girdle musculature. Unlike hypothyroidism, weakness may be severe. Winging of the scapula and wasting of the shoulder girdle may be seen. Patients complain of difficulty in combing their hair or raising their arms above their heads as well as trouble getting up from low chairs. In severe hyperthyroidism, distal and bulbar weakness may appear with ptosis, dysphagia, dysarthria, and even involvement of the respiratory muscles. Tendon reflexes are brisk and upper motor neuron (UMN) signs such as extensor plantar reflexes are seen rarely. Fasciculations and fine tremor are common.[54,55]

The CPK level may be normal in hyperthyroid myopathy and does not correlate well with the severity of the illness. EMGs demonstrate a shortening of the action potential and an increase in polyphasic activity. Muscle biopsy is nonspecific in both type I and type II atrophy.[14,46]

The diagnosis in cases where the usual signs of hyperthyroidism are present is not difficult. In elderly patients with masked or "apathetic" hyperthyroidism, the only manifestations may be weakness and cachexia. Motor neuron disease, carcinomatous neuromyopathy, or polymyositis may be considered in these patients.[56] Again, thyroid function tests and evaluation of both T_3 and T_4 should point to the diagnosis. Treatment of hyperthyroidism reverses all the muscle symptoms.[47]

Only some muscular conditions associated with thyroid disease will be mentioned. These include thyrotoxic periodic paralysis, which is seen in younger patients, usually in men who frequently have Oriental backgrounds. There is an association of hyperthyroidism with myasthenia.[46] This association appears to be indicative of the underlying immunologic dysfunction in both illnesses rather than a cause and effect. Both hypothyroidism and hyperthyroidism may aggravate MG. Manifestations of Grave's disease may include endocrine exophthalmos with ophthalmoplegia and proptosis. Increased thyroid hormone is not necessary for this manifestation as it may persist or worsen after treatment of hyperthyroidism.

Hyperparathyroidism, either primary from parathyroid adenoma or hyperplasia or secondary from prolonged hypocalcemic stimulation, may produce muscular symptoms. Early fatigability is an early complaint. Muscle pain and cramps are frequently present and can be severe enough to disturb function. Gait has been described as stiff, slow, and cautious. Weakness is usually mild and affects the proximal musculature with the lower extremities predominantly involved. In severe cases fasciculation of the tongue and bulbar weakness may be present. Deep tendon reflexes are usually brisk.[57,58]

The CPK level is usually normal. There appears to be no correlation between the serum or CSF calcium level, magnesium or phosphorus level, and the degree of myopathy.[59] The EMG shows short duration, low amplitude polyphasic potentials and decreased interference pattern. Muscle biopsy findings are equivocal and may include some type II fiber atrophy. Many biopsies are normal.

The differential diagnosis is one of ruling out other illnesses with muscle pain, cramps, and weakness. Polymyositis, polymyalgia rheumatica, and other endocrine myopathies must be ruled out. In severe cases with bulbar involvement and fasciculations, motor neuron disease may be considered. Calcium and phosphorus levels as well as parathyroid hormone (PTH) assays should suggest the diagnosis. Rarely muscle biopsy may be required to rule out other diagnoses.

Treatment of hyperparathyroidism reverses the manifestations of the illness.[57]

Hypoparathyroidism does not produce myopathy; however, with low calcium levels tetany can occur. Weakness, cramps, numbness of the hands and feet are common and, spontaneously or with hyperventilation, may progress to carpopedal spasm. Tetany may be severe, sudden, and lead to falls. Tetanic spasm of the respiratory and laryngeal muscles may cause respiratory insufficiency and death.

The CPK level may be mildly elevated. The EMG is either normal or may show spontaneous bursts and "doublets" or trains of motor unit potentials. The muscle biopsy is nonspecific. Serum calcium assays and the characteristic tetany with hyperventilation should allow diagnosis.[47]

Addison's disease or hypoadrenalism frequently produces weakness. However, weakness appears to be secondary to electrolyte disturbance and can be rapidly corrected with management of electrolyte levels. Primary hyperaldosteronism can produce periodic attacks of weakness that may last for hours to days. During an attack there is usually severe hypokalemia, alkalosis, hypernatremia, and hypertension.[60]

Glucocorticoid excess, whether the result of increased production or secondary to exogenous steroids, can produce muscular weakness, beginning from 3 to 20 months. The weakness is typically proximal and may be mild to moderate. The CPK level is usually mildly elevated to normal. EMG changes are nonspecific. Muscle biopsy shows selective type II atrophy in both Cushing's syndrome and steroid treated patients.[61] This change is nonspecific and may be seen with age or disuse. The differential diagnosis is made by the other associated findings of Cushing's syndrome and elevated cortisol levels. A more complicated problem is met when steroids are being administered to treat a disease in which muscular weakness is a manifestation, e.g., polymyositis. Serial urinary creatine excretion determination may be of value in differentiating the two conditions, although it is technically difficult to perform.[62] Using steroids with a shorter half-life, reducing the total dose, or every other day therapy may be helpful in reducing the severity of steroid myopathy when steroid administration cannot be stopped completely.

MOTOR NEURON DISEASE

Amyotrophic lateral sclerosis (ALS) is an illness in which motor neurons degenerate. The loss of lower motor neurons leads to atrophy of musculature, loss of the upper motor neurons, spasticity, and hyperreflexia. The most common form is sporadic and involves both upper and lower motor neuron disease. Its frequency in most series is in the range of 1 to 2 per 100,000, although some foci of increased incidence exist. Familial cases, sometimes with an autosomal dominant inheritance, may make up to 6% of the total. In the sporadic form the median age of incidence is in the late fifties and early sixties, but cases from the teens to the ninth decade can be seen.

Typically the disease is devastating. The course from first manifestation to death is about 3 years. Many patients do live longer, and reports of 20% 5-year survivals have been made.[63] Rosen[64] reported 40% to 60% 5-year survivals from the ALS case registry, but diagnoses in that series were not confirmed. Most studies have shown a slightly higher percentage of men than women with a ratio of 1.5:1 being typical. This sex difference, however, appears to decrease to 1:1 when onset is after age 60 and has not been as striking in recent series.[64,65]

Early symptoms include a patchy, frequently asymmetric onset of weakness, usually noted distally. The hands may become clumsy and stiff, and the patient notes difficulty in performing fine motor tasks. Increased tripping and falling may indicate early lower extremity distal weakness. Fasciculations may be noted early, although not usually before weakness is evident, and may disturb the patient at night. More bothersome and common as an early symptom are cramps, which frequently affect the muscles of the calf and thigh and can be painful and prolonged. Cramps frequently improve as the disease progresses. Spasticity and hyperreflexia usually occur at the same time as mucular weakness and may contribute to the loss of fine movement. Hyperreflexia may be severe enough to produce sustained clonus at the ankles, disturbing the patient's attempts to walk.

Bulbar weakness may lead to difficulty in speaking and swallowing and can be an early or dominant manifestation. The speech of a patient with ALS has features of both upper and lower motor neuron disease and is characteristically slow, forced, and monotonous in quality. With progression of the disease, swallowing can become increasingly difficult. At first, patients may report that food tends to "stick" in the pharynx; later, fluids become a problem, and saliva pools in the pharynx. Aspiration and poor nutrition result. Occasionally loss of upper motor neuron function may give rise to a pseudobulbar state with involuntary, inappropriate laughter and crying.

Sensory involvement is not primarily seen, although pressure palsies of peripheral nerves can be seen in bedridden patients. The extraocular muscles are not affected, and the presence of a gaze palsy may point to another diagnosis. Autonomic function is not affected, and bladder, bowel, and sexual dysfunction are not usually seen. In the common form, regardless of the initial manifestations, the disease will spread to almost all the skeletal muscles. Confinement to a wheelchair frequently occurs within 12 to 18 months. Death is usually caused by respiratory failure or pneumonia.[66,67]

Some variant clinical forms have been described. Progressive spinal muscular atrophy affects the spinal motor neuron with atrophy of the skeletal musculature. Bulbar weakness or signs of upper motor neuron dysfunction are not seen. The course is more benign that the classical form, and reports of survival for more than 10 years are common.[67]

Predominant involvement of the upper motor neuron is seen in primary lateral sclerosis. The initial manifestation in this form is the development of a slow, progressive, spastic paralysis of the legs that ascends to involve the trunk, arms, and, late in the course, bulbar musculature. Bowel, bladder, and sensory function are not affected. Prognosis for long survival is reportedly good.[67]

In progressive bulbar palsy, initial or more severe bulbar involvement is present. Prognosis is worse, with a median survival of 2 years and a 5-year survival rate of less than 20%.[64,67]

Focal motor neuron disease is a poorly characterized entity. Only one area of the body or muscle group is involved, with the shoulder girdle most frequently affected. The illness begins insidiously with fasciculations and wasting, progresses for a few months, and then may stabilize. Local nerve and cord disease must be ruled out in this form.[68-70]

The form of ALS seen in the high incidence areas of Guam, the Mariana islands, and Borneo appears to be identical to idiopathic ALS, although the age of onset may be somewhat earlier, and there may be some minor pathologic differences.[71] Pure forms of the previously mentioned variants are rare, and most researchers prefer to classify them under the general term ALS.

Hereditary ALS makes up approximately 6% of total cases. Inheritance sometimes appears to be autosomal dominant, although families may have recessive inheritance. Horton et al.[72] have divided reported cases into three varieties depending on course and mode of onset. However, there is considerable variability in the disease both within and between families.[73]

Laboratory studies are helpful in diagnosing the disease. The EMG shows widespread fibrillations, giant polyphasic potentials, and fasciculations. Nerve conduction velocities are usually normal. Muscle biopsy demonstrates changes characteristic of denervation with grouped atrophy and many small angulated fibers. Fiber type grouping sometimes reflects sprouting of axons and reinnervation of denervated muscle fibers. Much type grouping suggests a more chronic and more benign process. EMG and muscle biopsy changes are only diagnostic of ALS when widespread. Therefore when an arm is clinically symptomatic, a biopsy demonstrating denervation in the quadriceps will be of greater value in confirming the diagnosis than one with similar changes in the affected area.

Mild elevation of the CPK level, up to two to three times normal, is not uncommon. CSF studies are usually normal, although the protein level may be mildly elevated. Frequently seen glucose tolerance test (GTT) abnormalities probably represent reduced muscle mass.[74] HLA antigen typing studies have suggested increased representation of HLA-A3, HLA-BW-35, or HLA-B12 antigens although not consistently enough to help in the diagnosis.[75,76]

Differential diagnosis requires ruling out

treatable illnesses. Cervical cord lesions, particularly in elderly patients with degenerative diseases of the spine, can provide difficulties. These patients may have fasciculations and atrophy in the upper extremities and upper motor neuron signs in the lower extremities. Rarely may fasciculations be present in both upper and lower extremities with cervical cord lesions.[77] Other high cord lesions such as foramen magnum meningiomas, syringomyelia, and neurofibromas may be accompanied by symptoms suggestive of ALS and minimal sensory findings.

Because of diagnostic difficulty many physicians perform myelography to rule out mass lesions of the spinal cord when no evidence of involvement above the foramen magnum can be found. With the advent of the metrizamide cisternography with a CT scan, examination of the brain stem is being performed to rule out pathologic conditions of the brain stem in unusual cases.

Heavy metal intoxication has been reported to mimic idiopathic ALS. Lead,[78] mercury,[79] and selenium[80] intoxication have been implicated. Because of these rare cases many clinicians routinely perform 24-hour urine assays for heavy metal toxicity. Bone biopsy has been recommended for cases with suggestive histories.[81]

Some endocrinopathies may produce symptoms resembling motor neuron disease. Hyperparathyroidism may produce easy fatigability, muscle cramps, pain, and mild proximal weakness. In severe cases there may be bulbar involvement and tongue fasciculations. Serum calcium and PTH levels are elevated in most cases.[57,58] Hyperthyroidism may produce weakness, weight loss, fasciculations, and, rarely, corticospinal findings. The diagnosis is frequently more difficult in an elderly patient.[56] T_3 and T_4 will be elevated.

Chronic benign fasciculations and the "fasciculation with muscular pain" syndrome may be difficult to differentiate from early ALS. The course is nonprogressive, and weakness is not detected in the initial examination, unlike ALS in which weakness can be noted when fasciculations are present.[82-84]

Some heredito-familial disorders may be a source of confusion, particularly if the family history is not clear. These include the following: neuronal Charcot-Marie-Tooth disease in which the nerve conduction velocities are normal[85]; bulbospinal amyotrophy, which produces slowly progressive proximal limb muscle weakness with fasciculations in adults and has a much better prognosis[86]; and hereditary proximal neurogenic atrophy in adults.[87]

The cause of ALS is not known. The selective loss of motor neurons in the spinal cord, medulla, and cortex has stimulated a search for metabolic or structural characteristics that could explain their vulnerability. While some biochemical differences are present in motor neuron disease, none have been found to be related to the disease. No specific trophic factor has been found for motor neurons analogous to nerve growth factor for autonomic system neurons. While some features of the disease are mimicked by endocrine disturbances, these are not seen in most patients with ALS. Some abnormalities in calcium metabolism have been described, and patients with ALS appear to have more bone fractures than the general population, although the relationship to the development of ALS is not clear.[88,89] Speculations of a defect in androgen receptor function have been made but are not confirmed.[90]

Similarities between heavy metal toxicity and idiopathic ALS have led to examination of heavy metals or other toxins as causes of ALS. Lead exposure has been reported to be a frequent antecedent factor to ALS, and reports of elevated lead and manganese levels in the spinal cord tissue of patients with ALS have appeared.[91,92] However, no consistent pattern is yet evident.[93]

Slow virus infections are an intriguing possibility as a cause of ALS. The polio virus in humans is an example of a virus with an affinity for human anterior horn cells. Some studies have shown an increased incidence of a history of paralytic polio in patients who develop ALS.[94] Also a subgroup of patients with poliomyelitis can develop delayed slow progression of weakness with atrophy but few corticospinal signs and a more benign prognosis.[95,96] Kott et al.[97] have reported that a majority of patients with ALS have evidence of cell mediated immunity to polio virus, although their conclusions have been questioned.[98] However, no other evidence of slow virus infection by polio virus have been found. Polio virus titers are not elevated in ALS.[99] No transmission of virus from tissues of patients with ALS has been possible.[100,101] Cell fusion and nucleic acid hybridization studies have not revealed any latent virus infection.[102,103]

Other viruses may be implicated. An animal model has been reported in which a transmissible C-type murine retrovirus causes motor neuron disease in aging populations of wild mice.[104,105] Virus-like particles have been reported in the tissues of ALS patients, although their significance is unknown.[106]

Immunologic participation in the pathogenesis of ALS has been investigated. No abnormalities in serum complement or immunoglobulin levels are present. No consistent toxic components in serum or cell mediated immunities have been reported.[93] Oldstone et al.[107] reported immune complex formation in patients with rapidly progressive ALS, although the antigen was not determined. Histocompatibility studies have suggested increased representation of HLA-A3 and HLA-BW-35.[75,97]

Several other antecedent factors to ALS have been reported and are as diverse as excessive milk ingestion, athletic activity,[91] injuries,[108] and gastrectomy; while interesting, their relevance is not known.

Multiple therapeutic trials have been performed on ALS patients, none with reproducible documented improvement.[109] Recent negative trials include treatment with snake venom,[110,111] plasma exchange,[112] and transfer factor.[113]

At present treatment should be aimed at making the patient more comfortable and at palliating symptoms. Supportive psychologic and social care of the patient and family can be helpful. Mechanical devices such as braces, walkers, wheelchairs, raised toilet seats, or other orthotic devices may improve activities of daily living and warrant repeated rehabilitative evaluation as the disease progresses.[114] In patients with bulbar involvement, use of suction machines to relieve pooling of saliva in the pharynx may be helpful. Switching to a semisolid pureed diet may aid swallowing. Cricopharyngeal myotomy may be of help when cricopharyngeal spasm can be demonstrated and sometimes when it cannot. Meperidine, in low doses before eating, has been reported to help swallowing in some patients.[81] Cramps may be lessened by quinine, 180 to 300 mg per day. Rarely use of antispasticity agents such as diazepam or baclofen may be helpful.[115]

Respiratory insufficiency may produce hypoxemia, particularly at night, and may be alleviated by oxygen administration. Aspiration may lead to frequent episodes of pneumonia, which may require treatment.[116] As techniques for wheelchair life-support systems become more advanced, patients in whom respiratory failure has occurred may be managed with such a system over a long period of time. This approach presents many practical, philosophical, and ethical problems but may be increasingly used in the future.

INFLAMMATORY MYOPATHIES

Inflammatory myopathies continue to be a confusing area in the study of muscle disease. Bacterial and parasitic inflammatory diseases of muscle are common worldwide but are rarely seen in developed countries. If these are excluded, one is left with a variety of entities characterized by either clinical, laboratory, or, more controversially, therapeutic evidence of inflammation. Polymyositis dermatomyositis (PM-DM), although rare, remains one of the most common forms of acquired proximal weakness in adults, but the heterogeneity of the illness has complicated its study; today the cause, natural history, and treatment remain in question.

A useful classification suggested by Pearson and Bohan[117] subdivided polymyositis and its variants as follows:

Type I—polymyositis in adults	34%
Type II—typical dermatomyositis	29%
Type III—inflammatory myopathy associated with malignancy	8.5%
Type IV—childhood PM-DM	7%
Type V—myositis associated with collagen vascular disease	21%

Type I is the most common form. Typically it affects females in the third through the fifth decades. Type II has similar muscular manifestations and is accompanied by a characteristic skin rash of the face, neck, shoulders, and knuckles. Onset is from the second to seventh decade and is more common in women. Type III is separated by virtue of its association with neoplasia and may be accompanied by a rash or only by muscular manifestations. Neoplasia, in association with PM-DM, occurs with a frequency of 8% to 20%. It is not usually seen with the childhood form or that associated with collagen vascular disease. Childhood polymyositis is separated out because of the increasing frequency of vasculitic changes. Type V is frequently associated with Raynaud's phenomenon and sclerodermatous skin changes reminiscent of progressive systemic sclerosis or mixed connective tissue disease. Cases meeting criteria for systemic lupus erythematosus (SLE), rheumatoid arthritis (RA), or periarteritis nodosa are also seen.

Major evidence of motor neuron disease; evidence of a genetic or metabolic dystrophy; evidence of granulomatous changes such as may be seen with sarcoid or infection; use of drugs that may cause myopathies such as alcohol, endocrine myopathies, and myasthenia gravis would cast doubt on the diagnosis.[118]

The incidence of PM-DM is not really known but lies somewhere between five to ten patients per million. Any age may be affected, but most patients are in their fifth and sixth decades. Overall, females are affected twice as often as males. Typically the disease begins with a variety of systemic symptoms such as fever and malaise. Weakness may be acute and progress within days; more commonly, weakness comes on over a period of weeks. The distribution of weakness is proximal, and patients complain of difficulty in arising from a chair, climbing stairs, and lifting objects above their head. The anterior neck muscles are frequently affected. Facial weakness, while present occasionally, is rare. Dysphagia is a common feature and is caused by weakness of the striated posterior pharyngeal musculature. Dysphagia may be severe enough to make eating difficult, and the patient may require supplementation through a nasogastric tube. In more severe disease, weakness may involve any striated muscle of the body, and the patient may be bedridden or confined to a wheelchair.

The rash, if present, may occur before, after, or simultaneously with weakness and is seen in approximately 35% of patients.[117] The typical rash consists of dusky erythematous eruption on the face, frequently in a butterfly distribution. The eyelids may become discolored and assume a purple or lavender color. Edema may cause puffiness around the eys. An erythematous rash on the chest and neck is frequently seen, particularly in areas exposed to sunlight. The associated telangiectasia gives the rash an appearance reminiscent of that associated with irradiation. The skin over the elbows and knees may become thick and scaly; occasionally, nodules form, which may become necrotic. On the hands there are areas of erythema and thickening over the knuckles and interphalangeal joints. There is frequent erythema and scaling around the fingernails and finger pads. In severe cases, the rash may be diffuse, covering the whole body and producing severe atrophy and fragility of the skin. Such severe involvement is rare in adult dermatomyositis.[117]

While muscle pain is frequently thought to be a part of polymyositis, it is seen in only 25% to 40% of patients, and up to one third may have no symptoms of muscle pain whatsoever. Therefore its absence is no bar to the diagnosis of polymyositis, and most patients having aches and pain may have another diagnosis. When pain is present, it is described as a deep aching under the muscle, worsened by activity and improved by rest. The muscles may be swollen and tender to palpation. Raynaud's phenomenon may be seen in up to 20% of all patients and in up to 47% of patients with associated collagen vascular disease. Arthralgias are seen in all forms although again much more commonly in myositis associated with collagen vascular disease. Visceral involvement has been described. This may include interstitial fibrosis of the lung and intestinal manifestations, including hypomobility of the esophagus and small intestine similar to that seen in scleroderma. Cardiomyopathy and nonspecific rhythm abnormalities are occasionally seen.

The association of malignancy with PM-DM was described early, although the actual incidence is difficult to determine. Bohan et al.[119] noted in a series of 153 patients that 8.5% had an associated malignancy. DeVere and Bradley,[120] from a series of 118 patients, obtained a figure of 7.7%, two thirds of which were patients with dermatomyositis. When subgroups are examined, the incidence may be higher. If patients with PM-DM over the age of 50 are examined, the frequency of malignancy is 18% to 19%, with equal occurrence in men and women. While not strictly comparable, the incidence of malignancies in the series of Bohan et al. for all patients over 50 years was 19.2%. These figures can be contrasted with an estimated associated frequency of malignancy of 3.7% in patients with SLE and 0.59% in patients with RA.[121] The incidence of malignancy in children, in young patients, or in those in which the disease is associated with collagen vascular disease is much lower. The reverse figure, that is the number of patients with malignancy who develop PM-DM, is considerably lower. While no specific data is available, probably no more than 5% of patients with carcinoma develop any unexplained neuromuscular illness, and the percentage developing PM-DM is considerably smaller.[122]

PM-DM may be present in up to 60% of patients before the associated malignancy is diagnosed. However, extensive screening for malignancy has not proved helpful in most cases. Most health care workers would reserve simple screening (chest x-ray examination, stool guaiac test, urinalysis) to high risk groups with repeated evaluations at regular intervals. No specific neoplasms seem predisposed to association with PM-DM; the most common neoplasms were breast, lung, stomach, and gastrointestinal (GI) tract carcinomas, which are also most common in the general population.

The prognosis has also been difficult to establish. Estimates for PM-DM in adults have a rather wide range. In cases of polymyositis in which diagnosis required inflammatory changes in muscle biopsy to be present, Riddoch and Morgan-Hughs[123] found a mortality of 40%. DeVere and Bradley[120] found a mortality of 28% in a group of 118 patients, approximately four times higher than in an age-matched population. Polymyositis directly accounted for only 14% of all deaths in their series, carcinoma approximately 18%, and most of the rest were the result of coronary artery disease. The mortality in young patients was much less. In this same series the disability tended to stabilize after a few years, and the disease became "burned-out." Of the survivors, 66% had no functional disability after 3 or more years. The remainder were left with significant disability. In approximately 15%, the disease appeared to remain active.

There are multiple laboratory abnormalities described with PM-DM. Unfortunately, few are consistently abnormal, and none give good predictive information about the prognosis or activity of the disease. The CPK level is usually elevated in the serum as are the transaminases, particularly in the acute or subacute stages of the disease. In clinically inactive cases or in those in remission, the values are frequently normal. However, at any given time, regardless of the apparent course, the muscle enzymes may be normal. Up to 10% of all cases may have normal enzymes, even when other diagnostic criteria of myositis are present.[117] The erythrocyte sedimentation rate is frequently elevated in active disease but in a nonspecific and nonprognostic manner.[120] EMG abnormalities include short, low amplitude, polyphasic potentials and signs of muscle irritability, including bizarre repetitive discharges, fibrillations, and positive denervation potentials. Changes in the muscle biopsy have included variability in fiber size, focal or extensive degeneration of muscle fibers with necrosis, evidence of regeneration with prominent large fascicular nuclei, interstitial infiltrates of inflammatory cells, interstitial fibrosis, and perifascicular atrophy. While the degree of inflammation appears to correlate roughly with activity, approximately 75% of biopsies show inflammatory changes, implying that up to 25% do not, making inflammatory changes a helpful but not necessary change for diagnosis.[14,119]

Treatment of polymyositis with either steroids or immunosuppressants will reduce the inflammatory component but will not reduce the degree of necrosis and degeneration. A recent paper noted that the degree of type II atrophy decreased in patients that responded to treatment, while it increased in nonresponders. They suggested that a muscle biopsy showing increased type II atrophy without inflammation in a treated patient that was still weak would favor corticosteroid myopathy rather than further progression of the disease.[124] Other nonspecific abnormalities are seen. The antinuclear antibody factor (ANA) is positive in about 35% of all patients, although in only 2% when only patients with pure PM-DM are examined. Rheumatoid factor was elevated in approximately 20%. Approximately 40% have abnormal complement levels.[119]

The differential diagnosis is one of proximal muscle weakness appearing in adults. Important illnesses to exclude include the following: (1) late onset genetic dystrophies in adults. Although rare, this will be a problem in elderly patients. Both facioscapulohumeral dystrophy and limb girdle dystrophy may have late exacerbations and appear with "new" weakness in middle age. The medical history and muscle biopsy may be helpful in making this diagnosis. (2) Motor neuron disease may be accompanied by proximal weakness. (3) Granulomatous disease such as sarcoidosis or infections such as trichinosis, schistosomiasis, toxoplasmosis, or trypanosomiasis. (4) Use of toxins that may cause rhabdomyolysis or muscle inflammation. Paramount among these is alcohol. Alcohol induced rhabdomyolysis may present a similar picture to polymyositis; and biopsy appearance may also be similar. Other toxins to be considered include clofibrate, penicillamine, and aminoepsilon caproic acid. (5) Metabolic muscle disease such as McArdle's disease or carnitine deficiency. (6) Endocrine disorders including thyrotoxicosis, myxedema, hyperthyroidism and hypoparathyroidism, diabetic amyotrophy or neuropathies, or steroid myopathy.[118]

The cause is unknown but much evidence suggests that polymyositis is an autoimmune disease. An experimental model has been produced by injection of muscle extracts with complete Freund's adjuvant, the myofibrillar fraction producing more severe involvement.[125] The relationship of polymyositis to other autoallergic disorders has strengthened this belief. Both cellular and humoral immunity to muscle antigens has been reported.[126] In childhood PM-DM vasculitis has been reported, and complement abnormalities suggestive of antigen antibody complex formation have been seen in both childhood and adult polymyositis.[127,128] HLA studies have shown association with HLA-B8 in a substantial percentage of cases.[129]

Steroids and immunosuppressants have been the mainstay of therapy in PM-DM. However, no control studies are available to substantiate their effectiveness. Several recent studies reported improvement in serum enzymes and strength in patients treated with steroids.[119,120]

If steroids are to be used, they should not be used too late, nor in doses that are too small, nor should therapy be stopped too early. Appropriate dosage should initially be between 50 to 100 mg of prednisone daily and should be maintained for a trial of 2 to 4 months before steroid resistance is diagnosed. If response occurs, therapy should be slowly tapered or the treatment may be changed to every other day therapy. Complications have been relatively mild in most series. DeVere and Bradley[120] attributed 4% of the deaths in their cases to complications of steroids. Cataracts may be seen in up to 30% of patients in long-term steroid therapy.[130]

Immunosuppressants have been reported to work by themselves or as additives to steroids. Immunosuppressants used have included methotrexate, azathioprine, and cyclophosphamide. Again, no control studies are available on immunosuppressants alone. A recent study comparing prednisone treated patients to a prednisone and azathioprine treated group for the initial treatment of polymyositis showed no significant advantage to the group treated with both steroids and azathioprine. Both groups showed equivalent improvements.[131]

MYASTHENIA GRAVIS

More is known about the pathophysiology of MG than any of the other muscle diseases discussed in this chapter. The treatment of MG is also effective in reducing the severity of the disease and may even assist in the development of remissions. Clinically, MG is characterized by abnormal susceptibility of a patient's muscle to fatigue. The illness may occur at any age, although there are two periods of peak onset. One peak is in the third decade and the other is in the fifth and sixth decades. Most patients in the first group are women, those in the second group are mostly men,[132,133] although women develop the disease more often than men with a ratio of 3:2. Most cases are sporadic, although a familial tendency is seen in 2% to 5% of cases.[134,135]

Symptoms begin with weakness in one of three groups of muscles: the eyes, the bulbar musculature, or the limbs. In approximately one half of the patients the eyes are initially involved; in one third bulbar weakness is the initial symptom with trouble chewing, talking, or swallowing; and in about one fifth the predominant early symptom is generalized weakness of the limbs.

Ptosis is frequently an early sign and may be variable and asymmetric. Severity may vary from barely perceptible to severe and is often worse in the evening. The pupillary muscles are not affected but the external ocular muscles are frequently involved, producing a range of symptoms from mild blurring to bizarre, variable paralysis of gaze.

The facial muscles are often weak, particularly in the lower part of the face. Weakness of the palate and tongue can make speech difficult to understand. The patient's speech may be distinct at the beginning of a conversation only to become hollow, echoing, and without consonants. Difficulty swallowing and chewing is common. Weakness of the muscles of the neck is seen, usually at the neck extensors so the head tends to flop forward.

Weakness of the limbs and trunk is marked mainly by early fatigability, although there does appear to be more proximal involvement. The respiratory muscles are often involved, and respiratory distress and failure are the most serious complications of the illness.

A form of MG that carries a better prognosis is ocular myasthenia in which only the eye muscles are affected. Only 11% of these patients progress to develop other weaknesses.

The course of myasthenia is frequently relapsing and remitting. Approximately one third of patients improve, and of these, one half will be asymptomatic. The other two thirds will be unchanged or worse. Fluctuations in the severity of the disease may occur unpredictably. However, infection, viral or bacterial, regularly produces a worsening of the weakness in myasthenia and may be the most frequent cause of sudden exacerbation. Overuse of anticholinesterase medication, by producing a cholinergic crisis, may also worsen weakness although not often seen clinically.[136] Other exacerbating factors include hypothyroidism or hyperthyroidism, electrolyte imbalances, and occasionally pregnancy. Drugs such as quinine, quinidine, procainamide, propranolol, neomycin, streptomycin, aminoglycoside antibiotics, and phenytoin may also worsen the weakness in myasthenia.

The diagnosis is suggested by clinical evidence of pathologic fatigability. A fatigable ptosis is demonstrated by asking the patient to sustain upward gaze. With time, the eyelids begin to show a slow drift downwards. Fatigability of the limbs can be demonstrated by having the patient sit with outstretched arms and measuring the duration of the effort. Once pathologic fatigue is demonstrated, the effect of edrophonium may be tried. This anticholinesterase drug has a rapid onset of action, and its effect is over within 5 to 10 minutes. After measuring the degree of fatigue, a test injection of 1 mg is given intravenously. If no untoward effect is seen, 10 mg is then injected. Occasionally a control injection of saline solution is necessary. Particularly in elderly patients with heart disease the drug may cause arrhythmias and should be tried in an inpatient setting or with caution for an outpatient.

Thymoma is seen in as many as 10% of the patients with MG. It is reported to be more common in male patients with late onset,[137] but other reports suggest that the peak age of incidence for a thymoma patient is between the two peaks for the nontumor cases; there is no correlation with sex.[133] Prognosis for patients with thymoma is worse than for those without this tumor.[138]

MG can be clinically subtle in mild cases, and the diagnosis may be difficult. Electrical testing may be useful in the diagnosis. Repetitive stimulation of the motor nerve in normal subjects at frequencies below 10 cycles per second produces little change in the evoked potential. In MG there is, under similar conditions, a decrement in the evoked potential of greater than 10%. Not all msucles may be affected; proximal muscles are more likely to be affected than distal. Exercise, warming the muscle, or ischemia of the muscle cell may enhance decremental response.[139]

Single fiber EMG studies in MG also show increase "jitter," or variability, in the time interval between the depolarization of muscle fibers in the same motor unit. Other electrical tests employed include stapedius muscle reflex fatigability.[139]

The curare provocative test is occasionally of help in making the diagnosis. It is based on the increased sensitivity of patients with MG to curare, a postsynaptic blocking agent. Typically, one tenth of the usual curarizing dose is given; it will produce no weakness in the normal patient but severe weakness in the myasthenic patient. Because of its risk, including respiratory paralysis, a variant of the test involving only one limb, the regional curare test, is more frequently used.[140]

Muscle biopsy is not diagnostic unless the end plate is investigated by electron microscopy or intravital staining. Lymphorrhages are occasionally seen.

In MG there is a disorder of neuromuscular transmission in which normal nerve impulses and acetylcholine release activate only a small proportion of muscle fibers, producing weakness.[141,142] Studies using alpha-bungarotoxin, a polypeptide from the venom of Bungaris multicinctus, which irreversibly binds with acetylcholine receptors, have shown that the sera from patients with MG inhibits binding of the venom to normal muscle. The factor inhibiting alpha-bungarotoxin binding was identified as an immunoglobulin.[143] Binding of antibodies to the acetylcholine receptors of muscle end plates has been demonstrated and has been associated with receptor loss apparently from increased turnover and receptor degradation.[144]

The cause of the autoimmunity is not known. Some cell mediated immunity with sensitized lymphocytes has also been identified. HLA system studies have shown overrepresentation of HLA-A1, HLA-B8, and HLA-DW3, suggesting a defect in immunoregulation.[145]

Treatment of MG entails choices between the major forms of therapy available. These include anticholinesterase drugs, immunosuppressants (predominantly steroids), thymectomy, and most recently plasmaphoresis.

Anticholinesterase therapy for myasthenia remains one of the major forms of treatment. The dramatic response of weakness to edrophonium and frequently to the oral medications, neostigmine and pyridostigmine, make them attractive to physicians and patients. Pyridostigmine is the most widely used form since it has fewer cholinergic side effects and a longer duration of action. The drug takes effect within 30 minutes and lasts 4 to 6 hours. The dose must be adjusted to response, ranging from 30 mg every 6 hours to many times this dose.

Problems with anticholinergic medication include variability of effect, even within one patient; the possibility of overdosage, resulting in increased weakness; and poor response for some symptoms, predominantly extraocular muscle weakness. There is also a growing suspicion that chronic treatment with anticholinesterase agents may adversely affect acetylcholine receptor function.[147]

Steroids have become an increasingly popular therapy, with reports of improvement in function in 60% to 100% of patients.[142] Usual therapy at this time includes high doses (50 to 100 mg) of prednisone daily with conversion, if tolerated by the patient, to every other day therapy. A problem with initiation of high dose steroid therapy is a period of weakening early in the course that in patients who are already weak may precipitate respiratory distress. This can be partially prevented by a slow increase in dosage at the cost of a slower rate of improvement. Other steroid side effects that may cause problems include infection, hypertension, diabetes, and cataracts and must be managed individually. Most patients require indefinite continuation of steroids.

Thymectomy, particularly in younger patients, has become standard therapy for MG. Several studies have shown increased improvement and remission in patients undergoing thymectomy over untreated patients.[147] The role of thymectomy combined with other therapies is still unsettled, as is the advantages of early thymectomy versus waiting for failure of other therapy.[136]

In older patients there is also debate about whether thymectomy produces any improvement in symptoms. Morbidity from surgery is higher at this age, and thymic tissue may be absent in surgery.[148] Accordingly, many clinicians would defer thymectomy in patients over 50 until other therapeutic efforts have proved ineffective.

Other immunosuppressants, predominantly azathioprine and cytoxan, have been used in MG with reports of equivalent or better response than steroids, but their side effects have limited use to steroid "failures."

Plasmaphoresis is the latest technique employed in MG. The theoretical basis is removing or reducing plasma antibody levels. Titers of antibody to the acetylcholine receptor are reduced with plasmaphoresis, and improvement in symptoms has been reported, although it is difficult to predict a response in a given patient.[136,149] Most patients who have undergone plasmaphoresis were also receiving steroids and other immunosuppressants. The high cost and need for venous access have limited use to severe and unresponsive patients.

MUSCLE DISEASE AS REMOTE EFFECT OF CANCER

Nonmetastatic neuromuscular involvement in patients with neoplasia occurs in less than 5% of all cancer patients. However, in the United States cancer only follows heart disease as a cause of death, producing a large enough group of potentially susceptible patients to merit consideration. These paraneoplastic syndromes broadly referred to as *carcinomatous neuromyopathy* may include amyotrophy, myositis, conduction defects (MG and myasthenic syndrome), neuropathies, and motor neuron disease.[122] Some tumors appear to have a predilection for types of effects—thymoma for MG, small cell carcinoma of the lung for myasthenic syndrome—although the mechanisms involved are not fully understood. It is difficult in patients who are sick and treated with complicated and frequently toxic therapy to separate direct effects of the tumor from indirect effects caused by debility, malnutrition, or the effects of therapy. This has made identification and evaluation of the frequency and course of the muscular paraneoplastic syndromes difficult at times.[150]

Neuropathy

Many patients with remote neoplasm effects do not have a strictly classifiable syndrome. Rather, they have proximal muscle weakness and wasting and loss of tendon jerks. Studies of these patients suggest a mixed neuropathic-myopathic involvement. Shy and Silverstein,[151] in a survey of 1500 patients with malignancy, found 3.5% to have proximal weakness and decreased reflexes. Approximately 69% of these patients had muscle biopsy and/or EMG abnormalities. Muscle biopsy revealed frequent inflammatory responses and degenerating and regenerating fibers. EMGs revealed a mixture of myopathic and neuropathic findings. In patients with pulmonary carcinoma Campbell and Paty,[152] found approximately 50% to have evidence of proximal weakness (not all symptomatic); Trojaborg et al.,[153] found subclinical evidence of polyneuropathy in approximately 33%; Terarainen and Larsen[154] found some evidence of polyneuropathy in approximately 48%. Engel and Askansas[150] noted prominent type II atrophy in patients with carcinoma, frequently before evidence of cachexia or malnutrition was present, and suggested that a large component of the weakness was caused by this type II fiber loss.[155] They also noted some neurogenic changes in approximately 50% of the biopsies. The cause of the type II fiber loss is not clear. Type II fibers decrease selectively as a result of disuse, aging, and several endocrine disturbances.[15] Possible mechanisms in paraneoplastic involvement include the following: (1) production of primary neurotoxic or myotoxic factors; (2) alteration of endocrine functions secondarily affecting muscle; (3) competition for specific nutrients or factors required for normal neuromuscular function; and (4) stimulation of host mechanisms generating secondary neurotoxic or myotoxic reactions.

Eaton-Lambert or myasthenic syndrome may be an example of the first mechanism. Cushing's disease with type II atrophy is an example of the second form. The third form is an intriguing possibility since muscle protein represents a large amount of the stored energy available to the human organism; however, increased nutritional support does not usually reverse the findings in neoplastic cachexia. As has been frequently pointed out, a pregnant woman bears a metabolic burden that exceeds the burden of most tumors at the time that they cause the patient's death yet in contrast she suffers relatively little from it. The implication again is that more than just usage or competition of metabolic energy is involved. MG or polymyositis may represent examples of the fourth possibility.

Polymyositis

PM-DM is discussed in an earlier section of this chapter. Myositis in association with cancer is seen in approximately 8.5% of all patients with myositis, although the frequency is considerably higher in the age group over 50 years.

Myasthenia gravis

MG can be considered a perineoplastic syndrome because approximately 15% of patients, particularly older males, have a thymoma that may be malignant.[137] The illness is discussed in an earlier section in this chapter.

Myasthenic syndrome

In the early 1950s it was noted that some patients with malignancies showed an abnormal sensitivity to muscle relaxants administered during surgery. Studies of these patients allowed identification of a group with a neuromuscular conduction defect characterized by a block in transmission in rested muscle with facilitation on repetitive stimulation.[156]

Myasthenic syndrome occurs more frequently in men than in women by a factor of 5:1 and is usually found in individuals over the age of 40. Over 50% of the patients have an associated small cell carcinoma and up to 70% have some sort of malignancy. The symptoms may occur several months before the malignancy becomes evident. Initial symptoms are usually a feeling of weakness and tiredness around the hip, making rising from a chair or climbing stairs difficult. The weakness differs from that in MG in that it is worse in the morning and improves as the day goes on. While exercise may transiently increase strength, prolonged exercise causes early fatigability. The weakness may also involve the muscles of the legs, shoulders, and arms but rarely the muscles of the head and neck. Mild difficulty in swallowing is noted in about a third of patients; visual blurring and ptosis are rare.

The clinical examination may show mild weakness or no weakness. Occasional repetitive muscle testing may show increased strength although not always a consistent finding. Frequently the patients appear clumsy in addition to being weak, and the degree of disability may exceed what would be expected from muscle testing.[157]

The EMG shows a characteristic response pattern to repetitive stimulation. The initial amplitude of the evoked response is small. With repetitive stimulation at rates of 3 hertz or less, there is a further decrease in the amplitude of the evoked potential. However, with stimulation at 10 to 15 hertz there is a facilitation of response, which may become normal. Single fiber EMGs demonstrate a block that worsens after rest. The miniature end plate potentials (MEPP) recorded in the muscle are normal, but the end plate potentials produced by an evoked response are decreased. The postsynaptic membrane appears to have normal sensitivity to acetylcholine. All this suggests that the packet size and the response of the postsynaptic membrane are normal but that the release of acetylcholine is defective.[158,159] Muscle biopsy shows nonspecific findings with some type II atrophy. Electromicroscope studies seem to show overdevelopment of the postsynaptic region.[160]

The cause of myasthenic syndrome is not known. However, extracts from small cell bronchogenic carcinomas have reproduced a neuromuscular transmission defect in animal nerve-muscle preparations suggesting that a product from the tumor is responsible.[161] Some cases that have improved with treatment of the tumor add substance to this possibility.

Once diagnosis of this syndrome has been made, the high degree of association with malignancy requires that a search for malignancy be done if one is not already clinically evident. Since the symptoms may appear before the malignancy is apparent, repetitive evaluations are required. However, some cases have been reported that are not associated with any malignancy, even with long period of observation.[157] If a malignancy is present, treatment of the malignancy, if successful, will frequently improve symptoms of myasthenic syndrome. Guanidine has been suggested as an agent to improve strength by increasing acetylcholine release and has been used in doses up to 20 to 30 mg/kg given daily, divided in three doses; usually lower doses are required on initiation of therapy. Toxicity including nausea, vomiting, and dizziness plus hepatotoxicity in some patients has limited its usefulness.[162]

REFERENCES

1. Gutmann, E., and Hanzlikova, V.: Age changes in the neuromuscular system, Bristol, England, 1972, Scientechnical (Publishers), Ltd.
2. Burke, W.E., et al.:Relation of grip strength and grip-strength endurance to age, J. Appl. Physiol.**5**:628, 1953.
3. Anderson, W.F., and Cowan, N.R.: Hand grip pressure in older people, Br. J. Prev. Soc. Med. **20**:141, 1966.
4. MacLennan, W.J., Hall, M.R.P., Timothy, J.I., and Robinson, M.: Is weakness in old age due to muscle wasting? Age Ageing **9**:188, 1980.
5. Forbes, G.B., and Reina, J.C.: Adult lean body mass declines with age; some longitudinal observations, Metabolism **19**:653, 1970.
6. Häggmark, T.E., Jansson, E., and Svane, B.: Cross-sectional area of the thigh muscle in man measured by computed tomography, Scand. J. Clin. Lab. Invest. **38**:355, 1978.
7. Petrofsky, J.S., and Lind, A.R.: Aging, isometric strength and endurance, and cardiovascular responses to static effort, J. Appl. Physiol. **38**:91, 1975.
8. Larsson, L., and Karlsson, J.: Isometric and dynamic endurance as a function of age and skeletal muscle characteristics, Acta Physiol. Scand. **104**:129, 1978.
9. Ikai, M., and Steinhaus, A.H.: Some factors modifying the expression of human strength, J. Appl. Physiol. **16**:157, 1961.
10. Larsson, L.: Morphological and functional characteristics of the ageing skeletal muscle in man, Acta Physiol. Scand. (Suppl.)**457**:1, 1978.
11. Moritani, T., and deVries, H.A.: Potential for gross muscle hypertrophy in older men, J. Gerontol. **35**:672, 1980.
12. Campbell, M.J., McComas, A.J., and Petito, F.: Physiological changes in ageing muscles, J. Neurol. Neurosurg. Psychiatry **36**:174, 1973.
13. Caccia, M.R., Harris, J.B., and Johnson, M.A.: Morphology and physiology of skeletal muscle in aging rodents, Muscle Nerve **2**:202, 1979.
14. Dubowitz, V., and Brooke, M.H.: Muscle biopsy: a modern approach, Philadelphia, 1973, W.B. Saunders Co.
15. Engel, W.K.: Selective and nonselective susceptibility

of muscle fiber types, Arch. Neurol. **22:**97, 1970.

16. Sunderland, S.: Nerves and nerve injuries, Baltimore, 1969, The Williams & Wilkins Co.
17. Gollnick, P.D., et al.: Selective glycogen depletion in skeletal muscle fibres of man following sustained contractions, J. Physiol. (London) **241:**59, 1974.
18. Orlander, J., and Aniansson, A.: Effects of physical training on skeletal muscle metabolism and ultrastructure in 70 to 75-year-old men, Acta Physiol. Scand. **109:**149, 1980.
19. Hulten, B., et al.: Relationship between isometric endurance and fibre types in human leg muscles, Acta Physiol. Scand. **93:**135, 1975.
20. Tomonaga, M.: Histochemical and ultrastructural changes in senile human skeletal muscle, J. Am. Geriatr. Soc. **25:**125, 1977.
21. Jennekens, F.G.I., Tomlinson, B.E., and Walton, J.N.: Histochemical aspects of five limb muscles in old age: an autopsy study, J. Neurol. Sci. **14:**259, 1971.
22. Rebeiz, J., et al.: Variations in muscle status with age and systemic diseases, Acta Neuropathol. (Berlin) **22:**127, 1972.
23. Tomlinson, B.E., Walton, J.N., and Rebeiz, J.J.: The effects of ageing and of cachexia upon skeletal muscle: a histopathologic study, J. Neurol. Sci. **9:**321, 1969.
24. Ermini, M., and Verzár, F.: Decreased restitution of creatine phosphate in white and red skeletal muscles during aging, Experientia **24:**902, 1969.
25. Orlander, J., et al.: Skeletal muscle metabolism and ultrastructure in relation to age in sedentary men, Acta Physiol. Scand. **104:**249, 1978.
26. Shephard, R.: Physical activity and aging, London, 1978, Croom Helm, Ltd.
27. Saltin, B., and Grimby, G.: Physiological analysis of middle-aged and old former athletes, Circulation **38:**1104, 1968.
28. Annianson, A., et al.: Physical training in old men, Age Ageing **9:**186, 1980.
29. Suominen, H., and Heikkinen, E.: Enzyme activities in muscle and connective tissue of M. Vastus lateralis in habitually training and sedentary 33 to 70-year-old men, Eur. J. Appl. Physiol. **34:**249, 1975.
30. Welander, L.: Myopathia distalis tarda hereditaria: 249 examined cases in 72 pedigrees, Acta Med. Scand. (Suppl. 265)**141:**1, 1951.
31. Bautista, J., et al.: Hereditary distal myopathy with onset in early infancy: observation of a family, J. Neurol Sci. **37:**149, 1978.
32. Markesberry, W.R., et al.: Late onset hereditary distal myopathy, Neurology **24:**127, 1974.
33. Markesberry, W.R., Griggs, R.C., and Herr, B.: Distal myopathy: electron microscope and histochemical studies, Neurology **27:**727, 1977.
34. Welander, L.: Homozygous appearance of distal myopathy, Acta Genet. **7:**321, 1957.
35. Edström, L.: Histochemical and histopathological changes in skeletal muscle in late-onset hereditary distal myopathy, J. Neurol. Sci. **26:**147, 1975.
36. Kratz, R., and Brooke, M.H.: Distal myopathy. In Vinken, P.J., and Bruyn, G.W., editors: Handbook of clinical neurology, vol. 38, 1979, Elsevier North-Holland, Inc.
37. Barbeau, A.: The syndrome of late onset ptosis and dysphagia in French Canada. In Kuhn, E., editor: Progressive muscular dystrophy: myotonia myasthenia, Berlin, 1966, Springer-Verlag Berlin.
38. Montgomery, W.W., and Lynch, J.P.: Oculopharyngeal muscular dystrophy treated by inferior constrictor myotomy, Trans. Am. Acad. Ophthalmol. Otolaryngol. **75:**986, 1971.
39. Rebeiz, J.J., Caulfield, J.B., and Adams, R.D.: Ocularpharyngeal dystrophy, A presenescent myopathy, A clinico-pathological study. In Bronette, J.R., and Barbeau, A., editors: Progress in neuroophthalmology, Proceedings in the Second International Congress of Neurogenetics and Neuroophthalmology, vol. 2, Montreal, 1967, Excerpta Med.
40. Weitzner, S.: Changes in the pharyngeal and esophageal musculature in oculopharyngeal muscular dystrophy. Report of two cases, Am. J. Dig. Dis. **14:**805, 1969.
41. Bosch, P.E., Gowans, J.D.C., and Munsat, T.: Inflammatory myopathy in oculopharyngeal dystrophy, Muscle Nerve **2:**73, 1979.
42. Bethlem, J.: Myopathies, ed. 2, Amsterdam, 1980, Elsevier/North Holland Biomedical Press.
43. Turnbridge, W.M.G.: The epidemiology of hypothyroidism. In Evered, D., and Hall, R., editors: Clinics in endocrinology and metabolism **8:**21, 1979.
44. Morrow, L.B.: How thyroid disease presents in the elderly, Geriatrics **33**(4):42, 1978.
45. Bland, J.H., and Frymoyer, J.W.: Rheumatic syndromes of myxedema, N. Engl. J. Med. **282:**1171, 1970.
46. Ramsay, I.: Thyroid disease and muscle dysfunction, London, 1974, William Heinemann.
47. Stern, L.Z., and Fagan, J.M.: The endocrine myopathies. In Vinken, P.J., and Bruyn, G.W., editors: Handbook of clinical neurology, vol. 38, Amsterdam, 1979, Elsevier North-Holland, Inc.
48. Scarpalezos, S., et al.: Neural and muscular manifestations of hypothyroidism, Arch. Neurol. **29:**140, 1973.
49. Kudrjavcev, T.: Neurologic complications of thyroid dysfunction, Adv. Neurol. **19:**619, 1978.
50. Graig, F.A., and Smith, J.C.: Serum creatine phosphokinase activity in altered thyroid states, J. Clin. Endocrin. Metab. **25:**723, 1965.
51. McKeran, R.O., et al.: Muscle fibre type changes in hypothyroid myopathy, J. Clin. Pathol. **28:**659, 1975.
52. Wheeler, S.D., and Ochoa, J.: Probable hypothyroid myopathy: glycogen deficient Type 2B fibers, Muscle Nerve **1:**495, 1978.
53. Hochberg, M.C., et al.: Hypothyroidism presenting as a polymyositis-like syndrome, Arthritis Rheum. **19:**1363, 1976.
54. Ramsay, I.D.: Muscle dysfunction in hyperthyroidism, Lancet **2:**931, 1966.
55. Garcia, C.A., and Fleming, R.H.: Reversible corticospinal tract disease due to hyperthyroidism, Arch. Neurol. **34:**647, 1977.
56. Davis, P.J., and Davis, F.B.: Hyperthyroidism in patients over the age of 60 years: clinical features in 85 patients, Medicine **53:**161, 1974.
57. Patten, B.M., Bilezikian, J.P., and Malette, L.E.: Neuromuscular disease in primary hyperparathyroidism, Ann. Intern. Med. **80:**182, 1974.

58. Mallette, L.E., Patten, B.M., and Engel, W.K.: Neuromuscular disease in secondary hyperparathyroidism, Ann. Intern Med. **82**:471, 1975.
59. Cholod, E.J., et al.: Myopathy in primary familial hyperparathyroidism: clinical and morphological studies, Am. J. Med. **48**:700, 1970.
60. Conn, J.W., Knopf, R.F., and Nesbit, R.M.: Clinical characteristics of primary aldosteronism from an analysis of 145 cases, Am. J. Surg. **107**:159, 1964.
61. Pleasure, D.E., Walsh, G.O., and Engel, W.K.: Atrophy of skeletal muscle in patients with Cushing's syndrome, Arch. Neurol. **22**:118, 1970.
62. Askari, A., Vignos, P.J., and Moskowitz, R.W.: Steroid myopathy in connective tissue disease, Am. J. Med. **61**:485, 1976.
63. Mulder, D.W., and Howard, F.M., Jr.: Patient resistance and prognosis in amyotrophic lateral sclerosis, Mayo Clin. Proc. **51**:537, 1976.
64. Rosen, A.D.: Amyotrophic lateral sclerosis: clinical features and prognosis, Arch. Neurol. **35**:638, 1978.
65. Juergens, S.M., et al.: ALS in Rochester, Minnesota 1925-1977, Neurology **30**:463, 1980.
66. Bonduelle, M.: Amyotrophic lateral sclerosis. In Vinken, P.J., and Bruyn, G.W., editors: Handbook of clinical neurology, vol. 22, Amsterdam, 1975, Elsevier North-Holland, Inc., p. 281.
67. Norris, F.H., et al.: Old and new clinical problems in ALS. In Tsubaki, T., and Tokoyora, Y., editors: ALS: Proceedings of the International Symposium, Baltimore, 1978, University Park Press.
68. Norris, F.H.: Benign post-traumatic amyotrophy, Arch. Neurol. **27**:269, 1972.
69. Adornato, B.J., et al.: Benign focal amyotrophy, Neurology **28**:399, 1978.
70. Sobue, I., et al.: Juvenile type of distal and segmental muscular atrophy of upper extremities, Ann. Neurol. **3**:429, 1978.
71. Brody, J.A., Stanhope, J.M., and Kurland, L.T.: Patterns of ALS and parkinson-dementia on Guam. In Hernabrook, R.W., editor: Topics in tropical neurology, Philadelphia, 1977, F.A. Davis Co.
72. Horton, W.A., Eldridge, R., and Brody, J.A.: Familial motor neuron disease: evidence for at least three different types, Neurology **26**:460, 1976.
73. Hestness, A., and Melgren, S.I.: Familial amyotrophic lateral sclerosis: report of a family with predominant upper limb pareses and late onset, Acta Neurol. Scand. **61**:192, 1980.
74. Collis, W.J., and Engel, W.K.: Glucose metabolism in five neuromuscular disorders, Neurology **18**:915, 1968.
75. Antel, J.P., et al.: Histocompatibility typing in ALS, Arch. Neurol. **33**:423, 1976.
76. Pederson, L., et al.: HLA (SD and LD) in patients with myotrophic lateral sclerosis (ALS), J. Neurol. Sci. **31**:313, 1977.
77. King, R.B., and Stoops, W.L.: Cervical myelopathy with fasciculations in the lower extremities, J. Neurosurg. **20**:948, 1963.
78. Boothby, J.A., DeJesus, P.V., and Rowland, L.P.: Reversible forms of motor neuron disease; lead neuritis, Arch. Neurol. **31**:18, 1974.
79. Kantarjian, A.D.: A syndrome clinically resembling ALS following chronic mercurialism, Neurology **11**: 639, 1961.
80. Kilness, A.W., and Hochberg, F.H.: ALS in a high selenium environment, J.A.M.A. **237**:2843, 1977.
81. Norris, F.H., Denys, E.H., and U, K.S.: Differential diagnosis of adult motor neuron disease. In Mulder, D.W., editor: The diagnosis and treatment of amyotrophic lateral sclerosis, Boston, 1980, Houghton Mifflin Professional Publishers.
82. Troyaborg, W., and Bochtal, F.: Malignant and benign fasciculations, Acta Neurol. Scand. **41**:251, 1965.
83. Hudson, A.J., Brown, W.F., and Gilbert, J.J.: The muscular pain-fasciculation syndrome, Neurology **28**: 1105, 1978.
84. Greenhouse, A.H., et al.: Myotonia, myokymia, hyperhydrosis and wasting of muscle, Neurology **17**:263, 1967.
85. Dyck, P.J., and Lambert, E.H.: Lower motor and primary sensory neuron diseases with peroneal muscular atrophy II, Arch. Neurol. **18**:619, 1968.
86. Kennedy, W.H., Alter, M., and Sung, J.H.: Progressive proximal spinal and bulbar muscular atrophy of late onset, Neurology **18**:671, 1968.
87. Tsukagoshi, H., et al.: Hereditary proximal neurogenic muscular atrophy, Arch. Neurol. **12**:597, 1965.
88. Mallette, L.E., et al.: Calcium metabolism in amyotrophic lateral sclerosis, Dis. Nerv. Syst. 38:457, 1977.
89. Campbell, A.M., Williams, E.R., and Barltrop, D.: Motor neurone disease and exposure to lead, J. Neurol.Neurosurg. Psychiatry **33**:877, 1970.
90. Weiner, L.P.: Possible role of androgen receptors in ALS, Arch. Neurol. **37**:129, 1980.
91. Felmus, M.T., Patten, B.M., and Swanke, L.: Antecedent events in ALS, Neurology **26**:167, 1976.
92. Kurlander, H.M., and Patten, B.M.: Metals in spinal cord tissue of patients dying of motor neuron disease, Ann. Neurol. **6**:21, 1979.
93. Kondo, K.: Population dynamics of motor neuron disease. In Tsubaki, T., and Tokoyura, Y., editors: ALS: Proceedings of the International Symposium, Baltimore, 1978, University Park Press.
94. Norris, F.H.: Adult spinal motor neuron disease. In Vinken, P.J., and Bruyn, G.W., editors: Handbook of clinical neurology, vol. 22, Amsterdam, 1975, Elsevier North-Holland, Inc.
95. Mulder, D.W., Rosenbaum, R.A., and Layton, D.D.: Late progression of poliomyelitis or 'forme fruste' ALS, Mayo Clin. Proc. **47**:756, 1972.
96. Campbell, A.M.G., Williams, E.R., and Pearce, J.: Late motor neuron degeneration following poliomyelitis, Neurology **19**:1101, 1969.
97. Kott, E., et al.: Cell mediated immunity to polio and HLA antigens in ALS, Neurology **29**:1040, 1979.
98. Hoffman, P.M., and Robbins, D.S.: Cell mediated immunity to polio and HLA antigens in ALS, Neurology **30**:679, 1980.
99. Lehrich, J.R., Oger, J., and Arnason, B.G.W.: Neutralizing antibodies to poliovirus and mumps virus in amyotrophic lateral sclerosis, J. Neurol. Sci. **23**:537, 1974.
100. Cremer, N.E., et al.: Cultures of tissues from patients with ALS, Arch. Neurol. **29**:331, 1973.
101. Johnson, R.T.: Virologic studies of ALS, an overview.

In Andrews, J.M., Johnson, R.T., and Brazier, M.A.B., editors: Amyotrophic lateral sclerosis, recent research trends, New York, 1976, Academic Press, Inc.

102. Miller, J.R., et al.: ALS: search for poliovirus by nucleic acid hybridization, Neurology **30:**884, 1980.
103. Weiner, L.P., Stohlman, S.A., and Davis, R.L.: Attempts to demonstrate virus in ALS, Neurology **30:**1319, 1980.
104. Officer, J.E., Tecson, N., and Estes, J.D.: Isolation of a neurotrophic type C-virus, Science **181:**945, 1973.
105. Gardner, M.B., et al.: Lower motor neuron disease in wild mice caused by indigenous type C virus and search for a similar etiology in ALS. In Andrews, J.M., Johnson, R.T., and Brazier, M.A.B., editors: Amyotrophic lateral sclerosis, recent research trends, New York, 1976, Academic Press, Inc.
106. Pena, C.E.: Virus-like particles in ALS: EM study of a case, Ann. Neurol. **1:**290, 1977.
107. Oldstone, M.B.A., et al.: Evidence for immune complex formation in patients with ALS, Lancet **2:**169, 1976.
108. Kondo, K., and Tsubaki, T.: Case-control studies of motor neuron disease: association with mechanical injuries, Arch. Neurol. **38:**220, 1981.
109. Festoff, B.W., and Crigger, N.J.: Therapeutic trials in ALS, a review. In Mulder, D.W., editor: The diagnosis and treatment of ALS, Boston, 1980, H.M. Professional Publishers.
110. Tyler, H.R.: Double blind study of modified neurotoxin in motor neuron disease, Neurology **29:**77, 1979.
111. Rivera, V.M., et al.: Modified snake venom in ALS, Arch. Neurol. **37:**201, 1980.
112. Monstad, I., et al.: Plasma exchange in motor neuron disease, J. Neurol. **221:**59, 1979.
113. Olarte, M.R., et al.: Transfer factor is ineffective in ALS, Ann. Neurol. **5:**385, 1979.
114. Sinaki, M., and Mulder, D.W.: Rehabilitation techniques for patients with ALS, Mayo Clin. Proc. **53:**173, 1978.
115. Smith, R.A., Dawson, A., and Foroozan, P.: Pharmacologic and surgical modalities in ALS. In Mulder, D.W., editor: The diagnosis and treatment of amyotrophic lateral sclerosis, Boston, 1980, H.M. Professional Publishers.
116. Fallat, R.J., et al.: Spirometry in ALS, Arch. Neurol. **36:**74, 1979.
117. Pearson, C.M., and Bohan, A.: The spectrum of polymyositis and dermatomyositis, Med. Clin. North Am. **61**(2):439, 1977.
118. Bohan, A., and Peter, J.B.: Polymyositis and dermatomyositis. I. N. Engl. J. Med. **292:**344, 1975.
119. Bohan, A., et al.: A computer assisted analysis of 153 patients with polymyositis and dermatomyositis, Medicine **56:**255, 1977.
120. DeVere, R., and Bradley, W.G.: Polymyositis: its presentation, morbidity and mortality, Brain **98:**637, 1975.
121. Callen, J.P., et al.: The relationship of dermatomyositis and polymyositis to internal malignancy, Arch. Dermatol. **116:**295, 1980.
122. Kula, R.W.: Neuromuscular disorders associated with systemic neoplastic diseases. In Vinken, P.J., and Bruyn, G.W., editors: Handbook of clinical neurology, vol. 41, Amsterdam, 1979, Elsevier North-Holland, Inc.
123. Riddoch, D., and Morgan-Hughes, J.A.: Prognosis in adult polymyositis, J. Neurol. Sci. **26:**71, 1975.
124. Schwarz, H.A., et al.: Muscle biopsy in polymyositis and dermatomyositis, Ann. Rheum. Dis. **39:**500, 1980.
125. Manghani, D., Partridge, T.A., and Sloper, J.C.: The role of the myofibrillar fraction of skeletal muscle in the production of experimental polymyositis, J. Neurol. Sci. **23:**489, 1974.
126. Currie, S., et al.: Immunological aspects of polymyositis: the invitro activity of lymphocytes on incubation with muscle antigen and with muscle cultures, Q. J. Med. **40:**63, 1971.
127. Whitaker, J.N., and Engel, W.K.: Vascular deposits of immunoglobulin and complement in idiopathic inflammatory myopathy, N. Engl. J. Med. **286:**333, 1979.
128. Behan, W.M., and Behan, P.O.: Complement abnormalities in polymyositis, J. Neurol. Sci. **34:**241, 1977.
129. Behan, W., Behan, P.O., and Dick, H.A.: HLA-B8 in polymyositis, N. Engl. J. Med. **298:**1260, 1978.
130. Brooke, M.H.: A clinician's view of neuromuscular diseases, Baltimore, 1977, The Williams & Wilkins Co.
131. Bunch, T.W., et al.: Azathioprine with prednisone for polymyositis: a controlled, clinical trial, Ann. Intern. Med. **92:**365, 1980.
132. Osserman, K.E., and Genkins, G.: Studies in myasthenia gravis. A review of a 20 year experience in over 1,200 patients, Mt. Sinai J. Med. **38:**497, 1971.
133. Compston, D.A., Newsom-Davis, V., and Batchelor, J.R.: Clinical, pathologic, HLA antigen and immunological evidence for disease heterogeneity in myasthenia gravis, Brain **103:**579, 1980.
134. Hermann, C.: The familial occurrence of myasthenia gravis, Ann. N.Y. Acad. Sci. **183:**334, 1971.
135. Namba, T., et al.: Familial myasthenia gravis: report of 27 patients in 12 families and a review of 164 patients in 73 families, Arch. Neurol. **25:**49, 1971.
136. Rowland, L.P.: Controversies about the treatment of myasthenia gravis, J. Neurol. Neurosurg. Psychiatry **43:**644, 1980.
137. Castleman, B.: The pathology of the thymus gland in myasthenia gravis, Ann. N.Y. Acad. Sci. **135:**496, 1966.
138. Goldman, A.J., et al.: Myasthenia gravis and invasive thymoma: a 20-year-experience, Neurology **25:**1021, 1975.
139. Stalberg, E.: Clinical electrophysiology in myasthenia gravis, J. Neurol. Neurosurg. Psychiatry **43:**622, 1980.
140. Brown, J.C., and Charlton, J.E.: A study of sensitivity to curare in myasthenic disorders using a regional technique, J. Neurol. Neurosurg. Psychiatry **38:**27, 1975.
141. Drachman, D.B.: Myasthenia gravis I, N. Engl. J. Med. **298:**136, 1978.
142. Drachman, D.B.: Myasthenia gravis II, N. Engl. J. Med. **298:**186, 1978.
143. Vincent, A., and Newsom-Davis, J.: Anti-acetylcholine receptor antibodies, J. Neurol. Neurosurg. Psychiatry **43:**590, 1980.
144. Drachman, D.B., et al.: Mechanisms of acetylcholine receptor loss in myasthenia gravis, J. Neurol. Neurosurg. Psychiatry **43:**601, 1980.
145. Behan, P.O.: Immune disease and HLA associations

with myasthenia gravis, J. Neurol. Neurosurg. Psychiatry **43:**611, 1980.

146. Ward, M.D., Forbes, M.S., and Johns, T.R.: Neostigmine methylsulfate. Does it have a chronic effect as well as a transient one? Arch. Neurol. **32:**808, 1978.

147. Buckingham, J.M., Howard, F.M., and Bernatz, P.E.: The value of thymectomy in myasthenia gravis: a computer-assisted matched study, Ann. Surg. **184:**453, 1976.

148. Perlo, V.P., Arnason, B., and Castleman, B.: The thymus gland in elderly patients with myasthenia gravis, Neurology **25:**294, 1975.

149. Carter, B., et al.: Anti-acetylcholine receptor antibody titres in the sera of myasthenia patients treated with plasma exchange combined with immunosuppressive therapy, J. Neurol. Neurosurg. Psychiatry **43:**397, 1980.

150. Engel, W.K., and Askansas, V.: Remote effects of focal cancer on the neuromuscular system, Adv. Neurol. **15:**119, 1976.

151. Shy, G.M., and Silverstein, I.: A study of the effects upon the motor unit by remote malignancy, Brain **88:**515, 1965.

152. Campbell, M.J., and Paty, D.W.: Carcinomatous neuromyopathy. I. Electrophysiological studies: an electrophysiological and immunological study of patients with carcinoma of the lung, J. Neurol. Neurosurg. Psychiatry **37:**131, 1974.

153. Trojaborg, W., Frantzen, E., and Anderson, I.: Peripheral neuropathy and myopathy associated with carcinoma of the lung, Brain **92:**71, 1969.

154. Teräväinen, H., and Larsen, A.: Some features of the neuromuscular complications of pulmonary carcinoma, Ann. Neurol. **2:**495, 1977.

155. Warmolts, J.R., et al.: Type II muscle fiber atrophy: an early systemic effect of cancer, Neurology **25:**374, 1975.

156. Elmquist, D., and Lambert, E.H.: Detailed analysis of neuromuscular transmission in a patient with the myasthenic syndrome sometimes associated with bronchogenic carcinoma, Mayo Clin. Proc. **43:**689, 1968.

157. Brown, C.J., and Johns, R.: Diagnostic difficulties encountered in the myasthenic syndrome sometimes associated with carcinoma, J. Neurol. Neurosurg. Psychiatry **37:**1214, 1974.

158. Lambert, E.H., and Elmquist, D.: Quantal components of end-plate potentials in the myasthenic syndrome, Ann. N.Y. Acad. Sci. **183:**183, 1971.

159. Schwartz, M.S., and Stalberg, E.: Myasthenic syndrome studied with single fiber EMG, Arch. Neurol. **32:**815, 1975.

160. Engel, A.G., and Santa, T.: Histometric analysis of the ultrastructure of the neuromuscular junction in myasthenia gravis and in the myasthenic syndrome, Ann. N.Y. Acad. Sci. **183:**46, 1971.

161. Ishikawa, K., et al.: A neuromuscular transmission block produced by a cancer tissue extract derived from a patient with the myasthenic syndrome, Neurology **27:**140, 1977.

162. Kamenskaya, M.A., Elmquist, D., and Thesleff, S.: Guanidine and neuromuscular transmission, Arch. Neurol. **32:**505, 1975.

PART IV REHABILITATION

CHAPTER 32 · REHABILITATION MEDICINE

Franz U. Steinberg

The individual who through disease or injury has become physically disabled must learn anew how to cope with his environment. Everyday activities, previously performed with little effort or thought, become major undertakings. A short flight of stairs or a curbstone becomes an unsurmountable hurdle that denies the patient access to his place of work or to his home. Rehabilitation medicine is concerned with helping the disabled patient resume normal life in a familiar environment. It is the objective of rehabilitation to contain a physical disability and to keep it from becoming the cause of a social decline.

A successful rehabilitation program is predicated on a precise evaluation of the disability. The effect of the disability on the overall function of the individual must be identified. How does a given physical impairment affect the patient's ability to move about, to communicate, to live at home, or to return to gainful employment? The cause of the disability must also be identified, since it affects the prognosis for functional restoration. Therefore a thorough evaluation of the patient's physical and mental condition must form the basis of the rehabilitation program.

The rehabilitation of the aged disabled patient presents particular difficulties. Usually the disability has been caused by a disease process that has adverse effects on the patient's general health. The coexistence of several diseases, so common in the elderly, unfavorably influences the overall prognosis. Often the aged patient poorly tolerates the physical effort that is needed to carry out a rehabilitation program successfully. Also rehabilitation is a learning process, and the ability of an aged person to learn new techniques and to adapt to new situations often is impaired. For all these reasons the goals that the physician sets for an elderly disabled patient must be modest. Vocational rehabilitation usually need not be considered for this age group. The most common objective is to restore the patient to a level of function that will permit him to return to his home and family. A disabled aged patient generally can be managed at home if the following conditions are met:

1. He must be able to walk or at least transfer from bed to chair without having to be lifted.
2. He must have normal or nearly normal control of his excretory functions.
3. He should be able to take care of all, or at least an essential part, of his personal needs such as eating, dressing, and bathing.
4. His mental condition should be adequately clear.

The goal of returning an aged disabled patient to his home and community is well worth pursuing. Studies of nursing home populations have shown time and again that the confinement to a custodial institution could have been avoided for many persons had restorative care been available early in the course of their illness. It must be emphasized that rehabilitation must be initiated on time, concurrent with active medical or surgical care, to be effective. Prolonged inactivity may lead to a rapid physical and mental deconditioning that soon becomes irreversible. A patient who has been confined to a custodial institution for many months is a poor prospect for rehabilitation.[1]

Rehabilitation medicine attempts to restore lost function. If this is not possible, the patient is taught to function with his disability. He is provided with adaptive devices, and he must learn how to use them. He may need to acquire new means of locomotion.

In implementing a rehabilitation program, the physician works with a team of professionals with special skills: the rehabilitation nurse, the physical therapist, the occupational therapist, the social worker, the psychologist, the speech pathologist, and the orthotist. The members of this team must work closely together, consult with each other, and defer to each other concerning specialized knowledge and skills.

Rehabilitation is expensive, and trained personnel and rehabilitation facilities are in short supply. They should be used for all who can benefit from them, but they should not be misused. The physician with the assistance of the team must decide when maximum objectives have been reached and when rehabilitative care should be discontinued. To prolong care beyond this point wastes valuable resources and transforms a rehabilitation ward into a custodial facility. Rehabilitation means improvement of overall functions: being able to walk, being independent in the wheelchair, assuming responsibility for personal needs. To spend weeks or months in training the patient to perform a few movements that are too isolated and too weak to be of functional use is not rehabilitation; it is an expensive exercise in futility.

EVALUATION OF THE DISABLED PATIENT

Rehabilitation programs impose considerable physical demands on the patient. Exercise and gait training may overtax an aged patient who is no longer accustomed to physical effort. Therefore the general condition and particularly the status of the cardiac and pulmonary systems must be carefully evaluated. Furthermore, many of the disabilities of the aged person are the results of atherosclerosis. Before a rehabilitation program can be planned, the physician must know to what extent other vital organs have been affected by vascular disease. The evaluation begins, of course, with a thorough medical history and a physical examination. Urine examination, blood cell count, chemistry profile, and chest x-ray examination are part of the routine workup. An electrocardiogram must always be obtained. This is particularly important in the case of stroke patients, since clinically unrecognized myocardial infarctions not uncommonly precede strokes.[2] If the presence of obstructive emphysema is suspected, pulmonary function studies should be done. From the results of these examinations, the physician will be able to judge the patient's tolerance for physical effort.

Disabilities affect the organs of locomotion. Therefore the status of the skeletal and neuromuscular systems must be carefully assessed. Impairment of function must be described in detail, and quantitative methods should be used whenever feasible. The neurologist, whose main objective it is to make a diagnosis, may be satisfied with the general statement that the involved limb shows muscle weakness. The psychiatrist, who is concerned with retraining the patient to use the affected extremity, must know in detail which muscle groups are weak and which function adequately. The choice of an exercise program to be initiated or braces to be prescribed depends on these findings.

The following section will give a brief outline of the evaluation procedures commonly used in rehabilitation medicine. For details the reader should consult the appropriate textbooks.[3-5]

Joint range of motion

Joints have either one degree, two degrees or three degrees of freedom of motion. Hinge joints such as knees, elbows, or the interphalangeal joints of the fingers have one degree of freedom of motion; movements take place only about one axis. Pronation and supination of the forearm, which take place at the ulna-radial articulation, are also movements of one degree of freedom of motion. Joints that allow movements about two axes such as wrist and metacarpal phalangeal joints of fingers and thumb have two degrees of freedom. Ball and socket joints, which permit motion in three dimensions, such as shoulder and hip have three degrees of freedom. Joint range of motion is measured with a goniometer, the arms of which must have the appropriate length to assure maximal accuracy. Even then a fairly large margin of error remains. This subject has been recently reviewed by Moore.[6] The neutral resting position of a joint is designated as the zero baseline. Zero positions, for instance, are the positions of extension of hip, knee, elbow, and finger joints. The straight line position of hand to forearm is designated as the zero position of the wrist. Methods of joint range-of-motion measurements and normal values are given in a number of publications.[7,8]

Difficulties are encountered when joints such as the shoulder or the hip move in concert with other skeletal structures. Loss of range of motion at the hip joint can be obscured by associated movements of the pelvis and lumbar sacral spine. These movements can be eliminated by the Thomas maneuver by which the opposite hip is held in flexion over the abdomen; this position stabilizes the pelvis; and loss of hip extension, abduction or rotation range, will be brought to light. Clayson et al.[9] have described a method of measuring the extension of the hip joint by which associated lumbar sacral spine movements are eliminated.

Range of motion measurements may not be precise, but they give a good estimate of the impairment of joint function. Repeated measurements are valuable for gauging the progress of disease or the success of a treatment program.

Muscle strength

The strength of a muscle or group of muscles can be tested in two ways: either the patient performs a movement while the examiner gives resistance, or the examiner attempts to move a joint while the patient resists. The manual muscle test generally assesses the strength of composite movements, but with specific techniques it is possible to isolate the function of individual muscles. The techniques of manual muscle testing that are widely used by physical therapists have been described in monographs.[10,11] Muscle strength is classified in six grades: normal, good, fair, poor, trace, and zero, or in a numeric system from 5 to 0. Intermediate grades such as "fair plus" or "fair minus" are often used. "Fair minus," for instance, indicates that the segment of a limb can be moved against gravity but not through full range.

Manual muscle testing has significant limitations. The gauging of grades above the "fair" level becomes subject to considerable observer bias. Two examiners or the same examiner on different days may have considerable difficulties deciding whether a grade is "good" or "normal." Furthermore, muscles or muscle groups that test as normal may in fact not be strong enough to carry out their physiologic function. For instance, if a person stands on one leg, the hip abductors must generate a force of two to three times body weight to hold this position. These muscles may be normal on a manual muscle test and yet not be able to perform this important physiologic function. Therefore some muscles are best tested in a functional position. The gastrocnemius-soleus group is best tested by having the patient rise on tiptoes. The ability to stand on tiptoe with the knee flexed specificially tests the soleus. As mentioned before, the ability to stand on one leg is a good test for the hip abductors, specifically the gluteus medius. With the foot firmly on the ground, the hip abductors hold the center of gravity over the supporting leg.

For the geriatric patient without overt neurologic disease the manual muscle test is no more than a screening device. Patients may test normal in most groups and yet be unable to ascend steps or arise from a chair unaided. So-called "good" or "normal" muscles may simply not be strong enough to perform their natural functions. A functional assessment of strength may be more informative than a detailed manual muscle testing, a procedure which after all was designed for patients with lower motor neuron disease. In the future, the measuring of muscle strength with isokinetic equipment (Cybex) may turn out to be a most valuable tool.

Activities of daily living

In a rehabilitation program, much time is devoted to training the patient to care for his personal needs. A variety of systems has been developed to record the progress of these endeavors. These charts may list as many as 100 activities, and the examiner records whether a patient can perform these tasks independently, with adaptive devices, with supervision, with assistance, or not at all. Several writers have reduced the number of items to a few key activities to which arbitrary point values are assigned. In this way a numeric score is obtained by which progress or regression in self-care ability can be expressed. The most commonly used systems are the Barthel index,[12] which allows for a maximum of 100 points and operates in the decimal system and the Kenny scores.[13] The Kenny system uses six major functional subcategories: bed, transfers, locomotion, dressing, personal hygiene, and feeding activities. The patient is scored separately in each of these categories, which are equally weighted, and a total score with a maximum of 24 points is then obtained. The Katz index[14] classifies patients into one of seven groups. (Class A: the patient is independent in feeding, continence, transferring, toilet activities, dressing, and bathing; class B: the patient is independent in all but one of these functions; class C: the patient is independent in all but bathing and one additional function; etc.) The advantage of the Katz index lies in the avoidance of an arbitrary point system. On the other hand, its reliability is predicated on the assumption that various functions are restored in a definite chronologic order, for example, that patients will be able to feed themselves before they can bathe independently. Whenever this order is disrupted, the patient must be classified under "other" rather than in a specific group. Donaldson et al.[15] compared the Barthel index, Kenny scores, and Katz index; they found that the three systems showed simultaneous rises and falls in self-care ability in 68% of all cases. In the remaining 32% the scoring systems gave divergent results, the Katz index being the least sensitive of the three systems. They repeated this study for 138 Framingham Study stroke survivors and found all three systems to be satisfactory; in their experience the Barthel index provided certain advantages, such as greater sensitivity to change and completeness.[16]

It appears unavoidable, although unfortunate, that most rehabilitation facilities have developed their own systems of recording self-care ability. Because of this divergence it is often impossible to compare reports emanating from different institutions. However, different rehabilitation facilities serve different types of patients, and self-care scoring systems need to be adapted to the needs of a particular population. The Department of Rehabilitation at The Jewish Hospital of St. Louis uses a system which, similar to the Kenny Score, subdivides activities into eight categories that are scored separately and then averaged. Anybody who is tempted to devise an activities of daily living scoring system should consult a paper by Kelman and Willner,[17] which discusses the problems of performance evaluation in rehabilitation.

Sensory and perceptual evaluation

A sensory examination should be part of the general physical examination. Loss of touch, pain, temperature sensation, proprioception, and stereogenosis must be uncovered and recorded, since the loss of these sensory functions may have a good deal of bearing on the success of a rehabilitation program. Patients with cerebral cortical disease frequently exhibit more complex sensory deficits. Strokes involving the nondominant side of the body often cause an alienation of the affected extremities, which is due to a disturbed body image. The patient ignores the sensory input from the involved side. He does not use the extremity even if he has the muscle power to do so. This is a serious impairment that militates against successful retraining in self-care. A loss of vertical and horizontal space perception also is common in hemiplegic patients.[18] This loss of space perception must be recognized, since its presence jeopardizes the patient's ability to assume an upright position and immeasurably complicates gait training.

Impairment of vision, hearing, and speech is discussed in Chapters 27, 29, and 35.

Psychologic evaluation

An evaluation of a patient's mental status is important for diagnosis and for care planning. Cognitive functions should be assessed systematically and in a definite order. The examiner should evaluate the level of consciousness, general behavior, attention, memory, constructional ability, and abstract thinking. The methods used for a mental status examination in neurologically impaired patients have been described by Strub and Black[19] in a concise monograph, which should be consulted by all who deal with neurologically impaired patients. A well-planned mental status examination need not take more than 15 to 20 minutes; but it may give important information on the anatomic location of the lesion, and it will tell the examiner to what extent a patient will be able to cooperate with a rehabilitation program.

Somnolence and marked confusion are easily recognized but often a partial aphasia may be mistaken for confusion. In general, disorders of communication, that is, of speech or hearing will adversely affect mental function; they must be recognized and treated appropriately.[20]

The examiner should determine whether or not the patient is oriented to place and time. Past and recent memory can be tested with a few simple questions. To assess the ability to retain information, the examiner asks the patient to remember a number of digits. More complex mental functions are tested by having the patient perform simple arithmetic calculations or explain simple proverbs. Also abstract thinking can be evaluated by having the patient explain similarities and differences of objects or events, such as apple and pear, iron and silver, dwarf and child, and lie and mistake. Various forms of apraxia can be recognized when the patient performs simple tasks. The examiner should proceed from one-step to two-step and three-step instructions. If the patient is unable to perform simple tasks or to retain instructions from one day to the next, the prognosis in the rehabilitation program is poor.

Quantitative psychologic testing must be left to the clinical psychologist. A psychologic evaluation when there is aphasia presents a particular problem. The Peabody Picture Vocabulary is used in this instance.

The psychosocial evaluation must include information on the patient's premorbid personality. A passive individual who has always had difficulties in adapting to new situations and in relating to people will do less well in a rehabilitation program than a hard-driving, well-organized person. In spite of illness and possible brain damage, past good work habits may break through and may help the patient to adapt to his disability and to the demands made on him by the rehabilitation personnel.

The motivation of the patient is often considered the key to a successful rehabilitation program. Under the emotional impact of a serious disability, most patients are moderately depressed. Few patients appear highly motivated in the beginning. As a matter of fact, an excessive enthusiasm for the rehabilitation program may mask an unwillingness to face reality and may keep the patient from looking at his expectations and goals realistically. Few patients are so depressed and so poorly motivated that they fail to cooperate. Most patients accept the rehabilitation program without much enthusiasm, but they cooperate, and their motivation improves as they begin to see success.

THERAPEUTIC EXERCISE

The rehabilitation of the disabled patient usually involves the strengthening of weakened muscles, the improvement of endurance, the maintenance or increase of joint range of motion, the improvement of coordination of skilled movements, and the restoration of a functional gait. Therapeutic exercises are the most important tool that the therapist employs to meet these objectives.

Exercises should be prescribed by the physician. The prescription will depend on the objectives of the program and the general condition of the patient. Age as such is no limiting factor, but a thorough evaluation of the cardiovascular system must be done before an aged patient is started on an active exercise program. The therapist must understand the limitations that may be imposed by the patient's general condition. If there are risks entailed, the therapist must know about them and watch for early warning signs. Clear-cut instructions from the physician to the therapist enhance the chances for success and reduce the risks of inadvertently doing harm. (Details of therapeutic exercise programs are given in Chapter 33.)

Therapeutic exercises are either dynamic (isotonic), static (isometric), or isokinetic. During isokinetic exercise the speed of motion is kept constant. This has proved to be a very efficient method of strengthening weakened muscles, since the load on the muscle remains the same through the entire arc of motion. Isokinetic exercise requires special equipment and for this reason cannot be adapted for home use.[21]

Cardiopulmonary and metabolic effects of exercise

The energy for muscular contractions is provided through a chain of chemical reactions. The immediate source of energy for muscle contraction is adenosine triphosphate (ATP), which breaks down into adenosine diphosphate (ADP) and phosphate, releasing 7.6 kcal of energy per mole of ATP. Less than 1 second of muscular activity depletes the ATP stores. ATP must therefore be reconstituted from ADP and phosphates for muscular activity to continue. The energy for this reaction is provided by the breakdown of creatine phosphate. Tertiary energy supplies, needed to reconstitute creatine phosphate are furnished by the metabolism of carbohydrate and fat. During high intensity exercise carbohydrate (glycogen) is the main tertiary energy source. During low intensity long-term exercise fats provide a significant proportion of fuel. Carbohydrate and fats are in ample supply, but their utilization requires the steady supply of oxygen. Oxygen cannot be stored and must be provided as the muscular activity proceeds.[22]

The skeletal muscle mass makes up about 40% of the body weight. At rest the oxygen demand is about 3 ml per minute for 100 gm of muscle tissue. During exercise the oxygen consumption of muscle rises up to 100 times the resting value. For the adult with normal body weight the oxygen uptake at rest is about 250 ml per minute. This is equivalent to an energy cost of 1.25 gm calories or 1 Met.

The energy cost of various activities is determined by measuring the volume of the exhaled air and its oxygen content during activity and recovery. In this way the total oxygen cost for the work performance is determined.

During physical activity the blood flow through the muscle may increase 15 to 20 times the resting value. The blood flow through the abdominal organs is greatly reduced, whereas the coronary artery flow is increased. The heart rate rises, whereas the stroke volume increases very little. Pulmonary ventilation rises because of an increase both of the rate and tidal volume of respiration. The systolic blood pressure increases, whereas the diastolic pressure remains unchanged.

If the physical activity is moderate in intensity, the metabolic needs can be covered on a pay-as-you-go basis. Cardiac and respiratory rates remain at a tolerable level, and the activity can be carried on indefinitely. If the exercise is strenuous, heart rate and oxygen consumption rise steeply and reach a plateau within a few minutes. The oxygen supply lags behind the demand, and an oxygen debt develops. After cessation of the activity the oxygen consumption falls slowly to the preexercise level, which is not reached until the oxygen debt has been paid.

The measure of the aerobic capacity for a given individual is the maximum oxygen consumption ($\dot{V}O_2$ max) that can be achieved with intensive exercise. As exercise becomes more intense and prolonged, anaerobic metabolic processes are called into play to provide further fuel. During anaerobic metabolism carbohydrates are broken down with lactates as end-product, which accumulate in muscle and blood. Both muscle and blood lactate concentration begin to rise when the oxygen uptake is close to 60% of maximum. The eventual removal of lactic acid requires oxygen. The oxygen needed to complete this chemical process is called the *lactacid oxygen debt*.

As the effort increases, heart rate and oxygen consumption rise in parallel. Both maximal heart rate and maximal oxygen consumption decline with age in a linear fashion. A rough calculation of the maximum heart rate is given by the formula: 220 minus age. The exercise tolerance of an individual is best determined by measuring the maximal oxygen consumption and maximal heart rate. The great stress engendered by this procedure may make it unsafe for an older individual. For the sake of safety, stress tests have been developed that determine maximum heart rate and maximum aerobic oxygen consumption by extrapolation from submaximal tests.[23]

The decline of physical fitness with advancing years as demonstrated by the decrease of maximal oxygen consumption and maximal heart rate is related to the diminishing ability of the aging organism to take up and to transport oxygen. Tlustý[24] has shown that the ventilation equivalent and the oxygen pulse decline with age. More air needs to be exchanged to supply the body with a given amount of oxygen, and the heart needs to beat more frequently to distribute a given volume of oxygen throughout the body. Details of the changes of cardiovascular and respiratory function with age are presented in Chapter 1.

Exercise and physical fitness in the aged

Opinions vary to what extent the physical fitness of aged individuals can be improved by a training program. The many data reported in the medical literature are difficult to compare, since there is a great variation both in the methods and the duration of training and in the procedures employed to assess fitness.

As mentioned previously, the maximum oxygen consumption is the most reliable test of cardiovascular fitness; however, many investigators have shown an understandable reluctance to subject aged individuals to so stressful a procedure. Benestad[25] found no increase of $\dot{V}O_2$ max in men aged 70 to 81 years after 5 to 6 weeks of training. Barry,[26] on the other hand, reported an increase of $\dot{V}O_2$ max of 38% after a 3-month training program. There is a question, however, if the initial test conducted on deconditioned individuals who were confined to an institution was not unduly low and therefore not comparable to the later examination. A survey of the literature of a total of 203 observations showed an increase of the maximum oxygen uptake of 11.5% in 60-year-old individuals after fitness training compared to 16.7% in 30-year-old persons.[27] Other studies have shown that the $\dot{V}O_2$ max declines less with aging in those individuals who are engaged in a continuing training program[28] or in aging athletes.[29]

Other investigators have estimated the maximum oxygen intake from submaximal tests. DeVries[30] reported an increase of the estimated $\dot{V}O_2$ max of 8% after 42 weeks of training. Sidney and Shephard[31] reported a final gain of 24% after 1 year of training. Pollock et al.[32] were able to demonstrate an increase of $\dot{V}O_2$ max of 18% after 20 weeks of a walking and jogging training of sedentary men between the ages of 49 and 65 years.[32]

Additional effects of physical training are noteworthy. A systematic exercise program carried out for several weeks lowers the heart rate for a given submaximal work load. Recovery time is decreased, and the exercise systolic blood pressure rises to a lesser extent. Since the product of heart rate and systolic blood pressure parallels myocardial oxygen consumption, it may be concluded that after a physical training program the same work load imposes a lesser stress on the myocardium. DeVries,[30] working with 112 men of an average age of 69.5 years, found that training significantly improved those functions during the peak of activity which are involved with oxygen transport, such as oxygen pulse and minute volume of respiration. Physical work capacity, measured by the integrated watt minutes of work carried to the point when the heart rate rose to 85% of the maximum, was significantly improved. Physical training of women produced similar results.[33] Stamford[34] demonstrated that training of aged individuals reduced their exercise heart rate and systolic blood pressure. Barry et al.[26] reported a reduction of exercise heart rate, systolic blood pressure, and blood lactate concentration after a period of training. The individuals were also able to perform at a higher work load than before training.

Regardless of the effect of physical fitness training on measurable parameters of circulation and respiration, the beneficial effect on the physical and emotional well-being of healthy aged individuals cannot be questioned. Endurance is improved, and cardiopulmonary functions adapt better to exercise loads. Lean muscle mass is increased while a substantial amount of body fat is lost.[35] The self-image of aged individuals is improved by fitness training. The entire subject has been thoroughly reviewed by Shephard.[36]

Effort tolerance of disabled individuals

The effort tolerance of the aged individual must be taken into account when an exercise program for a physical disability is planned and executed. Most of the elderly patients who enter a rehabilitation program will not have been physically active for some time and will be out of condition. Muscle strengthening exercises, or the gait training of a hemiplegic patient or of an amputee, impose considerable stresses to which the patient is not accustomed. In addition, the patient is just recovering from a serious illness or operation that will have further reduced his stamina. These facts and the potential risks must be kept in mind by the physician and therapist.

The patient's response should be monitored carefully. Shortness of breath, cyanosis of the lips or nail beds, excessive perspiration, and complaints of dizziness and faintness are signs that the patient's effort capacity has been overtaxed. The therapist should watch for cardiac irregularities, determine the heart rate, and be aware of an excessive rise during activity or of the failure of the rate to drop to normal levels after cessation of the exercise. The systolic pressure rises during activity. An excessive increase or a drop below the resting level are signs of a compromised circulation.

The cardiovascular effects of isometric exercise need to be noted. The response of the heart and blood vessels depend not on the size of the exercised muscle but on the percentage of the maximal isometric contraction. Ramos et al.[37] showed that an isometric hand grip held for 5 minutes causes a considerable rise in blood pressure and heart rate. With increasing effort there is a considerable spread of activity to other muscles. The authors postulate that sustained isometric contractions, in contrast to dynamic exercise, are under constant conscious cerebral cortical control and cause a spread of the excitation to the vasomotor centers. In the aged and poorly conditioned individual isometric exercise carries particular risks.

Exercise of the patient at risk is best performed intermittently, allowing for adequate periods of rest. Sudden bursts of intensive activity should be avoided. The therapist should also see to it that the patient does not hold his breath during the exercise and thereby produce a Valsalva phenomenon.

The energy costs of various rehabilitation activities have been studied. Bard[38] found the metabolic cost of walking for hemiplegic patients to be elevated but still in an acceptable range. Spasticity increased the energy cost. Corcoran et al.[39] found the oxygen consumption of walking in hemiplegic patients to be 64% higher than in normal individuals. Braces did not lower the oxygen consumption but increased comfortable and maximum walking speeds. The literature on the energy cost of ambulation has been reviewed by Fisher and Gullickson.[40] The energy cost of propelling a wheelchair on level ground is lower than walking at equal speed, but the heart rate is higher.[41] The energy cost of walking with prostheses will be discussed later in this chapter.

Gait training

The ability to move about on one's own is a prerequisite to independence. In the aged, disturbances in ambulation must be attacked early, and corrective measures must be instituted before it is too late. Inability to walk can have many causes. The normal adult uses gravity and inertia efficiently during walking. He allows himself to fall forward; the elongating calf muscles control the rate of speed of the forward fall. The balance is recaptured by hyperextension of the lumbosacral spine, a motion which moves the center of gravity behind the hip joints. The aged may not have the coordination or flexibility necessary to recover the balance. Muscles become weaker and may respond less promptly. The lumbosacral spine may have lost range of motion due to arthritic changes and the capability to hyperextension and backward shift of the center of gravity may have been lost. The result of these changes is a reduction of stride length and walking speed. The swing phase to stance phase ratio is diminished. The vertical oscillations of the body are less pronounced, but the lateral oscillations are increased. Aged individuals frequently walk with a shorter but broader stride. Murray[44] who has exhaustively studied the gait of older persons states that old people often walk as if on a slippery surface or in the dark. An increasing stiffness of the lumbosacral spine forces the patient to walk with the trunk slightly flexed and over flexed hips and knees in order to keep the center of gravity over the point of support. The stiffness of the spine forces the aged person to use his muscles increasingly to retain and recapture his balance. Therefore the energy cost of walking is increased.

It is obvious that arthritic changes of low back and lower extremity joints will interfere with walking.

Gait disturbances due to arthritis of the hip or knee are treated with physical therapy. Ultrasound is particularly effective in applying heat to the hip joint. A cane in the hand on the side opposite the affected joint is most helpful, since it takes part of the pressure off the affected joint. If the patient is obese, he must be encouraged to lose weight. Denham[45] has shown that each additional pound of body weight adds 3 pounds of pressure to the hip joint during the stance phase of walking.

Even in the absence of significant arthritis the excusion of the hip joints during ambulation may be markedly reduced. Working with old men who walked with an apparently normal gait, Steinberg et al.[46] found a reduction of hip flexion of 75% and of hip extension of 81% compared to younger adults.

Hip extension deficits may be difficult to detect by the usual range-of-motion measurements. It causes the patient to walk with the hip and knee in slight flexion, and it forces him to use his hip extensor muscles to maintain his balance. This impairment is often compounded by weakness of the hip extensor muscles. Once the condition is recognized, it can be at least partly corrected by stretching the tight flexors and strengthening the hip extensor musculature. To this purpose we have found isokinetic exercises particularly helpful.

Various neurologic disorders such as stroke, Parkinson's disease, neuropathies, and combined system diseases may be causes of gait disorders.

Polymyositis and those types of muscular dystrophy that appear late in life affect the pelvic girdle muscles and cause the typical waddling gait of pelvic instability. A gait pattern characteristic of the very elderly person was first described by Petren[47] in 1900 and was called the "marche à petit pas." The patient walks with small shuffling steps accompanied by gross rowing movements of the arms. When the patient has to turn about, the steps become even smaller, and the leg movements are almost ineffectual. The neurologic basis for this gait pattern is not clear. Extrapyramidal elements obviously play a role. Meyer and Barron[48] have called this type of walking *apraxia of gait* and have found it associated with frontal lobe lesions. There is increasing evidence that apractic or ataxic gait disorders in the aged may be associated with normal pressure hydrocephalus.[49] Computerized tomography makes it possible to diagnose this condition without having to resort to invasive procedures.

Gait training is not effective for the patient with apraxia of gait. If the patient is made to concentrate, he can take a few normal steps, but there is no carry-over, and he quickly falls back to his small-step shuffle. He may need a mechanical aid, such as a wheeled walker, to be able to get about safely. A cane is usually not helpful and may add to the confusion pattern.

Whenever an elderly person begins to show difficulties in walking, the physician and therapist must search for the cause and take corrective measures when possible. If the cause cannot be corrected, mechanical aids must be employed to keep the patient ambulatory for as long as possible.

REHABILITATION OF SPECIFIC DISORDERS

Stroke[50,51]

Stroke is a major cause of disability in the geriatric age group, and the incidence rises sharply with advancing years. The annual incidence of stroke in the United States is 400,000. Approximately 60% survive the first month of illness and of these at least two thirds can be expected to have a permanent disability.[52] It is estimated that the population of the United States includes 2.5 million survivors of strokes with varying degrees of disability.

In general 80% of all who have survived the acute phase of a stroke can be rehabilitated to a level of self-sufficiency that will enable them to live at home. Only 20% remain so disabled that they must live in a custodial institution. However, surveys of the nursing home population show that these institutions house many stroke victims who could have been restored so that they could live in the community, if early and effective rehabilitative care had been available to them. Because of the sheer number of patients, rehabilitation of stroke victims is of foremost importance in the care of the geriatric population.

The rehabilitation must begin with a precise diagnosis so that surgically treatable lesions, such as brain tumors, subdural hematomas, and extracranial vascular lesions are recognized and treated. The early care must be concerned with lifesaving measures. The circulation must be supported. An adequate airway should be maintained. Fluid and electrolyte disorders must be corrected. Measures to lower elevated blood pressure should be undertaken with great caution to avoid a peripheral vascular collapse and a propagation of the intraarterial thrombosis. If an indwelling catheter is necessary, it should be removed as early as possible, before bladder infections and catheter dependence develop.

The large majority of strokes are caused by infarcts in the internal carotid artery system. The clinical syndrome arising from this type of infarct will be used as a model in discussing the rehabilitation of stroke patients. Pathogenesis, diagnosis, and medical therapy are discussed in Chapter 28.

The recovery of motor function follows a characteristic pattern. The paralyzed limb moves from a phase of flaccidity to spasticity and eventually to the restoration of normal muscle tone. From a phase of complete paralysis the motor function recovers in synergistic patterns (for instance when the patient attempts to flex the elbow the shoulder goes into abduction and internal rotation and the forearm into pronation); eventually the ability to move extremity segments separately is regained. Proximal muscles recover before distal muscles. In the lower extremity the extensors recover before the flexors. The reverse is true for the upper extremity. There are many exceptions to this pattern of recovery, partly dependent on the anatomic location of the infarct. The course of recovery can be arrested at any one particular point. The earlier the neurologic recovery comes to a halt, the more disabled the stroke patient will remain. Most of the recovery takes place during the first

6 weeks; the prognosis for further improvement is poor after 3 months, with the exception of speech, which can continue improving over a much longer time interval.

The rehabilitation of stroke patients must satisfy three objectives:

1. Prevention of secondary disabilities
2. Adaptation to the disability remaining
3. Restoration of function to whatever extent possible

The prevention of secondary disabilities includes the avoidance of physical and mental deconditioning. The older the patient, the sooner he or she will become dependent on others. For this reason activities should be initiated as early as possible. The patient should have physical and occupational therapy at bedside. Self-positioning, turning, coming to a sitting position, and so on should be taught the patient as soon as the general condition permits. The patient should be made to participate in his care as soon as possible. Catheters should be removed and bladder training be instituted as soon as the patient is able to cooperate. A bowel routine must be established early.

The development of contractures is a common although avoidable complication. Contractures may develop early due to faulty positioning. The hip, for example, may become contracted in external rotation because the paralyzed limb of a bedridden patient may turn outward by gravity. Positioning with sandbags or firm pillows at the outer aspect of the thigh can prevent this complication. An ankle splint will prevent the contracture of the heel cord. Careful positioning of the upper extremity will keep the shoulder from contracting. A small rolled-up towel placed in the paralyzed hand keeps the finger flexors from tightening. Once spasticity sets in, the tendency to develop contractures is enhanced. Passive exercises should be given at least once a day to prevent the permanent shortening of spastic muscles. The application of splints is of particular value. A long-term gentle stretch is often more effective than a forceful stretch applied once a day by a therapist. It needs to be emphasized that contractures develop more readily in limbs with impaired arterial circulation; particular care, therefore, must be given to paralyzed lower limbs with decreased arterial blood flow.

Particular attention must be given to a hemiplegic shoulder. Subluxated or contracted shoulder joints can become very painful, and this discomfort contributes significantly to both early and late total disability.

Under normal circumstances the humerus is held in the glenoid fossa by the fibers of the joint capsule reinforced by muscular contractions of the supraspinatus and posterior deltoid. These muscles respond to gravity loading of the arm by contracting, an activity which keeps the head of the humerus in place.[53] In flaccid hemiplegia this mechanism does not function; if the arm is permitted to hang down by gravity the capsule becomes stretched and the subluxation of the shoulder joint soon becomes permanent. Chaco and Wolf[54] have shown that the subluxation becomes irreversible after 3 weeks, even if supraspinatus function returns after that period of time. Furthermore, because of the slant of the glenoid fossa, abduction of the humerus enhances the tendency to subluxation. Therefore, during the early flaccid phase, the therapist should not passively abduct the shoulder past 45 degrees. The paralyzed arm should be supported by a sling to protect it against the effect of gravity.

When the extremity becomes spastic, contractures tend to develop in adduction and internal rotation. It is of course desirable to retain or restore as much range of motion as possible, but stretching should not exceed the point of pain. Caldwell et al.[55] have shown that the pain of a paralyzed spastic and contracted hemiplegic shoulder can be diminished if range of motion exercises are limited to 45 degrees of abduction, 45 degrees of flexion, and 10 degrees of rotation.[55]

A true reflex sympathetic dystrophy is seen in a small percentage of stroke patients. The hand appears swollen and glossy, and extension deformities develop in the metacarpophalangeal and interphalangeal joints rather than the usual flexion deformities. Stellate ganglion blocks may have to be employed if there is no response to the usual conservative therapy.

Peripheral nerve lesions may occur both in the upper and lower extremities superimposed on the upper motor neuron deficit of stroke. They are usually due to traction or pressure injuries contracted during long periods of coma. These secondary lesions may complicate the neurologic evaluation and affect recovery.[56]

A variety of surgical procedures are now available to correct the deformities caused by contractures.[57,58] A tight heel cord can be released, and contracted toe flexor tendons can be lengthened. A number of operations are available to improve upper extremity function. Surgical interventions should be delayed for several months to be certain that the patient's physical and mental condition and his motivation will allow him to benefit from surgical correction.

When muscle function returns, active exercises are added to the rehabilitation program. Both agonists and antagonists should be strengthened simultaneously if possible. If one group of muscles shows less return of function, the opposing muscle group must not be overexercised. As an example, the finger flexors usually show a better return of function than the extensors. The squeezing of a rubber ball enhances this imbalance and should be discouraged. Splints that support the wrist and fingers in moderate extension and the thumb in abduction may prevent deformities that may be caused by muscular imbalance.

As the next step the patient is taught to transfer from bed to chair by pivoting on the good leg. This is one of the most important achievements of stroke rehabilitation. If the patient learns to transfer with the assistance of one person, without having to be lifted, he can usually be managed at home even if no further improvement were to take place.

Spasticity of one muscle group may make opposing muscles ineffective. As pointed out before, spastic muscles are best stretched gently and slowly. A rapid jerking stretch elicits a stretch reflex and increases the spastic response. If splints are used, they should not overstretch the spastic muscle and stimulate reflex responses. If the spasticity is excessive and a hindrance to functional training, a phenol block of the motor nerve may produce temporary or permanent relaxation.[59] Muscle relaxants such as dantrolene sodium,[60] diazepam, or baclofen are helpful in relieving hemiplegic spasticity.

To most hemiplegic patients independent walking is the foremost goal. Ambulation is possible only if the affected leg can be propelled ahead of the trunk. This motion usually requires hip flexor action of adequate strength even though some stroke patients can manage to bring the leg forward by trunk rotation. Once the affected leg has been moved to a forward position, it has to support the body weight by itself until the sound leg has caught up with it. This is possible only if the hip extensors are strong enough to hold the trunk steady above the leg and if the knee can be kept from collapsing into flexion. Quadriceps action is not needed to keep the knee extended during level walking, provided the hip extensors and ankle plantar flexors are adequate (Figs. 32-1 and 32-2). If the ankle muscles are weak, a below-knee brace locked at the ankle can substitute for their action. There is no way to compensate for weak hip extensors by bracing.

Gait training begins between parallel bars. The patient is taught how to stand erect, to shift his weight from side to side, and to support himself on the involved leg. The hemiplegic patient should not be encouraged to take steps until the standing and weight-shifting phase of training has been successfully completed.

Whether or not a stroke patient can stand or walk cannot be predicted from a neurologic examination alone. The examiner may not be able to elicit any voluntary motion in the involved lower extremity, yet in a functional weight-bearing position sufficient muscle action may be recruited, possibly by reflex action.

Recovery of muscle group function usually proceeds from proximal to distal. In many cases the dorsiflexors and evertors of the ankle remain exceedingly weak while other muscle groups have recovered adequate strength. A below-knee brace can compensate for this impairment. A simple footdrop, especially if not associated with a good deal of plantar flexor muscle spasticity, can be corrected by a plastic footdrop brace. A more unstable ankle will require a brace with bilateral metal upright bars. Springs embodied in the ankle assembly substitute for dorsiflexor action. The inversion of the ankle can be corrected by a T-strap, attached to the lateral edge of the shoe and attached to the medial upright bar. If the plantar flexor muscles are also weak, the orthotic ankle needs to be provided with two channels, one to substitute for plantar flexion and one for dorsiflexion. The orthotic ankle can now be locked in a position of choice. The greatest degree of stability is achieved when the ankle is held in 10 degrees of plantar flexion.[61] Rounding the heel of the shoe further increases the stability. This type of brace should

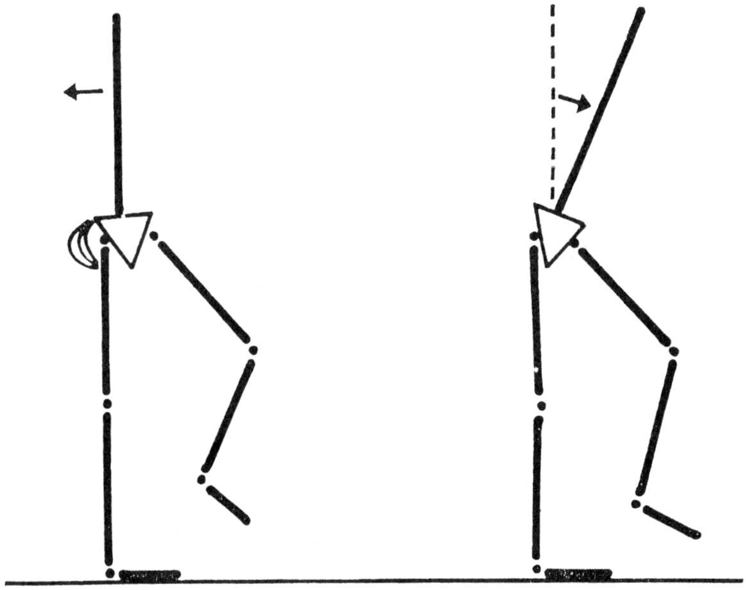

Fig. 32-1. Potential hemiplegic ambulation requires sufficient hip extension to hold the trunk over the involved leg during the stance phase (left). When insufficient thigh extension is present, the trunk will collapse in flexion over the pelvis (right). (From Mossman, P.M.: A problem oriented approach to stroke rehabilitation, Springfield, Ill., 1976. Courtesy of Charles C Thomas, Publisher.)

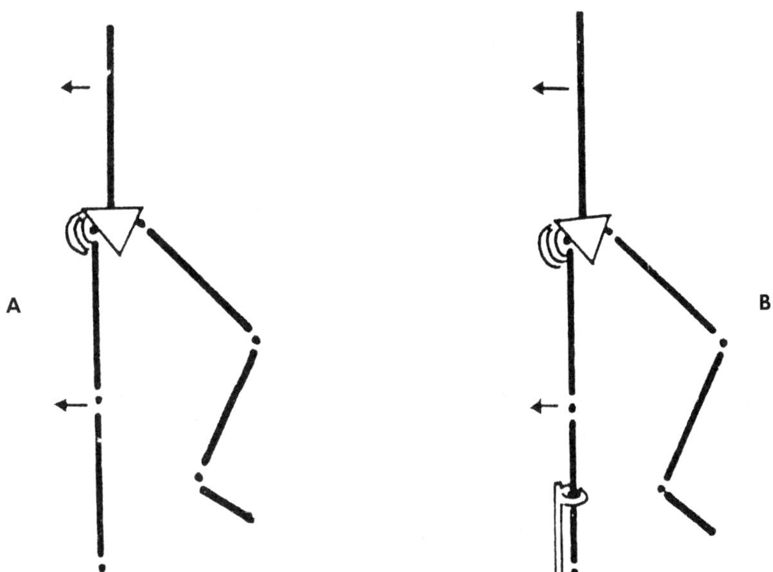

Fig. 32-2. A, During stance, adequate hip extension will keep trunk from collapsing into flexion and also maintain the knee extended, even in absence of good quadriceps mechanism. **B,** Furthermore, even with inadequate quadriceps mechanism, the knee cannot buckle if dorsiflexion of the ankle is prevented by a rigid ankle brace. Therefore, both mechanisms, adequate hip extension and controlled ankle dorsiflexion with a short leg brace, can prevent knee buckling, a long leg brace being redundant. (From Mossman, P.M.: A problem oriented approach to stroke rehabilitation, Springfield, Ill., 1976. Courtesy of Charles C Thomas, Publisher.)

be used if the knee extensors and/or flexors are weak, since the pressure of the calf band on the leg will keep the knee from buckling or from going into excessive hyperextension. Long leg braces are usually not indicated in the rehabilitation of stroke patients, since functioning hip extensors combined with a locked ankle brace are sufficient to maintain knee stability. Above-knee braces are heavy and difficult to apply, and if the hip extensor muscles are not functional the trunk will collapse into flexion over the top of such a brace.

The patient eventually will walk with a cane, a quadripod cane or a hemiwalker in the opposite hand. Gait training will be complete after the patient has learned to negotiate stairs and curbs. Even step length is of course desirable but it is not essential. Many stroke patients walk with a halting so-called "double step" gait in an attempt to use the involved leg for weight bearing for as short a period of time as possible. Safety is of prime importance.

The prognosis for regaining full use of the affected upper extremity is not favorable. Even though voluntary control of muscle activity may be present, the patient rarely regains the fine motor control and coordination essential to normal hand function. Nevertheless, active exercises should be initiated when recovery of motor function has begun to restore at least partial use of the involved upper extremity. Special perceptual training has not been shown to offer any advantages over conventional exercises.[62] It is imperative that the patient learn early to use the sound upper extremity to the fullest possible extent. This may be a difficult task, especially if the dominant extremity is affected. Adaptive devices are available that allow patients to perform activities which usually require the use of two hands with one hand. It is the task of the occupational therapist to train the patient in their use.

Sensory deficits, more often than not, complicate the rehabilitation program. Lack of proprioception, a distortion of the body image with autopagnosia in which the affected body parts are ignored, and inability to appreciate the vertical body position make functional retraining difficult. Visual field defects, usually in the form of a homonymous hemianopsia, are common in hemiplegics and are often not recognized by the patient. Pure motor hemiplegia without any sensory involvement or aphasia is actually rare and carries a better prognosis.[63] Disorders of communication are discussed in Chapter 35.

The rehabilitation procedures mentioned up to this point are designed to utilize returning motor and sensory function. Whether or not therapeutic measures can actually aid in the recovery of neurologic function remains questionable. Kottke[64,65] has discussed this subject in great detail, and a review of his writings is highly recommended. Most learned activities are automatic. Motor learning means the formation of engrams in subcortical centers; these engrams are volitionally activated if the individual wishes to perform certain motor acts. Furthermore, many motor activities are based on spinal reflexes, which are called into play and controlled by subcortical cerebral centers. A retraining of motor function needs to make use of these reflex patterns. Numerous repetitions of the same activity may restore the subcortical engram that had been lost due to the stroke. This principle may be effective in the restoration of more primitive activities such as gait. It is doubtful that it can be effective in the retraining of fine finger-hand function.

Over the years a number of facilitation techniques have been developed designed to restore lost motor-sensory function in stroke patients. Movements are facilitated by proprioceptive stimuli (Kabat-Knott), by cutaneous sensory input (Rood), or by techniques that inhibit unwanted motor activity (Bobath). These methods can be useful adjuncts to other rehabilitation procedures but should never become an end to themselves. Their effectiveness has not been proved.[66] Valuable time must not be spent to train a patient in using reflex maneuvers to perform a few weak isolated movements that do not contribute to the overall function.

In recent years biofeedback techniques have been used to facilitate motor function. These methods, which use electromyographic signals, are helpful in enforcing recovering but still feeble motor functions such as wrist extension or ankle dorsiflexion.[67,68] Since a stroke patient's proprioception is often impaired, biofeedback provides a substitute proprioceptive input which can be most helpful. Biofeedback can also be used to suppress unwanted movements, such as the shoulder abduction, which accompanies elbow flexion during the synergy phase of recovery.

The overall goal of rehabilitation of stroke patients is to make the patient as independent as possible. Time and energy should not be wasted on goals that have turned out to be unobtainable. If it appears that the patient will not be able to walk, the therapist should shift the emphasis to wheelchair independence and transfer activities. From the first possible moment the patient should take care of as many of his personal needs as possible. Nurses and occupational therapists must cooperate to train the patient in self-care. Adaptive devices are used whenever needed.

Before the patient is discharged, family members are instructed in the various techniques that will have to be applied at home. Exercises must be continued. Also the family must know what the patient can actually do, and how to assist in self-care. A coordinated home care program, if available, is extremely helpful for the period of transition from hospital to home. A number of publications, such as "Strike Back at Stroke" published by the United States Public Health Service and "Do It Yourself Again" published by the American Heart Association, will be invaluable to the families of stroke patients.

The negative attitude that many physicians exhibit toward stroke patients is to be deplored.[69] A good many stroke patients can achieve a significant measure of independence and live at home. A follow-up study of 107 stroke patients, consecutively admitted to the Jewish Hospital of St. Louis, showed that 70 were discharged to their own home and that after 12 months 47 were still living at home.[70] The timing of the rehabilitation program is of utmost importance. Newman[71] has shown that the neurologic recovery can take up to 12 weeks and that functional restoration runs in parallel. For this reason a rehabilitation program should not be arbitrarily discontinued after 3 weeks as long as the patient shows a steady although slow improvement. With a few exceptions stroke patients should not be confined to a custodial institution, unless they have first had an adequate trial with rehabilitation.

Careful observation of the patient will give the physician an indication of the prognosis and when the program is best discontinued. Persisting fecal incontinence is an indication of severe brain damage and denotes a poor prognosis. Stroke patients with hypertensive encephalopathy do not do well in rehabilitation programs. The achievements of patients with severe sensory and perceptual deficits are usually limited.

Parkinson's disease

Parkinson's disease is most commonly encountered in the geriatric age group even though it may occur earlier in life. The site of the disease process is in the basal ganglia, which have lost the ability to store and utilize dopamine. The incidence of the postencephalitic type, associated with the epidemic of 1917 to 1919, is decreasing rapidly.

The clinical picture is characterized by the following major groups of symptoms: (1) tremor, (2) impairment of voluntary motion caused by rigidity and bradykinesia, (3) dysfunction of the cranial nerves involving facial expressions, eye movements, dysphonia, and dysphagia, and (4) disorders of the autonomic nervous system. Rigidity and paucity of voluntary motion contribute most to the disability. The patient walks with a small-step shuffling gait. Arm swing is diminished. The patient walks with his back and hips flexed. The alternating back movements, necessary to maintain balance, are diminished. As a result, the gait becomes propulsive and often accelerates beyond control. At a later stage, the patient becomes unable to rise from a chair without assistance or to turn over in bed. Skilled movements such as writing become extremely difficult. The speech is monotonous and often close to being inaudible. Coarse resting tremor, excessive salivation, and difficulties in swallowing add greatly to the total disability.

The treatment of Parkinson's disease is medical. The most effective drug currently available is levodopa, the aminoacid corresponding to dopamine. It penetrates the blood-brain barrier and thus replenishes the reduced dopamine stores of the basal ganglia. The peripheral toxic effects of levodopa can be eliminated by combining it with carbidopa. This combination also permits the reduction of the amount of levodopa that needs to be administered. Levodopa-carbidopa (Sinemet) is now used almost exclusively for the levodopa therapy of Parkinson's disease. Levodopa has many side effects such as athetotic involuntary movements, postural instability, and dementia, and its administration must be carefully supervised. Its therapeutic effect appears to diminish after several years, but it does provide symptomatic relief for extended periods of time.[72,73] Other drugs used in the management of Parkinson's disease are bromocriptine, a dopamine agonist,[74] amantadine hydrochloride, and a variety of anticholinergic preparations.

In the early stages of the disease, there is no significant disability. The disabilities of the later stages are often compounded by inactivity and disuse, and their progress can be contained by rehabilitative measures.

The rigidity is controlled by active and passive exercises. The extremities and the back are stretched manually. Cervical traction is useful in stretching tight neck flexors, and a collar may help to correct head and neck posture. Active exercises are designed to improve mobility in general and to encourage reciprocal movements. A stationary bicycle and arm pulleys are helpful in accomplishing these purposes. The patient is exercised on the mat, on which he is taught to crawl, to turn over, and to come to a sitting position. Extremity exercises should be performed in diagonal patterns, and trunk rotation should be practiced. Breathing exercises are indicated if the respiration is affected. Gait training emphasizes long strides. The patient is made to step over obstacles to increase step length. Arm swing is practiced.

Exercises of the facial muscles and lips aid phonation. The patient must be made to speak loudly and with exaggerated phonation. In occupational therapy he will practice skilled activities chosen in accordance with his interests and functional goals.

Physical and occupational therapy cannot correct the neurophysiologic abnormalities of parkinsonism. However, therapy can prevent the deterioration engendered by lack of activity. Severe rigidity may lead to contractures. Certainly, all efforts should be made to prevent this secondary complication. The patient with parkinsonism becomes depressed by his inability to move, to speak clearly, and to show his emotions by facial expression. He withdraws into a shell, and often he appears mentally deteriorated, when he is only depressed. A program of well-planned activities delays the physical and mental decline and provides much emotional support.

Arthritis

The diagnosis and medical management of arthritis have been discussed in Chapter 4. Among elderly persons, osteoarthritis is the most common form of joint disease. The deterioration of the articular structures is caused by wear and tear on the aging cartilage, connective tissue, and bone. The joints most commonly affected are those that are subjected to the greatest stresses during a lifetime. The cervical and lumbar portions of the spine, the hips, and the knees are most frequently affected.

Mild degrees of arthritis are not incapacitating. However, if the deterioration of the joint structures is advanced and if the pain is severe, a significant disability ensues. Pain is relieved by medication and by application of heat. An intraarticular injection of corticosteroids can produce a dramatic improvement. Surgical treatment is discussed in Chapter 19.

A brief period of bed rest can tide the patient over an acute painful episode. For long-term management it is important to relieve the joint of part of the weight-bearing function. The use of a cane in the hand on the side opposite the affected lower extremity reduces the stress on an arthritic hip or knee. Obese patients should lose weight.[45] Occasionally, a brace must be prescribed to spare the affected joint. A chronic arthritis often is associated with weakness and atrophy of the muscles that move the joint. This association initiates a vicious circle. Muscles and their tendons physically support and stabilize joints. Furthermore, the contraction and slow relaxation of muscles act as a brake on joint motion. Therefore the deficient function of weak and atrophic muscles adds to the wear and tear on the joint structure. For this reason a program of active strengthening exercises is initiated once an acute painful phase has passed. Often isometric exercises have to be used, since the affected joint may not tolerate the repeated movements of isotonic exercise.

The physical treatment of an osteoarthritis of the spine is based on the same principles. The affected segment is temporarily immobilized by a cervical collar or a corset. Heat, exercise, and carefully employed traction are helpful. Because of the anatomic structure, nerve root irritation is a common complication of spinal osteoarthritis. Cinquegrana[75] has pointed out that a painful and stiff shoulder is often associated with an osteoarthritis of the cervical part of the spine. The pain in the shoulder is caused by an impingement of sensory and sympathetic nerve roots supplying the shoulder, and it can be relieved if the treatment is directed toward the neck.

Rheumatoid arthritis is not uncommon in the aged. Usually it constitutes a recurrence of this disease, which may have plagued the individual through much of his earlier life. The physical therapy does not differ materially from the program described for the patient with osteoarthritis. If the disease is active, there is considerable danger of a rapid joint destruction. Therefore the joints must be carefully protected against stress and traumas. Fingers and wrists may have to be immobilized by splints and cautiously exercised once a day to retain range of motion.

Amputations and prosthetics

Over the last two decades, considerable advances have been made both in the surgical techniques of amputations and in the design of substitute limbs. However, the criteria developed for the young or middle-aged amputee who has lost his limb because of injury are not automatically applicable to the geriatric amputee.

In the case of the aged patient, amputations are almost always the end result of obliterative arteriosclerosis, frequently associated with diabetes mellitus. Before deciding if the patient is suitable for prosthetic fitting, the physician must take into account the functional capacity of the patient's cardiovascular and pulmonary systems, the status of the remaining leg, and the patient's motivation and learning ability. Obviously, a patient who has led an almost sedentary life for months or years before the operation is not a suitable candidate. Coronary heart disease with angina pectoris on effort or advanced obstructive pulmonary disease are contraindications. The patient must be sufficiently alert to learn the technique of prosthetic walking. He will do poorly if he cannot retain instructions from one day to the next. If the other leg has severe vascular insufficiency and shows signs of impending gangrene, this process may be hastened by ambulation. In this situation the efforts should be directed toward preserving the remaining extremity. Some hardy, elderly double amputees may learn how to walk on two prostheses, and in Sakuma's series[76] one half of 53 geriatric bilateral amputees became ambulatory on two artificial limbs if at least one knee joint was preserved. In general, most geriatric double amputees depend on the wheelchair, even if they can take a few steps on their prostheses.

The aged amputee has a much better chance for successful prosthetic fitting if the knee joint is preserved. The sensory input from the knee greatly facilitates gait training. Many elderly amputees do not command the neuromuscular coordination needed to control a prosthetic knee.

The energy cost of walking with a prosthesis must also be taken into consideration. The oxygen consumption per distance covered is 2.2 times normal for the vascular amputee walking with an above-the-knee prosthesis, whereas it is only 1.6 times normal for the below-the-knee amputee.[77,78] On the other hand, the oxygen cost of walking when determined per unit time of walking varies little from normal, both for the below-the-knee and above-the-knee amputee. However, the above-the-knee amputee with prosthesis selects a walking speed of only 44% of normal, while the below-the-knee amputee walks with a speed of 55% of normal. It follows that the amputee with a prosthesis selects a walking speed that keeps the energy cost (per unit of time) at normal levels. The energy expenditure also depends on the length of the stump. If the stump is very short, the energy cost may be considerably higher.[79] Fortunately, newer surgical techniques allow for successful below-the-knee amputations, even when there is widespread vascular disease. Kihn et al.[80] reported that of 559 amputations, 200 were performed below the knee. Of these, 116 had no popliteal pulse, yet wound healing occurred in 73%. Of the below-the-knee stumps without bleeding at the time of operation, 69% healed eventually. Encouraged by these results, surgeons now attempt below-the-knee amputation much more frequently than in the past. Consequently, many more aged amputees can now be successfully furnished with prostheses.

The success or failure of prosthetic fitting often hinges on the early postoperative management. The development of hip flexion contractures in the above-the-knee amputee and of knee flexion contractures in the below-the-knee amputee must be avoided at all cost. The stump must be shrunk to the greatest possible extent with elastic bandages or with an air bag.

The use of an immediate postoperative prosthesis is still controversial. A plaster cast is applied to the stump on the operating table to which a pylon with a prosthetic foot can be attached when the patient is out of bed. The rigid dressing of the plaster cast reduces stump edema and postoperative pain and may facilitate wound healing.[81] Within a few days the patient will be able to stand and take a few steps. The cast is changed every 2 or 3 weeks. The stump must remain in the cast until the permanent prosthesis is ready for use. This method is contraindicated when there are wound infections or if the stump is anesthetic. If pain recurs, the cast must be removed promptly so that the wound can be inspected. The cast application should be undertaken only by those who have learned the elaborate technique. Malone et al.[82] reported that the use of an immediate postoperative prosthesis, allowing for an early mobilization of the patients, lowered the postoperative mortality from 16% to 0%. Kane et al.[83] found that the incidence of stump necrosis, reamputations at a higher level, and mortality were not affected by the use of the immediate postoperative prosthesis. However, 56% of the patients managed with an immediate postoperative prosthesis were eventually rehabilitated to the use of a definitive prosthesis compared to only 22% in the conventionally treated group. Earlier Warren et al.[84] had reported from a cooperative study of Boston hospitals and surgeons that the method was not harmful if properly applied but that it did not rehabilitate more amputees than other methods. However, it speeds rehabilitation by setting a definite timetable. It can be concluded that immediate postoperative fitting may be a valuable method if the appropriate patient is carefully selected and observed.

If immediate application of a plaster-socket prosthesis is not done, the fitting with a permanent prosthesis must wait until the incision has healed and stump shrinkage is close to being maximal. A patient who has learned to ambulate with a walker can usually manage a below-the-knee prosthesis. Crutch walking should not be a prerequisite. Many aged amputees do not have the coordination needed to walk on crutches, yet they do well with a below-the-knee prosthesis. If the stump is of adequate length, the patellar tendon–bearing prosthesis is preferred. However, for the elderly amputee it is advisable to make provisions for a thigh corset, which will increase stability.

The aged above-the-knee amputee has a less favorable outlook. To walk on an above-the-knee prosthesis is tiring, and the operation of the prosthetic knee is often difficult to learn. If the patient truly desires to have a prosthesis, if he has learned to walk with a walker, and if in the physician's opinion the heart can tolerate the effort, prosthetic fitting and training can be attempted. The longer the stump is, the better are the chances for success. An irreducible hip flexion contracture of more than 20 degrees is a contraindication. The above-the-knee socket is quadrilateral, and weight is born in the ischial tuberosity. A pelvic band suspension is preferred to a suction socket. Stability can be enhanced by a "safety knee," which prevents buckling. If the gait remains very unstable, an extension lock can be added. The patient then walks with a stiff knee; the lock is opened manually when he wishes to sit down.

The prosthetic components suitable for a given patient are best selected by an amputee clinic team, consisting of physicians, physical therapists, and prosthetists. The physician should not delegate the responsibility of the decision to the prosthetist alone, who cannot be familiar with the patient's overall problems. When the prosthesis has been constructed, the patient must be trained by the physical therapist. Elderly amputees are best admitted to a rehabilitation department for intensive training under close medical supervision.

If in the physician's best judgment the patient is not suitable for prosthetic walking, he must be told so as soon as this decision has been made. He should not be put off time after time because unrealistic hopes may be kept alive. He should made to understand that he can be independent even though he will not be able to walk. He should be provided with a wheelchair and trained in transfer techniques. Most patients will accept the physician's recommendation if the reasons are explained to them. An elderly amputee should never be refused a prosthesis because of age alone. Considerable numbers of geriatric amputees have become proficient in the use of below-the-knee, and even above-the-knee, artificial limbs and have used them for extended periods as their main mode of locomotion.[85-87] The decision must always be based on a thorough evaluation of the patient's general health, motivation, and social needs.

Cardiac rehabilitation

Over the last two decades cardiologists have loosened the constraints that had formerly kept patients with heart disease to a life of inactivity.

The 3 weeks of strict bed rest, once imposed on patients recovering from an uncomplicated myocardial infarction, were found not only to be unnecessary but actually added to the debility. It was found that a program of early and gradually increasing physical activity helped patients recovering from a myocardial infarction or from coronary artery bypass operations to regain strength and a sense of well-being. Several excellent monographs on cardiac rehabilitation have been published during the last few years.[88-90] A "Program Guide for Cardiac Rehabilitation" is available from the American Heart Association.[91]

During the recovery phase of a myocardial infarction the rehabilitation program progresses slowly from light bedside activities in the coronary care unit, including early ambulation, active and passive arm and leg movements, self care, sitting in bed or in a chair, and the use of a bedside commode. The intensity of early activities does not exceed 2 mets. Complications such as significant dysrhythmias, congestive heart failure, recurrent chest pain, or shock are obvious contraindications. At the time of discharge from the hospital and in the absence of complications, low level activities in the 2 to 3 met range are allowed. If these activities do not cause chest pain, tachycardia, dyspnea, dysrhythmias, or ST segment shifts on the monitor, the intensity can be increased cautiously. Isometric muscle contractions should be avoided at this stage; that means that the patient should not carry suitcases, attempt to open stuck windows, and so on.

A more formal program may be initiated several weeks after discharge from the hospital. These programs need to be conducted under medical supervision, and a cardiovascular nurse should be present during exercise. Submaximal exercise testing establishes the maximal heart rate. The therapeutic exercise should be conducted at 70% to 75% of the maximal heart rate. (The use of beta-blockers renders the monitoring of the exercise intensity by heart rate unreliable.) Exercises should be conducted for 20 to 30 minutes, preceded by a warm-up and followed by a cool-down period. The exercises should be aerobic and isotonic and involve large muscles both of the lower and upper extremities.[92] The intensity of exercise may be increased as tolerated, monitored by periodic submaximal stress testing. Contraindications to participation are unstable angina, severe ventricular dysfunction manifested by excessive dyspnea or a drop in systolic pressure during exercise, active cardiomyopathy during the preceding year, uncontrolled hypertension, complex dysrhythmias, second or third degree heart block, uncontrolled atrial fibrillation, substantial cardiomegaly and relevant valvular or congenital heart disease.[93] Various other noncardiac medical conditions or significant musculoskeletal impairments may also constitute contraindications.

After several months the patient may advance to a less supervised maintenance program, conducted either at home or in a physical education facility. This step may be taken when the patient has shown no inadvertent effects from the exercise, and if he has demonstrated an understanding of the overall problems and goals, including the limitations imposed by past medical events. The patient should be able to monitor his heart rate and detect irregularities of the heart beat.

The benefits of a cardiac rehabilitation program are an increase of work capacity, including an augmented oxygen extraction by the trained muscle groups; a lowering of the heart rate and systolic blood pressure, both at rest and at a given submaximal work load; and faster return both of heart rate and systolic pressure after termination of the exercise. The patient's well being and self-confidence are improved and anxieties are lessened. Adipose tissue may be reduced and the ratio of high density to low density lipoproteins may become more favorable. A recent study reported improvement of myocardial perfusion and function in five patients with coronary heart disease after exercise training, as demonstrated by improvement of the ejection fraction and of exercise thallium images.[94]

Whether or not the progress of coronary disease is retarded by a cardiac rehabilitation program, whether the collateral coronary circulation is improved, and whether there is a beneficial effect on the life expectancy have not been demonstrated even though the subject has remained controversial. In any case patients feel better and they lose the fears engendered by the sudden and dramatic "heart attack," which had so completely disrupted their life-style. The patients are able to return to work and their accustomed way of life sooner and with less anxiety.

REFERENCES

1. Muller, J.N.: Preventive rehabilitation: a study of nursing home residents, N.Y. State J. Med. **64:**1882, 1964.
2. Glathe, J.P., and Achor, R.W.: Frequency of cardiac disease in patients with strokes, Mayo Clin. Proc. **33:**417, 1958.
3. Krusen, F.H., Kottke, F.J., and Ellwood, P.M.: Handbook of physical medicine and rehabilitation, ed. 2, Philadelphia, 1971, W.B. Saunders Co.
4. Rusk, H.A.: Rehabilitation medicine, ed. 4, St. Louis, 1977, The C.V. Mosby Company Co.
5. Licht, S.: Rehabilitation and medicine, New Haven, Conn., 1968, Elizabeth Licht, Publisher.
6. Moore, M.L.: Clinical assessment of joint motion. In Basmajan, J.V., editor: Therapeutic exercise, ed. 3, Baltimore, 1978, The Williams & Wilkins Co.
7. American Academy of Orthopaedic Surgeons: Joint motion method of measuring and recording, Chicago, 1965, The Academy.
8. American Medical Association Committee on Rating of Mental and Physical Impairment: Guides to the evaluation of permanent impairment, Chicago, 1971, The American Medical Association.
9. Clayson, S.J., Mundale, M.O., and Kottke, F.J.: Goniometer adaptation for measuring hip extension, Arch. Phys. Med. Rehabil. **47:**255, 1966.
10. Daniels, L., and Worthingham, C.: Muscle testing, ed. 4, Philadelphia, 1980, W.B. Saunders Co.
11. Kendall, H.O., Kendall, F.M.P., and Wadsworth, G.E.: Muscle testing and function, ed. 2, Baltimore, 1971, The Williams & Wilkins Co.
12. Mahoney, F.I., and Barthel, D.W.: Functional evaluation. The Barthel index, Md. State Med. J. **14:**61, 1965.
13. Schoening, H.A., and Iversen, I.A.: Numerical scoring of self-care status: a study of the Kenny self-care evaluation, Arch. Phys. Med. Rehabil. **49:**221, 1968.
14. Katz, S., et al.: Studies of illness in the aged, J.A.M.A. **185:**94, 1963.
15. Donaldson, S.W., Wagner, C.C., and Gresham, G.E.: A unified ADL evaluation form, Arch. Phys. Med. Rehabil. **54:**175, 1973.
16. Gresham, G.E., Phillips, T.F., and Labi, M.L.C.: ADL status in stroke: relative merits of three indexes, Arch. Phys. Med. Rehabil. **61:**355, 1980.
17. Kelman, H.R., and Willner, A.: Problems in measurement and evaluation of rehabilitation, Arch. Phys. Med. Rehabil. **43:**172, 1962.
18. Bruell, J.H., and Peszczynski, M.: Perception of verticality in hemiplegic patients in relation to rehabilitation, Clin. Orthop. **12:**124, 1958.
19. Strub, R.L., and Black, F.W.: The Mental Status Examination in neurology, Philadelphia, 1977, F.A. Davis Co.
20. Schow, R.L., Christensen, J.M., Hutchinson, J.M., and Nerbonne, M.A.: Communication disorders of the aged, Baltimore, 1978, University Park Press.
21. Moffroid, M.T., et al.: Study of isokinetic exercise, Phys. Ther. **49:**735, 1969.
22. Soule, R.G.: Physiologic response to physical exercise. In Knuttgen, H.G.: Neuromuscular mechanisms for therapeutic and conditioning exercise, Baltimore, 1976, University Park Press.
23. Astrand, I.: Aerobic work capacity in men and women with special reference to age, Acta Physiol. Scand. **49:**(Suppl. 169), 1960.
24. Tlustý, L.: Physical fitness in old age, Respiration **26:**161, 1969.
25. Benestad, A.M.: Trainability of old men, Acta Med. Scand. **178:**321, 1965.
26. Barry, A.J., et al.: The effects of physical conditioning on older individuals. I. Work capacity, circulatory-respiratory function, and work electrocardiogram, J. Gerontol. **21:**182, 1966.
27. Hodgson, J.L., and Buskirk, E.R.: Physical fitness and old age, with emphasis on cardiovascular function in the elderly, J. Am. Geriatr. Soc. **25:**385, 1977.
28. Kash, F.W., and Wallace, J.P.: Physiological variables during 10 years of endurance training, Med. Sci. Sports **8:**5, 1976.
29. Bortz, W.A.: Effect of exercise on aging. Effect of aging on exercise, J. Am. Geriatr. Soc. **28:**49, 1980.
30. DeVries, H.A.: Physiological effects of an exercise training regime upon men aged 52 to 88, J. Gerontol. **25:**325, 1970.
31. Sidney, K.H., and Shephard, R.J.: Frequency and intensity of exercise training for elderly subjects, Med. Sci. Sports **10:**125, 1978.
32. Pollock, M.L., et al.: Physiologic responses of men 49 to 65 years of age to endurance training, J. Am. Geriatr. Soc. **24:**97, 1976.
33. Adams, G.M., and DeVries, H.A.: Physiological effects of a training regime on women aged 52 to 79, J. Gerontol. **28:**50, 1973.
34. Stamford, B.A.: Physiological effects of training upon institutionalized geriatric men, J. Gerontol. **27:**451, 1972.
35. Sidney, K.H., Shephard, R.J., and Harrison, J.E.: Endurance training and body composition of the elderly, Am. J. Clin. Nutr. **30:**326, 1977.
36. Shephard, R.J.: Physical activity and aging, Chicago, 1978, Year Book Medical Publishers, Inc.
37. Ramos, M.U., et al.: Cardiovascular effects of spread of excitation during prolonged isometric exercise, Arch. Phys. Med. Rehabil. **54:**496, 1973.
38. Bard, G.: Energy expenditure of hemiplegic subjects during walking, Arch. Phys. Med. Rehabil. **44:**368, 1963.
39. Corcoran, P.J., Jebsen, R.H., Brengelmann, G.L., and Simons, B.C.: Effects of plastic and metal leg braces on speed and energy cost of hemiparetic ambulation, Arch. Phys. Med. Rehabil. **51:**69, 1970.
40. Fisher, S.V., and Gullickson, G., Jr.: Energy cost of ambulation in health and disability: a literature review, Arch. Phys. Med. Rehabil. **59:**124, 1978.
41. Hildebrandt, G., et al.: Energy costs of propelling wheelchair at various speeds: cardiac response and effect on steering accuracy, Arch. Phys. Med. Rehabil. **51:**131, 1970.
42. Steinberg, F.U.: Gait disorders in old age, Geriatrics **21:**134, 1966.
43. Barron, R.E.: Disorders of gait related to the aging nervous system, Geriatrics **22:**113, 1967.

44. Murray, M.P., Kory, R.C., and Clarkson, B.H.: Walking patterns in healthy old men, J. Gerontol. **24**:169, 1969.
45. Denham, R.A.: Hip mechanics, J. Bone Joint Surg. **41-B**:550, 1959.
46. Steinberg, F.U., Roettger, R.F., and Baker, K.E.: A gait abnormality of old age: decrease of active hip motion, presented at the 40th Annual Meeting of American Academy of Physical Medicine and Rehabilitation, New Orleans, Nov. 13, 1978.
47. Petren, K.: Ueber den Zusammenhang zwischen anatomisch bedingter und funktioneller Gangstoerung im Greisenalter, Arch. Psych. Nervenkr. **33**:818, 1900.
48. Meyer, J.S., and Barron, D.W.: Apraxia of gait: a clinicophysiological study, Brain **83**:261, 1960.
49. Messert, B., and Wannamaker, B.B.: Reappraisal of the adult occult hydrocephalus syndrome, Neurology **24**: 224, 1974.
50. Licht, S., editor: Stroke and its rehabilitation, New Haven, 1975, Elizabeth Licht, Publisher.
51. Mossman, P.L.: A problem oriented approach to stroke rehabilitation, Springfield, Ill., 1976, Charles C Thomas, Publisher.
52. Feigenson, J.S.: Stroke rehabilitation. Outcome studies and guidelines for alternative levels of care, Stroke **12**:372, 1981.
53. Basmajan, J.V.: Muscles alive, ed. 4, Baltimore, 1978, The Williams & Wilkins Co.
54. Chaco, J., and Wolf, E.: Subluxation of the glenohumeral joint in hemiplegia, Am. J. Phys. Med. **50**:139, 1971.
55. Caldwell, C.B., Wilson, D.J., and Brown, R.M.: Evaluation and treatment of the upper extremity in the hemiplegic stroke patient, Clin. Orthop. **63**:69, 1969.
56. Kaplan, P.E., Meredith, J., Taft, G., and Betts, H.B.: Stroke and brachial plexus injury: a difficult problem, Arch. Phys. Med. Rehabil. **58**:415, 1977.
57. Waters, R.L., Perry, J., and Garland, D.: Surgical correction of gait abnormalities following stroke, Clin. Orthop. **131**:54, 1978.
58. Waters, R.L.: Upper extremity surgery in stroke patients, Clin. Orthop. **131**:30, 1978.
59. Khalili, A.A., and Betts, H.B.: Management of spasticity with phenol nerve blocks, RD 2529-M, Washington, D.C., 1970, U.S. Department of Health, Education and Welfare, Social Rehabilitation Services.
60. Steinberg, F.U., and Ferguson, K.L.: Effect of dantrolene sodium on spasticity associated with hemiplegia, J. Am. Geriatr. Soc. **23**:70, 1975.
61. Lehmann, J.F.: Biomechanics of ankle-foot orthoses: prescription and design, Arch. Phys. Med. Rehabil. **60**:200, 1979.
62. Taylor, M.M., Schaeffer, J.N., Blumenthal, F.S., and Grisell, J.L.: Perceptual training in patients with left hemiplegia, Arch. Phys. Med. Rehabil. **52**:163, 1971.
63. Fisher, C.M., and Curry, H.B.: Pure motor hemiplegia of vascular origin, Arch. Neurol. **13**:30, 1965.
64. Kottke, F.J.: Neurophysiologic therapy for stroke. In Licht, S., editor: Stroke and its rehabilitation, New Haven, 1975, Elizabeth Licht, Publisher.
65. Kottke, F.J.: From reflex to skill: the training of coordination, Arch. Phys. Med. Rehabil. **61**:551, 1980.
66. Stern, P.H., McDowell, F., Miller, J.M., and Robinson, M.: Effects of facilitation exercise techniques in stroke rehabilitation, Arch. Phys. Med. Rehabil. **51**:526, 1970.
67. Wolf, S.L., Baker, M.P., and Kelly, J.L.: EMG biofeedback in stroke: effect of patient characteristics, Arch. Phys. Med. Rehabil. **60**:96, 1979.
68. Basmajan, J.V., Kukulka, C.G., Narayan, M.G., and Tabeke, K.: Biofeedback treatment of foot-drop after stroke compared with standard rehabilitation technique: effects on voluntary control and strength, Arch. Phys. Med. Rehabil. **56**:231, 1975.
69. Anderson, T.P., and Kottke, F.J.: Stroke rehabilitation: a reconsideration of common attitudes, Arch. Phys. Med. Rehabil. **59**:175, 1978.
70. Steinberg, F.U.: The stroke registry: a prospective method of studying stroke, Arch. Phys. Med. Rehabil. **54**:31, 1973.
71. Newman, M.: The process of recovery after hemiplegia, Stroke **3**:702, 1972.
72. Sweet, R.D., and McDowell, F.H.: Five years' treatment of Parkinson's disease with levodopa, Ann. Intern. Med. **83**:456, 1975.
73. Boshes, B.: Sinemet and the treatment of parkinsonism, Ann. Intern. Med. **94**:364, 1981.
74. Hoehn, M.M.: Bromocriptine and its use in parkinsonism. J. Am. Geriatr. Soc. **29**:251, 1981.
75. Cinquegrana, O.D.: Chronic cervical radiculitis and its relationship to "chronic bursitis," Am. J. Phys. Med. **47**:23, 1968.
76. Sakuma, J., Hinterbuchner, C., Green, R.F., and Silber, M.: Rehabilitation of geriatric patients having bilateral lower extremity amputations, Arch. Phys. Med. Rehabil. **55**:101, 1974.
77. Waters, R.L., Perry, J., Antonelli, D., and Hislop, H.: Energy cost of walking of amputees: the influence of level of amputation, J. Bone Joint Surg. **58A**:42, 1976.
78. Sulzle, H., Pagliarulo, M., Rodgers, M., and Jordan, C.: Energetics of amputee gait, Orthop. Clin. North Am. **9**:2:358, 1978.
79. Gonzalez, E.G., Corcoran, P.J., and Reyes, R.L.: Energy expenditure in below-knee amputees: correlation with stump length, Arch. Phys. Med. Rehabil. **55**:111, 1974.
80. Kihn, R.B., Warren, R., and Beebe, G.W.: The "geriatric" amputee, Ann. Surg. **176**:305, 1972.
81. Burgess, E.M., and Romano, R.L.: The management of lower extremity amputees using immediate postsurgical prostheses, Clin. Orthop. **57**:137, 1968.
82. Malone, J.M., Moore, W.S., Goldstone, J., and Malone, S.J.: Therapeutic and economic impact of a modern amputation program, Ann. Surg. **189**:798, 1979.
83. Kane, T.J., III, and Pollak, E.W.: The rigid versus soft postoperative dressing controversy: a controlled study in vascular amputees, Am. Surg. **46**:244, 1980.
84. Warren, R., et al.: The Boston interhospital amputation study, Arch. Surg. **107**:861, 1973.
85. Kohn, K.H.: Use of lower-extremity prostheses in geriatric amputees, Arch. Phys. Med. Rehabil. **51**:99, 1970.
86. Steinberg, F.U., Garcia, W.J., Roettger, R.F., and Shelton, D.J.: Rehabilitation of the geriatric amputee, J. Am. Geriatr. Soc. **22**:62, 1974.
87. Steinberg, F.U., Sunwoo, I., and Roettger, R.F.: Advances in the rehabilitation of geriatric amputees, pre-

sented at the 12th International Congress of Gerontology, Hamburg, Germany, July 16, 1981.
88. Amsterdam, E.A., Wilmore, J.H., and DeMaria, A.: Exercise in cardiovascular health and disease, New York, 1977, Yorke Medical Books.
89. Wenger, N.K., and Hellerstein, H.K.: Rehabilitation of the coronary patient, New York, 1978, John Wiley & Sons, Inc.
90. Pollock, M.L., and Schmidt, D.H.: Heart disease and rehabilitation, Boston, 1979, Houghton Mifflin Co.
91. American Heart Association: Cardiac rehabilitation program guide, Dallas, 1977, American Heart Association.
92. Wenger, N.K.: Rehabilitation after myocardial infarction, J.A.M.A. **242:**2879, 1979.
93. A.M.A. Council on Scientific Affairs: Physician supervised exercise programs in patients with coronary heart disease, J.A.M.A. **245:**1463, 1981.
94. Froelicher, V., et al.: Cardiac rehabilitation: evidence of improvement in myocardial perfusion and function, Arch. Phys. Med. Rehabil. **61:**517, 1980.

CHAPTER 33 · PHYSICAL THERAPY

Robert J. Hickok

Physical therapy by definition, physis (natural) therapy (treatment), appears to be ideally suited to contribute to treatment programs designed for the disabled or well members of the aged population. Over the past two decades physical therapists have developed an in-depth knowledge of treatment procedures for managing neuromuscular-skeletal disabilities, locomotor problems, soft tissue injuries, or generalized nonspecific debilitation occurring from inactivity. Moving from a narrow heat, light, water, electricity concept of physical therapy, the physical therapist now focuses major attention on the assessment and correction of physical disability whatever the cause.

It is the physical therapist's ability to deal with problems and aberrations of movement that form the foundation for the practice of physical therapy as related to the aged population. The physical therapist's in-depth understanding of pathokinesiology, whether it be in the evaluation of an arm paralyzed by stroke or analysis of a pathologic gait resulting from Parkinson's disease, should provide an essential component to restorative programs for the aged. Another example would be the management of patients with intertrochanteric fractures of the hip. These patients would be seen for early mobilization to improve strength and range of motion as well as early ambulation. An effective physical therapy program for this type of patient, resulting from a sound referral relationship with a knowledgeable physician, might reduce the recovery period from a year to 3 months. A totally functional end product may result, with an aged patient (65 years and over) being able to function independently in whatever mode of living desired—an achievement that incidentally would reduce health care costs significantly.

In the past, physical therapists have not tended to become geriatric specialists. They have not written extensively about this age group (20 articles in *Physical Therapy* and its predecessor journals from 1921 to 1979) and to some extent have been resistant to becoming involved in a totally geriatric setting. In the main, treatment of the geriatric patient has been integrated into the total patient population being seen by physical therapists. The advent of medicare in 1966 altered the situation significantly. Physical therapists have moved in increasing numbers into skilled nursing facilities, nursing homes, and home health agencies in which the patient population is essentially over the age of 65 years. Thus the unique problems of the aged population are becoming increasingly important to physical therapists.

The role of the physical therapist in the care of the disabled aged might be considered paradoxical as well as essential. Individuals over 65 years of age represent the fastest growing group in the total population, numbering some 20 million; this number is six and one half times larger than it was in 1900. In fact, the most elderly of the aged population increased at an even greater rate, with the current median age of the above 65-year-old group being 71 years.[1,2] Society is faced, then, with a growing segment of the population with a greater need for services and the least capability to respond to those services. This places extraordinary responsibilities on those individuals (including physical therapists) who are responsible for initiating and carrying out restorative programs for the elderly. The variability among older individuals is startling. Certainly, genetic makeup and life-style play a prominent role in the physical condition of aged individuals. Those compulsive, disciplined people who pursued a sound ongoing exercise program that maintained muscular tone and skeletal flexibility should respond better to restorative programs necessitated by catastrophic disease or disability. Pessimism should not dominate in treating the aged. The evidence of effective restorative programs is rather extensive in the medical literature. For example, Steinberg et al.[3] and others have demonstrated that advancing technology in surgical techniques and prosthetic replacement of below-knee limbs has been effective in restoring a number of elderly patients with lower extremity amputations to an active ambulatory mode of living. These people previously would have been relegated to a wheelchair existence.

It is the purpose of this chapter to review briefly the value of physical therapy in the care of the aged. It is not intended to be a detailed treatise on physical therapy methodology.

EVALUATIVE PROCEDURES

Joint range-of-motion tests

A significant baseline test provided by the physical therapist is the measurement of joint ranges of motion. Characteristically with aging there is a gradual diminution of available joint motion. By way of example, some commonly seen changes that must be taken into account are as follows: (1) the increase in the normal thoracic kyphosis, with subsequent loss of forward flexion-elevation of the humerus; (2) a gradual tightening of the lumbosacral structures, the hamstrings, and in some cases the gastrocnemius-soleus group, thus compromising the ability to assume a long sitting position, and when extreme, to sit up straight in bed; and (3) hip flexor tightness with loss of the normal hip extensor mechanism is a common problem. These changes in joint range often represent poor postural habits, which contribute to the functional decline of the aged individual. With disease and subsequent inactivity, other changes frequently seen are loss of abduction of the thumb and straightening of the palmar arch, tightness at the metacarpophalangeal and interphalangeal joints, and wrist flexor tightness. In the lower extremity of special concern are tight external rotators of the hips, flexion contractures of the knees, and equinus deformities at the ankles. Loss of these key motions has a devastating effect on the residual functional capability of the elderly patient.

Accurate joint range measurement requires a definitive knowledge of basic principles of anatomy and kinesiology, that is, identification of joint centers, a thorough understanding of basic joint types, and expected normal joint range values. The simple protractor arthrometer (goniometer) continues to be a useful device, and if used carefully to screen out vicarious movements, can be accurate within 5 degrees. All physical therapists have extensive training in this technique and can administer the test and interpret the results effectively. The American Academy of Orthopaedic Surgeons periodically publishes a monograph describing techniques for joint range measurement and providing tables of normal values.[4]

Muscle testing

The techniques of manual muscle testing have been developed to a high state of efficiency by physical therapists. These techniques, carefully nurtured as an evaluative tool in the care of poliomyelitis patients, must be altered somewhat when used in the geriatric patient. The methods of grading muscle tests have been essentially unchanged for 50 years. In 1916 Lovett introduced a method of grading muscles from "gone" to normal.[5] Subsequent refinement in technique, whether using percentages to express levels of strength or other values, largely copied the earlier work of Lovett. Certainly a normal muscle for a geriatric patient varies somewhat from a younger norm. There have been attempts at quantitating strength levels in geriatric patients using strain gauges and electronic recording equipment. It has been suggested that a new set of values must be developed to establish more accurate bases for the interpretation of normal strength of the geriatric patient.[6] Also to be seriously questioned is the continued use of the classic muscle test in evaluating weakness in patients suffering from upper motor neuron disease. In such patients profound changes occur such as hyperreflexia, clonus, and spasticity, which render classic muscle testing inconclusive. Michels,[7] in a remarkably thorough paper, presented a functional method of testing the strength in the patient with upper motor neuron disease. These procedures should be a part of the armamentarium of a physical therapist practicing with geriatric patients.

Activities of daily living

Important to all patients, but critical to the elderly individual, is a total assessment of self-care needs. Setting an accurate baseline of self-care ability is perhaps the most sensitive barometer for measuring progress in rehabilitative patient care. As exercises improve strength, restore motion, or enhance coordination, the real proof of progress is reflected in the patient's ability to feed himself, dress, transfer from bed to wheelchair, and ultimately to walk. These techniques, developed and refined by Lawton[8] and others, use self-care charts listing up to 100 activities, which record whether a patient can accomplish a task independently, with supervision, with assistance, with adaptive equipment, or not at all. A more detailed discussion of activities of daily living are presented in Chapters 32 and 34.

RESPONSE TO EXERCISE

By far the most widely used procedures in caring for the elderly disabled individual by physical therapists is the selective use of a broad range of exercises. The term *exercise* is a general one, denoting activity directed toward strengthening muscles, improving endurance, maintaining and improving range of motion, and improving coordination. The adaptation of these procedures provides the keystone to restorative programs for the aged. The problems become more complex when viewed in the context of normal physiologic changes from aging, often compounded by the deconditioning of inactivity and complicated by disease and injury.

There is a gradual diminution of functional capability of specific organ systems as a result of aging, usually noticeable past the age of 40 years. This is particularly true for activity-dependent systems such as the cardiovascular system, the musculoskeletal system, and the autonomic nervous system. The most striking example of the effect of prolonged inactivity (bed rest) is muscular atrophy and the corollaries to this, weakness and decrease in endurance. In addition, atrophy of bone is often a resultant of inactivity. Gerontologists have long conjectured on the usefulness of exercise in the care of the aged. Some investigators have concluded that physical training in individuals past the age of 40 years is only modestly effective and past the age of 60 years has almost no observable effect.[9] However, others have shown significant improvement in physical work capacity from regulated exercise programs.[10]

Several years ago Perkins and Kaiser[11] compared the effectiveness of short-term isotonic and isometric exercise in persons over 60 years of age. A total of twenty individuals were used, ranging in age from 62 to 84 years, with the average age being 73.6 years. The standard 10 repetition maximum of DeLorme was used for the isotonic exercises. Isometric exercises consisted of 6-second holds in a test position repeated three times. Three muscle groups were included in the program: (1) plantar flexors of the ankle, (2) extensors of the knee, in a sitting position, and (3) extensors of the hip, in a supine position. The individuals exercised three times a week until a plateau in strength was noted, usually at the end of 6 weeks. The program resulted in an increase from a mean of 24.54 pounds to a mean of 38.50 pounds, a 56.88% increase for the isotonic group. The isometric group progressed from a mean of 28.92 pounds to a mean of 42.17 pounds, an increase of 45.82%. Of significance is that after 5 months the isotonic group held a mean of 43.11% more than their initial level, whereas the isometric group were able to hold a mean of 30.81% more than they could initially. The authors of this classic study conjectured that with such obviously significant gains in strength, it would appear wise to consider preventive resistive exercises for the aged populations of nursing homes as a means of retaining functional ability and reducing nursing care needs. For some obscure reason this project has not been repeated using a larger geriatric population.

More recently deVries[12] studied the physiologic effects of an exercise training regimen on men 52 and 88 years of age. In this study 112 white males voluntarily participated in a vigorous exercise program for varying periods of time, with 8 individuals completing 42 weeks of training.

After medical clearance a physiologic efficiency profile test was administered covering: (1) resting blood pressure; (2) skinfolds to estimate the percentage of body fat; (3) muscle relaxation using electromyographic methods; (4) muscle strength and girth; (5) maximal oxygen consumption; (6) oxygen pulse at a heart rate of 145 per minute; (7) pulmonary function; and (8) physical work capacity on the bicycle ergometer. This profile was readministered at regular intervals during the course of the study. The training program consisted of calisthenics, a walk-run program, stretching, and aquatics. The most significant findings related to the oxygen transport system. At a heart rate of 145 per minute the oxygen pulse increased by 29.4% and the minute volume of respired air by 35.2%. Arm strength improved by 11.9%. Significant decrease was noted in the percentage of body fat. Physical work capacity improved, as well as both systolic and diastolic blood pressure at rest. The control individuals showed no improvement when tested. The author concluded that the trainability of elderly men with respect to physcial work capacity is probably greater than had been suspected and does not depend on their having trained vigorously in youth as had been postulated by others. These studies strongly support the concept that deterioration of physical capabilities of the aged can be positively influenced by an appropriately conceived and professionally administered exercise program.

It is clear that the reasonably healthy aged, or even the aged individual with multiple chronic problems that reduce overall capability, can respond to graded activity. However, this response is greatly altered by diseases and disabilities such as arthritis, upper and lower motor neuron disease, fractures, myositis, disuse, or injury. In the face of disease or disability, safety margins are reduced, and caution becomes critical to the physical therapist treating the older patient. All exercises must be carried out with full understanding of inherent physical limitations and clear medical indications for activity.

THERAPEUTIC EXERCISES

Range-of-motion exercises

As noted previously, the normal aging process brings about an almost imperceptible diminution in normal joint motion and muscle strength. When compounded by active arthritis, an upper motor neuron lesion, injury, or an inflammatory process, muscles and joints become fibrotic and a rapid decline in joint mobility occurs. In many cases simple range-of-motion exercises can prevent or retard contractures from occurring. When possible, patient should be trained to carry out cardinal range-of-motion exercises independently. Active-assistive exercises may be used when moderate pain or spasticity is present, with the physical therapist ensuring full motion. In the face of more severe pain, limbs should passively be taken through as full a range of motion as tolerated. However, pain persisting for 6 to 12 hours indicates too vigorous an exercise bout. A key to the effectiveness of range-of-motion exercises is persistence in maintaining a daily exercise program. Obviously, the most effective flexibility exercises are carried out before the development of contractures.

The actual techniques of providing range-of-motion exercises skillfully requires close communication between the physical therapist and patient. For the upper extremities mild manual traction may be applied to the limbs to ensure effective proprioceptive response by the patient. Active and active-assistive exercises are preferable, and passive motion should be used only when necessary. In the lower extremities, because of the size of the limb segment, manual traction is often not possible, thus the limb must be handled skillfully to ensure acceptance by the patient. Care must be taken not to grasp the limbs over painful joints or to carry out motions not clearly understood by the patient. An excellent guide for correct technique in these exercises is contained in a series of monographs published by the federal government. "Strike Back at Stroke"[13] and "Strike Back at Arthritis"[14] are examples of these publications.

Stretching

Joint motion, once lost, is difficult to regain. This is particularly true for elderly patients for the multiple reasons previously stated. Indeed, in a joint such as the shoulder, loss of 85% of motion precludes the use of conservative measures to restore motion. In such cases manipulation, by a surgeon, under anesthesia, may be the treatment of choice. On the other hand, less severe contractures may be amenable to stretching. A well-trained physical therapist may restore motion by carrying an extremity through the available range-of-motion with a slow subtle stretch at the end of the arc of motion. Finger ladders, shoulder wheels, and overhead pulleys, although more time-honored than effective, may be used as assistive devices. For stretching well-established contractures in the lower extremities, such as seen in postfracture cases, the use of low-resistance stretching by means of a weighted pulley system, or sandbags, may be effective. This permits an extended period of stretch, more tolerable to the patient and frequently more effective than manually administered techniques.

One of the most commonly used forms of stretching (or traction) is that applied to the spine. The spinal column and adjacent soft tissues, which are vulnerable to osteoarthritis, intervertebral disc changes, and a variety of ill-defined soft tissue problems, can effectively be stretched by motorized traction units or simple over-door devices using sandbags or water bags for resistance. The intent of this stretching routine is either separation of the vertebral facets or stretch of the neighboring musculature.

The inappropriate application of stretching techniques can be hazardous. Ligaments, tendons, and muscles in the elderly are less elastic and therefore subject to injury. If the patient is in an advanced state of deconditioning, osteoporosis may be present, and overzealous stretching may induce a fracture.

As noted, attempts to stretch well-established contractures have equivocal results, thus emphasizing the need for preventive exercise programs. King and Herzig[15] described such a program for a generalized geriatric population, all of whom were over the age of 60 years. Simple range-of-motion exercises were carried out in groups for 5 minutes each day (with medical approval) as a means of maintaining and improving muscle strength and general flexibility.

Strengthening exercise

One of the critical elements of a therapeutic exercise program is the adaptation of existing techniques of strengthening exercises to the elderly individual. Exercises for improving strength are largely based on empiricism. It has been long accepted that muscles with appropriate nerve supply will respond to graded resistance by becoming stronger and in most cases hypertrophied. However, before considering exercise techniques, a review of basic muscle function from a kinesiologic standpoint is in order. Functionally, muscles can be classified as (1) prime movers or agonists, which are primarily responsible for a movement; (2) synergists, which assist prime movers; (3) antagonists; and (4) stabilizers. Muscles can perform any of these functions depending on the specific action required. Care must be taken to ensure appropriate balance between antagonists and agonists. The wrist flexors and extensors, in addition to their prime movements, act as stabilizers of the wrist. The continued exercising of a disproportionately strong wrist flexor, in face of a weak wrist extensor, would be inappropriate. Synergistic muscles should be excluded from an exercise set if the prime mover is the clear objective of the program. As an example, care must be taken to exclude the brachioradialis muscle if the goal of the exercise program is to strengthen the biceps muscle. However, in many cases total strength of a limb is the goal, and agonists and synergists are strengthened concurrently.

Of equal concern is the position assumed for exercise sets. The elderly patient should assume positions of comfort that provide maximum mechanical advantage. Conversely, exercise positions that place stress on adjacent structures should be avoided. If the objective of the exercise is to strengthen the hip flexor muscle, straight leg raising from the supine position with weights or a cable attachment to the foot should not be used, since this may cause a secondary strain on the lumbar spine and on the lower abdominal wall.

Strengthening exercises are inherently exercises requiring resistance and are usually classified in two major categories: isotonic, in which the muscle either shortens or lengthens as a limb moves through its range, or isometric, in which the muscle contracts without movement of the part being exercised. Resistance exercises, as noted previously, are more effective when the nerve supply is substantially intact. Weakness resulting from upper motor neuron lesions requires special consideration.

The effectiveness of isometric exercises compared with isotonic exercises is interesting but academic as it relates to their use in programs for the elderly. As noted by Liberson and Asa[16] in their excellent study in which isometric exercises, given to muscles at their normal resting length, appeared to be superior:

> Muscle training is an extremely complex and poorly understood process. In this process the increase in

muscle efficiency is due in part only to the changes in muscle tissue itself. A readjustment of mental attitudes, a re-coordination of the nervous centers, the adaptation of circulatory and metabolic processes—any of these extramuscular factors may play a dominant role. In our experiment these non-muscular forces must have been of great importance, since the increase of performance was both considerable and rapid.*

Thus it seems clear that the choice of an exercise program should be based on (1) the needs of the patient, (2) the setting in which the treatment will be given, and (3) the personnel available to provide the exercise; it should not be based on adherence to any classic system.

Manual resistance exercise given by the physical therapist has the advantage of being sensitively monitored throughout an arc of motion and adjusted to meet the needs of the patient, thus providing an extra measure of safety to the over 65-year-old patient. The major disadvantage, of course, is that resistance levels cannot be measured quantitatively. A second disadvantage is that the presence of a physical therapist is mandated. Certainly for home programs or other settings in which equipment is not available, manual resistance routines are a useful alternative.

In any discussion of isotonic resistance exercise in a medical setting, the work of DeLorme provides a significant bench mark. DeLorme formalized the low repetition-high resistance principle—using the ten resistive maximum (the amount of weight that can be lifted 10 times, but not 11) as the basic exercise standard. His classic routine called for the establishment of a ten resistive maximum (10 RM) each week, with a routine of one half 10 RM, three fourths 10 RM, and 10 RM (30 repetitions) to be carried out daily.[17] Modifications of this routine are widely used today. With many elderly patients, submaximal exercises may be used to avoid undue cardiac and pulmonary distress. Resistance for this type of exercise may be provided by an exercise table, conventional weights, weighted cuffs, saddle sandbags, or pulley-controlled wall weights. Wall weights have the advantage of being safe and quickly adaptable to a variety of arm and leg exercises. However, for lower extremities, particularly knee extensor and flexor muscles, a table equipped with a double lever system* provides a convenient and safe means of exercising.

Isometric exercises have been consistently shown by experimentation to be more efficient than isotonic exercises.[18] However, isometric exercises, when given with maximum effort using "static" holds lasting from 6 to 10 seconds, may cause cramping of the muscles and cause excessive stress on the older patient. As with other routines, submaximal isometric exercises may effectively be used and, indeed, may be the treatment of choice for strengthening muscles adjacent to an extremely painful joint. Here the period of time required to complete the program may be lengthened and smaller increments of improvement be accepted.

More recently, equipment has been developed that provides additional safety and comfort for the older patient carrying out resistive exercise. This equipment provides for a constant speed of motion (isokinetic), preset independently from the amount of force applied.[19] Isokinetic motion permits the patient to work at speeds at which he is comfortable, and to develop a smooth coordinated pattern throughout an arc of motion. Pain occurring at a point in the range of motion will signal the need for reduced force. Since these versatile devices can start, stop, or reverse at any spot in the range, they can be used to improve range of motion in addition to increased endurance or strength.

The physical therapist must constantly monitor the elderly patient's response to resistive exercises. Any sign of excessive or prolonged shortness of breath, cyanosis, or evidence of discomfort indicate excessive effort. The pulse rate should be monitored routinely and steps taken to avoid the Valsalva phenomenon. A more detailed discussion of physiologic response to exercise is included in Chapter 32.

Coordination and facilitation exercises

For the past 25 years physical therapists and others have been intrigued with the management of problems arising from lesions of the cortical and subcortical centers of the brain. In 1953 Kabat and Knott[20] stated: "A major change is occurring in physical therapy for overcoming pa-

*From Liberson, W.T.. In Basmajan, J.V., editor: Therapeutic exercise, ed. 3, Baltimore, 1978, The Williams & Wilkins Co.

*N-K Table.

ralysis. For many years, the treatment of paralysis was based on rest and a gradual increase in activity, with strict avoidance of fatigue, and routine progression in treatment from passive motion to assistive motion, through free motion with gravity eliminated, free motion against gravity, and finally, resistive exercise. Essential components of this treatment routine are careful isolation of motion to single muscles or single motions and avoidance of stretch of the muscles."* Kabat and Knott then went on to describe their proprioceptive neuromuscular facilitation technique with its diagonal patterns, maximal resistance, stretch and mass movement patterns. These authors stated emphatically that investigation of proprioceptive facilitation techniques for a number of years and their application in thousands of cases of paralysis of various types at the Kabat-Kaiser Institute demonstrated the practical value of these techniques in the treatment of paralysis. "This treatment program is, in our opinion, definitely superior to the older routine of treatment."*

Physical therapists have continued to study intensely the problems of central brain lesions. Brunnstrom,[21] in a brilliant series of papers starting in 1956, described with uncanny accuracy the associated reactions of the upper extremity in adult patients with hemiplegia. Later she published two equally thorough studies on walking preparation for adult patients with hemiplegia and the various recovery stages of hemiplegia.[22,23]

Rood, with her often bewilderingly complex system of treatment, emphasizes the need for increased sensory input in treatment. Stockmeyer[24] has stated, "The approach of Rood to neuromuscular dysfunction represents a philosophy of treatment which is concerned with the interaction of somatic, autonomic and psychic factors, and their role in the regulation of motion behavior."

Another widely used treatment technique is that espoused by the Bobaths[25] and presented as the neurodevelopmental treatment approach to the care of central nervous system disease. The treatment they have developed is directed toward disorders of movement and of postural tone, and derangements of the normal postural reflex mechanism. A fundamental principle of treatment is that abnormal postural patterns should be changed and normal postural reactions facilitated. This is effected by reflex-inhibiting patterns controlled at key points while automatic reactions are introduced.

Also having influence on this approach to treatment have been the principles of neuromuscular reflex therapy, as originally described by Fay.[26] Fay believed that human movements are based on primitive patterns of response which were evident in the amphibian, reptilian, and mammalian eras. Fay believed that reflexes are built-in exercises. It was his theory that reflexes are fragments of ancient motor behavior that emerge when higher and more recently developed centers are injured. His treatment procedures attempted to capture and refine the use of these primitive reflex patterns.

These treatment regimens are often used to the exclusion of other forms of treatment. However, Perry[27] takes a more conservative approach by combining the use of surgery, bracing, exercise, and phenol injection to implement her treatment program for the brain injured. She summarizes her program by stating:

> One must conclude that the basic concept behind the various treatment measures applicable to the hemiplegia patient is recognition that the fundamental lesion resides within the brain. Yet only periphery is available to the physical therapist and the physician. As a result the treatment program is channeled along three lines:
>
> 1. Minimization of the stimuli which initiate spasticity.
> 2. Use of reflex patterns and sensory substitutes to develop improved motor control.
> 3. Alterations of the patient's action patterns or the environment to overcome permanent losses.*

This combined approach may provide the best of two worlds, that is, recognition that central lesion problems are different but also including the use of surgery, bracing, and other forms of treatment to maximize treatment effectiveness.

These techniques, which appear to be similar in many ways, have brought about some thoughtful reappraisals of treatment methods. It is now recognized that the use of geometric cardinal range-of-motion exercises for the limbs is unnatural, and the use of diagonal movements

*From Kabat, H., and Knott, M.: Phys. Ther. Rev. **33**:53, 1953.

*From Perry, J.: Phys. Ther. **46**:345, 1966.

lends realism and effectiveness to exercise efforts. Perhaps most impressively from these various approaches has come an extremely accurate cataloging of the various stages of recovery from central lesions of the brain, particularly cerebral vascular accidents. This has resulted in the imaginative use of positional techniques to inhibit spasticity and in the discarding of unsound bracing methods that inappropriately applied resistance in the face of spasticity. The amount of literature produced describing these techniques is impressive. There is an absence, however, of objective studies documenting the effectiveness of these procedures for aged patients. The few that have been written were equivocal and, in one case, refuted the effectivensss of the techniques in treating stroke patients.[28] These procedures, when used, must be integrated into the total treatment plan and be judged both for their therapeutic and cost effectiveness. The often restricted rehabilitative potential of the elderly patient places a premium on the setting of reasonable goals for treatment and the selection of the most efficient way of achieving these goals.

Gait management

More than any other physical activity, walking provides clear insight to the decremental changes that occur with advancing age. Typically the aged show a classic flexion attitude while walking. The trunk assumes a position of mildly exaggerated dorsal kyphosis, the head and neck are forward, and the hips and knees are slightly flexed. Murray et al.[29] in a study of aged men, which largely corroborated findings of previous studies, found a slowing cadence, with shorter and broader stride dimensions and a lessening of the swing phase time compared with stance phase. The gradual dampening of the amplitudes of the compensatory mechanisms of the body during walking was pervasive. Decreases were noted in (1) the vertical oscillations of the head, (2) transverse rotation of the pelvis, (3) sagittal rotation of the hip, (4) ankle extension late in stance phase, (5) knee flexion and heel elevation early in the swing phase, (6) the forekick at the end of the swing phase, (7) the heel-floor angle at the instant of initial floor contact, and (8) shoulder flexion on the forward arc of the arm swing and less elbow extension on the backward arc. As expected, the amplitude of the lateral oscillations of the head increased in keeping with the broader base during stance phase. The elderly individuals also increased their foot-floor distances, despite the decrease in the amplitude of other gait factors analyzed. This appeared to be a subliminal need for security on their part, and in fact it was clear that the restrained nature of walking for the elderly individual, overall, was an attempt to secure maximum safety.

An understanding of these gait changes occurring in the healthy aged is fundamental to carrying out gait evaluations and gait management programs for elderly individuals suffering disabilities from musculoskeletal or neurologic causes. In gait evaluations, an altered set of determinants must be employed to provide a true picture of walking. The six gait determinants as described by Saunders, and co-workers[30] cannot be used successfully as a norm for the walking of the aged individual.

It is also significant that with an alteration in gait characteristics, the aged individual is more subject to falls than other age groups.[31] The cause of these falls has been attributed to several things—poor vision, vertigo, cerebral vascular accidents, postural hypotension, proprioceptive inadequacies, arthritis, and osteoporosis. Whatever the cause, concern about potential falls should provide a bench mark for the practicing physical therapist in setting up goals and choosing walking aids for the disabled elderly.

Gait training for the aged requires modification of techniques used for younger age groups. Time periods spent simply standing and relearning basic balance and gait techniques in the parallel bars may have to be lengthened. Choice of an appropriate walking aid requires considerable insight. The old rule of thumb that successful crutch walking using axillary crutches is a standard for upright ambulation should be discarded. The type of support chosen should carefully balance the residual functional capabilities of the patient, including problems of energy expenditure and basic safety. Older patients may find the use of a four-legged walk-aid a suitable assistive ambulation device, despite the fact that it requires an awkward nonrhythmic gait pattern. Use of the four-wheeled walker must be questioned because of safety problems; however, a walk-aid with wheels on the front casters only may provide an appropriate type of support for the Parkinson's disease patient who is unable to carry out a lift-step gait necessary in the standard walk-aid. An aged below-knee amputee awaiting the fitting of a tendon-bearing prosthesis may progress directly from a walk-aid to walking with a well-fitted prosthesis and opposite side support with a forearm crutch or a simple cane. Certainly aged patients, as for any patient group, should have the opportunity to use the minimal support necessary to permit safe walking. However, patient safety, of prime importance in all treatment programs, must be omnipresent when caring for the older individual.

A sense of confidence and patience must dominate gait training of the aged. The physical therapist must relate sensitively to the patient. An aged patient appearing aloof or seemingly confused may be responding to the "busy atmosphere" of a physical therapy or rehabilitation department. Shifting early training sessions to the privacy of a treatment room may prove beneficial in these situations.

USE OF PHYSICAL AGENTS

There has long been a strong association made by the lay public in the use of heat, cold, light, electricity, massage, and water in treating the degenerative problems of aging. This is unfortunate in that graded activity may be far more important. However, in most treatment settings an impressive array of physical agents is usually available. These may include whirlpool baths, both limb and full body emersion, hot packs (silica gel type), cold packs, paraffin baths, shortwave, and ultrasound diathermy, infrared, ultraviolet, and low-voltage electric stimulators, and massage. The physiologic effects of heat, cold, low-frequency electricity, and massage have been exhaustively discussed elsewhere and will not be included here.[32] Of importance is an understanding of the appropriate role of these agents in an aged population, both the well and disabled groups. The indiscriminate use of physical agents for long periods of time without clinical indication is not conscionable, and certainly is no replacement for a well-rounded rehabilitation program. First, it is very expensive; second, it is often unproductive; and third, the aged group is most vulnerable to injury. As Stillwell has pointed out, with impairment of cutaneous circulation, burns are more likely to be produced whether superficial or deep methods of heating are used. In addition, he questions the value of deep heating when circulation to the deeper structures is compromised, noting that little is to be gained by shunting what little blood is available from deep to superficial structures. Of concern as well is the possibility of impaired temperature or pain sensory mechanisms. As an example, there is no way of measuring the amount of energy being delivered to the tissues by shortwave or microwave diathermy, thus the sensation of the patient becomes critical. Combining these problems with the possibility of diminished cardiac and respiratory reserve in elderly individuals places obvious constraints on the use of physical agents. However, it should be noted that the judicious use of physical agents can be of value. It has been shown that the addition of ultrasound to a standard program for postoperative management of hip fractures statistically improved the range of motion and the subsequent ambulatory skills of the patients.[33] The study concluded that ultrasound could safely be used in the presence of metal implants and was the treatment of choice for joints such as the hip, which is covered by a thick layer of soft tissue. This illustrates that physical agents can be effectively used with a defined therapeutic end in mind.

Certainly the use of local heat applications for incipient generalized soft tissue and joint pain is valid if used with some discretion. If a choice of procedures is available, the simplified forms of heat such as hot packs (wool or silica gel), infrared, or localized whirlpool would be just as effective and have a greater safety margin.

Restraint should be exercised when low-voltage currents are used as a component of treatment. When used in the care of patients with stroke or other upper motion neuron lesions, this treatment frequently becomes a crutch both for the patient, who becomes addicted to seeing movement in an otherwise paralyzed upper extremity, and for the physical therapist, who uses it as a time filler that requires little attention other than attaching the electrodes. The treatment often continues long after the therapeutic intent has been forgotten.

Over the past decade, with the miniaturization of electrical stimulators, the use of electrical stimulation has broadened considerably. For example, many physical therapists and others have been in the forefront in the use of transcutaneous electrical nerve stimulation (TENS) as the treatment of choice in the management of pain. A review of the literature reveals a wealth of material that explains the neurophysiologic basis for response to TENS,[34,35] the use of TENS devices,[36] and case studies of treatment programs.[37] There is, however, little evidence of objective, double-blind studies evaluating TENS in relationship to other forms of treatment or placebos. Since chronic refractory pain is often a major problem for the aged, TENS should be considered with other forms of treatment. The subjective nature of the pain response requires that such treatment programs be evaluated in an austerely honest manner and stopped promptly if they are clearly not effective.

TREATMENT SETTINGS

The care of the aged patient by the physical therapist often requires an added dimension to be effective. That dimension is the inclusion of the home as a treatment center. It has been shown that a major defect in the treatment chain is at the point when a patient is discharged home from the hospital or rehabilitative facility.[38] Techniques in walking training, stair climbing, and activities of daily living laboriously learned in an institutional setting can be totally lost if provisions for home management are not included. This is true for several reasons:

1. Some elderly patients are often confused and frightened in an institutional setting and are thus uncooperative and subsequently not responsive to a treatment program.
2. Skills learned in an institutional setting cannot be accomplished in the altered environment of the home.
3. There is a feeling among some older people that rest is the panacea for all difficulties, and carefully learned skills are abandoned.
4. Many patients, particularly older ones, are more amenable to treatment in the familiar surroundings of their own home. They often do not adjust to the seemingly confused atmosphere of a busy physical therapy department.

Follow-up instruction, and in some cases more comprehensive programs, ensure that treatment goals achieved in the hospital are not lost on return home. This requires some adjustment on the part of the practicing physical therapist. In the home a premium is placed on improvisation and adaptation. The physical therapist must learn to function without the trappings of a well-equipped department and adjust the patient and the environment of the home into a workable setting. The concept that physical therapists should function only as consultants to home health agencies should be abandoned wherever possible. If an effective continuum of care is to be achieved, adding this element of care is essential.

CONCLUSION

Providing care for the aged places a special responsibility on the physical therapist. The advent of total joint replacement, improved prosthetic and orthotic devices, and more enlightened approaches to cardiac and pulmonary rehabilitation all require a superior technical competence when dealing with the most fragile component of society.

However, as pointed out by LeGuin,[39] it may be more important to understand the less tangible aspects of care, that is, (1) sensitive concern about the individuality of the patient, (2) patience and psychological reinforcement for small achievements to help restore lost self-confidence and favorable body image, (3) a realization that the geriatric patient may require more time for verbalization and more time for repetition of activities, (4) an appreciation for the variability that can exist, and (5) the establishment of reasonable goals.

In short, physical therapists must be flexible in their approach to treatment. As Mead[40] has indicated, the aged population represents those individuals who are the most fit to survive; they often show significant resources of courage and endurance. While metabolic processes slow down, disease processes slow down as well. Multiple diagnoses do not indicate cumulative disability. Each patient requires a careful assessment of residual physical and mental capabilities and a precisely designed restorative program to meet individual needs.

REFERENCES

1. United States Department of Commerce: Bureau of Census reports, Washington, D.C., 1970, U.S. Government Printing Office.
2. Brotman, H.L.: The fastest growing minority—the aging, speech presented to the 50th National Agricultural Conference, U.S., Department of Agriculture, February, 1972.
3. Steinberg, F.U., Garcia, W.J., Roettger, R.F., and Shelton, D.J.: Rehabilitation of the geriatric amputee, J. Am. Geriatr. Soc. **22:**2, 1974.
4. American Academy of Orthopaedic Surgeons: Joint mo-

tion: methods of measuring and recording, Chicago, 1965, The Academy.

5. Legg, A.T.: Physical therapy in infantile paralysis. In Mock, H.E., editor: Principles and practice of physical therapy, vol. 2, Hagerstown, Md., 1932, W.F. Prior Co., Inc.
6. deVries, H.A.: Exercise intensity threshold improvement of cardiovascular-respiratory function in older men, Geriatrics **26**(4):94, 1971.
7. Michels, E.: Evaluation of motor function in hemiplegia, Phys. Ther. Rev. **39**:589, 1959.
8. Lawton, E.B.: Physical rehabilitation for daily living, New York, 1952, McGraw-Hill Book Co.
9. Hollman, W.: Changes in the capacity for maximal and continuous effort in relation to age. In Jokl, E., and Simon, E., editors: International research in sport and physical education, Springfield, Ill., 1964, Charles C Thomas, publisher.
10. Skinner, J.S., Holloszy, J.O., and Cureton, T.K.: Effects of a program of endurance exercises on physical work—capacity and anthropometric measurements of fifteen middle aged men, Am. J. Cardiol. **14**:747, 1964.
11. Perkins, L.C., and Kaiser, H.L.: Results of short term isotonic and isometric exercise programs in persons over sixty, Phys. Ther. Rev. **41**:633, 1961.
12. deVries, H.: Physiological effects of an exercise training regime upon men aged 52-88, J. Gerontol. **25**:325, 1970.
13. United States Department of Health, Education and Welfare: Strike back at stroke, Washington, D.C., 1958, U.S. Government Printing Office.
14. United States Department of Health, Education and Welfare: Strike back at arthritis, Washington, D.C., 1963, U.S. Government Printing Office.
15. King, F., and Herzig, W.F.: Golden age exercises, New York, 1968, Crown Publishers, Inc.
16. Liberson, W.T.: Brief isometric exercises. In Basmajan, J.V., editor: Therapeutic exercise, ed. 3, Baltimore, 1978, The Williams & Wilkins Co.
17. DeLorme, T.L.: Restoration of muscle power by heavy resistance exercise, J. Bone Joint Surg. **27**:645, 1945.
18. Hettinger, T., and Muller, E.A.: Muskelleistung und Muskeltraining, Arbeitsphysiologie **15**:111, 1953.
19. Thistle, H.G., Hislop, H.J., Moffroid, M., and Lowman, E.W.: Isokinetic contraction—a new concept of resistive exercise, Arch. Phys. Med. Rehabil. **48**:279, 1967.
20. Kabat, H., and Knott, M.: Proprioceptive facilitation technics for treatment of paralysis, Phys. Ther. Rev. **33**:53, 1953.
21. Brunnstrom, S.: Associated reactions of the upper extremity in adult patients with hemiplegia, an approach to treatment, Phys. Ther. Rev. **36**:225, 1953.
22. Brunnstrom, S.: Recording gait patterns of adult hemiplegic patients, Phys. Ther. **44**:11, 1964.
23. Brunnstrom, S.: Motor testing procedures in hemiplegia based on recovery stages, Phys. Ther. **46**:357, 1966.
24. Stockmeyer, S.A.: An interpretation of the approach of Rood to the treatment of neuromuscular dysfunction. In Bouman, H.D., editor: Proceedings, exploratory and analytical survey of therapeutic exercise, Baltimore, 1967, The Waverly Press, Inc.
25. Bobath, K., and Bobath, B.: The facilitation of normal postural reactions and movements in the treatment of cerebral palsy, Physiotherapy **50**:246, 1964.
26. Fay, T.: Basic considerations regarding neuromuscular and reflex therapy, Spastics Q. **3**:5, 1954.
27. Perry, J.: Orthopedic management of the lower extremity in the hemiplegic patient, Phys. Ther. **46**:345, 1966.
28. Stern, P.H., et al.: Effects of facilitation exercise techniques in stroke rehabilitation, Arch. Phys. Med. Rehabil. **51**:526, 1970.
29. Murray, M.P., Kory, R.C., and Clarkson, B.H.: Walking patterns in healthy old men, J. Gerontol. **24**:169, 1969.
30. Saunders, J.B., Inman, V.T., and Eberhart, H.D.: The major determinants of normal and pathological gait, J. Bone Joint Surg. **35A**:543, 1953.
31. Fine, W.: Geriatric ergonomics, Gerontol. Clin. **14**:322, 1972.
32. Stillwell, G.K.: Therapeutic heat and cold. In Krusen, F.H., Kottke, F.J., and Elwood, P., editors: Handbook of physical medicine and rehabilitation, ed. 2, Philadelphia, 1971, W.B. Saunders Co.
33. Lehman, J.F., Fordyce, W.E., Rathbun, L.A., Larson, R.E., and Wood, D.H.: Clinical evaluation of a new approach in the treatment of contracture associated with hip fracture after internal fixation, Arch. Phys. Med. Rehabil. **42**:95, 1966.
34. Melzack, R., and Wall, P.: Pain mechanisms: a new theory, Science **150**:971, 1965.
35. Wolf, S.L.: Perspectives on central nervous system responsiveness to transcutaneous electrical nerve stimulation, Phys. Ther. **58**:1443, 1979.
36. Lampe, G.N.: Introduction to the use of transcutaneous electrical nerve stimulation devices, Phys. Ther. **58**:1450, 1979.
37. McDelvy, P.L.: Clinical report on the use of specific TENS units, Phys. Ther. **58**:1474, 1979.
38. Hickok, R.J.: The patient and the communication dilemma, Phys. Ther. **46**:1, 1966.
39. LeGuin, K.W.: Some aspects of gerontology: their importance to the physical therapist, Phys. Ther. **44**:348, 1964.
40. Mead, S.: Rehabilitation. In Cowdry, E.V., editor: The care of the geriatric patient, ed. 3, St. Louis, 1968, The C.V. Mosby Co.

CHAPTER 34 · OCCUPATIONAL THERAPY

William C. Mann

Occupational therapy is an essential component of a geriatric patient's treatment plan when the patient has lost the skills necessary for self-care. In addition, occupational therapy intervention is provided when a patient has suffered a disease or injury resulting in dysfunction in his role as a worker. A third area addressed by occupational therapy is the use of leisure time. In occupational therapy the goals of treatment reflect concern with the quality of life; optimal independent functioning is stressed in the areas of self-care, work, and leisure time.

The uniqueness of occupational therapy is that therapeutic goals are approached through involvement in activities. The term *activities* is defined as goal-directed use of a person's time. Cynkin has identified the distinctive features of activities:

> (1) They involve a series of manifest operations, carried out as part of the procedure of day to day living; (2) they involve a process of "doing"; (3) they are characteristic of and necessary to a human existence; (4) they are socioculturally regulated; (5) they delineate and differentiate an idiosyncratic style for each individual; (6) they can be learned.[1]

For occupational therapy treatment, the activity, in some cases, is identical with the goal. For instance, a patient who has suffered a stroke will learn new dressing techniques in occupational therapy by actually practicing dressing. In other cases, the goal of the activity is less apparent. A patient in occupational therapy completing a woodworking project could be increasing strength, joint range of motion, and coordination in preparation for a return to work.

Occupational therapy services are provided at four levels of intervention:

1. To provide preventive measures to protect the elderly individual's ability to perform within his occupational roles. Occupational therapists serve as consultants to senior centers and on committees and boards that develop social and economic policies regarding the elderly.[2,3]
2. To intervene early to minimize adverse effects resulting in dysfunction in the areas of self-care, work, and leisure time activities. Occupational therapists work in adult day care centers, day treatment centers, and early intervention home assistance programs where elderly persons are identified as functioning marginally in independent living.[4-7]
3. To provide rehabilitative treatment where functional limitations prevent the individual from performing in his occupational roles.[8]
4. To assist the dying patient in giving up occupational roles, working with both the patient and his family.[9,10] Occupational therapists work in hospitals, skilled nursing facilities,[11] health-related facilities, rehabilitation centers, and home health care programs[12] with geriatric patients who have suffered severe injury or disease.

This chapter is organized into sections, which reflect the temporal order of occupational therapy involvement in the care of a geriatric patient: referral, evaluation, treatment, and discharge. Fig. 34-1 illustrates the process of occupational therapy intervention.

REFERRAL

The occupational therapist receives and responds to referrals for evaluation and treatment of geriatric patients from many services: physicians, social workers, physical therapists, speech

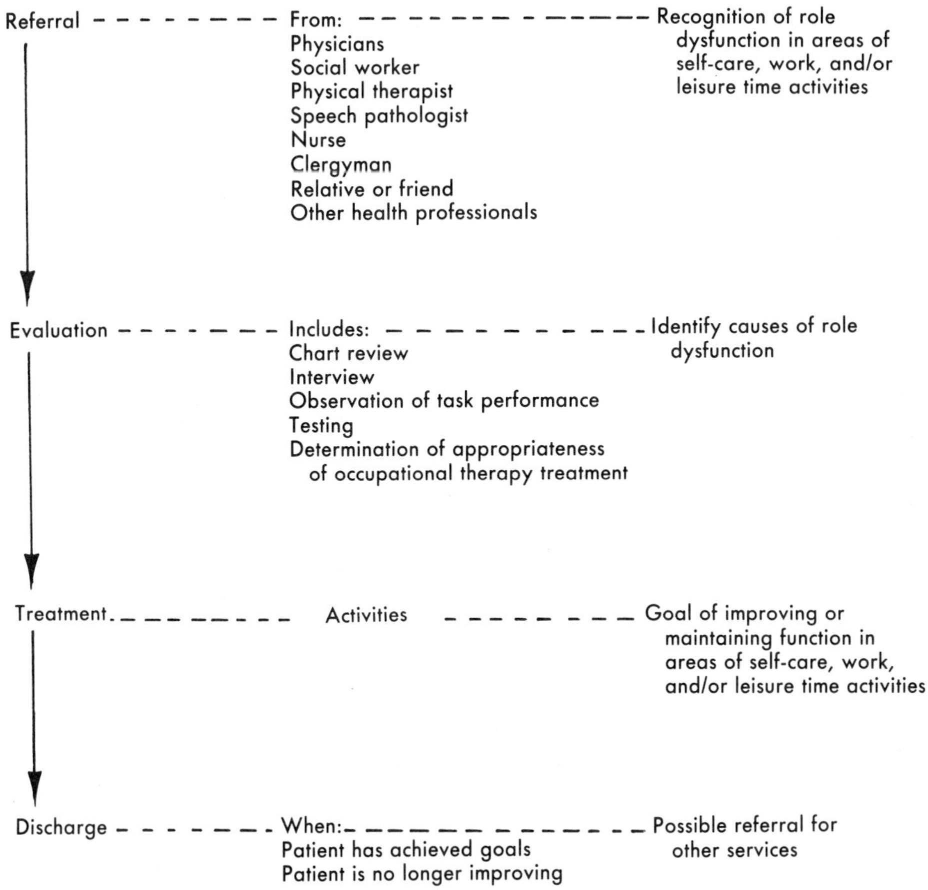

Fig. 34-1. Process of occupational therapy intervention.

pathologists, and others. Referrals include requests for evaluation of a patient's ability to function independently in the home situation, as well as evaluation and treatment within a 24-hour care facility.

The American Occupational Therapy Association has developed a Statement on Occupational Therapy Referral, which recognizes the physician as the person responsible for medical management of a patient. When an occupational therapist receives a referral that clearly requires medical management, the case is referred to a qualified physician. The occupational therapist responds to all referrals but provides services at his own professional discretion.[13]

EVALUATION

When a patient is referred for occupational therapy services and it has been determined that the patient is appropriately referred, an occupational therapy evaluation is carried out. The occupational therapy evaluation of a geriatric patient includes a data gathering process followed by a determination of need for occupational therapy intervention, type of treatment, and need for referral to other health professionals.

Information about the patient is gathered in several ways. First, the patient's chart is reviewed. Information on diagnoses, current health status, social history, and involvement of other health professionals is noted. Next, the patient is interviewed by the therapist to obtain an occupational history. The patient is asked questions concerning self-care, work, and use of leisure time. This may include use of an activity check list or activity configuration protocol.[14]

The area of self-care includes bathing, toileting, hair care, shaving, applying makeup, eating, dressing, functional mobility, and object manipulation. Each of these self-care role performance components requires specific skills. For instance, eating requires sucking, chewing, swallowing, and the use of appropriate utensils. Dressing requires choosing appropriate clothing, dressing in a sequential manner, and fastening and adjusting clothing. Object manipulation requires skills in using both small and large objects such as keys, doorknobs, packages, money, and calculators. The importance of being able to dial a telephone, an activity given little thought by those who have not lost the necessary skills, is not overlooked by the therapist.[15] Functional mobility includes the skills necessary for transferring from bed to chair, from toilet to chair, to move a wheelchair, to ambulate with or without adaptive aids, and use of public and private transportation. In the interview the patient is asked to identify any areas of self-care that have in the past or are currently causing problems. These areas may be explored later through observation of tasks.

Exploration of the role of worker is an important part of the occupational history. Although work refers to skills and performance in the areas of homemaking and home management, parenting, and employment, for the geriatric patient home management and homemaking are usually the most relevant. Specifically, this includes such things as meal planning, meal preparation and clean up, household chores, laundry, household repairs, budgeting, shopping, and home safety. For some geriatric patients, especially those in the young-old category, employment is also relevant to goals for returning to a job or finding a new job. For all patients, the occupational history addresses the role of worker, since past employment as well as home management will be a factor in determining the activity chosen for treatment, if occupational therapy is required.

The last area addressed in the interview is use of leisure time, which includes choosing and participating in activities for relaxation, enjoyment, amusement, and self-expression. Since the geriatric patient is at the time in his life when the opportunity for leisure activities is greatest, the interview focuses closely on this area. Again, the activity chosen for treatment will relate to the patient's patterns of use of leisure time.

Following the chart review and interview, the occupational therapist must decide what additional information about the patient is needed. Unless it has been determined that there are no limitations in the patient's ability to function independently in self-care, work, and leisure time activities, in which case no occupational therapy treatment would be recommended, those dysfunctional areas identified in the chart review and interview will be studied more closely. For example, why is it that this patient is unable to dress himself?

The therapist may choose one or more standardized tests or may select some specific task to determine why a patient has lost a skill. For a physical examination the therapist determines if there are any limitations of joint range of motion or of muscle strength, including grasp and pinch. Limitations in these areas could result in role dysfunction in any or all of the areas of self-care, work, and leisure time activities and could explain an inability to dress oneself. The therapist also tests for limitations in sitting and standing balance, gross and fine coordination, exteroception and proprioception, perceptual-motor skills, vision and hearing, and level of energy output.

A psychosocial evaluation may also provide explanations for dysfunctional performance in self-care, work, or leisure time activities. Again, the therapist may choose standardized tests or may have the patient complete a task, but much information is also gained during the interview. The therapist is concerned with determining alertness, judgment, comprehension, ability to retain directions, attention span, cooperation, motivation, expectations, reaction to illness, frustration tolerance, awareness of limitations, depression, regressed behavior, hostility, anxiety, memory loss, and orientation to person, place, and time.

On completion of the chart review, interview, and administration of specific tests, the occupational therapist makes a decision concerning appropriateness of occupational therapy for the patient. If the patient is dysfunctional in one or more of the three areas addressed by the therapist—self-care, work, and leisure time activities—then the patient has met the first criteria for treatment. Second, if the therapist can identify the reason for the dysfunction, and third, if therapy can alleviate the problem, then occupational therapy is recommended. In some cases, occupational therapy will be recommended when it has been determined that a patient has lost some function, and even though this is nonreversible, without therapy the patient's condition is likely to deteriorate further, causing additional dysfunction in the areas of self-care, work, and/or leisure time activities. Therapy provided when improvement is not a goal is termed maintenance occupational therapy in contrast to functional occupational therapy where improvement in role function is clearly a goal.

TREATMENT

Although occupational therapists provide treatment to patients with a wide range of functional limitations and to patients with almost every medical diagnosis, there is one aspect of occupational therapy which makes it different from any other therapy or treatment. This is the use of an activity for treatment. The choice of activity will relate to (1) nature of role dysfunction (Is it in one or more of the areas of self-care, work, or leisure time activities?); (2) cause of role dysfunction (Is it a physical problem resulting from injury or disease or a mental problem such as depression or confusion?); and (3) specific occupational history of patient (What was this patient's life-style prior to need for intervention?). Information gathered in the occupational therapy evaluation is used for treatment planning.

While the therapist must analyze the three points listed in the preceding paragraph before selecting an activity for treatment, the therapist must also analyze each activity to determine its therapeutic value for a particular patient. An activity such as clay modeling may provide muscle strengthening and active joint range of motion for an arthritic patient's hand, but if the patient is a retired clerk, who never enjoyed work or leisure time activities where his hands would get dirty, then the activity is inappropriate. The study of a particular activity for an individual patient is termed an activity analysis. Outlines for activity analysis have been provided by several authors.[1,16,17]

The possible activities for occupational therapy are as varied as the needs of the patient and the creativity of the therapist and are limited only by environmental factors. For dysfunction in the area of self-care, the activity most often selected is the actual activity the patient is having difficulty performing, including dressing, grooming, eating, and bathing. Ideally, the patient and therapist work right in the patient's living area in practicing techniques or use of adaptive equipment. Crafts are also used in occupational therapy for correcting dysfunction. The major crafts are weaving, woodworking, ceramics, and leatherwork. Other crafts include macrame, knitting, sewing, jewelry making, and mosaics. Other activities include dance, painting, drawing, sculpturing, cooking, cleaning, games, puzzles, gardening, and swimming. The importance of an activity is that it is uniquely suitable for an individual geriatric patient. For example, typing may be both therapeutic and enjoyable for one patient, while knitting might be the most appropriate activity for another patient. Activities can be further categorized as having components that are recreational, industrial, avocational, and educational.

To help clarify the approach of the occupational therapist, an example of a patient with role dysfunction in the area of self-care, a stroke patient, follows:

J.H. was a 68-year-old male who suffered a right cerebral vascular accident (CVA), resulting in left hemiplegia. Following the CVA, he was hospitalized, but had lived at home with his wife prior to the CVA. His wife was not strong enough to care for him unless he was independent in self-care. The occupational therapist evaluated J.H. and found that he could not dress himself, bathe himself, or transfer independently. For 6 weeks, J.H. received daily occupational therapy treatments, learned hemiplegic dressing techniques, practiced transferring between wheelchair and bed and toilet, and established a routine for washing and grooming. Following an evaluation of J.H.'s home, modifications were made for wheelchair mobility, the height of the bed was modified, and grab bars were installed in the bathroom. J.H. was successfully discharged to his home, no longer dysfunctional in the area of self-care.

A second example will demonstrate role dysfunction and occupational therapy intervention in the area of work:

R.D. was a 63-year-old man who had suffered a right hand injury. He had lived alone and had worked as a shipping clerk. This job required some lifting, and following his hand injury, he was unable to work. Evaluation by the occupational therapist established decreased strength and functional grasp of only 8 pounds with his right hand. R.D. was seen on an outpatient basis daily for 90 days. He enjoyed working with wood and was given a wood carving project to complete. This project required grasping a chisel with his right hand while hammering with his left hand. As his grasp strength improved, he began to hold the hammer with his right hand. R.D. also practiced lifting and moving packages, which were weighted, progressively more heavy, to simulate his work environment. On discharge from occupational therapy, R.D. returned to his former job.

A final example will illustrate occupational therapy intervention in the area of leisure time activities:

M.J. was a 70-year-old female who was hospitalized due to confusion and inability to care for herself at home. Following 2 weeks of hospitalization, she was transferred to a skilled nursing facility. Her condition improved, and she became less confused and more able to complete her self-care needs. The occupational therapy evaluation determined that M.J. was depressed and had been living reclusively and drinking heavily since her husband's death 5 years earlier. Prior to her husband's death she had been very active in church groups and enjoyed working with her hands, doing much of her family's tailoring as well as knitting, sewing, cooking, canning, etc. In occupational therapy M.J. began to knit, crochet, and cook, working with a group of alert patients doing similar activities. In 2 months, her mood became more elevated, and she looked forward each day to her activities in occupational therapy. M.J. was discharged to live in a senior citizen's apartment house. Prior to her discharge, the therapist arranged for M.J. to meet with the social club for the apartment house and with the women's group of the church in this neighborhood, where she could continue to have social contact and engage in the leisure time activities she enjoyed.

One disease frequently encountered by the occupational therapist deserves mention. While the occupational therapist approaches the geriatric patient from the perspective of ability to function rather than diagnosis, the symptoms of Parkinson's disease are such as to produce progressive disability and dysfunction.

Nonintention tremor, impairment of righting reflex, rigidity, a shuffle gait (short steps with no swinging of the arms), and difficulty in initiating movements (bradykinesia) are symptoms of Parkinson's disease, which can cause dysfunction in self-care, work, and leisure time activities. On evaluation of a patient with Parkinson's disease, if these symptoms are interfering with function, occupational therapy will be recommended. Short-term goals of treatment often include improved speed, coordination, and mobility; decreased rigidity; and reduction of tremor. Long-term goals involve higher levels of independence in self-care, work, and leisure time activities.

Treatment often involves an approach called proprioceptive neuromuscular facilitation (PNF). This approach uses resistance in movement patterns with passive and active range-of-motion exercise. The approach also stresses the importance of other stimuli including touch and verbal tones. Activities are used in occupational therapy treatment to stress active motion especially in rapid, rhythmic movements.

Blindness is another diagnosis that deserves special mention. Although blindness often appears as a single diagnosis, it frequently accompanies other diseases and even in cases where vision is not totally impaired can cause disruption of ability to function.

The major role of the occupational therapist with a blind patient is in assisting him to develop strategies to maintain an organized environment. In the home, the therapist would, for example, suggest placement of kitchen and eating utensils. Consistency in the placement of objects when tasks are completed is most important.

Systems also need to be developed for coordinating dressing activities. While blindness does not interfere with the ability to dress (dressing while blindfolded is not difficult), choosing appropriate styles and colors is more difficult. Selection of clothing should be done with the help of a sighted person, and clothes can be marked on the label for color.

There are many assistive devices for blind patients ranging from simple adaptations for a telephone keyboard to electronic measuring devices that emit audible signals for determining level of liquid in a cup or container while pouring.

Blindness alone should only result in temporary role dysfunction. However, blindness often occurs with other diseases that also interfere with function, and the therapist must determine appropriate short-term goals, which at first may not be directed toward blindness. For example, before a blind person with decreased strength can practice systems for dressing himself, he must first increase his strength.

The diversity of occupational therapy treatment for the geriatric patient is well documented in the literature. In the area of self-care, problems with swallowing during eating can be addressed with treatment techniques based on principles of neurophysiology.[18] Special techniques have been developed for working with confused patients, which include the use of reality orientation and life review.[19] For many geriatric patients vision is often impaired, and the therapist must address the impairment in planning treatment.[20,21] One of the largest diagnostic categories of geriatric patients receiving occupational therapy services is hemiplegia. Occupational therapy treatment techniques have been designed specifically for hemiplegic patients who are dysfunctional in one or more of the areas of self-care, work, and leisure time activities.[22,23] For regressed patients, sensory training, designed to stimulate each of the five senses, has been used successfully by occupational therapists.[16]

Two additional areas of expertise that occupational therapists possess should be discussed. The first is splinting. Occupational therapists can provide patients with splints to stabilize a joint or body part, most typically in the hand or wrist so that range of motion is maintained. This is frequently necessary for hemiplegic patients to prevent contractures. Splints are also used to substitute for muscle action that has been lost due to injury or disease. These dynamic splints can be constructed to provide wrist and finger flexion or extension. A patient, for example, who is able to flex his fingers but cannot extend them will regain the ability to grasp and release objects with a dynamic splint.

The second area of expertise is adaptive equipment. For many patients use of assistive devices makes the difference in being able to carry out self-care, work, or certain leisure time activities. There are many of these devices ranging from some as simple as a button hook or extended shoehorn to others as mechanically complex as an automatic book page turner. The occupational therapist, after carefully evaluating the patient, is able to determine not only if the patient could use certain assistive devices, but also determines if the device will be used and not left to collect dust on a shelf. There are several suppliers of adaptive equipment for handicapped individuals, and *The American Journal of Occupational Therapy* publishes a list of suppliers of such equipment annually.[25,26]

DISCHARGE

When a patient has achieved treatment goals or is no longer making progress and will not benefit from a maintenance program, he is discharged from occupational therapy. Often on discharge the occupational therapist will make a referral with specific recommendations to other health care providers. In a long-term care facility, this is often the nursing staff. For a patient being discharged to his home, referrals are frequently made to home health care agencies.

REFERENCES

1. Cynkin, S.: Occupational therapy: toward health through activities, Boston, 1979, Little, Brown & Co.
2. Hasselkaus, B.R.: A small group home for the elderly, Am. J. Occup. Ther. **31**:525, 1977.
3. Maguire, G.A.: Volunteer program to assist the elderly to remain in home settings, Am. J. Occup. Ther. **33**:98, 1979.
4. Kiernat, J.M.: Geriatric day hospitals: a golden opportunity for therapists, Am. J. Occup. Ther. **30**:285, 1976.
5. Aronson, R.A.: Programs I: the role of an occupational therapist in a geriatric day hospital setting—Maimonides Day Hospital, Am. J. Occup. Ther. **30**:290, 1976.
6. Williams, R.: Programs II: the day hospital at the Burke Rehabilitation Center, Am. J. Occup. Ther. **30**:293, 1976.
7. Menks, F., et al.: A psychogeriatric activity group in a rural community, Am. J. Occup. Ther. **31**:376, 1977.
8. Maloney, C.C.: The occupational therapist on a geriatric rehabilitation team, Am. J. Occup. Ther. **30**:300, 1976.
9. Gammage, S.L., McMahon, P.S., and Shanahan, P.M.: The occupational therapist and terminal illness: learning to cope with death, Am. J. Occup. Ther. **30**:294, 1976.
10. Oelrich, M.: The patient with a fatal illness, Am. J. Occup. Ther. **28**:429, 1974.
11. Seig, K.W.: The nursing home: occupational therapy services in an institution, Am. J. Occup. Ther. **31**:516, 1977.
12. Hasselkaus, B.R.: Relocation stress and the elderly, Am. J. Occup. Ther. **32**:631, 1978.
13. Manual on administration, Rockville, Md., 1978, American Occupational Therapy Association, pp. 76-77.
14. Matsutsuyu, J.S.: The interest check list, Am. J. Occup. Ther. **23**:323, 1969.
15. Leff, B.: Teaching stroke patients to dial the telephone, Am. J. Occup. Ther. **30**:313, 1976.
16. Fidler, G.S., and Fidler, J.W.: Occupational therapy: a commonwealth process in psychiatry, New York, 1963, Macmillan Inc., pp. 76-80.
17. Hopkins, H.L., Smith, H.D., and Tiffany, E.G.: The activity process. In Hopkins, N.L., and Smith, H.D., editors: Willard and Spackman's occupational therapy, ed. 5, Philadelphia, 1978, J.B. Lippincott Co.
18. Silverman, E.H., and Elfant, I.L.: Dysphagia: an evaluation and treatment program for the adult, Am. J. Occup. Ther. **33**:382, 1979.
19. Kiernat, K.W.: The use of life review activity with confused nursing home residents, Am. J. Occup. Ther. **33**:306, 1979.
20. Cristarella, M.C.: Visual functions of the elderly, Am. J. Occup. Ther. **31**:432, 1977.
21. Baker-Nobles, L., and Bink, M.P.: Sensory integration in the rehabilitation of blind adults, Am. J. Occup. Ther. **33**:559, 1979.

22. Trombly, C.A., and Scott, A.D.: Occupational therapy for physical dysfunction, Baltimore, 1977, The Williams & Wilkins Co.
23. Bouchard, V.C.: Hemiplegic exercise and discussion groups, Am. J. Occup. Ther. **26:**330, 1972.
24. Richman, L.: Sensory training for geriatric patients, Am. J. Occup. Ther. **23:**254, 1969.
25. American Occupational Therapy Association: Buyers guide '79, Am. J. Occup. Ther. **33:**137, 1979.
26. American Occupational Therapy Association: Buyers guide '80, Am. J. Occup. Ther. **34:**137, 1980.

CHAPTER 35 · SPEECH PATHOLOGY

Jacqueline Hartman

The geriatric patient is vulnerable to a number of conditions that can impair interpersonal and internal communication. Hearing loss diminishes awareness of environmental sounds and distorts the clarity of speech messages received. Reduced visual acuity may impair reading and also disrupt visual evaluation and monitoring of written expression. Difficulties with memory manifest themselves in inappropriate statements and even inappropriate behavior. Other alterations of mental status may result in the patient becoming easily confused. Motor disorders may impair writing and speech. Disorders of symbolization and association attributed to central nervous system changes may limit comprehension and expression of language.

Human communciation has many components, only a few of which have been mentioned and only some of which come to the attention of the speech pathologist involved in the rehabilitation of geriatric patients. All aspects are of concern in evaluating patients and planning their rehabilitation program, but this chapter will discuss only verbal communication, that is, speech and language.

DISTINCTION BETWEEN SPEECH AND LANGUAGE

The term *language* encompasses the symbols of verbal communciation. It represents grammar or syntax, vocabulary, and the complexity of sentence structure. Language involves the comprehension of these symbols, heard or read, and expression of these symbols, spoken or written.

Speech, on the other hand, refers to the mechanics of the production of only oral verbal communciation. In evaluating speech, one disregards vocabulary and syntax and considers how well the "machinery" is functioning in producing intelligible oral sounds.

One patient may have intact language but impairment of speech so that the listener cannot comprehend the ideas expressed. Another patient may have good ability to produce the sounds or phonemes (i.e., intact speech) but may have such language impairment that the patient cannot comprehend what has just been said and therefore cannot formulate an effective oral response. The patient cannot think of the intended word or cannot order words into a meaningful sequence.

Speech and language disorders are not mutually exclusive. Particularly with the elderly patient, components of both disorders often exist. Careful quantification of the extent of each component is vital to the physician in determining cause and prognosis and to the speech pathologist in planning a communication rehabilitation program.

LANGUAGE DISORDERS

Although senile dementia is certainly demonstrated as a communication problem and often is characterized by unusual language structures, discussion of its features are more pertinent to other sections of this book. A prominent language disorder in geriatric patients is *aphasia* or *dysphasia*. The latter term implies some degree of impairment of language, whereas the former implies complete loss of language. Dysphasia is semantically more appropriate to describe the impairment, but tradition has preserved the use of the term aphasia in American literature. The terms are generally used interchangeably.

Definition of aphasia

Aphasia is an impairment of the ability to comprehend, process, and/or express verbal language because of damage within the central nervous system. In older patients the primary cause is cerebral vascular disease, although tumor and head trauma are significant causative factors as well. "Aphasia," properly used, implies nothing about hearing sensitivity or motor function of the oral mechanism. It does imply some component of comprehension impairment as well as impairment of expression.

Evaluation of aphasia

Careful examination of receptive and expressive language abilities is perhaps best accomplished through the use of standardized tests for aphasia. The physician may not have access to these materials or time to administer and interpret them but may perform a cursory evaluation in the following manner:

1. Choose about five familiar objects such as a pen, a coin, a watch, a key, eyeglasses, and a spoon. Cards printed with the object's name should be available as should a pencil and paper for the patient.
2. Begin by testing expressive function.
   a. To test oral language:
      (1) Ask the patient to name the objects.
      (2) Ask the patient to repeat the names after you.
   b. To test written language:
      (1) Ask the patient to write the name of each object. Do not supply the name unless the patient is unable to do it alone, and note that this aid was given.
      (2) If even this is unsuccessful, ask the patient to copy the name from the card on which the name is written.
3. Test receptive language next.
   a. To test auditory comprehension: Tell the patient to point to the ________.
   b. To test reading comprehension: Ask the patient to match the word cards with the appropriate objects.

This quick screening method has several advantages over a more informal, less structured approach to evaluation. It is consistently reproducible, allowing the physician to compare patients and develop some idea of relative severity of the deficits should he or she choose to make this examination routine. It is sufficiently simple and the objects are sufficiently familiar so that the patient's level of education or intelligence should not interfere with performance on the test. Premorbidly illiterate patients, of course, cannot be expected to do well with the reading and writing tasks. It is possible to pick up effects of fatigue (more errors as the number of trials increase) or "tuning in" behavior (errors on initial trials, then accurate responses later) because several trials are given for each task.

Expressive skills of the aphasic patient are always more qualitatively impaired than receptive ones. With this testing format the skills most impaired are tested first. Thus the tasks should get easier for the patient as the evaluation progresses. This should compensate somewhat for the effects of tiring. The procedure is free from situational and contextual clues that might enable the patient to perform accurately despite severe language difficulty.

All the tasks just suggested are simple, and errors on any part should be interpreted as a significant indication of aphasia, with one exception: a patient's inability to say the names of the objects either spontaneously or in imitation may not be termed *expressive aphasia* without additonal evidence. The inability to speak may be a manifestation of some degree of speech, not language (i.e., aphasic), impairment. Further testing is imperative in such instances.

Since the preceding tasks are simple, the patient's performance must be considered not only in terms of the accuracy of response, but also the amount of time taken and number of repetitions needed to respond and any self-corrected errors. If the patient is unable to do any of the tasks accurately, the examiner should note whether the patient appears to be attempting the tasks, although making errors. The examiner should also observe if the patient has any verbal output and whether it is intelligible, unintelligible, or perseverative.

More comprehensive evaluation is essential in managing the aphasic patient. As explained earlier, aphasia by definition implies both receptive and expressive impairments. Although expressive difficulties are usually obvious, receptive ones can be quite subtle. DeRenzi and Vignoli[1] have developed a Token Test, which is especially sensitive to auditory comprehension problems and is easily administered by the physician. Others have modified this test. Among the modifications most easily employed in the clinical setting is that of Spellacy and Spreen.[2] The most comprehensive tests for aphasia now available are the Minnesota Test for Differential Diagnosis of Aphasia,[3] the Boston Diagnostic Aphasia Examination,[4] and the Porch Index of

Communicative Ability (PICA).[5] Of these tests, the PICA has the advantage of standard administration format, method for prediction of communicative ability at 6 months after onset of aphasia, and freedom from intellectual and educational variables. The PICA is especially valuable in detecting subtle changes in communication behavior. It has the relative disadvantages of any good psychometric tool in that it requires hours of supervised training to administer and interpret and regular practice in administration to ensure reliability. These factors make it somewhat impractical for the physician and for many speech pathologists who do not deal regularly with aphasic patients.

Many aphasiologists have attempted systems of classification to describe the behavior defined by the evaluation. A number of systems of nomenclature have resulted, and overwhelming confusion has developed. Most systems are based on the characteristics of the patient's spoken output and describe either a fluent or nonfluent aphasia. Patients with fluent aphasia produce inflected, well-articulated strings of words that are usually weak in content and grammatical structure. They exhibit impaired comprehension, little awareness of their deficit, and are described by some as having "receptive" aphasia. Patients with nonfluent aphasia demonstrate a paucity of speech, producing mostly content words in telegraphic patterns. They exhibit awareness of word finding problems, relatively better comprehension than fluent patients, and are sometimes described as showing "expressive" aphasia. The dichotomy of receptive and expressive aphasia is misleading, however, for it implies that the language problem is confined to only one modality. As stated before, both reception and expression are impaired in aphasia but in qualitatively different ways for fluent versus nonfluent aphasias. Until such time as one method of testing is standardized and accepted and one system of classification evolves from it, it is best for physicians and speech pathologists to describe the behavior observed when discussing communicaton disorders, rather than to provide labels.

Prognosis

The neurologically stable patient who has an uncomplicated course after the onset of aphasia is expected to show some spontaneous recovery. This spontaneous recovery period probably extends over the first year after a stroke and the first 2 years after cerebral trauma. The anticipated sequence of improvement is first in attention skills, second in comprehension, and third in expression. Listening and talking often improve more and faster than reading and writing. The patient with only mild to moderate receptive deficits in the early period regains more function than the patient who comprehends little. Automatic speech (counting, singing, responding "hi" and "okay" effortlessly) has little prognostic value regarding the level of eventual recovery of oral language.

It is not realistic to expect aged aphasic patients to recover the same communication levels attained before their illness, unless the aphasia is transient, lasting less than a few days. The damage to the central nervous system limits the reestablishment of the patient's former verbal dexterity. This is not to say that the patient will not regain functional language skills; it means only that verbal communication may not return to its original level of sophistication. It is often helpful to prepare the patient and the patient's family to temper their expectations early in the course of recovery by mutually setting realistic therapy goals.

The speech pathologist's role in rehabilitating the patient commences after careful consideration of prognosis, medical status, and the life situation and communication environment of the patient.

Language rehabilitation

The speech pathologist has an important role to play in comprehensive rehabilitation of the patient's communication status, although there is some spontaneous recovery to be expected.[6] The value of speech therapy in this period of spontaneous recovery has been difficult to demonstrate.[7] Current investigations of early versus delayed intervention by speech pathology services should provide guidelines as to the most cost-effective programs.

The goals should be to help the patient meet the most pressing communication needs with the most sophisticated skills available. It is not realistic to strive to retrain every patient as a functional speaker; it is realistic to expect needs to be expressed at least in a compensatory manner such as ringing a bell, pointing to a picture or word, writing a word, or speaking a telegraphic phrase. For the severely impaired patient with a poor prognosis for recovery of functional talking or writing, the formal language rehabilitation program will be short-term and may only involve teaching the patient some signal to summon help, such as ringing a bell or pressing a hospital call button.

Maximum involvement of the family by the speech pathologist, augmented by counseling by the social worker, is desirable for acceptance of limitations and optimal reinforcement of skills.

The program for elderly patients showing capability for more sophisticated performance should stress the development of functional comprehension before working on expression. Such a format will encourage awareness of errors and eventually the ability to self-correct them. Comprehension is vital to effective expression.

The speech pathologist should use actual materials, words, and phrases that the individual patient actually encounters in the environment. The patient should be trained to use these tools in tasks that are important to survival and that contribute to maximal resumption of family and community roles.

The literature in recent years has suggested the use of teaching machines and standard programs or workbooks in retraining the aphasic patient. This seems particularly inappropriate for the geriatric patient whose ability to generalize what is learned in a workbook to daily communication demands is limited. The communication needs of each individual are unique, and a conscientious therapist should design therapy activities to meet them. Rehabilitation is most effective when tailored to the particular patient, making maximal use of the environmental and situational contexts in which the patient will perform the skills emphasized. The patient and family are more motivated to practice and reinforce meaningful and functional activities than preprepared, standard drill material.[8] Aphasic patients should be trained by the speech pathologist to perform at least the following communication activities:

1. Some method of signaling attention. At simple levels this may mean ringing a bell. At more sophisticated levels the patient may call aloud for the desired person and state the need.
2. Ability to dial the telephone number of a neighbor or nearby family member who is alerted to the possibility of such a call and prepared to react appropriately.
3. A basic concept of money, such as coins needed to purchase candy or a newspaper from a vending machine or proper change needed for public transportation.
4. Ability to produce a signature or at least an "X" with the nondominant hand if necessary.
5. Ability to associate the day or date with the representation on the calendar.
6. Ability to associate railroad time (e.g., 9:15) with the clock face. This is particularly useful if patients are capable of administering their own medications. It is also useful for patients interested in specific television programs mentioned in the television schedule, for appointments, and so on.

The language rehabilitation program should be discontinued when the patient plateaus in the ability to perform more complex tasks. Monthly testing is optimal for detection of this plateau. If the physician and speech pathologist have explained the probable limitations of the disorder and goals of the program before it is begun, termination of intensive training should be easily accepted by the patient and family.

Aphasia groups and "stroke clubs" can provide opportunities for aphasic patients to reinforce their social communication skills and maintain a healthy adjustment to their deficits once individual therapy is discontinued.

Nonverbal means of communication have some limited application for the aphasic patient and will be discussed later in this chapter.

SPEECH DISORDERS

The functional integrity of the oral "machine" involves less complicated mechanisms than those associated with processing and use of symbols of verbal communication. Human speech is the result of precise coordination of the articulators (lips, tongue, soft palate), the respiratory system, and the larynx, all integrated by the central nervous system. In the geriatric population, the etiologic factors of speech disorders are mainly dysfunctions of the central nervous system or alterations of the laryngeal mechanism secondary to cancer therapy.

Laryngeal problems

A frequently encountered speech impairment is that resulting from laryngectomy. When patients have had total removal of the larynx, they become candidates for speech therapy.

Esophageal speech. The current method of choice in reestablishing oral communication is esophageal speech. This technique involves forcing air into the esophagus, trapping it there, and then audibly "belching." The bolus of air is used to form words with the lips, tongue, and soft palate in the same manner as before the operation. Mastery of esophageal voice is not always immediate. It may require several weeks of daily sessions before an audible belch or "charge" is produced. Training can then proceed in an orderly fashion from production of single syllable words to short phrases and finally to longer utterances that are produced effortlessly. The oral intake of air becomes less noticeable to listeners, and patients learn with practice to pace themselves and their sentence phrasing. No doubt the greatest practice is in daily social contacts. The speech pathologist should guide patients to attempt more syllables per charge as their ability permits, to utilize optimal phrasing, and to articulate as precisely as possible. Patients who are motivated to use this new technique will not need extended speech therapy once control and intelligibility are acquired.

Alternative methods of rehabilitation

Because of the extent of surgical intervention or because of failures to master esophageal voice, other methods of "voicing" may be attempted.

One involves surgical procedures to direct the tracheal air stream through the oral cavity. The Asai technique[9] and the LaBarge Voice-Bak procedures are examples. These techniques are used by otolaryngologists and extend beyond the scope of this chapter. Recent attention has been focused on a new technique of tracheoesophageal puncture, which uses a small valve-type prosthesis diverting tracheal air to the esophagus.[10] Although the technique appears to offer the patient immediate voicing and a minimum of complications, its long-term effectiveness is still under study.

Another alternative involves the use of mechanical devices. These are small instruments either held in the hand against the neck or held so as to be inserted in the mouth. They produce a hum or buzz, which the patient modifies with the articulators to form words. Audible speech by this method is usually mastered in a few sessions with the speech pathologist. It has the advantage over esophageal voice of providing the patient with an immediate means of oral communication. It has disadvantages of requiring the use of one hand for communication and producing an artificial monopitch "voice" that may be less intelligible than esophageal speech.

Speech disorders secondary to nervous system dysfunction

Speech disorders secondary to nervous system dysfunction are known as *dysarthrias*. The name implies impairment of movement or integration of movements because of neurologic or muscular dysfunction.

Cause. Dysarthrias in the geriatric patient often result from cerebral vascular disease. They are also manifested in neurologic disorders such as Parkinson's disease, multiple sclerosis, amyotrophic lateral sclerosis, ataxia of various causes, chorea, myasthenia gravis, Wilson's disease, and others. The speech symptoms vary with the severity and localization of the disorder.

Evaluation. Evaluation should be made of each of the systems involved in articulation. These include the following features:

1. Strength and range of motion of the lips
2. Strength, range of motion, protrusion, and lateral and vertical movements of the tongue
3. Elevation and symmetry of the soft palate on phonation
4. Presence of the gag reflex
5. Symmetric movement and adequate closing of the vocal folds (if visualized)
6. Adequate respiration

In the evaluation the speech pathologist will note the following:

1. Overall intelligibility of the patient's speech
2. Consistent misarticulation of specific sounds
3. Inability to sustain phonation
4. Presence of hypernasality or hyponasality
5. Difficulty in swallowing
6. Quality of phonation (harsh, hoarse, breathy, etc.)
7. Intensity of phonation
8. Ability to change pitch
9. Habitual pitch appropriate for age and sex
10. Effect of speed on articulation
11. Any deterioration of speech with sustained effort

12. Prosody of speech
13. Sensitivity of hearing

Dysarthria may be the presenting symptom of one of the aforementioned disorders and therefore, through speech evaluation, may lead to the diagnosis of the underlying disorder. Some of the distinctive patterns of the dysarthrias have been summarized by Darley et al.[11]

Prognosis and rehabilitation. Prognosis for recovery from dysarthria depends on its cause. Patients with dysarthria secondary to stroke often show spontaneous recovery in the first few weeks after onset. Short-term therapy is indicated to instruct the patient in strengthening exercises and in speaking slowly with attempts at exaggerated articulation.

An important prognostic factor in patients' abilities to monitor their speech is the integrity of their hearing, which should be examined carefully, and expectations for success tempered accordingly.

For the patient with dysarthria secondary to progressive neurologic disease, speech therapy can play a role in teaching the patient to self-monitor speech for maximal intelligibility. Goals of training include speaking in short phrases, the use of compensatory movements in lieu of traditional articulation, and striving for maximal loudness. Protracted therapy is usually not indicated in patients with progressive dysarthrias. Once patients can monitor their own best efforts and these are intelligible, the speech pathologist may discontinue regular sessions. The clinician's role is then one of providing periodic evaluations and suggestions for changes in monitoring as needed.

Many patients with progressive dysarthria have responded well to drug therapy. The improvement of the parkinsonian patient with the administration of levodopa is a good example. Such treatment may make a speech therapy program superfluous.

NONORAL COMMUNICATION

There are dysarthric patients and surgical patients who are incapable of intelligible speech. They are, nonetheless, candidates for some type of communciation therapy. They may be taught to express their needs by writing if they have good upper extremity control. However, this is time-consuming, and its effectiveness may be compromised by the patient's poor ability to spell (and embarrassment therefrom). An appealing alternative is the development of gesture language. One method is based on the gesture language of the deaf and sign language of the American Indian. It is versatile and can be fairly well interpreted by the naive observer. Those who have developed this Amerind sign language have even reported its usefulness in facilitating oral expression of the patient with verbal apraxia (or Broca's aphasia).[12]

Another means of nonverbal communciation is the communciation or language board. This is a large chart containing phrases, words, or at the simplest level, pictures to which the patient may point, thereby expressing needs or asking questions. There have been attempts to produce such charts commercially, but this nonverbal communication is probably more effective when made by the speech pathologist or patient's family to suit the unique needs of the patient. It may also be valuable to have available a large chart of the alphabet so that the literate patient can spell words that do not appear on the communication board.

The relatively recent development of small speech synthesizers may eventually make it possible for speech-impaired patients to press an appropriate button and have their needs stated aloud by a computer. This kind of device would be extremely useful for the patient who needs to use the telephone or intercom for communication. At this time, the expense of such instruments as the compact speech synthesizer is considerable and the decision for purchase should be based on indications for long-term need.

The use of such a device is restricted by the patient's ability to designate the correct button accurately and strength to press it or otherwise trigger the response signal. Most important of all, the individual must have the inner language and mental acuity to be aware of needs and how to effect their expression. These two factors often limit the use of nonverbal devices by the aphasic patient who, for reasons of dysarthria or of verbal symbolization problems, cannot talk. The patient may not be capable of learning to manipulate the device because of central nervous system dysfunction.

Training in the use of any of the nonverbal methods of communication should be discontinued when the patient is functionally expressing needs.

CONCLUSION

The communication disorders of geriatric patients are often the results of a condition that has implications for their life expectancies.

The long-term goal of a communciation rehabilitation program should be to retrain the patient to resume as many former roles as possible. Short-term goals should establish at every level of complexity some means of understanding or expressing needs. When the patient can comprehend or express with no greater complexity, despite the efforts of the speech pathologist, the program should be discontinued.

The family of the patient ought to be included in the program and counseled after each evaluation to accept both the limitations and potentials of the patient. This requires coordination of the entire rehabilitation team: the physical therapist to help patients become maximally mobile and increase the scope of their physical environment; the occupational therapist to encourage patients to be independent in activities of daily living; the speech pathologist to help patients to achieve optimal communication; the social worker to aid patients and their families in changes of roles, acceptance of the deficit, adjustments in financial matters, and, sometimes, institutional placement; and the physician to oversee and coordinate these efforts.

REFERENCES

1. DeRenzi, E., and Vignoli, L.A.: The Token Test: a sensitive test to detect receptive disturbances in aphasics, Brain **85:**655, 1962.
2. Spellacy, F., and Spreen, O.: A short form of the Token Test, Cortex **5:**390, 1969.
3. Schuell, H.: Minnesota Test for Differential Diagnosis of Aphasia, Minneapolis, 1965, University of Minnesota Press.
4. Goodglass, H., and Kaplan, E.: Aphasia and related disorders, Philadelphia, 1972, Lea & Febiger.
5. Porch, B.: The Porch Index of Communicative Ability, Palo Alto, Calif., 1967, Consulting Psychologists Press, Inc.
6. Hartman, J.: Measurement of early spontaneous recovery from aphasia with stroke, Ann. Neurol. **9:**89, 1980.
7. Wertz, R.T., et al.: VA Cooperative Study on Aphasia: preliminary report on a comparison of individual and group treatment, presented to the annual meeting of the American Association for the Advancement of Science, Washington, D.C., February, 1978.
8. Hartman, J., Swisher, L., and Kleffner, F.: The role of the speech pathologist with the chronic, home-bound CVA patient, presented before annual meeting of the American Speech and Hearing Association, Las Vegas, 1974.
9. Asai, R.: Asai's new voice production method: a substitution for human speech, presented before Eighth International Congress of Otorhinolaryngology, Tokyo, 1965.
10. Singer, M., and Blom, E.: An endoscopic technique for restoration of voice after laryngectomy, Ann. Otol. Rhinol. Laryngol. **89:**529, 1980.
11. Darley, F.L., Aronson, A.E., and Brown, J.R.: Motor speech signs in neurologic disease, Med. Clin. North Am. **52:**835, 1968.
12. Skelly, M., Schinsky, L., Smith, R., and Fust, R.: Amerind as a facilitator of verbalization of the oral verbal apraxic, J. Speech Hear. Disord. **39:**455, 1974.

PART IV SPECIAL ASPECTS OF GERIATRIC CARE

CHAPTER 36 · NURSING AND THE AGED

Irene Mortenson Burnside

Gerontological nursing is a growing field; it is one of the newest specialities in nursing. It will be useful at the beginning of this chapter to review the current state of the art. Although the terms *gerontological, gerontic,* and *geriatric nursing* are all currently used, the term *gerontological nursing*, adopted by the American Nurses' Association (ANA), will be used in this chapter.

GERONTOLOGICAL NURSING: STATE OF THE ART

Bates,[1] a physician herself, notes that physicians may be puzzled if they are asked to define nursing.

> Nursing is perceived as deliberate action of personal and assisting nature. The practice of nursing requires knowledge of: (1) normal growth and development; (2) basic human needs; (3) coping mechanisms used by individuals; (4) actual or potential health problems; (5) the effects of age, sex, cultural, religious, and racial factors on health needs; and (6) the ways by which nursing can assist individuals to maintain health and cope with health problems.

Individuals are viewed as having the right and responsibility to direct their own health-related activities. Even when self-direction is not possible individuals have a right to quality health care consistent with their individual and family beliefs.[2] The latter statement is especially important because many old people do not receive quality health care. The complexity of nursing care of the elderly was clearly described in the 1960s in the research of a famous British nurse, Doreen Norton.[3]

Cynthia Kelly reminds us that the health care of older persons provided by nursing "is not synonymous with medical care, but a much broader concept."[4] Nurses are expanding their practice; they practice preventive care and health maintenance and also focus on psychosocial aspects.

Yarling distinguishes between medical care and nursing care. "Most frequently, when nothing more can be done about a disease, a great deal more can be done for the patient. And characteristically it is the nurse who does it."[5] Helen Weber states

> The largest responsibility for geriatric care has been thrust upon the nursing profession. It has accepted the responsibility although it has very little authority for planning, financing, or evaluating the results. However, the profession of nursing is beginning to recognize its power, and the public must be made aware that better care would be possible if more decision-making power were allotted to nursing.[6]

NURSING EDUCATION AND RESEARCH

The demands of the expanded role for nurses require that nurses be more highly educated than ever before.

There are numerous[7] gerontological clinical specialist programs in the United States, and many of these nurses have master's degrees; others are in a continuing education program. Some nurses add the intensive work of a practitioner program to their existing education, which could be an associate degree, diploma, or a baccalaureate. At this writing the decision for gerontological nurse practitioners (GNP) to have master's degrees has not been made[8]; however, encouraging nurses to become practitioners with master's degrees does seem to be the direction the profession will take.

A nurse practitioner provides these services: (1) assessing health-illness status;[6,9] (2) entering a person into the health care system; (3) sustaining and supporting persons who are impaired, infirm, or ill during programs of diagnosis and therapy; (4) managing a care regimen for acutely and chronically ill patients within established standing orders;[10] (5) aiding and restoring persons to wellness and maximum level of functioning; (6) teaching and counseling persons about health and illness; (7) counseling and supporting persons in the aging process; (8) aiding patients and their survivors during the dying process.[11-14]

There is a desperate need for doctorally prepared nurses in gerontology, both for teaching positions in universities and for nursing research.[15,16]

The need for research in gerontological nursing is acute.[11,16] Miriam J. Hirshfeld, a leader in gerontological nursing in Israel, points out three ethical issues that must be considered in research: "(1) respect for persons; (2) adequate knowledge base for decision-making, (3) rethinking of the ethical issues related to quality of life, quality of death, distribution of limited resources, etc."[17] There currently exists an urgent need for clinical nursing research regarding the problems described in this chapter.

Gerontological nursing faces some of the same problems as medicine. The lack of content on aging in curricula has been well-documented both in medicine and in nursing.[15,18,19] The inclusion of gerontology and geriatric nursing has not been made mandatory for state board examinations. The enthusiasm and dedication of those already in the field can encourage others to gain that knowledge and experience.[20]

There are signs of growth in gerontological nursing. In 1974, the ANA delineated Standards for Gerontological Nursing Practice.[21] There are two professional journals: *Journal of Gerontological Nursing*, begun in 1975, and *Geriatric Nursing*, begun in 1980. Nurses now write their own protocols to provide the knowledge base needed to improve care. There are excellent books by nurses on geriatric protocols.[22,23]

Specific areas of practice and research that should concern nurses include the following: comprehensive physical and psychosocial assessment[9]: health maintenance, especially of the frail elderly[24,25]; early diagnosis of problems; patient mobility and safety, including prevention of falls; nutrition[26]; control of pain and sleep; confusion and disorientation; dementia; especially Alzheimer's disease, depression[27] and suicide risk; Sundowner's syndrome; drug monitoring; incontinence[28]; home assessment and home care (see Chapter 37); sexuality; economics; and crime against the elderly.

IMPORTANCE OF PSYCHOSOCIAL CARE

Dr. Barbara Bates states the important contributions nurses make in the psychosocial care of the elderly.

> Perhaps an even more difficult thing to do is to share our relationship with our patients. . . . Yet we must do this if we are to enable our nursing colleague to establish her own relationship and make her own contributions to patient care, especially in the psychologic realm. And once we have done so, we are apt to be surprised at how well things go.[1]

Nurses mainly care for the aged in three settings: (1) in nursing homes or long-term care units,[11,14,29] (2) in the community,[30-32] and (3) in acute care settings. In all three areas the nurse is expected to demonstrate skill in the physical and psychosocial assessment of aged persons. The nurse is expected to be able to differentiate normal aging changes and pathologic changes and also to understand the care of the frail elderly.[33]

NURSING AND THE AGED IN LONG-TERM CARE UNITS

There has been an increase in the literature about the gerontological nurse practitioner's role.[11,12,14,34] One study describes the effectiveness of gerontological nurses in a masters' program with aged clients in a nursing home.[11] Sister Schwab's devotion to high standards of excellence in long-term care are reflected in her writings.[29]

Most nursing directors of nursing homes do not have strong voices in the management and care of the elderly residents. There are few doctors who visit nursing homes, and often the nurses are subservient, not to the doctor but to the administrator. Nurses are in difficult positions to carve out strong and effective caring roles.

While nurse managers and directors in acute settings, colleges, and universities must have advanced education, nurses in nursing homes do not yet meet the same stringent requirements. We in nursing often fail to give them support and encouragement. They also must return to school to update their knowledge and skills in normal aging management and physical and psychosocial assessment of the older adult.

Nursing homes should be laboratories for student nurses at all levels of education. Recent awards by the Robert Woods Foundation will permit the beginning of teaching nursing homes.

Nurses work in retirement homes and may be employed in small nursing homes within a retirement home complex. These nurses are on call and available to residents who need assistance in their rooms and who need special diets, dressing changes, drugs monitored, or other health problems checked. Many retirement home persons are afraid that they will become a patient in the nursing home unit and try to stay in their independent quarters as long as possible. Residents often help one another so that they can manage in their own quarters. Their peer support system and their loyalty to their friends and confidantes are impressive. The value of confidantes described in the research by Lowenthal and Haven is still not widely incorporated into nursing care plans.[35]

CARE OF THE AGED IN ACUTE CARE SETTINGS

As one author wrote, "Remember, it is the chronically ill who constitute the bulk of the sick population in 'advanced' nations."[36] Health service needs correlate directly with age. Older people require more health services, have more difficulties when sick, and require more time to regain optimal health. Of people past the age of 65, 86% have one or more chronic disabilities.[37] The aged make frequent visits to physicians and hospitals, spanning months and years. For various reasons, the elderly often delay seeking medical attention for an illness, waiting until they are in critical condition. When they do enter an acute-care hospital they enter a setting that is oriented for short-term stays. Elderly patients stay longer than younger patients.[38] Consequently, the management of their illnesses is often fragmented and lacks continuity. During hospitalization, the older patient may become confused, depressed, and sometimes difficult to manage.

The elderly, indeed the public at large, demand health-care services that reflect the needs of the older patient. In answer to these demands, new services are being developed. In contrast to the team or functional approach, which is still the trend for care in most hospitals, primary nursing is an attempt by the nursing profession to alleviate fragmentation and to provide continuity of care.[39]

PRIMARY NURSING*

Primary nursing is described as nursing provided by one nurse so that the total care of an individual patient is the responsibility of one nurse, not many.[39] In contrast, team (or functional) nursing shares the responsibility for any one patient among several nurses on a single shift. Community-health nurses have been predicting the role of the primary nurse since the 1930s. At first, primary nursing was linked only to nurses with practitioner skills. The concept, however, as used here, is that the nurse is responsible for the patient 24 hours a day for the length of the patient's hospitalization. The nurse coordinates care and plans with the physician and auxiliary personnel for hospital care and postdischarge arrangements. The primary nurse assesses, plans, implements, and evaluates the care of 1 to 4 patients. The nurse is responsible for implementing the plan of care on a 24-hour basis. This, however, does not mean that the nurse is in constant attendance, any more than the physician who directs medical care is continually in attendance. But the primary nurse has the autonomy, authority, and the accountability to organize, implement, and direct the patient's nursing care. The primary nurse is in a sense a director of services who also delivers care. The nurse collaborates with others on the health team, for example, the physician, dietician, physical therapist, occupational therapist, and others so as to avoid fragmented care.

When a comparison is made between primary nursing and team nursing, the research findings verify that continuity of care seems to be increased by primary nursing, particularly in long-term care units. The question of whether the elderly can benefit more than others has not been studied, but primary nursing of the elderly has many possibilities.

*This portion of the chapter was written by Bobbye Gorenberg, R.N., M.S., Gerontological Nurse Specialist, San Jose State University, San Jose, Calif.

An elderly patient entering the acute setting is ill and unsure of the future. The transfer from either home or a long-term care facility is associated with a change in environment. The exacerbation of chronic illness in itself may trigger confusion and disorientation. The future is in doubt for the patient. While some studies have shown that mortality is not increased significantly by relocation, Miller and Lieberman[40] reported significant increases of physical and psychologic deterioration after relocation.

Case 1. Mr. S., a 65-year-old retired schoolteacher with cardiovascular disease, was admitted to the intensive care unit (ICU) of a large teaching hospital where the team nursing approach was used. He had sustained critical injuries in a car accident, and his wife was killed. He was transferred to a rehabilitation unit from the ICU. Shortly after the transfer, he was placed on complete enteric isolation. In the following 2 weeks, he was moved to a different room three times to provide better access to him for the nursing team. His confusion increased daily. When he first arrived on the unit, he knew his name and that his wife was dead. Each time he was moved he lost further contact with reality, until he did not know who he was or that his wife was dead. As nursing teams changed, his plan of care was changed. Familiar faces were replaced by strangers. He had no one with whom he could identify. He was finally discharged to a nursing home because rehabilitation seemed impossible.

Mr. S.'s needs were not identified by the team leaders. His isolation, coupled with constant relocation, indicated the fragmented care provided him.

Case 2. In contrast, Mrs. L., a widowed, retired schoolteacher, aged 72, was diagnosed as having breast cancer that had metastasized to the brain. She was admitted to an acute care hospital for radiation treatment and control of pain. The hospital used primary nursing. The primary nurse developed a plan of care that permitted Mrs. L. to remain in her room until she was transferred to a long-term care unit. Her plan of care was transferred to a primary nurse on the long-term care unit. As death approached, the nurses helped Mrs. L. fulfill her wish to die at home. The primary nurse coordinated plans with the physician, discharge planners, and Mrs. L.'s sister. Mrs. L. died at home approximately 2 weeks after she was discharged.

The coordination of care accomplished by the primary nurse is one example of the provision of comprehensive 24-hour care that can be developed for the elderly.

Grier believes that a major problem in providing care for the elderly is that many of them are in environments that are incongruent with their needs and that nurses may not be adequately involved in the selection of living arrangements.[41]

Accurate assessments of elderly persons' needs are often not made because there is no one person responsible for coordinating care from home to the acute care setting and back to the community. Most physicians conduct extraordinarily heavy practices and cannot be expected to carry this responsibility. Primary nursing is one method for providing care in a collaborative framework.

NURSING AND COMMUNITY-BASED ELDERLY CLIENTS

The ANA reminds us that the primary need of most persons requiring home care is for nursing services as evidenced by both historic and current experiences in nursing.[42]

There are several ways elderly people who have health problems can be maintained in their own homes. Some elderly persons can remain with their relatives if there is respite care available. One common form of respite care is the day-care center. A hospice care movement is currently sweeping the United States; it focuses primarily on caring for the dying person at home. Another means of keeping people in their homes is the use of health aides to perform chores and tasks for the frail or very sick elderly who are at home. Meals on Wheels may be the only support service an elderly person needs and may provide enough assistance and adequate nutrition to prevent institutionalization.

Still another support system that old people use is a senior center. Many of the outstanding multipurpose centers provide health screening clinics, annual health fairs, educational programs regarding health problems, and maximal social opportunities. Often there is a cafeteria or a meal program for the noon hour so that persons attending have one nutritious meal. It is not uncommon to hear them say that "it is the only good meal I have eaten all day."[26] The food program is a vital component of health care and socialization for many elderly persons. Transportation is usually a big problem for old people who wish to use these services but cannot drive. Transportation problems loom even larger with ever-increasing inflation and cost of gasoline.

Keeping old people in their homes, whether

they live alone or with others, requires strong support systems.[43] The careful monitoring of the aged client by a nurse, who coordinates all the various support systems that an elderly person might need, is perhaps the most important method of maintaining the aged in their homes. That role carries with it many more concerns and responsibilities if she is coordinating services for confused or demented elderly persons. In addition to coordinating all the support systems, the nurse must monitor the use of medications and prostheses, watch for health and nutritional problems (including malnutrition and dehydration), watch for psychologic problems such as "bereavement overload" (Kastenbaum's term) and relocation shock, and watch for withdrawal, loneliness, and depression.

One public health nurse has described the special needs of homebound clients who suffer from cardiovascular accident or arthritis.[10] Several writers have pointed out the nurse's various responsibilities for continuity of care for patients living at home.[32,43]

The nurse's first responsibility in working with the aged client at home is a comprehensive assessment of both the client and the environment. Family members often suffer stress in coping with incapacitated members and often do not know where to turn for help or even what resources are available. This is particularly true of family members of a person with Alzheimer's disease. Some are too proud to ask for help. The nurse can be instrumental in explaining the patient's problems and the services available to them and in reassuring them that they are not asking for charity, since health care is a right, not a privilege for a select few.

NURSE-MANAGED GERIATRIC DAY-CARE CENTERS

One exciting area for nurses to demonstrate leadership in the care of the aged is the management of, or participation in, day-care center programs.[30] Nurses are ideal for these positions because of their health care backgrounds and familiarity with disease processes. Such centers may delay the admission of the aged person to an institution for long-term care. A day-care center handles both the psychologic and physical problems that may beset the frail elderly. And not only does the center improve the quality of life for the older person but also for the family and caretakers. Even elderly persons who reside in board and care homes or in intermediate care facilities who are taken to a day-care center benefit from participation in a day-care program. An adult day-care center is not a "baby-sitting" service providing custodial care.

The focus of the day-care center should be on the positive and well aspects of the individual, rather than on the negative and the disease. Severely demented individuals can function quite well in a warm, structured, and safe environment. The caretaker must try many approaches with an individual and not give up easily.

The person who does not have a day-care center available in the area, is not ambulatory, or for some other reason cannot meet the criteria for a day-care center may be maintained at home with a network of support. Rossman has long advocated this and has pioneered work at Montefiore Hospital in New York City.[44]

CONCEPTS BASIC TO NURSING CARE OF OLDER PERSONS

Webster's Dictionary defines an intervention as "a state of coming or being between, interpositions . . . any interference in the affairs of others." Some older people do not see intervening as helpful. It is an important strategy for the nurse to try to establish immediate rapport with the older person. In the initial contact, the nurse tries to communicate to the person (even the most frightened and confused) that this is a friendly relationship. Some old people feel that they are more desperately in need of a friend than they are of a helper. A nurse may become a confidante or a pseudofamily member. It goes without saying that plans are mutually made and that the old person makes as many decisions about what is going to happen as is possible. This is one important aspect of care of the aged that is still blatantly ignored, not only by nurses but by other health professionals and families.

The problems that one must deal with in the aged patient can be frustrating; some even seem unsolvable. Areas of nursing concern include the following: abuse of medications; problems of dental care; skin problems resulting in decubitus ulcers; incontinence, both urinary and fecal are commonplace in care of the aged, particularly confused persons; and inadequate nutrition and fluid intake. The management of confused and disoriented patients usually falls in the realm of nursing. These frail elderly individuals may be sadly neglected; they require the most sensitive patient caretakers and exquisite nursing care.

MEDICATIONS AND THE ELDERLY

The monitoring of medications in the elderly person requires an interdisciplinary approach. The pharmacist can be a consultant, but we also need the astute observations of ancillary help who will report even the slightest behavioral change they see in a patient. Behavioral changes may be the first indication of a medication problem. Any agitation, combativeness, or confusion should be reported. The patient should not just be given a tranquilizer, even if one is prescribed. Rather the nurses must search for possible causes for the behavioral changes.

The forgetful client will have great difficulty in remembering what medications to take and when. This becomes a real concern for persons living at home or who reside in board and care homes where there may be minimal surveillance. It is not uncommon for one frail elderly person to be monitored by another frail elderly person who is also slightly confused and not dispensing medicines accurately.

One great area of concern is the use of hypotensive drugs. If patients are not properly educated about the drug, patients may get up suddenly, black out, fall to the floor, and subsequently may sustain hip fractures. Sometimes they receive a wrist fracture as they hold their arm out to break the fall.

The use of psychotropic medications must be carefully monitored. An elderly man in a psychiatric hospital was receiving chlorpromazine (Thorazine.) He forgot he was to wear a large-brimmed hat when he was outdoors in the sun. When his wife noted his red, swollen face, he told her that a bee had stung him. He was treated for a bee sting until an astute nurse realized the problem was photosensitivity.

Use and abuse of medications

Drugs must be given to the aged person with great caution and followed with close surveillance by nurses and others while the drug is being taken. This is true for the aged person either in or out of an institution. The adverse effects of drugs are well-known to health professionals.

Suggestions for interventions regarding medications

1. What are the specific instructions regarding the medication that the person is taking? Check to see that it is being taken with milk or after meals, and so on.
2. Devise a method of monitoring medications in the home setting.
3. Help slightly confused persons to remember their medications. Make up envelopes ahead of time with the medications inside to be taken daily or have someone call them and remind them.
4. Diuretics may cause marked dehydration and electrolyte imbalance in elderly clients. Check the fullness of the tongue because it is a constant and reliable sign of dehydration. A shrunken, furrowed tongue will indicate an advanced stage of dehydration.[45]
5. Monitor all antihypertensive drugs often, and double-check that the client is getting up slowly and carefully from supine and sitting positions.
6. Have a life vial in the refrigerator that explains the medications of the individual. It is kept in the refrigerator, and firemen, policemen, and caretakers should be instructed to look for this in case of emergency.
7. Offer the medication in a form most acceptable to the individual, that is, if an individual detests taking pills, try to find liquid medications when possible.
8. Write out instructions in large print using a black felt-tipped pen on white cards or paper. When anxiety is high, patients often do not hear or understand the instructions given by the doctor, nor can they read the fine print on medicine bottles.
9. The medication bottles designed to keep children out of the bottle also keep the elderly from getting medication because of poor instructions or arrows of the same color on the top that cannot be seen or lined up. Stiff arthritic hands cannot manipulate the plastic top of the bottle.
10. Instructions are often poorly given and must be checked constantly so that the older person understands the purpose of taking the medication, and why it is important to follow instructions. Sharing medications is common among aged persons living in the community.
11. An interdisciplinary approach is need-

ed—pharmacist, physician, nurse, dietician especially must work together in the area of medications.

SUBNUTRITION, MALNUTRITION, AND DEHYDRATION

The rising costs of food, transportation, and energy are playing havoc with the diets of the elderly. One only has to watch them push their carts through the food stores for an accurate picture of the food they consume. It is now common knowledge that many old people eat dog food because they cannot afford meat.

In the institution there are other problems related to poor nutrition. In mental hospitals, more aggressive patients often take food away from the frail elderly patients. Bland institutional food often does not appeal to the elderly, whose taste sensation may have diminished.

Meals on Wheels and dining facilities are important because of the social aspect involved in eating. Persons who deliver Meals on Wheels have reported that older individuals will eat more of their food if the deliverer of the meal will sit down and visit with them during the meal. The loneliness and bereavement of the newly widowed is another area for assessment. They often have no energy or desire to cook or to eat; some may begin drinking excessively instead of eating proper meals.

Since malnutrition and dehydration lead to states of confusion, it is crucial that the nurse carefully assesses how much food and fluids the aged person is taking. It is important to prevent water depletion in older persons. Dehydration is particularly serious during times of hot weather, since old people tolerate heat poorly. In a hospital during a hot spell or when an air conditioner malfunctions, old people can become dehydrated rapidly.

Nocturnal dehydration

Nocturnal dehydration is common in older people for several reasons. Many go to bed very early, some while it is still daylight. Some believe that they will have to get up during the night and go to the bathroom and so purposely avoid drinking fluids in the evening.

Suggestions to improve hydration in the elderly person

1. Make a special effort to give the client the type of food and fluids enjoyed. Cultural aspects are consistently ignored. An elderly Chicano may want tortillas instead of bread; the Japanese client may want rice for breakfast, and so on.
2. Allow a small glass of wine at bedtime. It is reported that this will induce sleep and may cut down on the need for sleeping medications. The social aspect of this could also be enhanced.
3. Carefully assess the loneliness, depression, and grief of the aged individual; efforts must be made to check food and fluid intake during these states.
4. Place patients together to eat instead of feeding them in isolation. One creative nurses' aide dressed the women in her care in their best clothes and once a week wheeled them to a lounge to have lunch. One woman acted as hostess each week and greeted the women as they were pushed to the doorway. This luncheon continued, even after the nurses' aide was transferred to another unit.
5. Suggest that students conduct reminiscing groups at meal time. Nurses have done this. I once had a supper hour and a reminiscing group with patients in a nursing home. All the members were nonagenarians. One feisty woman waited until her ninetieth birthday and wheeled herself into the group that day and said "I am 90. I can join." Such a group will permit the leader to observe eating habits, to encourage food intake, and to implement necessary changes with the dietary department.
6. Serve at least two glasses or cups of beverage at every group meeting to ensure adequate hydration. Begin a reality orientation class or a reminiscing group meeting with a glass of water. It is inexpensive and simple to do because many of the older people will use it to drink a toast. Explain to them why they need the water. They have dry skins, they may be taking medications that make their mouths dry, and they may not be drinking enough on their own. (They do not need to know that the leader is also hoping to prevent confusional states.)
7. Nighttime dehydration occurs from about 7 or 8 PM in institutions until about the same hours in the morning. As Cynthia Kelly says, "Elderly persons sabotage fluid balance with exquisite skill. Typically, an aged patient has been told by someone he trusts that if he does not

drink after 4 PM he will (may) not have to void (as often) during the night."[4]

Nutritional needs

Sister Marilyn Schwab[29] wrote, "I am less impressed by the nurse who can identify the patient who is throwing PVC's [premature ventricular contractions] than the nurse who can get a frightened, confused person to eat."

Suggestions for nurses to intervene in feeding problems with the elderly

1. In patients who have had a cardiovascular accident, check to see if there is hemianopsia, which might affect food intake, since these patients tend not to eat items that are on the half of the tray that they cannot see.
2. Carefully monitor the food and fluid intake of the confused person whether the person is at home, in a day-care center, or in an acute care hospital.
3. Use behavior modification strategies with patients who have Alzheimer's disease because they have to learn to eat.
4. Select in-service programs that heighten staff awareness about feeding problems.
5. Assist patients with mental health problems, for example, depression, loneliness, bereavement. Alleviating the mental health problem will usually help the feeding problem.
6. Intervene cautiously with paranoid individuals who think that you are poisoning the food. If someone can eat with them it may reduce their fears; giving them selected choice items, for example, chocolate, sweets, or milkshakes between meals is sometimes effective.
7. Pay attention to the circadian rhythm and life cycles of the elderly individual. Farmers who always rose at 5 AM do not appreciate a continental breakfast served at 8 AM.
8. When visiting the home, check the refrigerator. Look for moldy food, nonfood items in the refrigerator, or no food at all. Check pets; they sometimes eat better than the old person. Inability to care for the pet's needs may indicate that the elderly person cannot take care of his or her food needs.
9. Malnutrition may be a reason for poorly fitting dentures. As was stated earlier in the chapter, it is advisable to carefully check the nutritional status of all patients who come under the nurse's supervision. The symptoms complained of by the aged person says one dentist, are ". . . sore and inflamed aveolar ridge mucosa, a burning sensation of the tongue or palate, dryness of the mouth, soreness in the corners of the lips, and pain when attempting to masticate." (See Chapter 23.)[46]

ORAL HYGIENE NEEDS

Many older persons neglect the care of their mouth and do not see it as important. When they are ill, they may have bad breath and be unaware of it. They also may neglect to care for their dentures properly and need education in this area. Dentures present problems for nearly all of the persons who have them.

A questionnaire was sent to nurses about the most common problems they had with elderly clients who had glasses, dentures, wheelchairs, canes, and walkers. The problem areas with dentures the nurses identified in rank order were as follows: (1) poor fit; (2) labeling of the dentures; (3) lack of care of dentures; (4) refusal to wear dentures; and (5) loss of dentures. Nurses who worked in institutions felt that staff members did not spend enough time instructing or helping clients. Also there was little instruction of new staff members regarding dentures during orientation.[33]

Care of dentures

Bennett[47] has covered oral health maintenance in-depth, and his chapter is highly recommended. Bennett states that learning to live with dentures often can present many challenges to an older person; the replacement of old dentures with new dentures creates difficulties. The following suggestions by Bennett should be given to the person who is struggling with new dentures. The nurse may be the one who must instruct the patient.

- The dentures should be removed each night, cleaned and then placed in a glass of water.
- The dentures should be cleaned after every meal. They need to be scrubbed over a pan of water with a wash cloth at the bottom of the pan so they will not break if they are dropped.
- If sores appear in the mouth, the client should remove the dentures to give the mouth a rest.

- The fullness in lips and cheeks felt by patient is caused by plastic denture material replacing the bone. Learning to talk is a gradual process; encourage the client in his efforts.
- Soft tissue under the dentures must be kept in good health.
- If dentures becomes loose or ill fitting, they may need to be relined or remade for correct fit.

Further suggestions for care of dentures

1. Staff in-service classes are needed to teach nurses' aides about the proper care of dentures.
2. Instruct patients about the care and cleaning of dentures. If they are confused care of dentures must be taken over by the nursing staff.
3. Dentures must be labeled since they are often misplaced or lost by the confused elderly person. Sometimes they wear each other's dentures in the height of confusion.
4. Relatives get very upset about missing or lost dentures, so all that can be done to have relatives help in the care of the elderly person's dentures should be done.
5. Find out why a patient refuses to wear teeth; the dentures may not fit well.
6. Praise and reward persons who do wear their teeth.
7. Never embarrass or make fun of elderly persons and their dentures; many people are very sensitive about them and go to great lengths to pretend that they do not wear dentures.

Labeling dentures

Dentists do not routinely put names in dentures. This is a simple laboratory procedure and can be done when dentures are made. It would be advisable to have a family member take the dentures of an elderly member to a dentist, who can engrave the person's name or initials and then fill the engraving with a white plastic substance. It takes about a half hour for the plastic to set; it can then be polished.[33]

Some nurses in long-term care tell me they have purchased an electric needle to carve patients' initials into the dentures and then lightly sand the area to prevent rough areas from irritating the mouth.

Only after a nurse has searched for dentures in wardrobes, closets, clothing, and dirty linen hampers, can she appreciate well-marked dentures. Missing teeth also keep families perturbed about their loved one's care.

Effect of dentures on body image

Not enough attention is given to the effects of dentures on body image. I recall a middle-aged man once saying that his wife had no qualms about being seen in the nude but to be seen without her dentures in place mortified her. Patients going to surgery resist removing dentures and partial plates for as long as they possibly can. Preoperative procedures should allow for such concerns by not having the patient remove them too soon before the surgery.

CONTINENCE AND THE AGED PERSON

Wells and Brink[28] are two outstanding nurses who have studied urinary continence in the elderly. (Their urinary continence management nursing assessment guide is highly recommended to readers.)

Brocklehurst[48] advises that it is helpful to determine if the lack of urine control is considered to be transient or established and whether temporary or permanent. Hydration is important; the elderly person requires 2000 to 3000 ml of fluids per day, unless of course there is a serious medical condition, for example, cardiac or kidney failure.[49-51]

Drugs must be monitored since diuretics can cause loss of urine control, especially at night. Also drugs that cause drowsiness or confusion alter the aged person's ability to remain continent.

Wells and Brink[28] deplore environmental barriers, for example distances to toilets, the design of toilet chairs, and toilet sizes (e.g., accommodating wheelchairs). The correct urinal or bedpan for the type of individual problem must be considered.

Exercises also may be needed to develop the pelvic floor muscles. Another exercise, which is newer and not as well-developed, is called *bladder tolerance training*.

Prevention of urinary tract infections and dependence on urethral catheters should be studied more.

Responsibilities of nurse

1. Loss of urinary control is critical and immediate nursing action is needed.

2. Assess possible psychologic disturbances that aggravate urine control.

3. Maintain a milieu that promotes urine control.

4. Nursing excellence can improve even the most difficult case of urine control disability.

SKIN CARE OF THE AGED PERSON

Skin care is crucial in all elderly individuals since the loss of subcutaneous fat intensifies the production of wrinkles and the skin becomes lax, thinner, and often dry.

The older client should not be bathed too frequently; care should be taken to use mild soaps and emollients. Skin should not be rubbed after a bath. Because of the danger of slipping and falling in the tub, it is wise not to put ingredients into the bathtub water.

Protection from inclement weather is important, and older women should dress warmly and use lipstick.

Bed patients must be scrupulously monitored for redness and possible skin breakdown, especially those patients who are incontinent. Sheepskins can be useful for these persons.

USE AND ABUSE OF RESTRAINTS

The current concern over maltreatment of older persons includes concern over the use of restraints by families of older persons. Nurses in the community need to be alert for abuses of the aged. Cornelia Beck[52] has done work in this area.

However, health professionals still use restraints indiscriminately with aged patients. Often the patient is a "wanderer" or the staff is afraid of the person being injured in a fall. Restraints usually aggravate the aged person; even the tiniest person can fight and yell and create further disturbances.

The hazards of restraints must be considered because the patients can slide down and be caught in a Posey belt or in a wheelchair, for example. Patients in restraints must be checked frequently. Laws vary from state to state, so the nurse should know the legal implications.

Physical restraints are belittling and humiliating and should be considered only when all other attempts at intervention have failed. They can cause skin tears and cuts and can prevent the person from reaching a water pitcher, and the dangers and consequences of immobility can be serious.

NEEDS OF THE CONFUSED AND DISORIENTED INDIVIDUAL

Confusion and disorientation are commonplace in the elderly and may be caused by a variety of insults to the aged person. Medications are one common cause. Relocation can also be a cause, as described in the first case, p. 582. Malnutrition and dehydration are other causes.

Reality orientation is done both individually and in groups. Orienting an aged person to time, person, and place is part of the armamentarium of the nurse. There are three terms widely used, often incorrectly. *Reality orientation*, a specific group treatment modality for regressed, confused, disoriented patients, was begun in Tuscaloosa, Alabama, at the Veterans' Hospital in the early 1960s. It can be carried out on a 24-hour basis and should be used for the very confused. However, it must be done gently, and the orienter should back off if the aged person becomes agitated or hangs onto the denial mechanism.

The term *reality therapy*[54] is often used incorrectly. What is meant is reality orientation or reality testing. Reality therapy is a special form of psychotherapy and is conducted with juvenile delinquents. To date, Glaser has not worked with aged clients.

Reality testing is an ego function that provides the person with an objective evaluation and judgment of the world outside the ego or the self. Reality testing originates from psychiatric terminology, but it is part of nursing care of the elderly and must be discussed further. Reality testing must be considered a nursing responsibility and implemented in the following conditions:[55] (1) immediately following electroshock treatment; (2) during the transition from sleep to awakening (arousal from sleep); (3) during acute confusional states caused by anesthesia, surgery, acute illness, trauma, relocation shock, or dehydration; (4) during reactions from drugs or alcohol; (5) during hallucinations or delusions.

Suggestions for interventions regarding reality testing[55]

1. Reality testing is an urgent nursing task and must not be delayed, especially in crisis situations and in the ICU setting.

2. Explain all that is strange and different in the setting to the aged patient.

3. Be consistent. Reality orientation boards are often inaccurate and not updated. Staff members tell different stories—who is the old person to believe, the day nurse or the night nurse or relatives?

4. Give explanations with empathy and great patience.

5. Pace yourself so that you speak slowly and clearly, which can have a calming effect. Allow for sensory losses.

6. Allay fear and apprehension. Many aged persons (particularly Alzheimer's patients) cannot understand what is happening to them; they only know that it is different and terrible.

7. Touch the person during the reality testing process.

8. Help the aged to keep memorabilia with him or her. So often they are stripped of personal items that help them to maintain their identity.

9. Design interventions that will improve self-esteem. The confused may have low self-esteem. Aged people mirror society's negative view of them.

10. Do not argue when denial is rampant.

11. Encourage others to participate in reality testing, especially in hospital rooms or in group settings.

12. Have accurate information before you begin reality testing.

13. Record information on charts in detail and accurately. Most charting is inadequate. "Patient confused and disoriented" tells the reader nothing about the patient's actual behavior.

14. Take care of yourself so you do not become exhausted.

PREVENTION OF FALLS

Earlier in this chapter the serious consequences of falls in the elderly were mentioned. Because of the fragility of aged bones even a minor fall can be serious, and every effort must be made to provide a safe environment both in the institution and at home. The writer knows of a woman who lives in a retirement home. She has sustained three hip fractures, all from falls in the bathtub. Poorly lit and maintained stairways, slippery floors, icy walks, and uneven terrain are common hazards.

In institutions many patients fall from high beds, yet nurses are reluctant to lower the beds after they have finished bathing or giving care to the occupant. In Malaysia, I observed a home for the aged in which mattresses were placed on the floor to prevent falls.

Falls often occur during tests, in radiology or in the laboratory. The fall can be from a high table or during the process of getting on and off the table. The small stools often provided are hazardous. Some are rickety or the elderly may trip over them; they are not easily maneuvered by most frail elderly. Safe methods must be used during the transfer from and to the wheelchair.

Feist studied falls in a small nursing home and recommended that accident-prone individuals be identified to minimize unsafe activities.[3] As stated earlier, medications must be reviewed because tranquilizers may cause falls. Staffing should be increased during high risk time periods. One nurse commented that most hip fractures occurred during shift changes when reports were given and surveillance was at its lowest.

Keeping the confused and disoriented person in a safe milieu is most important. These individuals may have accidents other than falls, such as getting out onto highways or into rooms where there are faucets with hot water or dangerous equipment.

One must not take away all of the privileges and freedom from the aged person, yet their safety is a prime concern. A woman who has climbed ladders for 60 years to wash her own windows is indignant when reminded that she should give up that chore. One old man in Australia did not heed the advice of wife and children that at age 85 he might not need to trim the trees anymore. He trimmed as usual; he was lucky that when he fell he landed in a thick patch of undergrowth and plants that broke his fall.

These are only two instances. One must use great tact and have enormous patience in dealing with the feisty, independent elderly. It is a fine line to walk, both for the nurse who is caring for the individual and for the family.

SUMMARY

This chapter has presented the current state of the art of gerontological nursing.

An effort was made to combine a discussion of the state of the art and of the pertinent and perplexing problems we anticipate in caring for the elderly. Some problems require research by nurse clinicians. Psychosocial nursing care is a fertile area for research. Others may include the management of persons with Alzheimer's disease, abuse of the elderly, family support systems, prevention of burnout of the nursing staff and the family.

Some of these topics are covered in excellent current nursing textbooks. The reader is referred to a list at the end of this chapter.

The time that we have to work with an elderly person may be quite limited; therefore it is precious time to be well spent with that individual. The preciousness of the time should affect our decisions and mutual planning—there may not be a tomorrow to reminisce with them, to be their confidante, or to begin a rehabilitative program.

REFERENCES

1. Bates, B.: Changing roles of physicians and nurses, Wash. State J. Nurs. **1**:3, Spring, 1972.
2. California Board of Registered Nursing: Interim draft, No. 7B, Sacramento, Calif., 1979, p. 4.
3. Norton, D., McLaren R., and Exton-Smith, A.N.: An investigation of geriatric nursing problems in hospitals, New York, 1975, Churchill Livingston, Inc.
4. Kelly, C.H.: Nursing care. In Steinberg, F.U., editor: Cowdry's The care of the geriatric patient, ed. 5, St. Louis, 1976, The C.V. Mosby Co.
5. Yarling, R.R.: The sick aged, the nursing profession and the larger society, J. Gerontol. Nurs. **3**:42, 1977.
6. Weber, H.: Nursing the elderly patient, Reston, Va., 1980, Reston Publishing Co., Inc.
7. American Nurses' Association: Educational preparation for nurses caring for older adults in acute care settings, Resolution presented at ANA meeting, Houston, June, 1980.
8. Bahr, R.: Editorial, J. Gerontol. Nurs. **5**:66, February, 1980.
9. Lantz, J.M.: Assessment: a beginning to individualized care, J. Gerontol. Nurs. **2**:34, 1976.
10. Harris, B.: Coping with chronic disease. In Burnside, I.M., editor: Psychosocial nursing care of the aged, ed. 2, New York, 1980, McGraw-Hill Book Co.
11. Brody, S.J., Cole, L., Storey, P.B., and Wink, N.J.: The geriatric nurse practitioner: a new medical resource in the skilled nursing home, J. Chronic Dis. **29**:537, 1976.
12. Gerdes, J.W., and Pratt, S.C.: In anticipation of the geriatric nurse practitioner, Nurse Pract. **1**:14, 1978.
13. House of Representatives, 94th Congress, first session: Nurse Training Act of 1975, Report No. 94-143, 1975.
14. Loeb, P.M., and Robison, B.J.: Experience of a physician-nurse practitioner team in care of patients in skilled nursing facilities, J. Fam. Pract. **4**:727, 1977.
15. Gunter, L.M., and Estes, C.A.: Tomorrow's aged: impact of transgenerational trends on nursing education. In Power: nursing's challenge for change, Kansas City, Mo., 1979, American Nurses' Association.
16. Wells, T.J.: Nursing committed to the elderly. In Reinhardt, A.M., and Quinn, M.D., editors: Current practices in gerontological nursing, St. Louis, 1979, The C.V. Mosby Co.
17. Hirschfeld, M.J.: Research in nursing gerontology, J. Adv. Nurs. **4**:621, 1979.
18. Butler, R.N.: Medicine and aging: an assessment of opportunitites and neglect, testimony before the U.S. Senate Special Committee on Aging, October 13, 1976.
19. Butler, R.N.: The alliance of advocacy with science, Kent lecture, 1979, Gerontologist **20**:154, 1980.
20. Burnside, I.M.: Why work with the aged? Geriatric Nurs. **1**:28, 1980.
21. American Nurses' Association: Standards of Gerontological Nursing Practice, Kansas City, Missouri, 1978.
22. Hudak, C.M., Radstone, P.A., Hokanson, N.L., and Suzuki, I.E.: Clinical protocols, Philadelphia, 1976, J.B. Lippincott Co.
23. Pearson, L.J., and Kotthoff, M.E.: Geriatric clinical protocols, Philadelphia, 1971, J.B. Lippincott Co.
24. Blake, D.R.: Physical assessment of the aged: differentiating normal and abnormal changes. In Burnside, I.M., editor: Nursing and the aged, ed. 2, New York, 1981, McGraw-Hill Book Co.
25. Robison, B.J.: Assessment of the frail elderly. In Burnside, I.M., editor: Nursing and the aged, ed. 2, New York, 1981, McGraw-Hill Book Co.
26. Moehrlin, B.A., Wolanin, M.O., and Burnside, I.M.: Nutrition and the elderly. In Burnside, I.M., editor: Nursing and the aged, ed. 2, New York, 1981, McGraw-Hill Book Co.
27. Birren, J.E., and Sloan, R.B.: Handbook of mental health and aging, Englewood Cliffs, N.J., 1980, Prentice-Hall, Inc.
28. Wells, T.J., and Brink, C.A.: Urinary continence: assessment and management. In Burnside, I.M., editor: Nursing and the aged, ed. 2, New York, 1981, McGraw-Hill Book Co.
29. Schwab, M.: Implementation of standards of practice in gerontological nursing. In Burnside, I.M., editor: Psychosocial nursing care of the aged, ed. 2, New York, 1980, McGraw-Hill Book Co.
30. Dolan, M.B.: Day care for the elderly. In Burnside, I.M., editor: Psychosocial nursing care of the aged, ed. 2, New York, 1980, McGraw-Hill Book Co.
31. Eide, G.: Home care for the elderly. In Burnside, I.M., editor: Psychosocial nursing care of the aged, ed. 2, New York, 1980, McGraw-Hill Book Co.
32. Remnet, V.L.: The home assessment. In Burnside, I.M., editor: Nursing and the aged, ed. 2, 1980, New York, McGraw-Hill Book Co.
33. Burnside, I.M.: Accoutrements in aging, Nurs. Clin. North Am. **7**(2):29, 1972.
34. Pepper, C.A., Kane, R., and Teteberg, D.: Geriatric nurse practitioner in nursing homes, Am. J. Nurs. **76**:62, 1976.
35. Lowenthal, M., and Haven, C.: Interaction and adaptation: intimacy as a critical variable, Am. Sociol. Rev. **33**:20, 1968.
36. Strauss, A.L.: Chronic illness and the quality of life, St. Louis, 1975, The C.V. Mosby Co.

37. National Council on Aging: Fact book on aging: a profile of America's older population, Washington, D.C., 1978, National Council on Aging.
38. Introductory Report, Special Committee on Aging, U.S. Senate, 93rd Congress, Monograph No. 94, Washington, D.C., 1974, U.S. Government Printing Office.
39. Marram, G., Schlegel, M., and Bevis, E.: Primary nursing, a model for individualized nursing care, St. Louis, 1974, The C.V. Mosby Co., p. 125.
40. Miller, D., and Lieberman, M.A.: The relationship of affect state and adaptive capacity to reactions to stress, J. Gerontol. **20**:492, 1965.
41. Grier, M.: Living arrangement for the elderly, J. Gerontol. Nurs. **3**:19, 1977.
42. American Nurses' Association: Health care at home: an essential component of a national health policy, Kansas City, Mo., 1978, American Nurses' Association.
43. Burnside, I.M., and Moehrlin, B.: Maintaining the confused elderly in the community, Nurs. Clin. North Am. **15**(2): 389, 1980.
44. Rossman, I.: Environments of geriatric care. In Rossman, I., editor: Clinical geriatrics, ed. 2, Philadelphia, 1979, J.B. Lippincott Co.
45. Lapides, J., Bourne, R., and MacLean, L.: Clinical signs of dehydration and extracellular fluid loss, J.A.M.A. **191**:413, 1965.
46. Schabel, R.: Practical prosthetic treatment for chronically ill and aged patients, J. Calif. Dental Assoc. **44**(2), April, 1968.
47. Bennett, J.: Oral maintenance in the aged. In Carneral, D.L., and Patrick, M., editors: Nursing management for the elderly, Philadelphia, 1979, J.B. Lippincott Co., p. 111.
48. Brocklehurst, J.C., and Brocklehurst, S.: The management of indwelling catheters, Br. J. Urol. **50**(2):102, 1978.
49. Maney, J.: A behavioral therapy approach to bladder retraining, Nurs. Clin. North Am. **11**(1):179, 1976.
50. Kick, E.: Prescriptions for incontinence, ANA clinical sessions, Detroit, 1972, New York, 1973, Appleton-Century-Crofts.
51. Wells, T.: Promoting urinary continence in the elderly in the hospital, Nurs. Times **71**(48):1908, 1975.
52. Beck, C.: Abuse in the elderly, Paper presented at Western Gerontological Society Meeting, Seattle, Wash., April, 1981.
53. Taulbee, L.: Reality orientation: a therapeutic group activity for elderly persons. In Burnside, I.M., editor: Working with the elderly: group process and technique, North Scituate, Mass., 1978, Duxbury Press.
54. Glaser, W.: Reality therapy, New York, 1965, Harper and Row Publishers, Inc.
55. Burnside, I.M.: Reality-testing: an important concept, Assoc. Rehab. Nurs. **2**(3):7, 1977.

BIBLIOGRAPHY

Texts on gerontological nursing

Burnside, I.M.: Psychosocial nursing care of the aged, ed. 2, New York, 1980, McGraw-Hill Book Co.

Burnside, I.M.: Nursing and the aged, ed. 2, New York, 1980, McGraw-Hill Book Co.

Burnside, I.M.: Working with the elderly: group process and technique, North Scituate, Mass., 1978, Duxbury Press.

Mummah, H.R., and Smith, E.M.: The geriatric assistant, New York, 1981, McGraw-Hill Book Co.

Murray, R.B., Huelskoetter, M.M., and O'Driscoll, D.: The nursing process in later maturity, Englewood Cliffs, N.J., 1980, Prentice Hall, Inc.

Reinhardt, A.M., and Quinn, M.D.: Current practice in gerontological nursing, St. Louis, 1979, The C.V. Mosby Co.

Yurick, A.G., Robb, S.S., Spier, B.E., and Ebert, N.J.: The aged person and the nursing process, New York, 1980, Appleton-Century-Crofts.

Other books useful in caring for the aged person

Birren, J.B., and Sloan, H.B.: Handbook of mental health and aging, New York, 1980, Prentice Hall, Inc.

Harbert, A.S., and Ginsberg, L.H.: Human services for older adults: concepts and skills, Belmont, Calif., 1979, Wadsworth Publishing Co.

Wells, T.J.: Problems in geriatric nursing care, London, 1980, Churchill Livingstone, Inc.

Wolanin, M.O., and Phillips, L.R.F.: Confusion, St. Louis, 1981, The C.V. Mosby Co.

CHAPTER 37 · COORDINATED HOME CARE

Aaron Birenbaum
Marti Figlioli

HISTORICAL DEVELOPMENT

Home health care is presently in a stage of evolution, with both a fascinating history and an exciting future. Medical services to the sick in the home environment is not a new concept. Historically, medical care began in the home. As far back as 1796 the first home care program in the United States, the Boston Dispensary Program, was initiated to provide for the medical care of people in their home environment. At that time hospitals were reserved for the poor who could not afford the luxury of home care. Hospitals were viewed as pest houses where the poor went to die. The Boston Dispensary Program was inaugurated to relieve the sick poor of demeaning hospitalizations and "poor houses."

The next level of development of home care was the founding of the first voluntary agency, in 1885 in Buffalo, New York, which provided nursing care to the sick in their homes. In 1886 the concept of home nursing care spread to Boston and Philadelphia with the formation of voluntary agencies. As the need for medical and nursing services grew, Visiting Nurse Associations and official government health departments assumed the responsibility of delivering medical and nursing services to the community and began, in time, not only to expand in the number of agencies but also in the kinds of services available.

Home care since then has grown from the delivery of simple nursing tasks performed by volunteer lay persons for patients in their homes to its current definition:

> Home health service is that component of comprehensive health care whereby services are provided to individuals and families in their places of residence for the purpose of promoting, maintaining, or restoring health, or minimizing the effect of illness and disability. Services appropriate to the need of the individual patient and family are planned, coordinated, and made available by an agency or institution organized for the delivery of health care through the use of employed staff, contractual arrangements, or combination of administrative patterns. These services are provided under a plan of care which includes appropriate service components such as, but not limited to, medical care, dental care, nursing, physical therapy, speech therapy, occupational therapy, social work, nutrition, homemakers, home health aide, transportation, laboratory service, medical equipment and supplies.[1]

Until 1940 home care services were provided by official government agencies and Visiting Nurse Associations or community agencies organized in a similar fashion. In 1947 the first hospital-based agency was established in New York City at the Montefiore Hospital. This innovative program was designed to provide medical, nursing and social services specifically directed toward the care of the chronically ill. Later the Montefiore Program expanded to include physical therapy, occupational therapy, laboratory, x-ray, nutritional, and vocational rehabilitation services. This program became the model for other hospital programs. The Jewish Hospital of St. Louis, Missouri, for example initiated its Home Care Program in 1953 patterned after the Montefiore Program.[2]

Prior to 1966 the United States Public Health Service identified only 70 programs of coordinated home care in this country. With the advent of medicare and medicaid programs, under Titles XVIII and XIX of the Social Security Act, funding became available for selected home health care services. Federal agencies designed specific criteria and guidelines for agencies providing home care services and defined eligibility requirements for agencies and beneficiaries.[3] By 1977 there were 2496 agencies certified by the federal government for providing home health services and obtaining reimbursement from the funds allotted under the Social Security Act. The availability of federal money, then, removed home health care from the realm of charitable organizations for the poor or private for-profit organizations for the wealthy and made comprehensive health care available to a much greater portion of the population.

ORGANIZATION[4]

Home health agencies may be sponsored and financially supported by several systems. Of the 2496 certified agencies identified in 1977, 50% were sponsored by official health departments; 20% were sponsored by Visiting Nurse Associations; 11% were sponsored by hospital-based home care programs; 12% were sponsored by private nonprofit organizations; and the remainder were sponsored by combined government and voluntary agencies, prepaid health plans, extended care facilities, rehabilitation facilities, or independent agencies created for this purpose.

Whatever the organizational base, the central administration of the agency provides for the delivery of prescribed services. The home health system may provide all services following the prescription of the patient's private physician or may accept referrals of patients from physicians for additional medical care as well as all other services. The sponsoring agency assumes full responsibility for the smooth coordination of all services and the quality of the medical, nursing, social, therapeutic, and health-related services it provides.

The primary objectives of home care programs are as follows:

1. To furnish comprehensive medical, nursing, social, therapeutic, and health-related services to patients in their homes when the home environment is satisfactory to meet these needs
2. To provide more individualized or more consistent care for certain patients in their homes than could be provided in a hospital or extended care facility
3. To expedite recovery, prevent or postpone disability, and maintain personal dignity by restoring patients to normal family life and environment and to useful functional activity
4. To furnish comprehensive care to selected patients at a greatly reduced cost from hospital care by using the home as the center for delivery of health care
5. To shorten the length of hospital stay and prevent hospitalization or rehospitalization of selected patients
6. To improve utilization of existing hospital beds and reduce the need for additional inpatient facilities by suiting the health care services to the needs of the patient, that is providing only those services presently needed by the individual patient rather than housing the patient in a facility designed to meet comprehensive acute and chronic care needs including services that are not pertinent to the care of the individual patient
7. To provide for the needs of acutely ill, chronically ill, or terminally ill patients who can be adequately treated in the home rather than in an institutional setting

Home care interfaces and complements all other phases of the health care system including hospital care, nursing home or extended care facilities, day-care programs, rehabilitation facilities, and hospice care. For many patients, home care is a part of their health care at various stages of their lives, from the maternal-child health aspects of home care to the stage of acute or chronic illness as the individual ages, up to and including hospice home care during the terminal stages of illness and preparation for death. Home care then is a continuum of services for the community touching all aspects of health care at different stages and providing an essential companion set of services to all other institutional services.

TYPES OF SERVICES

The most comprehensive programs—government, community-based, or hospital-based—provide most or all of the following services: physician, nursing, dental, social work, physical therapy, occupational therapy, speech therapy, respiratory therapy, recreational therapy, homemaker, home health aide, nutritionist or dietician, laboratory, x-ray, transportation, medical equipment and supplies, music therapy, volunteer services, friendly visitors, pastoral care, and hospice care. All government certified agencies must provide nursing and one other service to patients. In the largest and most progressive home care programs, all the aforementioned services are available but not all services are reimbursable by medicare or medicaid and are paid for by charitable subsidies or underwritten by the sponsoring agency as part of the agency's commitment to the health of the community. Smaller agencies or those agencies in rural areas may provide only nursing service, social service, and home health aide services or only nursing and physical therapy.

It is important for the physician and the community to understand at least the basic roles of these various services and to be acquainted with the complementary functions of home health services.[5]

Nursing

Historically the registered nurse performed multiple functions in home care. In the past, and currently in a few rural agencies where no other skilled professional is available, the nurse filled not only the nursing role but the physical therapy, home health aide, dietician, social work, and laboratory roles as well. In a well-staffed agency however, the nurse should perform the nursing functions, and there should be qualified professionals from all other disciplines to provide the highest quality home health care to the patient.

With the development of related services and the specialization of therapeutic and social services, nursing remains the cornerstone of home health care and the one service required by federal law to qualify the agency as a certified home health agency.

Nursing has several distinct but related functions in home health care. These include direct nursing care, evaluation, monitoring, observation, instruction and supervision of patient and family in nursing care and communication with physicians, other disciplines, and other agencies. Depending on the size and organizational structure of the agency, the nurse may also be responsible for the coordination of other home care services.

Following referral by the physician of the patient to the home health agency, the initial evaluation that the patient receives is by a registered nurse who sees the patient in the home, the hospital, or the nursing home to assess the home care needs. The nurse discusses the patient's medical, nursing, and related care with the physician and begins the planning process for the patient's home health services. In large and progressive agencies, this is followed by an evaluation of the data by a multidiscipline team of nurse, physical therapist, social worker, and dietician or other combinations of disciplines to arrive at a comprehensive plan of carc for the individual patient. A written treatment plan is then drafted and authorized by the patient's physician.

Once the patient is at home, nursing care includes the entire nursing process of assessment, evaluation, monitoring, observation, reporting, teaching, supervision, and communication. Ideally this includes "hands-on" evaluation, monitoring, and observation of the patient and a review of the general condition, systems review, and measurement of vital signs. It also includes the evaluation of the nutritional, hydration, and mental status; the identification of immediate and long-term nursing needs; evaluation of home and family and of the caregiver's abilities and limitations; and assessment of the patient's progress, regression, or complications. This may require modification of the medical or nursing plan of treatment or the modification or addition of services to the patient.

Since home health care is not designed to replace the family but rather to supplement and support patient and family, one of the broad purposes of all services, especially nursing services, is teaching and supervision of the patient and family in performing the tasks necessary for maintaining health or for speeding the recovery process. This includes providing information concerning the nature and progress of the disease or recovery process and providing sufficient medical, nursing, and health care principles for the patient and family to become knowledgeable and capable of forming sound judgment about the patient's health or complications as well as becoming able to perform technical nursing functions. This teaching may range from assisting the patient or family to learn a simple dressing change of a wound or diabetic ulcer to performing intravenous hyperalimentation at home on a 24-hour basis.

Basic skilled nursing care is given by registered nurses in all certified home health agencies. In the more progressive agencies the talents and skills of the registered nurse may far exceed basic nursing functions. It is not unusual for the large home health agency to have Master's level prepared nurses and clinical practitioners in several specialty areas of community health. Traditionally, some treatments were performed only in institutional settings, for example, intravenous infusions, transfusions of packed cells, or hyperalimentation. With the additional skills that community health nurses have acquired and with the increasing need to use institutional beds for acute treatment, more of these sophisticated and complex treatments can be performed in the home environment. Of course this demands highly competent professionals and sound, thorough, administrative judgment and safeguards to adequately provide these services at home.

Of equal if not greater value is the skill of the registered nurse in observation and evaluation of the medical status of the patient. Accurately measuring, observing, and reporting cardiovascular function and complications, nutritional or fluid and electrolyte imbalances, complications of medications or treatments, healing status of wounds, and assessment of the patient's response to the treatment can often prevent major complications and help to keep the patient at home instead of returning to the hospital. The truly skilled public health nurse will, in time, and with a capable patient and family be able to impart these kinds of informed observational skills to the patient or caregivers and gradually assist the patient in becoming not only knowledgeable but more responsible for the quality of his health and his care.

Physical therapy

Next to skilled nursing services, supplemented by home health aide services, physical therapy is the most often prescribed service in the field of home health. In many instances the patient has begun a program of physical therapy while still in the hospital. The home program then becomes an extension of the in-hospital therapeutic regimen. As the patient progresses at home, the therapist adapts the treatment and objectives to suit the patient's changing needs and progress. Close communication with the patient's physician is essential so that the patient progresses at the maximum rate and achieves the highest level of functional independence.

Patients who have not been hospitalized prior to admission to home health programs can be evaluated for physical therapy needs at home by the physical therapist. After referral by the physician and the home evaluation, the plan of therapy is designed, taking into consideration both the patient's needs and the strengths and resources of the home environment.

Whether in the hospital or home, physical therapy is directed toward goals of restoring, improving, or maintaining maximum functional physical independence or of minimizing the effects of physical disability. The added dimension in the home situation is that of teaching and supervising the family members or caregivers in carrying out the therapeutic regimen on a daily basis. This supplements the direct intervention by the therapist and results in more rapid and more solid progress for the patient.

Since the home environment is unique to the individual patient, this is often a challenge to the imagination and resourcefulness of the individual therapist. The patient may respond quite well to instruction while walking along a broad, well-illuminated corridor or up and down conveniently located practice stairs in the hospital. The same patient, however, may be baffled by the differences in environment, physical obstacles, or unique floor plans in his home. The need for creativity, imagination, and improvisation on the part of the therapist is obvious. Special assistive devices, improvised equipment, and realistic planning with patient and family are necessary to make the home conducive to maximum therapeutic results for the patient. The encouragement, support, and resourcefulness of the therapist will often spell the difference between success and failure for the patient at home. The skilled therapist will assist the patient in making the necessary adaptations and reassure the patient that his home can be a safe and therapeutic environment for progress. Since the therapist is also teaching the family members to assist the patient, it is important to assure the patient that the family is capable of learning the skills and can safely assist in the treatment program.

The most frequently prescribed modalities of

physical therapy in the home environment are the following:

1. An exercise regimen that can vary from active, active assistive, resistive, or passive exercises, including stretching of shortened muscles
2. Gait training and all aspects of ambulation
3. Transferring activities; even for patients for whom no recovery or progress is anticipated, transfer skills for the caregivers make the home care safer and easier
4. The use of adaptive equipment such as ramps, overhead bars, footboards, overhead pulleys, and simple splinting devices
5. Preprosthetic and prosthetic training
6. Follow-up training in crutch walking and a variety of other modalities started in the in-hospital therapy program

Although the physical therapist is responsible for carrying out the prescribed regimen, the instruction and supervision of the family are essential in maintaining and if possible increasing the patient's function at a satisfactory level between therapy visits. Once the patient has made the initial adjustment to his home environment, it is not unusual for him to make greater progress at home than was demonstrated in the hospital. The direct care of the therapist, sound teaching of family members, and the desire to return to full participation in family activities often motivate the patient to participate fully in the therapeutic regimen, and thus the progress can be quite dramatic compared to his in-hospital status.

In contrast to the heavy and fixed equipment in the hospital physical therapy department, home equipment must be easily portable and often the therapist must improvise adaptive equipment for the patient's home. Much equipment is available now through retailers in the community. However, it is the task of the therapist to assist the physician, patient, and health care team to select the equipment that can be used by the patient in his particular home environment.

Occupational therapy

Occupational therapy is an important component of rehabilitation. Qualified occupational therapists, under medical prescription, use self-help, manual, creative, recreational, social, educational, prevocational, and industrial activities to gain from the patient the desired physical or mental response. The activities are prescribed by the patient's physician and are goal directed.

Once the evaluation is made, the occupational therapist designs and implements a variety of modalities directed at improving, maintaining, or stabilizing the patient's functional abilities in the home. Occupational therapy may be ordered for any of the following:

1. As a specific treatment for restoration of physical function; such as increasing joint range of motion, increasing muscle strength, or increasing hand-eye coordination
2. To assist in retraining of patients in all activities of daily living including bathing, dressing, eating, cooking, and activities that were a part of the patient's daily life before illness or injury
3. To teach the use of adaptive equipment in any of the aspects of activities of daily living
4. To make and instruct in the use of splints to correct or prevent deformity; usually these splints are constructed to treat some aspect of deformity of the upper extremities
5. To help the disabled patient, particularly the homemaker, readjust to the home routine and return to previous function with advice, instruction, and supervision in such areas as adaptation of home equipment, especially kitchen equipment, and in work simplification techniques
6. As a prevocational exploration to determine the patient's physical and mental capacity, social adjustment, interest, work habits, skills, and future employability
7. As a supportive measure to help the patient to accept and constructively utilize a prolonged period of convalescence
8. Where indicated, to assist in the redirection of the patient's vocational, avocational, and recreational interests.

Persons with perceptual or sensory motor problems often benefit from home treatment by the occupational therapist. Even if treatment in an ambulatory care setting is available, these patients may greatly profit by treatment at home, since they have difficulties translating learned skills from one setting to another, and the gains from an outpatient therapy treatment program may be quickly lost once the patient has returned to his home environment.

In a well-organized home health program, the physical therapist and occupational therapist will work together to define areas of modification in the home, ranging from the removal of environmental barriers to the construction or adaptation of assistive devices to obtain the best possible response from the patient in the home setting.

Input from the occupational therapist is essential in team conferences, particularly in the areas of the patient's progress and particular goals in activities of daily living. Well-intentioned family members and health team members may assist the patient in dressing or bathing when the occupational therapist has designed a program for the patient to be as independent as possible in these areas. Lack of communication or clarity regarding the fine points of the occupational therapy goals can result in team members being counterproductive in their interactions with the patient while they are carrying out another aspect of the home care program.

Occupational therapy is one of the most underused services in the home. Clients and health professionals are not well acquainted with the scope of occupational therapy services and therefore do not take full advantage of the talents and skills of this discipline. Occupational therapists have as their primary goal enabling the patient to become self-reliant in the performance of meaningful daily living activities. Secondarily, through staff and patient/family education, the occupational therapist can assure that home care patients are not seen in terms of their disabilities but rather in terms of their abilities and strengths and how these can be improved and enhanced to achieve maximum independence.

Social work

An understanding of "comprehensive home health" leads to the realization that treatment of patients if it is to be effective cannot focus on the physical aspects of illness or disability without concern for the individual's personal, social, psychologic, and emotional problems. The personal, emotional, social, financial, and environmental difficulties related to or resulting from the patient's illness are the particular concern of the social worker to the extent that such problems may further complicate the illness or hinder the maximum response to medical care and therapeutic treatment. The practice of social casework is then the primary function of the social worker in the home health setting.

It is easily demonstrated that emotional, social, and financial difficulties can affect the patient's ability to cooperate or participate in the therapeutic regimen in the home environment. The social worker directs his efforts toward alleviating or minimizing the impact of these difficulties on the patient's response to treatment.

Since emotional and environmental background and social circumstance have a major effect on the patient's general well-being and physical response, an adequate psychosocial study is essential at the point of application to the home health program. In the hospital-based agency with which we are most familiar, the medical social worker usually has had contact with the patient and family before discharge from the hospital and a thorough psychosocial study has been done before the patient is accepted in the home care program. In the community-based agency the social worker may make an initial home visit before acceptance in the program to accomplish this evaluation, or the patient may be accepted in the home care program and the social evaluation may be obtained by the social worker at the time of the first visit.

Through the techniques of social casework and the skill and compassionate assistance of the social worker, the patient and family are helped to identify and to understand some of the emotional responses to illness and disability. It has been repeatedly demonstrated that the presence and intervention of the social worker results in the prevention of crises in the home situation and in minimizing the effect of stress on the patient's response to medical care. The social worker is attuned to the emotional and psychosocial needs of the family as well as the patient. The social worker's expertise in facilitating family communication, strengthening family ties, and encouraging mutual understanding between patient and family is often the deciding factor in the quality of care the patient receives at home from the family members. Encouraging an atmosphere of warmth and genuine interest in the patient's difficulties and progress fosters a cooperative attitude, resulting in greater and more positive gains for the patient in the therapeutic aspects of his care.

The social worker plays an important role in assisting the other health team members in their understanding of the patient's emotional and psychologic response to illness or disability. All disciplines can use the social worker effectively to discern the most effective approach to the patient and family and to assist the patient and family in understanding and accepting a particular plan of treatment.

In many instances, the skilled social worker can assist the health team members in understanding their own emotional responses to be patient and thus provide for more effective intervention on the part of individual professionals in dealing with the patient's illness or disability.

Although all health team members have a responsibility to plan for the eventual discharge of the patient from home care, the social worker has a special role in facilitating and integrating the discharge planning. Whether the patient is fully recovered and returning to the activities of the community or the care of the patient has become unmanageable in the home and the patient must be readmitted to a hospital or extended care facility, the change of environment and the withdrawal of the support of the various health professionals will have an impact on the patient and family. Unless the patient and family understand the aspects of the anticipated change and can move easily and confidently into the new situation, the gains made by the patient under the supervision of the home health team can be rapidly lost. The social worker then maintains a caseworker relationship with the patient and family as long as necessary to ensure as much acceptance as possible for the different plan of care for the patient.

When the skills and talents of the social worker are combined with all other therapeutic disciplines, the patient has the best opportunity for accomplishing the goals of home treatment.

Home health aide and homemaker

Terms used to describe the services of home health aides, homemakers, and choreworkers are sometimes used interchangeably, although inaccurately. Describing their functions may be confusing as well, since functions differ in different agencies. In a certified home health agency, the term *home health aide* is used to define the nonprofessional person whose job it is to provide the following services to patients under the direction of a qualified professional, usually a registered nurse, but possibly a physical therapist or social worker: assist the patient with personal hygiene, including bathing in a tub, shower, or bed; shampoos; dressing; meal preparation; light housekeeping; grocery shopping; and similar tasks that will allow the patient to remain in the home environment. Usually the home health aide is assigned to assist a patient for 1 to 4 hours per day several times weekly, although this is extended to daily services in some cases.

In some large agencies, the home health aide may possess more technical skills, or the agency may have several classifications of home health aides performing increasingly complex personal care such as unsterile or sterile dressing changes, assistance with colostomy irrigations, and follow-through with the physical therapy program including range of motion exercises or walking with the patient. These additional responsibilities presuppose a degree of training and education of the home health aide by the professional staff and vary greatly with the agency and other services provided. In hospital-based agencies, the home health aide is often trained at the same level as the nurse's aide in the inpatient care system and may have more technical skills than the home health aide in a community-based agency. The converse may be true in rural agencies, since necessity may dictate that the home health aide have a greater proficiency in some areas and provide greater assistance to the professional nursing or therapy staff. Larger or more centrally located agencies might have sufficient professional staff that the home health aide can be utilized for personal care and homemaker activities only.

In some agencies the term *homemaker* is used to differentiate the functions of housekeeping, grocery shopping, meal preparation, and so on from the functions of personal care and assistance in the delivery of other professional services, which are performed by the home health aide. In still other agencies the actual job title of the person who performs any or all of the above defined functions is *Homemaker-Home Health Aide;* this is a kind of catch-all term that remains ill-defined.

Finally there are two additional terms, *choreworker* and *attendant,* which are used at times in the home health field and are confused with the terms *home health aide* and *homemaker*. Although the definitions of all vary with the sponsoring agency and area of the country, the most commonly accepted definitions are the following: the choreworker is a nonprofessional whose functions are usually limited to heavy housekeeping jobs, major marketing for the family, repair jobs needed to maintain the home environment, or routine housekeeping and household management on an ongoing basis; occasionally choreworkers will be placed in a home for an extended and unlimited length of time if the patients needs are such that the choreworker's presence spells the difference between the patient remaining at home or being placed in an institutional setting. The word *attendant* describes a person, either untrained or self-trained, employed by the patient or family for purposes of personal care, housekeeping, and general management of the patient in the home but not including skilled care.

Regardless of the title, most home health agencies do make available to patients at home a group of nonprofessional persons whose functions are to assist the patient with personal hygiene and activities of daily living and to provide an adjunctive service to the other professional services the patient is receiving on home care. In many instances it is the home health aide who teaches the family these basic skills as well and assists the family in becoming competent in caring for the acutely or chronically ill person at home. To reiterate, depending on the sponsoring agency, the home health aide may need a variety of complex skills to handle complicated home management for an entire family system or simple nursing skills to bathe, shave, and shampoo a home-bound patient three times a week. For best utilization of personnel, both professional and nonprofessional, the home health aide should be integral part of the home health care team and perform the nonskilled tasks needed to care for the patient at home.

Speech therapy

The services and skills of the speech pathologist are used in treating patients with varying degrees of impairment in communication. Depending on the kind, location, and sophistication of the agency the speech therapist might be used for treatment of patients who have aphasia resulting from cerebrovascular problems, patients who have undergone extensive facial and laryngeal surgery, or children with congenital speech impediments. The location of the agency and the patient population it serves will often determine the extent to which speech therapy services are needed and utilized. The functions of the speech therapist are treatment of the patient with the goal of returning the patient to normal speech and hearing functions, treatment with a goal of establishing alternate means of communication acceptable to the patient and family, or treatment with the goal of compensating for the loss of communciation due to injury, disease, or surgery. Treatment is based on a thorough evaluation of the speech or language problem, and the treatment plans are developed with the patient's physician and other members of the health care team.

Modalities of speech therapy are tailored to the specific needs of the individual patient and must be communicated to the other health team members. Because the field practice of the speech pathologist is highly specialized, the communication and education of family members and other health team members are essential if the treatment goals are to be understood and achieved.

Counseling and education of the family and home care staff are necessary so that all persons interacting with the patient will have an understanding about the nature of the communication problem the patient has and the best method of communicating with the patient. There is a general lack of understanding about speech and language difficulties, and the speech therapist may need to reassure the family and other team members that difficulties in communication do not necessarily reflect impairment of intelligence, deafness, or insanity. The inability to communicate effectively can be a source of frustration for the patient and an equal frustration for family members and the health care team. The skill of the speech pathologist becomes integral to accomplishing the total home health goals for the patient with communication difficulties.

Nutrition

The role of the nutritionist in home care includes both direct nutritional and dietary counseling of the patient and indirect counseling and assistance to the staff and family of the patient. The full-staffed home health agency should be able to design and assist the patient in implementing both normal and therapeutic diets. Again, the size, location, and sophistication of the agency may determine the scope of the nutritional services available to the patient.

Other professional services

A few other services are included in the scope of home health care, although not every agency has the ability to offer these additional services.

Patients who have needs related to the following services or physicians referring to home health agencies would do well to inquire if these services are available in their particular area. Many hospital-based agencies are able to offer additional medical services such as podiatry, pharmaceutical services, dental services, laboratory services, blood transfusion and related professional services unique to the nature of the hospital. Many progressive hospital-based and community-based agencies are now able to offer some forms of music therapy and recreational therapy, as well as respiratory therapy services through direct or contractual arrangements by the agency. Agencies, especially those which have a hospice home care program, may offer volunteer services, pastoral or spiritual counseling services, and legal services to selected home care patients.

Nonprofessional and other supportive services

Many agencies are able to offer some form of assistance to the home care patient in obtaining medical equipment, medical or surgical supplies, and assistance with transportation for medical or health-related appointments outside the home; and a few agencies maintain a transportation system for patients for nonhealth-related activities. Other support that may be offered by the home health agency directly or through arrangements in the community include home delivered meals, friendly visitor services, telephone contact services, and information and referral services to other adjunctive community service agencies.

Patient population

Experience in caring for patients in home health has provided us with knowledge and insight as to what type of patient is usually seen in home care programs. These patients can usually be classified into five main groups:

1. Patients recovering from acute illness
2. Patients who have acute exacerbations of chronic problems
3. Patients with terminal illness[6]
4. Maternal and child health patients
5. Patients with extensive physical disabilities[7,8]

Patients in the first group, those recovering from an acute illness, include persons recovering from an acute myocardial infarction, congestive heart failure, and cerebral vascular accident with paralysis, and new diabetic patients requiring instruction and supervision regarding insulin administration and diet. In addition, there are certain surgical patients who require follow-up, such as patients with hip fracture, patients with an ostomy, patients with postoperative wound infections, amputees and patients with acute pulmonary tuberculosis.

In the second group, those with acute exacerbation of chronic problems, one would see patients with chronic renal disease, and chronic obstructive pulmonary disease; diabetic patients with complications such as foot ulcers or amputations; patients with spinal cord injuries such as paraplegia or quadriplegia; patients with chronic neurologic problems such as multiple sclerosis, muscular dystrophy, Parkinson's disease, and amyotrophic lateral sclerosis; and patients disabled with severe rheumatoid arthritis, and malignant diseases.

In the third group, those with terminal illnesses, one would see patients with terminal malignancies requiring hospice care and those in terminal stages of renal, cardiac, or pulmonary disease.

In the fourth group, maternal and child health, one would see new baby follow-up and postpartum follow-up of mothers, and sick babies.

This is a partial list of the types of patients who are usually followed at home under the auspices of a home health program.

ADMINISTRATION/MANAGEMENT

Organization of the home health agency may take the form of traditional organizational structure with an administrative or advisory board as the top-level planning and regulating body. This is followed by descending authority of administrative and supervisory personnel, clinical supervisory personnel, and groups of professional and nonprofessional personnel engaged in the delivery of direct patient care. Another popular organizational form for home health agencies is a functional team concept system of organization with top management and administrative personnel involved in the overall planning and fiscal operation. In this system, groups of clinical supervisors in various disciplines work with an equally multidisciplinary team of nurses, therapists, home health aides, and social workers to cover a defined geographic area or a defined group of patients determined by diagnosis, age, or needs. There are still other agencies who use a system of organization that combines the traditional structure with a team concept and functional supervision of personnel.

Whatever the organizational structure, for home health care to be effective in achieving its purpose of delivering comprehensive health care in the home environment, the team approach must be used in day-to-day operations of the agency. Since by definition the home health system is a team of professionals and nonprofessionals delivering multifaceted services to the patient in the home, any system that works against team coordination and communication is self-defeating. The lack of coordination will become manifest in the quality of patient care.

Whatever the organizational system or structure employed and defined on paper, the following areas of administrative and clinical responsibility should be clearly defined in practice as well as in writing. Top administration should include overall planning and fiscal responsibility for the entire home health program. The administrator must be skilled in planning evaluation of the overall program, personnel management, and fiscal management. The administrator must know the legislative and developmental aspects of the program, including local, state, and national areas of home health. There should also be available personnel familiar with marketing and public relations aspects of the program with relationships to all other forms of health care delivery and community agencies whose purpose is complementary or supplementary to the provision of home health care. The size of the agency as well as the scope of services and geographic areas served will determine the administrative abilities needed, as well as the number of personnel in administrative positions. Middle management may be responsible for both administrative tasks as well as clinical supervision of personnel. There is an obvious need for all professional and non-professional disciplines to have clinical supervision in the actual delivery of health care services.

The need for multidisciplinary communication is essential to the smooth coordination of all home health services. This can be accomplished in a number of ways. Interdepartmental conferences, shared participation in the utilization review process of the agency, patient-team conferences, and case presentations may be used. A systemized sharing of written documentation of all pertinent patient data with the team members treating the individual patient is another method. Any combination of communication systems and tools that will effectively allow the professional and nonprofessional team members as well as the patient and family to know as much as possible about the patient's illness, prognosis, and treatment goals should be used to ensure success in accomplishing these goals. Without excellent communication and coordination of services, home care becomes an endless parade of professional and nonprofessional people, coming and going, treating different parts of the patient. It not only serves to confuse the patient and family, but discourages them as well. Thus comprehensive home health care becomes a nice sounding term in the textbook with no reality to back it up. Eventually the patient opts for institutional care because he can be assured of some continuity by the staff in the institutional setting.

COSTS AND REIMBURSEMENT[9]

Medicare/medicaid/private insurers

Medicare. Home Health Benefits are provided through Title XVIII (Medicare), Title XIX (Medicaid), Title XX (Social Services), private insurers (e.g., Blue Cross, Prudential, General American), philanthropic organizations and programs, and payment by private parties.

Medicare limits the provision of home health services to organizations certified as home health agencies. The agencies must meet the conditions of participation defined in Title XVIII of the Social Security Act and meet all federal, state, and local licensure and certification requirements. They must provide skilled nursing and at least one other home health service.

Medicare home health benefits are, by law,

oriented toward the need for skilled care and do not provide for coverage of care related to activities of daily living unless there are also skilled care needs. (There is ongoing discussion among agencies, fiscal intermediaries, and federal representatives as to the definition of skilled care. Over the past 10 years skilled care has an added dimension of a teaching and supervision component but is still not consistently defined. Often the issues fall under the broad category of professional judgment. For this reason there will be legitimate professional differences of opinion as to what activities and functions constitute skilled care.)

Under Title XVIII of the Social Security Act, the following are covered, or reimbursable services, under medicare:

1. Part-time or intermittent skilled nursing care provided by or under the direction of a registered professional nurse
2. Physical, occupational, or speech therapy
3. Medical social services
4. Home health aide services
5. Medical supplies (other than drugs) and use of durable medical equipment
6. Medical services provided by interns or residents under the teaching program of a hospital affiliated or under common control with a home health agency

The following adjunctive services are sometimes covered, depending on the patient's diagnosis and the quality of documentation by the home health agency: laboratory services, respiratory therapy, nutritional therapy or dietary counseling, and ambulance transportation in certain situations.

Medicare consists of two separate parts, A and B. Under Part A (hospital insurance). hospital, skilled nursing facility, and home health services are covered. Part B covers physician services, additional home health services, medical services, outpatient and laboratory services, pathology, and radiologic services. Participation in Part B of medicare is voluntary and paid for in part by the individual.

To receive home health services under medicare the beneficiary must be homebound, have the services prescribed and reviewed periodically by a physician, and need intermittent skilled nursing and/or physical, occupational, or speech therapy.

Medicaid. Title XIX of the Social Security Act (medicaid), has become the primary vehicle for financing health care services to low-income persons. Since medicaid is state administered under federal regulations, the services, amounts, and kinds of coverage, the documentation required, and the administrative details and "red tape" vary from state to state. Program costs are shared by the state and federal governments. States have broad discretion in determining eligibility criteria, reimbursement rates, and benefit packages.

Utilization of home health services under medicaid has been poor due to several factors: (1) varying regulations and interpretations of regulations from state to state; (2) reimbursement is usually lower than medicare reimbursement for similar services and often considerably less than the agency's actual cost of providing the service; (3) inadequately administered fiscal policy, which results in extended and unworkable delays for agencies in collecting any reimbursement from medicaid for services rendered to patients; and (4) cumbersome forms and restrictive criteria that are essentially contrary to the intent of the medicaid regulations.

Although home health services are mandatory benefits under medicaid, the actual definitions and restrictions are left to the discretion of individual states, and as a result medicaid beneficiaries rarely receive the kind and quantity of health care services that they need without subsidy from agencies themselves or from private organizations. Home health services presently mandated by Title XIX are nursing service, home health aide services, drugs, and equipment. However, states possess and have exercised their prerogative to place severely restrictive limitations on numbers of visits, restrictive criteria such as prior authorization for equipment (including cumbersome paperwork and unworkable time periods), and wide deviations in reimbursement.

Title XX is a grant-in-aid program instituted in 1975 and designed to assist states in providing monies for services directed to the population with the intended purposes of self-support; protection of children and vulnerable adults from abuse, neglect, or exploitation; prevention or reduction of institutional care by providing community or home based less intensive care; and appropriate institutional placement only when it is in the person's best interest.

Private insurers. Many major insurance companies now offer home health benefits as part of the insurance package of hospitalization and medical care. The amount of coverage varies greatly with the insurance carrier and may be as complete as 100% coverage for all home health services or as limited as none. However, most provide some coverage. Often there are limitations of services (nursing and physical therapy only), monies (70% to 80% of covered expenses), or visits (three home health visits for every unused hospital day under a hospitalization plan). In certain instances documentation in the clinical record must demonstrate that home care was in lieu of continued hospitalization and that services were of an intensive nature.

In general, private insurers have been slow to incorporate home health as an ordinary benefit of an insurance package. Currently, this is changing dramatically as insurers become aware that home care is a cost-saving method of providing medical and nursing care to large numbers of people.

WHY HOME CARE?

Home for most people is not only where they live, but "where the heart is." It is the place where we are most comfortable, most at ease, most able to be ourselves without fear of judgment, criticism, reproach, or threats to our well-being. Home then is the setting where, given the choice, most people would prefer to have their basic needs met, including health care needs as well as the other human needs of being fed, sheltered, and loved. Not all patients are able to be cared for at home. But far greater numbers of patients could be at home, with home health care services coming to them, than are now in home care programs. There are several reasons for the underutilization of home health programs. Inhome services now available are inadequate to meet the need of the population. Poor planning and fragmentation of services are frequent valid complaints against the home health system. Inadequate funding of home health programs accounts for many institutional beds being used for treatment of patients who could be treated at home. Many government and private funding mechanisms have a built-in institutional mentality if not an actual requirement for payment or reimbursement of legitimate patient care services. Or the payment for inpatient services may be higher than the payment for the same services rendered to the patient on a home care program or outpatient basis. Finally, there is limited awareness, experience, and appreciation of the value of home care by physicians, nurses, health professionals, and health care providers.

Much of the broad purpose in home health care is the teaching and supervision of the patient and family in all aspects of health care to accomplish the long-term goals of recovery, rehabilitation, minimizing disability, or enhancing the quality of life for the terminally ill patient. These goals cannot be achieved without the patient and family as essential members of the team. The "why" of the home care becomes apparent when we realize that people prefer to manage their affairs as well as they can for as long as they can. Many patients who do not manage their health care are either unable to do so physically or emotionally, or fears associated with technology, medical terms, and the mystique of the health care system convince the patient that he is not capable of managing his illness or rehabilitation process. Comprehensive home health care gives these abilities back to the patient and family as well as the responsibilities for the patient's health care and the decisions necessary to improve or maintain health. Most patients and family members not only are able to manage complex health-related tasks at home, but when given the opportunity, actually prefer to manage these tasks.

The scope of home care may depend on the talents and skills of the health professional involved. However, in addition, the success of home care, is directly dependent on the patient's or family's abilities and willingness to learn the skills and procedures necessary to provide quality patient care in the home environment.

Just as communication is the key to adequate coordination of services, the communication process and skills are also keys to motivating and supporting the patient and family in assuming responsibility for the health care given in the home on a 24-hour basis.

The most obvious reason for the existence of home care is that by its nature and philosophy the home care system is designed to treat the total patient, the whole person, in the environment in which that person functions most effectively already. The familiar environment, the support of caring, available family members, neighbors, and friends, and the talents and skills of a team of competent, caring health professionals is the best recipe for achieving the goal of healing the whole person. In home health, the definition of health is not simply the absence of illness. The concept of healing, of wholeness, extends beyond illness to areas of healing of both the actual injury or illness, and the sense of assisting and supporting people in healing relationships and in maintaining comfort and dignity despite a disease process that will end in the patient's death. Care in the home health system focuses on both the patient and the family and often, at least indirectly, extends into the area of healing the community. This may take the form of education, prevention of disease or disability, or assisting the community in initiating programs that will provide for the needs of the sick within the community.

REFERENCES

1. Hanlon, J.J., and Pickett, G.E.: Public health administration and practice, ed. 7, St. Louis, 1979, The C.V. Mosby Co., p. 645.
2. Littauer, D., Flance, I.J., and Wessen, A.F.: Home care, Hospital Monograph Series No. 9, Chicago, 1961, American Hospital Association.
3. Ryder, C.F., Stitt, P., and Elkin, W.F.: Home health services—past, present, future, Am. J. Public Health **59:**1720, 1969.
4. Stewart, J.E.: Home health care, St. Louis, 1979, The C.V. Mosby Co.
5. Development and use of home-care services: suggestions for physicians, J.A.M.A. **197:**129, 1966.
6. Rosenbaum, E.H., and Rosenbaum, I.R.: Principles of home care for the patient with advanced cancer, J.A.M.A. **244:**1484, 1980.
7. Steinberg, F.U., Birenbaum, A., and Stoddard, E.A.: Management at home of patients severely disabled by spinal cord lesions, Arch. Phys. Med. Rehabil. **49:**592, 1968.
8. Steinberg, F.U.: The management of patients with spinal cord injury by a hospital-based home care programme, Paraplegia **12:**246, 1975.
9. La Vor, J., and Callender, M.: Home health cost effectiveness: what are we measuring? Medical care **14:**866, 1976.

CHAPTER 38 · AGED IN THE COMMUNITY

Rodney M. Coe

The modern health practitioner understands very well that health cannot be divorced from environment and that individuals' physical well-being affects and is affected by their social well-being. For the physician this interrelationship of health and social well-being is a daily reality of medical practice. The physician knows that patients' situations in relation to the community—their roles, statuses, and relationships with others—can affect the course of their illnesses and the etiology, diagnosis, prognosis, and treatment.

The impact of community situations on illness is particularly evident among the aged, who are often subject to much greater stresses than younger persons and who often have fewer physical and material resources with which to withstand them. Many sources of these stresses are closely bound up with factors that tend to increase the aged individual's sense of isolation from the community. Reduced income, bereavement, retirement, diminished mobility, changes in the neighborhood ecology—these and other factors affect the aged persons' social situation and therefore physical and mental health.

The frequency with which these multifaceted problems are presented to physicians will continue to increase as the number of aging adults increases. In 1980, for example, there were an estimated 23 million adults age 65 or older, about 11% of the total population. By the year 2020 the proportion is expected to reach 16% to 18%. Moreover, the fastest growing segment of the elderly population are those age 75 and over; they also have the highest prevalence of chronic diseases and limitations of activity and use more physicians' services.[1] As is well known, chronic diseases are most susceptible to nonmedical influences such as social situation in the community. Many of the medical problems being presented to physicians for treatment will require nonmedical solutions.

Physicians then must deal with their patients' community problems along with their biologic disease. If they do not, they run the risk that their treatment will merely be palliative, since it will not remedy the basic problems that beset the patient. Moreover, patients' disabilities tend to aggravate the social factors that contribute to illness and that lie at the heart of their problems. To break this vicious circle physicians must alter patients' environments, and for this they will need the assistance of the community and its resources.

Thus physicians need to know what exists, or what can exist, in the community to assist them in dealing with the problems of the elderly patient. There often is far more help available than most physicians realize. Because physicians may not always know what services for the aged might be available in the community to help them, they often may fail to ask the right question of the right person. The purpose of this chapter is to provide a view not only of the influence of patients' community situations on their illness, but also of how that same community can assist the physician in dealing with patients' illnesses and problems.

COMMUNITY STATUS OF THE ELDERLY

The community situation of the aged population is as varied as the community itself.

Despite the variability among them, there are some stereotypes of the aged commonly held by the public and professionals alike. One of these depicts the elderly as sick and infirm. In fact, despite the presence of one or more chronic diseases, about 80% of the elderly are able to carry out their normal activities. Similarly, less than 15% of people age 65 or over have disabling mental disorders and even fewer are limited by senile dementia with organic bases.[2]

Another stereotype of the aged pictures them as dependent. In this stereotype they are seen as an institutional population, living in nursing homes, homes for the aged, mental institutions or with other members of their families. In fact, however, only 5% of the population 65 years of age and over live in institutions. Only 18% live with children or other relatives, and even within this group, the dependency roles may be reversed, with the children or other relatives dependent on the aged persons. With the growing number of four-generation families, it is not unusual to find aged persons living near children who themselves are in the so-called aged group, that is, over 65 years of age.[3]

A third stereotype describes the elderly as lonely and isolated. In fact, the elderly have approximately the same amount of contact with family members and friends as do persons under 65. Furthermore, loneliness was seen as "not a problem" by two thirds of a sample of elderly in a national survey.[4] In addition, about 13% of the elderly (19% of males and 8% of females) are still in the labor force.

Many of the stereotypes of the elderly are false nevertheless there are a number of social tendencies that have the effect of reducing the status of elderly persons in the community thereby influencing health status.

One major factor in the reduction of status is *lowered income*. Because material concerns such as food and housing must receive priority, for many of the elderly reduction of income means a reduction in social activities. For example, many elderly persons withdraw from participation in church or other groups because they believe that they cannot participate adequately without being financially contributing members. This withdrawal, in turn, diminishes aged individuals' interaction with others in the community and adds to their loss of role and status. It also means added problems in filling increased leisure time with satisfying activities.

Another major factor is *mobility*, since Americans are among the most highly mobile populations in the world. The children of aged parents move to take jobs; relatives and friends move to warmer climates; and the aged themselves frequently move for reasons of climate or to find better or cheaper living arrangements.

Bereavement is another factor that reduces the individual's status—the loss by death of spouse, siblings, children, or close friends. More women than men are affected by this problem. In the United States about 17% of men 65 years of age and older are widowed, whereas 55% of women 65 years of age or older are widowed.[1] It is estimated that these factors have caused most elderly persons to lose more than half their personal community at a time in their lives when it is extremely difficult for them to forge new personal communities.[5]

All these factors that reduce the status of elderly persons in the community become part of a chain reaction in which the factors act to limit the aged individual's participation in society. This limitation in turn reduces the number of stimuli that the individual receives from the environment. This *diminished social stimulation* in turn leads to a sense of *isolation* at the same time that the individual's resources to cope with problems—physical, emotional, material, and social—are reduced.

The chain is not yet complete. The elements that produce the sense of isolation also produce *stress*. Stress in turn contributes to *illness*.[6] If the illness is prolonged, it aggravates the community factors that produced the stress, thereby contributing still more to illness.

Aged people may find an escape from stress in the *role of illness*. Even among well persons, isolation exaggerates the perception of symptoms of illness. Therefore when elderly people become isolated, they may see themselves as ill. Furthermore, persons who are truly ill have a claim to the attention of others; even attendance at a medical clinic can be a social occasion. The community tends to see the aged as ill. This combination of self-image and of community image is often sufficient to push or to allow the aged individual to slip into the role of illness.

COMMUNITY ATTITUDES TOWARD AGING AND CHRONIC ILLNESS

The attitudes of the community, including those of the physician, toward aging and chronic illness are still another factor pulling the physician into the patient's community situation. The community tends to expect aged individuals to be sick and act out the role of illness.[4] Furthermore, the definition of illness has been broadened. Many problems that were once seen as "natural" consequences of growing old are now viewed as problems of illness and disability. Therefore the family and community as well as the aged individual expect the physician to be responsible for the aged patient and the patient's situation, even if the problem is not primarily medical.

The community, including the family of the patient, also tends to see the problems of the aged as irreversible and insoluble. The physician also tends to see the aged patient's problems as insoluble, especially since the technology of medicine is inadequate to reverse or to cure many of the conditions. Dramatic progress cannot be seen. The physician has been trained for total cure and finds it difficult to settle for less.[6]

Because both the family and the community tend to see the problems of the aged as insoluble, they often ignore or minimize them as long as possible. Prevention as a strategy for care of the elderly is thereby often overlooked.[7] When the problems become so severe that they can no longer be ignored, the family and the community are likely to reject the aged or to remove them from the community. This pattern of denial increases the isolation of aged patients, contributes further to their stress, and thereby increases the possibility of illness.

Disability and diminished function often tend to be confused with illness. Because large numbers of the aged manifest disability and diminished function, another situation is produced in which the community, the family, and the patient expect the physician to intervene. Thus the physician is called on again to deal with problems, not of illness alone but of community situation.

Again, it is a combination of stereotypes that pulls the physician into the community situation of the aged patient. First, the family and community may see old age as illness and therefore as compromising the patient's independent situation. Second, the family and community tend to equate disability with dependence. However, old age and disability in and of themselves may have little effect on day-by-day functioning. "It is really degree of fitness, rather than extent of pathology, that determines whether old people can manage by themselves and the amount of service they require from the community."[8] In the community situation of the elderly patient, then, the physician should not merely be concerned with the patient's deficits but is challenged to help the patient adjust to his potentials.

There are several principles contained in this brief description of community factors that influence the situation of the geriatric patient. Perhaps the most important of them may be summarized as follows:

1. Problems of aging and old age are usually defined in terms of disease and illness; thus physicians are often sought out as sources of advice.
2. Therefore physicians in the community are being called on to make decisions about health problems that are strongly influenced by essentially nonmedical factors.
3. Among these factors are environmental stress and a sense of isolation and their relationship to disease and illness. Hence there emerges a general principle that intervention in the social situation by doctors and other health professionals is necessary if the older person is to be helped to stay in the community.
4. The multifaceted problems of the elderly in the community require a multidisciplinary solution. Physicians are challenged to coordinate their skills with the services of other health professionals in the community to provide more comprehensive care to the elderly patient.

To meet the challenge, practicing physicians need to know more about the community resources available to them and how various factors affect the living arrangements for the aged in their community.

COMMUNITY RESOURCES AND THE PHYSICIAN

The family and the personal community

The family can be perhaps the most important and effective ally of physicians developing treatment programs for elderly patients. The stereotype that elderly people are isolated and socially alienated from the rest of the community is simply not borne out by the facts. Although most elderly persons prefer to live apart from their children, they continue to maintain close relationships.[3]

Many aged persons, often despite serious physical disabilities, are able to function effectively and to continue to maintain reasonably independent lives in the community because of the concern and devoted efforts of their families. In these efforts, what is important to the family is a sense of support by the physician. In many cases this support may take the simple form of assurance of the physician's availability to them by telephone. Given a feeling of support by the physician and furnished with information about other resources available to them, families can become the physician's most effective resource in the care of aged patients.[9]

As a resource to the physician, the family can provide a wide range of assistance. Their willingness to participate in the program of care is supportive to the aged patient and strengthens morale. The family can help the physician by assisting in the interpretation of instructions to the patient. The simple business of providing transportation to the physician's office or the clinic often makes the treatment program easier for both physician and patient. Giving financial assistance to the patient is another way in which the family can help, and of course many families can and do become direct collaborators in the treatment program by taking on the direct care of the aged patient.

Obviously the family can be used most effectively when the physician capitalizes on an established pattern of family organization and behavior instead of trying to change it. Thus if the family has functioned best by having the elderly and the young living separately, it would be best—assuming always that it is possible—for the aged patient to continue living apart from the family rather than, because it might be more convenient for all concerned, to move in with them. When there is tension between an aged parent and children, the role of the family might be limited to giving those forms of assistance that can be provided without much personal contact.

In addition to the family, other members of the aged patient's personal community are often useful resources to the physician. Neighbors sometimes are helpful. The church or lodge to which the patient may have belonged or still belongs frequently reaches out, informally or through organized programs, to its sick members. There are many senior citizen groups that have such reaching-out programs, especially if one of their own members is involved. There is beginning to be an increase in friendly visitor programs for the benefit of the elderly sick, some sponsored by community agencies and some organized, as already suggested, under the auspices of a church, lodge, or other group.[10]

This aspect of the personal community as a resource obviously is more effective in smaller communities in which relationship networks are visible. In larger communities, organized programs and services tend to take the place of these personal resources. Even in larger communities, however, it is important to make maximum use of those persons who are a part of the aged patient's immediate relationships. In fact, a major contribution often made by social workers and other professional persons working with the physician is finding out who belongs to the patient's personal community and helping the physician use these relationships in the patient's behalf.

An invaluable ally of the physician is the clergyman. Not only does the minister, priest, or rabbi meet the patient's spiritual needs in a period of stress but also is often an important source of information about the patient, about the patient's family, and about the community situation. The clergyman often fulfills the role of counselor and can be most useful in interpreting for the patient and family particular recommendations and orders of the physician as well as in helping to assure their implementation.

The larger community

In addition to the family and other members of the patient's personal community, the physician will often have access to more formalized sources of assistance in the larger community (as distinguished from the personal community). These agencies are found at all levels—federal, state, and local—and include a wide range of services, both direct and indirect, designed to help maintain the aged person in the community. Chief among them are associations of elderly adults in neighborhoods usually organized as senior citizen centers for expression of a variety of special interests and stimulating interaction. Beside voluntary health agencies, public health agencies, and private health insurance programs, there are a great many others. Some deliver services to patients in their own homes. Other provide services in more centralized community facilities.[11]

Organized home care programs. Organized home care programs may be based at a hospital, an outpatient service, a visiting nurse association, a health department, or an independent home care association. Comprehensive home care programs provide a full range of services: medical and nursing care, physical and occupational therapy, medical social service, home health aide or homemaker service, needed drugs and medical appliances, and access to hospital services when needed. Under certain conditions some of these services are covered by medicare.

Homemaker-housekeeper service. In the homemaker-housekeeper service the visiting homemaker or housekeeper assists or acts in place of the person such as the patient or a member of the patient's family, who would normally perform the duties of the home.

Home meal service. In a home meal service, sometimes known as Meals on Wheels, meals can be brought to the patient's home from a central point in the community, or if the patient lives in a senior citizen housing unit, meals may be delivered from the housing unit kitchen. Meals are sometimes available in senior citizen centers, too.

Friendly visiting service. The friendly visiting service is the result of an increasing number of organizations and agencies, as already described, training volunteers to visit with the aged sick who are homebound as well as with those who are living in institutions. Such visitors, especially if they come on a regular basis, can lessen feelings of isolation in the patient. Aged persons themselves volunteer for such programs.

Sheltered living facilities. In addition to serving the patient at home as described above, many communities have developed a range of services of varying types that can be applied for different lengths of time but all of which provide some social and environmental support. These range from regular but infrequent use of day-hospital and day-care centers to relatively permanent residence in congregate apartment complexes. Day hospitals provide various therapeutic modalities (e.g., physical, occupational, speech, etc.) plus meals, supervision of medication, and social stimulation during the day. At night, patients return home or to their regular living quarters. Day-care centers serve many of the same functions but generally have fewer therapeutic modalities and medical or nursing supervision. Other sheltered living facilities may include foster homes, special housing for the handicapped, and congregate residences that are designed to provide private living quarters and communal dining and recreation areas.

Related health practitioners. The foregoing description of community resources that may be available already suggests a large and growing number of related health practitioners on whom the physician can call for assistance in caring for elderly patients. Visiting nurses, physical therapists, occupational therapists, speech therapists, clinical psychologists, social workers, home health aides, practical nurses, and homemakers—all these are part of the health team.

Of course, not all the programs and services in this broad and varied spectrum are available to all who need them. In many communities, especially smaller ones, these programs and services do not exist at all. In too many communities in which these resources do exist, services are too expensive for the aged persons who require them, and most insurance programs do not include adequate coverage for ambulatory care as part of the benefits. Some of the programs are recent in origin and have been slow to be accepted because they are out of the mainstream of acute medical care services.

Nevertheless, substantial beginnings in the development and diversification of services for the aged have been made. Moreover, it can readily be seen that the first thrust of these programs is to assist older persons in maintaining themselves in the community. This gives rise to the second topic: determination of the particular living arrangement appropriate to the particular needs and situation of an individual patient. It is apparent that one must take into account a series of factors including preferences of the older person, what is known about the determinants of living arrangements, the types of housing available, and the kinds of services required. Collating these pieces of information should enable the physician to make a proper decision as to an appropriate residential setting for the geriatric patient.

PREFERRED LIVING ARRANGEMENTS

If one were to ask elderly persons what kind of living arrangements they preferred, the answer would most likely reflect a desire to be independent. Numerous surveys of aged citizens in communities of various sizes, as well as studies national in scope, have shown that the majority—ranging from 45% to 95% of these respondents—want to live independently of family or other relatives, usually in a self-owned, detached, single-family dwelling. There is some variation in this response depending on whether the respondent is widowed, whether there is family or other relatives, and whether financial resources are adequate. Generally, the second choice of aged respondents is to live with another person of the same age and sex but again independently of others. A third choice is to live near or with family or relatives. If compelled by circumstances to depend on relatives for support, most elderly people seem to prefer living *near* their relatives, and only as a last resort to live *with* them under the same roof. The last choice for most of these respondents is institutionalization in a facility for care of the aged, in other words, long-term care unit in a general hospital, chronic disease hospital, nursing home, or home for the aged. It should be noted, however, that some aged people prefer the institution to living with their family, especially under conditions in which they have a serious illness or disability from which they expect to recover.

DETERMINANTS OF HOUSING SUITABILITY

A survey of the literature on the factors affecting the choice of housing suggests a wide range of factors such as degree of physical disability, mental stability, loneliness, amount of income, accessibility to family members, personality makeup, and level of health. There is also a tendency to focus on one or at best two factors as the only ones to be considered. The relatively high degree of failure to accurately predict good adjustment or satisfaction with housing indicates that there is considerable interaction among several classes of variables, not just one or two factors.

Recently an attempt has been made to collate many of these factors into a theoretical framework that would improve design of residential environments to permit fulfillment of human needs. This is the *competence-press model*[12] which as the name suggests, describes behavior as a function of the competence of the individual and the environmental press of the situation. Competence is represented by characteristics of the individual such as physical and mental health, intellectual capacity, personality traits, resources, and so on. Environmental press is described by potential demands and/or limitations on the individual by features of the physical environment (character of residence, distance to needed resources such as the doctor, grocery store, etc.) and social environment (availability of and accessibility to others). The balance between these two dimensions represents degrees of adaptive behavior, while maladaptive behavior results from an imbalance, generally when competencies are inadequate to meet the demands of the environmental press. However, maladaptive behavior may also occur if the environmental press is so low that competencies are not tested, that is, there is a lack of stimulation.

To apply this competence-press model to choice of housing for the elderly the discussion will be limited to (1) physical capacities, (2) psychologic factors, (3) social factors, and to a lesser extent (4) economic resources.

The *physical capacity* of aged individuals varies considerably, but primarily, the category relates to the degree of disability of patients in terms of (1) their ability to get around unaided and to perform certain necessary tasks such as bathing, feeding, toileting, and other aspects of personal care or (2) degree of impairment of sight, hearing, and motor control.

The *psychologic factors* concerning the well-being of the elderly individual are most significantly related to mental health. For the most part, concern here is with the degree of deterioration of mental processes such as memory, but also with accuracy of perceptions and kinds of adjustments made to psychologic needs and to the environment. Another related factor is the degree of anxiety that may be aroused in the elderly person for a wide variety of reasons, not the least of which may be illness.

The inclusion of *social factors* involves some different features relating primarily to the nature and extent of the network of social relationships. Again, the research suggests a wide range of findings, ranging from concern for the social isolation of the aged to the advantages and disadvantages of large groups of elderly persons living in the same residence. Some studies have reported that older persons who remain in their own home in neighborhoods undergoing rapid change tend to become isolated, particularly if many or most of their friends have already died or moved elsewhere. Other reports have focused on what may be called congregate living, in which elderly people have private living quarters but share certain other facilities such as kitchens, dining rooms, or recreation areas. A new development here is the conversion of hotels to apartments for the aged. Another area of study has been retirement communities in which elderly people live more or less independently and privately in separate quarters but may have centralized community facilities. Finally, there are the formal institutions for the aged, such as hospitals and nursing homes.

Certain *economic factors* also must be taken into account. However, more must be considered than just the availability or unavailability of financial resources such as income, savings, investments, and Veterans Administration benefits. These are related to a more abstract concept of "style of living," which includes attitudes, values, expectations, and behaviors of the elderly that may or may not coincide with their actual financial resources. Nevertheless, it is known that a substantial proportion of elderly people have inadequate financial resources (15% have less than "poverty level" incomes) and at the same time have greater risk from a variety of health problems. Medicare, which was designed to alleviate a part of this problem by providing partial financing for some hospital charges and fees for physician services, has been unable to alter the general economic situation of the elderly. Thus the fact still remains that physicians must consider the elderly person's economic situation along with the preceding factors when determining the appropriate living arrangements.

TYPES OF HOUSING

One of the most confusing aspects of the literature on housing for the aged, at least in terms of conflicting recommendations, is in regard to the types of housing selected. As might be expected, there is a wide variation, from staying in the old homestead because of familiarity and memories to institutionalization. Between are recommendations for small, compact quarters, for ones with more space, for single-level facilities and split- or multiple-level dwellings, for special gimmicks to aid elderly persons and special designs so that they need not stoop over or reach too high. Other studies, however, have pointed out that these characteristics are less important than whether the housing is (1) integrated—in a neighborhood in which all age groups are represented, and specifically referring to the older person remaining in his own home; (2) segregated—in a situation in which large groups of aged people live together, at least in proximity if not in congregate style; or (3) isolated—in a residence in an institution.[13]

There are arguments both for and against each of these broad types of housing arrangements.[14] In the case of integrated housing, the positive factors include the following: life is in familiar surroundings, the home may already be paid for, all age groups act as the reference group, and neighborhood assistance may be available in time of need. On the other hand, it is often the case that the family home is too much for one person or one couple to manage alone, and in a highly mobile population the elderly person may, in effect, be isolated from the stream of events and become dependent on outside assistance.

There are some important and obvious advantages to some form of segregated communal life—whether congregate or in terms of proximity. Perhaps the most important of these is the ability to provide centralized, special services whether they are medical services, legal counseling, or friendly visiting. Furthermore, the centralization of older persons has the potential of bringing together many people who share the same interests and capabilities and who can serve as a resource for each other, often in significant social and psychologic ways. It is likely that people interested in living in this kind of setting would have much in common, such as amount of income and other resources, independence from parental roles, and interest in activities.

On the other hand, there is some evidence that elderly people who do not prefer congregate living, reject it because (1) being with other aged people constantly reminds them of their own status and tends to reinforce a generally negative attitude of self, such as "being old," and (2) illness and death of friends and neighbors is a particularly visible phenomenon, thus giving the setting a kind of "end of the road" perspective.

This perspective may be attributed in different degrees to different types of communal settings. That is, housing developments or retirement centers seem to have these characteristics only in a slight degree compared with isolated housing in formalized institutions such as chronic hospitals or nursing homes. It is in the institution that patients are exposed to maximum dependence on the institution for satisfaction of basic needs, but also they must accept a minimum of personal freedom. There is considerable evidence that both physical and mental capacities of patients deteriorate rapidly when they are placed in these settings. This deterioration is by no means caused by the characteristics of the institution alone, but it reflects a continuation or reinforcement of a physical or mental decline begun earlier and compounded by a number of social and psychologic factors.

SELECTION OF APPROPRIATE HOUSING

Some guidelines are presented here for collating the various factors discussed briefly in the preceding paragraphs. Initially, the assumption is made that of the four major dimensions—physical capacity, psychologic factors, social factors, and economic factors—the most influential is probably the degree of physical capacity ranging from "well," or not incapacitated, to fully incapacitated. With this one dimension the remaining three can be discussed in relation to it, resulting in several situations for which a type of housing or living arrangement is suggested, based on what is known from previous research.

The well aged person

If the elderly person has no physical incapacity, has no psychologic problems (about 80% of all elderly), prefers situations of frequent interaction and exchange, and has large or even modest economic resources, the selection of housing may well be left to the individual, since there really is no problem. It is included here more as a logical possibility rather than because physicians are likely to encounter this situation.

On the other hand, patients who have no physical incapacity but who exhibit some psychologic problems such as frequent loss of memory or temporary disorientation, and who have few or no economic resources, would probably be better served in some form of communal setting in which the patient is not far removed from interested others and in which certain minimal supporting services are readily available. Moreover, there are some types of communal settings designed to fit the reduced income levels of elderly persons and therefore are more appropriate than other types of housing. One exception is the well aged person who prefers living alone or at least not in close contact with many others. This person would probably be better off in a setting integrated with the rest of the general community, especially if an informal support network of neighbors and friends exists.[10]

The semi-incapacitated patient

For those patients who suffer some incapacity in mobility or functioning, but who have no significant psychologic or social deterioration, the segregated setting is likely to be the most appropriate. This choice is based largely on the availability of medical and social services commonly found in these settings. If, at the same time, older patients have sufficient economic resources to purchase these services—including transportation—separately, they could well remain in integrated housing. Persons of this latter type can often function adequately with occasional home care and homemaker services.

For patients who do reveal some deficiency in other dimensions—particularly psychologic problems and lack of interest in sustained interaction with others—some form of isolated housing might be a better choice. The form of communal housing must include a wide range of support services. Isolated or institutional housing presents a few more problems because of the variation in quality of care provided. Generally speaking, however, nonprofit agencies or small agencies sponsored by religious groups appear to give the best care.

The incapacitated patient

Fewer alternatives are available for the incapacitated patient, who represents less than 5% of all persons age 65 and over. Living at home in the general community is not a realistic choice except when there are rare conditions such as substantial economic resources and availability of around-the-clock personal services. However, some form of segregated housing may be feasible, especially if medical and support services are a part of the housing program (as distinct from readily available, but purchased separately). For the incapacitated patient who has other problems as well, the most appropriate setting is probably an institution in which close supervision may be exercised over the medical and supportive services that are required.

Although the discussion just presented oversimplifies the true complexities involved in evaluating the housing needs of elderly patients, it permits one to simultaneously take into account the major factors affecting decisions of this sort and relates them to types of housing as suggested by various reports of research. Much has been left unsaid; perhaps even more remains unknown. It is clear, however, that considerably more research effort will be required before more definitive answers are known.

CONCLUSION

In this chapter the major goals were (1) to indicate the importance of knowledge about the community and how its features can affect the health situation of elderly patients and (2) to provide some basic guidelines for physicians to help them determine the most appropriate residential setting for their elderly patients.

The first objective includes a brief discussion of various factors that alone or in conjunction with other factors tend to influence the health status of aged patients in the community. The principal conclusion was that the physician should make every effort to enable the aged person to continue living in the community.

To help patients with these problems, the physician must know about and collaborate with different sources of support. For example, there is the family as well as other members of the geriatric patient's personal community, such as clergymen, friends and neighbors, or club members. There is also a wide range of other more formal agencies that provide home care, day care, or meals on wheels, which the physician may also recommend.

All these services are designed to enable the elderly person to remain in the community. For this reason the physician must also know about and take into account some factors associated with different living arrangements for elderly patients. The main task of the physician is to consider the dimensions of physical capacity, social factors, psychologic factors, and to some extent, the economics of the patient's specific situation to arrive at the most realistic decision for helping geriatric patients cope with their problems.

REFERENCES

1. U.S. Bureau of Commerce: Statistical abstract of the United States, 1978, Washington, D.C., 1979, U.S. Government Printing Office.
2. Busse, E.W., and Pfeiffer, E.: Functional psychiatric disorders in old age. In Busse, E.W., and Pfeiffer, E., editors: Behavior and adaptation in late life, Boston, 1969, Little, Brown and Co.
3. Shanas, E.: Social myth as hypothesis: the case of family relations of old people, Gerontologist **19**:3, 1979.
4. Harris, L.: Myth and reality of aging in America, Washington, D.C., 1975, National Council on Aging.
5. Henry, J.: The personal community and its invariant properties, Am. Anthropol. **60**:827, 1958.
6. Eisdorfer, C., and Wilkie, F.: Stress, disease, aging and behavior. In Birren, J.E., and Schaie, K.W., editors: Handbook of the psychology of aging, New York, 1978, Van Nostrand Reinhold Co.
7. Coe, R.M., and Brehm, H.P.: Preventive health care for adults: a study of medical practice, New Haven, Conn., 1972, College & University Press.
8. Shanas, E., et al.: Old people in three industrial societies, New York, 1968, Atherton Press.
9. Maddox, G.L.: Families as context and resources in chronic illness. In Sherwood, S., editor: Long term care, New York, 1975, Spectrum Publishers.
10. Ehrlich, P.: Mutual help for the community elderly: the mutual help model, Carbondale, ILl., 1979, Southern Illinois University. (Mimeograph.)
11. Kahana, E., and Coe, R.M.: Alternatives in long term care. In Sherwood, S., editor: Long term care, New York, 1975, Spectrum Publishers.
12. Lawton, M.P.: An ecological theory of aging applied to elderly housing, J. Arch. Ed. **31**:8, 1977.
13. Rosow, I.: Social integration of the aged, New York, 1971, The Free Press.
14. Lawton, P., and Cohen, J.: The generality of housing impact on the well-being of the elderly, J. Gerontol. **29**:194, 1974.

CHAPTER 39 · EDUCATION IN GERIATRIC MEDICINE

Alvin J. Levenson

INTRODUCTION*

In 1978 the Institute of Medicine of the National Academy of Sciences published a study report entitled "Aging and Medical Education."[1] Among its recommendations the study suggested "that medical schools include appropriate content on aging in basic and clinical science courses" and that "preparation for care of the aged be included in clinical clerkship and in housestaff training programs, as well as in examinations for certification and licensure." The study committee further stated that

> Increasing specialization with its tendency to compartmentalize health care is often ill-suited to the care of people who have multiple, chronic medical problems. Health care reimbursement that overemphasizes acute care and the performance of procedures, while restricting length of hospital stay and the use of non-medical support services outside of acute care facilities, also can lead to inadequate or inappropriate care of the elderly.[1]

Since the report was issued, the interest of medical educators in the health care of the aged has increased. The American Geriatrics Society has established a section for teachers of geriatric medicine and has conducted annual interuniversity conferences on geriatric education.[2] The Gerontological Society has developed curricula on geriatric medicine for practicing physicians. Many schools of medicine have begun to implement the recommendations of the Institute of Medicine.[3]

There is a general consensus that geriatric medicine should not be a specialty with its own certifying board. The care of the aged patient best remains in the hands of internists or family practitioners. A large percentage of patients seen by internists in private practice is in the geriatric age group. This percentage will continue to grow as time goes on.

However, a special body of knowledge is required to adequately care for the aged patient, and neither our medical students nor our house staff have organized planned exposure to this material. The essentials of this body of knowledge can be summarized as follows:

1. There are a number of diseases that occur almost exclusively in older persons.
2. There are certain diseases that present a different clinical picture in old age. (Much of this has been discussed in the preceding chapters.)
3. Old people frequently exhibit several chronic disease processes at the same time. These processes interact and may present clinical pictures that are difficult to diagnose and evaluate.
4. Psychiatric problems are common in the aged, and many are treatable. A precise differential diagnosis is vital for proper management.
5. Proper care of the aged should include a functional evaluation. Physicians and their associates must be able to assess patients' ability to take care of their personal needs and to function in their environment.
6. Many of the conditions encountered in the aged are chronic and apt to cause physical disabilities. Many of these disabilities are at least

*Introduction written by Franz U. Steinberg.

partly correctable, and if properly managed need not lead to social or personal handicap. Therefore physical rehabilitation must be an important component of the care of the aged.

7. Proper care of the geriatric patient must be preventive. Malnutrition and misuse of medication are common causes of declining health of an aged person. Both are preventable. Many accidents that can lead to disabilities can be prevented by training older persons in safety precautions and by modifying their environment.

8. The physician must understand the social and psychologic problems specific to old age. These problems cannot be solved by medical means, yet the physician must be aware of them because they obviously interfere with a patient's health. The physician should know the social agencies to which patients can be referred for assistance.

This material can be presented to students without over burdening an already crowded curriculum. The following suggestions may be helpful.

1. Inhospital clerkships in medicine are well suited to teach the student about problems of old age. Many of the patients assigned to students will be in the geriatric age group. A skillful instructor will proceed from physical and laboratory findings and diagnosis and treatment of the acute phase of disease to the problems of long-range management, both medical and social.

2. A similar approach may be used in outpatient facilities, such as physicians' offices or the hospital's outpatient clinics.

3. A rotation through a home health service is most valuable. Students and residents will learn the problems and also the importance of providing medical care in the patient's home. To see patients in their natural environments will provide a better insight into social problems than lectures or seminars on this subject. The students will soon realize that unless good follow-up care and supervision are provided to seriously chronically ill patients they will soon be back in the hospital with the same problems for which they had been previously treated.

4. Some exposure to long-term care institutions is important. However, it needs to be emphasized that rotations through such facilities should come late in the training program. Patients in these institutions are frequently deteriorated beyond help, and they present a discouraging picture that is apt to turn students and young physicians away from the problems of the elderly.

5. Teaching by lectures should be kept to a minimum, but a few introductory lectures on the biology of aging and on the psychologic and sociologic aspects of aging will be valuable. It may be advisable to present these lectures in the freshman and sophomore years when students appear to be most receptive to social problems.

The organization of teaching of geriatric medicine will vary from medical school to medical school. In most instances the focus will be best placed in the departments of Internal Medicine or Family Medicine, even though in some cases other departments with strong specialized interests in old age, such as psychiatry, may assume leadership. In any case there will have to be one person to serve as a coordinator to make certain that all important aspects are covered and to prevent unnecessary duplication of curriculum material. The coordinator should see to it that all specialities and subspecialities assemble those data that are pertinent to the care of the aged and that they develop plans for incorporating these data into an overall teaching program.

The basic sciences, physiology, biochemistry, pathology, genetics, pharmacology, and so on, should be encouraged to emphasize problems of aging in their curricula where appropriate. The biology of aging is a fruitful field in basic sciences, and research in these areas should be encouraged. Some students, resident physicians, and fellows may become interested in participating in such research activities. However, care must be taken so that this does not become a form of seduction for the sole purpose of getting young physicians interested in the problems of old age. They should not look on the aged patient as a laboratory model instead of a human being in need of care.

Dr. Alvin J. Levenson's chapter, which follows, discusses the problems of education in gerontology and geriatrics from the vantage point of a psychiatrist, geriatrician, and educator. He examines the attitudes of society toward the aged and how these attitudes create obstacles to incorporating gerontology and geriatrics into teaching programs. He shows how these obstacles can be overcome.

MEDICAL SCHOOL EDUCATION IN GERONTOLOGY AND GERIATRICS

Medical care of the elderly in the United States has been characterized by negativism, defeatism, and professional antipathy. Ageism, a bias against the elderly based predominantly on their age, is believed to be the major cause. While the roots of ageism are many, self-perceived clinical ineptness, borne largely of inadequate education and lack of role models, is significant. Such self-perceptions tend to produce avoidance of the unpleasant stimulus. Haphazard efforts to establish educational programs in gerontology and geriatrics, however, may result in their premature demise. Suboptimal education for service providers will have a negative impact on the elderly.

Certain requirements must be soundly established and perpetuated for a medical school's undergraduate, graduate, and continuing education programs in aging to survive. First, the purpose of the programs must be clearly delineated and substantiated. Second, the curricula must be designed to accomplish this purpose. Third, the design of the curriculum must conform to well accepted educational theory and practice. Fourth, the faculty must be willing to serve as role models, particularly in the more applied aspects of the program. Fifth, pertinent characteristics of the student population must be respected during curriculum development and implementation. Sixth, potential obstacles to incorporation of the curriculum into existing programs require address and solution. Seventh, the programs must be administered by a stable organizational component.

Program purpose

The overall purpose of the medical school's undergraduate, graduate, and continuing education programs must be the improvement of health care of the elderly. Not only is the development, dissemination, and application of clinical knowledge the medical school's traditional responsibility, but enhanced service is clearly one of the elderly's most pressing needs. There is a considerable quantitative and qualitative deficit in health care delivery to the aged. Quantitatively, for example, only 43% of the elderly with arthritis consulted a physician for this potentially debilitating condition in 1977. Despite the fact that 86% of the aged have at least one chronic illness and 50% have two or more illnesses with acute exacerbations that require intensive treatment, 83% of them reported no hospitalization in 1977. This is compared to 89% of the total population who reported no hospitalization in the same year. Approximately three fourths of the elderly do not use preventive care services. In 1977, only 29% had an electrocardiogram, 25% a glaucoma test, and 32% a chest x-ray examination. Currently, 80% to 93% of the 2.5 to 5.5 million psychiatrically ill elderly in the United States are not having their mental health needs met through existing services. The aged use a disproportionately high amount of psychiatric inpatient services (three times that of younger populations) despite a rational imperative to halt unnecessary hospitalization and often consequent institutionalization. While state hospitals have been discharging large numbers of these patients to be treated in clinics, little provision has been made to accommodate them. To wit, practicing American psychiatrists currently spend less than 2% of their time seeing the elderly, and less than 4% of community mental health center rosters are represented by the mentally ill aged. Overall, the geriatric population uses 2.3% of outpatient psychiatric services.

Qualitatively, a therapeutic nihilism often pervades treatment of elderly patients. Since old age tends to be viewed as "irreversible," many perceive late life illness as likewise beyond significant assistance. It has been noted that the aged are usually referred for "disposal" rather than disposition. In that light, terms such as "gomer," "crock," and "nursing home dump" are frequently associated with such treatment. Attitudes such as these prompt palliation and control measures. Minimal emphasis is placed on the production of remission of otherwise reversible states, on rehabilitation for the future, on the individuality of the aging process, and hence on the need for individualized treatment. This approach tends to produce suboptimal therapeutic results, to significantly increase the risk of iatrogenic disease, to elevate the likelihood of recidivism, and to reduce opportunities for potentially productive futures.

Relationship of curriculum to purpose

The desired educational outcome of the curriculum is to promote the health care provider's competence, confidence, and comfort in the assessment and treatment of the ill elderly and in the prevention of unnecessary disease and institutionalization. That is not to indicate that the health professional must "love" each and every elderly person or the aged in general. It implies, however, that the health care provider will feel a sense of commitment to offer the older individual every opportunity to live as healthy and productive a life as possible. The principle educational effort is, therefore, to build an adequate basic and clinical sciences foundation via the requirements for optimal health care to the elderly. The author's conception of some of these health care requirements are summarized.

First, there must be an appreciation of the fact that the geriatric years represent the last stage of life, which render them unique to any other period of the life cycle. Any stage that is the last, however, implies that the individual innately desires a sense of satisfaction from life thus far, so that death may be preceded by a sense of relative equanimity and calm. Therefore, these issues must be addressed where problematic.

Second, in the presence of a progressive decline in physiologic and psychologic reserves to withstand stress, as well as an increase in stress, assessment must yield and treatment be directed toward removal of obstacles to restoring balance and reapproximating or reattaining the individual's premorbid baseline. The baseline includes proclivities toward engagement in and quality of such things as interpersonal relationships, education, work, recreation, religion, nutrition, health, skilled and basic activities of daily living, and personality. The premorbid baseline is an important treatment consideration and goal for several reasons. It represents the major life areas in which gratification was sought to produce and maintain psychologic comfort (the absence of persistent or intolerable anxiety)—the essence of life—thereby forming an apt treatment goal regardless of the health care provider's speciality or discipline. Knowledge of the patient's baseline guides the clinician in individually tailoring a therapeutic approach and avoiding unnecessary iatrogenic problems. For example, if the individual has been essentially nonpathologically introverted most of his or her adult life, iatrogenic induced stress may arise if the patient is "coerced" into "socialization" activities. The premorbid baseline assists the clinician in evaluating total improvement vis-à-vis premorbidity reattainment of reapproximation and in avoiding the pitfalls of judging the patient's involvement in standard ward or clinic activities (in which he or she has never engaged) as indicative of treatment outcome.

The removal of obstacles to attaining premorbidity baseline is best accomplished by optimal geriatric technique, defined as the application of optimal practice for younger adults modified by special aging and late life related factors. Suboptimal technique with younger populations will likely be continued with the elderly, however, with greater potential consequences. This issue is exemplified by the use of psychotropic medications. For example, later and late life physiologic changes (e.g., reductions in plasma protein binding, hepatic function, skeletal muscle mass, and renal function) require lower doses of many medications for the aged. When standard younger adult dosages are prescribed, the risks of untoward reactions and disease precipitation rise. Furthermore, if the clinician is unaware of these agents' indications and contraindications (both factors pertinent to optimal technique), negative therapeutic effects often result, for example, the absence of remission of the acute state and the production of greater than minimal side effects.

Third, treatment must be preceded by optimal assessment. This assessment seeks to delineate the following factors. First, an accurate inventory of the patient's premorbid baseline must be gathered. This inventory should include components such as interpersonal relationships (e.g., grooming and other aspects of personal hygiene and care); skilled activities of daily living (e.g., driving, household bookkeeping, grocery shopping, food preparation, etc.); education; work; recreation; nutrition; religion; health attitudes; and personality. When assessing these premorbidity or preproblem areas, the clinician must examine them for the individual's proclivity and involvement in each. For example, while it is important to determine that the patient ceased his or her formal education on completion of the tenth grade, it is more crucial to know the significance of education to the person in terms of its impact on the production of psychologic comfort. Were education important in that regard, a premature departure from formal education would not indicate necessarily the absence of a desire to continue. When considering, for example, the area of nutrition, it is important to evaluate such factors as caloric intake, as well as preferences for meal size and specific foods, seasonings, and so on. However, it is equally important to be cognizant of the emotional significance of food and activities surrounding it. Exemplary of the latter issue would be the importance of serving, being served, the dining partner's role, and so on. The second facet of the assessment process includes delineating and evaluating obstacles impeding reattainment or reapproximation of premorbid baseline. These obstacles may be of many types; for example, illness; normal age-related impairments (no evidence of a causal disease), decreased hearing or vision; disrupted family conditions; economic loss, and so on. Regardless, these factors assume import by virtue of their significance to the particular individual. A person who had never invested emotionally in family would tend not to miss it. Likewise, one who received little psychologic comfort from work and who looked forward to retirement would likely not bemoan a departure from the work force. One who, for example, received much enjoyment and emotional support from reading or handwork (such as sewing) would greatly miss adequate visual acuity. It is important to assess these life events through the eyes of the individual patient or client and not through those of the health care provider. Not everyone who loses grieves the loss! Furthermore, the quality of the individual's response to these losses is patterned in great part by predominant personality traits, stress coping ability, and replacement alternatives.

Fourth, treatment should consist of specific plans designed to remove obstacles impeding reattainment or reapproximation of the patient's premorbid baseline. Conceptually, plans may be of two major types—treatment of specific disease states and problems as well as therapies designed to stimulate reengagement in baseline activities.

Regarding treatment of specific disease states, one must be alert to the presence of late life physiologic dysfunction and its correction. Of the elderly 86% have at least one chronic illness and 50% have two or more—all of which may exacerbate into acute illnesses or predispose the individual to others. Not uncommonly, physical illness or toxin-induced disease states have an impact on brain function and produce reversible psychiatric illness (nonfunctional psychopathology). Therefore psychiatrically ill elderly patients should always receive a thorough physiologic evaluation.

While prevalence rates vary somewhat, the characteristics of late life psychiatric illness are essentially the same as those occurring in younger populations. Barring coincidental catastrophe, nothing magical happens overnight between the sixty-fourth and sixty-fifth birthdays. What is reversible before is likewise reversible after. The same treatment modalities (including indications and contraindications) available to younger adults are available and efficacious for the geriatric population. As mentioned previously, however, optimal geriatric technique requires the application of optimal technique for younger adults modified for special age-related factors.

Fifth, assessment and treatment updates should be performed frequently in an effort to measure reapproximation or attainment of premorbidity baseline. Regimen modifications should be launched as indicated.

Sixth, since the individual is multifaceted, assessment and treatment are best rendered by a multidisciplinary team. This group should be composed of members from those disciplines having expertise in the major areas of the patient or client's past, present, and future. Few disciplines are skilled and trained to cover extradiscipline areas adequately. For example, most physicians would not qualify to perform a religious assessment; most social workers are not prepared to render a physiologic assessment, and so on.

Curriculum compliance with educational theory and practice

The educational course or program should be ideally based on well-founded educational principles of curriculum design and implementation. Educational goals must first be determined. An educational goal is a broad statement of general knowledge, skills, and attitudes to be accomplished by the curriculum. For example, the goal of this chapter (which might be considered a course in teaching education to educators) is to assist in improving health care to the elderly by introducing the reader to the generalities of gerontologic/geriatric educational program design, its establishment and its perpetuation. Based on these goals, educational objectives must be delineated. These objectives are specific measureable skills that should result from having taken the course or program. An example of objectives for this chapter might be as follows: At the completion of this chapter, the reader should be able to demonstrate, in writing, a working knowledge of the following:

1. A major reason for impoverished health care delivery to the aged in the United States
2. Five requirements that must be met to assure that medical school courses on programs in aging will be soundly established and perpetuated
3. The overall purpose of medical school courses or programs in aging

The next step in design is to develop content that will meet the curriculum's educational goals and objectives. All too frequently content is planned in advance of goals and objectives, precluding a well planned frame of reference and means of evaluating performance outcome.

One must plan the vehicles by which curriculum content will be imparted to the students. It is essential that these formats be planned to maximize learning. Considerations include such factors as whether the curriculum should be offered in block format, as one course, several courses, or diffused throughout the entire curriculum; elective or required; time of day to be taught; on-the-job instruction or, didactic, and so on.

One must also determine the means by which the student's performance on meeting the educational objectives will be assessed. Factors to consider include what constitutes a passing score; written or oral examination or a combination of both; time of day examination given, and so on. Regardless, the examination must be based on reinforcing the curriculum's goals and objectives.

Faculty as role models

Student's attitudes are influenced greatly by their educators. Several reports have indicated that educators have negative attitudes about the aged, the intensity of their attitudes exceeding that of their students. Studies have further revealed that students begin their 4-year undergraduate medical school curriculum with positive attitudes toward aging and the aged. After 3 years of exposure to their educators, their attitudes have deteriorated. A relatively recent report indicated that medical students' prejudice toward the elderly is exceeded only by prejudice against color.

Ageism is prejudice. Prejudice is borne of self-perceived threats to psychologic comfort. The elderly threaten many. An understanding, enthusiastic, knowledgeable, and supportive role model has great potential for reducing fear, enhancing the knowledge and self-esteem of the student, and hence lessening the risk of prejudice as he or she "walks the student through" the experience of assessing and treating the aged.

Characteristics of student populations

Formal and empirical observations reveal certain characteristics of medical student populations. First, as mentioned earlier, most students enter medical school with a philosophical, altruistic, and esthetic bent. This continues to flourish best when education is presented in such a way that promotes high levels of self-esteem, often threatened by the uncertainty of the newness of medical school examination and clinical faculty assessment. Self-esteem is maintained when students receive material in a structured and highly organized format, a format that can be implemented relatively easily in the clinical setting. Esoteric or other information that neither helps to accomplish this nor to place that information in perspective by giving its existence a rationale tends to dampen positive attitudes.

The field of aging's place in the medical school curriculum and in the minds of the students remains tentative. Therefore the educator must respect these student characteristics when planning curricula. Sloppy work tends to produce similar results, an issue of even more critical significance in aging education.

Obstacles to incorporation of curricula

Cognizance of potential obstacles to incorporating gerontology and geriatrics into existing educational programs is fundamental to their avoidance and solution. Although other possibilities exist, three obstacles are delineated for consideration.

The first is negative attitudes toward aging and the aged, which has already been covered in some detail. As an obstacle, however, the negativism of the teacher, the individual most often responsible for the design and implementation of curricula, may actually defeat the incorporation of curricula in aging. A recent national survey of senior medical students and their educators found that only 2% of the student cohort felt that geriatrics should not be incorporated as opposed to 10% of the educators. A similar query was made of senior residents in psychiatry and their educators with respect to the same question. None of the residents rejected the incorporation of geriatrics in contrast to 18% of the faculty.

A sound educational program; experiencing the relatively well elderly in the community; rotating through acute as well as chronic care facilities; successfully treating reversible illness; learning methods of improving the quality of life in irreversible states; viewing the patient as a person and not a "medical museum"; and working under the leadership and supervision of an enthusiastic, devoted, and competent role model have been cited as means of offsetting negative attitudes.

The second potential obstacle is health care delivery problems attendant to serving the elderly. Several reasons exist for this difficulty. Time-consuming social service tasks are often involved in serving these individuals. For example, seeking the assistance of attorneys to obtain conservatorships and other protective devices are often necessary to decrease injustice possibly incumbent on the older person. Numerous phone calls and correspondence are commonly required to provide financial services sufficient to maintain the barest subsistence levels for the aged.

Another problem within this category revolves around the trainee's ability to accommodate the different styles of service delivery to the elderly. The student or resident may be threatened by collaboration with other team professionals when discovering that they may possess more knowledge and experience in the geriatric patient's care.

It is crucial in the education of the medical student and resident that they be exposed to the theoretical concepts and practical applications of other professions in the delivery of health care and social services. Lectures by representatives of various professions and community organizations can broaden the trainee's knowledge of the intricacies and benefits of the team and community support system. Actual supervised practice and role model support in the case conference setting has also been found helpful.

A third obstacle is the uncertainty on the part of educators as to the construction and implementation of a curriculum. Contrary to the commonly held notion that there is very little material on the subject, a knowledge base exists. Vacillation on the part of educators in developing curricula could be alleviated by duplicating, with appropriate modifications, the successful efforts of others.

Stability of administrative component

If the adminsitrative matrix in which the educational program resides is unstable and poorly grounded in appropriate perspectives, the educational program will suffer. The integrity and perpetuation of a medical school component's educational programs are in part dependent on the component's fulfillment of certain requirements. There must be clearly delineated needs for its establishment and acknowledgement of these needs by key segments within society and the institution establishing the program. Ideally the person heading the component should be aware of these needs, should be highly motivated to assist in offsetting them, should be committed to an academic existence, since it is the matrix in which the program is to be established, and should serve as a role model. The component's programs must be designed to both communicate and offset these needs. The departmental component should be represented as a composite and integrated unit; however, it must have access to and engagement with similar components or individuals in other departments and institutions. The foundation activity of the component should be patient care, since this is the most pressing need within the geriatric population and the most significant need to which any medical school component should direct its attention. Patient care should conform to the requirements for optimal health care of the elderly for that particular specialty or discipline. All additional programs developed by the component should serve that end. The staff of the component must have sufficient daily time to accomplish these tasks. Last of all, functioning of the component must have clear lines of authority, avoiding administrative entanglements that hamper performance and dampen positive attitudes.

REFERENCES

1. Institute of Medicine, National Academy of Sciences: Aging and medical education, report of a study, Washington, D.C., 1978, National Academy of Sciences.
2. Steel, K., editor: Geriatric education, Lexington, Mass., 1981, The Collamore Press.
3. Libow, L.S., and Sherman, F.T.: The core of geriatric medicine: a guide for students and practitioners, St. Louis, 1981, The C.V. Mosby Co.

BIBLIOGRAPHY

Cohen G.C.: Mental health services and the elderly: needs and options, Am. J. Psychiatry **133**:65, 1976.

Eisdorfer, C.: Aging and mental health: an introduction, Generations **3**(4):4, 1979.

Gayne, B.M., and Briggs, L.J.: Principles of instructional design, New York, 1974, Holt, Rinehart & Winston.

Levenson, A.J.: Gerontologic and geriatric training at the University of Texas Medical School, World J. Psychosynthesis **12**:32, 1980.

Levenson, A.J.: Aging and mental health, Health Values **5**:70, 1980.

Levenson, A.J., and Felkins, F.J.: Tertiary psychiatric prevention: a model service, Proceedings of the annual scientific meeting of the American Geriatric Society, 1979.

Levenson, A.J., and Porter, D.M.: The section on geriatric psychiatry: theory and practice, J. Psychiatr. Treatment and Evaluation **2**:269, 1980.

National Council on Aging: Fact book on aging: a profile of America's older population, Washington, D.C., 1978, National Council on Aging.

Spence, D.L., Feigenbaum, E., Fritzgerald, F., and Roth, J.: Medical student's attitudes toward the geriatric patient, J. Am. Geriatr. Soc. **16**(9):976, 1968.

Task panel reports submitted to the President's Commission on Mental Health, vol. 3 appendix, Washington D.C., 1978, U.S. Government Printing office.

U.S. Bureau of the Census: Statistical abstract of the United States, 1979, ed. 100, Washington, D.C., 1979, U.S. Government Printing Office.

U.S. Senate Committee on Aging: Developments in aging: 1978, Washington, D.C., 1979, U.S. Government Printing Office.

INDEX*

*T = table; italicized numbers indicate illustrations.

B

D

O

S

Wild Flowers of Northern Oman

Text by James P. Mandaville, Jr.

Illustrations by Dorothy Bovey

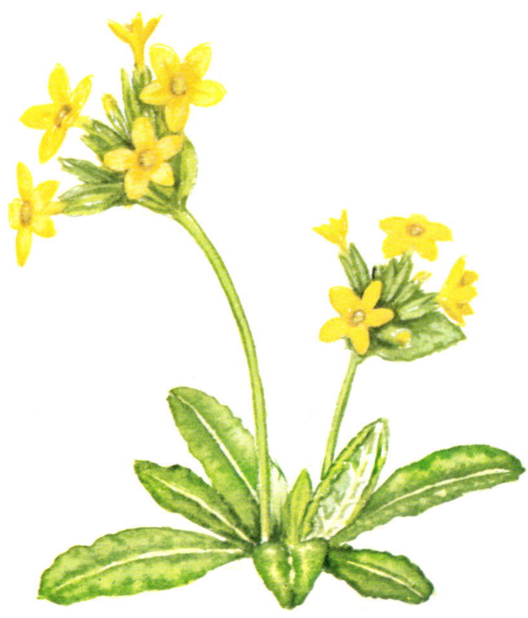

Dionysia mira

Bartholomew Books, London

The cover picture shows *Nerium mascatense* (see p.40)

ISBN 0 7028 10789

Produced and published in Great Britain 1978 by
John Bartholomew and Son Ltd.,
216 High Street, Bromley, Kent. BR1 IPW.
in collaboration with
The Office of the Government Adviser
for the Conservation and Development of
the Environment.
Sultanate of Oman.

Printed and bound in Great Britain by
Hazell Watson & Viney Ltd,
Aylesbury, Bucks

بسم الله الرحمن الرحيم

FOREWORD

It gives me great pleasure to write the Foreword for this book about the wild flowers of our beloved country.

The people of Oman have for many generations understood the value and usefulness of wild flowers and plants as a source of medicine and food for man as well as livestock. Not only are the wild plants a beautiful part of our natural environment but an important natural resource which, together with our other gifts from Nature, should be protected and used with wisdom.

His Majesty Sultan Qaboos bin Said has said in the Foreword to the Special Report of the 1977 Journal of Oman Studies: 'Disease on a wide scale, quite apart from its direct danger to mankind, could destroy entire species of food plants and food animals. In the wild lie the sources from which new food stocks could be produced. For this reason alone it is important for us to learn all we can about the wild flora and fauna of all parts of the earth's surface'.

I hope that 'Wild Flowers of Northern Oman' will help the students in our schools to learn to enjoy and appreciate our country's wild flowers and to extend this interest to our national heritage as a whole. Additionally, I am sure that this little book will give pleasure not only to those who are already familiar with our flowers but also to those who perhaps had not before realised that there is so much of interest and beauty in Oman right at our feet; even among the barren rocks.

Take this book with you into the mountains, valleys and plains of Oman and learn about some of our wild flowers; come back wanting to know more. There is much more to tell and it is my hope that this will soon be done. The more we know about our environment the better we will understand its uses and needs.

I wish to thank the author and artist for helping to bring to us all, countrymen and visitors alike, a new appreciation of our heritage.

Muscat,
September 1978

Faisal Bin Ali Al-Said
Minister of National Heritage

Introduction

The importance of learning more about the plant life of northern Oman began to be appreciated well over 100 years ago, after the French botanist-explorer P. Aucher-Eloy made available to the scientific world the plant specimens which he had collected there in 1838. It was soon realised that the flora of this region was in many ways unique, providing important links between the basically African flora of southern Arabia and the Asiatic plant communities across the Gulf to the east. The isolated mountains of Oman had also seen the evolution of plant species which were not to be found elsewhere. For the most part, however, the land remained outside the reach of detailed scientific study until the present decade when, under the leadership of His Majesty Sultan Qaboos bin Said, the Government of Oman embarked on its sweeping programme of social and economic development. Appreciating that a detailed knowledge of natural resources is indispensable to improving the quality of life, His Majesty ordered work to be started on surveying and describing the wildlife of the country.

It was natural that northern Oman's unique topographical feature—the highland massif of Jabal al-Akhdar—should be given priority attention in any such study, and the Flora and Fauna Survey of Oman began work there in 1975. The scientific results of this survey were published in March 1977 in the *Journal of Oman Studies Special Report.* Those of us who had the privilege of participating in this venture soon began to appreciate that the results could have broader application. The people of Oman are anxious to learn more about the resources and natural products of their country, parts of which—long isolated by rugged terrain—are now being linked by better means of communication. Also, visitors in Oman, struck by the beautiful and unusual wildlife of the country, are asking 'What is that flower, that bird, that animal'? It was to meet this need that the Ministry of Diwan Affairs environmental office conceived the idea of putting some of the Survey's findings into more popular form by producing illustrated guides to the wildlife of the region. This book is the first of a series.

This Book: Purpose and Arrangement

The aim of this small volume is to provide, through the illustrations so accurately and beautifully executed by the botanical artist, Dorothy Bovey, a means for the student and non-specialist visitor to identify those wild flowers of northern Oman that are commonly encountered.

Virtually all of Mrs Bovey's paintings were drawn from living specimens, which were then pressed and forwarded to the British Museum (Natural History) to confirm the scientific identification and nomenclature of each species. Miss Dorothy Hillcoat, who specialises in studies of the Arabian flora at the Museum, performed this work, and her expert assistance greatly helped assure the scientific accuracy of this guide.

The plants chosen for inclusion are of two categories: those that have showy flowers or are of otherwise special visual interest, and others which are major components of the dominant vegetation and thus important to an understanding of regional ecology. Thus, although designed primarily as a wild flower guide for the layman, it is hoped that the book will prove useful to the more serious student of the Oman flora as well as to visiting specialists who need to make a quick acquaintance with the dominant mountain plants. It should be noted, however, that some important groups, such as the grasses, have not been included.

The geographical area referred to here as 'northern Oman' is centred on Jabal al-Akhdar and its surrounding lowlands, as opposed to the southern deserts of the country and the Southern Region of Dhofar, which to various degrees have different floras. It does not by design extend to the far northern parts of the country, north of the 25th parallel, although the guide may be partially useful in those areas.

The plants are arranged by family in the traditional Bentham and Hooker sequence, in order to show anatomical and family relationships for the student.

The identifications to species of a few plants illustrated had not been museum-confirmed at press time. Several of these may be undescribed species. They are included, nevertheless, because they are likely to be encountered by travellers and visitors who will be interested to know their generic names even though the formal and sometimes complex process of scientific naming may not have been completed.

Arabic Plant Names

The Arabic names provided for plants in this book were taken almost exclusively from the field notes of the 1975 Oman Flora and Fauna Survey expedition. They have the virtue, therefore, of coming from informants using the living language. The expedition, however, was limited in the geographical area that it could cover and by the time which it had available, and its members were obviously unable to collect all local variations in popular plant names. Names vary among different tribes and geographical areas. The users of this guide, therefore, should expect to encounter some good vernacular names that differ from those listed here. Users should also remember that as in all countries, individuals differ greatly in their knowledge of plant names and plant lore. Sometimes an eagerness to please overshadows the strict accuracy of villagers' botanical information.

Many vernacular names of plants in Oman, as in other Arab lands, are well established in classical Arabic literature dating back to the 9th Century A.D. Some of these early compositions, such as the famour *Book of Plants* of Abū Ḥanīfah ad-Dīnawarī (d.895 A.D.), to beyond the scope of mere name lists and are valuable descriptive botanical works.

Presenting Arabic names in English for readers without any knowledge of the language is always a problem. There is no system of transliteration that can provide much more than a rough approximation of the pronunciation of most names. For those who know the Arabic alphabet and the rudiments of the sound system, there are various well established methods of indicating spelling and pronunciation in Roman script. Rather than attempting a purely phonetic system for the non-Arabic speaker—one that will certainly be only half successful—we have adopted the standard classical transliteration system of the Permanent Committee on Geographical Names (London). Oman plant names have been checked with classical Arabic references, and spellings used in those works are generally followed unless the Omani vernacular clearly differs in grammatical form. Readers without experience in Arabic should find these spellings recognisable in most cases, although colloquial soundings of some consonants sometimes vary from classical norms. For example, *'k'* is sometimes pronounced as 'ch'; *'j'* sometimes as hard 'g'. Stress normally falls on syllables containing the long vowels (ā, ī, ū, pronounced as in father, machine and blue) or diphthongs (*aw,* often sounded as 'o'; and *ay*). Names without long vowels are often stressed on the first syllable. The plant names are given in their collective forms; the singulars are regularly formed by the addition of the suffix *-ah*.

Geography, Climate and Vegetation Zones

The main mountain massif of northern Oman, the Hajar Range, is the most prominent landform feature of northern Oman. The highest part, Jabal al-Akhdar, reaches a height of about 3,050 metres. This block has extremely steep northern faces, while slopes on the south side are more gradual. The steep terrain has allowed for little soil development, although alluvial silts in lower mountain valleys are often deep. The higher parts of the mountains have a climate distinctly cooler and somewhat more moist than the lowlands, but the whole range must be classed as having an arid or semi-arid climate. Annual rainfall, even on the higher peaks, probably does not exceed 375 millimetres. When rains do occur, however, they may be torrential, causing flash floods in the *wadis* and short-lived but spectacular waterfalls on the northern cliff faces. There are few permanent streams, although valley gravels carry subterranean flows that are visible on the surface in some areas. Temperatures in the higher mountains sometimes fall to freezing during the winter, but they are best described as warm to hot during much of the year. The lowlands south of the mountain country are true—often extreme—desert, with annual rainfall of 75 millimetres or less.

Much of northern Oman's plant life at lower and middle altitudes is largely African in character and origin. This is not surprising, in view of the fact that the Arabian Peninsula is geologically a part of the African continent, from which it was separated by the Red Sea Rift only recently in geological time. The African vegetation, marked by conspicuously dominant *Acacia* trees, apparently spread into Arabia before this separation, and even the casual traveller will notice the resemblance between Oman's lowland *Acacia* country and parts of the East African savanna. Oman is considerably more arid than most of East Africa, however, and this has inhibited development of the true savanna grasslands. Many of the Oman desert plants are short-lived annuals, which evade the extreme temperatures and dessication of the desert environment by assuming the form of drought-resistant seeds for most of the year. They grow quickly, flowering and fruiting within a few weeks after the infrequent rains, and many have evolved unusual chemical and physical means of sensing the amount of moisture available to avoid germinating under 'false alarm' conditions of insufficient rainfall. Those plants which do live year-round have developed means of reducing their water losses by shedding leaves or other parts and by suspending their growth until the rains again bring moisture. The very successful *Acacias* and some other larger trees have long roots which can tap subterranean water that is available even during summer at deeper levels, beyond the reach of other plants.

Another plant zone of northern Oman lies in the mountain valleys, or *wadis,* at elevations of about 350 to 1,050 metres above sea level. Some of the larger lowland trees, such as *Acacia, Ziziphus* and *Prosopis,* extend into this zone. The rockier soil and more abundant moisture, however, give the vegetation a distinctive character. Here, where water is near the surface in valley gravels, are found dense groves of Oman's native oleander, *Nerium mascatense,* while rocky *wadi* walls bear well developed wild fig trees. Irrigation channels near cultivated plots are lined with maidenhair and *Pteris* ferns. The golden-flowered *Tecomella* tree is a rarer find in these habitats, while other woody shrubs with showy flowers, such as *Acridocarpus,* begin to be seen.

The steep slopes and rocky soil of the hillsides above the mountain *wadis* bring another major change in the vegetation. *Acacias,* where still present, become stunted and wider spaced, and a new and unusual shrub becomes dominant. This is the leafless, fleshy *Euphorbia larica,* conspicuous with its many erect, light green branches and sticky white sap that flows from the slightest wound. It is a good example of a succulent, water conserving, arid zone perennial. Here also appear several low species of *Convolvulus* and the violet-flowered lavender, *Lavandula subnuda.* The caper, with its showy white flowers, is common here among the rocks.

One enters yet another zone around 1,200–1,300 metres elevation on the north face of Jabal al-Akhdar. Here one may begin to see the woodland of *Reptonia (būt)* and wild olive trees *('utm)* so characteristic of much of the highland country. In protected ravines, the vegetation begins to take the character of true forest, with shrubs and trees up to 8 metres high. The juniper tree appears about 1,500 metres above sea level, but it is better developed in the higher summit areas. Important shrubs in this woodland zone include *Sageretia spiciflora (nimt),* with its edible fruits; the bright yellow-flowered composite, *Euryops;* the striking red and yellow-flowered *Ebenus;* and *Dodonaea.* The dwarf fern, *Cheilanthes,* grows in the shade of boulders, while the open ground begins to bear a richer cover and variety of perennial grasses. Two special prizes to be sought by the wild flower photographer in this zone are the diminutive wild violet, *Viola cinerea,* and *Dionysia mira,* a bright yellow-flowered, *Primula*-like, cliff dweller.

Above about 2,300 metres elevation, on open, rocky and windswept ground along the ridge lines, lies the juniper summit zone, where junipers grow as hemispherical trees up to 10 metres tall, with tussock grasses and shrublets on the rocky ground between.

The mountain plant communities above about 1,000 metres altitude, are of special scientific interest because many of the important plants are known to be of Asiatic origin, with close relatives across the Gulf in southern Iran and even in the Himalayas. This evidence of early connections between eastern Arabia and mainland Asia is reinforced by the presence of a number of animals in northern Oman related to those on the mainland. A dry land connection probably existed between Arabia and the lands across the present Arabian Gulf as recently as 20,000 years ago. An exchange of plant and animal life could have occurred then, under more temperate climatic conditions. As extreme arid conditions began to prevail in Arabia, these species survived in isolation in Oman's cooler highlands.

Near vertical north face of Jabal al-Akhdar, as seen from the wadi bed near the village of al-Nid. The summit, left of centre, is over 3,000 metres above sea level. ▼

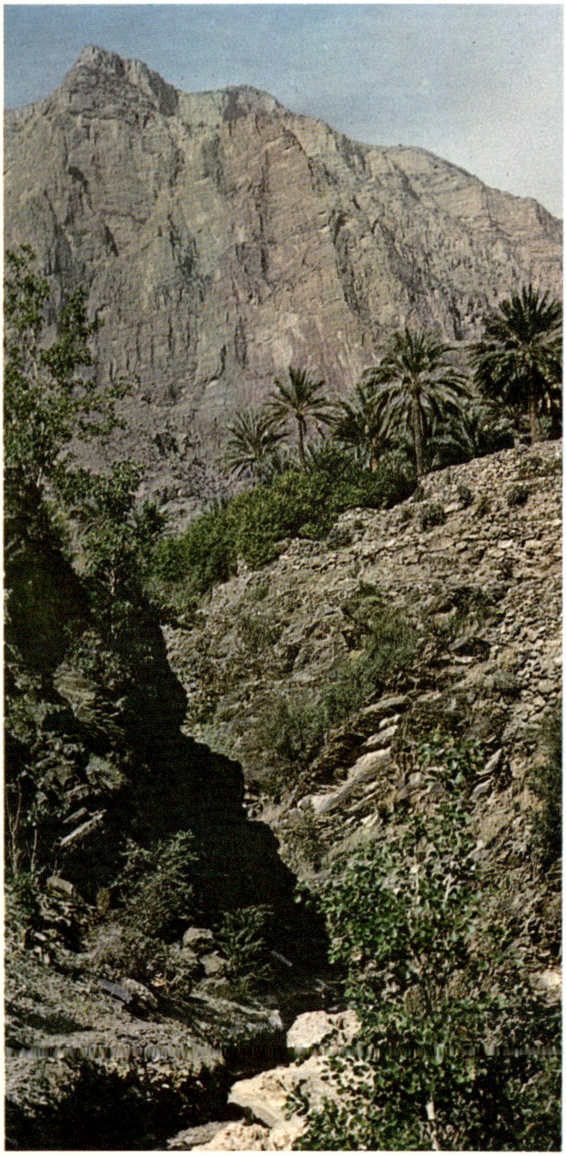

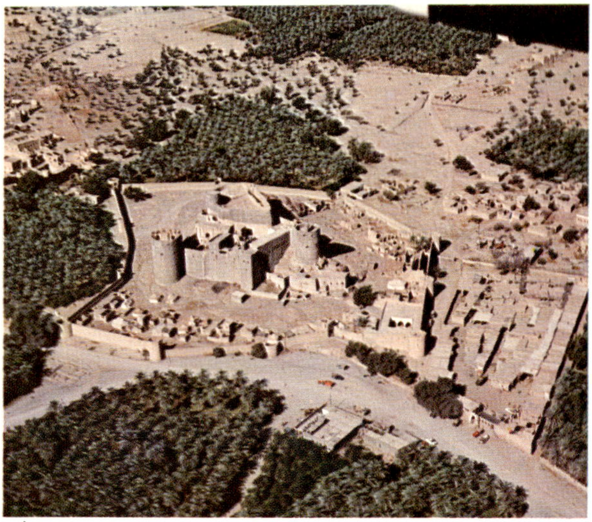

▲ The fort at al-Rustaq. Situated in palm gardens in the lowlands, al-Rustaq is an important and historical town, one of the main approaches to Jabal al-Akhdar.

Juniper trees in the Jabal al-Akdhar summit zone, elevation 2,650 metres. Seemingly dwarfed here by the broad vista, these junipers are about 7 metres high and often as wide. The small shrublets are *Dodonaea.* ▼

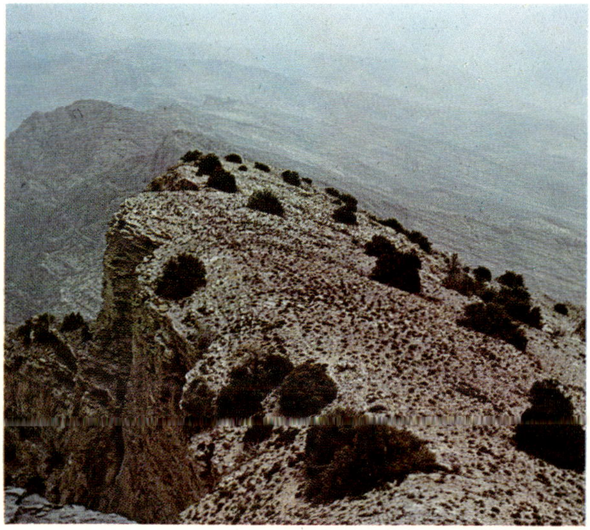

Conservation of Plant Life

One of the encouraging finds of the 1975 Flora and Fauna Survey was that the wild vegetation in the higher zones of Jabal al-Akhdar was in essentially natural condition and not—except in the plateau country around Sayq—greatly disturbed or changed by man and his domesticated animals. It is undoubtedly the extremely steep and difficult nature of the mountain terrain that has provided this degree of natural protection.

The well established unity of Oman today, the opening up of previously isolated parts of the country to mechanised transport, as well as the growing emphasis on rural economic development—all positive and essential steps in their own right—will also lead to increased exposure of the mountain vegetation to disturbance. This, fortunately, has already been recognised by the Government, which is taking steps to plan for a series of national parks or reserves where Oman's flora and fauna can be protected from disturbance and possible extinction.

Visitors and students who take an interest in studying wild plants in Oman should remember that the vegetation in such an arid country is under continual pressure, not only from the extreme natural environment, but from the expanding activities of man. Plants in the higher mountains may appear to be isolated and secure, but travellers in those parts are largely restricted to a limited number of trails and passes, and wild flowers along those routes will soon disappear if visitors pick and carry away specimens. Those studying wild flowers in any area, therefore, are strongly urged to do their collecting with a camera, or as drawings, rather than by taking plants or their parts; this will help ensure the future enjoyment of others and protect plants which may be rare world-wide or unique in Oman.

James P. Mandaville, Jr.

Glossary of Technical Terms Used in the Text

achene — a small, dry, non-opening fruit with a single seed free from the fruit wall.
alkaloid — a nitrogenous compound occurring in some plants, often medicinally active or poisonous.
annual — a plant which completes its life cycle and dies in one year or less.
awn — a bristle-like appendage usually at the top of a plant part, such as the floral parts of grasses.
bloom — in reference to plant surfaces, a fine waxy, sometimes powdery covering on fruits, stems or leaves.
bract — a (usually small) leaf-like structure growing beneath a flower or flower cluster.
calyx — the outermost circle of parts of a flower, often composed of several green sepals (q.v.).
capsule — a simple dry fruit developing from a compound pistil and splitting along two or more lines.
carpel — a simple pistil (the female, seed-bearing, organ of a flower including the ovary, style and stigma) or one unit of a compound pistil.
chlorophyll — the green colouring matter in plants; the chemical substance that enables green plants to utilize the energy of sunlight in manufacturing high-energy nutrients.
composite — (noun) a plant belonging to the Compositae (composite family), such as a daisy, sunflower.
compound leaf — one leaf consisting of two or more blades, each called a leaflet (q.v.).
corolla — the second (from outside) circle of flower parts, often composed of coloured petals (q.v.) but sometimes absent.
crown — in a shrub or tree, the base at ground level from which the trunk or main branches spring; also, the upper leafy part of a tree as opposed to the naked trunk or bole.
elliptical — shaped like an ellipse; widest in centre and tapering equally to each rounded end.
filiform — thread-like; fine and slender.
floret — one of the individual flowers in a head (q.v.); also, the basic floral unit in grasses.

fruit — the mature ovary, or seed-bearing structure of a plant. *Note:* This is often not a fleshy or edible body, as implied by the non-technical use of the term.
glabrous — smooth without any form of hair.
head — a dense rounded or flattened group of unstalked flowers or florets growing on a common supporting structure (the receptacle); the characteristic inflorescence of the composite family.
latex — the milk-like, white, sticky juice of some plants; characteristic of the milkweed family.
leaflet — one division of a compound leaf.
legume — a member of the legume family, Leguminosae; also, the one-celled, usually two valved and pod-like fruit often characteristic of that family.
ligulate — pertaining to the florets (q.v.) with strap-shaped limbs found in flowers of the composite family; also, referring to a composite inflorescence having only that kind (and not tubular) florets.
ovate — egg-shaped in outline, with broader end towards the base.
palmate — (usually of leaves) having lobes spreading from a central area, like fingers on a hand.
panicle — a many-branched, usually open, arrangement of flowers.
peduncle — a flower stalk supporting a single flower or a cluster of flowers.
perennial — (noun) a plant which continues to live from year to year.
petal — one of the individual parts of the corolla (q.v.) of the flower, often leaf-shaped and coloured as contrasted with the sepal (q.v.) which is often green. In some flowers, the petals may be fused or absent altogether.
photosynthetic — (adj.) pertaining to photosynthesis, the process by which green plants use light energy in manufacturing carbohydrates from water and atmospheric carbon dioxide.
pinnae — (sing. pinna) a first or main division of a pinnately compound leaf.
plumose — feather-like, with many (usually fine) hairs borne along a central column.
pod — an elongated fruit that dries and splits open lengthwise.
prostrate — lying flat on the ground.
rosette — a cluster or circle of spreading leaves at the base of a plant.
sepal — one of the separate parts of a flower's calyx (q.v.), often green as contrasted with the often coloured petals and borne below and outside the petals.
serrate — with forward-pointing tooth-like projections on the edges, as in some leaves.
spike — a group of sessile (unstalked) flowers with the central stem upon which they are borne.
spores — the microscopic single-celled reproductive bodies in ferns.
stamen — the pollen-bearing male organ of the flower.
stipular — pertaining to, or derived from, stipules, the small paired appendages borne at the base of the leaf in some plants.
succulent — fleshy, with much juice.
valve — one of the parts or segments into which a pod or other fruit splits or divides.
vein — a strand of nutrient and water conducting tissue in a leaf or other flat organ.

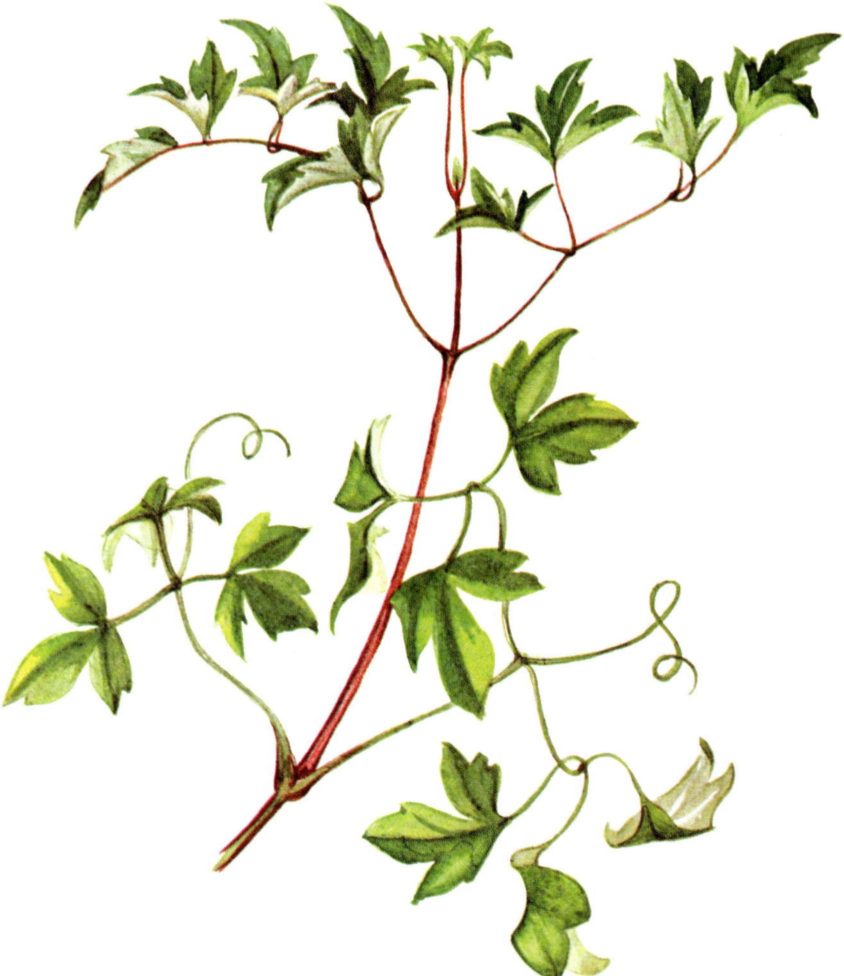

Clematis orientalis

Clematis orientalis L.
Ranunculaceae (Buttercup Family)

This climber is widespread in the northern Oman mountains above about 2,000 metres elevation, where it is usually seen growing on other shrubs or trees. Its specific identity remains to be confirmed by museum study of flowering specimens, but it will most probably be found to belong to the rather variable species *orientalis.* The flowers of *Clematis* are without petals, but they have white or near-white petal-like sepals. The clustered seed-bearing achenes have long, feathery awns. *Clematis* is well known among mountain tribesmen by the name *khaymarān.* In some parts of southern Arabia *Clematis* has been known to bloom in January and February; in Oman it may be found to be a summer or fall bloomer.

Diplotaxis harra (Forssk.) Boiss.
Cruciferae (Mustard Family)

Diplotaxis harra is widespread in Middle Eastern deserts and can grow either as a perennial or as an annual, depending on local moisture conditions. Young plants first form a basal rosette of leaves, then extend a central stalk that may reach a height of 30 centimetres or more, sometimes branching. Lowland desert plants are usually rough hairy, but those found on cliff faces of Jabal al-Akhdar and known to the highland Arabs as *khawshyān* may be nearly glabrous. This highland form may be classifiable as a separate variety or subspecies.

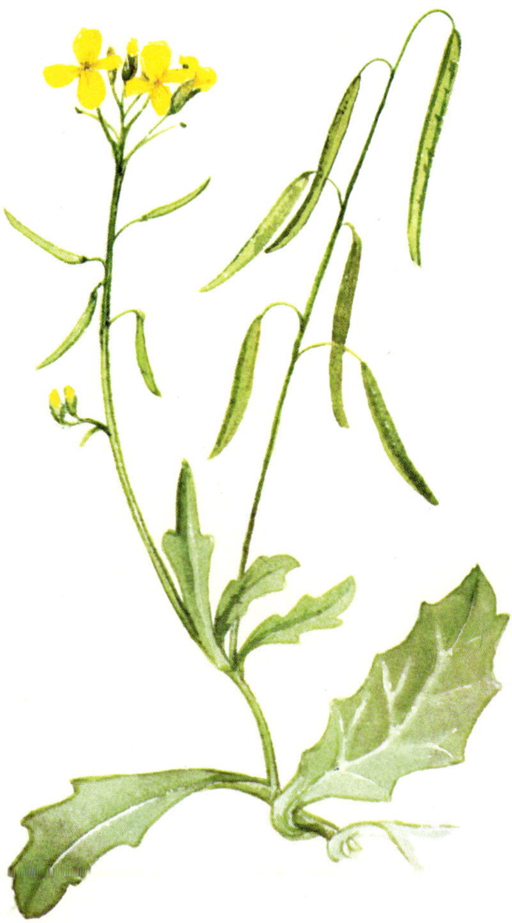

Diplotaxis harra

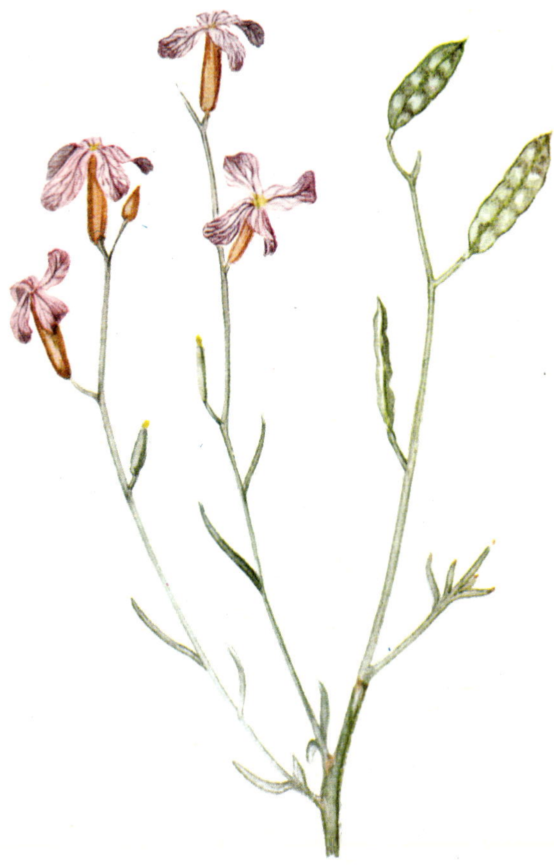

Farsetia aegyptia

Farsetia aegyptia Turra
Cruciferae (Mustard Family)

A tough, more or less woody grey shrublet up to 80 centimetres high, *Farsetia aegyptia* has a wide distribution in arid and semi-arid zones of the Middle East. Its covering of fine hairs is probably an adaptation to the desert environment, reflecting radiant heat and slowing water losses. The flower colour varies from a dull, leaden grey tinged with pink or yellow to shades of pink or blue. In Oman it has a wide altitudinal range, and some specimens seen at 2,200 metres on Jabal al-Akhdar were particularly robust with bright, clear blue flowers. The Arabic name, *masharrī,* has been applied to *Farsetia* in the highlands, but that probably better belongs to *Chrozophora,* which it somewhat resembles in texture and colour.

Physorrhynchus chamaerapistum (Boiss.) Boiss.
Cruciferae (Mustard Family)

This unusually stout member of the mustard family grows man-high or sometimes taller. It is a lowland or mid-altitude species often seen on the alluvium of *wadis* emerging from the northern mountain slopes. Known in Oman as *khafīj* or *khawfīj, Physorrhynchus* is an eastern genus distributed across the Gulf from southern Iran to north-western India.

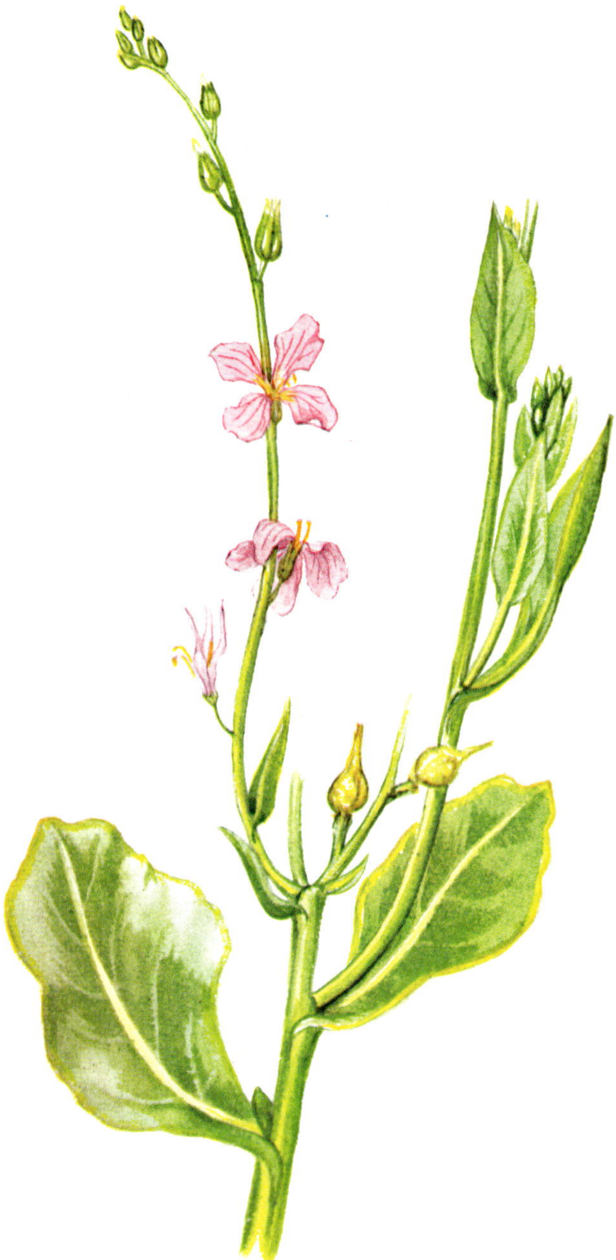

Physorrhynchus chaemarapistum

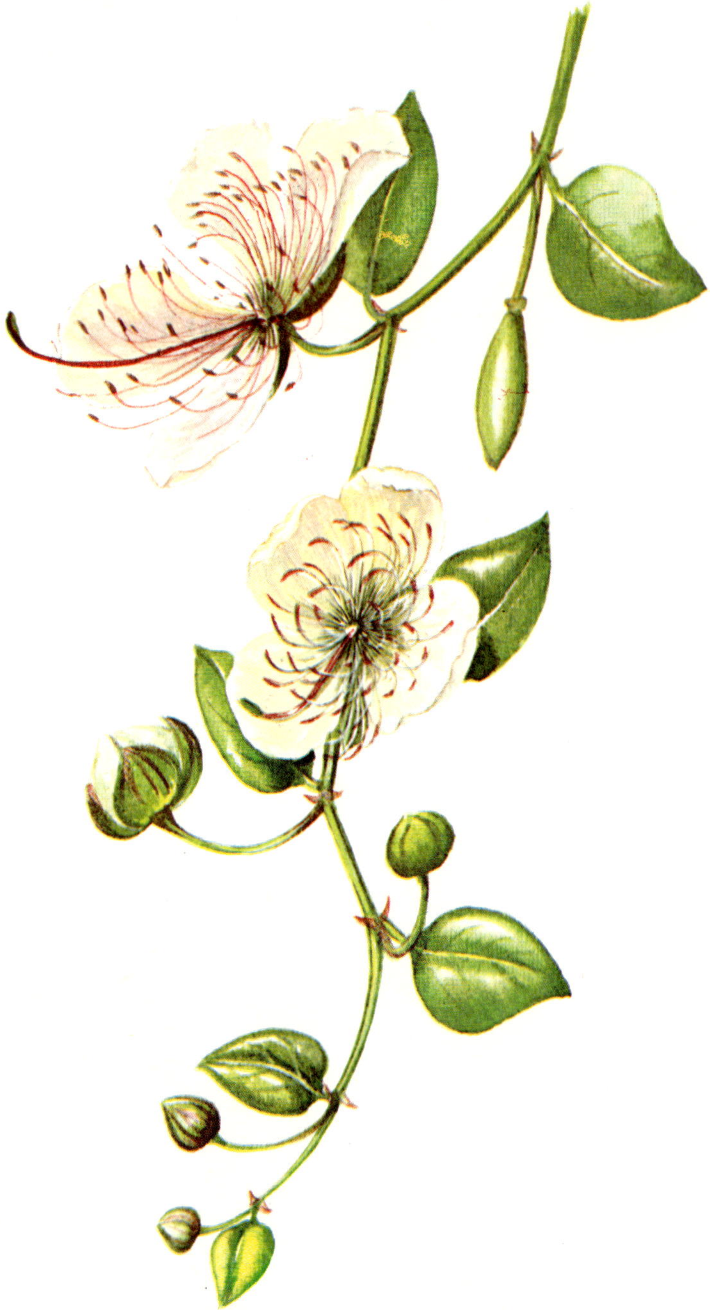

Capparis mucronifolia Boiss.
Capparidaceae (Caper Family)

At least two species of caper are known in northern Oman, both called by their classical Arabic name, *liṣāf*. The one not pictured here (although very similar in appearance) is *Capparis spinosa,* which is widespread in the Middle East and cultivated in southern France for its flower buds, which are pickled to produce the capers of commerce. *Liṣāf* shrublets are almost always found in rocky habitats. Its many-stamened flowers are showy but wilt quickly, while its hooked prickles are particularly vicious; once engaged they are very difficult to remove.

Capparis mucronifolia

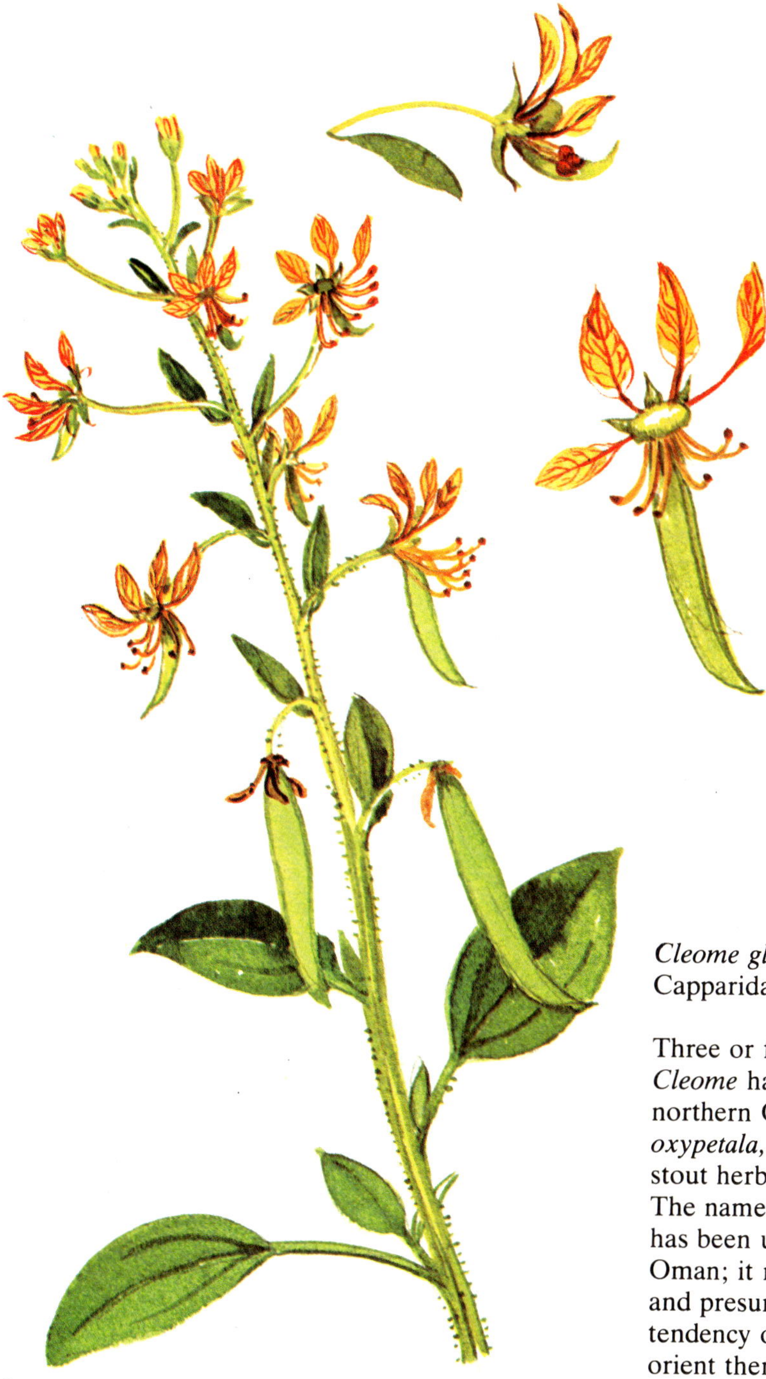

Cleome glaucescens

Cleome glaucescens DC. *forma*
Capparidaceae (Caper Family)

Three or four species of *Cleome* have been found in northern Oman, including *C. oxypetala, C. scaposa,* and the stout herb illustrated here. The name *muqaybil ash shams* has been used for *Cleome* in Oman; it means 'sun facer' and presumably refers to a tendency of the leaves to orient themselves towards the sun.

Maerua crassifolia

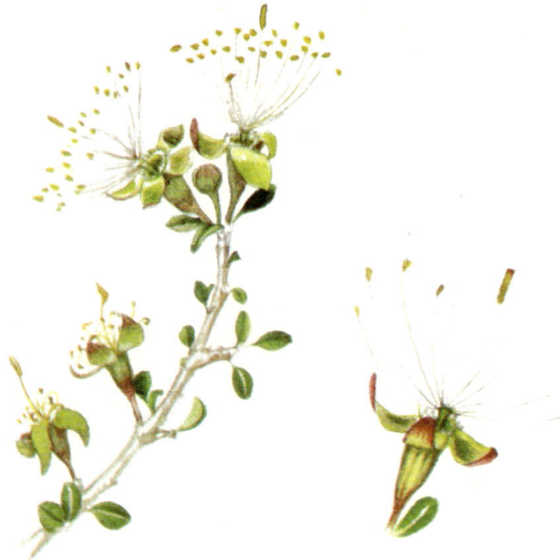

Maerua crassifolia Forssk.
Capparidaceae (Caper Family)

Maerua, known throughout tropical Arabia as *sarḥ,* is a small tree, often stunted and gnarled, of rocky hillsides and ravines. The smaller branches sometimes harden into pointed spines. The greenish flowers have no petals; their spreading parts are the sepals, divided above into four parts, but growing together as a tube below.

Helianthemum lippii (L.) Pers.
Cistaceae (Rock Rose Family)

The bright yellow flowers with numerous stamens and the elliptical leaves with rolled-under edges are the keys to recognising this rock rose, known in Oman as *bīqān.* It is a dwarf shrublet, seldom more than about 30 centimetres high, and is frequently seen along rocky mountain trails. It also occurs in the lowlands in rocky habitats. In central and northern Arabia this is one of a number of *Helianthemum* species, known collectively as *ruqrūq,* that mark for the Bedouins the soils favourable for growth of the desert truffle.

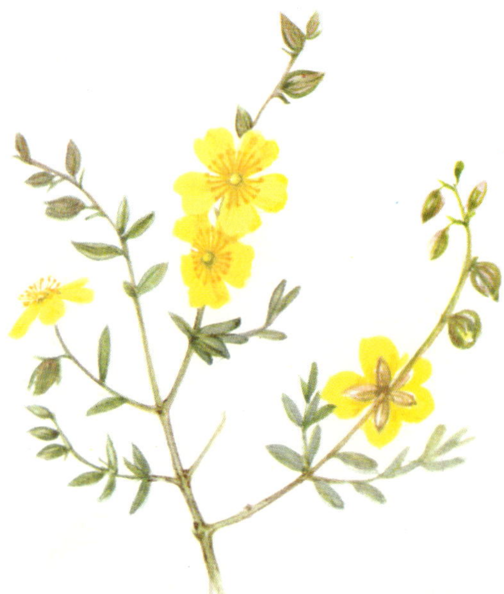

Helianthemum lippii

Viola cinerea Boiss.
Violaceae (Violet Family)

Oman's diminutive violet, often not more than 5 centimetres high, is most often seen growing in cracks in limestone on mountain-sides between 450 and 2,500 metres elevation. It tolerates habitats that are rocky and dry, only reducing its size in more rigorous exposures. Found also in mountain Iran, this is one of several plants that give evidence of links in earlier geologic times between the floras of south-eastern Arabia and mainland Asia.

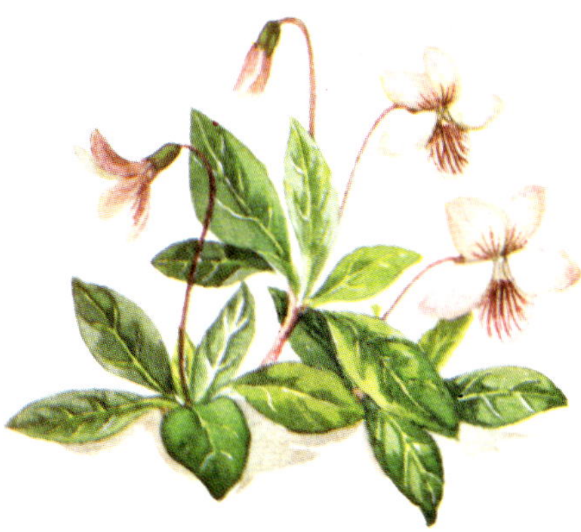

Viola cinerea

Silene schweinfurthii Rohrb.
Caryophyllaceae (Pink Family)

This campion, usually found at elevations above 1,600 metres, where it is known to mountain tribesmen as *yawtın,* grows about 50 centimetres high. It normally has one or more slender, erect stems and is an inconspicuous plant, but one with delicately structured flowers that repay closer inspection. Like many other *Silenes,* the flowers of *yawtın* are sensitive to the heat of the midday sun. In strong sunlight the petals roll inward and contract almost to a knot; they can thus be best appreciated in early morning, in the evening, or on overcast days, when they make a fine subject for close-up photography.

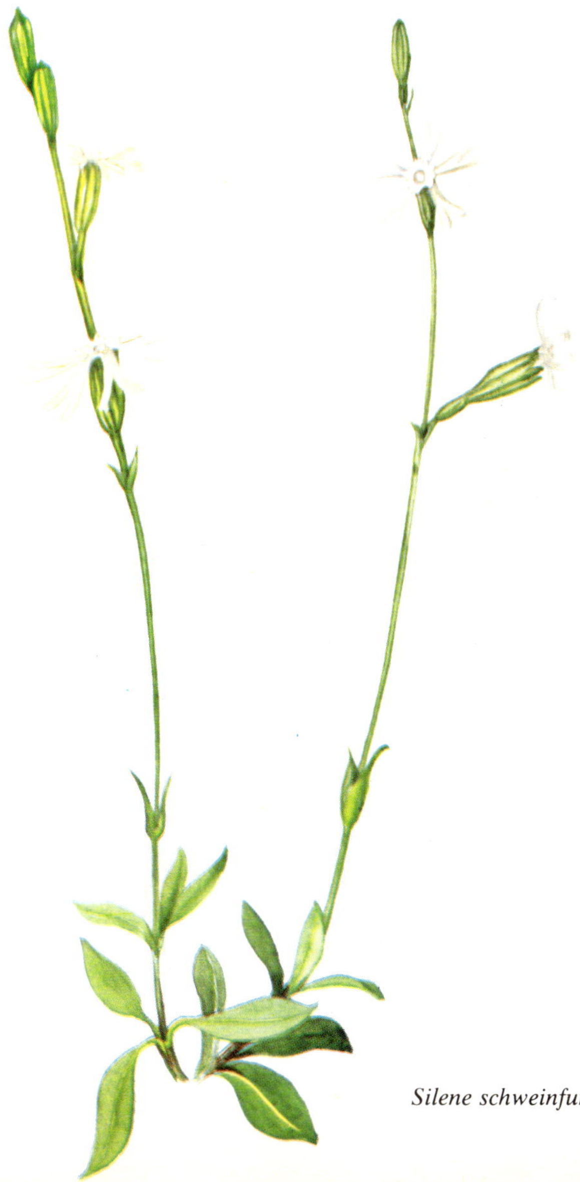

Silene schweinfurthii

Abutilon pannosum (Forst.f.) Schlecht.
Malvaceae (Mallow Family)

Munaqqā', as this shrubby, sometimes man-high *Abutilon* is sometimes called, has flattened, ear-like seed-bearing carpels packed 20–30 per fruit. A fibre is derived from this plant in some Asiatic countries, while Bedouins in the Dead Sea area, Jordan, have been known to eat its seeds. *Abutilon* is most often seen on disturbed ground, around cultivated areas.

Malva neglecta Wallr.
Malvaceae (Mallow Family)

Malva neglecta, or dwarf mallow, is a European weed usually seen as a procumbent annual along road-sides or on waste ground. It may grow to about 40 centimetres high, but is usually lower. The name *khubbayz,* 'little baker' is given to *Malva* in some Arabian Gulf countries because the disc-like fruits resemble flattened round loaves of bread. This species is reported to contain tannin, and it is used in folk medicine in some countries as a purgative and to reduce inflammation. A similar species, *Malva parviflora,* is also known as a weed in northern Oman and may be more common. Its fruit segments are wrinkled, rather than smooth as in *M. neglecta.*

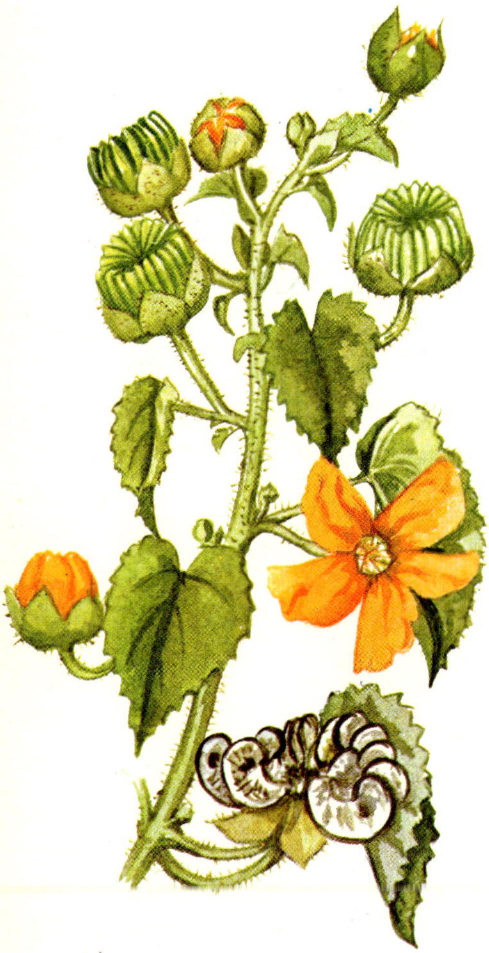

Abutilon pannosum

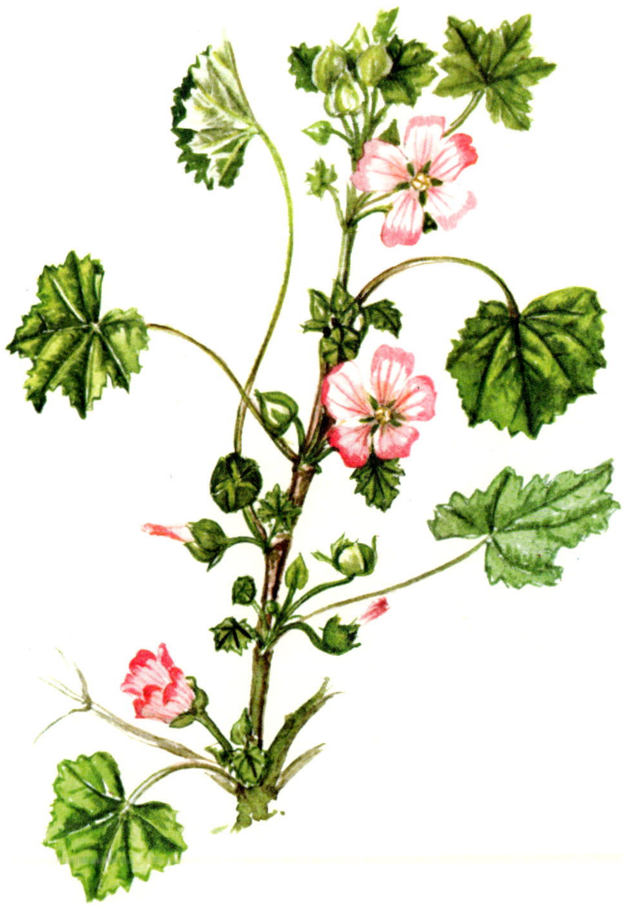

Malva neglecta

Grewia erythraea Schweinf.
Tiliaceae (Linden Family)

This low tough shrub, known to all highland Omanis as *sharḥam,* is distinguished by its small but attractive white flowers and its red, berry-like edible fruits, growing in four-parted clusters. It thrives on wind-blown, rocky mountain-sides.

Linum usitatissimum L.
Linaceae (Flax Family)

This slender annual, which may grow up to 80 centimetres high, has been collected on the highland plateau around Sayq. It is the well-known cultivated flax, known in Egypt as *kattān,* and may have escaped from cultivation in Oman or have been introduced with crop seeds from other lands. It is the source of linen and linseed oil, both important commercial products.

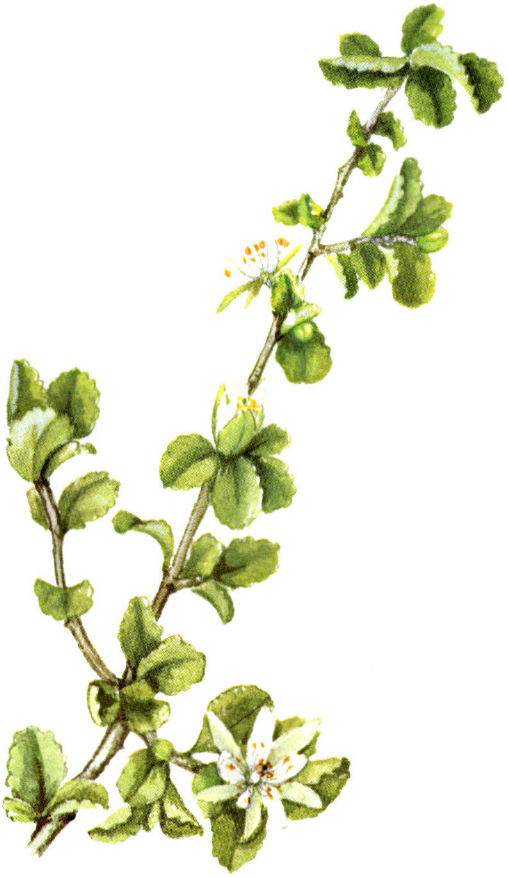

Grewia erythraea

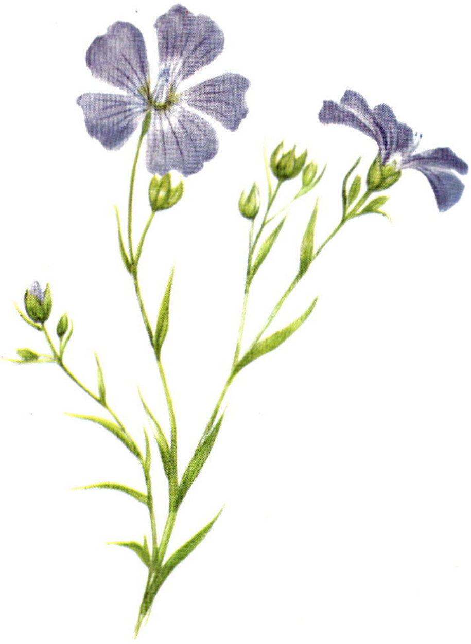

Linum usitatissimum

Malpighiaceae (Malpighia Family)

Zygophyllaceae (Caltrop Family)

Acridocarpus orientalis

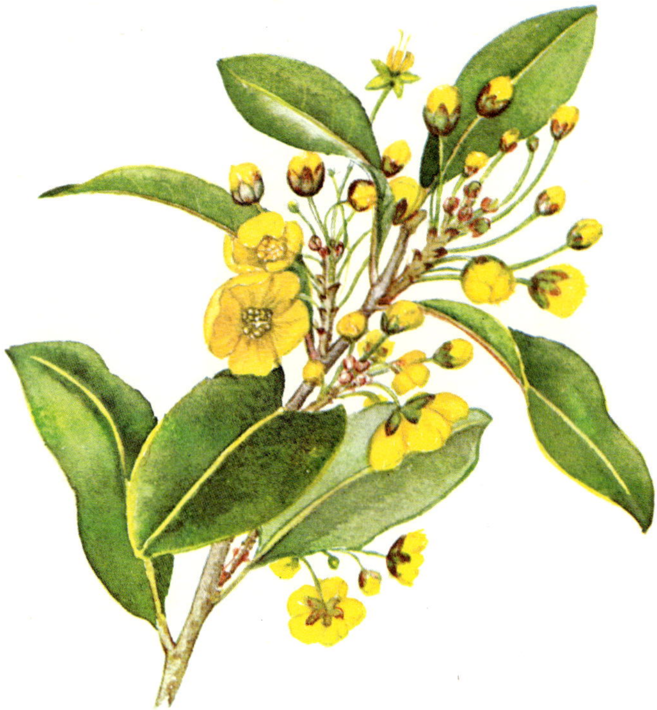

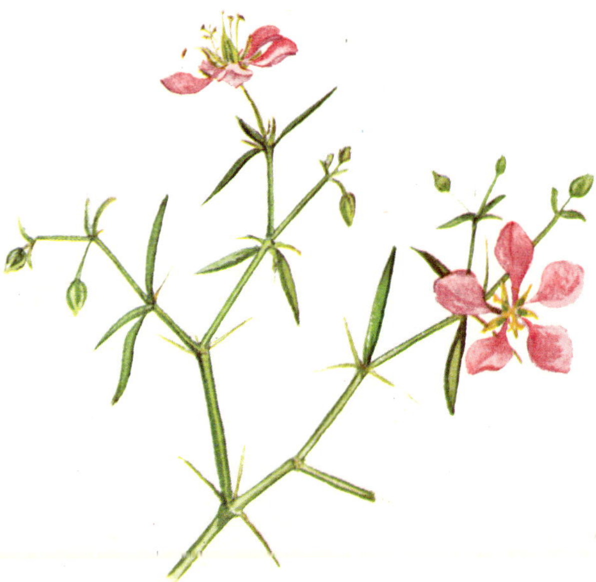

Fagonia indica

Acridocarpus orientalis A. Juss.
Malpighiaceae (Malpighia Family)

The showy flowers of this large, broad shrub are sure to catch the eye of travellers along the banks of *wadis* draining the northern flanks of Jabal al-Akhdar or on mountain-sides at higher altitudes. *Qafaṣ,* as it is called in Arabic, has fruits with peculiar wings, reminiscent of those of the maple. These probably serve as a dispersal mechanism.

Fagonia indica Burm. f.
Zygophyllaceae (Caltrop Family)

Mushikkā' (often pronounced *'mshichchạ̄'a'* in Omani colloquial dialect) is a very common small shrublet of rocky mountain slopes at low to medium altitudes. It is well armed with sharp stipular spines and has small five-angled capsules as fruits. The 9th Century Arabic botanical book of Abū Hanifah ad-Dīnawarī describes the plant accurately and calls it *shukā'á,* an earlier name based on the same Arabic root.

Erodium laciniatum (Cav.) Willd. Geraniaceae (Geranium Family)

The leaves of this storksbill are deeply cut, but do not have the finer fringe-like divisions of *Erodium cicutarium.* Both of these winter annuals are relished by livestock. In Saudi Arabia it is called *raqm.*

Erodium cicutarium

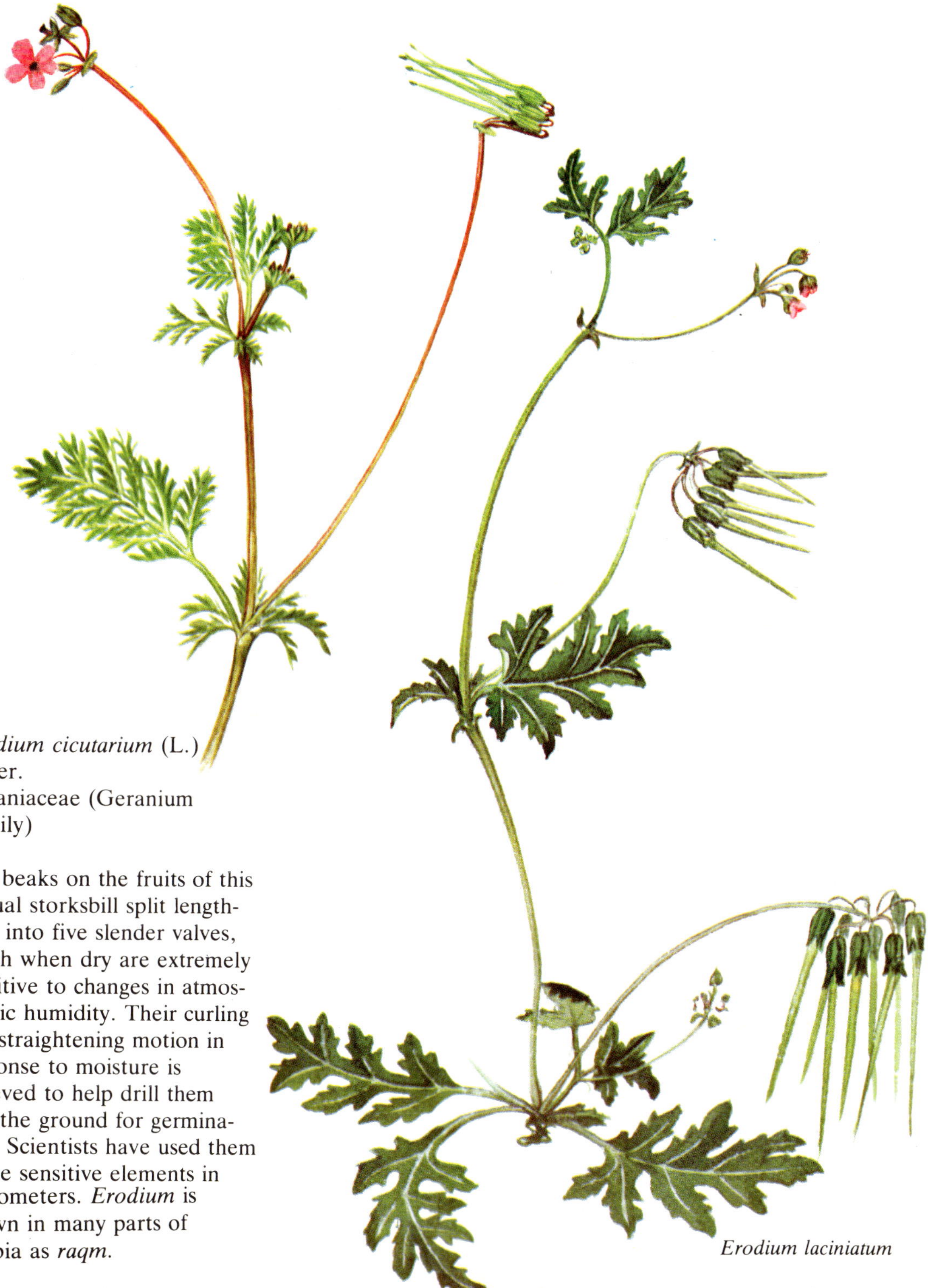

Erodium cicutarium (L.) L'Her.
Geraniaceae (Geranium Family)

The beaks on the fruits of this annual storksbill split lengthwise into five slender valves, which when dry are extremely sensitive to changes in atmospheric humidity. Their curling and straightening motion in response to moisture is believed to help drill them into the ground for germination. Scientists have used them as the sensitive elements in hygrometers. *Erodium* is known in many parts of Arabia as *raqm*.

Erodium laciniatum

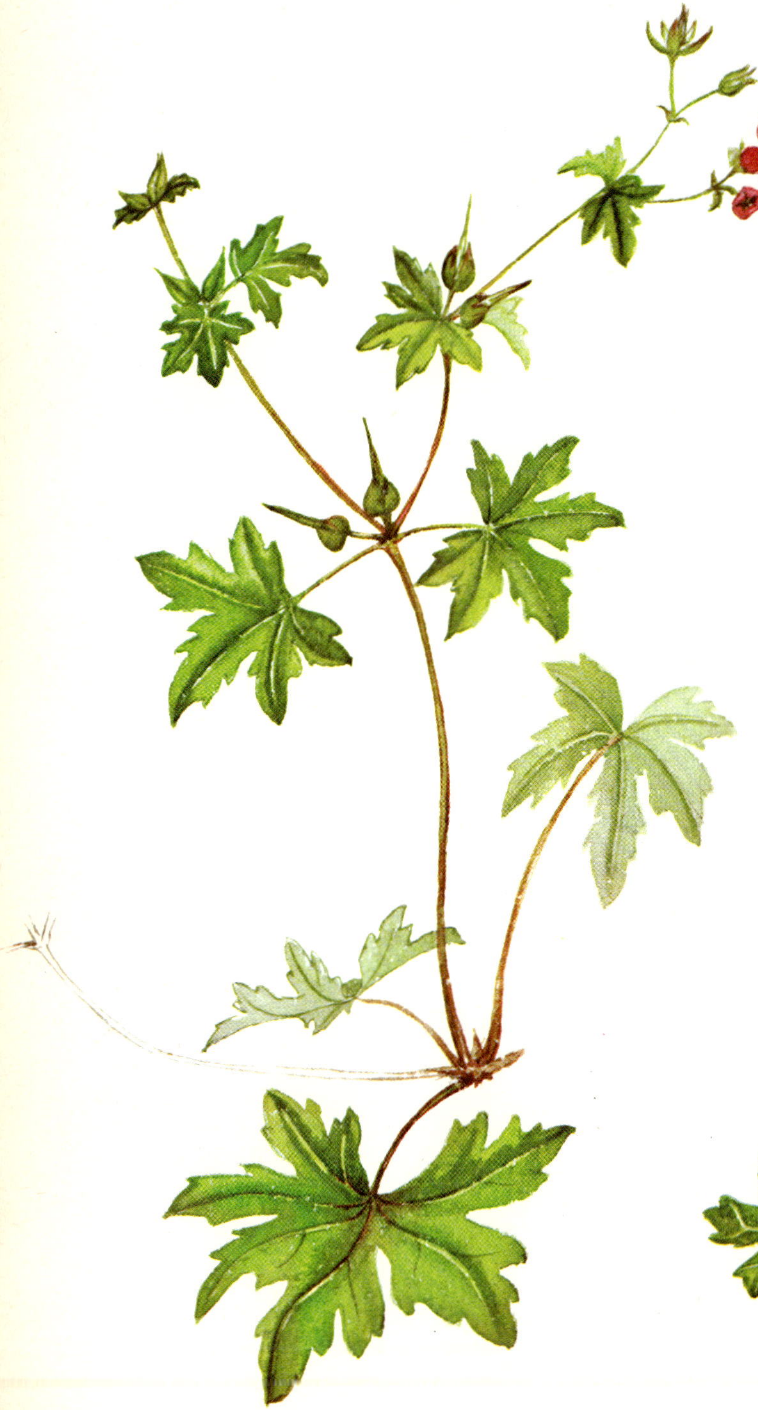

Geranium mascatense Boiss.
Geraniaceae (Geranium Family)

This wild *Geranium* was discovered as a new species by the French plant explorer Aucher-Eloy, who crossed Jabal al-Akhdar in March, 1838. The name of the capital, Mascat, was then often applied by Europeans to the country as a whole, and several new mountain plant species were thus given the specific name *mascatensis.* Sometimes called in Arabic *shuwayb al-ḥamām,* this is a plant of cooler, shaded habitats, and is often seen on disturbed ground around mountain farmlands.

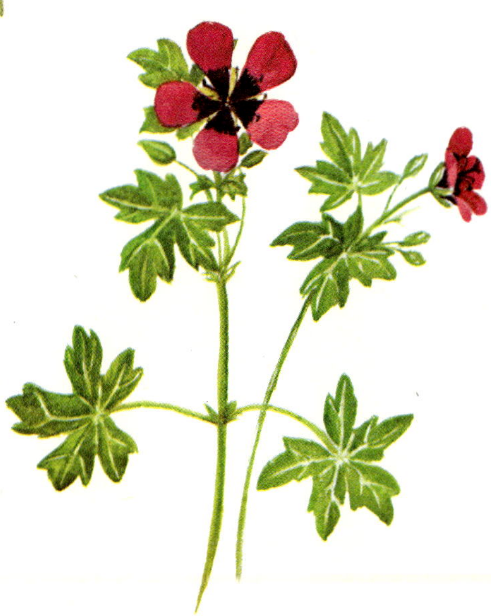

Geranium mascatense

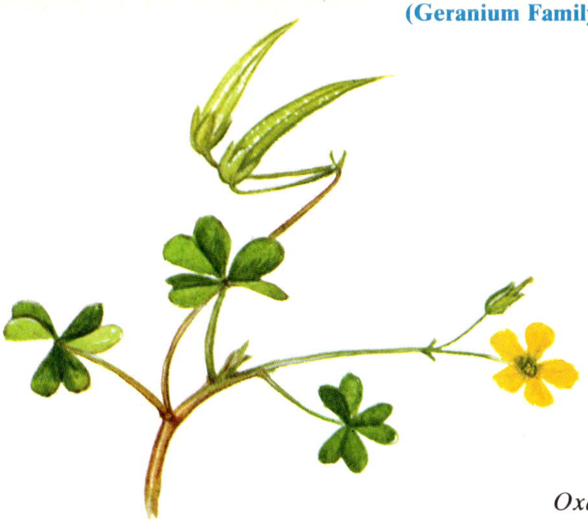

Oxalis corniculata

Ruta chalepensis

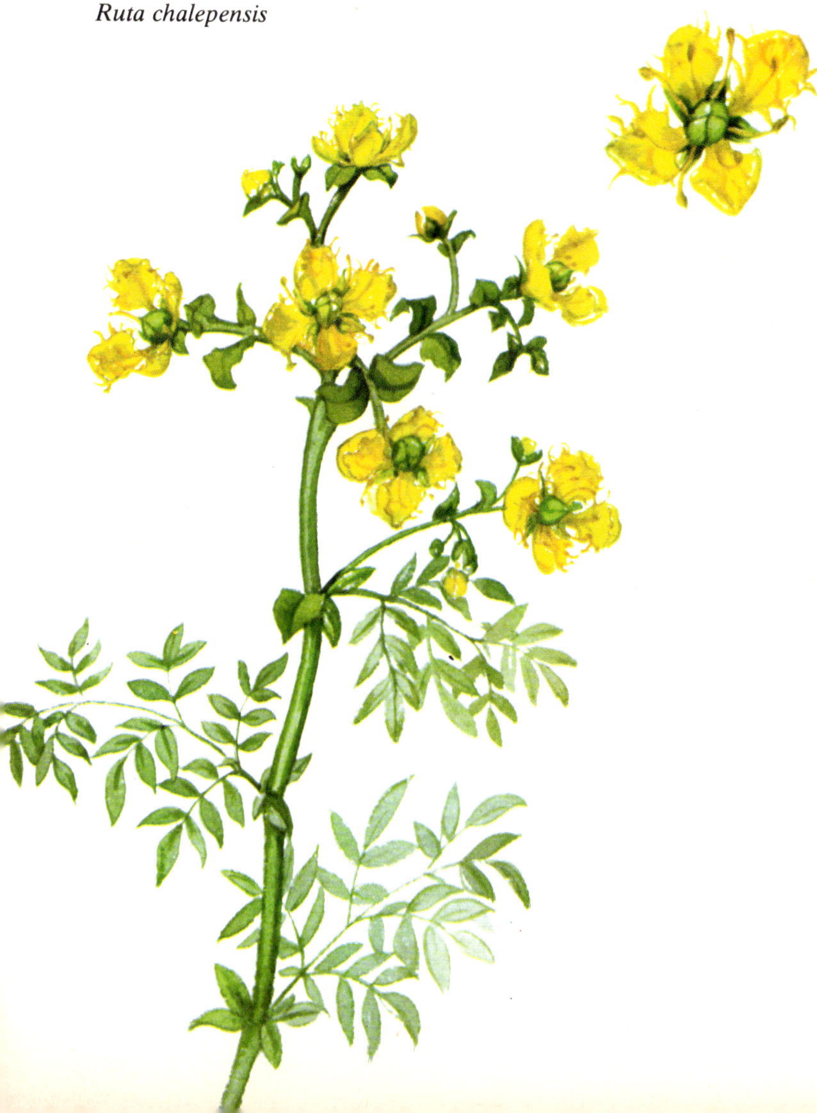

Oxalis corniculata L.
Geraniaceae (Geranium Family)

This common sorrel is often seen as a weed in gardens. It also occurs in natural habitats, but usually where the ground has been disturbed. It prefers shade and grows as a creeper, rooting at intervals and sending up green stems a few centimetres high. Because of its sour taste, it is known as *ḥummāḍ* or *muḥummāḍ,* the same name that is applied to wild dock, *Rumex,* and which is derived from an Arabic word meaning 'sour'. In India, *Oxalis* is used as a folk remedy for fevers and to treat skin ailments.

Ruta chalepensis var. *bracteosa* (DC.) Boiss.
Rutaceae (Rue Family)

The fringe-petalled rue, a Mediterranean shrublet that may grow up to 0.7 metre high, is usually found as a weed along paths, garden edges or other disturbed habitats. Its pungent odour comes from a volatile oil which is in the leaves and which has a wide spectrum of uses in folk medicine in all countries where the plant is found. The name *khiḍf* has been recorded for rue in the Jabal al-Akhdar area.

Rhamnaceae (Buckthorn Family)

Sageretia spiciflora (A. Rich.) Hutch. & Bruce
Rhamnaceae (Buckthorn Family)

Nimt is one of a half-dozen wild plants that have an especially close association with mountain Oman, and like several others of this group, it is an eastern plant whose range in Arabia is restricted to the mountains of al-Ḥajar. *Nimt* is a large shrub that sometimes achieves the stature of a small tree. It is never really dominant in the vegetation, but is very well-known for its sweet, berry-like fruits that provide a refreshing mouthful for passing herdsmen or travellers. The fruits would probably also make a successful base for jams or jellies. *Nimt* is most often seen at higher altitudes above about 2,000 metres.

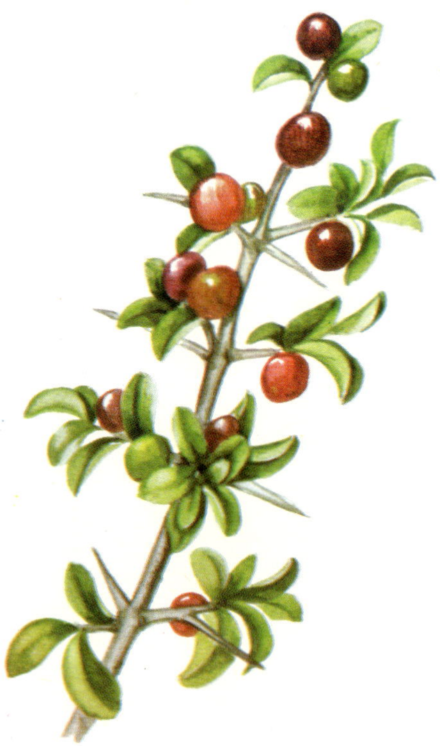

Sageretia spiciflora

Ziziphus spina-christi (L.) Willd.
Rhamnaceae (Buckthorn Family)

The *sidr,* or Christ-thorn tree, has a wide distribution in Arabia, growing wild in *wadis* draining mountainous regions in the south of the Peninsula and cultivated even in the central and northern desert regions. In Oman it is one of the most prominent trees found along *wadi* banks, reaching relatively great stature, and it is easily recognised by its ovate leaves, each with three prominent, almost parallel, veins. *Sidr* is closely related to the jujube and itself has cherry-sized edible fruits, known as *nabaq,* that are not unlike apple in texture and flavour. The small yellowish flowers attract large numbers of flies, which probably serve as pollinators. Wild trees bear spines of variable size, but these are reduced or absent in the cultivated form which has somewhat larger fruits. A related tree, with similar leaves but of different growth form, is found on higher mountain slopes. Known in Oman as *qaṣam,* its precise scientific identity is yet to be confirmed.

Ziziphus spina-christi (cult.)

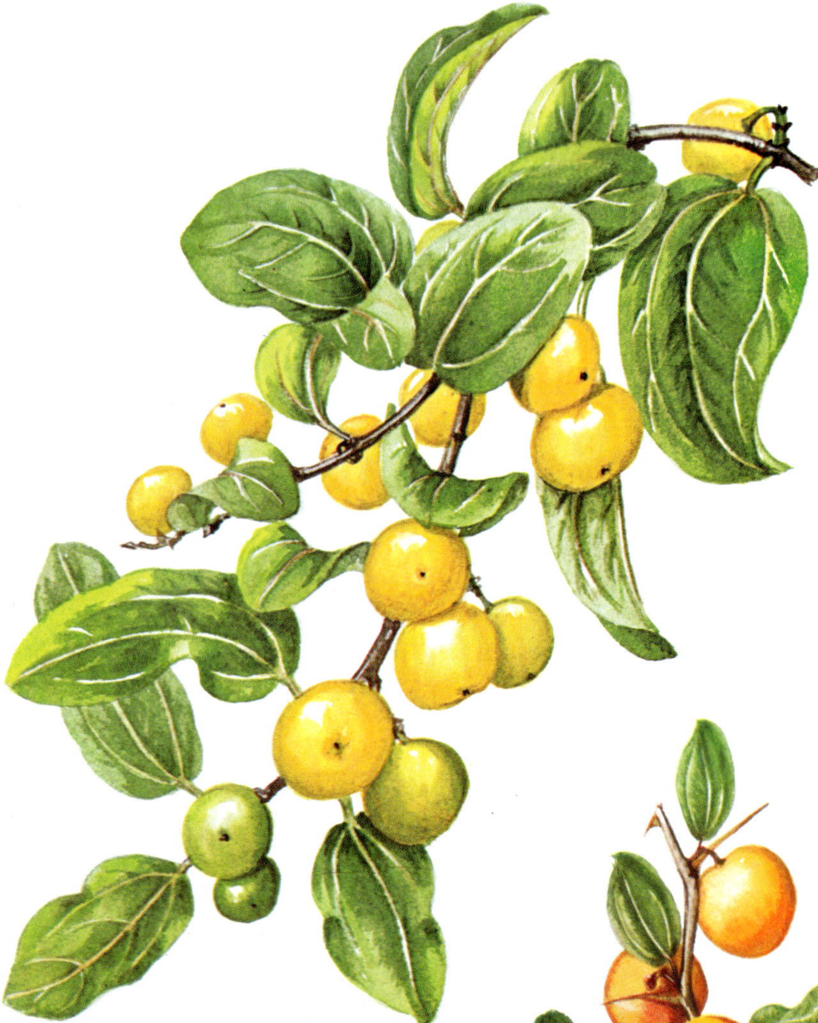

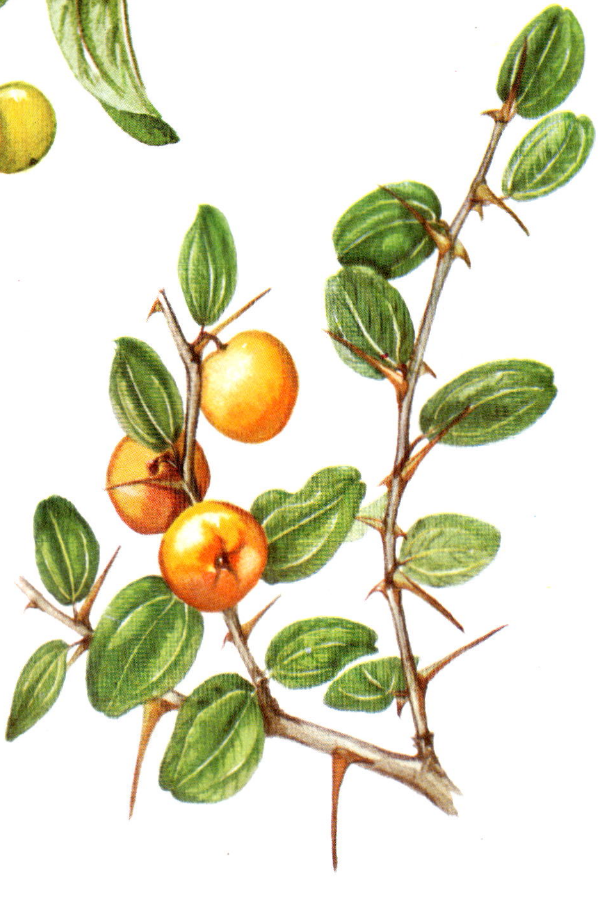

Ziziphus spina-christi (wild)

Dodonaea viscosa Jacq.
Sapindaceae (Soapberry Family)

A mountain shrub most often found at altitudes above 1,700 metres, *Dodonaea* has a wide tropical distribution including mountainous parts of south and west Arabia. It grows 1–2 metres high, with bright green elongated leaves, tapering at the base, that are glossy, as if coated with lacquer. The winged fruits are also distinctive. The shrub is cultivated as a hedge plant in some countries, and in India its close-grained wood is used for tool handles. *Dodonaea* is called *shaḥs* in Oman.

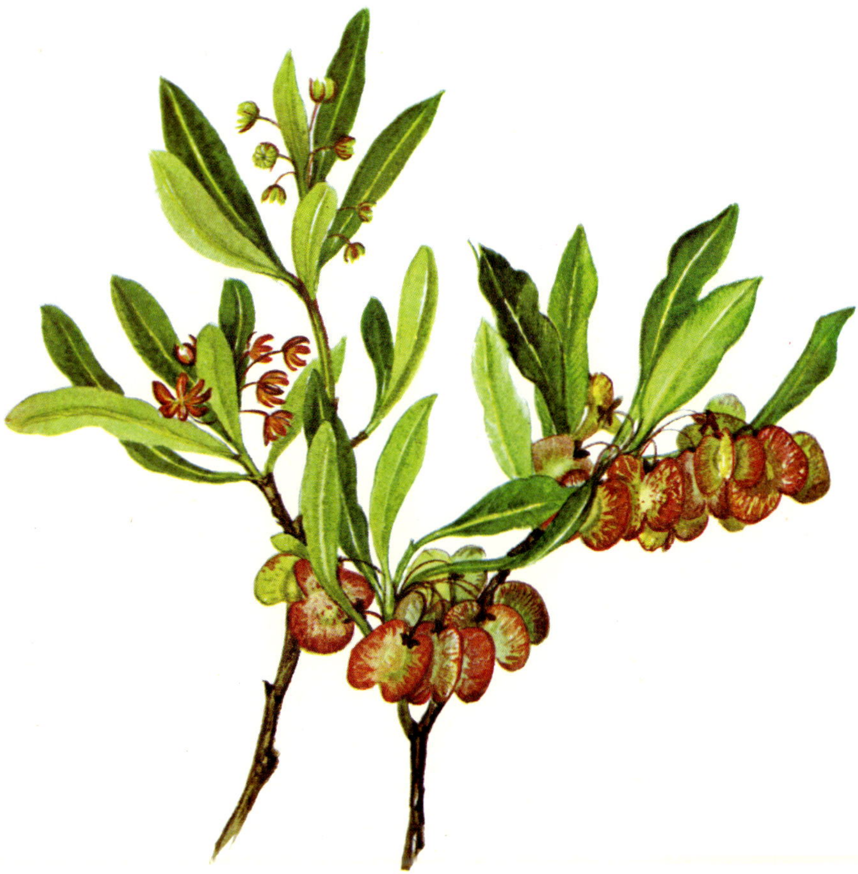

Dodonaea viscosa

Acacia ehrenbergiana Hayne
Leguminosae (Pea Family)

Acacias are the dominant trees over much of lowland northern Oman, and their flat-topped forms account for the African savanna look of the vegetation. Africa is the centre of dispersal of the genus, and the Arabian populations are derived from ancestors that migrated across the land bridge that connected Arabia with Africa until recently in geologic history.

By far the most common lowland *Acacia* in northern Oman is a variety of *Acacia tortilis,* known to all desert Arabs as *samur.* Among these, however, are frequently found a few shrubs or small trees of *salam,* or *Acacia ehrenbergiana,* the species pictured here. The two species can be distinguished by counting the number of pinnae, or stalks bearing the tiny leaflets, in each compound leaf. *Salam* has only one or two pairs of opposed pinnae; *samur* has three to four or more.

Acacia ehrenbergiana is a shrub or small tree, usually only 2–6 metres high. Its fragrant, ball-like flower heads appear in spring, around April, while *samur* blooms in early summer. Both Acacias are armed with sharp, almost metal-hard spines. The camel does not, as some travellers tales have it, devour Acacia branches spines and all. His delicate, prehensile lips in fact avoid the harder spines by working around and between them, while artfully stripping off the tender leaflets.

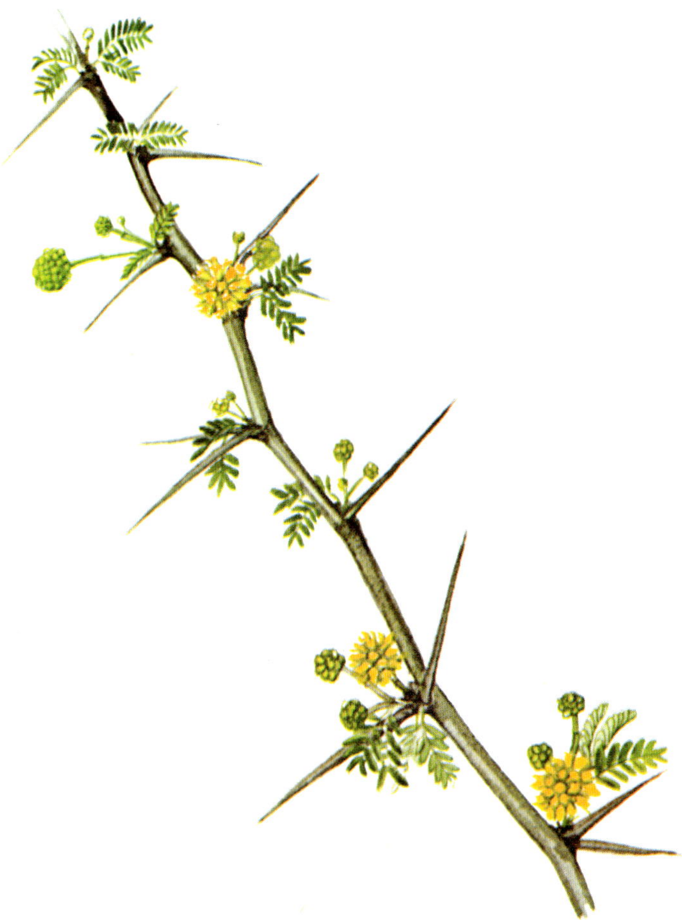

Acacia ehrenbergiana

Cassia italica

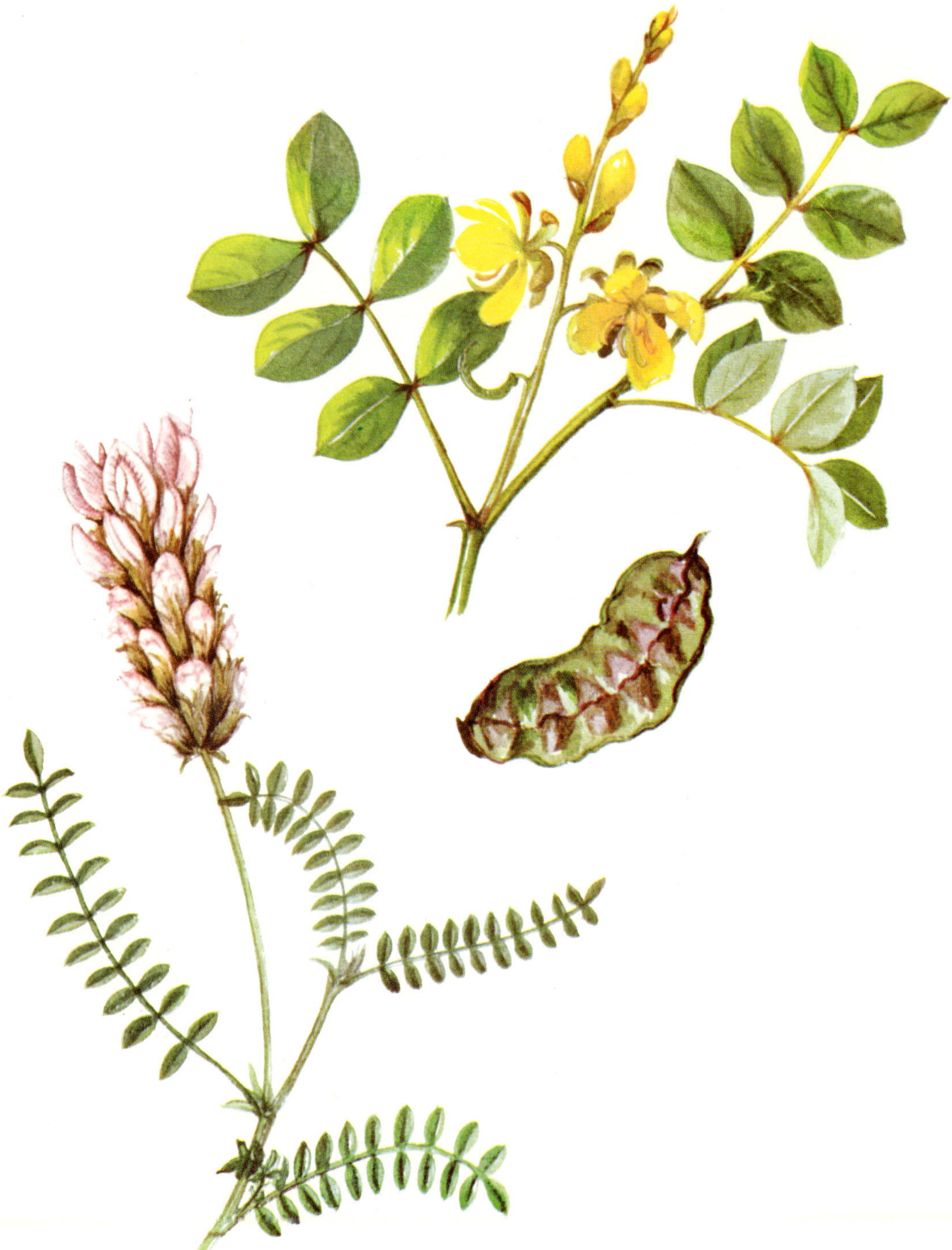

Astragalus sp.

Astragalus sp.
Leguminosae (Pea Family)

This large flowered, low-growing vetch, known to highlanders of the Jabal Aswad area as *farrākh al ḥuṣaynī,* or 'fox's sprout', is likely to be seen only in the higher plateau country, where it seems to favour level silt-filled basins and flats. It is common in the vicinity of Sayq, and is included here as a plant likely to be seen by mountain visitors although herbarium studies required to assign it a specific name had not been completed by press time.

Ebenus stellata Boiss.
Leguminosae (Pea Family)

Ebenus stellata, a dense spiny shrub growing about 1 metre high, is one of the more showy members of the pea family in mountain areas above about 1,600 metres elevation. It sometimes occurs in dense populations on exposed flats between ravines or in rocky plateau country. The flowers, with red petals tinged with yellow, are in head-like spikes. The plumose, filiform teeth of the calyx give the inflorescence a soft, delicate appearance, but the effectiveness of the plant's armament will be appreciated by those who would carry away a bouquet. Flowers of two colour forms are known in Oman. Predominantly red ones are seen in the Jabal al-Akhdar massif, while an isolated population on Jabal Aswad, 45 kilometres south-southwest of Muscat, has yellow as the base flower colour and is only tinged with red. In Oman, *Ebenus* is called *kalbān,* or *kum'il.*

Cassia italica (Mill.) Lam.
Leguminosae (Pea Family)

This low, shrubby *Cassia* is widespread in the Middle East and in Arab countries, including Oman, and is known as *'ishriq*. Its bluish-green leaflets grow in 3–7 pairs, while the fruit is a flat, angled pod with a series of raised crests on each side. *'Ishriq* has long been an important folk remedy, serving as an effective purgative without the cramping effects of colocynth. It was formerly important in the international drug trade as a source of senna, but it has recently been supplanted in commerce by Indian senna, from *Cassia angustifolia.*

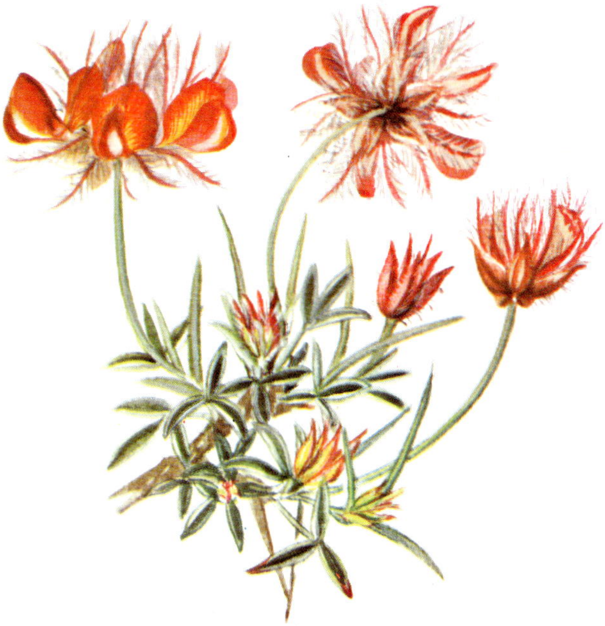

Ebenus stellata

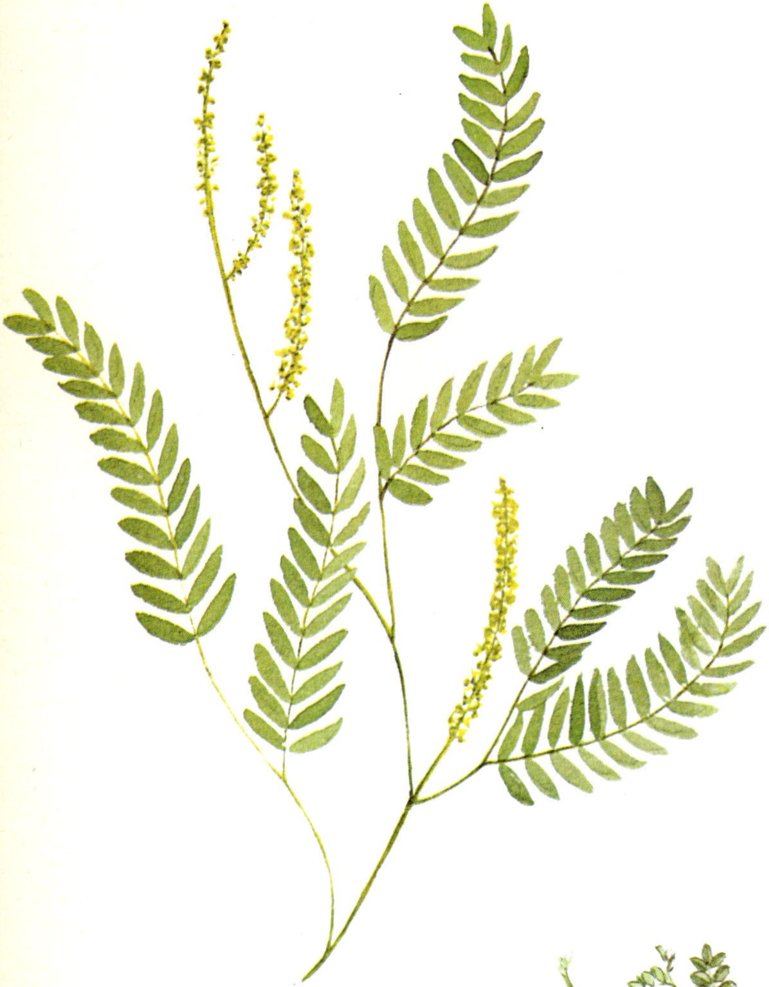

Prosopis cineraria

Prosopis cineraria (L.) Druce
Leguminosae (Pea Family)

Ghāf is one of the biggest wild trees of Oman and is found along *wadi* channels from the coastal plain inland as far as the edge of the Rub' al-Khālī sands. It has a dense, often rounded crown that provides fine shade, while its elongated pods are consumed by livestock. It is easily recognised as a large tree with *Acacia*-like compound leaves, but without the stout spines of *Acacia*.

Indigofera intricata Boiss.
Leguminosae (Pea Family)

A low-growing, sometimes prostrate plant, usually seen on the coastal sands, and one of six species of *Indigofera* recorded from northern Oman. All are related to the cultivated indigo, still grown in Oman as a source of the well-known blue dye.

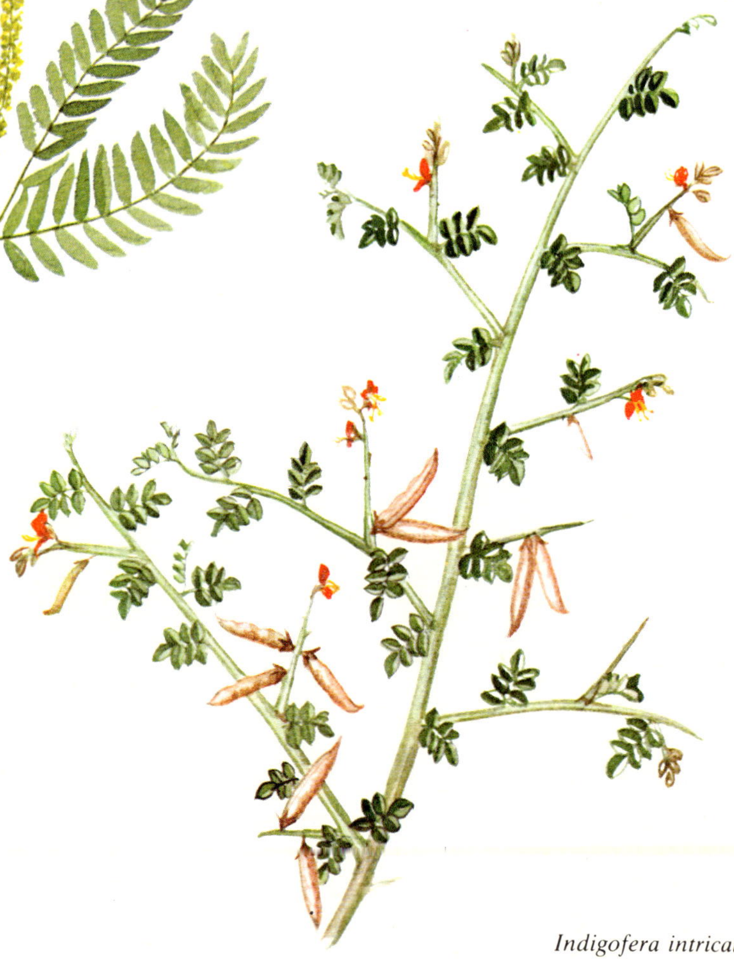

Indigofera intricata

Taverniera glabra Boiss.
Leguminosae (Pea Family)

The genus *Taverniera,* named after the French traveller in the Orient, Jean Tavernier (1605–1689), includes seven species of shrubby legumes found in the Middle East. The Oman plant is characteristic of the lower Gulf area, being found also in southern Iran. It grows 0.7–1 metre high and, like other members of its genus, is most likely to be seen in saline coastal habitats.

Taverniera may be recognised by the form of its pod, which consists of two or three flattened, rounded, connected joints, often bearing short bristles. Its Arabic name is *'aṣmaṭ.*

Tephrosia haussknechtii Bornm.
Leguminosae (Pea Family)

This bright-flowered shrublet of rocky, lower altitude hill-sides is the most common of the five *Tephrosia* species known from northern Oman.

It is called *ḍafrā'* in Arabic. One of the others, *Tephrosia purpurea,* is known by the same vernacular name and is unusual in being a species that occurs in tropical countries of both the Old and New Worlds. In Asia it is used as a fish poison, while the Seminole Indians of America used a decoction of it as a specific for nose bleeding. A third Oman species, *Tephrosia nubica,* is called *'aytimān* in Oman and is reported to have local medicinal uses.

Taverniera glabra

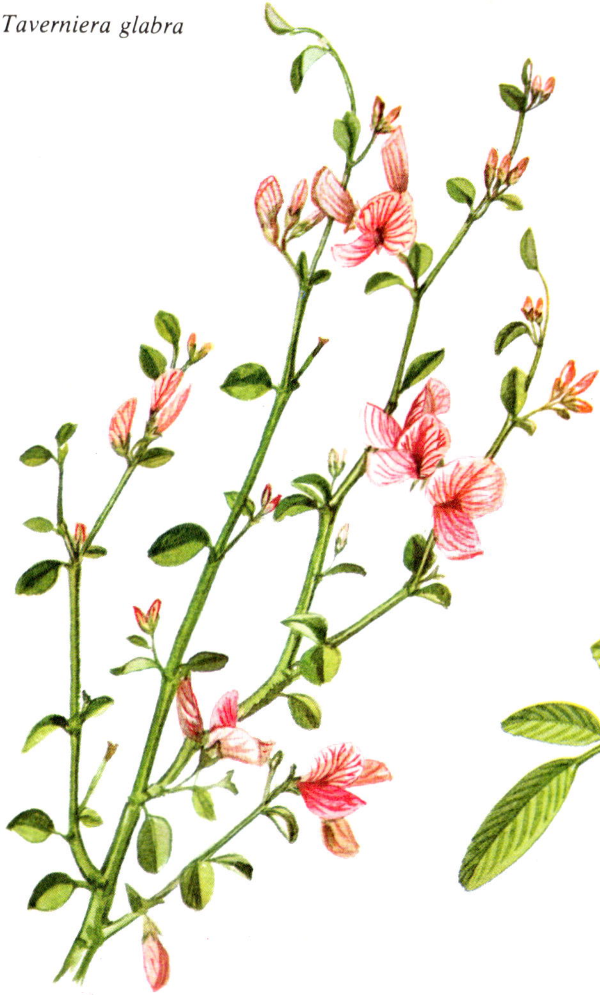

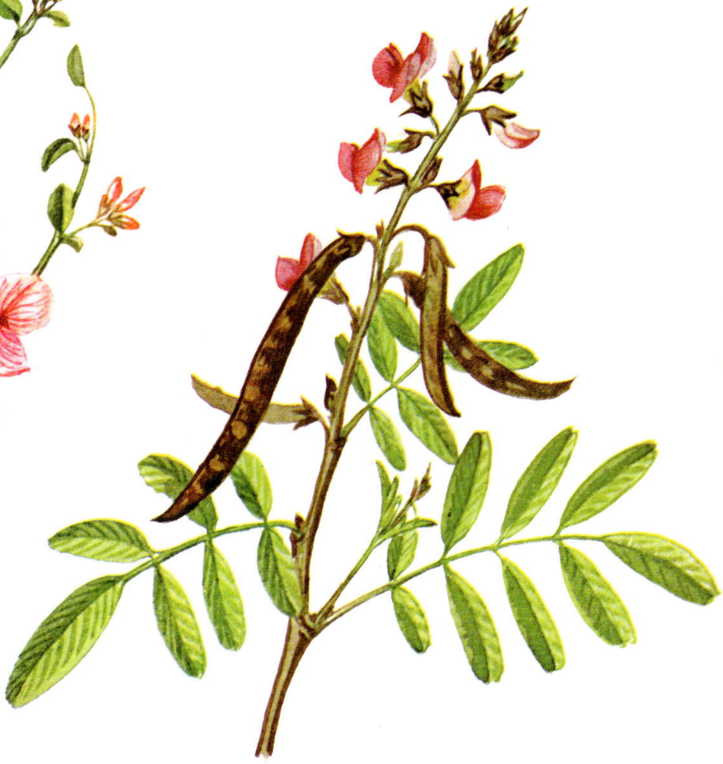

Tephrosia hausknechtii

Myrtus communis L.
Myrtaceae (Myrtle Family)

This aromatic shrub or small tree is the myrtle so well-known since ancient times and which figured in classical mythology. It is a native of the Mediterranean region and may have been introduced in Oman, now usually being found in the vicinity of mountain villages. Myrtle is a dense evergreen shrub, growing up to 3 metres high, that bears many-stamened white flowers and rounded berries that ripen blue-black. The leaves contain an aromatic oil that is distilled as an essence in some countries. Villagers collect the leaves in Oman, dry them, and beat them to a powder that is used for its aromatic properties. The classical Arabic name for the myrtle is *ās*. In Oman it is called *yās*.

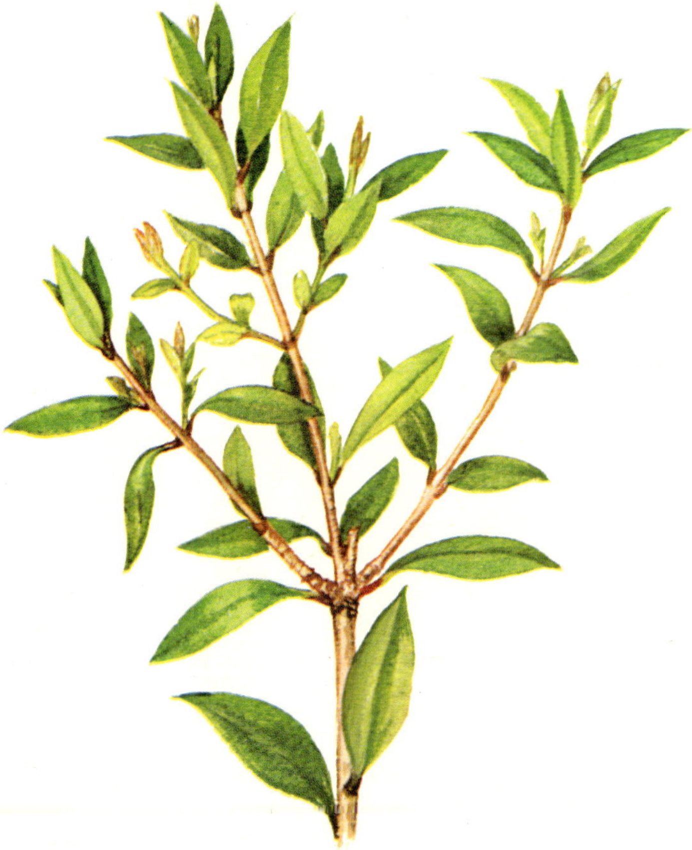

Myrtus communis

Carthamus tinctorius L.
Compositae (Composite Family)

This safflower, or 'false saffron', is strictly speaking a cultivated plant. It is a common escape around farm areas, however, and it is sometimes seen growing apparently naturally in wild surroundings. It is an annual, growing to 0.7–1.2 metres high, with very bright orange to red flowers. Once widely cultivated as a source of yellow and red dyes, it is now economically important in many countries as a source of edible oil, which is pressed from the seeds. In Oman, as in other parts of southern Arabia, safflower is still grown for its colouring matter and is used as a cosmetic by village women. A yellow pigment in the flowers is extracted with water. The red compound also present requires more processing, dissolving in alkaline solutions and reprecipitating with the addition of acid. Safflower is known in Oman as *shawrān*.

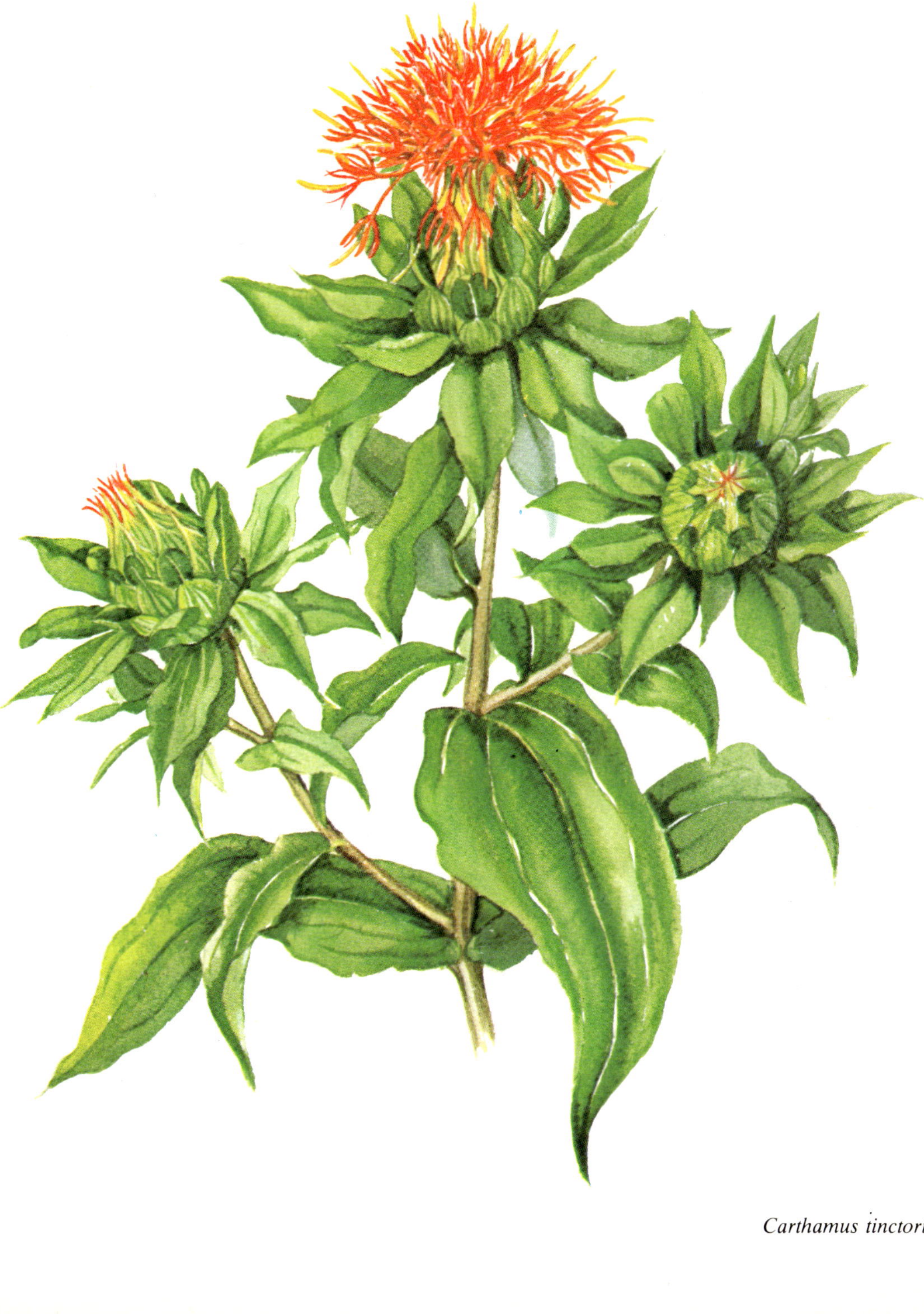

Carthamus tinctorius

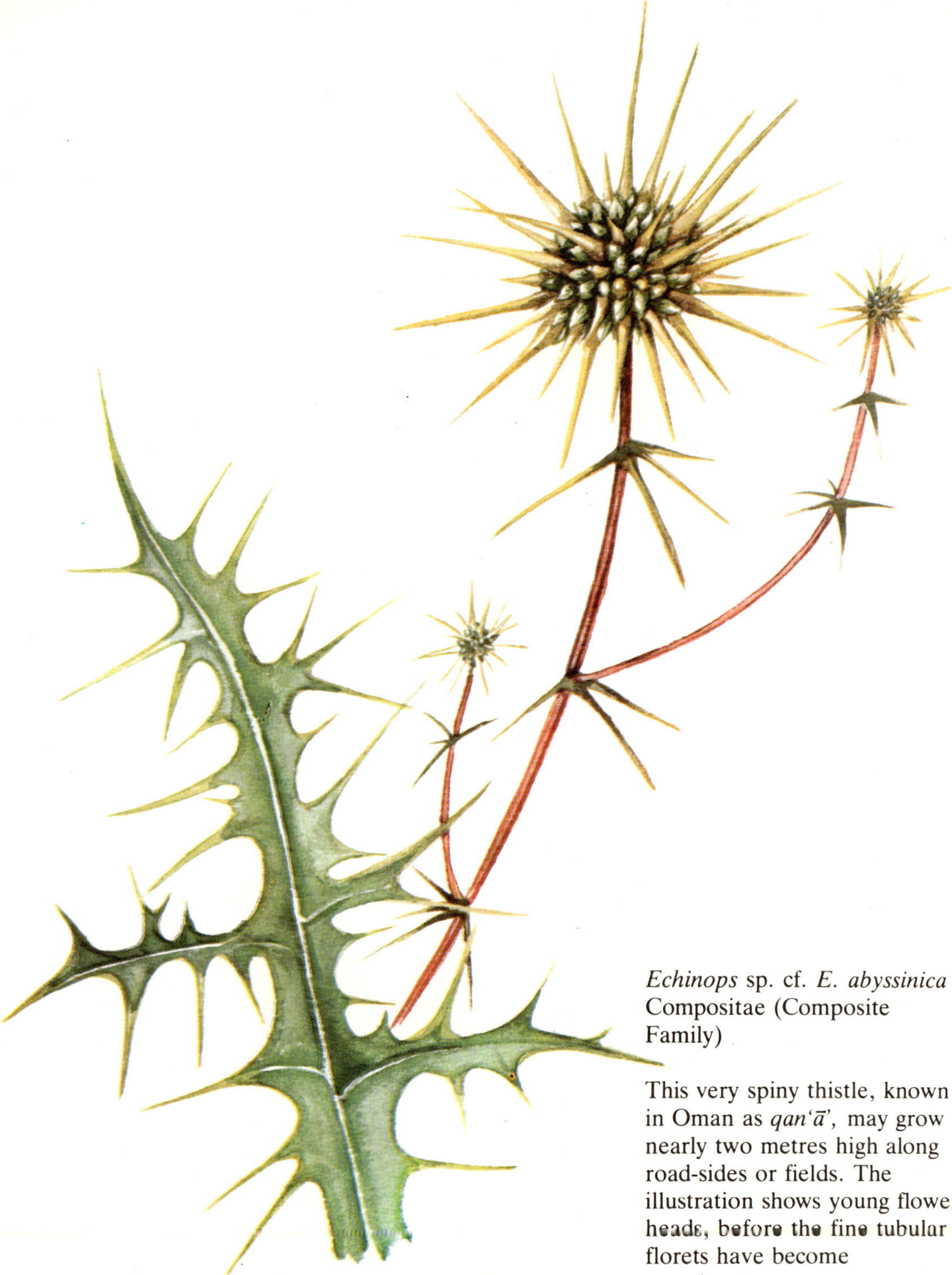

Echinops sp.

Echinops sp. cf. *E. abyssinica*
Compositae (Composite Family)

This very spiny thistle, known in Oman as *qan'ā'*, may grow nearly two metres high along road-sides or fields. The illustration shows young flower heads, before the fine tubular florets have become prominent.

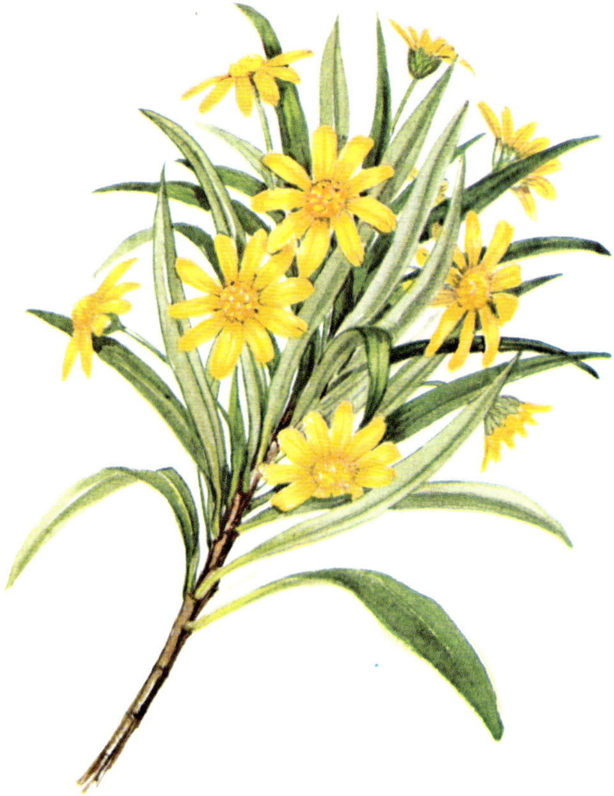

Euryops pinifolius

Euryops pinifolius A. Rich.
Compositae (Composite Family)

This bright-flowered shrublet, known in Oman as *ḥanqalān* or *ḥayqalān,* grows to about 1 metre high. Branched at the base with several to many ascending stems, it is usually found at altitudes above 1,500 metres. A series of *Euryops* species is distributed from southern and eastern Africa across highland south Arabia.

Helichrysum sp.
Compositae (Composite Family)

This pink-tinged everlasting, about 25 centimetres high and often seen in rocky habitats at higher mountain levels, is called *shajarat al babaw,* or *'bulbul's bush'* by some highland tribesmen. It is one of several plants collected by the 1975 Oman Flora and Fauna Survey that are still undergoing herbarium study for the assignment of specific names.

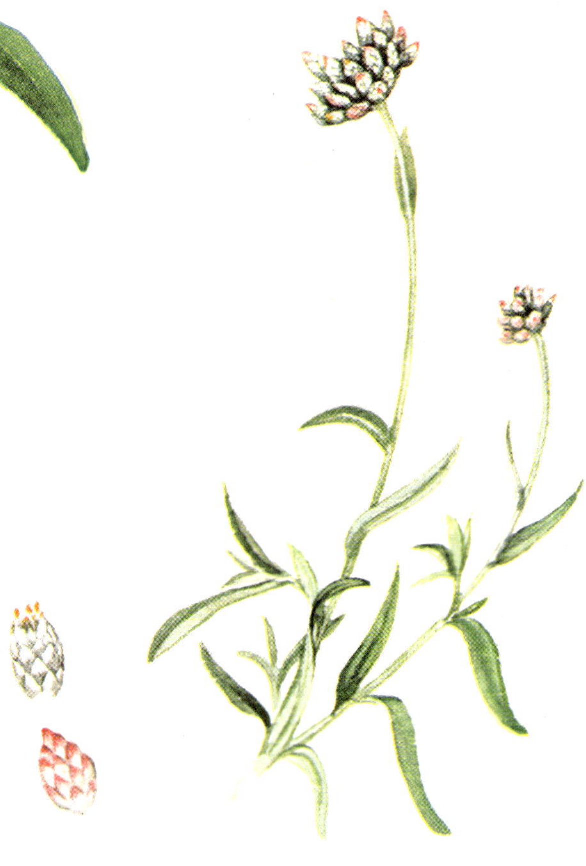

Helichrysum sp.

Compositae (Composite Family)

Osteospermum vaillantii (Decne.) T. Norl. Compositae (Composite Family)

The best aid to identifying this marigold-like plant are its unusual winged, seed-bearing achenes. After flowering, they hang together in a pendulous structure resembling a Chinese lantern. *Osteospermum* in Oman may be seen from the lowlands up to subalpine habitats above 2,500 metres. In North Yemen this plant is called *yahdab.*

Phagnalon viridifolium Decne. Compositae (Composite Family)

Shrublets of the genus *Phagnalon* are well-known for their preference for rocky habitats. This Oman species is most likely to be seen on steep hill-sides—even cliffs—bending upright from its base rooted in the cleft of a nearly vertical rock face. The name *janānat an nāqah* is used in Egypt.

Osteospermum vaillanti

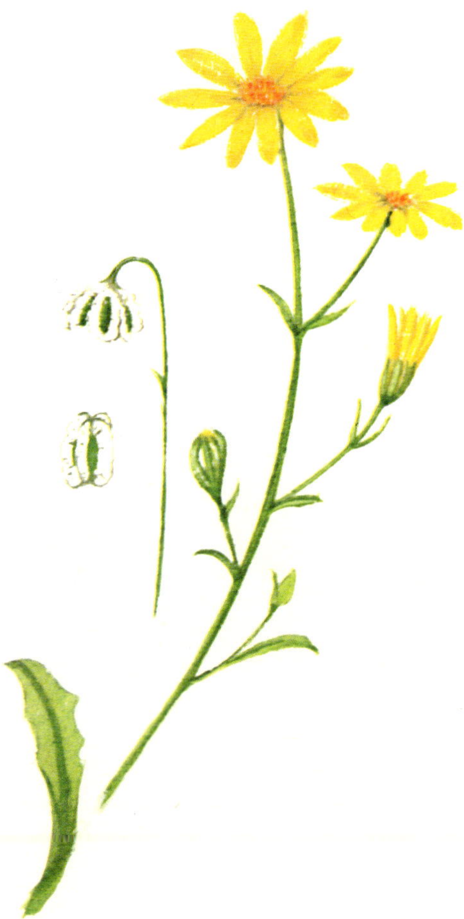

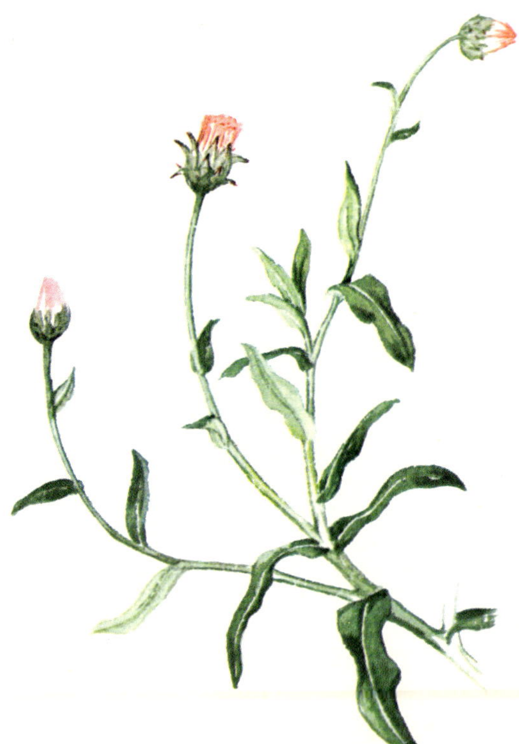

Phagnalon viridifolium

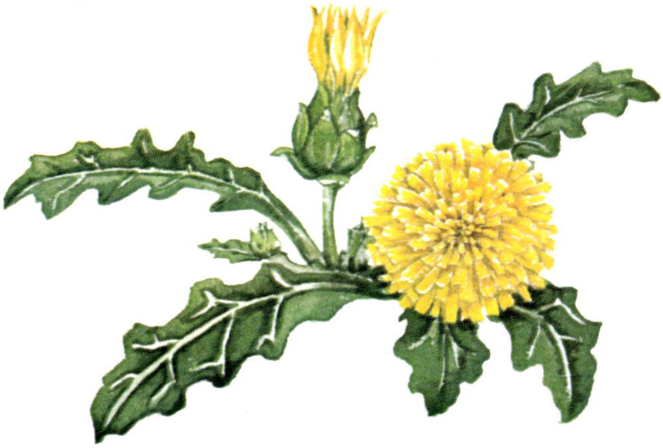

Reichardia tingitana (L.) Roth.
Compositae (Composite Family)

This dandelion relative may be found from the lowland desert to intermediate mountain slopes. The reddish tinge on the leaves is variable, tending to occur more often in plants on drier soil. The Arabic name, *ḥuwwāʔ* is often applied to this plant, as it is to *Launaea* and other composites with ligulate flower heads.

Reichardia tingitana

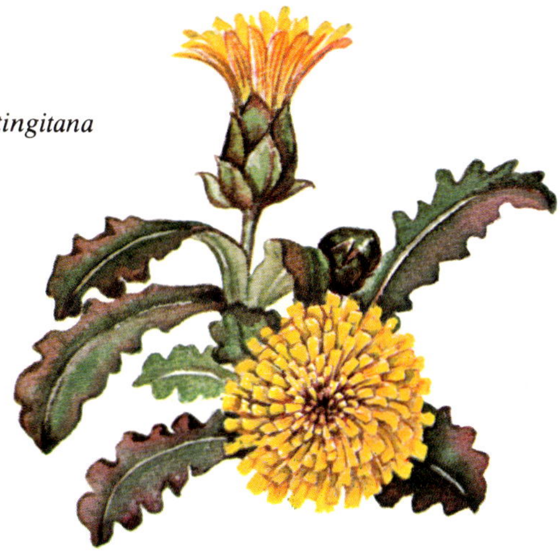

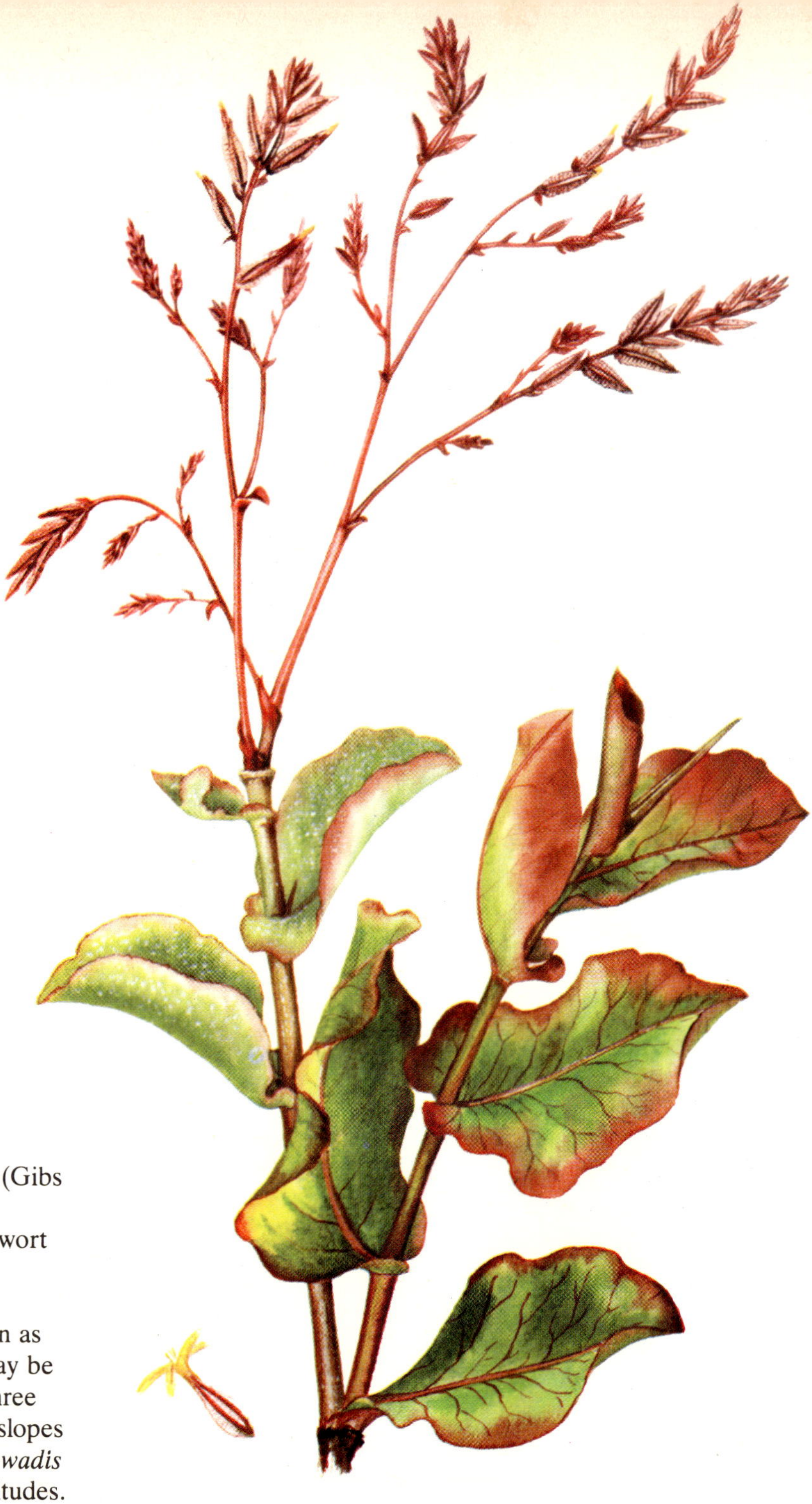

Dyerophytum indicum (Gibs ex Wight) Kuntze
Plumbaginaceae (Leadwort Family)

Widely known in Oman as *maliḥlāḥ,* this shrub may be found growing up to three metres high on rocky slopes above lower mountain *wadis* as well as at higher altitudes. The leathery leaves are often covered with a whitish or greyish powdery bloom.

Dyerophytum indicum

Anagallis arvensis L.
Primulaceae (Primula Family)

The blue pimpernel, illustrated here, and the scarlet pimpernel are generally considered to be colour variants of one species. In Oman, the blue-flowered variety appears to be by far the more common. It is a small herb, usually growing singly, that is a weed in both temperate and tropical parts of the world. In Oman it is common enough in the oases and around gardens, but it also occurs in natural habitats in the lowlands and up to at least medium elevations in the mountains. The seeds are contained in a globular capsule that splits circumferentially, the top portion opening as a lid. In Saudi Arabia this flower is called *'uwaynah.*

Dionysia mira Wendelbo
Primulaceae (Primula Family)

A bright-flowered, cliff-dwelling perennial which by name and tradition is closely associated with a unique Oman animal, the tahr, which frequents the same high-altitude rock faces. Jabal al-Akhdar tribesmen call it *shajarat al wa'l,* or 'tahr bush', because that rare wild goat is said to be especially fond of it. *Dionysia* grows up to 50 centimetres high in rock clefts. Its flowers and leaves have a peculiar slightly bitter medicinal odour. The sight of a fine specimen in full flower is a mountain naturalist's prize, and it is an excellent subject for photographs. It deserves special protection and attention from conservationists; wild mountain plants should never be cut or uprooted for the sake of short-lived bouquets or probably unsuccessful garden transplants.

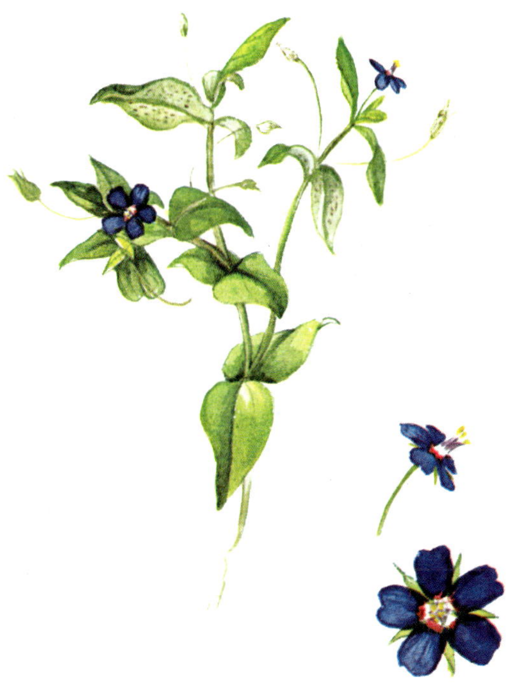

Anagallis arvensis

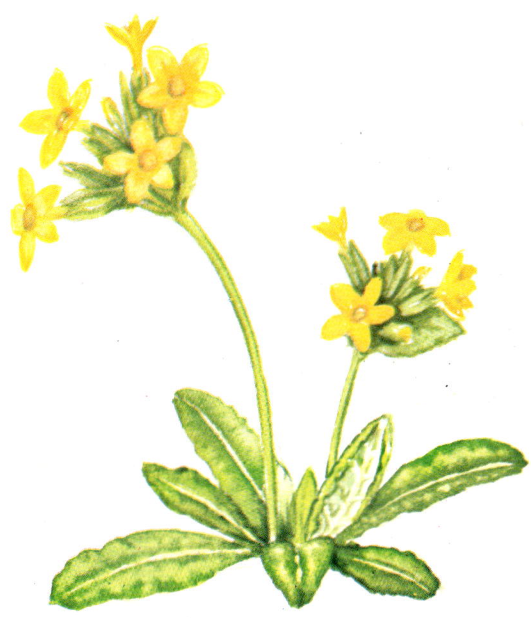

Dionysia mira

Sapotaceae (Sapote Family)

Reptonia mascatensis (A. Db.) Radlk. ex Schwartz
Sapotaceae (Sapote Family)

This 4–6 metre-high tree is one of the most important components of the woodland vegetation found on Jabal al-Akhdar in the 1,350–2,300 metre altitude zone, where it forms bits of dense forest in protected ravines. It is a plant peculiar to Oman, its nearest relative occurring in the mountains of east Afghanistan. Well-known to all highland Omanis by its classical name, *būt, Reptonia* was described by Arab writers in the 9th Century A.D. as a 'mountain tree with edible berries, ripening black, that blacken the mouth of the eater'. The fruits are gathered today by mountain villagers and herdsmen. *Būt,* like a few other trees or shrubs found predominantly or uniquely in Oman, is something of a national botanical symbol. Oman historical writers list it as one of the characteristic and useful plants of their highlands.

Oleaceae (Olive Family)

Olea africana Mill.
Oleaceae (Olive Family)

This wild olive, in Arabic *'utm,* is one of the larger trees of Jabal al-Akhdar and is an important constituent of the *Reptonia-Olea* woodland plant community of the 1,350–2,300 metre altitude zone. It usually grows to between 5 and 10 metres high and is best developed in the

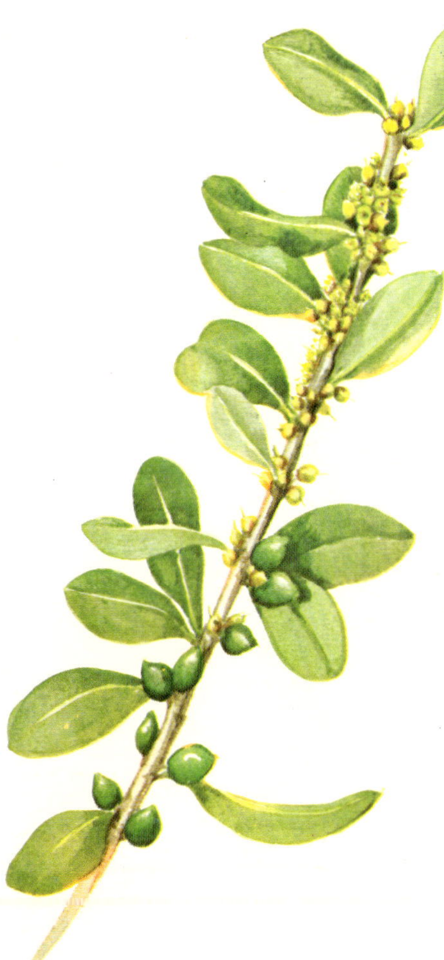

Reptonia mascatensis

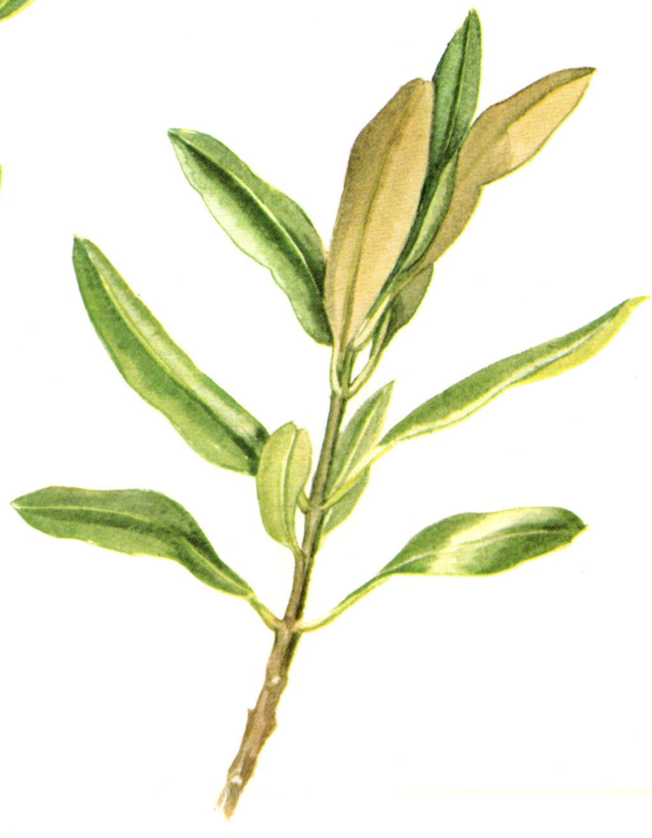

Olea africana

partially protected ravines draining to the steep northern face of the mountains, where water flow is concentrated. This olive is a plant of African origin, and its distribution can be traced eastward through Yemen and 'Asīr, across to Oman, and into Iran. The very small fruits are not eaten, but are used by highland Bedouins and villagers in poultices to treat livestock sores and wounds. In south-western Arabia wild olive wood is used in making rakes and other simple agricultural implements.

Salvadora persica L.
Salvadoraceae (Salvadora Family)

This shrub, *rāk* or *arāk* in Arabic and often called the 'tooth-brush tree' in English, is well-known throughout the Arabian Peninsula and in Africa as the source of the twigs used by both nomads and townspeople as simple but very effective tooth-brushes *(masāwīk,* singular: *miswāk). Salvadora* varies greatly in stature, sometimes being a single shrub about a metre high and sometimes growing in thickets two or three metres high with many separate rootstocks. The flowers have a coffee-like odour, and the fruits are small reddish berries. Branches or roots 1–2 centimetres thick are cut into lengths of about 20 centi-metres, scraped clean, washed and dried. The tooth-brush is prepared for use by cutting away about 1.5 centimetres of

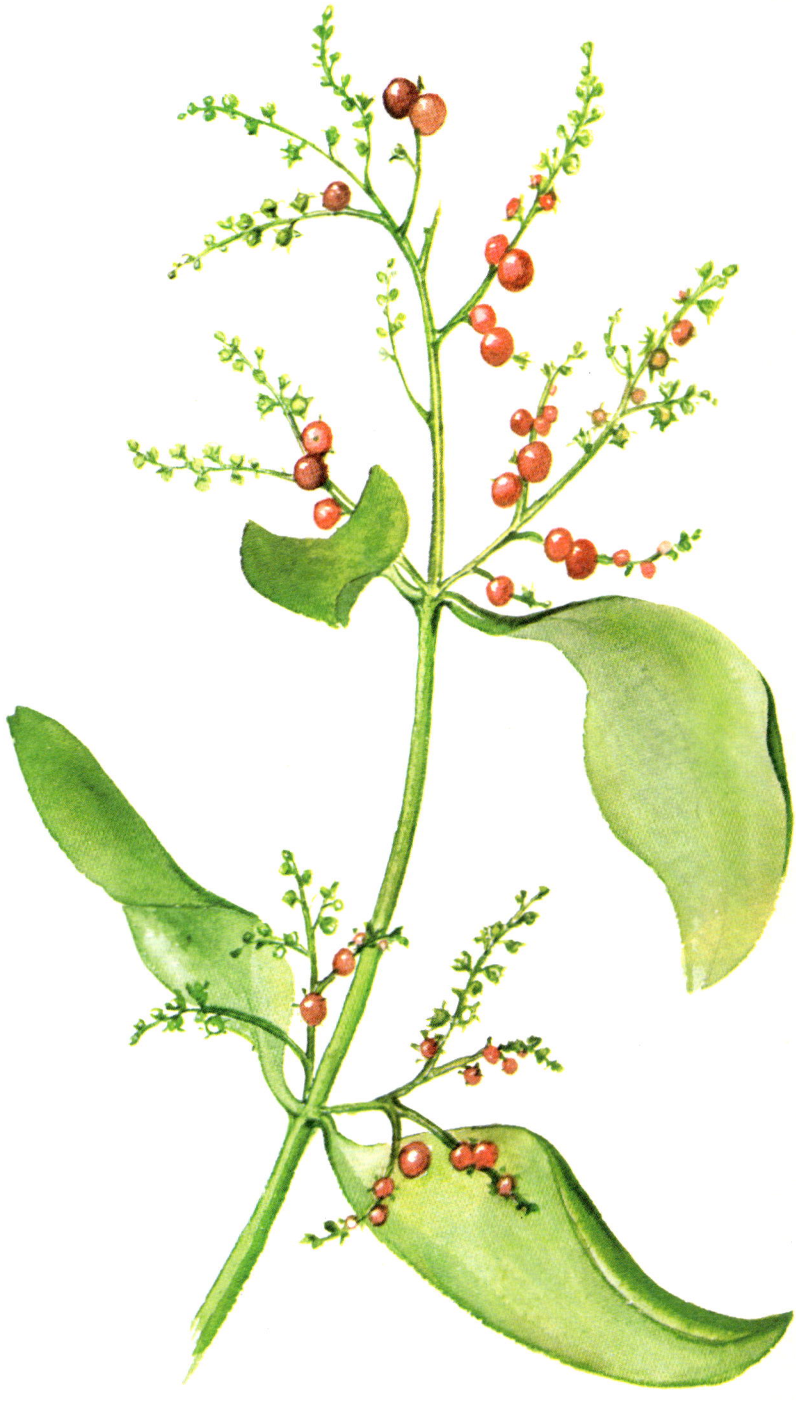

Salvadora persica

bark all around at one end, then working or chewing the fibrous central part of the stem into a brush-like tip. The wood contains a slightly bitter and astringent substance that provides an effective natural dentifrice. In northern Oman, *rāk* may be seen along and above the banks of mountain *wadis* and sometimes on rocky hill-sides. It may also be found in the coastal sands.

Nerium mascatense DC.
Apocynaceae (Dogbane Family)

The oleander is known in Oman as *ḥaban*, and classical Arabic works on plant lore prove that this name has been used in the country for at least a thousand years. Closely resembling the garden oleander widely cultivated in tropical parts of the world, the Omani plant is a distinct species that has evolved in this geographically isolated part of the Arabian Peninsula. It grows in dense clumps, sometimes higher than a man, in gravelly *wadi* bottoms where water runs at or near the surface. It is strongly poisonous, but animals avoid its bitter leaves, and livestock losses are rare.

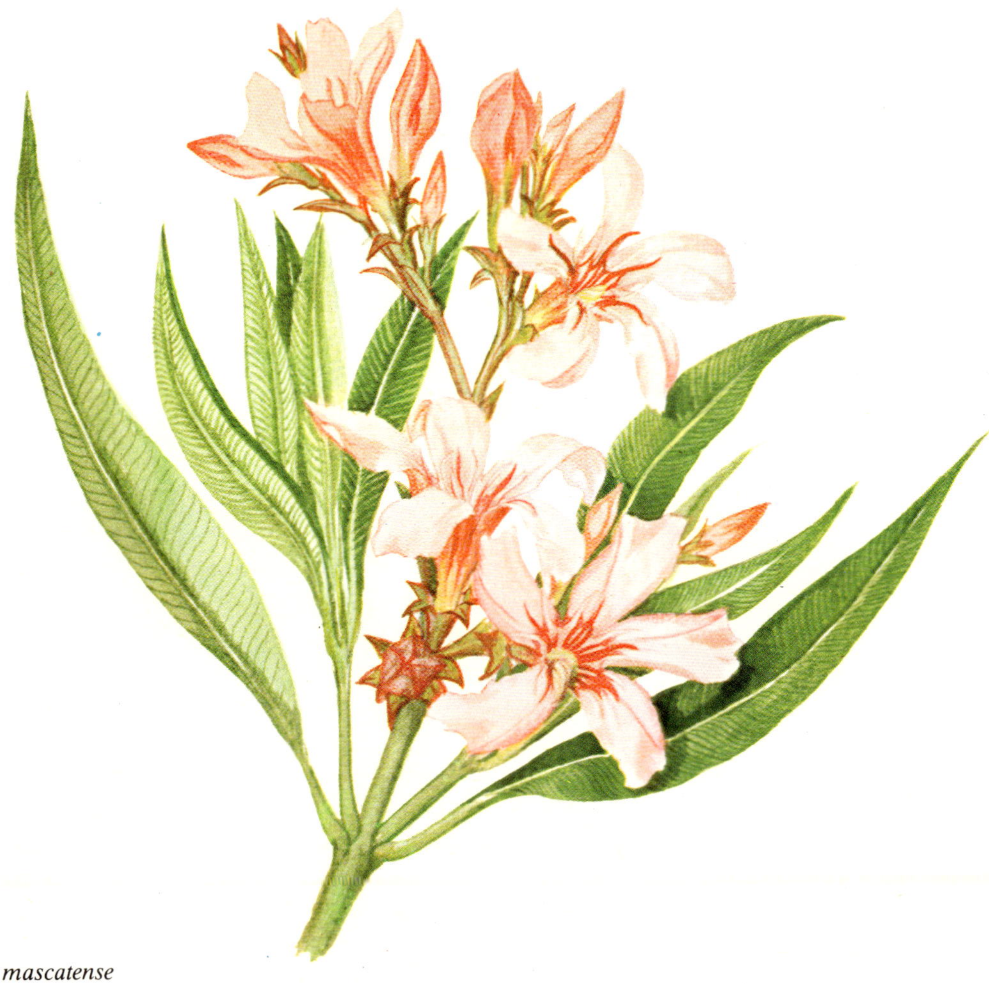

Nerium mascatense

Rhazya stricta Decne.
Apocynaceae (Dogbane Family)

The flower and fruit structures of this undershrub, known throughout Arabia as *ḥarmal,* prove its close relationship with the oleander. *Ḥarmal* grows to about 1 metre high on silty flatlands in lower altitudes. Like the oleander, it is to some degree poisonous and normally is avoided by grazing animals. In some parts of Arabia it has been used in folk medicine as a remedy for respiratory ailments or fevers, smoke from the ignited dry leaves being inhaled from a pipe.

Pergularia tomentosa L.
Asclepiadaceae (Milkweed Family)

The heart-shaped leaves, twining habit, and thick white sap of this milkweed relative make it easy to recognise. Sometimes growing alone as a small bush, it is more commonly seen climbing on other shrubs. The flowers are whitish, and the fruits are inflated, tapering to the tip, and covered with spine-like tubercles. The proper Arabic name for *Pergularia* is *ghalqah;* it is also called *shajarat al julūd.* This means 'hides bush' and refers to its use in removing the hair from hides in preparation for tanning. Early Arab writers described the Abyssinians' use of this plant in making arrow poisons.

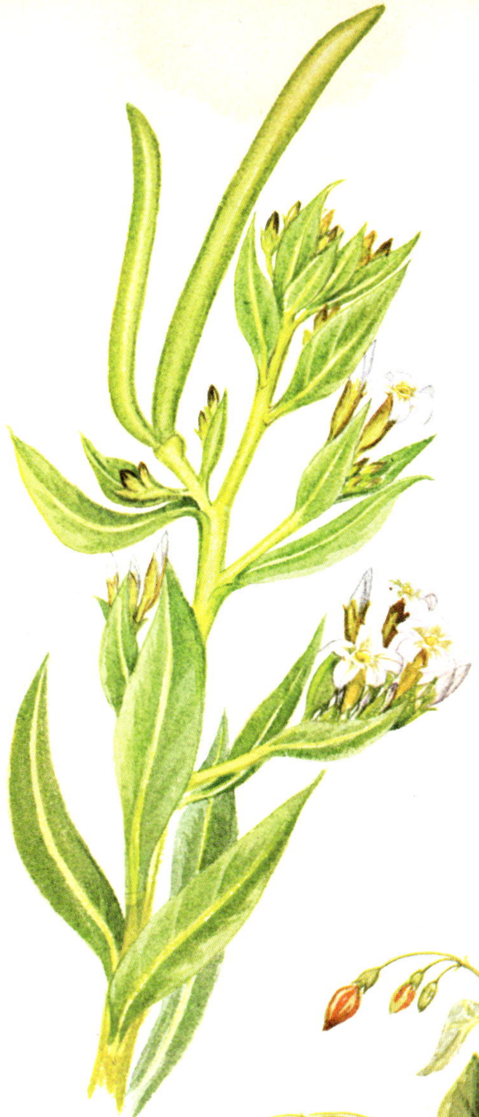

Rhazya stricta

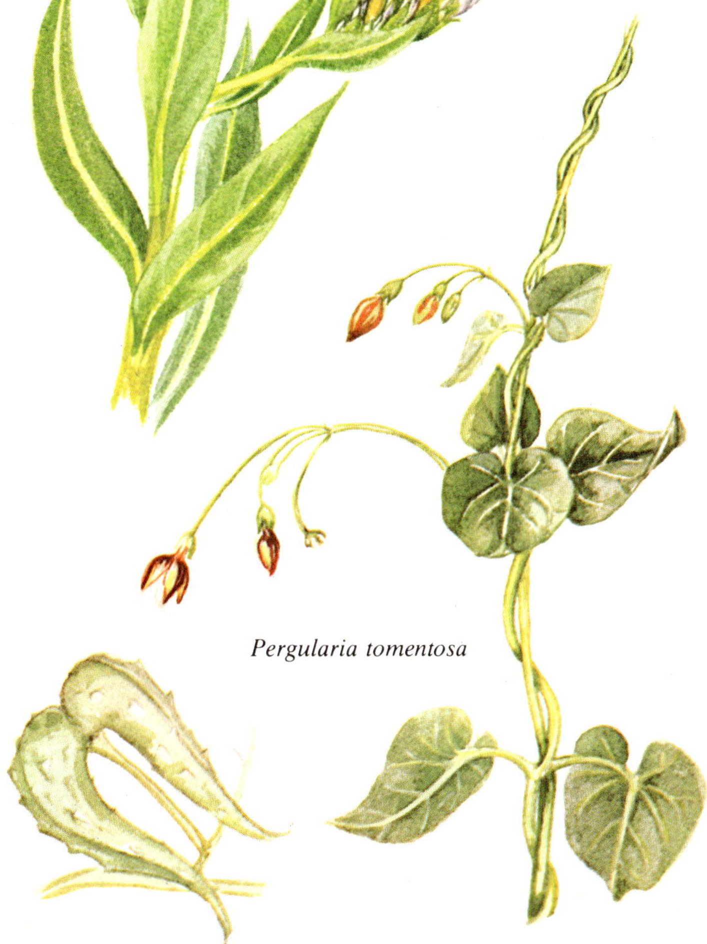

Pergularia tomentosa

Calotropis procera (Ait.) Ait. f.
Asclepiadaceäe (Milkweed Family)

This 2–5 metre-high lowland shrub or small tree, called *shakhr* in Oman, is better known in other parts of Arabia under the name *'ushar*. Like other members of the milkweed family, it bleeds copious white sap or latex when cut. Also like other milkweeds, it contains toxic compounds with medicinal uses. Its poisonous white sap has been used in some parts of the Middle East to treat camel mange. In India, an extract of the roots was used to make an arrow poison.

The leaves of *shakhr* are broad, smooth, somewhat fleshy and grey-green. The unripe fruits are smooth green and apple-like, with a spongy inside texture. The ripe seeds are covered with fine white floss. *Calotropis* was well-known among earlier generations of Arabs for its wood and bark which, when burned, provided the finest charcoal for making gunpowder. The plant is found ranging from Africa, across Arabia to Iran and India.

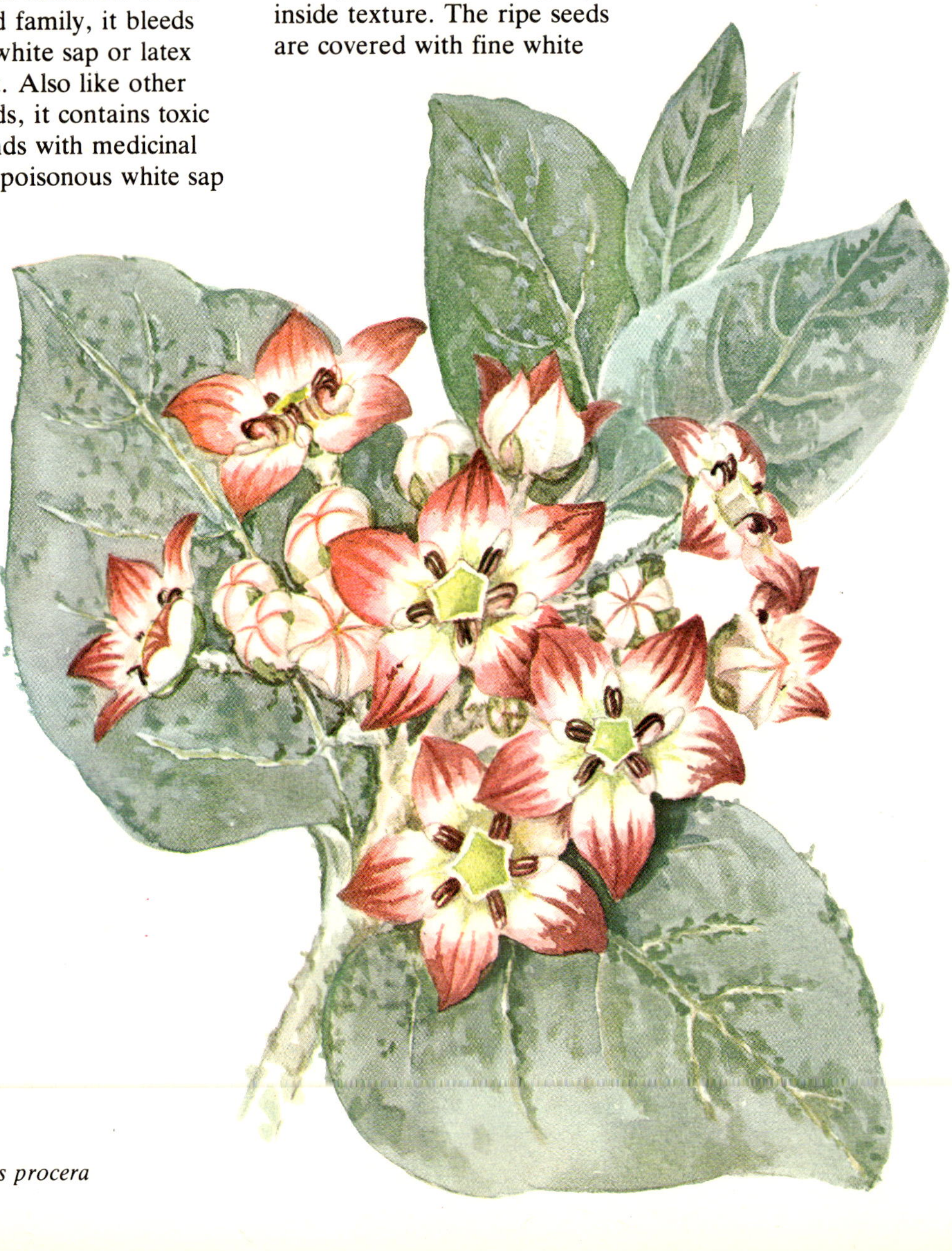

Calotropis procera

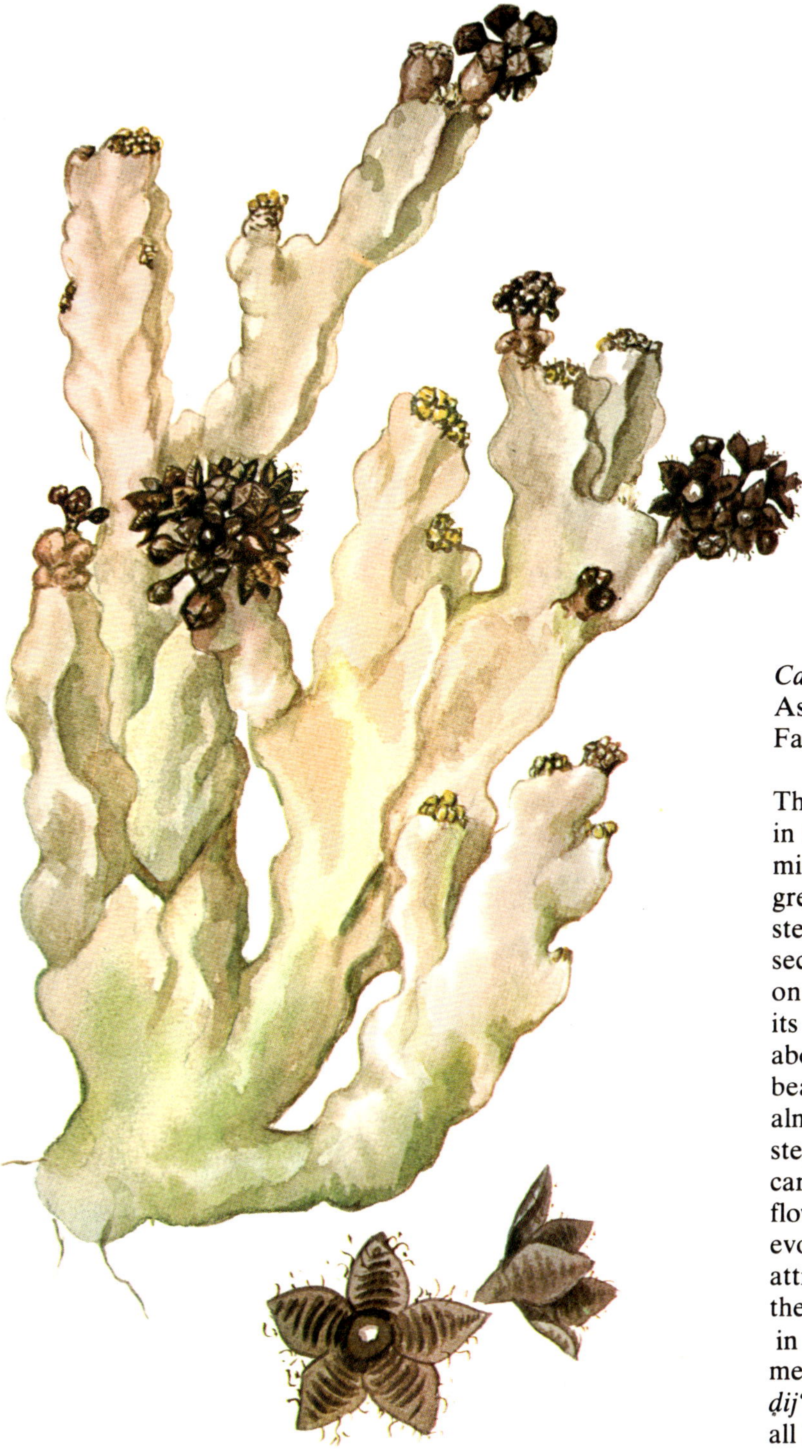

Caralluma sp.

Caralluma sp.
Asclepiadaceae (Milkweed Family)

This plant, at least when not in flower, is very likely to be mistaken for a stone. Its greyish, leafless, succulent stems, roughly square in cross-section, are easily overlooked on the rocky hill-sides that are its favoured habitat. It is about 25 centimetres high and bears clusters of dark red, almost black, flowers at the stem tips. The unpleasant carrion-like odour of the flowers is not just an evolutionary accident; it attracts flies which pollinate the plant. The seeds are borne in narrow pods about 5 centimetres long. *Caralluma,* called *ḍij*ʻ in Oman, is well-known to all hill folk, who pound up the stems and prepare a tea said to be good for liver ailments.

Centaurium pulchellum

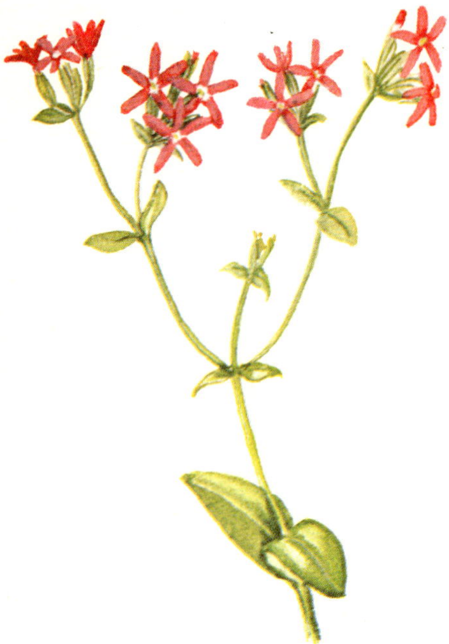

Centaurium pulchellum (Sw.) Druce
Gentianaceae (Gentian Family)

Probably the most common of the Middle Eastern centauries, this slender herb grows as a weed around inhabited and cultivated areas. It is often found near springs or water channels. The closely related *Centaurium spicatum* is called *khifjī* in Saudi Arabia.

Periploca aphylla Decne.
Asclepiadaceae (Milkweed Family)

This leafless or near-leafless mountain shrub, called *ḥandabūb,* has small but striking dark purple flowers about 1 centimetre wide. The corolla lobes are thickly bearded along the edges with white hairs. The narrow, pointed fruits are borne in spreading pairs, and the seeds are covered with fine silky hairs for windborne dispersal. The buds of *ḥandabūb* are edible.

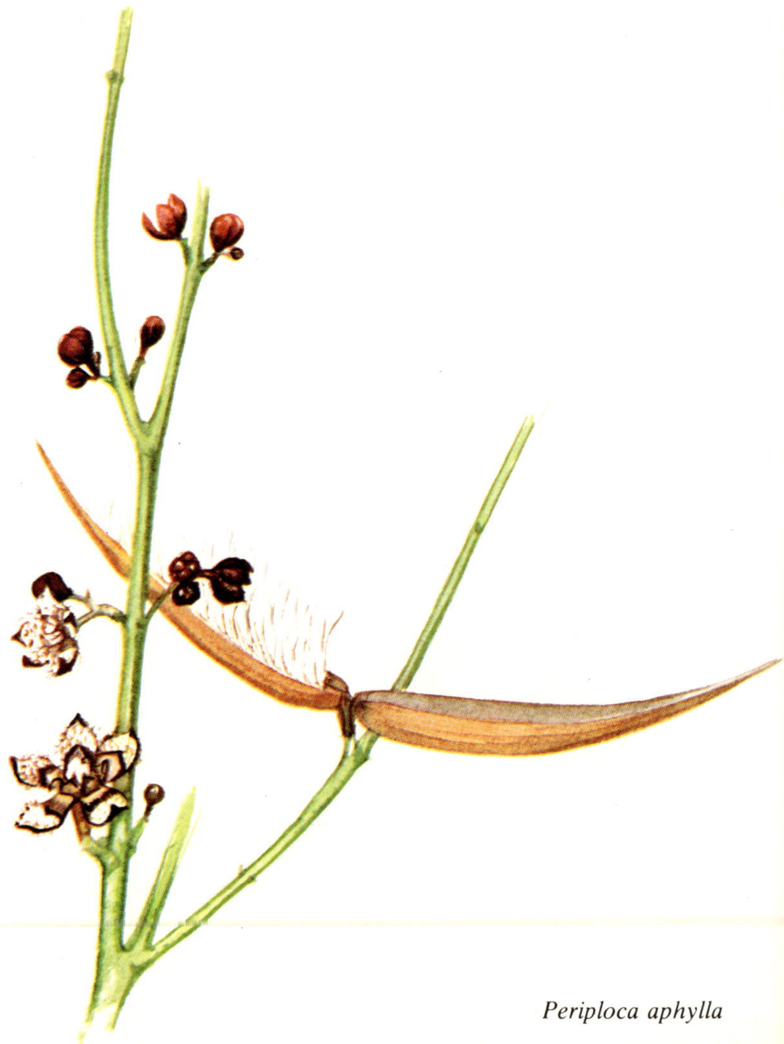

Periploca aphylla

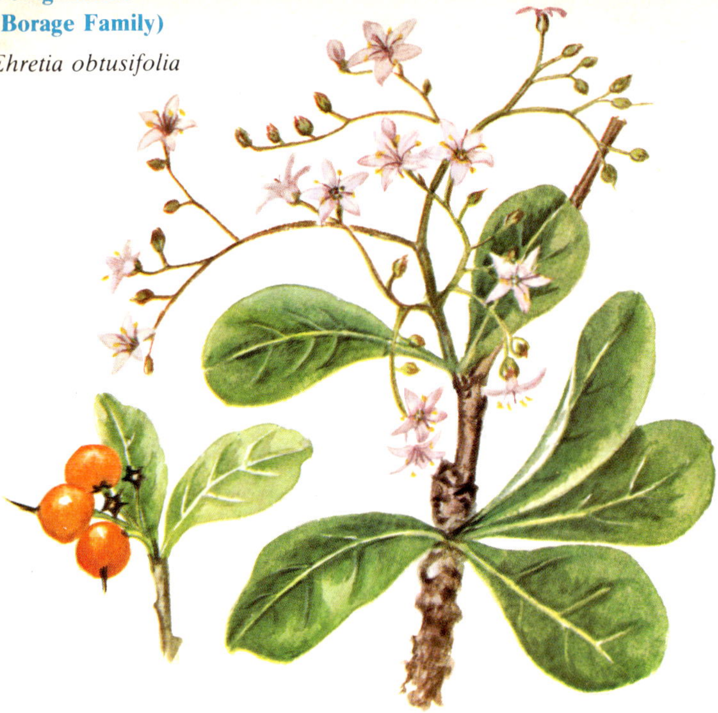

Ehretia obtusifolia

Ehretia obtusifolia Hochst. ex DC.
Boraginaceae (Borage Family)

Ehretia is an Old World tropical genus, some species of which are cultivated as ornamentals. This shrub is found from north-east Africa, across southern Arabia to Pakistan. In North Yemen it is called *misk.* It has been seen growing up to 2 metres high along water channels near Sayq in Oman.

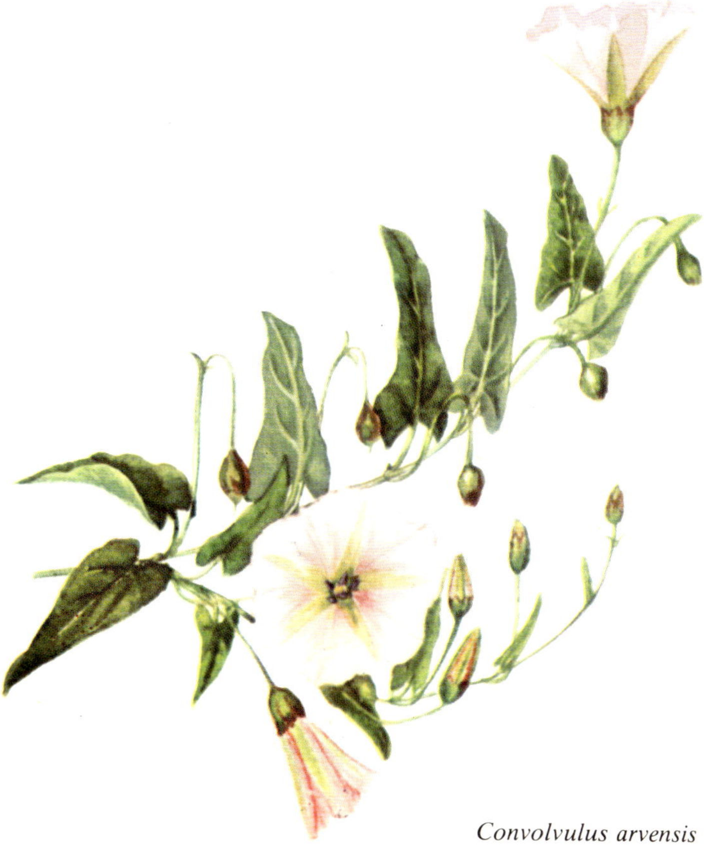

Convolvulus arvensis

Convolvulus arvensis L.
Convolvulaceae (Morning Glory Family)

This field bindweed is commonly seen in and around cultivated fields and gardens, where it is sometimes a serious pest. Climbing and twining over crop plants—seemingly choking them to death—it is very difficult to eradicate once established. It is nevertheless an attractive plant, with rather showy flowers that may vary in colour from pure white to pinkish. The root is known to be a powerful cathartic, and it is used as such in some countries. This is a species that has an almost worldwide distribution. In Oman it is sometimes called *mulawwiyah,* which means ‘twister’ or ‘twiner’.

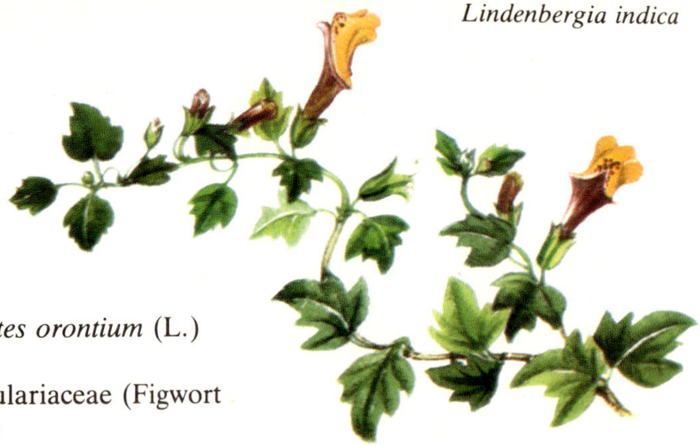

Lindenbergia indica

Lindenbergia indica O. Kuntz
Scrophulariaceae (Figwort Family)

Lindenbergia is a tropical genus distributed from Africa to east Asia. This species, in Oman, is likely to be seen in rocky habitats. The Arabic name *suqqayt* has been recorded for a closely related species in Sinai.

Misopates orontium (L.) Rafin.
Scrophulariaceae (Figwort Family)

Usually seen as a weed around gardens or fields, this annual is sometimes classed as a member of the genus *Antirrhinum*. In Syria it is called *sīsim*.

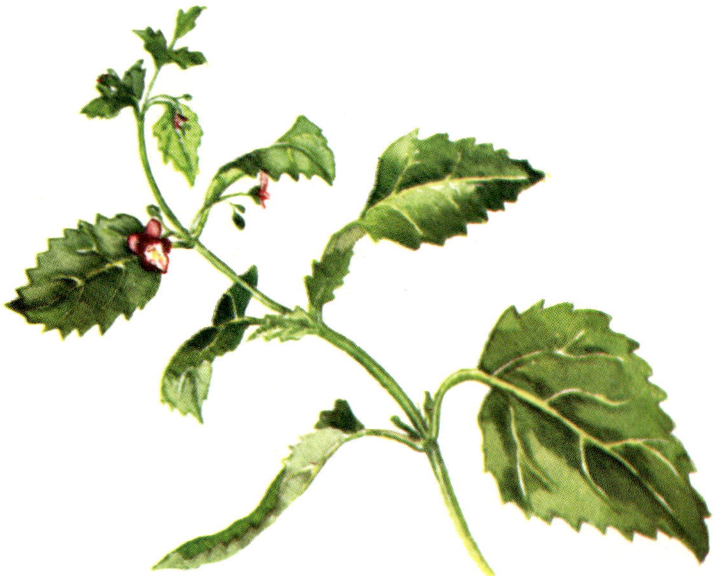

Scrophularia arguta

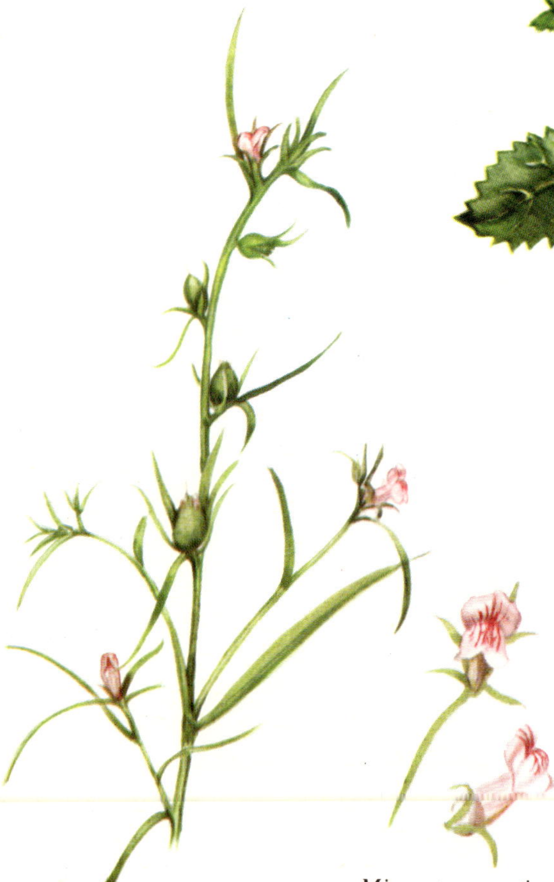

Misopates orontium

Scrophularia arguta Ait.
Scrophulariaceae (Figwort Family)

This annual figwort may be recognised by its serrate leaves and deep red flowers. It is known as *malīsah* in Egypt.

Verbascum cedreti Boiss. var.
Scrophulariaceae (Figwort Family)

This showy mullein, 30–80 centimetres high, is a lowland plant in Oman, but is closely related to a variety found in alpine habitats in Lebanon, and in Egypt it is called *būṣīr*.

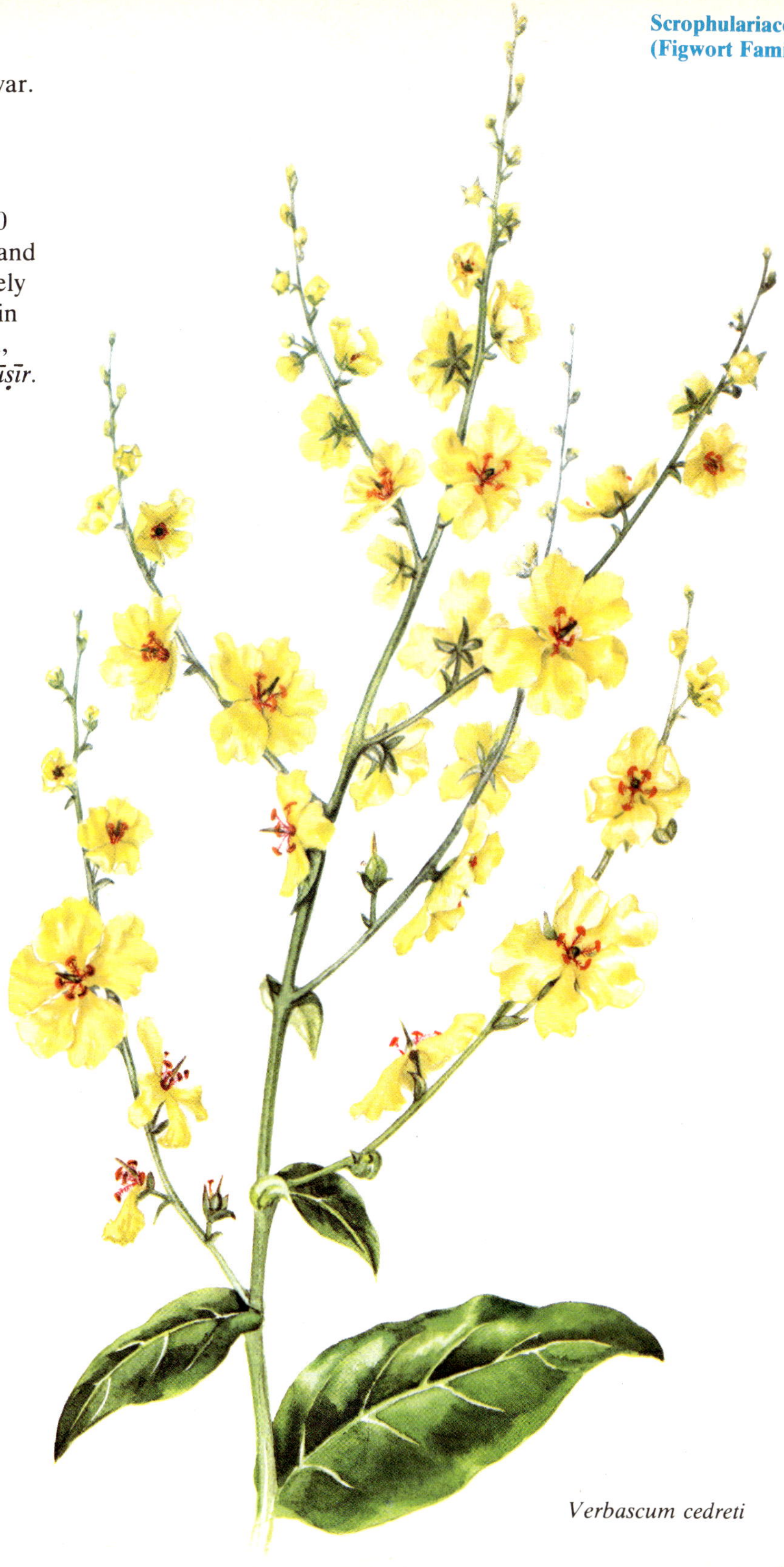

Verbascum cedreti

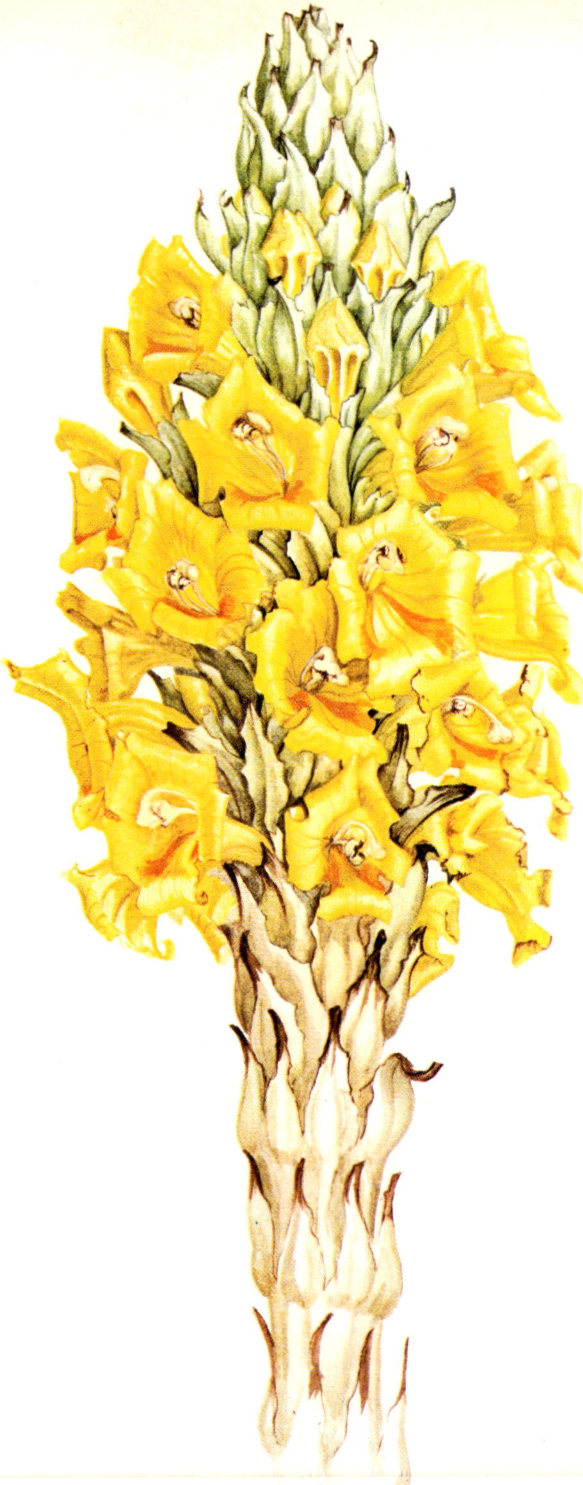

Cistanche phelypaea

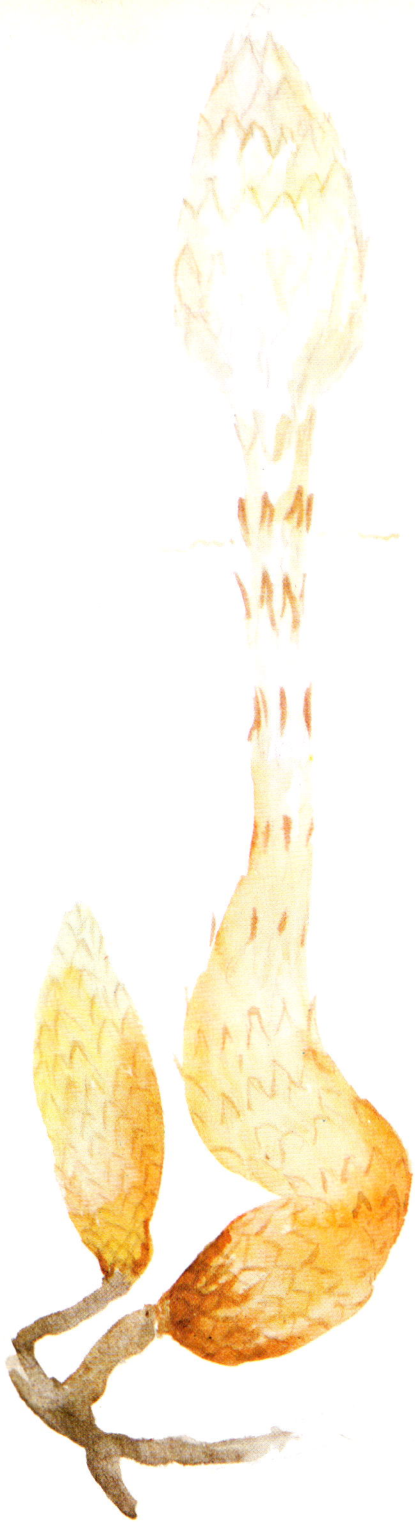

Cistanche phelypaea (L.) Cout.
Orobanchaceae (Broomrape Family)

This striking fragrant spike of flowers is the reproductive structure of a root parasite, widespread in the Middle East, and known in many Arab countries by the name *dhānūn*. Foreign residents sometimes call it 'desert candle'. It is leafless, lacking chlorophyll, and dependent on the photosynthetic powers of other plants for its nourishment. Its club-like underground stem attaches itself to the roots of other plants—often member of the saltbush group—by a thread-like connection that can be seen and traced after careful excavation. *Cistanche* reproduces by seeds, and young plants are capable of some growth, probably depending on nourishment stored in the seed, before finding a host. *Cistanche* spikes emerge from the ground almost overnight near their host shrubs after rains. With plentiful moisture and 'stolen' foodstuffs, they may grow up to a metre high.

Tecomella undulata (G. Don.) Seem.
Bignoniaceae (Bignonia Family)

This tall shrub, or small tree, usually 3–5 metres high, is sometimes cultivated in Oman for its bright showy flowers. It may also be seen along the gravelly beds of larger *wadis*, sometimes at some distance from inhabited areas, and its precise status—whether a naturalised introduction or an Oman native—is not clear. According to local tradition it is a wild shrub of the country, and its occurrence wild in Baluchistan, Pakistan and parts of India with a climate and flora similar to that of Oman, suggests that it could well occur naturally here. The tree is said to be easily propagated from cuttings. *Tecomella* is called *farfār* in Arabic, and it appears to have been known in Arabia at least as early as the 9th Century A.D., when the botanist-lexicographer Abū Ḥanīfah ad Dīnawarī described it as a tree with 'leaves like those of the almond and flowers like roses'

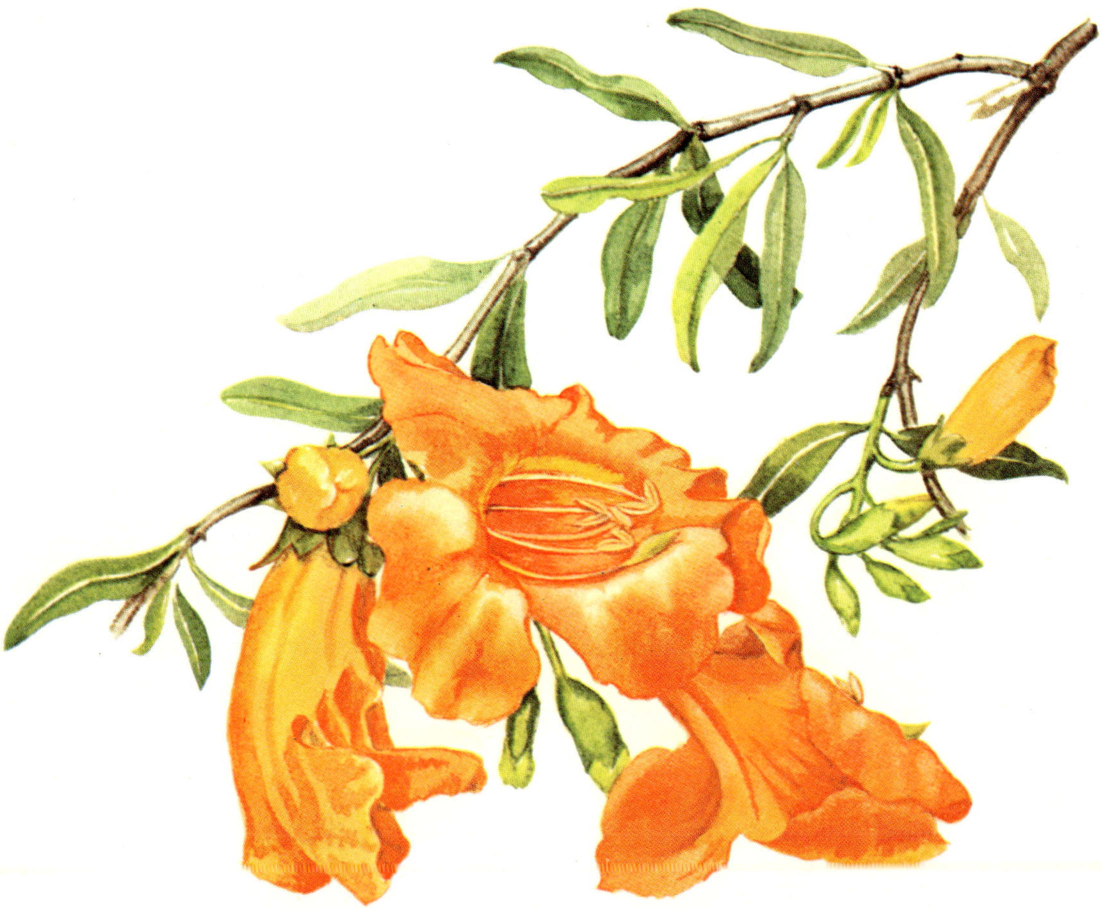

Tecomella undulata

Ecbolium viride (Forssk.) Alston
Acanthaceae (Acanthus Family)

A coarse, shrubby herb, sometimes a metre high, often seen along the banks of *wadis,* along walls, or in other disturbed habitats. The dense, spike-like inflorescence is conspicuous by its bright green over-lapping bracts. The slender protruding corollas, which are of a delicately bluish or yellowish tint, soon wither. This is a common plant in India. In Oman it is called *thawmah.*

Lantana petitiana A. Rich
Verbenaceae (Verbena Family)

This close relative of the *Lantana* so widely cultivated for ornamental use in warmer parts of the world is a small mountain shrub in Oman, usually found above 2,000 metres elevation. As in the cultivated plant, the small flowers, often of differing colour, are borne in dense, head-like spikes. There appears to be no well-known Arabic name for wild *Lantana,* a plant of little economic importance. It has been called *sifsif.*

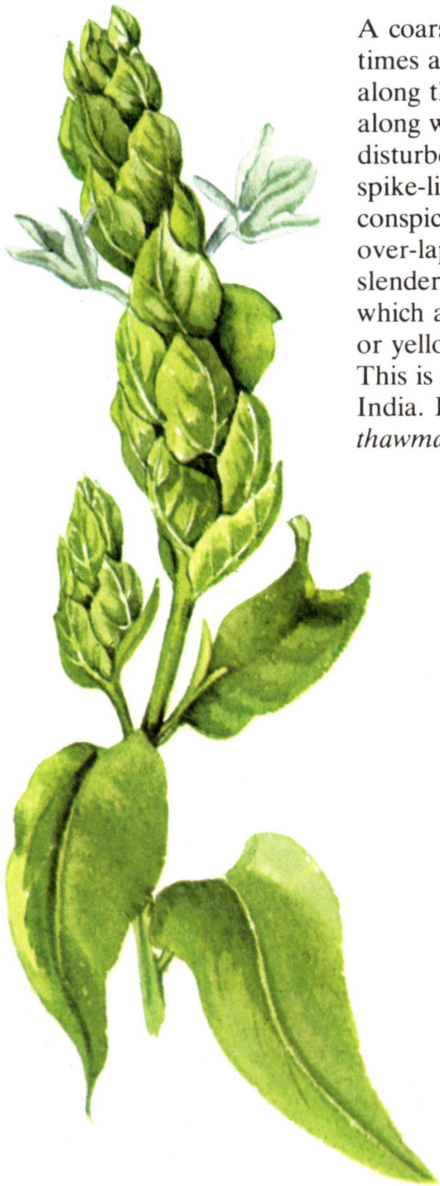

Ecbolium viride

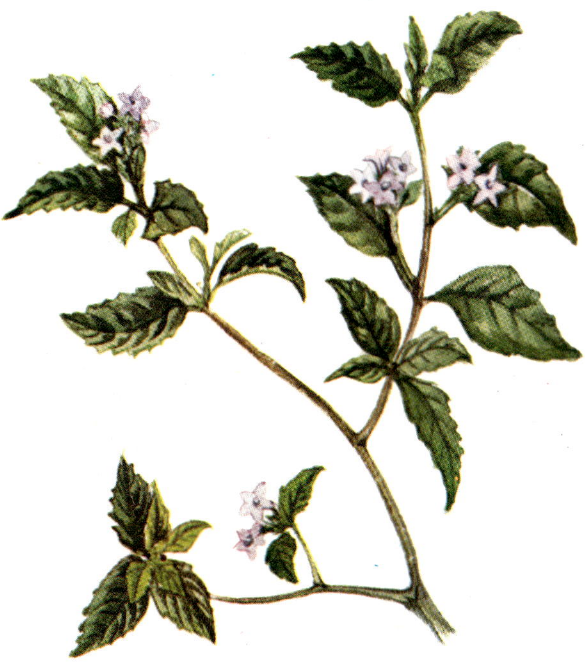

Lantana petitiana

Halopeplis perfoliata (Forssk.) Bge. ex Schweinf.
Chenopodiaceae (Goosefoot Family)

Like other members of the Goosefoot family that have adapted to saline habitats, this plant has evolved into a highly succulent form. Its leaves are thick fleshy structures encircling the stem, and this, with the plant's often marked red pigmentation, have led to its being called *khurrayz*—from a word meaning 'glass beads'—in other Arabian Gulf countries where it is common. The flowers are almost invisible, petal-less structures embedded in groups of three in the stem, which may grow about 60 centimetres high. *Halopeplis* may be found along coastal salt flats, growing just above the inter-tidal mud level.

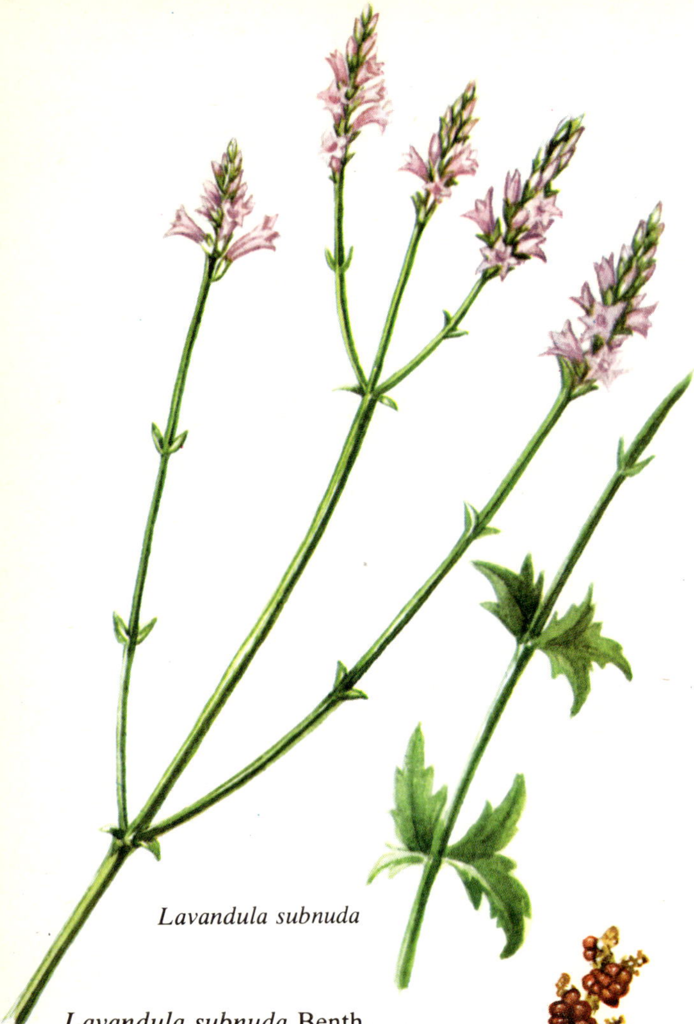

Lavandula subnuda

Lavandula subnuda Benth.
Labiatae (Mint Family)

The square stems and flower structure of this perennial mark it as a member of the mint family, but unlike most lavenders and other mint relatives, it has little aromatic quality. The erect stems of the plant, which is known in Oman as *haraq* or *ṣawmar,* are usually almost leafless and about 1 metre high. They may be seen among rocks, particularly on steep hill-sides above mountain *wadis.*

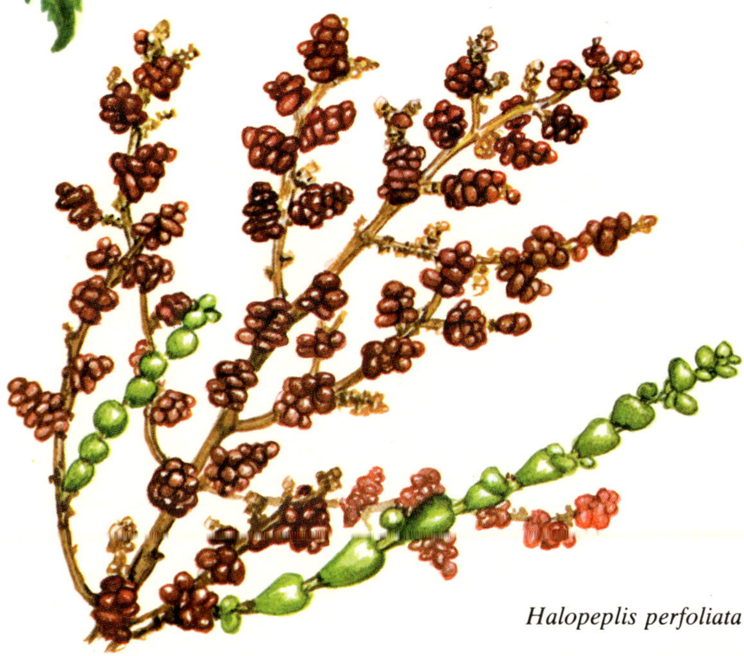

Halopeplis perfoliata

Salvia aegyptiaca

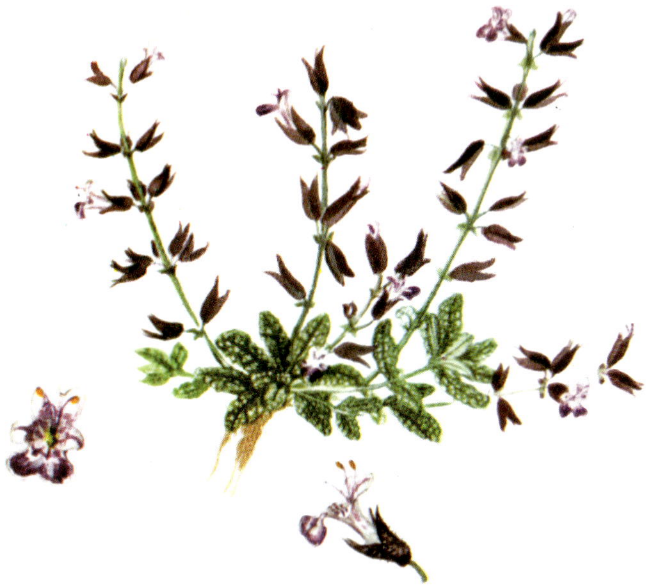

Salvia aegyptiaca L.
Labiatae (Mint Family)

This narrow-leaved, non-aromatic sage, known as *ra'al* in Egypt, is found in rocky habitats, where it grows about 20 centimetres high. The *Salvias* may be distinguished from other mint family members of the area by their flowers having only two (rather than four) stamens. Two other species, *Salvia schimperi* and *Salvia macilenta,* have also been recorded from northern Oman.

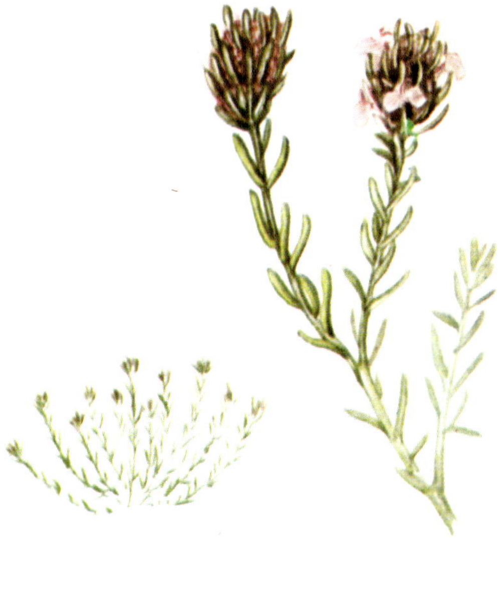

Teucrium mascatense

Teucrium mascatense Boiss.
Labiatae (Mint Family)

An aromatic perennial, a native of Oman, which grows about 25 centimetres high on rocky hill and mountain slopes. It bears the same Arabic name—*ja'dah*—that is applied to the closely related *Teucrium polium,* famous throughout the Middle East for its use in traditional medicine as a fever remedy. Another member of the genus, *Teucrium stocksii,* has also been collected in mountain Oman.

Nyctaginaceae (Four o'clock Family)

Boerhavia elegans Choisy
Nyctaginaceae (Four-O'Clock Family)

This plant, the most conspicuous of the three species of *Boerhavia* known from northern Oman, is sometimes seen along roadsides, appearing as a puff of purplish smoke among the rocks. Its Arabic name, *ḥadimdām* or *liḥdimdām* (with an apparently fused definite article), is derived from a root verb meaning 'to be hot' or 'red like fire' and apparently refers to the striking reddish colouration of the whole plant. The small flowers are borne on fine, almost hair-like peduncles in large, leafless panicles.

Amaranthaceae (Amaranth Family)

Aerva javanica (Burm. f.) Spreng.
Amaranthaceae (Amaranth Family)

This densely woolly, grey to white shrublet is essentially a plant of the lowlands and lower hills. It grows to about 1 metre high and is widely known by its classical Arabic name, *ra'*. The soft fleecy flower spikes are sometimes collected by villagers in Oman, as in other countries where the plant is found, and used to stuff pillows and saddle pads.

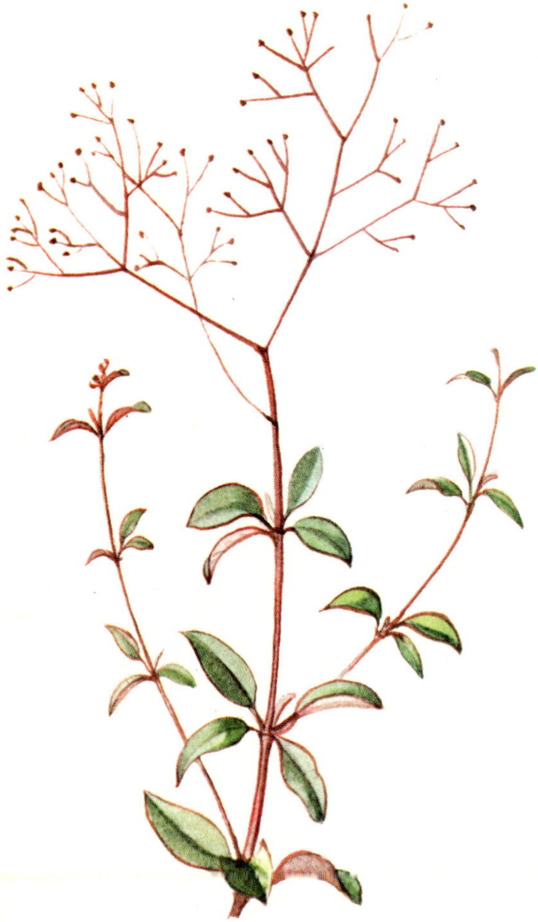

Boerhavia elegans

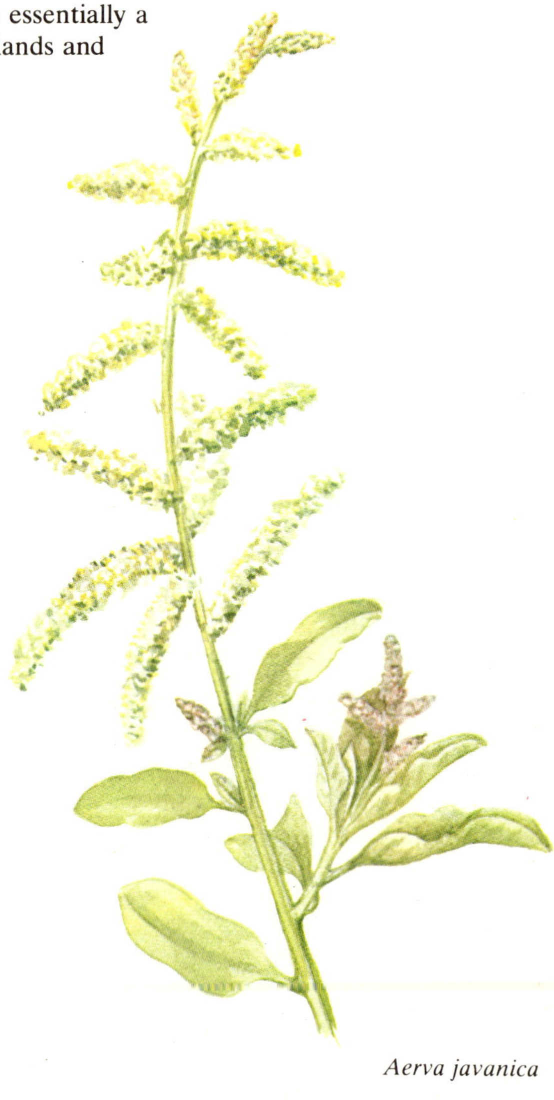

Aerva javanica

Calligonum sp.

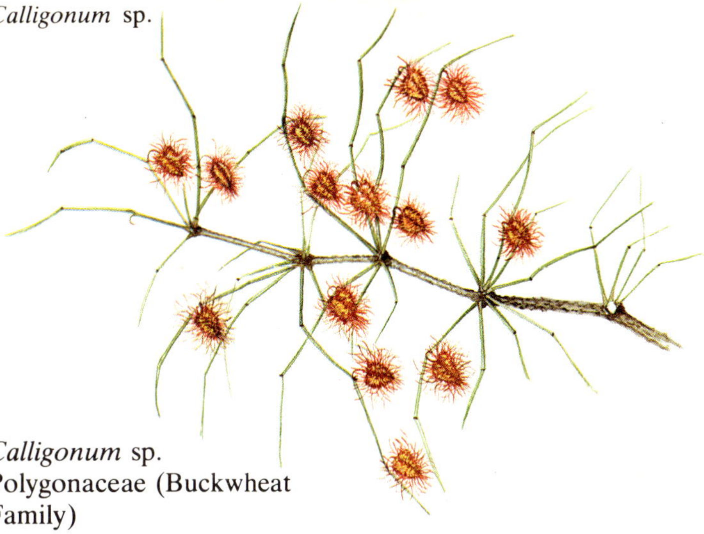

Calligonum sp.
Polygonaceae (Buckwheat Family)

Calligonum, represented by several species in Arabia, is a well-known shrub of sandy habitats in the Peninsula. One of them is an important woody plant of the deep Rub' al-Khāli. Around Muscat it is most likely to be seen in the coastal sands, where it grows as a leafless, or nearly leafless shrub, up to a metre or more high, with stiff, whitish branches. In the inland sand deserts, the Bedouins prize it as firewood that burns with a clear long-lasting flame. It is also used as a source of tannin in curing hides. As is often the case in other members of the buckwheat family, the fruiting structures of *Calligonum* are more showy than its flowers. Here it is the bright red, hair-tufted coverings of the fruits which attract attention. They appear soon after flowering in spring. In many parts of Arabia, the shrub is known as *arṭa.* Bedouins of the Rub' al-Khālī and adjacent steppes, however, know it as *'abal.*

Pteropyrum scoparium Jaub. & Spach
Polygonaceae (Buckwheat Family)

A narrow-leaved shrublet which grows in dense stands in the flood channels of *wadıs* flowing out of Jabal al-Akhdar and other mountain areas. It is usually 1–1½ metres high. *Sīdāf,* as it is known in Oman, is one of those Asiatic species whose range extends across the Gulf. Parts of the plant are eaten by some tribesmen, who describe it as 'a blood purifying tonic'.

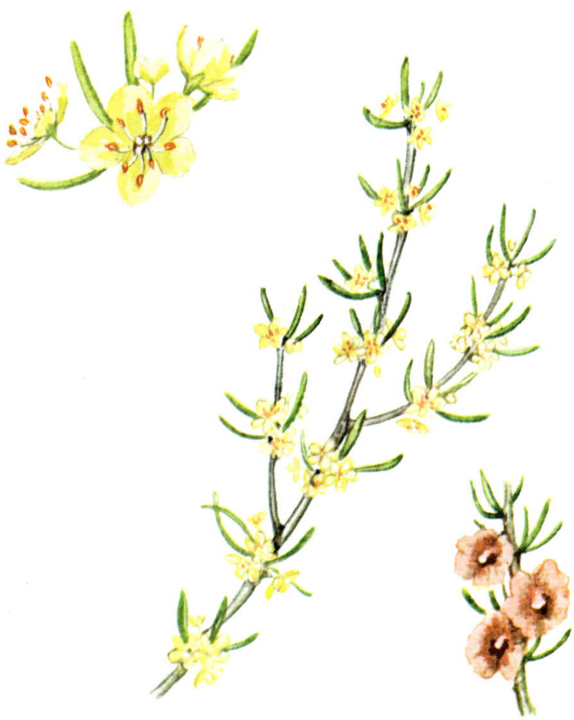

Pteropyrum scoparium

Polygonaceae (Buckwheat Family)

Rumex vesicarius L.
Polygonaceae (Buckwheat Family)

This wild dock, whose Arabic name *ḥummāḍ* is derived from an adjective meaning 'bitter' or 'sour', can be found both in the lowland deserts and in the mountains. In either zone it is often associated with rocky habitats. *Ḥummāḍ* is recognised in many parts of Arabia as an edible plant, and in earlier times of famine was eaten raw or cooked. Now it is more often just a juicy, astringent tidbit nibbled by Bedouin tribesmen as a mouth freshener. The flowers of *Rumex,* a few of which are shown in this illustration, are small and inconspicuous. The showy, pinkish-veined structures are the membranous wings which enclose the developing fruits.

Chrozophora oblongifolia A. Juss.
Euphorbiaceae (Spurge Family)

Chrozophora, a greyish-green woolly shrublet, may grow to about 1 metre high. The flowers, which are inconspicuous, are followed by fruits in the form of small scaly capsules. Known in Oman as *mashariyah* (or *masharriyah),* it has a juice which stains blue-black, the colour intensifying upon exposure to air. This was used in Arab lands in the preparation of ink before the commercial product became available.

Euphorbiaceae (Spurge Family)

Rumex vesicarius

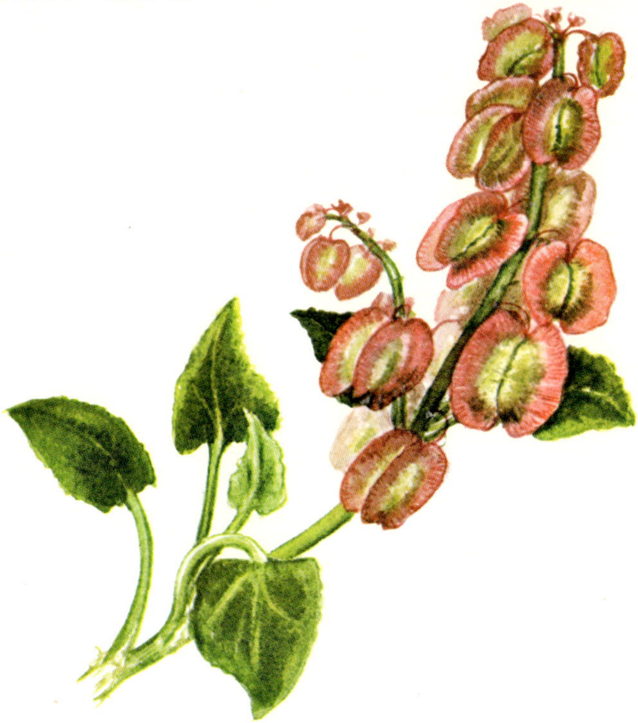

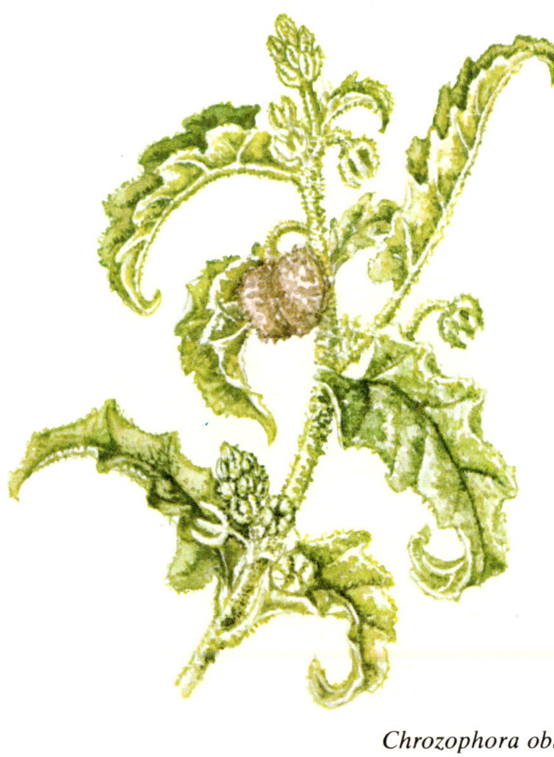

Chrozophora oblongifolia

Euphorbia larica

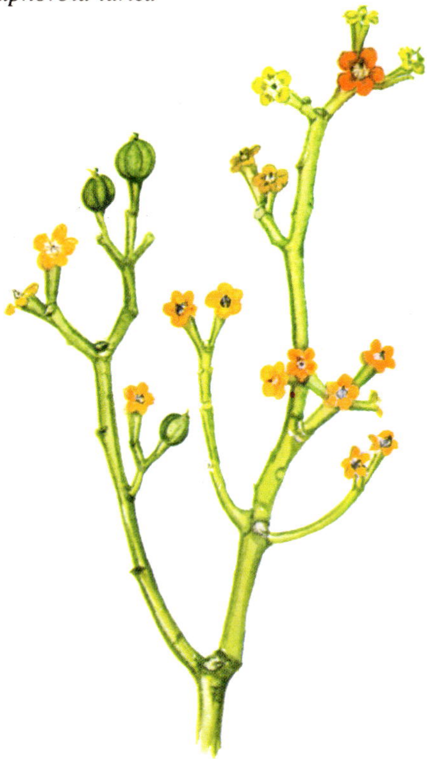

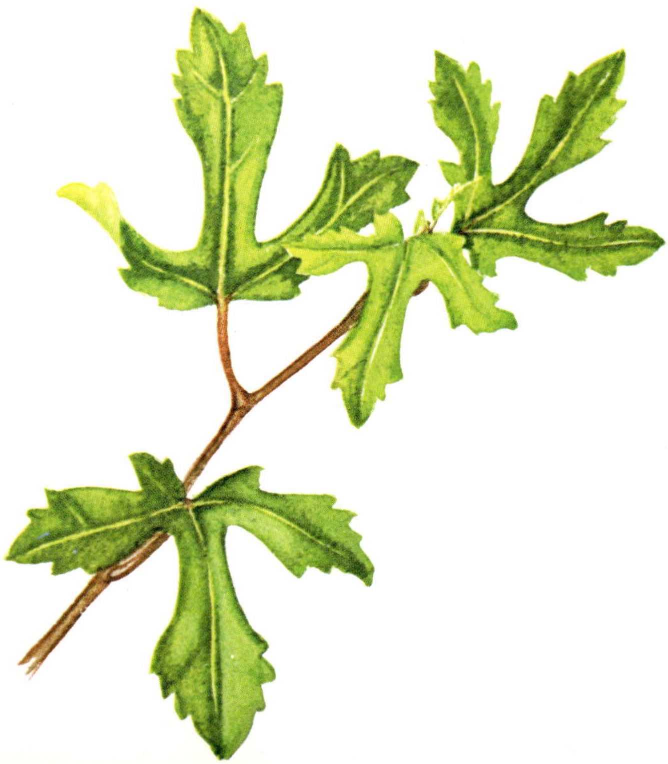

Euphorbia larica Boiss.
Euphorbiaceae (Spurge Family)

Euphorbia larica, known in Oman as *isbaq,* is a virtually leafless shrub whose striking appearance will certainly attract the attention of even the casual traveller. Its smooth, light yellow-green, succulent stems grow erect, candelabra-like and sometimes man-high from the root crown. The yellow flowers at the branch tips are succeeded by round green fruits. Large quantities of thick, milky latex flood out of any cut in the fleshy stem. It is probably poisonous. *Isbaq* is a dominant shrub on steep rocky mountain-sides between about 400 and 1,300 metres elevation. It may also be found on rocky ground at lower altitudes towards the coast.

Ficus palmata Forssk.
Moraceae (Mulberry Family)

Two species of wild fig are common in northern Oman: the palmate fig, illustrated here and known by various colloquial name variants including *siqab, isqab,* and *thiqab;* and the willow-leaved fig, *Ficus salicifolia* Vahl, which has long, narrow leaves and is called *lithab.* Both are large shrubs or small to medium-sized trees conspicuous along the rocky banks of *wadis* and ravines in the hot mountain foot-hills. They may also be seen occasionally at higher elevations up to about 1,500 metres. Neither tree is of direct economic importance, but they are of considerable ecological value, helping control flood erosion and providing important cover for birds and other wildlife.

Forskohlea tenacissima L.
Urticaceae (Nettle Family)

The Arabic name of this low bushy plant, *lazzāq*, may be translated as 'stick-tight'. Its most noticeable characteristic is, indeed, the fine hooked hairs that cover it and provide hold-fasts to the hair of passing animals or the clothing of foot travellers—much as in the manner of 'velcro' fastenings on astronauts' space suits. *Lazzāq* sometimes grows nearly prostrate and often has red-flushed stems. The leaves are whitish woolly beneath, and the flowers are inconspicuous. The scientific name *Forskohlea* was given by Linnaeus to commemorate its European discoverer, the Swedish botanist Per Forsskal (1732–1763), who died in Yemen on a collecting expedition.

Juniperus macropoda Boiss.
Coniferae (Conifer Family)

This most striking tree of upper Jabal al-Akhdar is the Indian juniper or Himalayan pencil cedar. It may be seen from about 1,450 metres elevation on the north face of the Jabal up to the highest

Forskohlea tenacissima

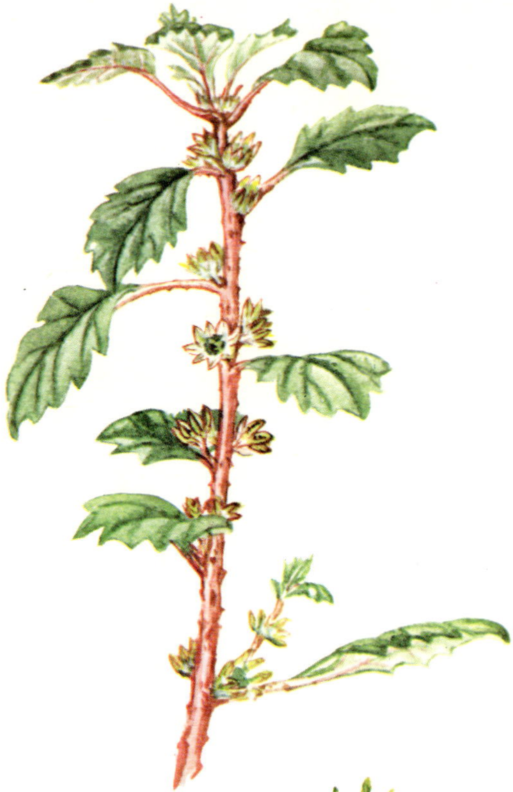

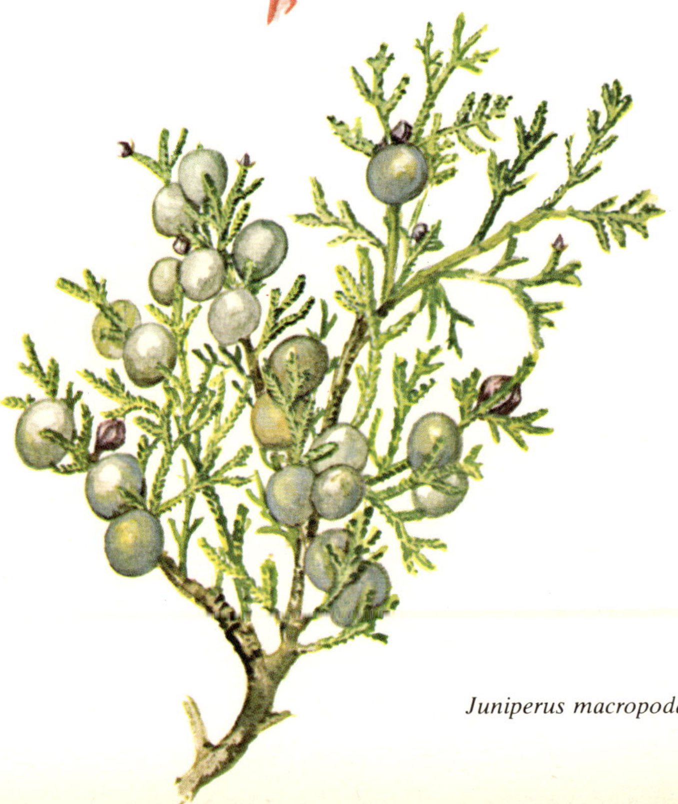

Juniperus macropoda

summits near 3,000 metres. In the summit area it is dominant, growing widely spaced as a great hemispherical tree some 10 metres high. Unlike the few other trees found in this high zone, which are best developed in the ravines, juniper may grow on fully exposed limestone flats on very shallow soil. This tree is an eastern species and is common in the drier mountain ranges of Pakistan and India at similar altitudes. Its wood is used there for making pencils, and distillation of the shavings provides an aromatic oil. The tribesmen of Jabal al-Akhdar call the juniper *'al'alān*. In south-western Arabia it is known by its classical name, *'ar'ar*.

Aloe barbadense Mill.
Liliaceae (Lily Family)

This *Aloe* is a native of Mediterranean North Africa, and several varieties of it have long been cultivated in the tropics as a source of the drug, aloes. The Oman plants, sometimes seen along rocky farm embankments or walls, are certainly introduced. Here it is known as *isqal* or *isqill*. The drug is obtained by collecting and drying the thick bitter sap that exudes from the cut leaves. Village Omanis use it to prepare 'a cooling eye ointment', and it is probably also used internally as in other countries as a purgative and vermifuge. The plant grows up to about a metre high, and the flowers are borne on a stalk from the centre of the leaf rosette. The outside of the flower segments are coral with greenish brown margins; inside they are yellow. *Aloe*, with its smaller, toothed leaves, should not be confused with the much larger *Agave*, which grows along *wadis* near farms and is called *masad*. *Agave* has somewhat similar leaves but without toothed edges.

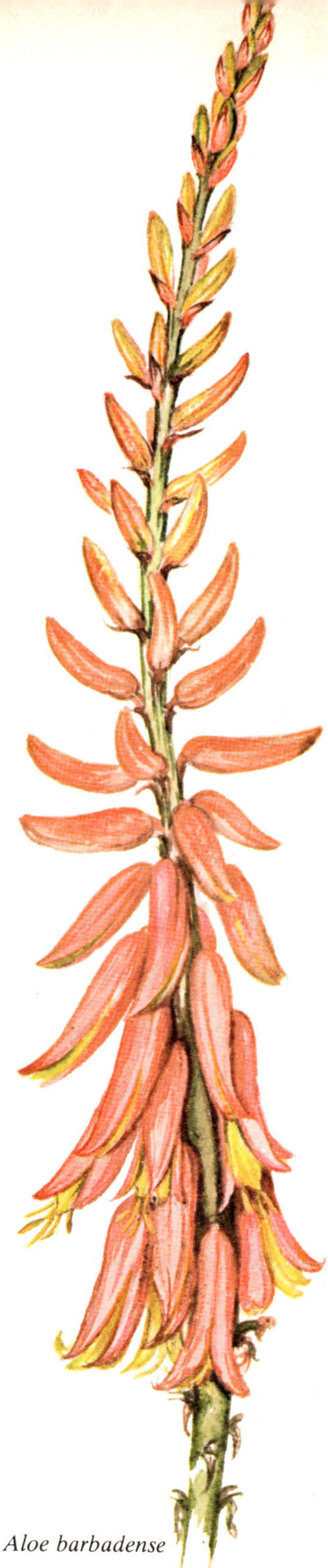

Aloe barbadense

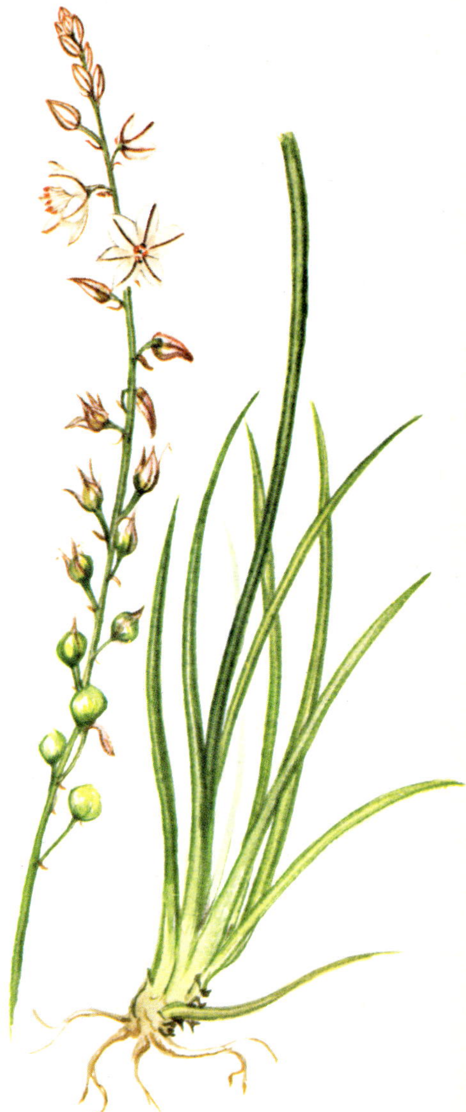

Asphodelus fistulosus

Liliaceae (Lily Family)

Asphodelus fistulosus (Cav.) Baker
Liliaceae (Lily Family)

This asphodel, called in Oman *buṣaylī* or 'little onion', is one of the most common annuals in both the lowlands and higher altitudes. It varies greatly in size, depending on local soil and moisture conditions; many may be seen 0.3 to 1 metre high. It is also common in other Middle Eastern countries.

Polpodiaceae (Polypody Family)

Pteris vittata

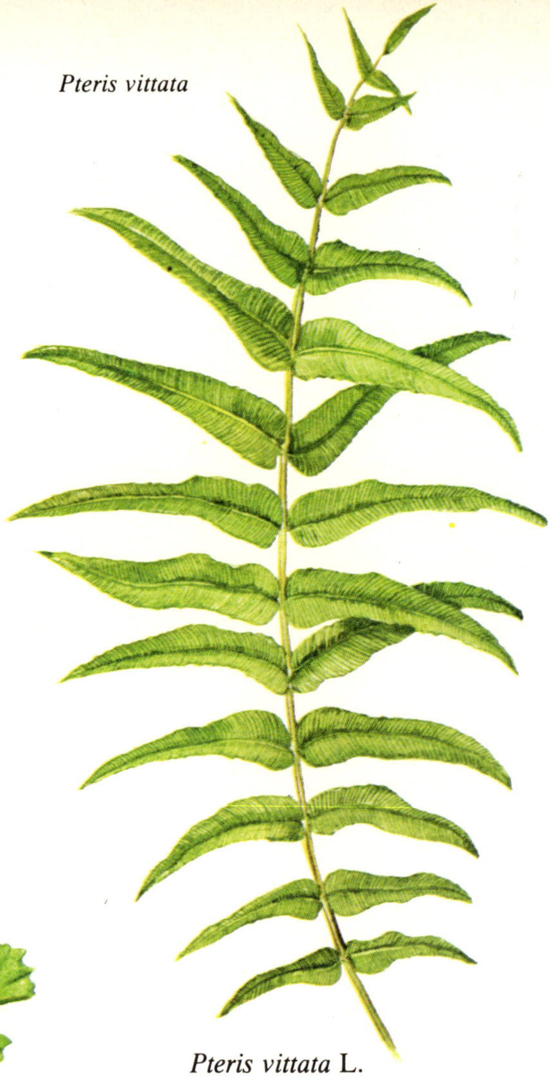

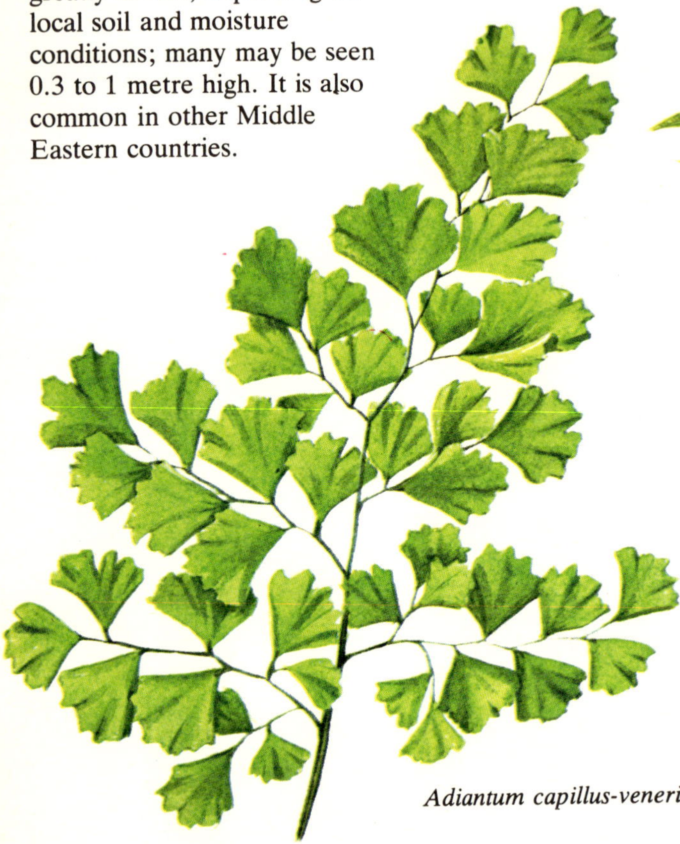

Adiantum capillus-veneris L.

Adiantum capillus-veneris L.
Polypodiaceae (Polypody Family)

This is the well-known maidenhair fern. Known in Oman as *khuwaysat mā'* 'little water frond', it is very common along water channels and in other shady wet places, such as near mountain springs.

The fronds may grow 30–40 centimetres long, but are usually shorter. The spore-bearing organs are on the leaflet undersides, near the tips.

Pteris vittata L.
Polypodiaceae (Polypody Family)

Khawṣat mā', literally 'water frond', is the name usually given to this attractive fern. It is very common along irrigation channels in gardens and along small aquaducts built along *wadi* banks. Like other ferns, it reproduces by microscopic spores released from spore cases on the undersides of the leaves and does not bear flowers. *Pteris* may grow 75 centimetres high in favourable habitats.

INDEX

Index of Arabic Plant Names Used in the Text